**Understanding
Medical Education**

EVIDENCE, THEORY AND PRACTICE

Understanding Medical Education

EVIDENCE, THEORY AND PRACTICE

Second edition

EDITED BY

Professor Tim Swanwick

Dean of Postgraduate Medical Education
Health Education North Central and East London
London, UK

WILEY Blackwell

This edition first published 2014 © 2010, 2014 by The Association for the Study of Medical Education

Registered office: John Wiley & Sons, Ltd, The Atrium, Southern Gate, Chichester, West Sussex, PO19 8SQ, UK

Editorial offices: 9600 Garsington Road, Oxford, OX4 2DQ, UK
The Atrium, Southern Gate, Chichester, West Sussex, PO19 8SQ, UK
350 Main Street, Malden, MA 02148-5020, USA

For details of our global editorial offices, for customer services and for information about how to apply for permission to reuse the copyright material in this book please see our website at www.wiley.com/wiley-blackwell

Library of Congress Cataloging-in-Publication Data
Understanding medical education
    Understanding medical education : evidence, theory, and practice / edited by Professor Tim Swanwick. – Second edition.
        p. ; cm.
    Includes bibliographical references and index.
    ISBN 978-1-118-47240-8 (pbk.)
    I. Swanwick, Tim, editor of compilation.   II. Association for the Study of Medical Education, sponsoring body.   III. Title.
    [DNLM: 1. Education, Medical–methods–Collected Works.   2. Education, Medical–organization & administration–Collected Works.   W 18]
    R845
    610.76–dc23
                        2013019854

A catalogue record for this book is available from the British Library.

Wiley also publishes its books in a variety of electronic formats. Some content that appears in print may not be available in electronic books.

Cover image: ©iStockphoto
Cover design by Visual Philosophy Design Ltd

Set in 9/11pt Palatino by Toppan Best-set Premedia Limited
Printed and bound in Malaysia by Vivar Printing Sdn Bhd

1 2014

Contents

Contributors

Mark A Albanese
Professor Emeritus
Population Health and Educational Psychology
University of Wisconsin
Madison, WI, USA

Antony Americano
Chapter written whilst Director of Corporate Services,
London Deanery, University of London
Current: Employer Liaison Advisor, General Medical Council
London, UK

Dinesh Bhugra
Professor of Mental Health and Cultural Diversity
Institute of Psychiatry, King's College London;
Honorary Consultant at the Maudsley Hospital
London, UK

David Blaney
Senior Educationalist
Medical Protection Society
London, UK;
Honorary Professor Health Sciences
University of York
York, UK

Alan Bleakley
Professor of Medical Education
Peninsula Medical School
Plymouth, UK

Nicole J Borges
Assistant Dean, Medical Education Research and Evaluation
Office of Academic Affairs;
Professor, Department of Community Health
Wright State University Boonshoft School of Medicine
Dayton, OH, USA

Katharine AM Boursicot
Reader in Medical Education and Head of Assessment
St George's, University of London
London, UK

Paul Bradley
Professor of Clinical Skills and Simulation
Institute of Medical Education
University of Swansea
Swansea, UK

Julie Browne
External Relations Manager
Wales Deanery
Cardiff University
Cardiff, UK

Alison Bullock
Professor of Medical and Dental Education
Cardiff University School of Social Sciences
Cardiff, UK

William P Burdick
Associate Vice President for Education
Foundation for Advancement of International Medical Education and
Research (FAIMER);
Clinical Professor of Emergency Medicine
Drexel University College of Medicine
Philadelphia, PA, USA

Deborah Cohen OBE
Senior Medical Research Fellow
Individual Support Programme
Centre for Psychosocial and Disability Research
Institute of Primary Care and Public Health
School of Medicine
Cardiff University
Cardiff, UK

Ian Cooper
Language and Communications Specialist
Individual Support Programme
Institute of Primary Care and Public Health
School of Medicine
Cardiff University
Cardiff, UK

Laura C Dast
Curriculum Development Manager
University of Wisconsin School of Medicine and Public Health
Madison, WI, USA

André F De Champlain
Acting Director
Research and Development
Medical Council of Canada
Ottawa, Canada

Erik Driessen
Associate Professor of Medical Education
Maastricht University
Maastricht, The Netherlands

Kate Ellis
Academic Standards and Policy Officer
Plymouth University
Plymouth, UK

Caroline Elton
Head of Careers Support and Planning
Professional Support Unit
Shared Services – Working on behalf of Health Education North Central
and East London
Health Education North West London and Health Education
South London
London, UK

Kevin W Eva
Senior Scientist
Centre for Health Education Scholarship;
Professor
Director of Education Research & Scholarship
Department of Medicine
University of British Columbia
Vancouver, Canada

H Martyn Evans
Professor of Humanities in Medicine
School of Medicine and Health
Durham University
Durham, UK

Joseph C Fantone
Senior Associate Dean for Educational Affairs
Professor of Pathology
University of Florida College of Medicine
Gainesville, FL, USA

Eamonn Ferguson
Professor of Health Psychology
University of Nottingham
Nottingham, UK

Della Freeth
Professor of Professional Education
Centre for Medical Education
Queen Mary University of London
London, UK

J Jill Gordon
Associate Professor
University of Sydney
Sydney, Australia

Janet Grant
Emerita Professor, The Open University;
Honorary Professor, University College London Medical School;
Director, Centre for Medical Education in Context
London, UK;
Honorary Professor
Plymouth University Peninsula Schools of Medicine and Dentistry
Plymouth, UK

Larry D Gruppen
Josiah Macy Jr, Professor of Medical Education
Chair, Department of Medical Education
University of Michigan Medical School
Ann Arbor, MI, USA

Jan Illing
Professor of Medical Education
Centre for Medical Education Research
Durham University
Durham, UK

Brian Jolly
Professor of Medical Education
University of Newcastle
NSW, Australia

Peter GM de Jong
Adviser for Educational Technology
Center for Innovation in Medical Education
Leiden University Medical Center
Leiden, The Netherlands

David M Kaufman
Professor
Faculty of Education
Simon Fraser University
Burnaby, Canada

Tara J Kennedy
Developmental Pediatrician and Clinical Leader
Pediatric Autism Rehabilitation Services
Stan Cassidy Centre for Rehabilitation
Fredericton, New Brunswick, Canada

Jean Ker
Professor of Medical Education
Director of Clinical Skills Education
College of Medicine, Dentistry and Nursing
University of Dundee
Dundee, UK

Alec L Knight
Consultant Psychologist
Work Psychology Group
Derby, UK

John Launer
Associate Dean for Faculty Development
Professional Development
Health Education South London
London, UK

Lorelei Lingard
Director and Professor
Centre for Education Research & Innovation
Department of Medicine
Schulich School of Medicine & Dentistry
Western University, London, ON, Canada

Bridget Lock
Deputy Director of Medical Education
South London Healthcare NHS Trust
London, UK

Andrew Long
Vice President (Education)
Royal College of Paediatrics and Child Health;
Honorary Senior Lecturer
University College, London
Consultant Paediatrician
Great Ormond Street Hospital
London, UK

Chris Lovato
Professor, School of Population & Public Health
Director, Evaluation Studies Unit, Faculty of Medicine
University of British Columbia
Vancouver, Canada

Karen V Mann
Professor Emeritus
Division of Medical Education
Faculty of Medicine
Dalhousie University
Halifax, Canada

Peter McCrorie
Professor of Medical Education
St George's University of London
London, UK

Jean McKendree
Senior Lecturer in Medical Education
Associate Dean for Assessment
Hull York Medical School
York, UK

Judy McKimm
Professor and Dean of Medical Education
College of Medicine
Swansea University
Swansea, UK

Clare Morris
Head of Department
Clinical Education and Leadership
University of Bedfordshire
Luton, UK

Stella Ng
Director of Research
Centre for Faculty Development
Li Ka Shing Knowledge Institute
St. Michael's Hospital;
Education Scientist
Centre for Ambulatory Care Education
Women's College Hospital
Faculty of Medicine
University of Toronto
Toronto, ON, Canada

John J Norcini
President and CEO
Foundation for Advancement of International Medical Education and
Research (FAIMER)
Philadelphia, PA, USA

Geoff Norman
Professor
Clinical Epidemiology and Biostatistics
McMaster University
Hamilton, Canada

Fiona Patterson
Principal Researcher
University of Cambridge
Cambridge, UK

Melody Rhydderch
Senior Occupational Psychologist
Individual Support Programme
Centre for Psychosocial and Disability Research
Institute of Primary Care and Public Health
School of Medicine
Cardiff University
Cardiff, UK

Scott Rice
Honorary Lecturer in Medical Education
University College London
London, UK

Trudie E Roberts
Director of Leeds Institute of Medical Education
Chair of the Association for the Study of Medical Education
University of Leeds
Leeds, UK

Lambert WT Schuwirth
Professor of Medical Education
Flinders Innovation in Clinical Education
Flinders University
Adelaide, Australia

John Spencer
Professor of Primary Care and Clinical Education
Newcastle University
Newcastle, UK

Yvonne Steinert
Professor of Family Medicine
Richard and Sylvia Cruess Chair in Medical Education;
Director, Centre for Medical Education
Faculty of Medicine
McGill University
Montreal, Quebec, Canada

Tim Swanwick
Dean of Postgraduate Medical Education
Health Education North Central and East London
London, UK

Jan van Tartwijk
Professor of Education
Utrecht University
Utrecht, The Netherlands

Cees PM van der Vleuten
Scientific Director
School of Health Professions Education
University of Maastricht
Maastricht, The Netherlands

David Wall
Deputy Regional Postgraduate Dean
West Midlands Deanery
Birmingham, UK

Casey B White
Associate Dean for Medical Education, Research and Instruction
University of Virginia School of Medicine
Charlottesville, VA, USA

Diana F Wood
Director of Medical Education and Clinical Dean
University of Cambridge School of Clinical Medicine
Cambridge, UK

Foreword to the second edition

Understanding Medical Education is a synopsis of educational theory and practice (almost 500 pages, including an index) that is easily navigated and covers a variety of topics and themes that are timely and crucial in health professions education. It contains cutting-edge information presented in simple language and applicable across the entire spectrum of health professions education, from undergraduate to postgraduate to continuing professional development and training. It crosses all geographic boundaries and cultures, touches on many global educational issues, and is applicable to all. It moves beyond presenting a European or a North American perspective, and sensitizes the reader to the cultural nuances that exist in different learning communities, educational environments, continents and countries around the world. Because of all these characteristics, the book fills a unique niche among textbooks of health professions education.

The first edition was a brilliant initiative by the Association for the Study of Medical Education (ASME), collating a comprehensive and well-researched suite of monographs on a range of educational topics. This volume builds wonderfully on it, making changes with respect to both organization, and the breadth and depth of topics. It covers several additional areas and is organized into five main sections. Part 1, *'Foundations'*, provides a strong grounding in medical education, with chapters on teaching and learning, principles of curriculum design, and quality in medical education. Part 2 *,'Educational Strategies'*, is the longest of the five parts and covers a variety of teaching strategies, such as problem-based learning, work-based learning, teaching and learning in small and large groups, technology-enhanced learning, and e-learning. It also explores issues related to self-regulated learning, learning medicine from the humanities, and patient involvement in medical education. Part 3, *'Assessment'*, focuses entirely on principles and methods of written and performance assessment when used for formative and summative purposes. It also provides a menu and examples for standard setting methods. Part 4, *'Research and Evaluation'*, completely covers quantitative and qualitative research methods in medical education, and concludes with program evaluation. Part 5, *'Staff and Students'*, deals with student selection, career progression, and issues related to remediation and diversity; it ends with an in-depth overview of educational management and leadership.

Many unique features distinguish this book from others that are available. In terms of language and style, it is clear and simple, promoting understanding rather than accumulation of facts. Many complex concepts, theories and models are beautifully illustrated and further elaborated through case studies and rich examples. A number of innovations, guiding principles, latest advances, conceptual frameworks, best practices, perspectives, and methodologies are introduced, supported by evidence and implementation strategies. Whenever suitable, issues related to practicality,

feasibility, generalizability, and impact are considered. Additionally, each chapter contains several boxes, highlighting the main concepts, making it easier to read, understand, use and remember. In addition to a regular reference list, some chapters also contain web links for further information, continuous professional development websites, content repositories, further readings and other online tools. The authors of these chapters are prominent, internationally known experts in their fields. The input from these authors has tremendously enriched the perspectives, scope, and diversity of examples presented in this volume.

Educating health professionals in the twenty-first century is a challenging endeavor. A number of factors, such as differences in culture, religion, social fabric, economics, information technology, changes in governmental structures, national priority shifts, availability and distribution of resources, integration of health care delivery and medical education, and population health, have started to significantly influence education programs and outcomes. The Flexnerian curriculum, based on an evaluation of the educational system in the early twentieth century, had a great impact in eliminating undesirable and dysfunctional aspects of education, to such an extent that it forced many medical schools to close their doors. However, in the contemporary world with the current wave of educational reform, the demands and the dynamic interplay of many of these factors have created an unsettled environment. Health professions education institutions are required to meet the demand of regulators, such as the certification, licensure, and accreditation bodies, while still graduating competent and safe professionals and practitioners. To support these changes, institutions are in dire need of faculty development and there is a great shortage of experts who can deliver such training. Clear evidence of the shortage of medical education leaders is the exponential growth of Masters Programs in health professions education. Whereas, in 1997, there were only 7 programs worldwide granting a Master's degree in health professions education, after only 15 years, in 2013, the number has increased to 131 and it is still growing.

In this day and age, busy professionals do not have enough time to review the literature, read journal articles, and book chapters in their own disciplines let alone education. They quickly search the Internet, and sometimes scan seemingly relevant abstracts. *Understanding Medical Education* is a "one-stop" approach to solving this problem. The latest, most relevant and essential material in health professions education is synthesized, illustrated, and presented in a single volume. This could be the single best companion for medical educators, health professionals, physicians, nurses, allied health professionals, program directors, health practitioners, and students in certificate and Masters' programs in health professions education. It will be useful to students, teaching faculty, department heads, deans, administrators for academic programs, and leaders of health professions education institutions, organizations, associations, and agencies irrespective of their rank or position. This book will provide an efficient and cost-effective approach to searching and acquiring the knowledge that one needs for health professions education leadership. *Understanding Medical Education* is a significant milestone in the history of publications in medical education. It synthesizes the latest knowledge, evidence, and best practices and intersects with the broader perspectives of theory, practice and evidence, thus making it one of the best reference books on the market. This volume should be on the desk of every health professions education educator and on the shelf of every health sciences library, worldwide.

Ara Tekian
Professor of Medical Education
Director, International Affairs
Department of Medical Education
Associate Dean, Office of International Education
College of Medicine
University of Illinois at Chicago
Chicago, IL, USA

Preface

Understanding Medical Education was launched as a series of monographs in September 2006, and was the brainchild of the Association of Medical Education's then Chief Executive, Frank Smith. It proved an outstanding success, selling tens of thousands of copies worldwide and in 2010 the Association brought the series together into a single core textbook, providing a comprehensive guide to the theoretical and academic bases to modern medical education practice. Contributors include experts from all walks of medical education from across the world. As well as providing practical guidance for clinicians, teachers and researchers, *Understanding Medical Education* is designed to meet the needs of all newcomers to medical education, including those studying at certificate, diploma or master's level, providing an accessible and contemporary reference. Most importantly, *Understanding Medical Education* aims to be both accessible and useful to the reader. The intention is that after reading one of the chapters the reader will not only be better informed about their field of interest, but able to assimilate their new knowledge into their clinical teaching or academic activities.

This second edition sees major updates of all existing chapters but also some completely new ones, including chapters on technology-enhanced learning, standard-setting in assessment and career support. The second edition also comes with a new foreword from Ara Tekian, Professor of Medical Education at the University of Illinois and winner of the 2012 ASME Gold Medal Award.

Understanding Medical Education remains the first port of call for anyone engaged in medical education as an academic discipline. The book is a unique resource which should prove invaluable for anyone involved in the development of health care professionals, in whatever discipline, wherever they are in the world.

An online edition of the complete book together with individual chapter downloads is available at http://onlinelibrary.wiley.com/

Editor: Professor Tim Swanwick

Tim Swanwick MA FRCGP MA(Ed) FAcadMEd has a broad range of experience in medical education and is based in the UK in London, where he is Postgraduate Dean of Medical Education for Health Education North Central and East London. Tim is also a Visiting Professor at the University of Bedfordshire and an Honorary Senior Lecturer at Imperial College and has researched and published widely, particularly in the fields of faculty and leadership development.

Association for the Study of Medical Education

The Association for the Study of Medical Education (ASME) seeks to improve the quality of medical education by bringing together individuals and organisations with interests and responsibilities in medical and health care education. The association is unique in that it draws its members from all areas of medical education and from all specialties. It provides a forum for debate and the exchange of information, and an international network for the promotion of knowledge and expertise in medical education.

Acknowledgements

Producing a textbook such as this is a team effort, and thanks for this second edition must go to the ASME Executive and *Understanding Medical Education* advisory board for their guidance, Nicky Pender and the ASME team for their administrative support and also to Martin Davies and Karen Moore at Wiley Blackwell for helping to make the second edition of *Understanding Medical Education* such an impressive and attractive volume.

ICONS

Throughout the *Understanding Medical Education* series readers will come across a number of icons in the margin. These graphic devices serve to highlight certain insert boxes where the author wishes to take the reader off into a particular area in greater detail (Focus on), explore the evidence behind a particular concept (Where's the evidence), provide practical advice (How to) or summarise the main points of the paper (Key messages).

FOCUS ON

WHERE'S THE EVIDENCE?

HOW TO

KEY MESSAGES

Part 1
Foundations

1 Understanding medical education

Tim Swanwick
Health Education North Central and East London, UK

It was the nuclear physicist and father of the hydrogen bomb, Edmund Teller, who once wrote (perhaps rather alarmingly) 'Confusion is no bad thing; it is the first step towards understanding'.(1, p. 79) Newcomers to the field of medical education could be forgiven for being confused. Medical education is a busy, clamorous place, where a host of pedagogical practices, educational philosophies and conceptual frameworks collide. It is a place where academic journals vie for attention, institutions and professional bodies compete for political leverage, and the wheel of reform and 'improvement' revolves faster than, and often independently of, the cycle of evaluation and research. And it is a place of increasing accountability and regulation because of its proximity to one of the prime socio-political concerns of government, that of the health of its people.

It was the desire to develop evidence-based policy and practice in this complex arena that led to the establishment of the Association for the Study of Medical Education (ASME) in 1957. The past 50 years have seen a burgeoning of literature in the field. This is both a help and a challenge to the clinician taking on responsibilities for teaching, assessment and educational supervision. The range and diversity of relevant theory and research are now almost overwhelming, and in 2006 ASME recognised the need for a succinct yet comprehensive guide to the vast literature now underpinning best practice in medical education. *Understanding Medical Education* aims to be that guide.

What is medical education?

Medical education as we know it today spans three sectors: undergraduate, postgraduate and the continuing professional development of established clinicians. However, it has not always been that way, and Abraham Flexner – whose seminal report on the transformation of the American medical school system was celebrated earlier this decade(2) – would not have recognised the attention currently given to the design, management and quality assurance of structured training in the postgraduate years, still less the need to instigate regulatory systems to ensure the ongoing personal and professional development of practising clinicians.

Medical education's ultimate aim is to supply society with a knowledgeable, skilled and up-to-date cadre of professionals who put patient care above self-interest, and undertake to maintain and develop their expertise over the course of a lifelong career. Medicine has a privileged position in society and, as a result, medical education is itself set apart from the main body of higher education. In many countries it luxuriates in separate funding streams and higher rates of remuneration for its clinical teachers; is the beneficiary of status and patronage through its colleges, academies and professional institutions; and is a formidably powerful, and predominantly conservative, political lobby, more than occasionally a source of frustration for those who seek to modernise health services.

Within the confines of this academic and political preserve lies the discipline of medical education; although one could question whether medical education is a discipline in its own right, or an idiosyncratic collection of concepts appropriated from other educational fields and perfused with a technical rationality borne out of the dominance of bioscience within medicine.(3,4) There are certainly a number of predominant educational assumptions, such as experiential learning and reflective practice, and favoured curricular approaches borrowed from other fields – witness the transplantation of competency-based education from vocational training. But medical education is not just a 'magpie' and has made, and continues to make, its own significant advances and contributions to the wider educational literature. Many of these unique and major developments are expounded within this book: problem-based learning, simulation, structured assessments of clinical competence, supervision and the use of technology to enhance learning, to name but a few.

Challenges and preoccupations

Another characteristic of medical education is that it is, as Cooke and her colleagues note, 'in a perpetual state of unrest'.(5, p. 1339) A constant stream of reports issues from regulators, commissions, inquiries and task forces urging reform. This may just reflect the sluggish response to change and innate conservatism of the profession and its educational institutions. This is not, as it happens, a new phenomenon. In the UK, George Pickering, writing as far back in 1956, offers us the wry observation that 'no country has produced so many excellent analyses of the present defects of medical education as has Britain, and no country has done less to implement them'.(6) Britain is not alone in this regard and from the other side of the Atlantic, Warren Anderson – in a special centenary 'Flexner' edition of *Medical Education* – questions 'whether the current proliferation of literature about reforms in medical education can lead to real change, or whether it constitutes a self referential agitation that, in the aggregate, holds little promise'.

Understanding Medical Education: Evidence, Theory and Practice, Second Edition. Edited by Tim Swanwick.
© 2014 The Association for the Study of Medical Education. Published 2014 by John Wiley & Sons, Ltd.

(7, p.29) Despite such reservations, the frequency of such reports increases, and the clarion calls to action grow ever louder. So what are the current preoccupations of medical education and society's expectations of it?

To begin at the beginning, getting the right students and later on the right trainees training in the right specialty is crucial. In a competitive and litigious environment, the importance of having demonstrably fair selection processes is unarguable. Good person–job fit is essential to productivity, quality and job satisfaction. In Chapter 28, Fiona Patterson and her colleagues identify just how difficult getting all this right can be. Predicting who will make a good doctor is critically dependent on what the role of the doctor will be 10–15 years into the future, something that is increasingly uncertain. So are there generic attributes that we can select for? What selection methods should we use? And to encourage the recruitment of well-rounded practitioners, should entry to medical school be graduate only?

Having selected the right students and, with luck, matched the right trainees to the most suitable postgraduate training programme, how and what are they to learn, and how can the *quality* of their education and training be ensured? An array of educational approaches are described in the central section of this book, framed by a discussion by Janet Grant on approaches to curriculum design and the importance of its context (Chapter 3). A concise summary of relevant, and guiding, educational theory is provided by David Kauffman and Karen Mann in Chapter 2, and in Chapter 4, Alan Bleakley and colleagues discuss the prevailing, and some alternative discourses surrounding the thorny concept of quality.

It was Flexner's mentor, William Osler, who brought students and patients closer together through his educational philosophy that medicine was 'learned by the bedside and not in the classroom',(8, p. 188) and the practical introduction of residency programmes. Both are now threatened by concerns over patient safety, expansion of medical student numbers, regulatory requirements on working hours and a staggeringly accelerated patient throughput. Patients undergoing gall bladder operations in Osler's day were in hospital for several weeks – the procedure now is carried out on a day-patient basis. At almost every stage of training, learners see fewer patients, do less to them and as a consequence find themselves increasingly unprepared for practice.(9) This, as Clare Morris and David Blaney highlight in Chapter 7, and John Launer in Chapter 8, requires new ways of thinking about work-based learning and the role of the trainer or supervisor.

A related concern is patient safety. Medicine is not only faster-paced, it is also more hazardous. As Cyril Chantler has succinctly put it: 'Medicine used to be simple, ineffective and relatively safe. Now it is complex, effective and potentially dangerous'.(10, p. 1178)

One of the responses to reduced opportunities for contact with patients and more hazardous interventions has been the widespread adoption of simulation across all fields and stages of medical education. The availability of sophisticated technologies now enables high-fidelity reproduction of complex patient scenarios. Students and doctors in training no longer need to carry out procedures for the first time on real patients – the skills of ophthalmoscopy, venepuncture and catheterisation can all be learned in the skills laboratory. Full-immersion scenarios also offer the opportunity to work on non-technical areas such as team working, leadership and situational awareness. However, questions remain about transfer to the authentic setting – an issue that is explored in depth by Jean Ker and Paul Bradley in Chapter 13.

Growing concerns over patient safety have influenced not only the way medicine is practised – with the widespread introduction of protocols, checks and audit – but also the degree to which doctors are now publicly accountable. In the UK, high-profile cases such as Bristol,(11) Alder Hey,(12) and Shipman(13) and more recently the Francis Inquiries (14,15) have ushered in a new era of accountability, and 2013 sees the introduction of relicensing for all medical practitioners in Britain, with regulators coming under increasing and critical pressure. Patient safety issues also permeate undergraduate medicine. Protecting patients within a teaching and learning environment, while producing competent doctors who will maintain their knowledge, attitudes and skills, is a major challenge for those who design undergraduate curricula.

Increasing accountability is just one facet of a new social compact with patients; a compact, no longer based on blind and unquestioning trust, but on true partnership. As John Spencer, writing with Judy McKimm, highlights in Chapter 17, we see increased patient involvement across the board in both teaching and learning, and also in decision-making about how medical education is organised, governed and its resources allocated. Patients are now also intimately involved in the selection and assessment of both undergraduate students and postgraduate trainees, and feedback from patients is a routine feature of continuing professional development and reaccreditation processes.

One of the corollaries of the above is that there is a growing recognition of the need to professionalise clinical teaching.(16) The pressures for this are channelled through professional bodies, but also arise from an increase in the expectations of students and doctors in training about the quality of the learning opportunities they are afforded. Clinical teachers and others with responsibilities for medical education increasingly look for academic support and accreditation of their expertise, and one of the target groups of *Understanding Medical Education* are newcomers to medical education, whether undergraduate or postgraduate, including those studying at certificate, diploma and master's levels. As Yvonne Steinert describes in Chapter 32 – on faculty development – such professional credentialing of medical educators is a burgeoning industry in Europe and North America and reflects a more general trend of the 'professionalisation' of medical education. Professionalisation has produced a new breed of scholarly educators and, coming as they do from a bioscientific background, a desire for evidence-informed medical education practice.

This raises questions about the nature of medical education research and again, as is highlighted in the four chapters on research and evaluation (Chapters 24–27), we see worlds colliding. In a recent exchange in ASME's academic journal, *Medical Education,* a series of articles considered whether it is helpful to construe medical education as a medical or a social science.(17,18) Monrouxe and Rees capture the essence of the debate:

> Medical education research has benefited from its association with 'hard' medical science in that this has encouraged the engagement of clinicians in research activities. However, this gain is offset by a particular loss represented by the failure (of some) to understand that medical education is about people, and the way we think, act and interact in the world. Medical education research is not a poor relation of medical research; it belongs to a different family altogether.(18, p. 198)

Curriculum design continues to evolve, with problem-based learning, discussed in detail in Chapter 5, now influencing the majority of medical school courses. Postgraduate medical education is also in the throes of curricular change, with many specialties formerly taught to implicit and informal curricula now articulating explicit and public curriculum statements for the first time. Curriculum delivery is also challenged by the emerging possibilities of technology, many of which are addressed by Scott Rice and Jean McKendree in Chapter 12, and in a new chapter by Alison Bullock and Peter de Jong on the relationship between technology and learning (Chapter 11).

There are macro-political concerns too, around the commissioning of medical education and its responsiveness to service needs. The demographics are changing: at the beginning of the 21st century the developed countries are already experiencing the demands of an increasingly elderly population with complex health care needs, and across the increasingly interdependent world, we see a health inequalities gap that shows no signs of narrowing, with health care systems struggling to cope.(19) Rising patient expectations and an ease of access to information present challenges not only in how care is delivered, but where and by whom. Managers within all health care systems are waking up to the fact that the majority of their future employees already work in their health services and that significant investment may need to be diverted from training new and inexperienced practitioners into developing and supporting their existing workforce.

Finally, there is the vexed question of 'what is a doctor?' (or any other health care professional, for that matter). With significant overlaps in knowledge and skills developing, what unique features does a doctor bring to the bedside or office, and what do we mean by a professional in the 21st century? Friedson argues that the professions, societal groups based on expertise, altruism and self-scrutiny, will never disappear, but will merely shrink in size, as much of their work is taken on by a deprofession-alised operating core of medical technicians.(20) Others, such as Donald Berwick, disagree and see 'the reinvention of professionalism in a world on new terms of engagement; complexity, interdependence, pervasive hazard, a changing distribution of power and control and borne on the back of technology, distributed, democratised capacities . . .'(21, p. 130)

What is certain is that at no point in the past has the medical profession had to engage so actively with these debates, and the question 'What are we educating for?' has never been so important.

Scholarship and the pursuit of excellence

Understanding Medical Education began life as a series of free-standing monographs. The aim of the series was to provide an authoritative, up-to-date and comprehensive resource summarising the theoretical and academic bases to modern medical education practice. It is now a best-selling textbook worldwide and although its expert authors come from Europe, Australasia and North America, it offers a global perspective on contemporary practice and scholarship.

Boyer's expanded definition of 'scholarship' takes us beyond the narrow confines of research to consider the need to recognise and reward not only the scholarship of 'discovery' but also that of integration of new knowledge, its application to social practice and teaching.(22) This is a hugely important distinction for medical education, as the vast majority of medical educators are not researchers, nor indeed do they have the opportunity to work across disciplinary boundaries to integrate new knowledge. What they can be, and often are, are excellent teachers and scholarly agents of change and improvement within medical education. This highlights a perennial problem in medical education, namely that funding for academic institutions, either through grants or vehicles such as the UK's Research Excellence Framework(23) is linked strongly to research output. Similarly, teaching in clinical settings usually plays 'second fiddle' to clinical productivity. This has led to a situation where both academic and service institutions continue to emphasise staff involvement in activities other than teaching, an activity that remains largely unrewarded and unrecognised, and a challenge that new professional bodies such as the UK's Academy of Medical Educators have set out to address.(24)

Medical education is complicated, contested and highly political. In a complex and uncertain world we need to make the best decisions about education, training and development that we can. For that, we need both scholarly medical educators *and* educational scholars. I hope that this book may contribute to their development.

References

1 Teller E, Teller W and Talley W (1991) Hypotheses non fingo, Chapter 5. In: *Conversations on the Dark Secrets of Physics*. Perseus Publishing, Cambridge, MA.

2 Lexner A (1910) *Medical Education in the United States and Canada: A Report to the Carnegie Foundation for the Advancement of Teaching*. Carnegie Foundation for the Advancement of Teaching, New York.

3 Swanwick T (2013) Doctors, science and society. *Medical Education*. **47**: 7–9.

4 Whitehead C (2013) Scientist or science-stuffed? Discourses of science in North American Medical Education. *Medical Education*. **47**: 26–32.

5 Cooke M, Irby DM, Sullivan W and Ludmerer KM (2006) American medical education 100 years after the Flexner Report. *New England Journal of Medicine*. **355**: 1339–44.

6 Pickering GW (1956) The purpose of medical education. *British Medical Journal*. **2**(4968): 113–6.

7 Anderson W (2011) Outside looking in: observations on medical education since the Flexner Report. *Medical Education*. **45**: 29–35.

8 Osler W (2003) Quoted. In: Silverman ME, Murray TJ and Bryan CS (eds) *The Quotable Osler*. American College of Physicians – American Society for Internal Medicine, Philadelphia, PA.

9 Illing J, Davies C and Bauldauf B (2008) *How Prepared are Medical Graduates to Begin Practice. A comparison of three diverse medical schools. Report to Education Committee of the General Medical Council.* General Medical Council, London.

10 Chantler C (1999) The role and education of doctors in the delivery of healthcare. *Lancet.* **353**: 1178–81.

11 Bristol Royal Infirmary Enquiry (2001) Learning from Bristol: the report of the public inquiry into children's heart surgery at the Bristol Royal Infirmary 1984–1995. (http://www.bristol-inquiry.org.uk; accessed June 2009).

12 Redfern M (2001) The Royal Liverpool Children's Inquiry Report (The Alder Hey report). (http://www.rlcinquiry.org.uk; accessed June 2009).

13 Smith J (2005) Shipman Fifth Report. Safeguarding Patients: lessons from the past – proposals for the future. (http://www.the-shipman-inquiry.org.uk; accessed June 2009).

14 Francis R (2010) The Mid Staffordshire NHS Foundation Trust Inquiry. (http://www.dh.gov.uk/en/Publicationsandstatistics/Publications/PublicationsPolicyAndGuidance/DH_113018; accessed 11 January 2013).

15 Francis R (2013) The Francis Inquiry [due out Feb 2013 – add in at page proof stage].

16 Swanwick T (2009) Teaching the teachers – no longer an optional extra. *British Journal of Hospital Medicine.* **70**: 176–7.

17 Bligh J and Brice J (2008) What is the value of good medical education research? *Medical Education.* **42**(7): 652–3.

18 Monrouxe LV and Rees CE (2009) Picking up the gauntlet: constructing medical education as a social science. *Medical Education.* **43**: 196–8.

19 Frenk J, Chen L, Bhutta ZA *et al.* (2010) Health professionals for a new century: transforming education to strengthen health systems in an interdependent world. *Lancet.* **376**: 1923–58.

20 Friedson E (1988) *Profession of Medicine: A Study of the Sociology of Applied Knowledge.* University of Chicago Press, Chicago, IL.

21 Berwick D (2009) The epitaph of profession. *British Journal of General Practice.* **59**: 128–31.

22 Boyer EL (1997) *Scholarship Reconsidered: Priorities of the Professoriate.* Jossey-Bass, San Francisco, CA.

23 Higher Education Funding Council for England, Scottish Funding Council, Higher Education Funding Council for Wales, Department for Employment and Learning NI. (2012) Research Evaluation Framework 2014. (http://www.ref.ac.uk/; accessed 11 January 2013).

24 Bligh J and Brice J (2007) The Academy of Medical Educators: a professional home for medical educators in the UK. *Medical Education.* **41**: 625–7.

2 Teaching and learning in medical education: How theory can inform practice

David M Kaufman[1] and Karen V Mann[2]

[1]Faculty of Education, Simon Fraser University, Canada
[2]Faculty of Medicine, Dalhousie University, Canada

 KEY MESSAGES

- Understanding educational theory can enhance both teaching and learning.
- The learner is an active contributor in the educational process.
- Learners interact actively with curricula, patients and teachers in a complex, changing environment.
- The entire context of learning is important, rather than any single variable, and includes interactions of all the variables.
- Values, attitudes and the culture of the profession are often learned implicitly and without explicit teaching or awareness of learning.
- Learning is enhanced when it is relevant, particularly to the solution and understanding of real-life problems and practice.

- Individuals' past experience and knowledge are critical to how they learn.
- Learning has a significant emotional aspect to it that is often under-recognised.
- Individual learners are capable of self-regulation, that is, setting goals, planning strategies and monitoring their progress.
- The ability to reflect on one's practice (performance) is critical to lifelong, self-directed learning.
- Learning occurs collectively as well as individually as individuals construct shared knowledge and understanding through their work together.

Introduction

The frequently identified gap between theory and practice has led practitioners in many professions to conclude that theory belongs in its ivory tower, neither useful nor relevant to those in practice. Education is no exception.(1) However, as the processes that underpin educational practice are better understood, it is clear that theory has the potential both to inform practice and to be informed by it.

Our purpose in this chapter is to describe eight selected approaches to education theory and explore their implications for the practice of medical education. We use the term 'theory' in a general sense, that is, as a set of assumptions and ideas that help to explain some phenomenon. Knowles put this succinctly more than 25 years ago, defining a theory as: 'a comprehensive, coherent, and internally consistent system of ideas about a set of phenomena'.(2, p. 5)

Each of the theoretical approaches we describe is consistent with Knowles' definition. The eight theoretical approaches discussed are:
- adult learning principles(3)
- social cognitive theory(4)
- reflective practice(5, pp. 57–60)
- transformative learning(6)
- self-directed learning(7)
- experiential learning(8)
- situated learning(9)
- learning in communities of practice.(10)

We selected these because we believe them to be particularly useful in the context of the issues facing medical education today. We will describe each theoretical formulation, highlighting its major constructs, and present implications of the theory for educational practice. We will conclude with a consideration of the connections and commonalities among the eight theories, so that readers may make these connections within their own practice.

Adult learning principles

The purpose of adult education has been the subject of a number of typologies.(11–15) In general, they accord with a list proposed by Darkenwald and Merriam,(15, pp. 43–64) namely:
- cultivation of the intellect
- individual self-actualisation
- personal and social improvement
- social transformation
- organisational effectiveness.

Understanding Medical Education: Evidence, Theory and Practice, Second Edition. Edited by Tim Swanwick.
© 2014 The Association for the Study of Medical Education. Published 2014 by John Wiley & Sons, Ltd.

A number of theoretical frameworks have developed around these functions, which Merriam[16] has grouped into three categories. The first category is based on *adult learning characteristics*, in which the best-known framework is 'andragogy'.[3] Also in this group is Cross's[17] 'Characteristics of Adults as Learners' model, based on differences between adults and children across personal and situational characteristics. The second category emphasises the *adult's life situation*. Two theories have been proposed in this category, Knox's Proficiency Theory[18] and McClusky's Theory of Margin.[19] The third category focuses on *changes in consciousness*. Several models in this category emphasise reflection upon experience and environment of which Mezirow's Perspective Transformation[20] (discussed later) and Freire's Theory of Conscientisation[21] are the best-developed models.

Merriam, Caffarella, and Baugartner[22] have provided an excellent summary of the various theory-building efforts in adult learning. They conclude that no single theory fares well when judged by the criteria of comprehensiveness (i.e. includes all types of learning), practicality and universality of its application. They also assert that a phenomenon as complex as adult learning will probably never be adequately explained by a single theory. Although these theoretical frameworks provide implications for practice, few have actually been applied widely in adult education practice. Knowles' andragogy[3] is the exception. The remainder of this section therefore focuses on andragogy, and its implications for practice and provides an example of its use in undergraduate medical education.

Andragogy

Malcolm Knowles[3] first introduced the term 'andragogy' to North America, defining it as 'the art and science of helping adults learn'. Knowles did not present andragogy as an empirically based theory, but simply as a set of four assumptions,[3] to which a fifth and sixth were later added. The six assumptions underlying andragogy, as theorised by Knowles, are that: (1) adult self-concept is well-developed; (2) adults bring considerable experience to learning; (3) readiness to learn depends on need; (4) adults tend to have a problem-centered focus; (5) adults are generally internally motivated; and (6) adults need to know why they need to know something. *See* Box 2.1.[22–24]

Andragogy has its roots in humanistic psychology through the work of Maslow[25] and Rogers.[26] The core basis of andragogy is that the attainment of adulthood is marked by adults coming to view themselves as self-directed individuals. Knowles' 'model of assumptions' has given adult education a 'badge of identity' that distinguishes the field from other areas of education, for example, childhood schooling.[27] Bard has asserted that andragogy 'probably more than any other force, has changed the role of the learner in adult education and in human resource development'[28, p. xi]. However, it has also caused enormous controversy, debate and criticism. The early criticism led Knowles to later modify his model by describing andragogy and pedagogy as a continuum, and suggesting that the use of both teaching methods is appropriate at different times in different situations, regardless of the learner's age.[23]

BOX 2.1 Andragogical assumptions[3,23]

1 *Self-concept*. Adults typically want to choose what they want to learn, when they want to learn it, and how they want to learn.

2 *Experience*. Adult learners have a wealth of life experiences that they bring with them into new learning experiences, and they can contribute richness to learning from and with each other.

3 *Readiness to learn depends on need*. Adults are ready to learn when they see what they need to know will help them to deal with life situations.

4 *Problem-centred focus*. Adults need to see the immediate application of learning, so they seek learning opportunities that will enable them to solve problems.

5 *Internal motivation*. Adults seek learning opportunities due to external motivators, but the more potent motivators, such as self-esteem, better quality of life, and self-actualisation, are internal.

6 *Adults need to know why they need to learn something*. Adults need to know how they will benefit from this new knowledge, for example, to solve a problem or apply immediately.

It is widely accepted that andragogy is not really a theory of *how* adults learn, the assumptions being merely descriptions of the adult learner.[29] Furthermore, even the assumptions have been questioned as prescriptions for practice. The general critique is that andragogy lacks the fundamental characteristics of a science because of limited empirical evidence produced.[22,30,31] Others argue that andragogy may in time become a theory, but through empirical studies of the assumptions. Knowles resigned himself to explaining andragogy as less of a theory of adult learning than a 'model of assumptions about learning or a conceptual framework that serves as a basis for emergent theory'.[3, p. 112] At the least, andragogy captures general characteristics of adult learners and offers guidelines for planning instruction with learners who tend to be at least somewhat independent and self-directed.[32]

Implications for educational practice

There are several implications for practice that can be derived from the theories of adult learning which have at their heart the fact that an adult's life situation is quite different from that of a child. Merriam *et al.*[22] discuss the differences between adults' and children's' learning in three areas: context, learner and learning process.

Context

Children are dependent on others for their well-being, while adults have assumed responsibility for managing their own lives. Typically, being a learner is only one of several roles played concurrently by adults. Additionally, the principles that have guided approaches to teaching children, and which have been applied to learners of all ages, have focused on generalised learning in the school setting.(33) In contrast, adults generally learn and function in settings where situation-specific skills are required to resolve relevant problems.

Learner

As Knowles(3) has described, there are significant differences between adults and children that must be addressed in the learning process. These include the need of adults to be self-directing, their large reservoir of experience, the relationship of their readiness to learn to their social role, their desire for knowledge that can be immediately applied to current relevant problems and their internal motivation to learn.

Learning process

Three non-cognitive factors have been shown to affect adult learning:(22)
- pacing
- meaningfulness
- motivation.

Pacing of learning, through deadlines or other external pressure, may adversely affect learning, since adults have many competing demands. Also, adults tend to perform poorly on learning tasks that are not meaningful, or which do not fall within their domain of interest.

A teacher using andragogical principles focuses more on being a facilitator of learning rather than a transmitter of knowledge and evaluator.(34) Vella(35) lists 12 major steps that should be addressed with adult learners. These include a needs assessment of what is to be learned; a feeling of safety for the learner in the environment; sound relationships between the facilitator and the learners; the sequence of the content presented and its reinforcement; the use of praxis; the establishment of respect for learners as decision makers; the understanding of the learners' ideas, feelings, and actions; immediacy of the learning; clearly established roles on the part of the facilitator and learners; the use of teamwork; the engagement of learners, and accountability.

The ideas presented thus far can be formulated as a set of principles to guide adult learning activities. Several writers have proposed principles or 'tips' for practitioners.(23,36) Knowles(23) himself drew seven principles from the assumptions of andragogy, which are presented here (*see* Box 2.2).

Social cognitive theory

Social cognitive theory belongs to the family of social learning theories, which acknowledge that our learning is social in nature: we learn from and in interaction with others and with our environment. Social cognitive theory,(4) formerly social learning theory, was developed by Bandura(37) and unites two approaches to our understanding of learning. These are the behaviourist approach, which emphasises the influence of the environment on our actions, and the cognitive approach, which emphasises the importance of cognition in mediating our learning and functioning.

> **BOX 2.2 Principles of adult learning(23)**
>
> 1 An effective learning climate should be established. Learners should be comfortable, both physically and emotionally. They should feel safe and free to express themselves without judgement or ridicule.
>
> 2 Learners should be involved in mutual planning of methods and curricular directions. Involvement will help assure that collaboration occurs in the content and learning process. It will also increase the relevance to learners' needs.
>
> 3 Learners should be involved in diagnosing their own learning needs. Once again, this will help to ensure meaningfulness and will trigger learners' internal (intrinsic) motivation. It will also promote self-assessment and reflection, and effective integration of learning.
>
> 4 Learners should be encouraged to formulate their own learning objectives. The rationale for this is the same as for 3, above. Learners are thus encouraged to take control of their learning.
>
> 5 Learners should be encouraged to identify resources and to devise strategies for using them to accomplish their objectives. This principle connects adult learning needs to practical resources for meeting their objectives, and also provides motivation for using such resources for a specific and focused purpose.
>
> 6 Learners should be helped to carry out their learning plans. One of the key elements of motivation is expectancy of success. Learners will become discouraged and lose their motivation, if a learning task is too difficult. Also, too much pressure without support can lead to a decrement in learning.
>
> 7 Learners should be involved in evaluating their own learning. This is an essential step in a self-directed learning process that requires critical reflection on experience.

These two approaches are united in a basic tenet of social cognitive theory, which posits that our actions, learning and functioning are the result of a continuous, dynamic, reciprocal interaction among three sets of determinants: personal, environmental (situational) and behavioural. Personal factors include the individual's attitudes, perceptions, values, goals, knowledge and all previous experience. Environmental factors encompass all those influences that may enable or hinder actions and the achievement of goals. Bandura notes explicitly that 'personal and environmental influences do not function as independent determinants; rather, they affect each other. People create, alter and destroy environments. The changes they produce in environmental conditions, in turn, affect them personally.'(4, p. 23) Bandura further states that behaviour, rather than being a 'detached by-product' of persons and situations, is itself an interacting determinant in the process. Figure 2.1 shows the interactions schematically and how these might apply to medical education.

Bandura asserts that the relative influences exerted by each of the three sets of factors will vary for different

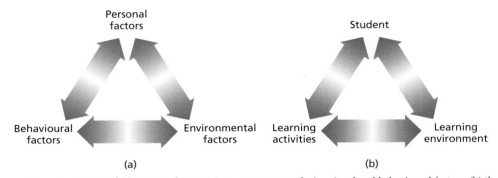

Figure 2.1 Diagrammatic representation of (a) reciprocal interaction among personal, situational and behavioural factors; (b) the same factors using a medical education example.

activities, different individuals and different circumstances. For example, when environmental conditions exert a powerful influence, they will prevail. In a medical education example, when trainees are thrust into the busy environment of a clinical ward, they will do what is required to 'get the job done' and to meet expectations. In other cases, the behaviour and its feedback will be a major influence. For instance, when students are learning and practising a new skill, the feedback from this will have a strong influence. Finally, in those instances where situational influences are relatively weak, personal factors will exert the strongest regulatory influence. To complete our example, when not pressed by powerful environmental forces students may choose to learn a new skill or to learn more about talking with patients. These choices will be affected by the student's own values, perceived needs and individual goals. There may also be interaction within each factor (for example, conflicting values within and individual). The simple example provided here is not intended to convey lack of complexity; rather, it is to emphasise the ongoing, dynamic nature of our interaction with our environment.

Environmental influences can affect people in ways other than their behaviour, as when thoughts and feelings are modified through observing others' behaviour (modelling), or through teaching or social persuasion. Our thoughts do not arise in a vacuum. Individual perceptions and understandings are developed and verified through both direct and vicarious experience, judgements of others and by inference from what is already known.(4, p. 27)

Basic human capabilities

Bandura views humans as possessing five basic capabilities that underpin our learning and functioning in all situations. These capabilities are particularly important when we consider the processes of learning in medical and health professional education.

Symbolising capability

Almost every aspect of our lives is touched by our remarkable ability to use symbols to transform our experience into a form that can be internalised and serve as a guide to future actions. This ability enables us, when confronted with a new problem, to test possible solutions symbolically, rather than laboriously trying out each alternative.

Forethought capability

Most of our behaviour is regulated by thought. We anticipate the likely outcomes of our actions and plan goals for ourselves and courses of action to maximise the likelihood of obtaining them. Also, as noted, images of desirable future events, such as achieving our goals, can become motivators of our current behaviour.

Vicarious capability

If learning occurred only through performing actions and experiencing their effects, learning and development would be slow, tedious and enormously inefficient. Fortunately, much learning that can be acquired through direct experience can also be acquired or facilitated vicariously through observation of other people's actions and their consequences. This applies to social development, especially where, in some situations, new behaviours can only be conveyed effectively by modelling. Even if learning can occur in other ways, the ability to learn vicariously distinctly shortens the process.

Self-regulatory capability

In social cognitive theory, the capability for self-regulation is central. Much of our behaviour is regulated primarily by our internal standards and our evaluative reactions to our own actions. Any discrepancies between our actions and those standards activate a self-evaluation, which will influence our subsequent behaviour. Self-evaluation is our personal guidance system for action. We exercise self-regulation or self-directedness by arranging facilitative environmental conditions for ourselves, using our images of future events as guides and creating incentives for our efforts.

Self-reflective capability

Perhaps the most distinctive is the capability for self-reflection, whereby we can look critically at our experiences and think about our thought processes. Cognitive theorists refer to this as metacognitive capability. Through self-reflection we gain understanding about ourselves, our behaviour and the world around us. (Reflection and reflective practice will be addressed later in the chapter.)

Self-efficacy

A central concept in social cognitive theory is *self-efficacy*; the individual's judgement about his or her ability to carry out a specific task or activity, and to produce certain attainments. It is not a global perception, but is more specific to a domain of activity. These beliefs influence the courses of action we pursue; the challenges and goals we set, and our commitment to them; the level and difficulty of the goals we set; the effort we invest, and how long we persist in the face of obstacles; our resilience to adversity, the life choices we make, and what we can achieve.(38) In 2006, Bandura noted that self-efficacy beliefs affect not just our behaviour, but our goals and aspirations: they also determine what barriers and opportunities we see in the environment (*see* Box 2.3).(39)

 BOX 2.3 FOCUS ON: Self-efficacy(40)

According to Bandura,(4) a central type of thought that affects action is people's judgements of their capabilities to deal with different realities, or their self-efficacy. This judgement influences what people choose to do, how much effort they invest in activities, how long they persist in the face of disappointment and whether tasks are approached anxiously or assuredly. Judgements about our personal efficacy, whether accurate of faulty, arise from four main information sources, as follows.

- *Performance attainments* – our own performance is the most influential source of efficacy because it is based on authentic experience of mastery. Successes raise our efficacy appraisals; failures generally have a lowering effect, especially if they occur early in the learning and they do not reflect lack of effort or difficult situations. Once strong positive efficacy perceptions are developed, occasional failures do not have a marked effect. Feelings of capability are generally task-specific, though they can generalise to other, similar tasks.

- *Vicarious experience* – observing other similar people perform successfully can raise our own beliefs that we can perform similar tasks. This source of information is particularly effective when people encounter new tasks and have little experience on which to base their perceptions. Learning from role models is an excellent example of vicarious learning.

- *Verbal persuasion* – we have all had the experience of trying to convince people that they possess capabilities that will enable them to achieve what they seek. If the heightened efficacy that the persuasion is attempting to achieve is realistic, it can be influential, particularly in affecting the amount of effort individuals put into a task.

- *Physiological state* – people often judge their capability based on the messages received about their physiological states. We frequently interpret arousal in taxing situations as an ominous sign of vulnerability, and tend to expect more success when we are not tense and aroused.

Implications for educational practice

Understanding the concepts of ongoing dynamic interactions, basic human capabilities and how people form perceptions of their abilities allows us to plan a learning environment that is most conducive to maximising each individual's development. We will consider some implications of this theory for effective teaching and learning; in particular, five learning processes (that build on the basic capabilities) that can be brought to bear in medical education:

- formulation of a clear objective, goal or desired outcome
- modelling or demonstration
- provision of task-relevant knowledge
- guided practice and feedback
- opportunities for learners to reflect on their learning.

A *clear objective*, goal or image of the desired outcome enhances learning. It builds on our capability for forethought, providing a guidepost for monitoring and directing our progress appropriately. Awareness of the goal also increases the energy and effort expended and stimulates the development of strategies to reach the goal. Encouraging learners to set their own goals builds on this basic capability.

Modelling or demonstration of the desired process or skill facilitates vicarious learning through observation. This opportunity not only shortens the learning process, it is often essential when new skills are being acquired. Demonstration can help students to form an image of the desired skill/behaviour, which can be used as a guide for action and as a standard of performance against which to monitor their personal progress. Finally, learner perceptions of efficacy are increased by observing someone else perform successfully.

Learners require *task-relevant knowledge*. Learners must have the basic building blocks to use as a foundation for newly acquired knowledge and skills. It may be knowledge related to content or to process, but it must be relevant to the individual's prior knowledge and skills, and to the current learning goal. Further, learners may need stimulation and assistance to activate prior knowledge and to relate it to the new learning. This knowledge promotes students' views of themselves as capable of the task. Otherwise, their perceptions of their efficacy are likely to be low, which will affect both developing efficacy perceptions and their future performance.

Guided practice of a new skill with feedback allows learners to develop positive efficacy perceptions about the task, and to experience successes rather than failures in the crucial early learning period. Practice promotes the internalisation of personal standards, which can then be used in self-regulation and self-evaluation. Corrective, formative feedback is integral to effective learning. Without feedback, the level of performance achieved is lower. Similarly, feedback is less effective in improving performance when it is not related to a goal or desired level of achievement.(40) A large literature exists about feedback and factors that influence its provision, its acceptance and its incorporation and use for improvement. Feedback is central to effective self-direction, setting of goals and internal standards, and self-assessment.

Finally, and arguably most critically, learners require *opportunities to reflect* on their learning, to consider their strategies, to determine whether new approaches are required to achieve their goals and to draw lessons for future learning. Reflection also allows the integration of new experiences into existing experience and knowledge. Finally, it allows the learner to build accurate and positive perceptions of efficacy, based on their experience.

Understanding that learning occurs through observation (i.e. 'vicariously') has important connections to and implications for our practice. This is particularly so when we consider ourselves as role-models. The literature continues to support role-modelling as a pervasive means of teaching and a powerful means of learning. Teachers model knowledge, attitudes, behaviours, approaches to problems, applications of knowledge and skill, and interactions with colleagues, learners, other health professionals, patients, and families. Modelling occurs both when we are aware of it and when we are not. Further, the meaning and intent of what learners observe may not always be clear to them. This suggests the importance of being willing to reflect openly in appropriate situations to allow the meaning to be understood. It is this process of 'making the implicit explicit' that promotes learners to reflect on what they have learned and integrate it into their growing knowledge, skill and developing professional identity. Recognising our roles as models and reflecting on the ways in which we teach through this method can raise our awareness and allow us to be more mindful of ourselves as models.

In summary, social cognitive theory provides us with several important constructs that may inform our educational practice. They include the central concept that learners are constantly interacting with their environment and their actions and consequences. Many of the characteristics that we seek in our learners are present as basic capabilities common to all. Rather than creating these characteristics, learning opportunities can be created to develop and build on them. Finally, we can have some confidence that people are inherently self-directed. Given the appropriate conditions and support, they will set goals, develop strategies to attain them and monitor their progress regularly.

Reflection and reflective practice

The concepts of *reflection* and the *reflective practitioner* are at the centre of the epistemology of professional practice. They borrow from, and link, three previously well-established epistemologies or worldviews about the nature of knowledge and how we can know and understand our world: positivism, interpretive theory and critical theory.(5,41) The positivistic view of science assumes that theory is a scholarly pursuit that may be unrelated to practice. It is the predictive value of theory that is of practical value. Reflection in professional practice extends this view by proposing that theory and practice inform each other. It is a basic premise of reflection that we can learn from our experience in an ongoing iterative process. As knowledge is embedded in practice, practitioners are positioned to test and revise theories through practice. They do so by reflection and action. The reflective process, as such, serves as a bridge in the theory-practice relationship.

Reflection is also related to the interpretive model, which proposes that theory is interpreted in light of personal current and past experiences. Theory guides or enlightens action and understanding. Lastly, the concept of reflective practice shares with critical theory the observation that theory is intimately linked to practice through a process of critical thinking and examination. This process permits professionals to break free from established paradigms and reformulate the ways in which practice, problems and problem solving are viewed. This reframing is part of learning and change. It is how practice helps organise theory.(5,42) Reflective practice then becomes a vehicle for learning effectively.

Several definitions and approaches to reflection and reflective practice are found in the educational literature. Boud, Keogh and Walker defined reflection as 'a generic term for those intellectual and affective activities in which individuals engage to explore their experiences in order to lead to a new understanding and appreciation'.(43, p. 19) With respect to clinical education for medical students, Branch and Paranjape described reflection as 'consideration of the larger context, the meaning and the implications of an experience or action'(44, p. 1185). Lastly, Moon describes reflection as 'a basic mental process with a purpose, an outcome, or both, applied in situations in which material is unstructured or uncertain and where there is no obvious solution'.(45, p.10)

Models of reflective practice

Donald Schön has arguably been the most influential thinker in our understanding of reflective practice among professionals. Schön(5,46) summarises the need for a new scholarship that recognises knowing-in-action, on-the-spot experimentation (reflection-in-action) and action research. Schön's writings about reflective practice(5,46,47) are based on the study of a range of practice professions. He argued that formal theoretical knowledge, such as that acquired in the course of professional preparation, is often not useful to the solution of the 'messy, indeterminate' problems of real-life practice. Central to his premise is the need for professional scholarship and the recognition of an epistemology of professional practice. The reflective practitioner incorporates these principles by relating professional knowledge to practical competence and professional activity. By linking theory to practice, both can inform each other.

Professionals develop zones of mastery around areas of competence. They practise within these areas almost automatically. Schön terms this a professional's 'knowing-in-action'. Indeed, practising one's profession has been likened to riding a bicycle. Occasionally the bicycle skids.(48) This occurs in response to a surprise or to the unexpected. Two types of reflection are triggered at this time: 'reflection-in-action' and 'reflection-on-action'.(5)

Reflection-in-action occurs during the course of an experience; it involves three activities of: (a) reframing and reworking the problem from different perspectives; (b) establishing where the problem fits into learned schema (i.e. already existing knowledge and expertise), and (c) understanding the elements and implications present in the problem, its solution and consequences. *Reflection-on-action*, which occurs after an event, is a process of thinking back on what has happened in the situation to determine what may have contributed to the unexpected, and how what has been learned from this situation may affect future practice. Both are iterative processes whereby insights and learning from one experience may be incorporated into future 'knowing-in-action'.(5,46)

Other approaches to reflection and learning from experience have also been influential.(48–50) Boud *et al.*(43) also outline an iterative process comprising three main phases, beginning with the *experience*. The second phase involves *returning to the experience* and, through reflective processes, dealing with both negative and positive feelings about it, and re-evaluating it. The last aspect of the process Boud *et al.* labelled *outcomes*, in which new perspectives on experience can lead to a change in behaviour and a readiness for application and commitment to action. These authors view reflection as the key to learning effectively. They also emphasise the importance of recognising the emotional aspects of experience that accompany effective learning from experience.

Moon(45) views reflection as the catalyst that moves surface learning to deep learning. Deep learning can be integrated with current experience and knowledge, resulting in rich cognitive networks that the individual can draw on in practice. More recently, reflection has been described as a multifactorial approach that can bring a more systematic method to understanding situations and problems of practice.(51)

Similar characteristics are found across a number of models of reflection, as follows:
- reflection is described as an iterative process
- levels of reflection are defined, from the superficial to the deep
- deeper reflective levels are generally regarded as more difficult to achieve, although they hold greater potential for learning and growth.

There also appears to be a dynamic relationship between reflective practice and self-assessment, both explicitly and implicitly. The ability to self-assess depends on the ability to reflect accurately on one's practice, and the ability to reflect effectively relies heavily on accurate self-assessment.(52,53)

In the workplace, professionals are known for their ability for on-the-spot experimentation and improvisation, their commitment to ongoing practice-based learning and their self-directed reflective learning skills. It is these collective skills that permit professionals to continually and subtly learn from practice, adapt to change and maintain their competence. The core capabilities of professionals are tied to a number of essential skills. Professionals recognise and value the traditional form of knowledge that is gained in school or in study, as well as experiential knowledge that is gained through experience and practice. In the context of their practice, professionals use both these forms of knowledge to continually reshape their approach to problems, solutions, actions and outcomes. This creative process,

sometimes called wisdom or artistry, occurs in response to new meanings, insights and perspectives gained through reflection on current and past experiences. It leads to continued learning and ongoing competence within a profession.(5)

Reflection has frequently been viewed as an individual professional activity. In some cases, reflecting inadequately or inaccurately on one's performance can result in circular, 'single-loop' learning, which can often lead to confirmation of current behaviours, rather than to questioning and identifying areas for learning.(54) For this reason, reflection is increasingly suggested as a collective activity whereby individuals can share individual insights and reflections, and increase their collective and individual learning.(55) Collective reflection is also proposed as a vehicle for developing collective norms and values.(56) The growing evidence surrounding reflective practice is summarised in Box 2.4.

BOX 2.4 WHERE'S THE EVIDENCE: Reflective practice

Despite the observation that reflection has been described in several different fields, and much has been written about it in the respective literatures, the research literature in the field is relatively early in its development. A review(49) of the research across medicine, nursing and other health professions suggests the following.

- Reflective thinking is seen in practising professionals and in students across a variety of heath professions, including nursing, dentistry, medicine and health sciences.
- Reflection appears to serve a number of purposes. In medicine, it appears to occur most naturally in response to complex and new problems.(50) However, it is also demonstrated in anticipation of challenging situations.(57)
- The phenomenon of reflection is not unitary. Several elements and aspects of reflection have been demonstrated. The tendency to reflect and reflective ability vary across individuals and across situations.
- Attempts to measure and classify reflective thinking have resulted in validated instruments which demonstrate that differences exist and are measurable. Generally, it seems that deeper levels of reflection are achieved less often and are more difficult to achieve.
- It appears that reflective ability can be developed. Strategies associated with reported changes in reflective ability used small group resources and activities such as portfolio and journal-keeping.
- Several factors appear to constantly influence reflection, both negatively and positively. These include environment, time, maturity, effective guidance and supervision, and the organisational culture.
- Reflective practice appears to be linked to learning, particularly to deep learning, the development of self-regulated learning and the development of professional identity.(45)

Implications for educational practice

Reflection and reflective practice have become an expected capability of practising professionals. This expectation is stated explicitly in goal statements and definitions of competence. For example, Epstein and Hundert define competence as 'the habitual and judicious use of communication, knowledge, technical skills, clinical reasoning, emotions, values, and reflection in daily practice for the benefit of the individual and community being served'.(58, p. 226) In their definition, reflection becomes a 'habit of mind'.

Reflective practitioners are able to assess a situation from the perspectives of both theoretical background and practical experience. They must be able to bridge successfully the theory–practice gap and apply both aspects of learning, while examining the situation from all perspectives. They must also be able to use their reflective skills to review their practice critically and to inform their self-assessment, based on the feedback they receive. Reflectivity in practice is a learned skill of critical thinking and situation analysis. Deliberate critical reflection on practice may stimulate a new way of thinking about one's practice and lead to the development of adaptive expertise.(59)

While some individuals may be more oriented to reflection than others, reflection, practice-based learning and action based on these are all skills to be learned and applied, and opportunities to acquire them must be made available. The skills required for reflection can be developed in professional courses within our undergraduate, graduate, clinical and continuing medical education areas. Initially, the mentor or teacher models, shares and demonstrates the skills. He or she facilitates the learners' abilities to perceive options and alternatives, to frame and reframe problems, and also assists the learners to reflect on the actions and options they have chosen, and on the knowledge and values that may have influenced their choice. Finally, teachers assist learners to consider critically what they have learned and integrate it into their existing knowledge.

Once the learner has gained sufficient experience and insight into the profession, the teacher's role becomes one of facilitating systematic experiential learning, on-the-spot experimentation and reflection. Teachers observe, provide feedback and help to make explicit those situations in which the learner's reframing has occurred.(48) This helps the learner to become consciously aware of the process of reflection.

However, reflection and how it may enhance learning may not be clear to all learners. Modelling the process becomes very important. This is a challenge for clinicians, as reflection may be a tacit process for many practitioners. Teaching reflection requires making the implicit process explicit. Faculty development programmes developed to enhance the teaching of humanistic skills report success in helping faculty learners to use reflection on their own experience as a source of learning.(60,61) Also, studies of distinguished clinician teachers revealed that they use reflection deliberately, both to improve their own practice and to foster it in their learners.(61)

Several authors have explored how reflection may be taught and incorporated into practice. Slotnick(49) linked Schön's work to how physicians learn in practice. He emphasised the importance of thinking while solving problems (reflection-in-action) and thinking after problem-solving (reflection-on-action). These two activities are required for clinicians to gain new insights and perspectives around practice-based problems, problem solving and practice itself. Slotnick(49) also outlined related principles and implications for learners and teachers in practice. Shapiro and Talbot(48) applied the reflective practice model to family medicine. They proposed that open learning environments encourage a continual reshaping of practice-based learning, along with the development of continuous competence. Lockyer *et al.*(55) explored how reflection could be used in both classrooms and practice to enhance the integration of knowledge and its translation into professional practice.

Other authors have addressed specific areas of teaching, learning and curriculum. Clift *et al.*(62) analysed issues and programmes that encourage reflective practice in education. Palmer *et al.*(57) addressed curriculum design issues specific to professional education and reflection in nursing. They described roles for lecturer-practitioners, mentors (coaches) and mentees. Based on a review by Atkins and Murphy,(52) they identified five skills as essential to partake in reflection: self-awareness, description, critical analysis, synthesis, and evaluation. Crandall(50) demonstrated through clinical teacher interviews that stages of Schön's model occur during effective clinical learning events and offered strategies for using the model to implement reflective practice across the medical education continuum.

Westberg and Jason(63) also offer practical approaches for fostering reflection in medical education, before, during and following experience. They emphasise the importance of the learning environment in effectively fostering reflection. Lastly, Moon(64) proposes a process of reflection to promote transfer of new learning to practice.

Several authors(42,65–70) have linked reflective practice to adult learning theory, deep approaches to learning, developing professional identity and self-directed learning. It appears that reflection may be most useful when it is seen as a strategy to enhance learning. Reflection can help learners to integrate new learning into their existing experience from the beginning of their professional education and throughout their practice. However, learners may require a structure to support them as they acquire these skills. To foster the development of these skills, learners may need feedback on both the content and process of their reflection. Guidance and supervision are critical to this process. The literature documents many varied approaches to incorporating reflection and reflective learning into professional curricula. These include various reflective exercises, reflective writing and portfolio keeping.

There are challenges in the assessment of learning from reflection. There are validated scales that have been developed to measure and assess learners' reflection. Two that have been validated with medical student learners are the Self-reflection and Insight Scale(71) and the Reflection In Learning Scale.(72) These scales can be useful for both learners and teachers in understanding students' readiness for and use of reflection in their learning and its development over time. Palmer *et al.*(57) provided guidance specific to assessing reflective learning. Wald *et al.*(73) have recently developed and validated a rubric for fostering and evaluating reflective capacity in medical learners. Assessment of reflection raises the tension between public and private reflection, which students perceive as a challenge.(74)

As evidence to support the importance of reflection continues to grow, there has been a notable effort to incorporate more reflective activities at all levels of medical education. However, it challenges us to select strategies that will both facilitate active development of reflective capacity and be relevant to learning and practice. A further challenge in the professional context involves helping learners to appreciate the relevance of these activities to their development as competent professionals. A learning environment that values and supports critical reflection is essential.

Transformative learning

Mezirow's concept of transformative learning has developed over 30 years into a comprehensive and complex theory.(6,65,68) Transformative learning theory defines learning as the social process of constructing and internalising a new or revised interpretation of the meaning of one's experience as a guide to action. In other words, transformative learning involves helping adults to elaborate, create and transform their meaning schemes (beliefs, feelings, interpretations, decisions) through reflection on their content, the process by which they were learned and their premises (social context, history and consequences).(68) Transformative learning can be contrasted with conventional learning that simply elaborates the learner's existing paradigm, systems of thinking, feeling or doing, relative to the topic. Although learning is increased, the learner's fundamental structure is maintained. Transformative learning changes the learner's paradigm so radically that, although it may retain the old perspective, it is actually a new creation. Critical reflection and rational discourse are the primary processes used in learning. The core of transformative learning in Mezirow's(68) view is the uncovering of distorted assumptions or errors in learning.

Empowerment of learners is both a goal and a condition for transformative learning. An empowered learner is able to participate fully and freely in critical discourse and the resulting action. This requires freedom and equality, as well as the ability to assess evidence and engage in critical reflection.(65) Reflection is a key concept in transformative learning theory. Mezirow(68) defines it as the process of critically assessing the content, process or premises of our efforts to interpret and give meaning to an experience. He distinguishes among three types of reflection:
- *content* reflection – examination of the content or description of a problem
- *process* reflection – examination of the problem-solving strategies being used
- *premise* reflection – questioning the problem itself, which may lead to a transformation of belief systems.

Perspective transformation may be the result of a major event in one's life, or the cumulative result of related transformations in concepts, beliefs, judgements or feelings. The most significant learning involves critical reflection around premises about oneself. This kind of learning is triggered by a disorienting dilemma that invokes self-examination and a critical assessment of assumptions. Through a process of exploring options for new roles, relationships and actions, new knowledge and skills are acquired. This leads to planning and implementing a new course of action, provisionally trying new roles, renegotiating relationships and forming new ones, and building competence and self-confidence.

Mezirow(6) explains that discourse is a crucial process, and refers to a special kind of dialogue in which the focus is on content and attempting to justify beliefs by giving and defending reasons, and by examining the evidence for and against competing viewpoints.

Transformative learning is a complicated, emotional process requiring significant knowledge and skill to implement effectively.(70) A new paradigm emerges only after the old one becomes dysfunctional, and it is the task of the transformative educator to challenge the learner's current perspective. A paradigm shift will occur only if the learner perceives the existing paradigm to be significantly inadequate in explaining his or her experience. However, the new paradigm appears only after a period of disorientation during which no clear paradigm remains. It is typical for the learner to resist letting go of the old paradigm and beginning the transition to the new one. During this process, the teacher–learner relationship may intensify enormously because the learner may begin to resent the teacher or feel anger towards him or her. Often learners feel a complex love–hate for the teacher who intentionally assisted in the collapse of their existing paradigm.

Successful transformative learning questions assumptions (this is a key to the process), provides support from others in a safe environment, presents challenge, examines alternative perspectives and provides feedback. New assumptions are tested in the authentic settings or in discussion with others.

At present, it can be argued that there are a variety of alternative conceptions of transformative learning theory that refer to similar ideas and address factors often overlooked in the dominant theory of transformation (Mezirow's), such as the role of spirituality, positionality, emancipatory learning and neurobiology. The exciting part of this diversity of theoretical perspectives is that it has the potential to offer a more diverse interpretation of transformative learning and to have significant implications for practice.(75)

One new perspective is a distinctive neurobiologically-based pathway to transformative learning. From this perspective, learning is seen as 'volitional, curiosity-based, discovery-driven, and mentor-assisted' and most effective at higher cognitive levels.(76, p. 144) Furthermore, a neurobiological approach suggests that transformative learning: (1) requires discomfort prior to discovery; (2) is rooted in students' experiences, needs and interests; (3) is strengthened by emotive, sensory and kinaesthetic experiences; (4) appreciates differences in learning between males and females; and (5) demands that educators acquire an understanding of a unique discourse and knowledge base of neurobiological systems. Other perspectives have been described by Taylor,(75) and these are appropriate for application to a variety of contexts.

Transformative learning theory continues to be a growing area of study of adult learning and has important implications for the practice of teaching adults. The growth is so significant that it seems to have replaced andragogy as the dominant educational philosophy of adult education, offering teaching practices grounded in empirical research. Taylor reminds educators that the body of research and alternative perspectives implies that fostering transformative learning is much more than implementing a series of instructional strategies with adult learners. Transformative learning is first and foremost about educating from a particular worldview, i.e. a particular educational philosophy. It is not an easy way to teach. It means asking oneself, 'Am I willing to transform in the process of helping my students transform?'. Without developing a deeper awareness of our own frames of reference and how they shape practice, there is little likelihood that we can foster change in others.

Patricia Cranton, author of several books on the application of transformative learning summarises:

> Transformative learning can occur when students encounter alternative points of view and perspectives. Exposure to alternatives encourages students to critically question their assumptions, beliefs, and values, and when this leads to a shift in the way they see themselves or things in the world, they have engaged in transformative learning. Transformative learning can be promoted by using any strategy, activity, or resource that presents students with an alternative point of view. Readings from different perspectives, field experiences, videos, role plays, simulations, and asking challenging questions all have the potential to lead to transformative learning. The educator needs to create an environment in which critical reflection and questioning norms is supported and encouraged.(77)

Implications for educational practice

How can educators promote and support transformative learning? First, as educators, we need to take a reformist perspective, rather than a subject-centred or consumer-oriented perspective.(78) In a subject-centred perspective, the educator is the expert authority figure and designer of instruction. In a learner- or consumer-oriented perspective, the educator is a facilitator and resource person. In a reformist perspective, essential to transformative learning, the educator is a co-learner and provocateur; they challenge, stimulate and provoke critical thinking.(70) Box 2.5 illustrates Cranton's(70) stages before, during and following transformative learning.

Cranton(70) provides the following guidelines for transformative educators:
- Promote rational discourse, a fundamental component of transformative learning and part of the process of empowering learners.
- Promote equal participation in discourse by stimulating discussion through a provocative incident or controversial statement.
- Develop discourse procedures (e.g. stay on topic, summarise) and avoid using own position to make dismissive statements.

BOX 2.5 Stages of change in transformative learning(70)

Stage of change	Through
Initial learner development	Freedom to participate
	Comfort
	Learner decision-making
Learner critical self-reflection	Questioning assumptions
	Consciousness-raising
	Challenging assumptions
Transformative learning	Revision of assumptions
	Educator support
	Learner networks
	Action
Increased empowerment	Critical self-reflection
	Transformative learning
	Autonomy

- Develop group facilitation skills (e.g. dominant participant, silent participant).
- Encourage decision making by learners, by making the process open and explicit.
- Encourage critical self-reflection through challenging learners, asking critical questions and proposing discrepancies between learners' experiences and new or conflicting information. To be successful here, a climate of openness and supportiveness needs to be established.
- Consider individual differences among learners. Learners should be assisted in becoming more aware of their own learning styles and preferences. The educator needs to develop a strong awareness of how learners vary in the way they think, act, feel and see possibilities.
- Employ various teaching/learning strategies. Many strategies are effective, for example: role-playing (with skilful debriefing), simulations and games, life histories or biographies, exposure to new knowledge, journal writing (with self or others' feedback) and critical incidents arising in the practice setting.

Self-directed learning

Self-directed, lifelong learning (SDL) is increasingly essential in the development and maintenance of professional competence. It is integral to the process of self-regulation. Those responsible for professional education, including that of physicians, are challenged to create curricula that ensure the development of these skills as well as the assessment methods needed to ascertain their achievement.

The literature on SDL has developed along two overlapping pathways. The first has framed self-direction as a goal towards which individuals strive, reflecting a humanistic orientation such as that described by Maslow(79) and Brockett and Hiemstra.(80) These models imply achievement of a level of self-actualisation, along with the acceptance of personal responsibility for learning, personal autonomy and individual choice.

The second line of development has framed SDL as a method of organising learning and instruction, with the tasks of learning left primarily in the learner's control. Early development included linear models, where learners moved through a series of steps to reach their learning goals (e.g. Knowles(81)). Later models have described the self-directed learning process as more interactive, involving opportunities in the environment, the personal characteristics of learners, cognitive processes, the context of learning and opportunities to validate and confirm self-directed learning collaboratively. Examples of this are seen in several models clearly described by Merriam *et al.*(22) This line of development also includes models of instruction such as those of Grow(82) and Hammond and Collins,(83) which present frameworks for integrating self-directed learning into formal educational settings.

Candy(7) clarified the field of SDL significantly, bringing educators closer to understanding the specific characteristics to identify, develop and evaluate in the self-directed learner. He identified approximately 100 traits associated with self-direction, clustered around four dimensions:
- self-directedness, including personal autonomy
- self-management in learning
- learner control of instruction
- the independent pursuit of learning.

Although these characteristics were identified in 1991, their relevance is unchanged.

Self-directed learning is an integral aspect of several theoretical approaches, including the cognitive, social learning, humanist and constructivist. As noted earlier in the chapter, the social learning approach views individuals as inherently self-regulating, with self-direction as a natural activity. The humanist approach views self-direction as evidence of higher levels of individual development. The cognitive perspective recognises the need to build rich, interconnecting knowledge structures, based on existing knowledge, which allow continuing incorporation of new learning. The constructivist perspective recognises the unique personal and social construction of knowledge that occurs in different learners. Self-directed learning elements can also be seen in the ability to learn from experience through critical reflection, which allows learners to identify their personal learning needs and to be aware of, monitor and direct the growth of their knowledge, skills and expertise.

Generally, self-direction is a natural human process that can occur both within and/or outside of formal settings. SDL does not exclude formal activities such as lectures or courses. It is the learner's choice of activities to meet and manage a particular learning goal that denotes self-direction. A number of factors in the learner and in the environment will affect the learner's ability to be self-directing, as follows.
- The learners' view of themselves as learners is an influencing factor. Learners who view themselves as competent, with the skills to learn in a variety of situations, are more likely to be self-directed and independent.
- Sometimes the demands of the learning situation influence the capacity for self-direction. Where the situation demands that certain (particular) knowledge and skills

are non-negotiable, or where the situation requires the learner to reproduce exactly what has been taught, the capacity for self-direction may be obscured.
- Self-direction is, to some degree, a function of subject matter mastery. As the learner builds a base of relevant knowledge and skills, the capacity to be self-directed is enhanced. This basic knowledge is held by some to be essential for effective SDL. Others who promote learning based on activation of prior knowledge tell us that there are few learning situations where the learner is completely lacking in relevant knowledge to engage a learning task. Part of enhancing self-direction is helping learners to identify their relevant knowledge and experience.
- Much of professional learning is situated learning; that is, the learning is inseparable from the situation in which the knowledge is used. Similarly, professional knowledge and acumen become embedded in practice, and part of the professional's 'knowing-in-action'.(46) Learners may require help in understanding the way knowledge is structured and used, in order to understand fully the range of learning opportunities available to them. They also benefit from opportunities to participate in their community of practice and the knowledge embedded in it.(22,81)
- Knowledge is also socially constructed, in that it is built from mutually understood perceptions and assumptions. Learners' participation in the social construction of knowledge through discussion and participation provides a cultural basis for their self-direction.
- Knowledge is dependent on context for its meaning, its structure in memory and its availability. Understanding and experience of a broad range of discipline-relevant contexts encourage self-direction in transferring knowledge to other appropriate contexts.

Comprehensive measures of self-directedness are few. Two scales have been used sufficiently to have achieved validation.(84,85) The Self-Directed Learning Readiness Scale (SDLRS) was developed by Guglielmino(84) as a tool to assess the degree to which people perceive themselves as possessing the skills and attitudes conventionally associated with SDL. The Oddi(85) Continuing Learning Inventory is a 26-item scale that purports to identify clusters of personality characteristics that relate to initiative and persistence in learning over time, through a variety of learning modes. The Self-reflection and Insight Scale (SRIS) developed by Roberts and Stark(71) explores reflection as an activity basic to making self-directed change, thus uniting these two important elements of self-regulation.

The ability to self-assess is critical to effective self-directed learning. To properly direct one's ongoing learning, and to assess where and what learning is required, the individual must be able to assess his or her current practice with reasonable accuracy. A recent review of the self-assessment literature suggests that our current understanding of self-assessment is insufficient and that our ability to assess our own performance accurately is limited. Eva and Regehr (86) suggest that accurate self-assessment requires a knowledge of what constitutes appropriate performance, and of the criteria by which to judge it. They further suggest that several sources of information may be necessary for accurate self-assessment, including feedback from others about one's performance. It is also important to better understand the cognitive, affective and psychomotor bases of self-assessment to effectively promote the development of self-assessment capacity. Several authors have explored self-assessment further and the processes and conditions which influence it.(87)

A more detailed look at self-assessment and self-regulated learning is provided in Chapter 15.

Implications for educational practice

There are a number of important implications for curricula, teaching and learning in medical education, all of which are facilitated by the creation of a supportive learning environment where learners feel safe to ask questions and to admit to not understanding. Learners must have the opportunity to develop and practise skills that directly enhance effective SDL. These include competency at asking questions, seeking relevant information and a critical appraisal of new information.

Learners also need to acquire multiple approaches to learning, along with the ability to decide when each is appropriate. For ongoing SDL, however, deep *learning skills*,(88) which involve understanding principles and concepts, and elaborating the relationships among them, are most likely to support self-direction. Making use of learners' existing knowledge structures, and assisting them to add to and enrich those structures and understand similarities and dissimilarities, encourage the individual to understand his or her knowledge base and to identify gaps. A fundamental skill in self-direction is that of critical reflection on one's own learning and experience. Learners must practise and develop skills at reflecting on all aspects of their learning to determine additional learning needs and to set goals accordingly. Miflin *et al.*(89) describe an attempt to introduce SDL into graduate medical education in a university in Australia. Lack of clarity among teachers and students of what constitutes self-direction forced a reconsideration of the curriculum.

Critical to the achievement of both explicit and implicit curriculum goals are congruence and alignment (90) among the goals, the educational strategies and the assessment methods.(19) Assessment will invariably drive learning and give the strongest messages to learners about the real goals of the curriculum. Although there are genuine attempts to do otherwise, too frequently assessment methods reward teacher-directed, fact-oriented learning, and do not reward or evaluate the learner's achievement of self-directed learning.

Experiential learning

Kolb's experiential learning theory(8) is derived from the work of Kurt Lewin,(91) John Dewey(92) and Jean Piaget.(93) Lewin's(91) work in social psychology, group dynamics and action research concluded that learning is best achieved in an environment that considers both concrete experiences and conceptual models. Dewey(92) constructed guidelines for programmes of experiential learning in higher educa-

tion. He noted the necessity of integrating the processes of actual experience and education in learning. Piaget's(93) research regarding cognitive development processes constituted the theory of how experience is used to model intelligence. Abstract thinking, including the use of symbols, is closely linked to learners' adaptation to their environment. Fenwick(94) offered a summary of five contemporary perspectives on experiential learning – constructivist, psychoanalytic, situative, critical/cultural, and enactivist – that have emerged in recent scholarly writing addressing experiential learning and cognition. She compared these five currents along the following eight dimensions: focus, basic explanatory schemata, view of knowledge, view of relation of knower to object and situation of knowing, view of learning process, view of learning goals and outcomes, view of the nature of power in experience and knowing, and view of the educator's role, if any, in learning. In this important theoretical article, Fenwick(94) presented a different understanding of the positioning of educators, learners and learning, and of the relationship between theory of learning and the practice of teaching. However, Kolb's experiential learning theory is more useful as a model of learning from an applied perspective. It can be used as a framework in interpreting and diagnosing individual learners, as well as designing learning environments.(95) Kolb's four learning environments are:

- affectively oriented (feeling)
- symbolically oriented (thinking)
- perceptually oriented (watching)
- behaviourally oriented (doing).(96)

Within these environments, grasping and transforming experiences are the two constituent activities of learning tasks.(97) There are two components of the grasping phenomena: concrete experience, which filters directly through the senses, and abstract conceptualisation, which is indirect and symbolic. The transforming experience also consists of two processes: reflection and action. One, or a combination of the four activities (concrete experience, abstract conceptualisation, reflection and action) may be used in learning.(8) Learning is enhanced if students are encouraged to use all four components (*see* Figure 2.2).

The next section explores Kolb's learning environments in more depth by presenting practical implications for planners of educational programmes, teachers and learners. Educational formats for delivering experiential learning activities are also included.

Implications for educational practice

Programme planning

Kolb provides us with three major guideposts for directing experiential instructional activities.(98) First, experiential learning methods and procedures are bridges connecting a learner's existing level of understanding, philosophies, affective characteristics and experiences with a new set of knowledge, abilities, beliefs and values. Second, in experiential learning the learner adopts a more assertive role in assuming responsibility for his or her own learning. This leads to a shift in the power structure from the traditional relationship between teacher and learner. Last, experiential

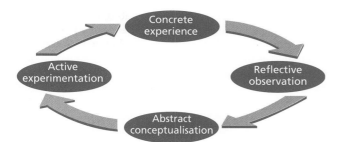

Figure 2.2 Kolb learning cycle.

learning involves the transfer of learning from an academic mode to one that involves more practical content.

More specifically, in the affectively oriented environment, learners experience activities as though they were professional practitioners.(8,97) The learner's existing values and experience generate information. In the symbolically oriented environment, the learner uses experiences to develop skills or concepts that can provide the right answer or the best solution to a problem.(8,97) The source of information is primarily conceptual. In the perceptually oriented environment, the learner views concepts and relationships from different perspectives such as watching, thinking, and feeling.(8,9) Behaviourally oriented activities focus on specific problems or practices to which learners apply their competencies.(8,99)

Teaching

The roles and actions of teachers depend on the particular learning context.(8,99) In the affectively oriented environment they act as role models and relate to the learner as friendly advisors. They deliver information quickly and tailor it to the needs and objectives of individual learners. Teachers monitor progress by encouraging ongoing discussion and critique without constricting guidelines to inhibit students.

In the symbolically oriented environment, the teacher's role is that of a content expert, as well as a facilitator in order for the learner to reach a solution or a goal.(8,99) Success is compared against the correct or best solution by objective criteria. The teacher provides guidelines regarding terminology and rules.

In the perceptually oriented environment, teachers act as process facilitators, emphasising process rather than solution. They also direct and outline connections between discussions. Learners evaluate answers and define concepts individually. Performance is not measured against rigid criteria but by how well learners use predetermined professional criteria.

In the behaviourally oriented environment, teachers act as mentors and reflect on their background when giving counsel. There are few guidelines. Learners manage their own time and focus on 'doing'.(8,99) It is essential that the learner complete the task using professional standards.

Learning

In the affectively oriented environment the learner must work with people, be perceptive to encompassing values and feelings, and become engaged in a learning group in a concrete experience.

In the symbolically oriented environment learners study quantitative data to test their theories and postulations.(97,99) Using unique ideas and action plans, learners develop and conceptualise their experiences and models. This relates to the experience of abstract conceptualisation.

The perceptually oriented environment encourages the learner to analyse and manage data with an open mind.(97,99) The learner must learn to see things with a broad point of view, compose complete plans of action and conjecture about the implications of ambiguous circumstances. The learner undergoes the transformative experience of reflective observation by openly approaching the learning activity.

In the behaviourally oriented environment learners must make their own choices in order to locate and exploit potential opportunities, committing themselves to meet predetermined goals and objectives. They are encouraged to adapt to uncertainty and shifting circumstances, and to guide others. This relates to the transforming experience of active experimentation.

Caffarella(98) describes a number of formats for experiential learning activities in medical education in a variety of settings, from practical clinical environments to strictly academic arenas. Depending on the format, the teacher may form a strict regimental relationship with the learner or may foster a caring bond.

Learners along the medical educational continuum use various experiential learning methods. These may include apprenticeship, internship or practicum, mentoring, clinical supervision, on-the-job training, clinics and case study research. For maximum benefits, it is important that they continue to cycle through the four learning environments described in Kolb's model.

Situated learning

Situated learning belongs to those theories of learning that have a sociocultural basis, which view learning and development as occurring via transformation through participation in community activities. Learners transform their understanding, roles and responsibilities as they participate.(9,99,100)

Sfard(101) described two metaphors for learning that may be helpful: *acquisition* and *participation*. In the *acquisition* metaphor, learning is seen as the acquisition of knowledge, skills and attributes which belong to or are 'owned' by the individual. This is a very prominent metaphor especially in older writings. However, most of the theories discussed to date in this chapter could be seen as fitting that metaphor. In contrast, the participation metaphor sees learning as becoming a member of a community, by participating in the activities of that community.

Situated learning is about *participation*. Learning occurs through collaboration with other learners and more senior community members in carrying out activities with purposes connected explicitly with the history and current practices of the community.(102) New learners enter the community of practice at the edge of the community and learn through a process of legitimate peripheral participation in which they observe and perform the less vital tasks of the community. As they take on more responsibility in the community, learners move towards the centre. As they participate increasingly in the community's practice, they come to understand the particular knowledge that distinguishes that community from others.

A central tenet of situated learning is that learning occurs through social interaction. It emphasises the learning that occurs through the interaction with and bonds between members of the community. Learners acquire knowledge from all aspects of their participation in the community. A powerful source of learning is the 'discourse' or 'talk' of the community.(103) Discourse may be thought of as the way we talk about our work and other aspects of our world. The discourse or 'talk' both reflects the way we see our world, and frames the way we view it. Through participation in talk, learners begin to participate in the community. The community offers a wide variety of relationships and exemplars from whom to learn, including masters, more advanced apprentices and peers. Learners learn how more senior members of the community walk, talk and conduct their lives; observe what other learners are doing and what is needed to become part of the community. Through this participation they learn about the values and shared knowledge and practices of the community. They learn how people in the community 'collaborate, collude and collide, and what they enjoy, dislike, respect and admire'.(102)

For Lave and Wenger, who introduced the notion of situated learning in communities of practice, the opportunity to learn around relationships with other apprentices and to observe the masters' (senior practitioners) practice creates the curriculum in the broadest sense. Learners can develop a view of what the whole enterprise is about, and what there is to learn. 'Engaging in practice, rather than its object, may be a condition for the effectiveness of learning'.(102)

It is useful to consider the relationship of situated learning to other learning theories. Situated learning allows a broad view of learning that relates to several other conceptions of learning, both long-standing and more recent.

Situated learning shares with social cognitive theory(4) the view that learning occurs in a dynamic interaction between the learner and the environment. Situated learning suggests that learning is not separate from social influences. The context in which teaching and learning occur is critical to learning itself, and learning is culturally and contextually specific.(104) Learning occurs within social relations and the practices that occur there.

Situated learning also holds that some knowledge related to a task is only present in the context or location of the task. Brown *et al.*(105) described *situated cognition* and emphasised the idea of cognitive apprenticeship. Cognitive apprenticeship supports learning in a domain by enabling students to acquire, develop and use cognitive tools in authentic domain activity. This happens in practice as teachers guide learners through processes of framing problems and applying disciplinary knowledge to their solu-

tion. In the process, teachers provide a scaffold for the learner's development, which can be withdrawn gradually as the learner gains more knowledge and experience.

Situated learning as described by Lave and Wenger(9) extends beyond the acquisition of concepts and structures by the individual and includes all of the learning in the learning environment. It views the community and learning opportunities as a way of structuring learning resources, with pedagogical activity (teaching) as only one resource among many.

Situated learning theory was originally a means for studying the learning that occurs through apprenticeship.(9) Traditionally, apprenticeship has been viewed as a relationship between a master or senior practitioner and the novice or learner. Through apprenticeship, the learner comes to understand the content and process of professional practice. Situated learning provides a way of understanding the process whereby apprentices acquire knowledge and skills through following and attempting to be like the teacher or expert practitioner. In the situated learning model, the learner's apprenticeship is actually to the whole community, and much of the learning occurs in the relationships between people, rather than inside the individual learner's head. Brown *et al.* emphasise the idea of cognitive apprenticeship: 'Cognitive apprenticeship supports learning in a domain by enabling students to acquire, develop and use cognitive tools in authentic domain activity'(105, p. 39). Cognitive apprenticeship means that the learner observes the thinking process, and not just the actions, of experts and other participants in the community.

Situated learning also relates closely to our growing understanding of informal learning. According to Eraut,(106) informal learning is a significant dimension of the learning that occurs in the course of our work. He suggests that it is implicit, unintended, opportunistic and unstructured, and often occurs in the absence of a teacher. Learning about how things are done, exposure to a variety of different approaches and practical approaches to problems occur daily. There is still much to understand about it; however, the evidence that informal learning and learning from others in the workplace occurs is convincing. This is in contrast to the image of independent learners that is embedded in much of formal medical education.

Informal learning with its corollaries of implicit learning – 'the acquisition of knowledge independent of conscious attempts to learn and in the absence of explicit knowledge about what was learned'(107) – and tacit knowledge – 'that which we know but cannot tell'(108) – will be covered in more detail in the context of the medical apprentice elsewhere in this book (Chapter 7).

Situated learning also relates to experiential learning, or learning by doing. Experiential learning has as its goal the integration of conceptual models and concrete experience,(8) and of authentic experience and formal education. Again, situated learning extends the concept to include the experiential learning as occurring within a context. It also extends the idea of experiential learning beyond the individual learner, as it views the learner as contributing to, and participating in, the shared experience of the community.

In addition to all the above theoretical relationships, situated learning is entirely in keeping with constructivism. Constructivism views learning as a process of active participation in problem-solving and critical thinking. Through these processes, learners construct their own knowledge and understanding of the world based on their previous knowledge and experience. Knowledge is integrated into previously existing concepts and schemata, which gradually become richer and more connected.

Postmodern constructivist approaches do not view the locus of knowledge as in the individual. Rather they view learning as a social constructivist process. Learning and understanding are social; cultural activities and tools are essential to conceptual development that will allow learners to develop the skills and standards that are valued by the community.(104) In the context of situated learning, knowledge may be constructed not only individually, but jointly by communities and the individuals who are members of those communities.

Implications for educational practice

Situated learning is relevant to medical education in many ways and at all levels of the continuum of education. Apprenticeship remains a pervasive teaching and learning method in physician learning. Learners in undergraduate and postgraduate medical education programmes are assigned to various clinical and community sites where they are immersed, to a greater or lesser degree, in the work of the community, performing minor tasks and striving to learn from the more advanced learners and mentors in the community. Authentic activity is important for learners because it is the only way they gain access to the standpoint that enables practitioners to act meaningfully and purposefully. It is activity that shapes or sharpens their tools.(105) However, there is another important aspect of situated learning, namely socialisation.

Increasingly, medical and health professional education are recognised as a process of professional socialisation. In that process, learners are developing their professional identity. Their experiences, knowledge, interactions, and informal and formal learning all contribute to the professional identity that each individual constructs. The recent Carnegie Foundation report on physician education(109) suggests that a focus on learners' development of professional identity is one of four fundamental principles for reforming physician education.

Hafferty and Franks (110) articulated the notion of three levels of curriculum as including formal, informal and hidden. These may be helpful in thinking about the environment or community in which our learners are placed. The *formal curriculum* represents that which is stated. The *informal curriculum* may include both explicit and serendipitous goals, and is found in the interaction between teachers and learners, and clinical environments, other students, personal interests and goals. Part of the informal curriculum may also be what Hafferty and Franks termed the *hidden curriculum*, which may be seen in the practices and routines of the community, particularly in relation to how its members cope and thrive. The hidden curriculum often teaches values and moral judgements and may be found especially in the institutional policies, language, assessment strategies and allocation of resources of an institution. Clearly, these curricula all exist and are enacted in the context of situated learning in medicine. Importantly, not all messages of the hidden curriculum are negative. Both negative and positive aspects have been described. Often these are unintentionally imparted through actions, discussions and relationships among members of the community. This relates the notion of situated learning closely to role modelling, as the senior members of the community enact through their behaviours, both tacitly and explicitly, how problems of the discipline are approached, how colleagues are regarded and how knowledge is built and used.

When learners are involved in clinical placements, participation in the actual daily round of activities is important in enhancing the effectiveness of their learning. Clearly, the longer the engagement in a community, the greater the opportunity to participate meaningfully. Where attachments are short, learners may remain at the periphery and experience little feeling of participation in the community. Special attention may be needed to identify how their participation can be ensured and enhanced.

Faculty (teachers) enact several roles concurrently. As in the perspective of social learning theory, they are modelling skills, knowledge, values and attitudes that learners observe, along with how those actions are received in the community. Beyond role modelling, faculty are also demonstrating how knowledge is built, understood and how practices evolve. This aspect of talk offers both challenges and advantages. Learners who participate in and listen to the talk of the community are able to learn in a contextualised way. However, the nature and content of the talk become important considerations. As teachers, being mindful of our talk and open to reflecting on it with learners is important. Learning through observation is also vulnerable to misunderstanding, as learners will interpret what they observe in light of their current experience and understanding.(111) It is important to find opportunities and demonstrate willingness to discuss and reflect on experience with learners.(112)

Participation in the work of the clinical site or community is a key to this understanding of learning. Situated learning suggests that all members of the community are involved. In the case of medical education this means that more senior learners and other health professionals can all enhance the newer learners' participation.

Different fields of medicine have distinct knowledge and skill bases. However, there will still be some aspects that are common to all, including communication with patients, ethical approaches and grounding of actions, basic clinical skills, learning in interprofessional teams, etc. in which learners can participate across their fields of experience As teachers, we can think carefully about how we can promote participation among learners.

Building on the advantage of situated learning, we have the opportunity to rethink our students' experience and consider all the ways we have available to promote their learning. However, this involves thinking of learners as contributing members of our learning environment, rather than as temporary adjuncts to it.

Learning in communities of practice

In the previous section on situated learning, we discussed the concept of community as a place where participants are socialised and develop a professional identity. In this section on communities of practice, we expand this concept to include knowledge transmission, construction and translation. Lave and Wenger(9) first proposed the term *community of practice* (CoP) to capture the importance of activity in integrating individuals within a community, and of a community in legitimising individual practices. Within this context, they described a trajectory in which learners move from legitimate peripheral participant to full participation in the CoP. The concept of legitimate peripheral participation means that access to a CoP, its resources and activities provides a means for newcomers to learn through observation and gradually deepen their relationship to the CoP. Barab *et al.*(113) defined a CoP as 'a persistent, sustaining social network of individuals who share and develop an overlapping knowledge base, set of beliefs, values, history and experiences focused on a common practice and/or mutual enterprise'.

Wenger defined CoPs more simply as: 'Communities of practice are groups of people who share a concern or a passion for something they do and learn how to do it better as they interact regularly'.(114)

He proposed three constituent parts of a CoP: *mutual engagement, joint enterprise* and a *shared repertoire*. Mutual engagement involves both work-related and sociocultural activities, achieved by interaction, shared tasks and opportunities for peripheral participation. Joint enterprise refers to the need for the group to respond to a mandate for itself, and not simply an external mandate. Finally, a shared repertoire involves the 'routines, words, tools, ways of doing things, stories, gestures, symbols, genres, actions or concepts that the community has adopted in the course of its existence'.(10) Wenger summarised his conceptual framework for a social theory of learning comprising four components that are 'deeply interconnected and mutually defining'.(10) All of these should be present in a true CoP. The components include the following.

- *Meaning* – learning as experience. Members talk about their experience and create shared meaning.
- *Practice* – learning as doing. Members talk about the shared ideas and resources that can sustain action.
- *Community* – learning as belonging. Members talk about the community process and how they are learning and developing competence.
- *Identity* – learning as becoming. Members talk about how learning changes who they are.

Therefore, we can see that the concept of a CoP is complex and multidimensional, serving multiple purposes both for individuals and for the subcommunities that participate in the full community.

Wenger(114) provides a description of typical activities in CoPs. These are shown in Box 2.6 with examples to reflect medical settings.

The primary purpose of CoPs in this conception is knowledge translation. Knowledge translation has been defined as 'the exchange, synthesis and ethically sound

---

BOX 2.6 Typical activities in communities of practice

Activity	Example from medical practice
Problem-solving	'Can we discuss this patient and brainstorm some ideas? I'm stuck.'
Requests for information	'Does anyone know a good website about treatment of Chagas disease?'
Seeking experience	'Has anyone dealt with a patient in this situation?'
Reusing assets	'I have a proposal for a new clinic that I wrote for our hospital last year. I can send it to you and you can easily tweak it for your situation.'
Coordination and synergy	'Can we combine our purchases to achieve bulk discounts?'
Discussing developments	'What do you think of the new patient information system? Does it really help?'
Documentation projects	'We have faced this problem five times now. Let us write it down once and for all.'
Visits	'Can we come and see your clinic? We need to establish one in our city.'
Mapping knowledge and identifying gaps	'Who knows what are we missing? What other groups should we connect with?'

---

application of knowledge – within a complex system of interactions among researchers and users – to accelerate the capture of the benefits of research . . . through improved health, more effective services and products, and a strengthened health care system'.(115)

More recently, other terms have been proposed for essentially the same broad concept. These terms include knowledge mobilisation,(116) knowledge utilisation,(117) knowledge exchange,(118) knowledge management (119) and knowledge brokering,(120) all of which involve an active exchange of information among various stakeholders, such as researchers, healthcare providers, policy makers, administrators, private sector organisations, patient groups and the general public. Partnerships are at the heart of all knowledge translation activity,(115) and effective knowledge translation is dependent on meaningful exchanges among network members for the purpose of using the most timely and relevant evidence-based, or experience-based, information for practice or decision-making.

In the field of continuing medical education, the limitations of traditional workshop/presentation models are becoming apparent.(121) It is now recognised that there is a need for continuous learning to occur in the context of the workplace, and for reflection-in-practice and reflection-on-practice to be supported.(5) Knowledge translation is essential to shortening the path from evidence to application of that evidence in practice, and CoPs provide an opportunity to embed learning within a clinical context. A highly effective way to learn about complex issues is through experience, application and discussion with mentors and peers in the same or similar contexts. Relevant learning occurs when the participants in the CoP raise questions or perceive a need for new knowledge. Using internet technology enables these discussions to occur in a timely manner, and records of these can be archived for later review or by those who missed the discussion.

There are a number of key factors that influence the development, functioning and maintenance of CoPs.(122) The legitimacy of the initial membership is important. Commitment to the desired goals of the CoP, relevance to members and enthusiasm about the potential of the CoP to have an impact on practice are also key. On the practical side, a strong infrastructure and resources, such as good information technology, useful library resources, databases and human support, are essential attributes.

The benefit for being involved in a CoP is increased expertise and skills. Intrinsic motivation for participation can be viewed as the following.

- *Anticipated reciprocity.* A member is motivated to contribute to the community in the expectation that he or she will receive useful help and/or information in return.
- *Increased recognition.* The desire for prestige is a key motivation for an individuals' contribution to a learning community.
- *Sense of efficacy.* The act of contribution results in a sense that the individual has had some effect on the community.(123)

Skill in accessing and appraising the knowledge sources is important, as is the skill in bridging this knowledge to practice. Providing the above-mentioned key factors requires strong, committed and flexible leaders who can help guide the natural evolution of the CoP. If professional learning is to flourish, it is critical that a blame-free culture is established in which community members can learn from positive and negative experiences.(124)

Some writers have outlined some key questions to address in establishing a CoP.(125)

- How will the community be formed and evolve?
- How and when will members join?
- What do members do and how will they interact?
- How will the CoP be supported by the members' organisation(s)?
- What value will members and their organisations receive?

Others have suggested principles for cultivating CoPs.(126) CoPs are dynamic entities and need to be designed for adaptability and large growth. They should combine the perspectives of both insider members and outsider participants, and all members should be valued, regardless of their level of participation. Both public and private spaces are necessary and need to be related. A critical principle is that the CoP must provide value to its members, otherwise participation will be minimal or absent. Although familiarity is important, challenge and excitement need to be provided to keep the energy high. Finally, CoPs have a rhythm they need to settle into, one that works for its members (*see* Box 2.7).

Virtual communities of practice

Virtual (online) communities play a socialisation role to the same extent as real communities do.(127) The theoretical

BOX 2.7 HOW TO: Build a successful community of practice

Lave and Wenger (9) suggest that the success of a community of practice depends on the following five factors:

- the existence and sharing by the community of a common goal
- the existence and use of knowledge to achieve that goal
- the nature and importance of relationships formed among community members
- the relationships between the community and those outside it
- the relationship between the work of the community and the value of the activity.

Wenger(10) later added the idea that achieving the shared goals of the community requires a shared repertoire of common resources – for example, language, stories and practices.

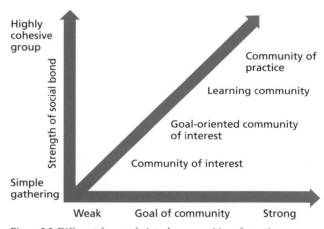

Figure 2.3 Different forms of virtual communities of practice according to their context of emergence. Adapted from Henri and Pudelko(128, p. 476).

foundation of virtual communities is based on social cognitive theory and situated learning. Henri and Pudelko(128) have proposed three components of the social context of activity in virtual communities – the goal of the community, the methods of initial group creation, and the temporal evolution of both the goals and the methods of the group – leading to the development of four different types of community. Figure 2.3 illustrates that a CoP requires a highly cohesive group with a clear goal.

Box 2.8 dissects the characteristics of these four types of community further. It demonstrates that although many types of virtual community can exist, they may not be true CoPs. The virtual CoP generally arises from an existing, face-to-face CoP in which professional practice is developed through sharing knowledge among members. Through this interaction, new practices may be developed and identification with the community can occur.

BOX 2.8 Principal descriptors of the four types of virtual communities (adapted from Henri and Pudelko)(128, p. 485)

	Community of interest	Goal-oriented community	Learning community	Community of practice
Purpose	Gathering around a common topic of interest	Created to carry out a specific task	Pedagogical activity proposed by the instructor	Stems from an existing, real community
Activity	Information exchange	Sharing of diverse perspectives and production of objects commissioned by the mandate	Participation in discussions of collective topics	Professional practice development through sharing knowledge among members
Learning	Knowledge construction for individual use	Knowledge construction from diverse knowledge systems towards collective use	Knowledge construction by carrying out social situated activities	Appropriation of new practices and development of involvement

Some writers have distinguished 'soft' from 'hard' knowledge.(129) Soft knowledge can be gathered in a domain through sharing solutions to a particularly difficult problem, describing idiosyncrasies of particular tools, equipment or processes, and recounting and reflecting on challenging events (i.e. recounting war stories). This refers to the implicit or tacit knowledge in a domain. CoPs are central to the creation and maintenance of soft knowledge. Hard knowledge, in contrast, is stored in databases and documents. It is highly explicit and codified. A key question is whether a virtual CoP can effectively share soft knowledge, which tends to be situated in specific contexts. This is a question that requires further research.

There are currently a number of large virtual CoPs, such as http://www.doctors.net.uk/, http://www.doctorslounge.com/, and http://www.medhelp.org/ to name a few. However, virtual CoPs are a relatively recent phenomenon, and few studies on their effectiveness to enhance learning have been carried out. Parboosingh(130) advocates conducting evaluation studies that focus on how the CoP takes advantage of the technology, rather than how the technology affects the CoP. Resources are available for assisting with this,(131) and many methods are available to evaluators. Examples include the following.

- *Case study.* You can investigate, for example, what changes happened within a particular project/organisation as a result of a member's participation in the CoP). http://www.cgiar-ilac.org/content/case-study
- *Contribution analysis.* To what extent are observed results due to programme activities, rather than other factors? http://www.cgiar-ilac.org/content/contribution-analysis
- *Horizontal evaluation.* Combines self-assessment and users.
- *Institutional histories.* Records new ways of working creating more effective ways to achieve goals; can be used at the CoP co-ordination team's organisation.
- *Institutional linkage diagram.* Illustrates the extent to which individuals, organisations, projects or services

interact with each other; it can be used to illustrate how individuals and organisations who never engaged before are now in contact because of the platform.

Implications for educational practice

This section of the chapter integrates the concepts of knowledge translation and CoPs. These ideas have many obvious applications in the medical education arena, and a number of these CoPs are emerging in various specialties. The application outlined in this section is a CoP for palliative care practitioners and students. This is an excellent application because palliative care is a truly interdisciplinary field that involves subcommunities of various specialties, including oncologists, family physicians, nurses and social workers. These subcommunities need to interact in CoPs, but the various professional groups also need to interact with each other around specific topics and cases. This provides an excellent model for continuing medical education, and also provides an environment for training residents, interns and medical students. Since many participants are acquiring and applying new knowledge in this field, scaffolding learners through an evolving continuum from simulation to participation to co-determined interactions is an effective instructional approach.(132) For example, family physicians, residents and nurses who have trained with oncology specialists may begin with simulated cases. They then learn to participate in real cases supported by learning materials and/or clinicians, until they are able to operate as full participants. The scaffolding process proposed here uses a staged approach for bridging from a learner (knowledge) identity to a participant (practitioner) identity. This approach is consistent with the constructivist (127) view of learning, which espouses the learner as central in the educational process. The advantages of the situated learning approach over the traditional didactic approach, are discussed above in the section on situated learning.

A CoP implemented in a community-based learning environment could include specialist and non-specialist practitioners in palliative care, as well as residents and medical students (clerks). It would aspire to achieve a number of different aims, based on the challenges by Richardson and Cooper.(133)

- Engage all trainees in a research culture (i.e. encourage evidence-based practice).
- Provide an opportunity for participants to identify with their peers and supervisors.
- Encourage cross-site discussion to explore shared theory, methodological and practical issues.
- Provide a forum for discussion and a recognised channel for communication and collaboration.
- Facilitate high-quality supervision to ensure adequate access to teaching and learning for all practitioners.
- Foster scholarly interaction and good supervisory practice to stimulate dialogue among students and supervisors across sites.

CoPs provide a critical resource to professionals who want and need recommendations, pointers, tips and tricks, best practices, insights and innovations. Part of what makes a community practice strong is the aggregation of relevance; that is, people and information related to a coherent set of topics which certain people will find interesting, useful, and potentially profitable. We are asserting that linking medical students, their community preceptors and medical school specialists in an online CoP can greatly enhance the learning and practice experience of all participants. A recent study(134) demonstrated that students assigned to community practices for their paediatric clerkship perform as well as, or better than, students assigned to academic medical centres in written examinations. Other studies have demonstrated similar outcomes. An online CoP approach can build on this positive finding and perhaps provide an even more effective community experience for medical students. A side-benefit could be the improvement in teaching and supervisory methods used by their preceptors.

Connections

In this chapter, we have presented eight theoretical approaches to learning, each of which has the potential to inform our practice as educators. For each theoretical approach we have set out the underlying framework and principles and provided examples of its application. The application of educational theory to practice has always been somewhat eclectic. This is not unusual in applied sciences such as education. Wilson and Myers(135) have argued that practitioners tend to be opportunistic with respect to theoretical conceptions; they might try viewing a problem from one perspective, then another, and compare results. This stance might be termed 'grab-bag', but we prefer to think of it as problem- or practitioner-centered. People, rather than ideologies, are in control. The needs of the situation rise above rules, models, or even sets of values. Although this could be described as pragmatic, we prefer a more integrative approach. To make this exposition of theory as useful as possible to our educational practice, we believe it is helpful to consider the relationships among the theoretical frameworks, and the consistency of mes-

sages and themes that can be drawn from all of them to inform teaching and learning. Some of these common themes are presented here.

All theoretical frameworks view the learner as an active contributor in the learning process. In each of the theoretical approaches discussed here the learner actively interacts with a changing, complex environment. The curriculum can no longer be viewed as something that is transmitted to, or acts upon, the students – be they undergraduate, postgraduate or practising physicians. There is an important element of human agency. Moreover, in practice, the physician–learner is stimulated to learn through interactions in the practice environment.

The entire context of learning is more important than any one variable alone. The learning environment is complex. It includes learners, faculty, patients, colleagues, resources and other workers. It is both the interacting and the independent effect of all these variables that result in a learning environment, that is experienced by learners at all levels. Learning is accomplished both through direct experience and vicariously, and from many interactions in this complex system. Consequently, we must analyse as many factors in the environment as possible when planning, implementing and evaluating our educational programmes. In learning from practice, physicians solve complex problems that occur in the environment of the patient, family, physician and community. All of these influence the effectiveness, nature and outcomes of learning.

Learning is integrally related to the solution and understanding of real-life problems. For adult learners, learning is most effective and motivating when it is relevant to the solution of real-life needs or problems. This is obvious in the learning that occurs in reflective practice, where the new learning is triggered by the surprise encountered in a problem in practice. Experiential learning in real-life problems leads to ongoing mastery and competence. Similarly, learning around clinical problems, both in the clinic and in the classroom, represents learning to solve the authentic tasks of the profession and of future professional practice.

Individuals' past experience and knowledge are critical in learning, in actions and in acquiring new knowledge. At all levels, learning must be connected to relevant experience, or compatible with the learner's existing knowledge. Past experience and knowledge will affect perceptions of self-efficacy, which will, in turn, affect the choice of new experiences and goals. Learners' past experience is important in providing a framework for acquisition of new knowledge. In practice, the new learning opportunities identified will depend substantially on the individual's existing experience and knowledge.

Learners' values, attitudes and beliefs influence their learning and actions, and building learners' self-awareness in this area is important for their development. These values, attitudes and beliefs are central to learners' willingness to attempt new actions. They affect virtually everything that learners think, as well as their interactions with mentors, peers and patients. Self-awareness is critically important in the development of professional identity. Various processes exist to modify these, such as reflective observation, perspective transformation, role-modelling and feedback on action.

Individuals as learners are capable of self-regulation, that is, of setting goals, planning strategies and evaluating their progress. Adult learners are viewed as self-motivated and directed, pursuing those learning objectives relevant to personal goals. They are inherently self-regulating, and the process of reflection implies a learning that arises directly out of experience. In planning learning experiences we must regard these not as skills we have to teach students, but as skills and abilities that need to be developed and enhanced.

The ability to reflect on one's practice (performance) is critical to lifelong, self-directed learning. At the heart of all these theoretical approaches is the belief that we can learn from our experience, incorporating it into our existing knowledge and skills. This opportunity for reflection requires an early introduction to a systematic approach to facilitate reflection. Reflection is not merely description of experience, but analysis of it. It is not a natural and intuitive ability, and it must be developed through practice. It is critical to becoming an effective lifelong learner, as it also enables learners to develop and apply standards to their performance, decide what further learning needs to occur, and continue their learning over a professional lifetime.

Learning occurs not only individually, but in collaboration with others. These theories support the learning that occurs in interacting with others in a dynamic way; they also recognise that learning can occur collectively as individuals share experiences, knowledge and perspectives. The result of this is that knowledge and understanding are constructed collaboratively or mutually, and that all members of the group can contribute to that growth. Applying these theories to medical education requires reflection and practice. As medical educators we can benefit from reading and considering relevant literature to better understand these theories, and from participation in a community of peers who have a common interest in this area. Through the process of practising the application of each theory, receiving feedback from learners and peer observers, and reflecting on practice, medical educators will continue to improve in their teaching role. Through their participation in the community, they will contribute to the construction of shared knowledge and understanding and to the transformation of medical education.

Acknowledgement

We would like to acknowledge Dr Penny Jennett in the Faculty of Medicine of the University of Calgary for her co-authorship of the first version of this ASME monograph, on which the section on Reflective Practice is based.

References

1 Tripp D (1993) *Critical Incidents in Teaching. Developing Professional Judgement.* Routledge, London.

2 Knowles M (1973) *The Adult Learner: A Neglected Species.* Gulf Publishing, Houston, TX.

3 Knowles MS (1980) *The Modern Practice of Adult Education: From Pedagogy to Andragogy* (2e). Cambridge Books, New York, NY.

4 Bandura A (1986) *Social Foundations of Thought and Action. A Social Cognitive Theory.* Prentice-Hall, Englewood Cliffs, NJ.

5 Schön DA (1983) *The Reflective Practitioner: How Professionals Think in Action.* Basic Books, New York, NY.

6 Mezirow J (1994) Understanding transformation theory. *Adult Education Quarterly.* **44**(4): 222–44.

7 Candy PC (1991) *Self-Direction in Lifelong Learning.* Jossey-Bass, San Francisco, CA.

8 Kolb DA (1984) *Experiential Learning: Experience as the Source of Learning and Development.* Prentice Hall, Englewood Cliffs, NJ.

9 Lave J and Wenger E (1991) *Situated Learning: Legitimate Peripheral Participation.* Cambridge University Press, New York, NY.

10 Wenger E (1998) *Communities of Practice: Learning, Meaning, and Identity.* Cambridge University Press, New York, NY.

11 Selman G and Dampier P (1990) *The Foundations of Adult Education in Canada.* Thompson Educational Publishing, Toronto, ON.

12 Hallenbeck W (1960) The function and place of adult education in American society. In: Knowles MS (ed.) *Handbook of Adult Education in the United States* pp. 29–38. Adult Education Association of the USA, Chicago, IL.

13 Verner C and Booth A (1964) *Adult Education.* Centre for Applied Research in Education, New York, NY.

14 Jarvis P (1985) *The Sociology of Adult and Continuing Education.* Croom Helm, London.

15 Darkenwald G and Merriam SB (1982) *Adult Education: Foundations of Practice.* Harper & Row, New York, NY.

16 Merriam SB (1987) Adult learning and theory building: a review. *Adult Education Quarterly.* **37**(4): 187–98.

17 Cross KP (1981) *Adults as Learners.* Jossey-Bass, San Francisco, CA.

18 Knox AB (1980) Proficiency theory of adult learning. *Contemporary Educational Psychology* **5**: 378–404.

19 McClusky HY (1970) An approach to a differential psychology of the adult potential. In: Grabowski SM (ed.) *Adult Learning and Instruction* pp. 80–95. ERIC Clearinghouse on Adult Education, Syracuse, NY.

20 Mezirow J (1981) A critical theory of adult learning and education. *Adult Education.* **32**: 3–27.

21 Freire P (1970) *Pedagogy of the Oppressed.* Herder and Herder, New York NY.

22 Merriam SB, Caffarella RS and Baumgartner LM (2007) *Learning in Adulthood: A Comprehensive Guide* (3e). Jossey-Bass, San Francisco, CA.

23 Knowles MS (1984) *Andragogy in Action: Applying Modern Principles of Adult Learning.* Jossey-Bass, San Fransisco, CA.

24 Knowles M, Holton EF III and Swanson RA (2005) *The adult Learner* (6e). Elsevier, Burlington, MA.

25 Maslow AH (1970) *Motivation and Personality* (2e). Harper & Row, New York, NY.

26 Rogers C (1968) *Freedom to Learn.* Charles E Merrill, Columbus, OH.

27 Brookfield S (1986) *Understanding and Facilitating Adult Learning.* Jossey-Bass, San Francisco, CA.

28 Bard R (1984) Foreword. In: Knowles MS. *Andragogy in Action* p. xi. Jossey-Bass, San Francisco, CA.

29 Hartree A (1981) Malcolm Knowles' theory of andragogy: a critique. *International Journal of Lifelong Education.* **3**(3): 203–10.

30 Pratt DD (1993) Andragogy after twenty-five years. *New Directions for Adult and Continuing Education.* **57**: 15–23.

31 Rachal JR (2002) Andragogy's detectives: a critique of the present and a proposal for the future. *Adult Education Quarterly.* **52**(3): 210–27.

32 Merriam SB (1996) Updating our knowledge of adult learning. *Journal of Continuing Education in the Health Professions.* **16**(3): 136–43.

33 Resnick LB (1987) Learning in school and out. *Educational Researcher*. **16**: 13–20.

34 Taylor B and Kroth M (2009) Andragogy's transition into the future: meta analysis of andragogy and its search for a measurable instrument. *Journal of Adult Education*. **38**(1): 1–11.

35 Vella J (2002) Quantum learning: teaching as dialogue. *New Directions for Adult and Continuing Education*. **93**: 78–84.

36 Zemke R and Zemke S (1981) 30 things we know for sure about adult learning. *Training (New York, N.Y.)*. **18**: 45–9.

37 Bandura A (1977) *Social Learning Theory*. Prentice-Hall, Englewood Cliffs, NJ.

38 Cervone D (2000) Thinking about self-efficacy. *Behaviour Modification*. **24**(1): 30–56.

39 Bandura A (2006) Guide for constructing self-efficacy scales. In: Pajares F and Urdan T (eds) *Self-Efficacy Beliefs of Adolescents* (vol. 5), pp. 307–37. Information Age Publishing, Greenwich, CT.

40 Bandura A (1997) *Self-Efficacy: The Exercise of Control*. WH Freeman, New York, NY.

41 Carr W and Kemmis S (1983) *Becoming Critical: Knowing Through Action Research*. Deakin University Press, Geelong, Victoria, AU.

42 Al-Shehri A, Stanley I and Thomas P (1993) Continuing education for general practice. Systematic learning from experience. *British Journal of General Practice*. **43**: 249–53.

43 Boud D, Keogh R and Walker D (eds) (1985) *Reflection: Turning Experience into Learning*. Kogan Page, London.

44 Branch W and Paranjape A (2002) Feedback and reflection: teaching methods for clinical settings. *Academic Medicine*. **77**: 1185–8.

45 Moon J (1999) *Reflection in Learning and Professional Development*. Kogan Page, London.

46 Schön DA (1987) *Educating the Reflective Practitioner: Toward a New Design for Teaching and Learning in the Professions*. Jossey-Bass, San Francisco, CA.

47 Schön DA (1995) The new scholarship requires a new epistemology. *Change*. **27**(6): 26–34.

48 Shapiro J and Talbot Y (1991) Applying the concept of the reflective practitioner to understanding and teaching family medicine. *Family Medicine*. **23**(6): 450–6.

49 Slotnick HB (1996) How doctors learn: the role of clinical problems across the medical school-to-practice continuum. *Academic Medicine*. **71**(1): 28–34.

50 Crandall S (1993) How expert clinical educators teach what they know. *Journal of Continuing Education in the Health Professions*. **13**: 85–98.

51 Mamede S, Schmidt H and Penaforte J (2008) Effects of reflective practice on the accuracy of medical diagnoses. *Medical Education*. **42**: 468–75.

52 Atkins S and Murphy K (1993) Reflection: a review of the literature. *Journal of Advanced Nursing*. **18**(8): 1188–92.

53 Mann K, Gordon J and MacLeod A (2009) Reflection and reflective practice in health professions education: a systematic review. *Adv in Health Sciences Educ*. **14**: 595–621.

54 Jennett PA, Lockyer JM, Maes W, ParboosinghI J and Lawson D (1990) Providing relevant information on rural practitioners: a study of a medical information system. *Teaching and Learning in Medicine*. **2**(4): 200–4.

55 Lockyer J, Gondocz ST and Thivierge RL (2004) Knowledge translation: the role and place of practice reflection. *Journal of Continuing Education in the Health Professions*. **24**(1): 50–6.

56 Frankford DM, Patterson MA and Konrad TR (2000) Transforming practice organizations to foster lifelong learning and commitment to medical professionalism. *Acadaemic Medicine*. **75**(7): 708–17.

57 Palmer A, Burns S and Bulman C (eds) (1994) *Reflective Practice in Nursing: The Growth of the Professional Practitioner*. Blackwell Scientific Publications, Oxford.

58 Epstein RM and Hundert EM (2002) Defining and assessing professional competence. *Journal of the American Medical Association*. **287**(2): 226–35.

59 Regehr G and Mylopolous M (2008) Maintaining competence in the field: learning about practice, from practice, in practice. *Journal of Continuing Education in the Health Professions*. **28**(Suppl 1): S19–23.

60 Branch Jr WT, Frankel R, Gracey CF *et al.* (2009) A good clinician and a caring person: longitudinal faculty development and the enhancement of the human dimensions of care. *Academic Medicine*. **84**(1), 117–26.

61 Weissmann PF, Branch WT, Gracey CF, Haidet P and Frankel RM (2006) Role-modeling humanistic behavior: learning bedside manner from the experts. *Academic Medicine*. **81**(7): 661–7.

62 Clift R, Houst WR and Pugach M (eds) (1990) *Encouraging Reflective Practice in Education: An Analysis of Issues and Programs*. Teachers College Press, New York, NY.

63 Westberg J and Jason H (2001) *Fostering Reflection and Providing Feedback. Helping Others Learn from Experience*. Springer Series on Medical Education. Springer, New York, NY.

64 Moon J (2004) Using reflective learning to improve the impact of short courses and workshops. *Journal of Continuing Education in the Health Professions*. **24**: 4–11.

65 Mezirow J (1991) *Transformative Dimensions of Adult Learning*. Jossey-Bass, San Francisco, CA.

66 Lockyer J, Woloschuk W, Hayden A, McCombs B and Toews J (1994) Faculty perceptions of their role as consultants to practising physicians. *Academic Medicine*. **69**(10): S13–5.

67 Beecher A, Lindemann J, Morzinski J and Simpson D (1997) Use of the educator's portfolio to stimulate reflective practice among medical educators. *Teaching and Learning in Medicine*. **9**(1): 56–9.

68 Mezirow J and associates (eds) (1990) *Fostering Critical Reflection in Adulthood*. Jossey-Bass, San Francisco, CA.

69 Jennett PA, Parboosingh IJ, Maes WR, Lockyer JM and Lawson D (1990) A medical information networking system between practitioners. *Journal of Continuing Education in the Health Professions*. **10**(3): 237–43.

70 Cranton P (1994) *Understanding and Promoting Transformative Learning: A Guide For educators of Adults*. Jossey-Bass, San Francisco, CA.

71 Roberts C and Stark P (2008) Readiness for self-directed change in professional behaviours: factorial validation of the Self-reflection and Insight scale. *Medical Education*. **42**: 1054–63.

72 Sobral D (2005) Mindset for reflective learning: a revalidation of the reflection –in-learning scale. *Advances in Health Sciences Education*. **10**: 303–14.

73 Wald H, Borkan JM, Taylor JS, Anthony D and Reis SP (2012) Fostering and evaluating reflective capacity in medical education: developing the REFLECT rubric for assessing reflective writing. *Academic Medicine*. **87**: 41–50.

74 Vivekananda-Schmidt V, Marshall M, Stark P, Mckendree J, Sandars J and Smithson S (2011) Lessons from medical students' perceptions of learning reflective skills: a multi-institutional study. *Medical Teacher*. **33**: 846–50.

75 Taylor EW (2008) Transformative Learning Theory. *New Directions for Adult and Continuing Education*. **119**: 5–15.

76 Janik DS (2005) *Unlock the genius within*. Rowman and Littlefield Education, Lanham, MD.

77 Kelly R (2009) Transformative learning Q & A with Patricia Cranton. *Faculty Focus*. (http://www.facultyfocus.com/articles/instructional-design/transformative-learning-qa-with-patricia-cranton/; accessed 2 December 2012).

78 Brookfield SD (1990) *The Skillful Teacher: On Technique, Trust and Responsiveness in the Classroom*. Jossey-Bass, San Francisco, CA.

79 Maslow AH (1968) *Toward a Psychology of Being* (2e). Van Nostrand Reinhold, New York, NY.

80 Brockett RG and Hiemstra R (1991) *Self-Direction in Adult Learning: Perspectives on Theory, Research and Practice.* Routledge, New York, NY.

81 Knowles MS (1975) *Self-Directed Learning: A Guide for Learners and Teachers.* Association Press, New York, NY.

82 Grow G (1991) Teaching learners to be self-directed: a stage approach. *Adult Education Quarterly.* **41**(3): 125–49.

83 Hammond M and Collins R (1991) *Self-Directed Learning: Critical Practice.* Nichols/GP Publishing, New York, NY.

84 Gugliemino LM (1977) *Development of the self-directed learning readiness scale.* Unpublished doctoral dissertation. University of Georgia, Athens, GA.

85 Oddi LF (1986) Development and validation of an instrument to identify self-directed continuing learners. *Adult Education Quarterly.* **36**(2): 97–107.

86 Eva KW and Regehr G (2005) Self-assessment in the health professions: a reformulation and research agenda. *Academic Medicine.* **80**: 547–54.

87 Sargeant J, Armson H, Chesluk B *et al.* (2010) The processes and dimensions of informed self-assessment: a conceptual model. *Acad Med.* **85**: 1212–20.

88 Entwistle N and Ramsden R (1983) *Understanding Student Learning.* Croom Helm, London.

89 Miflin B, Campbell CB and Price DA (1999) A lesson from the introduction of a problem-based graduate entry course: the effects and different views of self-direction. *Medical Education.* **33**: 801–7.

90 Biggs J (2003) *Teaching for Quality Learning at University* (2e). Open University Press, Bury St. Edmonds.

91 Lewin K (1951) *Field Theory in Social Sciences.* Harper & Row, New York, NY.

92 Dewey J (1938) *Experience and Education.* Kappa Delta Phi, Touchstone, New York, NY.

93 Piaget J (1971) *Psychology and Epistemology.* Penguin Books, Harmondsworth, UK.

94 Fenwick T (2000) Conceptions of experiential learning: a review of the five contemporary perspectives on cognition. *Adult Education Quarterly.* **50**(4): 243–72.

95 Holzer SM and Andruet RH (1998) A multimedia workshop learning environment for statics. Workshop presented at ASEE Conference and Exposition, Seattle, WA. Virginia Polytechnic Institute and State University, Blacksburg, VA.

96 Lee P and Caffarella RS (1994) Methods and techniques for engaging learners in experiential learning activities. *New Directions for Adult and Continuing Education.* **62**: 43–54.

97 Fry R and Kolb B (1979) Experiential learning theory and learning experiences in liberal arts education. *New Directions for Experiential Learning.* **6**: 79–92.

98 Caffarella RS (1992) *Psychological Development of Women: Linkages to the Practice of Teaching and Learning in Adult Education.* ERIC Clearinghouse on Adult, Career and Vocational Education, Columbus, OH.

99 Rogoff B, Matusov E and White C (1996) Models of teaching and learning: participation in a community of learners. In: Olsen DR and Torrance N (eds) *The Handbook of Education and Human Development: New Models of Learning, Teaching, and Schoolingpp,* pp. 388–415. Blackwell, Oxford.

100 Rogoff B (2003) *The Cultural Nature of Human Development.* Oxford University Press, New York, NY.

101 Sfard A (1998) On two metaphors for learning and the dangers of choosing just one. *Educational Researcher.* **27**: 4–13.

102 Lave J and Wenger E (2002) Legitimate peripheral participation in communities of practice. In: Harrison R, Reeve F, Hanson A and Clarke J (eds) *Supporting Lifelong Learning. Perspectives on Learning,* pp. 1111–26. Routledge Farmer, London.

103 Borg E (2003) Discourse community. *The ELT Journal.* **57**(4): 398–400.

104 Palinscar AS (1998) Social constructivist perspectives on teaching and learning. *Annual Review of Psychology.* **49**: 345–75.

105 Brown JS, Collins A and Duguid P (1989) Situated cognition and the culture of learning. *Educational Researcher.* **18**(1): 32–42.

106 Eraut M (2000) Non-formal learning and tacit knowledge in professional work. *British Journal of Educational Psychology.* **70**: 113–36.

107 Reber A (1995) *Implicit Learning and Tacit Knowledge: An Essay on the Cognitive Unconscious.* Oxford University Press, New York, NY.

108 Polyani M (1958) *Personal Knowledge: Towards a Post-Critical Philosophy.* Routledge and Kegan Paul, London.

109 Cooke M, Irby D and O'Brien B (2010) *Educating Physicians: A Call for Reform of Medical School and Residency.* Jossey-Bass, San Francisco, CA.

110 Hafferty F and Franks R (1994) The hidden curriculum, ethics teaching and the structure of medical education. *Academic Medicine.* **69**: 861–71.

111 Coulehan J and Williams PC (2001) Vanquishing virtue: the impact of medical education. *Academic Medicine.* **76**: 598–605.

112 Dornan T, Boshuizen H, King N and Scherpbier A (2007) Experience-based learning: a model linking the processes and outcomes of medical students' workplace learning. *Medical Education.* **41**(1): 84–91.

113 Barab SA, Barnett M and Squire K (2002) Developing an empirical account of a community of practice: characterizing the essential tensions. *The Journal of the Learning Sciences.* **11**(4): 489–542.

114 Wenger E (2006) Communities of practice: a brief introduction. (http://www.ewenger.com/theory/communities_of_practice_intro.htm; accessed 2 December 2012).

115 Canadian Institutes of Health Research (CIHR) (2004) *Knowledge Translation Strategy: 2004–2009: Innovation in Action.* CIHR, Ottawa, ON.

116 Phipps D (2012) Knowledge mobilisation and why does it matter to universities *Guardian Profesional* 9th March 2012 (http://www.guardian.co.uk/higher-education-network/blog/2012/mar/09/introduction-to-knowledge-mobilisation; accessed 2 December 2012).

117 Caplan N (1978) The two communities theory and knowledge utilization. *American Behavioral Scientist.* **22**: 459–70.

118 Oftek E and Sarvary M (2002) Knowledge exchange and knowledge creation: should the emphasis shift in a competitive environment (working paper). INSEAD, Fontainebleau, France.

119 World Health Organization (WHO) (2006) Bridging the 'know–do' gap in global health (http://www.who.int/kms/en/; accessed 6 October 2006).

120 Canadian Health Services Research Foundation (CHSRF) (2003) *The Theory and Practice of Knowledge Brokering in Canada's Health System. A Report Based on a CHSRF Consultation and a Literature Review.* CHSRF, Ottawa, ON.

121 Davis DA, Thomson MA, Oxman AD and Haynes RB (1992) Evidence for the effectiveness of CME. A review of 50 randomized controlled trials. *Journal of the American Medical Association.* **268**: 1111–7.

122 Lathlean J and LeMay A (2002) Communities of practice: an opportunity for interagency working. *Journal of Clinical Nursing.* **11**: 394–8.

123 Gerstein J (2011) Learning communities: the future (the Now?) of education. (http://usergeneratededucation.wordpress.com/2011/08/29/learning-communities-the-future-the-now-of-education/; accessed 2 December 2012).

124 Triggs P and John P (2004) From transaction to transformation: information and communication technology, professional development and the formation of communities of practice. *Journal of Computer Assisted Learning.* **20**: 426–39.

125 Millen DR, Fontaine MA and Muller MJ (2002) Understanding the benefits and costs of communities of practice. *Communications of the ACM.* **45**(4): 69–73.

126 Wenger E, McDermott R and Snyder W (2002) *Cultivating Communities of Practice: A Guide to Managing Knowledge*. Harvard Business School Press, Boston, MA.

127 Vygotsky LS (1978) *Mind in Society: The Development of Higher Psychological Processes*. Harvard University Press, Cambridge, MA.

128 Henri F and Pudelko B (2003) Understanding and analyzing activity and learning in virtual communities. *Journal of Computer-Assisted Learning*. **19**: 474–87.

129 Kimble C, Hildreth P and Wright P (2001) Communities of practice: going virtual, In: Malhotra Y (ed.) *Knowledge Management and Business Model Innovation*, p. 220. Idea Group Publishing, Hershey, PA.

130 Parboosingh JT (2002) Physician communities of practice: where learning and practice are inseparable. *Journal of Continuing Education in the Health Professions*. **22**: 230–6.

131 CGX2.0 (n.d.) Evaluating communities of practice. Evaluating a platform after some time. (https://sites.google.com/a/cgxchange.org/evaluation-cop/home/evaluating-phase; accessed 15 June 2013).

132 Hung D and Tan SC (2004) Bridging between practice fields and real communities through instructional technology. *International Journal of Instructional Media*. **31**(2): 1–8.

133 Richardson B and Cooper N (2003) Developing a virtual interdisciplinary research community in higher education. *Journal of Interprofessional Care*. **17**(2): 173–82.

134 White CB and Thomas AM (2004) Students assigned to community practices for their pediatric clerkship perform as well or better on written examinations as students assigned to academic medical centers. *Teaching and Learning in Medicine*. **16**(3): 250–4.

135 Wilson BG and Myers KM (1999) Situated cognition in theoretical and practical contexts. In: Jonassen D and Land S (eds) *Theoretical Foundations of Learning Environments*, pp. 57–88. Lawrence Erlbaum, Mahwah, NJ. [eBook]

3 Principles of curriculum design

Janet Grant

The Open University, UK; University College London Medical School, UK; Centre for Medical Education in Context, UK; Peninsula Schools of Medicine and Dentistry, UK

 KEY MESSAGES

- A curriculum is an ideological, social and aspirational document that must reflect local circumstances and needs.

- The curriculum is made up of all the experiences learners will have that enable them to reach their intended achievements from the course.

- A curriculum statement should enable learners, teachers and managers to know and fulfil their obligations in relation to the course. It should describe intended learner achievements, content to be covered (the syllabus), teaching, learning, supervision, feedback and assessment processes, entry requirements and course structure.

- A syllabus is simply a list of the main topics of a course of study. This is only part of the curriculum.

- The way in which a curriculum for medical education is constructed depends on the designers' views about how students learn, how medicine is practised, issues of social responsibility and accountability, the role of the knowledge base, professional values and health service development.

- The curriculum design process should ask what is the purpose of the educational programme, how the programme will be organised, what experiences will further these purposes and how we can determine whether the purposes are being attained.

There is no body of evidence that shows that there is one best choice for framing a curriculum as a whole or any of it parts. A curriculum should simply be fit for the purpose and context of its place and day.

Introduction

My bookshelves carry an ever-expanding history of medical education, so I chose some books at random to determine whether the years had produced different ideas about curriculum design. Partially they had, and partially they had not. For instance, in 1961,(1) curriculum debates centred on instructional skills and ideas about how students learn. The curriculum was to be made up of objectives and experiences with relatively traditional divisions of content, but all based on the health needs of society, the philosophy of scientific thinking and the professional characteristics of physicians. In 1972,(2) the advice was to define aims and objectives in behavioural terms (not so different from today's preoccupation with competences, perhaps), and also that curricula should offer what the student and community require – not what is convenient for medical school staff to offer. Teachers were advised to try to integrate their teaching more effectively and give students some choice over what they learn. By 1982(3) and 1983,(4) a systems approach to educational design was advocated, with an emphasis on teaching methods aimed at delivering the learning objectives in the belief that active student involve-

ment in learning was a likely effective strategy. By 1989,(5) it seemed reasonable to devote entire books to the question of how the curriculum might be structured to facilitate learning appropriate to clinical practice. In the journals, there is the constant revived and revisited theme of social accountability,(6) incongruously placed alongside the equally powerful, and contradictory, rhetoric of the 'post-colonial dilemma' of globalisation.(7)

We can see from this snapshot that ideas develop according to economic and social imperatives but continue to have roots in previous thinking. Ideas of integration, a focus on students' learning rather than teachers' teaching, a need for teachers to learn how to do their job well, a focus on outcomes, albeit expressed as objectives or even competences, and a recognition of the responsibility of the school to respond to societal need and to prepare the student for professional practice have been current for many years. But the same ideas can give rise to different curriculum designs and to different processes of reaching that design. The design principles that we have now are based on the professional choices that curriculum designers make. Those choices are informed by the theories, the dominant rhetoric and social conditions of the day, and by the values and experiences of the medical profession doing its best to produce the next generation of doctors fit for its changing purpose.

And there is an enduring truth, expressed by Michael Apple,(8) that a curriculum is an ideological statement, expressing values, beliefs and aspirations. It cannot be a

---

neutral document, but must reflect relevant values deriving from the local political, cultural, professional and social context. This is even more so, as globalisation is the catchword of the day which threatens to homogenise curricula to standards not derived from local contexts.

Jolly and Rees recognise that there is a need for rational, open and accountable curriculum design processes. They eloquently describe the accompanying lack of evidential basis for how best to do this, but conclude that: 'Although curriculum design is an imprecise and arbitrary rubric, such a code is needed: systematic and arbitrary is somewhat better than capricious'(9, p. 22).

Curriculum design in medical education is an arena in which many battles are fought. There are many different views about, for example, what medical students should learn, how they should learn it, what qualities we want them to develop, where the science base stands, where skills of communication and examination should be acquired, how long it should all take and whether we want to frame their task in terms of outcomes or competences. The call for management, leadership and teaching skills to be included in the curriculum persists,(10) as, apparently in contradiction, the debate about curriculum overload continues, albeit without substantial research evidence.

There are equally as many views about how a curriculum should be developed and structured. And given that in education it is often difficult to find incontrovertible research findings on which to base decisions, there are no evidence-based approaches to curriculum design that we could meaningfully quote. This means that vogues in curriculum design ebb and flow in response to the dominant concerns of society and the professions, just as they ebb and flow in relation to teaching and learning methods, curriculum evaluation and even assessment of learning.

All these factors make a heady cocktail, which ensures that the business of curriculum design, development and review will never close. Eisner(11) talks of 'curriculum ideologies', which are 'the value premises from which decisions about practical educational matters are made'. These can be very strong, so that, as Toohey says, 'Alternative views are literally "unthinkable"'(12, p. 44). And so zealousness for a particular curriculum model develops, as she says, on beliefs that are 'so commonly held in the discipline, that they are accepted without question'. Integration, learner-centredness, and adult learning theories probably come into this category of belief. So because curriculum theory is based largely in ideology rather than evidence, this continuing spiral of changing views will never cease.

To muddy the pool even further, predominant concerns in curriculum design at the basic (medical school), postgraduate and continuing education levels are very different. In medical school, we have students who have everything to learn and a school that has the responsibility and opportunity to ensure that they do and the right to call on the student's time and fill it with activities that reflect the school's view of curriculum.

At the postgraduate level, learning occurs in the context of clinical practice. Our student now is a young doctor who still has much to learn and examinations to pass, but also has clinical duties to fulfil. Much of the learning is dependent on the clinical work that is experienced, and teachers and curriculum planners only have limited power to organise the days of a postgraduate trainee.

At the stage of continuing professional development, every doctor has become an autonomous professional, each with a unique history of experience and many with unique learning needs arising out of their professional practice. For most, there is little protected time and minimal finance for learning. At this point, the idea of a set curriculum might seem to be an unworkable irrelevance. This, in turn, renders the standardised assessment of practising physicians highly problematical.(13) Instead, we might simply guide senior doctors to identify their own learning needs, design their own learning and reinforce that in their own practice.(14)

Here, therefore, the principles of curriculum design are discussed only as they apply to undergraduate medical education and postgraduate training. Enduring principles are presented that will stand the test of time, changes of fashion and the many different contexts across the world in which medical curricula are applied. The principles outlined should be flexible enough to yield different types of curricula in different hands. The curriculum must be appropriate to its context, not a slave to abstract, if well meaning, intent. Effective education must be contextual, rooted in its own culture and conditions.

What is curriculum?

Educators and philosophers have addressed the question of what to teach and how to teach at least since Plato wrote *The Republic* in about 360 BCE. It might seem surprising, then, that it is only relatively recently that curriculum design has become a topic of debate in its own right, although the initial concerns about the nature of curricula arose with the advent of mass schooling in the late 19th century.(15) Until that point, curricula were defined by elite and specialist groups, and a curriculum statement (whether explicit or implicit) might contain only the content to be studied, and perhaps the time to be taken and the teaching method to be used.

Nowadays, however, this will not do. For reasons discussed in the next section, a curriculum statement now would be regarded as satisfactory only if it addresses the wider experience of the learner and the context of learning as well as the content and quality control of the enterprise. The curriculum should guide the learner, the teacher and educational managers. At the same time, it should leave room in its implementation for the creative and individual professionalism of the teacher, and for the individual preferences of the learner, given that both are clear about what is to be achieved.

The specification of intended curriculum outcomes (expressed in whatever terms) is, in almost all cases, nonnegotiable, not least because the curriculum is the basis for planning and developing the assessment system. If there is no agreed curriculum, how can we develop an objective, representative, valid and reliable assessment system? Simply, we cannot.

Many countries have some kind of guidance in relation to curricula at all stages. But few set actual standards for how a curriculum should be stated, what its component parts should be, and how it should be developed, implemented and used. In some countries, curricula are set by the state; in others they are set by regulatory or professional bodies. In the USA, the Liaison Committee on Medical Education sets accreditation standards that contain guidance on many key aspects of curriculum, but not on how to frame the curriculum statement itself. The UK offers a similar statement at the undergraduate level(16) and specific standards for curriculum design at the postgraduate level,(17) which allow the development of different curriculum statements that meet those set standards. Increasingly, medical educators at all levels are comparing their own curricula and medical education and training processes with the standards set by the World Federation for Medical Education.(18)

Definition

Although much is written about curriculum, definitions are few and far between. Accordingly, on the basis of a review of curriculum theories, the context of medical education, and the needs of teachers, trainers and regulators, a definition of curriculum was developed and adopted by the UK's General Medical Council (*see* Box 3.1). Curricula that comply with this definition will offer all stakeholders a clear description of requirements and expectations. The definition, although developed for postgraduate training, is appropriate to all levels.

However, this statement is possibly not enough, given the tension between increasing prominence of ideas of globalisation, and the articulated, but perhaps less acted on, imperative for a curriculum which reflects local needs. The requirements of the health care service and of communities are concrete. The best way of structuring a curriculum is theoretical, until it is decided on the basis of those local needs and resources. A curriculum must be contextual.(19)

BOX 3.1 What is a curriculum?

A statement of the intended aims and objectives, content, experiences, outcomes and processes of an educational programme, including the following:

- a description of the training structure (entry requirements, length and organisation of the programme, including its flexibilities, and assessment system)
- a description of expected methods of learning, teaching, feedback and supervision.

The curriculum should cover both generic professional and speciality-specific areas.

The syllabus content of the curriculum should be stated in terms of what knowledge, skills, attitudes and expertise the learner will achieve.

Source: UK General Medical Council

Standards for design

Curriculum standards address more than simply the syllabus content of the course. For example, the guidance in the GMC's *Tomorrow's Doctors*(16) – which forms the basis of quality inspections of medical schools in the United Kingdom – addresses a wide range of issues from the core knowledge, skills and attitudes expected of students on graduation, to systems of assessment and arrangements to ensure the health and safety of patients.

In the USA, the Liaison Committee on Medical Education sets similar accreditation standards for American Medical Schools(20) as a condition for licensure of their graduates. Not surprisingly, among the accreditation standards are some fundamental curriculum issues such as the following:

- educational objectives
- curriculum structure and design
- content
- teaching and assessment
- curriculum management
- roles and responsibilities
- evaluation of curriculum effectiveness

In the UK's postgraduate arena, the General Medical Council, sets out specific standards against which all postgraduate curricula are formally judged and approved before implementation.(17) These standards themselves reflect the view taken of the learning process, and the key contexts and factors that influence medical education. These are discussed further in the next section. Although the standards shown in Box 3.2 were developed for curricula in postgraduate medical education, there is no reason why they should not equally be applied to any level of medical education and training in any location.

Such standards try to decrease the distance between the three coexisting types of curriculum identified by Coles:(21)

- the curriculum on paper
- the curriculum in action
- the curriculum the learner experiences.

Further afield, the World Federation for Medical Education (WFME) has set, piloted and evaluated quality improvement standards for all aspects of medical education at all stages to 'provide a mechanism for quality improvement in medical education, in a global context, to be applied by institutions, organisations and national authorities responsible for medical education'.(18) These are all aspects of curriculum. The WFME standards(18) address:

- mission and outcomes
- the educational programme
- the learning and training process
- assessment of learning
- students and trainee characteristics and needs
- staffing and faculty
- educational resources and training settings
- evaluation of the educational programme and process
- governance and administration
- curriculum renewal.

These standards are already widely used for self-studies within medical schools and for accreditation purposes. They support the view that curriculum design must encompass

BOX 3.2 Standards for postgraduate medical curricula

1 The purpose of the curriculum must be stated, including linkages to previous and subsequent stages of the trainees' training and education. The appropriateness of the stated curriculum to the stage of learning and to the specialty in question must be described.

2 The overall purpose of the assessment system must be documented and in the public domain.

3 The curriculum must set out the general, professional, and specialty-specific content to be mastered.

4 Assessments must systematically sample the entire content, appropriate to the stage of training, with reference to the common and important clinical problems that the trainee will encounter in the workplace and to the wider base of knowledge, skills and attitudes demonstrated through behaviours that doctors require.

5 Indication should be given of how curriculum implementation will be managed and assured locally and within approved programmes.

6 The curriculum must describe the model of learning appropriate to the specialty and stage of training.

7 Recommended learning experiences must be described which allow a diversity of methods . . .

8 The choice of assessment method(s) should be appropriate to the content and purpose of that element of the curriculum.

9 Mechanisms for supervision of the trainee should be set out.

10 Assessors/examiners will be recruited against criteria for performing the tasks they undertake.

11 Assessments must provide relevant feedback to the trainees.

12 The methods used to set standards for classification of trainees' performance/competence must be transparent and in the public domain.

13 Documentation will record the results and consequences of assessments and the trainee's progress through the assessment system.

14 Plans for curriculum review, including curriculum evaluation and monitoring, must be set out.

15 Resources and infrastructure will be available to support trainee learning and assessment at all levels.

16 There will be lay and patient input in the development and implementation of assessments.

17 The curriculum should state its compliance with equal opportunities and anti-discriminatory practice.

Source: UK General Medical Council(17)

---

much more than a statement of the content to be covered in the course.

A note of caution

The standards cited all require the curriculum designer to think about the intended product and character of the course, its rationale, values or mission. Without these elements, standard setting for curricula becomes a dangerous and instrumental undertaking, apt to serve only political or economic purposes. 'Aims-talk', as Noddings(22) calls it, is the first and most important element of curriculum design and its most important standard whereby local relevance can be assured.

Curriculum in context

The most powerful emerging influence on thinking about curriculum concerns the role of local context, and the dangers of importation of curriculum models from different cultures and systems,(7) even as the international trade in curriculum as a transferable commodity flourishes. And yet there is no evidence that western models (for the flow of ideas is invariably from west to east) are any better in their outcomes than other models.(7,23,24) A phenomenon has been noted, namely the 'apologetic stance taken by authors in the east about their slowness in adopting western methods, even though . . . those methods will demand an "intense re-socialisation of learners into metropolitan Western mindsets"'.(7, p. 177)

But this is not simply an east-west diversification. Differences in educational and assessment culture have been shown in medical education, even within and between western countries.(25–27) So a contextual curriculum will not place its emphasis narrowly on educational method and the search for the most effective methods of teaching and learning, for which there is no robust differentiating evidence base. Instead, the emphasis must be on context, on health benefits and benefits to the scientific and cultural basis of medicine. In a contextual curriculum, the 'medical education' decisions become secondary.

Before we go on to think about curriculum in more general terms, we should be clear about the necessary components of a curriculum designed to be sensitive to the local context. Some of these will be true for any curriculum, but some will not. These include the following.

- Consideration of the body of knowledge, skill and experience necessary for the practice of medicine in the local context. This may be derived from the scientific base as commonly used and understood but must be done so consciously and on the basis of analysis.
- Prioritisation of health problems, which will yield very different results from location to location.
- Contextualisation of knowledge, appropriate to the local setting which will allow not only appropriate understanding of the context of health and illness, but also of the approach to communication and clinical decision-making.
- Awareness of the diversity of medical practice, according to which, even the classification of disease, its manifesta-

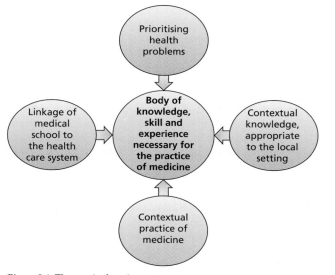

Figure 3.1 The curriculum in context.

tion and treatment are all linked to the local context. Thus the content of the curriculum is affected by the context, at every level. In the era of globalisation, universal truth is hard to find.(28,29)

• Linkage of medical school inputs, processes and outputs to the health care system without which contextualisation of learning is severely compromised.

We can represent this as shown in Figure 3.1.

In summary, a curriculum must be contextual to be meaningful. Bearing this in mind, we can now consider the more traditional views of curriculum.

Factors that influence curriculum design

It can be seen from the GMC curriculum definition and standards cited that a comprehensive curriculum is much more than a syllabus statement, which simply sets out the topic headings or content of a course or a programme. Writing a curriculum is a process that demands consideration of values, beliefs and choices. It deserves a review of evidence and a development process, which sends out messages about quality assurance and recognition of all the stakeholders.

The days when subject experts or workforce managers alone wrote down what was to be learnt are now past. These days, curriculum design encompasses many other factors that derive from the democratisation of social processes, the development of educational theory, political imperatives and economic concerns. Box 3.3 highlights some influences on modern medical curricula and their areas of effect. Each of the influences cited here has had its effect, and the residue of each of those effects remains to become incorporated into the new generation of curricula, making each new reformulation richer than the previous models.

The evolution of curriculum models and learning theories is addressed below. But the other factors, which are not

part of the academic discourse, are equally as important in shaping ideas about curriculum. Some of these factors affect the content of the curriculum, and some affect its design. For example, theories of professional practice have arisen around the sorts of ideas that are embodied in the UK General Medical Council's statement on *Good Medical Practice*, which defines a set of common content for professional behaviour and values.(30) This document covers such issues as professional standards for clinical care, maintaining good medical practice, educational activity, and relationships with patients, colleagues and teams. It is a professional statement that influences curriculum guidance.(16)

Another highly influential statement is that of the Royal College of Physicians and Surgeons of Canada(31) on the essential roles and key competencies of specialist physicians (CanMEDS). This statement addresses the qualities of a doctor that every educational programme should facilitate:

• medical expert
• communicator
• collaborator
• manager
• health advocate
• scholar
• professional.

Such statements not only contribute to the vision that an organisation has of its intended product, but will also affect directly the content and style of the curriculum. On the other hand, social drivers for accountability and transparency have determined the use of clear outcomes, amenable to peer or lay input and review. Political imperatives have often pushed curricula to be more aware of issues of the cost and speed of workforce production. From this, we should be aware that choice of curriculum design or model is not an objective entity but is socially, professionally, academically and politically constructed.

At any one point, curriculum design is a child of its time.

Curriculum models

Curriculum models have been the subject of academic and management theory since the mid-20th century, when Tyler first put forward the idea that: '. . . it is very necessary to have some conception of the goals that are being aimed at. These educational objectives become the criteria by which materials are selected, content is outlined, instructional procedures are developed and tests and examinations are prepared'.(32, p. 52)

Although Tyler adopted a relaxed view of how objectives should be framed, this approach still allowed a 'transmission model'(33) of learning, which focuses on the teacher's rather than the learner's activity. Despite Mager coining the subsequent term 'instructional objectives', and taking a harder line on expressing objectives in measurable terms, his simultaneous intention was to change that focus and emphasise the importance of student achievement rather than teacher activity.(34) At the same time, he was much more prescriptive about exactly how those achievements should be specified: in behavioural, observable terms that were amenable to assessment. And so the use of the curriculum as the foundation of assessment became a central tenet.

There followed a raft of curriculum theorists who found that the Mager and Tyler models did not encompass all types of valued learning. So, for example, Eisner(11) introduced the idea of problem-solving and expressive objectives or expressive outcomes, leading us on to a current dominant view of curriculum formulation. Some theorists tried to break free from curriculum models that specified outcomes in whatever form. Stenhouse,(35) for example, proposed a process model that focused on the processes of acquiring, using and evaluating the knowledge of the discipline. Outcomes, then, would be truly learner centred, rather than having the contradictory position of a learner-centred rhetoric aimed at their achievement of outcomes specified by others.

This contradiction has been compounded in more recent times, during which the cultural hegemony of a competence-based curriculum model, which was originally introduced in practical vocational subjects, has held sway. Its suitability as a basis for assessments, its common-sense appeal, its apparent analytical basis and its implicit message that if we could define competences, we can ensure that learners acquire them and be assured by relevant testing that this is so, all make a competence model attractive. I have myself argued that competences alone cannot describe even the skills, much less the performance, of a profession.(36) Some prominent writers, such as Hyland, have suggested that the competence movement in curriculum design is little more than an economically driven derivative of the behavioural school: 'This attempt to specify exactly what is to be achieved and measured is, of course, nothing more than reconstituted behaviourism . . . Constructed out of a 'fusion

of behavioural objectives and accountability' . . . the movement provided irresistible appeal to those seeking accountability and input–output efficiency in the new economic realism of the 1980s'.(37, p.49) Perhaps this does 'ring some bells' today.

The twin factors of accountability and efficiency of education or training appeal to medicine, which has become increasingly concerned about demonstrating transparency and public accountability in times of increasing litigation. The contextual climate of a hard-pressed health service, limited resources, and managerial and political imperatives has made the appeal of the model very alluring. On the other hand, the rise of competency-based models has possibly increased the tendency to 'teach-to-the-test' along with a more instrumental, less creative, approach to learning on the part of the students.(38)

We can see from these examples of curriculum models that their use can be a function of instrumental pragmatism, values and vision, political, social and managerial imperatives, and of the ideas that are current about how people learn. This means that selection of a curriculum model is a process that requires careful thought and open justification. That justification is unlikely to be in terms of research evidence; it will be in terms of ideology.

Theories of learning

An important factor in the development of new curriculum models has been the burgeoning field of learning research and theory. Not unexpectedly, there is a symbiotic relationship between learning theory and curriculum models. While objectives-based curriculum models were predominant, so was behavioural theory. While behavioural theory has declined, however, assessment theory and managerial imperatives have taken over to ensure that the behavioural aspects of curriculum definition still remain, albeit in new guises.

Learning theory has entirely changed its stance on effective pedagogy during the past half century. As with every other aspect of education, learning theory and consequent pedagogical practice is a never-ending work in progress. Ideas change. So, we have seen that at the time of the objectives-based curriculum models, behavioural theory was also in its prime, and the role of the teacher in shaping behaviour was a main focus. High on the best-seller list were books that explained how to teach, not how students learn. But even those books, and some were excellent, strayed into recognising the students' responsibility for learning.(39)

However, things have changed, and in the past 20–30 years, the focus has moved away from teaching and towards learning. Nicol explains that nowadays, the teacher: '. . . encourages participation, dialogue and interaction by students with course materials and with each other. The teacher should function as a facilitator of learning, intellectually critical, stimulating and challenging, but within a learning context that emphasises support and mutual respect'.(40)

Surely in this we can see the roots of curriculum models such as problem-based learning, and the brief phase when it seemed unacceptable to use the word 'teacher' or any word derived from it. And just as educational theory develops and enfolds the whole range of education, we have seen problem-based learning applied, and then gradually retreating, in such diverse arenas as design, chemical engineering and the arts. So learning theories, even when they are simply that, are powerful in their practical effects on educational practice.

Around this current view of effective learning requiring activity on the part of the learner has developed a panoply of ideas about the components of this approach. So in medical education, as in every other form of education, we have seen a considerable body of published work on approaches to learning, on learning styles, group work and the social context, on the trainer–learner relationship and the value system in which learning occurs. Such ideas, even when they do not progress beyond being simply declamatory, have a direct effect on curricula and the models of curriculum that are adopted.

Specific theories of learning are too many and varied to report, although there are some key ideas that have persisted and have influenced curriculum design. Adult learning theory,(41) which promotes active self-directed learning towards personally relevant goals, despite its lack of evidence base, seems to have an intuitive or social appeal and has been widely cited as the basis for curriculum and course design. For example, the University of New Mexico School of Medicine, in its own words, 'gained national and international recognition for its constantly evolving curricular innovations which are aimed at adapting adult learning theory to medical education'.(42)

Other key theoretical frameworks that medical education has chosen to embrace include the dichotomy between deep and surface-level approaches to learning.(43) The former is characterised by an active concern in the student to seek the underlying meaning, the wider picture, the relationship between different information and experiences, the logic of the argument, and the need to question and understand. Surface-level processors, on the other hand, are said to take a passive approach and seek to learn the content, acquire the knowledge and get the right answers. But a surface characterisation of learning styles can fail to illuminate the deep strategic thinking that is actually occurring, and can be culturally determined.(44)

Our knowledge of learning styles and approaches has clear implications for curriculum design in terms of teaching skills and methods, learning opportunities and assessment.(45) Curricula that dissuade students from apparently simple rote learning (although this might actually be productive repetitive learning) and encourage apparently deep processing (although this can only occur in the presence of acquired knowledge) have now become the dominant form. And curricula can affect a learner's approach to learning. So McManus *et al.* put forward the opinion that:

> Formal education, particularly effective formal education, can also alter study habits and learning styles . . . Intercalated degrees increase deep and strategic learning and decrease surface learning at medical school . . . Deep and strategic learning also relate to the clinical experience gained by medical students, making it possible that greater patient involvement during undergraduate clinical training, rather than mere reliance on textbook learning to pass exams, a

characteristic of surface learners, will also reduce surface-disorganised approaches to work.(46)

The learning theories that inform today's curriculum design seem to be very far from the ideas of behavioural theories of learning, and from the idea that the knowledge base of the discipline must first be learnt before its application can be attempted. Today's trajectory of learning is flatter, with integration being the hallmark throughout the course, and deep learning in the context of practice its aim.

Yet at the same time as these developments, we also have seen the rise of competence-based curriculum frameworks, which seem strangely to hark back to the days when curricula were based on the attainment of set objectives and the underlying theory was distinctly behavioural. This contradiction remains unresolved in the competence-based curricula of today, which simultaneously claim to rely on student-centred learning methods. And the acquisition of a large body of knowledge still lies at the heart of medicine, as it does in any profession.

Theory and practice of the discipline

Integration

Of course it is not only theories of how students learn that affect the design of curricula. Theories about the discipline of medicine itself have also been paramount in changing the face of curricula. As the Case Western Reserve University School of Medicine describe their own history: 'Already a leading educational institution for more than a century, the School of Medicine in 1952 initiated the most advanced medical curriculum in the country, integrating the basic and clinical sciences, focusing on organ systems and featuring an introduction to patients and clinical work in the first year. Many other medical schools followed suit'.(47)

Today it seems almost universally accepted that the practice of medicine requires this integration of its component parts: of science and clinical experience, knowledge, skills and attitudes, judgement and problem-solving, even of continuing to learn through reflection on practice. So whereas in former times a curriculum for medicine might have offered in sequence its component constituents of science, clinical skills and experience to facilitate clinical judgement, leaving the integration of these to the learner, this learning trajectory has been superseded and the integrated context of practice now is reflected in the integrated nature of curricula. The curriculum is increasingly for practice,(48) rather than simply to acquire the elements of professional knowledge, skills and attitudes for later application.

Trajectories of learning

It might seem surprising, then, that a traditional curriculum is more effective in encouraging clinical problem-solving skills.(49) On the other hand, educational psychology would tell us that a well-structured knowledge base is a good springboard towards freedom of creative thought.(50) In an environment which demands constant new problem-solving, as each new patient does demand, it a strong and structured base of knowledge, tuned through experience and supported by skills, that is the essential component. The most effective trajectory of learning, therefore, will initially ensure well-structured knowledge which is almost independent of problems or situations and relates to the learner's stage of mastery of concepts. Such knowledge is therefore transferable, and can be followed or accompanied by its contextual application. But the knowledge must come first and must have its own coherent organisation. It is that which ensures transferability. This might suggest that learning the basic sciences while having the contextual background that, for example, early clinical exposure offers, would indeed yield more effective clinical problem-solvers.

The use of learning trajectories to structure the curriculum has been successfully used at all levels of learning. For example, the approach has been explained convincingly in relation to early childhood mathematics.(51) The three components of goals, the developmental path and instructional activities to link the two, leading to increasingly higher levels of thinking, will be familiar to many medical teachers.

Team working

A further aspect of professional practice that has influenced curriculum design is the advent of team working in medicine. As health care has become more complex, working practices have changed and health care managers seek more cost-effective ways of delivering high-quality care. So, many medical schools (such as Southampton) have developed their curricula to offer prospective students: '. . . the opportunity to develop the attitudes, skills and knowledge you need to become a skilled practitioner in a modern, changing health service, capable of following a career in a wide range of specialities . . .'(52)

Professionalism

Very recently, the whole question of professionalism and how it is acquired has gripped the profession and its educational institutions worldwide. Such issues have arisen from a series of trigger crises that the profession itself experienced in standards of practice and in changing practices, as well as in the changing role of doctors in society, market forces and accountability within the health care system, and society's changing relationship with the professions in the light of greater universal education and wider access to previously protected knowledge. Each of these ideas has its direct effect on the design of curricula. It has already been suggested by one key working group(53) that medical schools should 'consider introducing professional values early into the undergraduate medical course . . .' and that '. . . each student's professional values should be assessed throughout their training to ensure their fitness to practise'.

Another major influence on curriculum design has been the move of health service provision into the community, along with the realisation that medical schools themselves have a social responsibility.

Curriculum design then, is subject to a wide variety of influences in relation to the profession of medicine, the health care service and society as a whole. Each curriculum design team must decide for themselves which of these they will choose to characterise their own work (*see* Box 3.4).

BOX 3.4 WHERE'S THE EVIDENCE: For comparative curriculum design

Although there is much research published about different curriculum models, and teaching and learning strategies, there is no evidence to suggest that there is a 'best' template for curriculum design. This is partly because a curriculum is made up of many components and there is little evidence to suggest that even for any one of these there is a 'best choice' for all circumstances. Curricula have many different specific purposes and therefore many different designs. Their effectiveness can only be judged against their intended purposes. And few share exactly the same purpose, beyond intending to produce safe and responsible doctors.

This makes comparative or controlled research almost impossible.

So each curriculum designer must decide on the purpose of the curriculum and then search the literature for the relevant evidence about the likely effect of each curriculum component in serving that purpose. Convincing evidence may sometimes be difficult to find. So curriculum designers will often rely on their professional judgement and values and should always seek to gather their own evidence about the effects of their own curriculum.

The purpose and components of curriculum design

Curriculum design has two components: the structure of the curriculum, and its content. Battles are fought and choices made in both arenas on the basis of the values, vision and assumptions of the curriculum designers and their institutions, or their social, economic, political and cultural influences.

Prior to the 1960s, curriculum change was best described as unplanned 'drift'(54) although even before that time, curriculum ideology was informed by dominant social ideologies and imperatives. For example, the need to reconstruct the world after the Second World War certainly gave rise to the management by objectives movement and so to objectives based curricula, in the race to normalise as quickly and efficiently as possible. But from that point, Kelly(55) records that educationalists recognised the need for planned innovation to keep pace with societal changes, while maintaining standards and values, and taking advantage of new theoretical underpinnings. At the same time, the idea of the curriculum as a total description of the intentions, mechanisms, context and outcomes of education took hold. The curriculum must explain and justify itself, describe the intended learning experiences and their rationale and explore the likely effects of the students' exposure to them.

A curriculum is therefore a document that must:

- tell the learner exactly what to expect including the methods of student support

- advise the teacher what to do to deliver the content and support the learners in their task of personal and professional development
- help the institution to set appropriate assessments of student learning and implement relevant evaluations of the educational provision
- tell society how the school is executing its social responsibilities.

The curriculum should present a reasoned picture of the subject to be studied and define the teaching and learning processes, and the intended outcomes of that study. But all curriculum decisions must be made on the basis of a prior statement of vision or mission or values. And that statement must be made for the local context. General statements are of limited value. Contextual statements expressed in concrete terms will drive useful change at all levels.

It can be seen that the curriculum is a powerful tool and for that reason is often the focus of battles for power and control. The major theorists of our time have seen that curriculum is the instrument for a more humane and socially accountable society. In medicine, the current trend for greater involvement of the community and its health care needs, and of patients and their families in curriculum development is a reflection of this tenet.

Steps in curriculum design

Despite the differences of view that have existed over the years and between different practitioners and theorists, all are generally agreed that the process of curriculum design must answer the following central questions, originally set out by Tyler in 1949.(32)
- What is the purpose of the educational programme?
- How will the programme be organised?
- What experiences will further these purposes?
- How can we determine whether the purposes are being attained?

The curriculum designer must make choices about how to answer each of these questions. We have seen that those choices are influenced by a number of contextual factors, but what are the options that are available at each stage? The next sections set out some of those options.

It must be said, however, that although these steps and their subsections are discussed below serially, in real life, many such decisions occur in parallel, or in a different order, because they are so tightly interdependent and are a function of local conditions. Figure 3.2 summarises the steps that most curriculum writers agree should be undertaken in the process of curriculum design and lists the sorts of options that the curriculum designer must choose between at each stage. In addition are presented the factors that are required to make the curriculum responsive to its own context.

How do we express the overall purpose of an educational programme?

The purpose of a programme is often based on a set of aims, or a mission statement, such as the WFME standards require, or a statement of professional values such as that

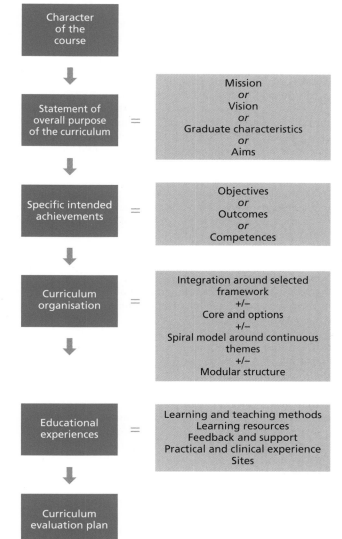

Figure 3.2 Steps and options in curriculum design.

of the CanMEDS project mentioned above, or a 'vision statement' such as that developed by the University of Sheffield Medical School, which encompassed the general intentions, values and characteristics of the curriculum. For example, the Sheffield vision statement dealt with:
- the qualities of the intended graduates
- the method of expressing the intentions of the curriculum (outcomes-based)
- the curriculum structure (integrated, patient contact, community experience, facilitating student learning and student choice)
- curriculum organisation (based on body systems, progressively presenting undifferentiated patient problems)
- the instructional approach (a spine of problem, case- and patient-based integrated learning activities complemented by a range of other teaching and learning activities, with an increase in systematic teaching of some components to ensure competence in key areas)

- student learning approach (progressively more self-directed, supported by information technology resources, distance learning and activities)
- the assessment system (formative and summative based on the defined outcomes)
- the curriculum management system and team
- the curriculum monitoring and improvement system.

Thus a vision statement addresses all the central curriculum design issues and must be the result of extensive discussion and consultation with all the relevant stakeholders and experts. Such consultation is fundamental to a properly managed change process,(56) and in Sheffield, it took nearly a year to complete.(57)

On another level, Brown University School of Medicine (58) chose to think about the intended achievements of its curriculum in terms of the abilities of successful doctors. It derived, through consultation, nine such abilities, as follows:

1 Effective communication
2 Basic clinical skills
3 Using basic sciences in the practice of medicine
4 Diagnosis, management and prevention
5 Lifelong learning
6 Self-awareness, self-care and personal growth
7 The social and community contexts of health care
8 Moral reasoning and clinical ethics
9 Problem-solving.

In the end, a comparison of the statements of different types shows that they express very similar ideas. What is important is that the statement of purpose of the programme is made to suit the local context. Figure 3.1 shows that this would include reflection on social, academic and professional issues, as well as a local prioritisation of health problems.

How does the curriculum design allow for local choice?

Underpinning the overall purposes of the curriculum will be a set of values that pervade the thinking or the aspirations of the school. Many years ago, these value choices were set out in the SPICES(59) model (Figure 3.3) as a series of dimensions between two extremes. But this analysis has perhaps been superseded by both a lack of subsequent evidence to underpin either its dimensions or its hierarchy, and a more recent value set that suggests that curriculum

purpose and context, have primacy over curriculum organisation. We should be clear that no automatic value judgements should be attached to either dimension; for example, apprenticeship learning is still regarded as fundamental to medical training, and the potential narrow instrumentality of a planned systematic approach is recognised as having its dangers in professional training.

How can we describe specific intended achievements?

There are many ways to express what it is that a curriculum is intended to achieve. We have seen that the choice of how to express this is often as much a function of social context and educational fashion or belief as it is of any objective evidence of effect. The importance of this stage of planning is twofold; it will:

- define the content of the course
- be the basis of the assessment blueprint.(60)

Not surprisingly, this is another contentious area: every department and teacher will want to have their own subject properly represented in the curriculum, and a team-based approach that matches the organisation of the curriculum is advisable, with iterative consultations following a properly managed change process.(56)

Essentially, what the curriculum intends to achieve is most commonly expressed in one of the following ways.

- As *objectives*, expressed as the specific knowledge, skills and attitudes that the student will display at the end of the course. As we have seen, the objectives model became predominant after the Second World War, when reconstruction was most efficiently tackled in a managerial way, leading to observable and measurable changes, after the chaos of the preceding period.
- As *intended outcomes*, stated in clear and precise terms, which will allow the designer to specify the learning experiences that will facilitate achievement of the stated outcomes. For many, this is a return to Tyler's original idea of objectives.(61)
- As *competences* to be achieved and assessed, again expressed in terms that bear similarity to objectives but are often thought of in relation to the ultimate intended performance that the competences underpin.

There has been and still is a furious debate around the use of these terms, and what they mean, how they differ, what they imply and how they are used. It has been argued that

Innovative approaches	Traditional strategies
1 Student-centred	Teacher-centred
2 Problem-based	Information gathering
3 Integrated	Discipline-based
4 Community-based	Hospital-based
5 Electives	Standard programme
6 Systematic	Apprenticeship-based

Figure 3.3 Educational strategies in curriculum development: the SPICES model.

a simple statement of competences alone cannot reflect the complex nature of a profession or the central skill of professional judgement.(36) It was Stenhouse's belief that a statement of behavioural objectives cannot address socialisation and problem-solving,(62) which are processes fundamental to a profession.

It has also been argued that such 'product-oriented curricula' are disempowering for the learners and take control of learning away from the learner,(63) and possibly disempower teachers similarly. In this, an outcomes-based curriculum would be incompatible with a learner-centred approach to learning, yet the two, in many curricula, attempt to coexist.

Specific guidance on the specification of outcomes has been offered and makes its similarity to the objectives-based model clear. In outcome-based education:

> Decisions about the curriculum are driven by the outcomes the students should display at the end of the course. In outcome-based education, product defines process. [It] ... can be summed up as "results-orientated thinking" and is the opposite of "input-based education" where the emphasis is on the educational process and where we are happy to accept whatever is the result. In outcome-based education, the outcomes agreed for the curriculum guide what is taught and what is assessed.(64, p. 8)

It is not surprising that the instrumental nature of this approach has given rise to some controversy. Key writers have sometimes opted to use these terms interchangeably,(58) equating outcome-based and competency-based as the same thing in practical terms.(65) We could equally say that objectives are not very different. An outcome might be: 'Obtains history in relation to possible underlying causes including cardiovascular and non-organic causes'.(57)

It would be difficult to say in what way this is different from a competence or an objective. And it really does not matter, because statements such as this are fit for purpose. It is a debate with no conclusion, and perhaps the answer really does not matter. What is important is fitness for purpose, and the main purposes of stating the intended achievements of the curriculum are:

- to inform learners of what they should achieve
- to inform teachers of what they should help the learners to achieve
- to be the basis of the assessment system, so that everyone knows what will be assessed
- to reflect accurately the nature of the profession into which the learner is being inducted and the professional characteristics that must be acquired.

Regardless of the rhetoric surrounding these different ways of describing what a curriculum should achieve, the important point is that this is done in terms specific enough to guide planning, assessment and review, and to give students and teachers appropriate expectations. Perhaps it is high time that medicine found a new and more appropriate way of describing its qualities (*see* Box 3.5).

How will the programme be organised?

Once the overall intentions of the curriculum and its more specific intended achievements are defined and agreed, the curriculum must be written to reflect the

---

 BOX 3.5 FOCUS ON: Competence and competency

The terms 'competence' and 'competency' seem to be the focus of concern and debate. But in education, preoccupation with definition of terms is, perhaps, to miss the point. In dictionary terms, these are alternative words with the same meaning. Both simply mean 'the ability to do something; the ability to perform a given task'. So there is no contest between competence and competency – it is simply a matter of which word you care to use. But this definitional fact does not stop a semantic debate raging.

It seems that in common curriculum parlance, a competence is a specific, measurable entity (knowledge, skill, behaviour) that the learner should display by the end of the programme. But this does not mean that the possessor of the competences will translate these into performance. And so, in education, the term 'competency' sometimes seems to be used to suggest the underlying propensity to turn competence into performance.

The underlying pedagogical theory seems to be that if we can define the competences that make up professional performance, then we can aim the teaching programme at them and make it more efficient and effective. This theory is flawed.

If the acquisition of competences in turn leads to competency to perform, this will be because the separate competences have been used repeatedly in concert in the context of complex professional practice to gather information, to process it, to make judgements and decisions, to solve problems, to make interventions, to deal with and interact with peers, colleagues and patients, and to think in multidimensional terms about personal, interpersonal, ethical, financial, managerial, multiprofessional and evidence-based factors.

So a curriculum that bases itself on the specification of competences is only recognising the first step on a path that leads to the competency that is the precursor of the ultimate complex professional performance. And if we spend too long on debating definition, perhaps we are no more than sublimating our energies and closing our eyes to more difficult questions.

---

intended organisation of the course. The main current organisational models are:

- integration
- core and options
- spiral model
- modular.

These options are not mutually exclusive and many curricula display elements of them all. So an integrated curriculum with a modular core of mandatory content and student-selected options, which contain topics that are revisited in increasing depth at successive stages of the curriculum, is quite possible and possibly the most common approach among new curricula.

Integrated

A curriculum based primarily on separate disciplines is probably not integrated. Although, as we have seen, a traditional curriculum accompanied by early clinical exposure may well be seen as being integrated. In general, however, in a discipline-based curriculum, the knowledge and skills are presented in silos and the integration has to occur entirely in the student's head through use in practice. There is no robust evidence that this is a flawed strategy. An integrated curriculum, however, organises the material to be learnt around an entity that is more related to practice.

Curriculum integration can be managed as either horizontal integration between different subject areas or vertical integration between the clinical and basic sciences. Integrated curricula in medical schools across the globe are now too numerous to mention and it seems likely that, in time, curricula worldwide will adopt both vertical and horizontal integration. This can be a threatening development for some departments, especially in basic sciences, which often feel that they are likely to lose their identity. But if integration is properly managed, and the curriculum content properly defined, every department should be able to track its own contribution to the curriculum as a whole.

It is a common and strong view(66) that the early clinical experience vertical integration offers students is beneficial to their motivation and satisfaction, their acclimatisation and professional induction, and their valuing and contextualisation of the scientific base. It might strengthen and broaden learning and intensify the relevance of the course to ultimate clinical practice. However, these assertions still only attain the status of claims. Despite the widening adoption of integration as the basis of curriculum organisation, there is still no robust evidence base that shows its actual effects. As with most changes in education, the innovation occurs as a result of belief rather than evidence and gains credibility only through custom and practice.

The adoption of integration implies a significant reorganisation of the curriculum and so decisions must be made about the basis for that integration. In other words, what will be the framework around which the content of the curriculum will be arranged? There are many choices.
- In Sheffield, the curriculum was designed around an agreed list of presenting clinical problems derived from published sources and other curricula, added to locally and then rated by clinical teachers for their importance. A blueprint for each problem was then constructed, which defined the curriculum content and outcomes.(57)
- In Manchester,(67) the core problem-based curriculum was organised around index clinical situations (ICSs) for which new graduates must have a required level of competence. These ICSs were derived in consultation with primary and secondary care clinicians, who then defined the knowledge and skills base for each one in a variety of specific domains, including technical, contextual, intellectual and interpersonal.

Equally, the basis for integration could be bodily systems, age, patient cases or any other grouping. Each approach has its advantages and disadvantages. Within the chosen framework, however, the specific content to be covered can be specified in terms of repeated and consistent curriculum themes that run vertically through the whole course. This is described further below in relation to modular design.

Core and options

This specification of mandatory and optional sections of the curriculum was a response to the perceived (if not proven) problem of content overload in medical education. Given that this is the central, mandatory content of the curriculum, 'core' can mean different things in different contexts. But if a core and options model is chosen, then the basis on which the core is selected must be known and agreed. To date, there is no adequate evidence base to suggest that one way of identifying the core is better than any other.(68) Harden and Davis(69) set out the possibilities:
- the essential aspects of each subject or discipline
- the essential competencies for practice
- areas of study relevant to many disciplines.

A fourth possibility is a study of only those disciplines deemed essential, but this approach 'has caused great alarm among some teachers, and justifiably so'.(69) At medical school, it is generally thought that students must gain knowledge and experience of all major disciplines since they are being prepared for any one of these.

There are many ways of determining the content of the core curriculum, ranging from modified Delphi processes (70,71) and other formal consultations, to statistical and epidemiological methods, critical incident techniques and more informal consultative and team-based work. Whatever method is chosen, it should be well understood and publicised, and properly managed according to a timescale. It should involve all interested parties and stakeholders and bear in mind the vision of the school.

Options can then be built around the core and given timetabled slots or blocks to offer students choices in their learning and career development, and the opportunity for more self-directed study. Some guidance can be given: for example, options can be provided in different categories such as basic sciences, core extension studies, laboratory specialties, social and community sciences, education and management. Students may then be required to undertake options in a variety of these areas.

Some medical schools have an 'options bank', which departments and teachers add to and students then select from. These would normally be well-defined elements with a specific assessment plan, each of which would be able to accommodate a limited number of students. It is also possible to allow students to design their own options, either within certain headings or freely but according to set criteria about planning, process and outcomes against which the option can be marked and assessed.

Spiral

The principle of the spiral curriculum, first elaborated by the titan educationalist Jerome Bruner,(72) is that students should revisit material at increasing levels of complexity as they progress through the course. This is almost unavoidable, in practice. Thus, for example, the themes of clinical methods, ethics and health promotion, and their accompanying attitudes, knowledge and skills, were designed into the Dundee curriculum(73) to be revisited in more complex ways during the four main stages of the course, which dealt with normal structure, function and behaviour, then abnormal structure, function and behaviour, then clinical practice and, finally, on-the-job-learning.

Thus the features of the spiral curriculum, which might seem not unlike many other types of curricula, and might even seem unavoidable in practical terms, are that:(74)

- topics, themes or subjects are revisited on a number of occasions throughout the course
- there are increasing levels of difficulty
- new learning is related to previous learning
- the competence of the learner increases.

Modular

A module is a self-contained unit of study. It should have its own outcomes (however expressed), activities and assessments. Students tend to take more than one module of study at a time. Modules are planned according to the curriculum framework selected. In an integrated course, modules will tend to have similar structures, with the vertical themes of the course that spiral through the curriculum being addressed in each module. So, for example, a module on cardiovascular disease might have its content decided in relation to curriculum themes of:

- clinical sciences
- basic sciences
- behavioural sciences
- population sciences
- clinical skills
- interpersonal skills and professional behaviours.

The module might then be taught around a number of index cases, which illustrate these themes and the necessary content. It is in the nature of modules that there is some flexibility in the order in which they are taught.

How do we determine the experiences that will further those purposes?

The experiences that students have will be selected on the basis of the planning and design work that has been carried out in the previous steps. The choices that must be made are in relation to:

- learning and teaching methods, including learning resources, feedback and support
- practical and clinical experience, including sites.

Learning and teaching methods, including learning resources, feedback and support

Decisions about learning and teaching methods will flow from the planning of previous stages. But there is no one-to-one relationship between course intentions and teaching and learning methods. Every curriculum designer has a range of choices that could lead to the same outcomes. And although it might be true, for example, that problem-based learning fosters active learning and encourages deep learning and integration (recognising that all these concepts are difficult to pin down in practice), it is not the only way of achieving those aims. And every strength of any one teaching or learning method is accompanied by weaknesses. There is no pedagogical silver bullet or panacea.

Likewise, although problem-based learning can be an entire curriculum approach, more frequently it is used for just part of a curriculum – either in the first couple of years or as just one type of teaching and learning method as part of a curriculum that also includes other approaches. Problem-based learning, which might now be seen as having passed its zenith, does itself contain a variety of learning methods, and although there is now no commonly agreed definition of problem-based learning,(75) all definitions do tend to emphasise small group learning, authentic problems that stimulate the self-directed learning process (often carefully defined), and acquisition of knowledge and problem-solving skills.

The curriculum designer can choose from the following, at a minimum – each of which has a positive role to play:

- clinical skills laboratories, including communication skills training
- clinical experience, inpatient, ambulatory and community
- study guides describing what is to be learnt and relating this to available learning opportunities(76)
- lectures
- seminars and tutorials
- independent or guided group work
- simulations
- practicals
- resource-based learning, including e-learning and library work
- formative assessment, appraisal and feedback on learning.

The curriculum designer should state what balance of these methods might be desirable and expected. But the method selected alone will not determine effect on learning unless it is used in an appropriate manner. Thus problem-based learning has variable effects on the acquisition of knowledge,(77) and any teaching or learning method, whether apparently learner-centred or not, which has a heavy workload, high contact hours, excessive material or an emphasis on coverage, is likely to push students towards a surface approach to learning.(78) Likewise, any educational method that displays an appropriate motivational context, a high degree of learner activity, interaction with peers and teachers, and a well-structured knowledge base may encourage a deep approach.(79) But this is not to set any value on a deep approach as opposed to a surface approach. Both have their value. Even rote learning suggests some inner cognitive activity and is passionately defended in some disciples and cultures. We have no evidence-based reason to demur.(80)

The role of assessment as an instrument of learning, especially if used formatively for that purpose only, should not be overlooked and might be considered with other interventions such as appraisal and regular structured and supportive feedback sessions.

Practical and clinical experience, including sites

In basic medical education, and perhaps even beyond, a wide range of knowledge, skills and attitudes can be acquired as effectively in the community as in hospital settings.(81) So if the curriculum has the intention of producing graduates with an interest in practice in the community,(82,83) then primary care might be developed as a major provider of teaching, learning and experience, offering effective integrated teaching.(84) Four types of community-based teaching have been identified:(85)

- community-orientated teaching: teaching in and about the community
- agency-based teaching: teaching involving community health care providers other than primary care physicians
- general practice-based teaching: either specific clinical teaching or an attachment in primary care
- specialist teaching in the community: specialist subjects taught by hospital practitioners in a community setting.

Equally, such knowledge and skills might also be achieved in hospital settings. The choice of location is to be decided by curriculum designers in the light of previous steps. Finally, the role of skills laboratories in helping students to acquire basic and more advanced clinical and communication skills in a safe, structured environment before using these with patients should also be considered as part of the curriculum design process.

How can we determine whether the purposes are being attained?

Whether the purposes of the curriculum are attained might be measured in two ways. First, a robust assessment system that is properly blueprinted on to the curriculum will measure students' attainment of the intended learning outcomes of the programme. Second, a curriculum evaluation strategy that addresses the views and experiences of all stakeholders will offer information about how the curriculum in practice fulfils or does not fulfil its purposes. On the basis of assessment and evaluation findings, the curriculum can be reviewed and renewed to ensure that it remains fit for purpose. The assessment of student learning, evaluation of the curriculum in practice and approaches to curriculum renewal are topics for other chapters in this book.

Throughout all the steps outlined above, and in relation to all the considerations and judgements that are brought to bear in designing a curriculum, there is one principle that must hold sway. And that is the principle of purpose. And purpose must derive from context. That context does not preclude the design of a curriculum that will produce researchers and academics – they also have a key role in determining the scientific and practice basis of medicine; it does not preclude the production of doctors for secondary, or even tertiary care – they too are needed. A contextual curriculum can produce all these. But it does so by recognising local need and circumstances, and not by benchmarking to external contexts which derive from other cultures and practices.

References

1 Miller G (ed.) (1961) *Teaching and Learning in Medical School.* Harvard University Press, Cambridge, MA.
2 Simpson MA (1972) *Medical Education. A Critical Approach.* Butterworths, London.
3 Cox KR and Ewan CE (eds) (1982) *The Medical Teacher.* Churchill Livingstone, Edinburgh.
4 Newble D and Cannon R (1983) *A Handbook for Clinical Teachers.* MTP Press, Boston, MA.
5 Balla JI, Gibson M and Chang AM (1989) *Learning in Medical School. A Model for the Clinical Professions.* Hong Kong University Press, Hong Kong.
6 Boelen C and Woollard B (2009) Social accountability and accreditation: a new frontier for educational institutions. *Medical Education.* 43(9): 887–94.
7 Bleakley A, Bligh J and Browne J (2011) *Medical Education for the Future. Identity, Power and Location.* Springer, London.
8 Apple MW (2004) *Ideology and Curriculum* (3e). Routledge Falmer, London.
9 Jolly B and Rees L (eds) (1998) *Medical Education in the Millennium.* Oxford University Press, Oxford.
10 Gillam S (2011) Teaching doctors in training about management and leadership. *British Medical Journal.* 343: d5672.
11 Eisner EW (1994) *The Educational Imagination: on the Design and Evaluation of School Programs* (3e). Macmillan, New York, NY.
12 Toohey S (1999) *Designing Courses for Higher Education.* Society for Research into Higher Education and Open University Press, Buckingham.
13 Norcross WA, Henzel TR, Freeman K, Milner-Mares J and Hawkins RE (2009) Toward meeting the challenge of physician competence assessment: the University of California, San Diego Physician Assessment and Clinical Education (PACE) Program. *Academic Medicine.* 84(8): 1008–14.
14 Grant J (2012) *The Good CPD Guide.* (2e). Radcliffe, Oxford.
15 Flinders DJ and Thornton SJ (2004) *The Curriculum Studies Reader* (2e). Routledge Falmer, New York, NY.
16 General Medical Council (2009) *Tomorrow's Doctors. Outcomes and Standards for Undergraduate Medical Education.* General Medical Council, London.
17 General Medical Council (2010) Standards for curricula and assessment systems. (http://www.gmc-uk.org/education/postgraduate/standards_for_curricula_and_assessment_systems.asp; accessed 27 December 2012).
18 World Federation for Medical Education (2012) WFME global standards for quality improvement. WFME Office: University of Copenhagen, Denmark (http://www.wfme.org/standards; accessed 28 December 2012).
19 Grant J, Abdelrahman M and Zachariah A (2013) Curriculum design in context. In: Walsh K (ed.) *Oxford Textbook of Medical Education.* Oxford University Press, Oxford.
20 Association of American Medical Colleges Liaison Committee on Medical Education (2011) *Functions and Structure of a Medical School. Standards for Accreditation of Medical Education Programs Leading to the M.D. Degree.* (http://www.lcme.org/functions2011may.pdf; accessed 28 December 2012).
21 Coles CR and Gale Grant J (1985) ASME Medical Education Research Booklet No 1. Curriculum evaluation in medical and health-care education. *Medical Education.* 19(5): 405–22.
22 Noddings N (2003) *Happiness and Education.* Cambridge University Press, Cambridge.
23 Rao KH and Rao RH (2007) Reflections on the state of medical education in Japan. *The Keio Journal of Medicine.* 55: 41–51.
24 Rao RH (2006) Perspectives in medical education. Implementing a more integrated, interactive and interesting curriculum to improve Japanese medical education. *The Keio Journal of Medicine.* 56: 75–84.
25 Segouin C and Hodges BD (2005) Educating physicians in France and Canada: are the differences based on evidence or history? *Medical Education.* 39: 1205–12.
26 Hodges BD, Maniate JM, Martimianakis MA, Alsuwadan M and Segouin C (2009) Cracks and crevices: globalisation discourse and medical education. *Medical Teacher.* 31(10): 910–7.
27 Jippes M and Majoor GD (2008) Influence of national culture on the adoption of integrated and problem-based curricula in Europe. *Medical Education.* 42(3): 279–85.

28 Tharyan P (2005) Traumatic bereavement and the Asian Tsunami: perspectives from Tamil Nadu, India. *Bereavement Care*. **24**(2): 23–5.

29 Tharu S (2010) Medicine and government: histories of the present. In: Zachariah A, Srivatsan R and Tharu S (eds) *Towards a Critical Medical Practice. Reflections on the Dilemmas of Medical Culture Today*. Orient, Hyderabad.

30 General Medical Council (2013) *Good Medical Practice* (2e). General Medical Council, London.

31 Frank JR (ed.) (2005) *The CanMEDS 2005 Physician Competency Framework. Better Standards. Better Physicians. Better Care*. The Royal College of Physicians and Surgeons of Canada, Ottawa, ON.

32 Tyler RW (1949) *Basic Principles of Curriculum and Instruction*. University of Chicago Press, Chicago.

33 Jacques D (2000) *Learning in Groups. A Handbook for Improving Group Work* (3e). Routledge Falmer, London.

34 Mager R (1975) *Preparing Instructional Objectives* (2e). Fearon-Pitman Publishers, Belmont, CA.

35 Stenhouse L (1975) *An Introduction to Curriculum Research and Development*. Heinemann, Oxford.

36 Grant J (2000) The incapacitating effects of competence. A critique. *Journal of Health Sciences Education*. **4**(3): 271–7.

37 Hyland T (1995) *Competence, Education and NVQs*. Continuum International Publishing Group Ltd, London.

38 Schwartz B and Sharpe K (2010) *Practical Wisdom*. Riverhead Books, New York.

39 McKeachie WJ (1951–69) *Teaching Tips. A Guidebook for the Beginning College Teacher* (1–6e). DC Heath and Company, Lexington, MA.

40 Nicol D (1997) Research on Learning and Higher Education Teaching. UCoSDA briefing paper 45. Universities and Colleges Staff Development Agency, Sheffield.

41 Knowles M (1979) *The Adult Learner: A Neglected Species?* Gulf, Houston, TX.

42 University of New Mexico School of Medicine (2012) *Office of Student Admissions. Curriculum Overview*. (http://hsc.unm.edu/som/admissions/curriculumover.shtml; accessed 28 December 2012).

43 Marton F and Säljo R (1976) On qualitative differences in learning I and II. *British Journal of Educational Psychology*. **46**(1/2): 4–11, 128–48.

44 Kee-Kuok Wong J (2004) Are the learning styles of Asian international students Culturally or contextually based? *International Education Journal*. **4**(4): 154–66.

45 Newble DI and Entwhistle NJ (1980) Learning styles and approaches: implications for medical education. *Medical Education*. **20**(3): 162–75.

46 McManus IC, Keeling A and Paice E (2004) Stress, burnout and doctors' attitudes to work are determined by personality and learning style: a twelve-year longitudinal study of UK medical graduates. *BioMed Central Medicine*. **2**(29). Available at: http://www.biomedcentral.com/1741-7015/2/29

47 Case Western Reserve University School of Medicine (2012) Bulletin. (http://bulletin.case.edu/schoolofmedicine/; accessed 28 December 2012).

48 Fish D and Coles C (2005) *Medical Education: Developing a Curriculum for Practice*. Open University Press, Maidenhead.

49 Goss B, Reid K, Dodds A and McColl G (2011) Comparison of medical students' diagnostic reasoning skills in a traditional and a problem-based learning curriculum. *International Journal of Medical Education*. **2**: 87–93.

50 Cholowsk KM and Chan LKS (2001) Prior knowledge in student and experienced nurses' clinical problem Solving. *Australian Journal of Educational & Developmental Psychology*. **1**: 10–21.

51 Clements DH and Sarama JA (2009) *Learning and Teaching Early Math: The Learning Trajectories Approach (Studies in Mathematical Thinking and Learning Series)*. Routledge, New York, NY.

52 University of Southampton School of Medicine website. (http://www.southampton.ac.uk/medicine/undergraduate/index.page?; accessed 28 December 2012).

53 Royal College of Physicians (2005) *Doctors in Society. Medical Professionalism in a Changing World*. Royal College of Physicians of London, London.

54 Hoyle E (1971) How does the curriculum change? In: Hooper R (ed.) *The Curriculum: Context, Design and Development*. Oliver and Boyd in association with The Open University Press, Edinburgh.

55 Kelly AV (1999) *The Curriculum. Theory and Practice*. Paul Chapman Publishing, London.

56 Gale R and Grant J (1997) Managing change in a medical context: guidelines for action. AMEE guide no. 10. *Medical Teacher*. **19**: 239–49.

57 Newble D, Stark P, Bax N and Lawson M (2005) Developing an outcome-focused core curriculum. *Medical Education*. **39**: 680–7.

58 Smith SR and Dollase R (1999) AMEE guide no. 14. Outcome-based education. Part 2 – planning, implementing and evaluating a competency-based curriculum. *Medical Teacher*. **21**(1): 15–22.

59 Harden RM, Sowden S and Dunn WR (1984) Educational strategies in curriculum development: the SPICES model. *Medical Education*. **18**: 284–97.

60 Newble D, Jolly B and Wakeford R (eds) (1994) *The Certification and Recertification of Doctors*. Cambridge University Press, Cambridge.

61 Prideaux D (2000) Emperor's new clothes: from objectives to outcomes. *Medical Education*. **34**: 168–9.

62 Stenhouse L (1975) *An Introduction to Curriculum Research and Development*. Heinemann, London.

63 Rees C (2004) The problem with outcomes-based curricula in medical education: insights from educational theory. *Medical Education*. **38**: 593–8.

64 Harden RM, Crosby JR and Davis MH (1999) AMEE guide no. 14. Outcome-based education. Part 1 – an introduction to outcome-based education. *Medical Teacher*. **21**(1): 7–14.

65 Harden RM, Crosby JR, Davis MH and Friedman M (1999) AMEE guide no. 14. Outcome-based education. Part 5 – from competency to meta-competency: a model for the specification of learning outcomes. *Medical Teacher*. **21**(6): 546–52.

66 Dornan T, Litttlewood S, Margolis SA, Spencer J and Ypinazar V (2006) BEME guide. How can experience in clinical and community settings contribute to early medical education? A BEME systematic review. *Medical Teacher*. **28**(1): 3–18.

67 O'Neill PA, Metcalfe D and David TJ (1999) The core content of the undergraduate curriculum in Manchester. *Medical Education*. **33**(2): 114–20.

68 D'Eon M and Crawford R (2005) The elusive content of the medical school curriculum: a method to the madness. *Medical Teacher*. **27**(8): 699–703.

69 Harden RM and Davis MH (1995) AMEE guide no. 5. The core curriculum with options or special study modules. *Medical Teacher*. **17**(2): 125–48.

70 Alahlafi A and Burge S (2005) What should undergraduate medical students know about psoriasis? Involving patients in curriculum development: modified Delphi technique. *British Medical Journal*. **330**: 633–6.

71 Syme-Grant J, Stewart C and Ker J (2005) How we developed a core curriculum in clinical skills. *Medical Teacher*. **27**(2): 103–6.

72 Bruner J (1977) *The Process of Education* (2e). Harvard University Press, Cambridge, MA.

73 Harden RM, Davis MH and Crosby J (1997) The new Dundee medical curriculum: a whole that is greater than the sum of the parts. *Medical Education*. **31**: 264–71.

74 Harden RM and Stamper N (1999) What is a spiral curriculum? *Medical Teacher*. **21**(2): 141–3.

75 Gijbels D, Docht F, Van den Bossche P and Segers M (2005) Effects of problem-based learning: a meta-analysis from the angle of assessment. *Review of Educational Research*. **75**(1): 27–61.

76 Harden RM, Laidlaw JM, Hesketh EA and AMEE guide No. 16 (1999) Study guides – their use and preparation. *Medical Teacher.* **21**(3): 248–65.

77 Albanese MA and Mitchell S (1993) Problem-based learning: a review of the literature on its outcomes and implementation issues. *Academic Medicine.* **68**: 52–81.

78 Gibbs G (1992) Improving the quality of student learning through course design. In: Barnett R (ed.) *Learning to Effect.* SRHE and Open University Press, Buckingham.

79 Biggs JB (1989) Approaches to the enhancement of tertiary teaching. *Higher Education Research and Development.* **8**(1): 7–25.

80 Larsen-Freemen D (2012) On the roles of repetition in language teaching and learning. *Applied Linguistics Review.* **3**(2): 195–210.

81 Murray E, Jolly B and Modell MA (1999) A comparison of the educational opportunities on junior medical attachments in general practice and in teaching hospital: a questionnaire study. *Medical Education.* **317**: 170–6.

82 Bligh J (1999) Is it time for a community-based medical school? *Medical Education.* **33**(5): 315.

83 Nazareth I and Kaya M (1999) Medical education in the community – the UNITRA experience. *Medical Education.* **33**: 722–4.

84 Worley P, Silagy C, Prideaux D, Newble D and Jones A (2000) The Parallel Rural Community Curriculum: an integrated clinical curriculum based in rural general practice. *Medical Education.* **34**: 558–65.

85 McCrorie P, Lefford F and Perrin F (1994) *Medical Undergraduate Community-Based Teaching: A Survey for ASME on Current and Proposed Teaching in the Community and in General Practice in UK Universities.* ASME occasional publication no. 3. Association for the Study of Medical Education, Edinburgh.

4 Quality in medical education

Alan Bleakley[1], Julie Browne[2] and Kate Ellis[3]
[1]Peninsula Medical School, UK
[2]Cardiff University, UK
[3]Plymouth University, UK

 KEY MESSAGES

- High-quality medical education is a vital prerequisite for high-quality patient care.
- Continuous quality improvement is the responsibility of all medical educators.
- Quality improvement is a dynamic and continuous process whose aim is the achievement of excellence rather than mere fitness for purpose or competence.
- While protocols, regulation and standards are important tools for quality assurance, they may have unintended

negative consequences, particularly if introduced without consideration of the context and culture in which they will be implemented.

- Quality may be considered in terms of discourses: managerial, economic, scientific, aesthetic, ethical, professional, social and political. It is important for medical educators to be aware of these discourses if they are to be proactive and imaginative in developing a culture of quality in their own fields of practice.

What is quality?

In discussing what is meant by 'quality', Aristotle took the example of a knife: 'An examination of a knife would reveal that its distinctive quality is to cut, and from this we can conclude that a good knife would be a knife that cuts well.'(1) However, as Zhuangi, a late 3rd to early 4th century BCE Chinese philosopher, reminds us: 'A good butcher changes his knife once a year, because he slices flesh. A mediocre butcher changes his knife once a month, because he hacks at bone.'(2)

Thus, an expert can bring out and maintain the quality of a good knife, but for a novice the knife may be handled badly, never revealing ultimate quality. Quality is then a transaction, rather than an intrinsic property – quality mechanisms subject to poor or inappropriate use will not capture quality. Thus, while medical education has its quality processes – primarily Quality Assurance (QA) and Quality Improvement (QI) – these processes are also subject to quality assurance and improvement! The quality of quality processes depends upon the users, not just the tools. Further, it is only through ownership of quality processes by stakeholders that a quality *culture* emerges, essential for continuous improvement of quality.(3) Stakeholders in this activity include both those who provide quality services and those who benefit from such services. Box 4.1 attempts to summarise and define various quality processes. Box 4.2 lists the proliferating body of quality guidelines, protocols and standards for medical education, in what has become a veritable industry.

Quality can be described in this transactional sense as something that is fit for purpose, where 'fitness for purpose

focuses on whether a product or service meets customers' needs or the mission of the institute'.(5) The 'customers' of a medical school and postgraduate education are medical students and junior doctors, but of course the ultimate customers of their services are patients. We must then judge the quality of medical education by its effective translation into patient care. This is why medical education research is so important – to build an evidence base for what may translate from innovative pedagogy into effective patient care.

In short, quality sets something apart from the run of the mill, or separates the extraordinary from the ordinary. We all want a high-quality medical education, but we are not agreed on what that might mean. Outwardly, QA and QI processes facilitate communication around standard setting in all areas of a curriculum – they are tools that promise transparency, accountability, examination or measurement, inspection, regulation, revalidation, evaluation, remediation, censure and penalties, and support continuing professional development, including curriculum design, course accreditation, and portfolio recording. Again, these tools are only as good as the individuals and communities of practice who employ them, and they must be employed selectively and critically to avoid unintended negative consequences.

A critical approach to quality

In this chapter, we address the following clusters of questions:
- Why is there such an intense current interest in quality frameworks and guidelines? What are they used for? What forces shape and drive such initiatives?

Understanding Medical Education: Evidence, Theory and Practice, Second Edition. Edited by Tim Swanwick.
© 2014 The Association for the Study of Medical Education. Published 2014 by John Wiley & Sons, Ltd.

BOX 4.1 HOW TO: Define quality and quality processes

QUALITY: The authors see quality as an attribute (the extraordinary, separated from the ordinary) assessed by a process (quality assurance). Ensuring quality entails the translation of certain values into practices (quality enhancement).

The following definitions are adapted from the *European Student Handbook on Quality Assurance in Higher Education*.(4)

QUALITY ASSURANCE: The anticipatory means by which an institution can guarantee with confidence and certainty that the standards and quality of awards granted in their name are being maintained and enhanced.

QUALITY CONTROL: The verification procedures (both formal and informal) used by institutions at the point of delivery in order to monitor quality and standards to a satisfactory standard and as intended.

QUALITY ENHANCEMENT/IMPROVEMENT: The process of positively changing or evolving activities in order to provide for a continuous improvement in the quality of institutional provision.

QUALITY ASSESSMENT: The process of external evaluation, undertaken by an external body, of the quality of educational provisions in institutions, in particular the quality of the student experience.

QUALITY AUDIT: The process of examining institutional procedures for assuring quality and standards, and whether the arrangements are implemented effectively and achieve stated objectives.

STANDARDS: Describe prescribed levels of attainment against which performance may be measured. Attainment of a standard usually implies a measure of fitness for a defined purpose.

QUALITY CULTURE: The creation of a high level of internal institutional quality assessment mechanisms and the ongoing implementation of the results. The ability of the institution, programme, and so forth to develop quality assurance implicitly in the day-to-day work of the institution and marks a move away from periodic assessment to ingrained quality assurance.

ACCREDITATION: The endorsement of an education programme or institution after a process of review, as recognition that a programme or institution fulfils certain quality standards.

BOX 4.2 HOW TO: Find quality assurance frameworks

Quality assurance frameworks abound in medical education. Here are just a few:

1. Academy of Medical Educators Professional Standards www.medicaleducators.org
2. World Federation for Medical Education Global Standards for Medical Education www.wfme.org/standards
3. World Federation for Medical Education Global Standards for Quality Improvement in Medical Education: European Specifications www.wfme.org/standards/european-specifications
4. General Medical Council Quality Improvement Framework www.gmc-uk.org/Quality_Improvement_Framework.pdf_39623044.pdf
5. Committee on Accreditation of Canadian Medical Schools (CACMS) Accreditation Standards for Continuing Medical Education http://www.afmc.ca/cacme-accreditation-e.php
6. Joint Committee on Standards for Educational Evaluation: Program Evaluation Standards www.jcsee.org/program-evaluation-standards
7. Quality Assurance Agency for Higher Education: Framework for Higher Education Qualifications www.qaa.ac.uk/Publications/InformationAndGuidance/Pages/The-framework-for-higher-education-qualifications-in-England-Wales-and-Northern-Ireland.aspx
8. Quality Assurance Agency for Higher Education: Subject Benchmark Statement for Medicine www.qaa.ac.uk/Publications/InformationAndGuidance/Pages/Subject-benchmark-statement-Medicine.aspx
9. Australian Medical Council Standards (Basic Medical Education and Specialist Medical Education and Training) www.amc.org.au
10. Liaison Committee for Medical Education (US and Canada) Standards for Accreditation of Medical Education Programs leading to MD Degree www.lcme.org/functions.pdf
11. European Student Handbook on Quality Assurance in Higher Education www.vss-unes.ch/typo3/fileadmin/vss_dateien/Dossiers/Akkreditierungspool/ESIB_QA_handbook_2003.pdf
12. UK Professional Standards Framework www.heacademy.ac.uk

- How might we recognise, maintain and enhance quality?
- How does quality in education translate into clinical practice? Who are the stakeholders and how are they represented?
- What are the possible negative unintended consequences of quality assurance protocols?

We do not promise definitive answers to these complex questions – in fact, we studiously avoid this. We will not, however, leave readers suspended, but offer some positive conclusions. We set out core debates, noting what has been evidenced, what remains speculation and what may have lasting value in a rapidly changing, or 'liquid',(6) world of health care in a 'risk society',(7) whose chief characteristic is dialogue between risk and regulation.(8,9)

Our purpose is to look critically at the recent explosion of interest in quality frameworks in medical education to

BOX 4.3 WHERE'S THE EVIDENCE:
Does training in quality improvement
improve patient care?

In this case study, Atkins and Handal(10) show how
paediatric residents improved quality of service through
education in practice-based learning and systems-based
assessment (group projects) with measured patient outcomes.
The study implemented a series of QI projects over three
years, participation in which was mandatory to all residents.
Residents recorded their experiences in their portfolios, which
were monitored quarterly by the Programme Director. The
study found that the use of QI methodology enabled
residents to:

– improve management of children with obesity
– achieve high compliance with the national patient safety
  goals
– improve the paediatric hotline service
– implement better patient flow in resident continuity clinics

Based on their experiences, Atkins and Handal conclude that
to implement QI projects in residency programmes
successfully, QI techniques must be formally taught, the
opportunities for resident participation must be multiple and
diverse, and QI outcomes should be incorporated in resident
training and assessment so that they experience the benefits
of the QI intervention.

ask what dilemmas and paradoxes this new wave of interest brings, and how we may face these paradoxes resource-
fully to provide the best possible care for patients. We are
impressed by studies such as that of Atkins and Handal
(10) (summarised in Box 4.3), who show how focus on
improvement of quality of medical education for a clinical
specialty improved patient outcomes.

This chapter does not expound on what is readily
available in the literature, but sets out to expand our
understanding of that literature. In moving beyond the
descriptive, we aim to offer an original contribution by
critically engaging with quality debates. We develop an
argument that points to what we see as a worrying drift in
interpretations and expressions of QA and QI in medical
education, and how this may be countered. This drift is
towards a representation of quality as:

• a form of business rather than education
• uni-dimensional, rather than the product of multiple,
  competing discourses
• shaped by a risk-averse, rather than a risk-aware,
  agenda
• subject to a prescriptive, rather than a conversational,
  approach.

When we say that we are taking a critical, rather than
descriptive, approach to quality in medical education, what
do we mean? Let us take an illustrative example. A key text
on quality in higher education is the 2002 *European Student
Handbook on Quality Assurance in Higher Education*(4) (referenced in Box 4.2). This framework is part of the wider

Bologna process of standardising higher education across
Europe for purposes of comparability and transfer.

A close reading of this text reveals a distinct (and unac-
knowledged) tension in values. The document opens with
a set of 'Aims and Objectives for the National Unions of
Students in Europe'. These are largely about human rights,
status and welfare of students, including equality of opportunity and equal access to educational resources. These
frame quality of higher education in terms of ethical and
political values. However, in considering students as
primary stakeholders in quality assurance of higher education, the document takes on a different tone, drawing on
metaphors and values from the world of business and economics and framing education as a competitive rather than
collaborative enterprise:

> Quality Assurance (QA) has always been of utmost impor-
> tance, originally, in business but now also in education and
> other public services sectors. Quality remains the most
> important attribute that creates value about the product/
> service for the receiver. It is also the means by which business/
> service providers differentiate themselves from their com-
> petitors. Since businesses are leaders in quality assurance,
> non-business organisations such as educational institutions
> can benefit from the important lessons learnt by business.(4)

Such business orientations may privilege economic (value
for money) values rather than ethico-political (democratic)
values – the latter ensuring that quality is the delivery of
agreed standards in such a way that no learner is treated
unfairly, where quality embraces equality.

As a further example of business values shaping quality
processes, Da Dalt *et al.*(11) freely use obfuscating business-
speak in describing QA and QI implementation for postgraduate medical education in Europe, based on an example
from paediatrics:

> For the ISO 9001:2000 standard, the curriculum was managed
> as a series of interrelated processes and their level of function
> was monitored by ad hoc elaborated objective indicators. . . .
> The training programme was fragmented in 19 interlinked
> processes, 15 related procedures and 24 working instruc-
> tions . . . Based on the measurable indicators developed to
> monitor some of the processes, areas of weakness of the
> system were objectively identified and consequently QI
> actions implemented. The appropriateness of all this allowed
> the programme to finally achieve an official ISO 9000:2001
> certification.(11)

For those with a more expansive view of quality, this is
credentialing as electrical wiring. In the example above we
feel a long way from the human face of health care. Such
'quality' vocabulary can create the impression that something important is happening when it may not be so.
Quality processes, however, need not be constrained by an
instrumental business discourse. There are several other
discourses of quality to be explored.

Discourses of quality

While quality is valued and processes introduced in good
faith, because of their complexity such projects can lead
to negative unintended consequences, as well as positive

intended consequences. In Box 4.4, we provide an example of a quality protocol introduced into surgical environments that, despite being developed through research evidence, introduces unintended consequences that compromise quality, as well as its intentions to enhance and assure quality.

Qualifiers of quality such as 'enhancement', 'assurance' and 'control' offer a powerful rhetoric – they have a reassuring ring of certainty and mastery. Such 'quality' vocabulary can create the impression that something important is happening when it may not be so. What we mean by quality, its assurance and improvement is not a transcendental injunction set in stone, but changes according to historical periods and socio-cultural influences.

In this section, we demonstrate that no one way of thinking about quality is right – rather notions of quality are legitimated in any one period of history through culturally specific ways of thinking in which a set of values is predominant. We describe how claims to quality gain legitimacy through the adoption of particular forms of 'discourse'. Discourses are culturally legitimated ways of knowing and doing, described by Michel Foucault(12) as practices that systematically form their objects of interest. Importantly, a dominant or legitimating view of what we mean by 'quality' will surface at any one time and will come to marginalise other views.

Notions of 'quality' change historically. For example, a contemporary approach to quality assurance that engages with equality of opportunity, such as gender balance and widening access to medicine, was not in the frame of quality thinking in the late 19th century, with its 'ideal of the "gentleman-physician" well versed in the classic liberal arts'.(13) This notion of the doctor with the 'right stuff' has lingered. As late as 1975 the UK Royal College of Physicians felt it important to say that its membership examination requirement 'remains partly a test of culture, although knowledge of Latin, Greek, French and German is no longer required'.(14)

What was considered a quality medical education before the time of Flexner's(15,16) ground-breaking 1910 report changed radically as a result of that report, and what would be considered a quality medical education now is different from Flexner's time. Flexner's main concern with medical education at the time was the absence of quality control. Schools differed wildly from one another with no overriding framework for comparability and standardisation.

For many years before Flexner, doctors from the USA had travelled to German medical schools, where a sophisticated core science curriculum had developed, including preclinical study that focused on laboratory science and learning anatomy through dissection under careful tuition.(17) Flexner's vision was to develop a rigorous, standardised preclinical science-based curriculum prior to medical students gaining clinical experience. However, a series of unintended negative consequences flowed from Flexner's well-intentioned quality assurance initiatives. Many medical schools in North America were closed because they provided inadequate preparation for clinical practice and could not afford to set up more sophisticated laboratory and anatomy facilities. Unfortunately, some of

---

BOX 4.4 FOCUS ON: Are protocols the answer?

In this case study we examine the paradoxes in implementing a quality assurance protocol. The WHO Surgical Safety Checklist was launched in 2008 as part of a global patient safety initiative *Safe Surgery Saves Lives*. The checklist can be found at www.who.int/patientsafety/safesurgery/ss_checklist/en/index.html.

Checklists are useful where activity and decision-making are too complex to rely on memory alone. Half of all medical errors occur in surgical settings and over half are avoidable through improving teamwork. While an initial international study found that use of the protocol dramatically reduced surgical error, paradoxes remain.

1. Use of the checklist is now mandated. Quality assurance may work best when it is offered as a guideline rather than mandated (which tends to produce resistance particularly from surgeons, who historically have had a high degree of autonomy). The checklist is a classic 'administrative control' – an attempt to standardise certain work processes through prescribed actions linked to monitoring of adherence. The alternative is intensive use of social and self-controls to guide safe behaviour – or, developing a safety culture.

2. Simply introducing a quality control checklist does not take into account *process* issues of implementation such as rollout, embedding, evolved modifications and the quality of, and variations in, embedded use; as well as patients' understanding of, and involvement in, such use.

3. Protocols are accepted and sustained (or resist decay) only as they become embedded in a wider, supportive cultural process. Mindful use of the checklist requires a pre-existing, developed safety culture. A decrease for compliance with protocols over time is common – this may be because protocols are sometimes adopted instrumentally rather than mindfully. Adherence decays because the protocol is not internalised as part of the cultural fabric and the practitioner's mindset.

4. Focus on cognition in use of the checklist does not address affective and interpersonal elements of surgical work that may have consequences for patient safety.

5. Checklists may paradoxically generate, or make visible, inconsistencies in implementation practices within teams and differences in motives for use. For example, nurses may utilise protocols to promote more democratic patterns of teamwork and proactivity towards patient safety. Surgeons, however, may use protocols as a rhetorical device to increase individual advocacy and resist democratic teamwork.

8. The protocol is limited to the operating theatre and anaesthetic room, whereas over 50 per cent of incidents occur outside the operating room (such as the recovery room).

In summary, quality assurance through protocols is necessarily limited. This does not mean that we abandon quality assurance protocols, but that we design them thoughtfully and refine them through iterative use.

these schools were the only ones providing places for minority and women students.(18)

Also, Flexner's initial report appeared at a time when quality was becoming dissociated from its roots in individual craft to become associated with industrial production. The major effect of this shift was to place less emphasis on the qualities of the individual (the craftsman) and more on the qualities of the organisation, where workers became components in a 'Total Quality Management' approach that still infects health care today, as we have seen from our business-oriented examples above. Quality after the craft era was about efficiency and productivity, rather than innovation or originality. It can be argued that this emphasis has remained, so that the quality of medical education is about maintaining efficiency and generalised comparative standards rather than originality. The quality frameworks listed in Box 4.2 confirm this bias.

In the sections that follow we explore the different discourses of quality that have held sway over time and continue to pervade quality debates and practice in medical education today. We first describe a cluster of dominant functional discourses – managerial, economic, political and scientific – and then a cluster relating to the 'form' of quality – aesthetic, ethical or professional – that tend to be marginalised but provide a valuable counterpoise.

Managerial

Quality as efficiency rather than uniqueness is associated with a certain kind of managerial discourse, where factors such as 'throughput' are vital to the running of health services as businesses. In medical education, quality is often conceived as governed by managerial processes, including evaluation of curricula and appraisal of faculty members. A negative unintended consequence of a dominant managerial discourse of quality is that it is driven by efficiency and output rather than inputs such as humane and social values (especially in recognition of the needs of deprived populations). Where social values are displaced by managerial efficiency (usually driven by economic values, as below), clinicians will often complain that patient care is compromised.

Economic

Managerial and business discourses are intimately bound to economic discourses where the main question is: 'What does quality cost?' Quality for the budget holders must be cost-effective. But 'value for money' may be mistaken for quality, or what is ultimately best for patients. Doctors are reminded that allocation of resources must be an important part of their decision-making processes. This is commonplace experience for general (family) practitioners, who now run practices as businesses. It is acute where pressure is placed on medicine to utilise expensive, technologically sophisticated approaches that may only benefit relatively few, but high-profile, cases. Doctors have to be aware that a quality practice is also a fair practice in terms of limited resource allocation.

The world of medical education has necessarily been subjected to the demands of the marketplace, and these may undermine drives for improvement in quality. Economic discourses on the quality of education inevitably impose boundaries on its potential. Marketisation, governance and working conditions are forces that challenge the higher education sector and have an inevitable international impact. Of these, perhaps the most pertinent to maintaining high-quality medical education is marketisation, in which the temptation to 'package' medical training for a global market, to global standards, may actually serve to lower standards, producing a negative unintended consequence. This has been recognised to a certain extent, with international and national regulatory bodies recommending both minimum standards and what constitutes excellence (enhancement and improvement), such as the World Federation for Medical Education's(18) quality improvement framework which delineates between: '*Basic standards*: The standards that must be met by every medical school and fulfilment demonstrated during evaluation of the school. Basic standards are expressed by a "must"', and: '*Standards for quality development*: Standards set in accordance with international consensus about best practice for medical schools and basic medical education . . . Fulfilment of these standards will vary with the stage of development of the medical schools, their resources and educational policy. Even the most advanced schools might not comply with all standards. Standards for quality development are expressed by a "should"'.(18)

Political

Political discourses concerning quality centre on issues of power, equality and inequality. Given that most universities, medical schools and providers of health care around the world are at least in part state-funded, it is not surprising the political discourse should shape medical education. In the UK, where most health care is provided by the State, the Government has been influential in shaping medical education. *Modernising Medical Careers*,(19) for example, was a government-led programme of reform with the aim of 'improving medical education' and providing 'a transparent and efficient career path for doctors'. The education of doctors, and quality issues that arise from this such as registration and revalidation, are no longer the sole province of the medical profession and medical schools.(20)

Scientific

Judgements of quality are now largely led by a scientific approach of measurement and evidence. Because quality is multi-factorial, context-dependent and transactional, measuring quality is difficult. In arguing for the value of developing a quality culture over inevitably piecemeal measurement, Vroeijenstijn(21) suggests that 'Quality depends not on measurement instruments and tools but rather on the spread of quality awareness among faculty, staff, and students.' This challenges the claim of Dolmans *et al.*(5) that 'The first step in quality assurance is to make measurements' – where the authors argue for the use of batteries of reliable and valid instruments, for example, to measure the effectiveness of tutors.

One problem with measuring quality is just how many measurements you need to judge that a culture of medical education is one of quality. Further, are you measuring the right things? For example, the quality of an education may rest as much in the hidden curriculum as it does in explicit pedagogy and management of programmes. Finally, how do we measure the negative unintended consequences of QI and QA, such as managerial throughput emphasis in clinical settings reducing the opportunity for quality educational contact between experts and novices?(22)

Aesthetic

Paradoxically, as we saw above, the quality of education is often measured using quantitative methodologies. However, as Eisner(23) has shown, viewing an educational culture from an aesthetically inclined viewpoint can provide a more generous conception of the practice of education. Medicine has long been considered both science and art, and an aesthetic discourse on the 'quality' of medical education may view educational practice as a form of 'connoisseurship'.(23) At root, 'aesthetic' means 'sense impression', and an important aspect of medical education is to educate the senses as the basis for expert clinical judgement.(24)

In contrast to scientific measurement, here, the art of QA and QI is embodied in the culture of conversational 'expert review'. It is common in medical education research to garner the views of high-profile figures in the field on a topic such as 'what makes a "good" doctor?'.(25) Such qualitative approaches may be subjective, but the subjects are experts collectively offering a discriminating power lacking in quantitative evaluations.

Ethical

The practice of medicine is seen as an ethical endeavour requiring the highest possible standards in professionalism. Nevertheless, ethical discourse often presumes a fixed set of ethical standards that can be universally applied. Patients and communities vary in their needs, and hold different cultural values and norms of health. We might assume that ethics quality is the same across all health care organisations, but as Wynia(26) observes, 'anyone who's worked in more than one healthcare organization knows that the ethical culture of different organizations can vary dramatically'. Wynia(26) questions, for example, whether concern for justice is more important than concern for autonomy, or whether it is ethically more commendable to fulfil a duty to community or to special relations.

Ethical standards are not based on universal, fixed objective principles but, rather, reflect the values of a given society. Fox and Swazey(27) argue that the conceptual framework of bioethics as espoused within medical schools' curricula has accorded paramount status to the value-complex of individualism, underscoring the principles of individual rights, autonomy and self-determination. After their 1981 visit to hospitals and clinics in China, they argued that the team of bioethicists who had previously visited, and had mistakenly concluded that there were 'no medical ethics in China', were simply blinded by their own ethnocentricity. Indeed, they demonstrated that the kind of medical morality being practised by doctors and nurses in China was one that focused on sensitivity to the interdependency and relatedness of their patients to others.

The same argument applies to the exportation of pedagogies based on individualistic learning theories to collectivist cultures, and collaborative pedagogies such as small-group learning to authority-led cultures, as forms of neo-colonialism.(28) How can we be sure that modern global initiatives in medical education – including quality frameworks – which are largely advocated and funded by those in the modern, metropolitan West who have the resources and influence to drive them through, are not just another type of domination by the advanced country over the developing nation?

Professional

A discourse of professionalism has come to the fore in recent years, and, as part of QI and QA, 'professionalism' is now measured, bringing it within the fold of instrumental discourses about quality.(29) Medicine as a profession has long been identified with a series of traits and characteristic practices that include an altruistic orientation towards those served by the profession, and a code of ethics through which to define and monitor that service. However, during the 1970s and 1980s, Freidson(30) developed a critique of professional dominance. He argued that medicine, in common with other professions, is an organised occupation that seeks to control the conditions of its own work by developing and defining a relevant body of knowledge, and by educating, testing and credentialing practitioners.

The medical profession is thus able to exercise autonomy over work undertaken by its members, control and manage the work of others in the health care field, evoke deference from patients and the wider public, and exercise institutional power, maintaining cultural and legal authority over its jurisdiction. Freidson(30) further argued that it was the ability of the medical profession to persuade successive governments to support it (for example, through legal recognition of the American Medical Association in the USA, and the General Medical Council (GMC) in the UK) that helped it to secure its dominant position.

Having enjoyed high autonomy, the medical profession has responded to criticisms of lack of transparency and accountability by setting in place more robust regulation mechanisms, ensuring that:

- Errant doctors are detected and prevented from practising.
- Doctors are appraised and revalidated for practice to maintain high standards of current practice.
- The public is informed about litigation procedures.
- Measures are set in place to ensure the high-quality education of all doctors.
- Professionalism is explicitly taught, to encourage the internalisation of the value systems of the good (not just the good enough) doctor.

In the UK, the Royal College of Physicians(31) has abandoned previous aspects of professionalism, in particular the notions of 'mastery, autonomy, and privilege, and self-regulation', replacing them with increased emphasis on the patient, doctor–patient interaction and on securing public trust. This echoes Kenneth Ludmerer's(32) suggestion that restoring trust between medicine and the wider community is a pressing issue for medical education for the 21st century.

A challenge for the future is the shift in doctors' roles and identities in a new 'liquid'(6) world. Doctors are now both medical professionals and inter-professional clinical team members. They are expected to adopt identities of scientist, clinician, teacher, counsellor, advocate, witness to patient suffering and manager.(33) This widening of expertise poses new challenges for quality frameworks.

Quality and safety: risk and regulation

As quoted earlier, Vroeijenstijn(21) could write with confidence in 1995 that: 'Quality depends not on measurement instruments and tools but rather on the spread of quality awareness among faculty, staff, and students.' The emphasis here is on continuous development of a quality *culture* – a QI approach that is proactive. However, in what Voss *et al.*(34) call 'changing conversations' about quality in medical education, quality is now tied up with avoidance of medical errors through patient safety(21,35,36) – an approach that is reactive.

Where Voss *et al.*(34) note: 'Improving patient safety and quality in health care is one of medicine's most pressing challenges. Residency training programs have a unique opportunity to meet this challenge by training physicians in the science and methods of patient safety and quality improvement', the twinning of quality and safety has been naturalised. It has perhaps even become institutionalised in the title of the major BMJ group publication *Quality and Safety*, that brings the two strands together as natural bedfellows. QI education is now focused upon educating undergraduates and postgraduates in issues such as how to carry out a root cause analysis, and appreciating systems-based safety issues.(35,36) A recent Canadian systematic review(36) of teaching QI to both medical students and postgraduate trainees twins this with teaching patient safety, again as if the two naturally occurred together.

In speculating on future directions for QI in medical education, Wong *et al.*(22) also link improvement of the quality of patient care to preventing 'the occurrence of avoidable (medical) errors'. The authors conclude that 'we must refocus our attention at all levels of training and instil fundamental, collaborative, open-minded behaviours so that future clinicians are primed to promote a culture of safer, higher-quality care'. But, from a quality point of view, movement from the individual out to the culture may be back to front. We have indicated that establishing QI is a cultural challenge. Changing the culture of medicine through medical education is not just about changing the safety behaviours of individual clinicians, but about conversations between clinicians, health care colleagues, patients, academic medical educators, politicians, managers, and other stakeholders in reviewing ingrained values of medical culture – such as heroic individualism – that prevent quality change.

Patient safety awareness is part of a wider 'risk discourse'(8) – talk and activity surrounding risk – that has become central to thinking about quality. Ulrich Beck(7) described post-industrial cultures as 'risk societies' – while prone to risk, late modern cultures have also become risk-averse, as 'safety cultures'. Welchman(8) notes that contemporary life is caught up in a seemingly ever-expanding network of both proactive and reactive strategies for the 'management' of risk, and that art can provide a touchstone for debate concerning risk. For some, the dialogue between risk and regulation shapes identity and lifestyle, where risk is aestheticised.(8) Thus, while we are increasingly concerned about regulating health, individuals continue to gain pleasure through risky activities such as extreme sports. For others, risk is not a choice – war, conflict, poverty, famine, exploitation and living conditions worldwide create uninvited risk daily, especially for women and children.(37)

Risk discourse has infected thinking about what it is to be both intelligent and healthy in contemporary culture. Thus, Howard Gardner(38) claimed that human intelligence could not be reduced to one dimension and described eight. In the 1990s, Daniel Goleman(39) added a ninth dimension – emotional intelligence. This reflected a growing concern with excessive self-interest at the expense of sociability, and correlated with labelling of varieties of autism, especially Asperger's syndrome. Recently, Dylan Evans(40) has suggested a tenth dimension – risk intelligence, where it is 'intelligent' to tolerate uncertainty, estimate probabilities and accept reasonable levels of risk. The 'discovery' of 'risk intelligence' can be read rather as the social construction of a dimension to intelligence shaped by a current cultural fascination with risk. Public health has become a focus for risk aversion with emphasis in particular upon quality of diet and lifestyle.

Through the implementation of safety protocols, industries such as nuclear, oil, aviation and the railways have shifted from high risk to high reliability, while much of medicine, especially surgery, remains high risk.(41) This is due to a historical refusal of uncertainty, and the lack of recognition that medical error is largely grounded in systems-based miscommunications, where the basic system is the clinical team.(42) With reference to medical students, Ludmerer(32) points out that throughout the century since Flexner, 'medical faculties had done poorly at teaching learners how to manage uncertainty'. Uncertainty was typically hidden from patients and is now managed clinically through proliferation of diagnostic testing. Conventional medical education currently aims to transform medicine from high risk to high reliability. For example, where students once learned clinical skills *in vivo*, for safety reasons these are now learned *in vitro*, under conditions of simulation. While medical education is firmly embedded in the risk discourse, it is also moving towards the risk aversion end of the spectrum.

In the context of North American medical education, Ludmerer(32) traces two processes that, by the 1980s, had led to the erosion of high autonomy or self-governance and the introduction of other stakeholders into quality control. Dissatisfaction among patients with the quality of care that doctors were offering led to greater patient involvement in how doctors are educated and behave in practice. Doctors, however, pointed out that throughput-driven approaches had compromised quality of patient care and opportunities for education of students and juniors. In the UK, a series of scandals in the late 1990s – unacceptable levels of death in paediatric heart surgery at the Bristol Royal Infirmary, organ retention at Alder Hay in Liverpool, and failure to investigate early signs of the activities of the rogue GP Harold Shipman, who was the most prolific serial murderer in recorded history – led to a public outcry for greater transparency and accountability in medicine.

A deal was struck whereby quality assurance would involve collaboration between stakeholders. While medicine would still retain a degree of autonomy, regulating bodies such as the General Medical Council, patients, managers and politicians representing the public would collectively assure quality. Systems such as tighter control of medical school curricula outcomes, and appraisal and revalidation of doctors, would be developed as quality processes.

This new deal is based on a 'risk-based regulation' approach to quality assurance – for example, the UK General Medical Council's(43) quality assurance framework states that 'The GMC accepts and endorses the principle of risk-based regulation'. Here, those deemed to be at risk are scrutinised more closely by governing bodies than those deemed to be at less risk. While it was clear that quality assurance in medicine and medical education should involve all stakeholders and aim for high transparency and accountability, in the early 2000s there was a collective effort to avoid excessive regulation and coercion, or what King(44) calls 'compliance models', that can be contrasted with risk-based regulation:

> Risk-based regulation implies that some risks are tolerable and to be expected – but politicians, media, consumers, and even the public may have other ideas. Scandal or failure can quickly turn such stakeholders away from risk-based regulation and back towards more uniform and standardized compliance models.(44)

From self-regulation to watchdog compliance

The development of interest in risk-based regulation within QA and QI introduces two main paradoxes for medical education. Firstly, one of the main aims in higher education, stimulated by values of equity and equality of opportunity, has been to widen access to medical education. This includes gender balance, adequate representation from minority groups, support for students with physical and learning disabilities, opportunity for mature students and those who have worked in health care or professions allied to medicine to convert to a medical education, and opportunities for humanities and social science graduates to enter medicine through science conversion programmes. However, the paradox is that such students may then be placed 'at risk' within programmes, where 'support' can easily slip into regulation.

Secondly, while 'risk-based regulation' focuses upon quality issues for 'at risk' medical schools, what about successful schools who thrive *because of* risk, such as innovations in pedagogy? Historical examples of this include the introduction of problem-based learning, the Objective Structured Clinical Examination, longitudinal integrated clerkships (LICs), learning clinical and communication skills through simulation, and cumulative progress testing, rather than 'Big Bang' examinations in assessment. Evidence on the outcomes of such large pedagogic innovations is equivocal, largely because the interventions are complex and then very difficult to evaluate, or because they are relatively new (progress testing, LICs) and have not yet developed an evidence base.

Despite its good initial intentions, risk-based regulation in medical education is in danger of slipping into a 'watchdog' mentality. On a sliding scale, quality frameworks can be employed in either a facilitative way – helping practitioners to improve quality from within their own cultures and resources – or in an authoritative and punitive way, to regulate practice from outside, demanding compliance. The *European Student Handbook on Quality Assurance in Higher Education*(45) reminds us of a lingering historical bias in health care services:

> Within the industrial/business setting the philosophy over the past 50 years has focused on the training of employees to prevent problems, strengthening organisational systems, and continually improving performance. While within public service areas such as health and education the philosophy has been based on taking a watchdog approach, relying on government controls, professional credentials, internal audits, and, more recently, external inspections to maintain standards, weed out poor performers, and solve problems.(45)

Our fear is that medical education has become a regulated body, where sensitivity to risk is outrunning pedagogic innovation and paradoxically compromising quality. Ivan Illich(46) famously noted that the professionalisation of medicine in less industrially 'developed' countries led to a deskilling of the ordinary citizen's power to help and care for others. Lupton(47) noted that public health initiatives had come to regulate populations not because they are necessarily technically correct, but because they act as moral imperatives. Further, such imperatives are grounded in a risk discourse. Quality of public health services is judged by how well the 'at risk' groups are targeted by services, returning us to the risk-based regulation model for QA described earlier. However, as noted earlier, quality of life for many in privileged contexts is defined precisely by at-risk behaviour – such as engaging in challenging sports, 'workaholic' behaviour leading to stress, drinking alcohol, taking recreational drugs, or adopting unhealthy eating habits.

We noted earlier that medicine is becoming a more stringently regulated profession largely because of focus upon patient safety. While patient safety is undoubtedly important, 'medical error' may have become a folk devil, causing a moral panic. We suggest again that the result of this may be a movement towards over-policing or regulating quality of medical education from outside, rather than encouraging self-regulation and peer monitoring from within the medical education constituency, particularly through the patient-centred movement in which quality is defined by the nature of dialogue between doctors and patients. Despite the promise of light touch, 'risk-based regulation' medicine and medical education are increasingly subject to stronger forms of governance, including standardisation of curricula that stifles pedagogical innovation intended as positive risk.

What was once an invitation has perhaps become a finger-wagging imperative, where 'quality' has moved away from an ethical and aesthetic base to a political one, invoking issues of power. Foucault(48) described how we are entering an era of 'governmentality'. Invitations become prescriptions that inscribe the characters of those involved as 'the controlled' and 'the controlling'. Regulation may be advertised as hands off – 'light touch' and 'open dialogue', but can disguise a new form of imperialism. In the face of such surveillance,(49) and attempts to control, forms of resistance may develop from within the medical education community, although these are often subtly displayed as 'sly civility' – tactics of resistance where the outward smile and deference covers an inward dislike.

This slippage from negotiated quality to tighter regulation matters for two main reasons. Firstly, as noted above, what constitutes quality in medical education is contested. Regulation of quality may say more about issues of 'regulation' than it does about issues of 'quality'. Again, power issues may be occluding the quality debate. Secondly, in displacing self-review informed through quality frameworks by mandatory regulatory devices, quality assurance becomes undemocratic. Not only does this potentially stifle the voice of the main stakeholders – medical educators and patients – but also serves to deskill medical educators as they are removed from direct involvement in quality decisions.

From assembly to monitory democracy

The shift towards other-directed regulatory quality assurance, rather than self- and peer-directed conversation with guidelines, mirrors a wider, historical cultural shift in forms of democracy from assembly (direct involvement) to monitory (regulatory) governance.(50) Medical schools globally have largely turned to highly democratic, participatory forms of learning such as small group work and work-based learning involving patient partnership, on the basis of evidence from educational studies that these forums provide quality education. Such participatory forms of learning also provide a forum for 'assembly' democracy,(50) the original ancient Greek form of democracy, where a group of people collect together, debate and vote. In a clinical context, a team briefing and debriefing serves as an assembly democracy, ensuring quality of service to patients. Where assemblies get large (populations), while a referendum is possible, democracy switches mainly to 'representative' forms,(50) where we elect politicians through a majority vote. Medical schools have lecture formats for learning, student representatives, and hospitals have clinical directors sitting on decision-making executive boards.

Assembly and representative structures of democracy, however, are giving way to 'monitory'(50) forms as quality assurance for all (or the maintenance of a civil society) through monitoring: surveillance, laws, rules, regulations,

protocols and procedures. Quality frameworks in medical education are typical forms of monitory democracy, bypassing face-to-face and 'parliamentary' debate (assembly and representative democracy). As we peruse the list of sample quality frameworks in Box 4.2, we should ask ourselves, as medical educators, 'What part did I play in producing this set of quality regulations'?

This chapter then acts as a warning against what we see as a slippage from democratic to more autocratic processes of quality assurance – from negotiation and self-review to finger-wagging governance. We suggest that a productive balance can be achieved between invitation and injunction – precisely the issue that doctors face, as their prescriptions engage with varying levels of patient compliance.

How well do quality frameworks evaluate the quality of pedagogy?

Quality frameworks provide a ladder that we must all climb, aspiring to excellence in medical education. But what if the ladder is against the wrong wall? While sophisticated quality frameworks may ensure standards in terms of agreed outcomes, there is wide disagreement as to how those outcomes shall be achieved – or on the quality of a wide variety of teaching and learning methods within contested curriculum structures. 'Best' practice in medical education might be measured once such practice is agreed, but there is lack of both research evidence and expert opinion consensus on how we should decide on what pedagogies offer quality practices within medical education.

Commonly used contemporary pedagogies such as problem-based learning, the OSCE, learning clinical and communication skills through simulation, and scaffolded work-based learning, have equivocal evidence bases, and have been challenged for their cultural, ideological and instrumental biases. This can be extended to learning anatomy through dissection, which continues largely because of tradition rather than evidence of lasting effect.(51) In turn, innovative educational strategies – such as learning anatomy without dissection, through surface and living modes;(52) assessment through progress testing rather than 'big bang' examinations;(53) longitudinal integrated clerkships;(54) authentic simulation;(55) and the medical humanities in the core curriculum(56) – are only just beginning to gather evidence for efficacy.

Again, while quality frameworks now clearly set out what must be achieved at the end of a course of study in terms of outcomes, competences or capabilities for knowledge, skills and attitudes/values and how such outcomes are achieved is left largely to individual medical schools or postgraduate institutions. The latter – the world of pedagogy or learning theory, curriculum design, assessment models, and so forth – is quality unassured!

William Pinar(57) notes that the learning objectives or outcomes movement in education generally has now become a dominant form. It is almost heresy to challenge the notion that learning should not be driven by assessment, the latter based around meeting learning outcomes at various levels. However, Pinar(57) notes that Ralph

Tyler's legacy of forming learning and teaching strategies around assessed outcomes led to a culture of focusing on 'what students had failed to learn', rather than their successes. Importantly, the whole art of teaching itself, now recast around achieving pre-formulated objectives, became formulaic or lost its art, where teaching became 'implementation'. This simple but devastating demotion eradicates academic – intellectual – freedom, one indispensable prerequisite for teaching. The ends (attainments) serve the means (educational experiences, innovations and insights) so that the tail of assessment comes to wag the dog of learning, the latter now cast as 'instruction'. As Pinar(57) suggests, outcomes-based learning can 'restrict the educational imagination'. Curiosity and desire become replaced by functional orientations as assessment comes to drive learning. A high-quality medical education is surely not one in which students learn only what they need to know for examinations.

The GMC(43) has set out quality frameworks for UK undergraduate and postgraduate medical education that do not define 'quality' per se, but say that quality is achieved through meeting the standards and outcomes set by the GMC for graduates from medical school and for doctors in the early stages of postgraduate training. However, again such standards and outcomes are divorced from discussion of the best pedagogies by which such standards and outcomes may be met.

This does not mean that we should abandon outcomes-based approaches, which have obvious strengths of signposting for learning, and forming frameworks for assessment. A 'quality' medical education is about bringing outcomes frameworks and imaginative pedagogies into alignment. However, while the latter remain a contested field, this alignment is complicated. Indeed, there is a basic incompatibility between outcomes based learning and process-oriented pedagogy, where outcomes can constrain innovation and experimentation. Educationalists often puzzle at the slow uptake of pedagogical innovations in medical education, while they may applaud the strides forward that have been made in developing outcomes-based quality frameworks. Quality is compromised while this paradox remains unaddressed.

For example, it is strange that an exciting educational innovation – curriculum reconceptualisation,(58) in which curricula are described as differing kinds of 'texts' (historical, political, economic, phenomenological, aesthetic, ethical, gendered, and so forth) – has made no impact in medical education.(59) This model, for example, helps to make sense of why a curriculum written technically, merely as a syllabus, is often quite displaced from the experienced curriculum that students describe (the curriculum as a phenomenological text). Without considering the curriculum as a gendered text (mostly written by male medical educators and clinicians in a dominant patriarchal climate, even though women now constitute the majority of medical students globally and will soon form the majority of working doctors), how can we claim that we are seriously considering the 'quality' of a medical education? Such text-based approaches to the curriculum parallel the plural discourses approach to quality that we described earlier.

Given that the majority of a medical education is work-based, it is again strange that the 'fit for purpose' collection of learning theories that best explain work-based, collaborative learning – sociocultural theories(60) – has only in very recent years gained traction in medical education. Our point, again, is that while quality frameworks and mechanisms proliferate, quality issues concerned with pedagogy – the processes of education – lag behind. In improving quality, there is an urgent need for the medical education community to become conversant with cutting-edge educational theory.

With reference to the value of work-based learning, and returning to our earlier point about excessive patient safety awareness potentially stifling the enhancement of quality through greater risk taking, we will give an example of an innovative pedagogy that addresses these issues head on. In an account of innovations in surgical education, Roger Kneebone(55) asks how we can 'allow learners to "experience danger safely"'. His answer is to create effective simulation taking into account research evidence. We know from research on learning theory that context is key, and that transfer from a learning context to a practice context is readily frustrated.(61) Kneebone(62) approaches this dilemma by setting up 'authentic simulations' for learning interventionist clinical skills; firstly, using real patients or actor patients in combination with prostheses so that students learn in an authentic setting but without risk of harm to persons; and secondly, by increasing the authenticity of simulated settings by using better scripted scenarios and more realistic props, as 'immersive' learning. Quality is then an informed and inventive conversation between persons, scripts and artefacts.

Where quality guidelines make reference to, for example, medical schools making informed choices about curriculum models and pedagogical approaches, this is often in the form of highly generalised and woolly prescription, such as in this extract (again) from the WFME Global Standards:

> *Quality development:* The curriculum and instructional methods should ensure that students have responsibility for their learning process and should prepare them for life-long, self-directed learning . . .
> - Curriculum models would include models based on discipline, system, problem and community, etc.
> - Instructional methods encompass teaching and learning methods.
> - The curriculum and instructional methods should be based on sound learning principles and should foster the ability to participate in the scientific development of medicine as professionals and future colleagues.(63)

We do not suggest that pedagogies should be prescribed, but that 'fit for purpose' pedagogies can be recommended. While the quality framework example above talks of pedagogies and processes, it does not critically engage with educational theory, such as work-based learning approaches informing the development of longitudinal integrated curricula such as clerkships (or placements). We are not at all sure where the 'quality' debate is here. Phrases such as 'instructional methods encompass teaching and learning methods' as a quality development imperative (a 'should') are vacuous and circular. Why the document does not discuss specifics (for example: sociocultural learning theories are 'fit for purpose' when it comes to explaining collaborative, work-based learning) is presumably because the field of pedagogical research is still so highly contested. It is extremely difficult to map out clear evidence for any one practice.

In the quality frameworks we have listed (Box 4.2), there is no mention of the central pedagogical value of a medical education to democratise medical practice, where the latter is still governed by traditional authoritarian structures and hierarchies. Yet such democratisation is central to the patient safety agenda, in developing effective teamwork.(64) Further, there is no mention of 'quality' concerns in medical education's key task of identity construction, where a 21ˢᵗ century doctor is not only, as we mentioned earlier, scientist and clinician, but also humanitarian, counsellor, advocate, witness to patient suffering, educator, manager and leader. Paradoxically, in one area of medical pedagogy where we have a very strong evidence base – how clinical reasoning and judgement develop(65) – outcomes frameworks do not explicitly state that this is what must (and not what should) be learned.

Finally, if we test a quality assurance framework against pedagogical practices, what emerges can be nonsense. For example, consider the extract below from the Association of Faculties of Medicine of Canada Committee on the Accreditation of Continuing Medical Education.(66) This offers four levels for judgement:

Non-compliance: The variety of educational activities and services is so limited that the office could meet few, if any, educational needs of identified target audiences.

Partial compliance: The variety of educational activities and services is limited but could meet some educational needs of identified target audiences.

Compliance: There is a good variety of educational activities and services that are able to meet a wide range of educational needs of indentified target audiences.

Exemplary compliance: In addition to meeting the criteria for compliance, the CME/CPD office reaches out to other CPD providers, especially within the Faculty of Medicine / Health Sciences, to collaborate and to offer its services as an expert educational resource.

How will we examine and regulate levels of compliance as we scan the range of pedagogies that are core to more innovative medical schools, such as learning of anatomy through surface and living modes, authentic simulation for learning clinical and communication skills, problem-based learning with actual patients, longitudinal integrated clerkships, and progress testing? What are the criteria for compliance, especially where the evidence base from research studies is equivocal, contested, or in its infancy?

Conclusions

In raising issues such as unresolved conundrums, paradoxes, negative unintended consequences and contested implications of quality frameworks, we do not set out to muddy the waters of QI and QA for the sake of it. Rather, we point to what must now be attended to as a priority in setting out quality frameworks and processes in medical education. As a result of reading this chapter we hope that you will:

- Retain commitment to quality assurance and improvement.
- See yourself as a proactive member of a quality culture as a distinct community of practice, getting involved in decision-making and pushing for assembly democracy, where you do not abrogate responsibility or power, and do not allow yourselves to be deskilled.
- Maintain a critical perspective on quality debates.

In engaging critically with quality debates and pointing to paradoxes and complications, we recommend that:

- Quality should be engaged with as a conceptual as well as a practical issue.
- Quality is practised as a transaction between informed persons.
- Key stakeholders become familiar with the emerging vocabulary of quality, so that nothing is lost in translation.
- Quality is engaged with as a plural set of discourses, some dominant or legitimate and some acting as points of resistance, where the dominant business/managerial discourse in particular is challenged for its biases.
- Ways of measuring quality are understood, but limitations are also noted, where quality exceeds measurement.
- A supposed natural association between quality and safety in medicine is challenged.
- The risk-based regulation approach to quality is critically engaged with, in the context of a wider risk discourse. This suggests close examination of the balance between maintaining patient safety while exercising risk, for example through imaginative pedagogies such as 'authentic simulation'.
- A perceived drift towards over-regulation (a watchdog mentality) is challenged, with a view to restoring regulation as a conversation between key stakeholders, where the medical education culture has a primary holding.
- Quality cultures in medical education encourage wide membership to include all stakeholders in decision-making. Further, a drift towards monitory democracy is challenged through active participation in assembly democracy opportunities such as briefing and debriefing in clinical teams as a quality activity.
- Quality frameworks engage directly with suggestions concerning fit for purpose pedagogies without slipping into prescribing pedagogies.
- Approaches to quality engage with processes as well as outcomes of learning.
- The quality discussion engages in particular with how both QA and QI translate into effective patient care, bolstered by evidence of improved patient outcomes.

This last point is our most important, opening up a challenging field of inquiry where studies into the quality of health care begin to engage with medical education research.

References

1 Aristotle (2000) *Nicomachean Ethics*. Cambridge University Press, Cambridge.

2 Quoted in: Bleakley A, Bligh J and Browne J (2011) *Medical Education for the Future: Identity, Power and Location*, p. 33. Springer, Dordrecht.

3 Spencer-Matthews S (2001) Enforced Cultural Change in Academe. A Practical Case Study: implementing quality management systems in higher education. *Assessment & Evaluation in Higher Education*. **26**: 51–9.

4 The National Unions of Students of Europe (2002) European Student Handbook on Quality Assurance in Higher Education.9. (http://www.vss-unes.ch/typo3/fileadmin/vss_dateien/Dossiers/Akkreditierungspool/ESIB_QA_handbook_2003.pdf; accessed 16 November 2012).

5 Dolmans D, Stalmeijer R, van Berkel H and Wolfhagen I (2011) Quality assurance of teaching and learning: enhancing the quality culture. In: Dornan T, Mann K, Scherpbier A and Spencer J (eds) *Medical Education: Theory and Practice*, pp.258–9. Churchill Livingstone/Elsevier, Edinburgh.

6 Bauman Z (2007) *Liquid Times: Living in an Age of Uncertainty*. Polity, Cambridge.

7 Beck U (1992) *Risk Society: Towards a New Modernity*. Sage, London.

8 Welchman JC (ed.) (2008) *The Aesthetics of Risk*. JRP/Ringier, San Diego, CA.

9 Hutter BM (2005) The Attractions of Risk-based Regulation: accounting for the emergence of risk ideas in regulation. London: Economic and Social Research Council. (http://www2.lse.ac.uk/researchAndExpertise/units/CARR/pdf/DPs/Disspaper33.pdf; accessed 16 November 2012).

10 Atkins RB and Handal GA (2009) Utilizing quality improvement methods to improve patient care outcomes in a pediatric residency program. *Journal of Graduate Medical Education*.**1**: 299–303.

11 Da Dalt L, Callegaro S, Mazzi A *et al.* (2010) A model of quality assurance and quality improvement for post-graduate medical education in Europe. *Medical Teacher*. **32**: e57–64.

12 Foucault M (1972) *The Archaeology of Knowledge*. Tavistock Publications, New York, London.

13 Warner JH (2011) The humanising power of medical history: responses to biomedicine in the 20th century United States. *Medical Humanities*. **37**: 91–6, 92.

14 McManus IC (1995) Humanity and the medical humanities. *The Lancet*. **346**: 1143–5, 1144.

15 Flexner A (2010) *Medical Education in the United States and Canada*. Carnegie Foundation, New York.

16 Barr DA (2011) Revolution or evolution? Putting the *Flexner Report* in context. *Medical Education*. **45**: 17–22.

17 Hodges B (2005) The many and conflicting histories of medical education in Canada and the USA: an introduction to the paradigm wars. *Medical Education*. **39**: 613–21.

18 World Federation for Medical Education (2003) *Basic Medical Education: WFME Global Standards for Quality Improvement*. University of Copenhagen, Denmark: WFME, 8.

19 National Health Service (2008) Modernising Medical Careers. (http://www.mmc.nhs.uk; accessed 16 November 2012).

20 Corrigan OP and Pinchen I (2010) Tomorrow's doctors, a changing profession: reformation in the UK medical education system. In: Bronson C and Turner B (eds) *Handbook of the Sociology of Medical Education*, pp. 242–60. Taylor and Francis, Oxford.

21 Vroeijenstijn AI (1995) Quality assurance in medical education. *Academic Medicine*. **70**: s59–67, S59.

22 Wong BM, Levinson W and Shojania KG (2012) Quality improvement in medical education: current state and future directions. *Medical Education*. **46**: 107–19.

23 Eisner EW (2004) What can education learn from the arts about the practice of education? *International Journal of Education and the Arts*. **5**: 1–13.

24 Bleakley A, Farrow R, Gould D and Marshall R (2003) Making sense of clinical reasoning: judgement and the evidence of the senses. *Medical Education*. **37**: 544–52.

25 Mylopoulos M, Lohfeld L, Norman GR, Dhaliwal G and Eva KW (2012) Renowned physicians' perceptions of expert diagnostic practice. *Academic Medicine*. **87**: 1413–7.

26 Wynia MK (2006) Who is measuring the ethical quality of care in American medicine? No one, yet. *Medscape General Medicine*.**8**.

27 Fox R and Swazey J (1984) Medical morality is not bioethics – medical ethics in China and the United States. *Perspectives in Biology and Medicine*. **27**: 337–61.

28 Bleakley A, Brice J and Bligh J (2008) Thinking the post-colonial in medical education. *Medical Education*. **42**: 266–70.

29 Stern DT (ed.) (2006) *Measuring Medical Professionalism*. Oxford University Press, Oxford.

30 Freidson E (1970) *Profession of Medicine: A Study of the Sociology of Applied Knowledge*. Dodd, Mead, New York.

31 Royal College of Physicians UK (2005) *Doctors in Society: Medical Professionalism in a Changing World*. Royal College of Physicians, London.

32 Ludmerer KM (1999) *Time to Heal: American Medical Education from the Turn of the Century to the Era of Managed Care*, p. 325. Oxford University Press, Oxford.

33 Heath I (2008) *Matters of Life and Death: Key Writings*. Radcliffe, Abingdon.

34 Voss JD, May NB, Schorling JB *et al.* (2008) Changing conversations: teaching safety and quality in residency training. *Academic Medicine*. **83**: 1080–7.

35 Day I and Lin A (2012) Quality assurance in postgraduate medical education: implications for dermatology residency training programs. *Journal of Cutaneous Medicine and Surgery*. **16**: 5–10.

36 Wong BM, Etchells EE, Kuper A, Levinson W and Shojania KG (2010) Teaching quality improvement and patient safety to trainees: a systematic review. *Academic Medicine*. **85**: 1425–39.

37 Vollmann WT (2007) *Poor People*. Harper Perennial, New York.

38 Gardner H (1993) *Frames of Mind: The Theory of Multiple Intelligences*. Fontana Press, London.

39 Goleman D (1996) *Emotional Intelligence: Why it can Matter More Than IQ*. Bloomsbury, London.

40 Evans D (2012) *Risk Intelligence: How to Live with Uncertainty*. Atlantic Books, London.

41 Amalberti R, Auroy Y, Berwick D and Barach P (2005) Five system barriers to achieving ultrasafe health care. *Annals of Internal Medicine*. **142**: 756–64.

42 Xyrichis A and Ream E (2008) Teamwork: a concept analysis. *Journal of Advanced Nursing*. **61**: 232–41.

43 General Medical Council (2010) *Quality Improvement Framework for Undergraduate and Postgraduate Medical Education and Training in the UK*, p.12. GMC, London. (http://www.gmc-uk.org/education/assuring_quality.asp; accessed 16th November 2012).

44 King R (2011) The risks of risk-based regulation: the regulatory challenges of the Higher Education *White Paper for England*. London, 3. (http://www.hepi.ac.uk/files/Main%20Report.pdf; accessed 16 November 2012).

45 The National Unions of Students of Europe (2002) European Student Handbook on Quality Assurance in Higher Education. 10. (http://www.vss-unes.ch/typo3/fileadmin/vss_dateien/Dossiers/Akkreditierungspool/ESIB_QA_handbook_2003.pdf; accessed 16 November 2012).

46 Illich I (1977) *Limits to Medicine: Medical Nemesis – the Expropriation of Health*. Penguin, Harmondsworth.

47 Deborah L (1995) *The Imperative of Health: Public Health and the Regulated Body*. Sage, London.

48 Foucault M (1991) Governmentality. In: Burchell G, Gordon C and Miller P (eds) *The Foucault Effect: Studies in Governmentality*, pp. 87–104. University of Chicago Press, Chicago, IL.

49 Pecora VR (2002) The culture of surveillance. *Qualitative Sociology.* **25**: 345–58.

50 Keane J (2009) *The Life and Death of Democracy.* Simon & Schuster, New York.

51 Guttmann GD, Drake RL and Trelease RN (2004) To what extent is cadaver dissection necessary to learn medical gross anatomy? A debate forum. *Anatomical record. Part B, New Anatomist.* **281B**: 2–3.

52 Collett T, Kirvell D, Nakom A and McLachlan J (2009) The role of living models in the teaching of surface anatomy: some experiences from a UK Medical School. *Medical Teacher.* **31**: e90–6.

53 Freeman A and Ricketts C (2006) The Progress Test at the Peninsula Medical School. (www.medev.ac.uk/.../156; accessed as Word File online 17 November 2012).

54 Norris TE, Schaad DC, DeWitt D, Ogur B and Hunt DD (2009) Longitudinal integrated clerkships for medical students: an innovation adopted by medical schools in Australia, Canada, South Africa, and the United States. *Academic Medicine.* **84**: 902–7.

55 Kneebone R (2011) Simulation. In: Fry H and Kneebone R (eds) *Surgical Education: Theorising an Emerging Domain*, pp. 37–54. Springer, Dordrecht.

56 Bleakley A, Marshall R and Brömer R (2006) Toward an aesthetic medicine: Developing a core medical humanities undergraduate curriculum. *Journal of Medical Humanities.* **27**: 197–214.

57 Pinar WF (2011) *The Character of Curriculum Studies: Bildung, Currere, and the Recurring Question of the Subject*, p. 84. Palgrave Macmillan, Basingstoke.

58 Pinar WF, Reynolds WM, Slattery P and Taubman PM (1995) *Understanding Curriculum: An Introduction to Historical and Contemporary Curriculum Discourses.* Peter Lang, New York.

59 Bleakley A (2009) Curriculum as conversation. *Advances in Health Sciences Education: Theory and Practice.* **14**: 297–301.

60 Bleakley A (2006) Broadening conceptions of learning in medical education: the message from teamworking. *Medical Education.* **40**: 150–7.

61 Koens F, Mann KV, Custers EJ and Ten Cate OT (2005) Analysing the concept of context in medical education. *Medical Education.* **39**: 1243–9.

62 Kneebone R (2010) Simulation, safety and surgery. *Quality and Safety in Health Care.* **19**: i47–52.

63 World Federation for Medical Education (2003) *Basic Medical Education: WFME Global Standards for Quality Improvement (Standard 2.1)* Copenhagen: WFME.

64 Bleakley A (2013) Working in 'teams' in an era of 'liquid' healthcare: What is the use of theory? *Journal of Interprofessional Care.* **27.1**: 18–26.

65 Norman GR, Young ME and Brooks LR (2007) Non-analytical models of clinical reasoning: the role of experience. *Medical Education.* **41**: 1140–5.

66 Association of Faculties of Medicine of Canada (2010) Canadian Committee on the Accreditation of Continuing Medical Education Accreditation Standards. (http://www.afmc.ca/accreditation-cacme-e.php; accessed 16 November 2012).

Part 2
Educational Strategies

5 Problem-based learning

Mark A Albanese[1] and Laura C Dast[2]
[1] Population Health and Educational Psychology, University of Wisconsin, USA
[2] University of Wisconsin School of Medicine and Public Health, USA

 KEY MESSAGES

- Problem-based learning (PBL) has become one of the dominant forms of undergraduate medical education in the world.
- Universal features of PBL are:
  - a patient problem serving as the stimulus for learning
  - small group instruction
  - instructors serving as facilitators/tutors.
- PBL problems are critical to the process and need to meet specific criteria.
- PBL facilitators/tutors need to be instructed in how to fulfil their role.
- PBL requires planning for physical and instructional resources to be available.
- Recent implementations of PBL curricula show a trend towards hybridisation, with lectures providing cognitive scaffolding for basic sciences in support of PBL.

- Implementation of PBL in the clinical years can homogenise the experience to meet competencies, but care should be exercised that it does not supplant patient contact.
- Assessments of PBL have been fraught with methodological problems but PBL has generally shown high student and faculty satisfaction, and a trend towards improved clinical knowledge and functioning.
- Recent assessments of PBL have suggested that hybrid curricula produce increases in performance in both the basic science and clinical years in the order of a small to medium effect size. There is also evidence that there may be a differential effect in which some students who have performed relatively poorly in previous schooling do well, and those who have done well in the past do relatively poorly, indicating that there may be a need to tailor instruction to students' needs.

What is problem-based learning?

Problem-based learning (PBL) began at McMaster University, when it opened in 1969. In designing the curriculum for the newly opened university, the originators borrowed heavily from different disciplines, including case studies from business.(1) Howard Barrows and Victor Neufeld both came to McMaster in 1970, an event that would lead to the two being largely responsible for PBL being exported throughout the world. In an effort to clarify what exactly PBL is, Barrows published a taxonomy of PBL in 1986.(2) This taxonomy was anchored at one end by what has been called case-based learning, in which a completely digested patient case is presented by an instructor, and at the other end by what Barrows refers to as 'reiterative' PBL.

PBL can be characterised as an instructional method that uses patient problems as a context for students to acquire knowledge about the basic and clinical sciences. 'The basic outline of the PBL process is: encountering the problem first, problem-solving with clinical reasoning skills and identifying learning needs in an interactive process, self-study, applying newly gained knowledge to the problem, and summarizing what has been learned.'(3, p. 15) In

Barrows' original reiterative form, the PBL process concludes with students evaluating the information resources they used and then analysing how they might have better managed the patient problem. In recent years, other methods of PBL have been developed, and the Maastricht 7-Step method,(4) a 'how to do it' list of instructions to the tutor and student, has become increasingly popular (*see* Box 5.1).

In reiterative PBL:
- The process begins with a patient problem. Resources accompanying the problem included detailed objectives, print materials (originally primarily book chapters), audiovisual resources (originally slide-tape shows), multiple-choice self-assessment exercises and resource faculty.
- Students work in small groups, sometimes called 'tutorial groups'. Six to eight students per group are often recommended.
- The small groups are moderated by one or more faculty facilitators (sometimes called 'tutors').
- Students determine their own learning needs to address the problem, make assignments to each other to obtain necessary information, and then return to report what they have learnt and continue with the problem. This

Understanding Medical Education: Evidence, Theory and Practice, Second Edition. Edited by Tim Swanwick.
© 2014 The Association for the Study of Medical Education. Published 2014 by John Wiley & Sons, Ltd.

BOX 5.1 HOW TO: Organise a PBL tutorial using the Maastricht 7-step method(4)

Step 1: Identify and clarify unfamiliar terms presented in the scenario; scribe lists those that remain unexplained after discussion.

Step 2: Define the problem or problems to be discussed; students may have different views on the issues, but all should be considered; scribe records a list of agreed problems.

Step 3: 'Brainstorming' session to discuss the problem(s), suggesting possible explanations on the basis of prior knowledge; students draw on each other's knowledge and identify area of incomplete knowledge; scribe records all discussion.

Step 4: Review Steps 2 and 3 and arrange explanations into tentative solutions; scribe organises the explanations and restructures if necessary.

Step 5: Formulate learning objectives; group reaches consensus on the learning objectives; tutor ensures learning objectives are focused, achievable, comprehensive and appropriate.

Step 6: Private study (all students gather information related to each learning objective).

Step 7: Group shares results of private study (students identify their learning resources and share their results); tutor checks learning and may assess the group.

happens repeatedly as students secure more information and keep probing deeper into the problem.
- Students return for a final debriefing and analyse the approach they took after receiving feedback on their case report.
- Student evaluation occurs in a small group session and is derived from input from self, peers and facilitators.

There are many derivatives of these approaches that have been used and called PBL. Dolmans *et al*. indicate, 'Although PBL differs in various schools, three characteristics can be considered as essential: problems as a stimulus for learning, tutors as facilitators and group work as stimulus for interaction'(5, p. 735). While the 'McMaster Philosophy' had three key features – self-directed, problem-based and small group tutorial learning – the only characteristic that cuts across all of what has passed as PBL since then is that learning is based on a patient problem. While purists probably consider such variations on PBL to be corruptions of the basic PBL process, I think it is important to explore how the various elements of PBL continue to make the learning experience valuable. Who knows, we may ultimately find that the only thing that is really important is for learning to be structured around patient cases and that the small-group elements and facilitating tutors are incidental. However, it will take time and creative research to determine how these differing elements of PBL interact to achieve the goals of PBL.

Problems

Characteristics of problems

There are seven qualities required of an appropriate PBL problem. It should:
- present a common problem that graduates would be expected to be able to handle, and be prototypical of that problem
- be serious or potentially serious – where appropriate management might affect the outcome
- have implications for prevention
- provide interdisciplinary input and cover a broad content area
- lead to an encounter of faculty members' objectives
- present an actual (concrete) task
- have a degree of complexity appropriate for students' prior knowledge.(6)

The structure or format of the problem, sometimes called a 'case', provides room for variability. It can range from brief paragraphs describing a symptom or set of symptoms (e.g. chest pain), to elaborate paper or computer simulations or even the use of simulated patients. It can be relatively unorganised, unsynthesised and open-ended – a form that Barrows(2) suggests promotes the application of clinical reasoning skills, structuring of knowledge in useful contexts and the development of self-directed learning, and will also be more motivating. One example of this type of format are problem-based learning modules (PBLMs), a specialised written simulation that provides flexibility for students to pursue almost unlimited types of enquiry. There are other forms that provide more structure. The Focal Problem, developed at Michigan State University, for example, starts with a written narrative of a clinical problem as it unfolds in a real-life setting. In this design, after descriptions of significant developments occur, 'stop and think' questions are inserted for students to ponder. This approach helps students to focus on the steps in the decision-making process used in solving problems that may have more than one viable solution.(7–9)

These varied problem designs and computer-based variants may all have a role at some point in a PBL curriculum. More structured formats might be better placed early in the curriculum when students will be challenged by even the simplest clinical scenarios, while the less structured formats may be more effective after students gain clinical experience and comfort with the PBL method. However, this recommendation is based more on theory and intuition than on any specific research.

Sources of problems

There are a number of resources from which PBL cases can be obtained. MedEdPORTAL is a resource developed by the Association of American Medical Colleges (www.mededportal.org/) as a repository of peer-reviewed materials for medical education, facilitating the dissemination of educational scholarship. Cases submitted for review are evaluated by peers for their quality, and contact information is made available in a searchable database. Anyone interested in using a case can then contact the authors to work out an arrangement for using the case.

The PBLMs described earlier are available from Southern Illinois University (www.pbli.org/shopping/ePBLM.htm). PBLMs are actual patient cases in a book format that permits free enquiry. The learner can ask the patient any question in any sequence and get the patient's response, and perform any item of the physical examination in any sequence and learn the result as in the real clinical situation. Any laboratory and diagnostic test can be ordered in any sequence as well. Whatever can be done with the real-life patient in terms of history taking, physical examination and the ordering of laboratory tests can be done with the PBLM. A separate *User's Guide* provided with each PBLM can be used with any of the PBLMs in the series and provides the key for free enquiry. There is also a section in the PBLM that allows learners to follow the course of the patient under the care of the physicians responsible for the actual case. PBLMs are copyrighted and cannot be reproduced. The Tutorial Process Videotape set demonstrates the proper use of a PBLM in a tutorial group.

There is also the Health Education Assets Library (HEAL; www.healcentral.org), which is a repository of peer-reviewed materials for medical education, facilitating the dissemination of educational scholarship. HEAL is a collaborative university-based project started in 2000 by three universities. It is committed to open access to high-quality resources in perpetuity worldwide and to sharing developed tools in an open-source environment.

Problem selection

In a PBL curriculum, the problems are the central feature of the curriculum. It is essential that the problems provide a developmentally appropriate sequence that addresses key skills and abilities that lead students to developing competence. Any given case can address a multitude of objectives besides the medical content, such as population health, epidemiology, communication skills, health literacy, spousal abuse and prevention. The challenge is to ensure that the cases meet their stated objectives and that the pathway that students take through the case invariably leads to their achieving the case objectives. This is more difficult to achieve than one might think. Hays(10) warns of biases in PBL problems towards more acute problems in the younger age groups, urban health care and dominant culture issues. He further elaborates that many problems that have objectives pertaining to rural health describe poor health care in rural settings and patients having to be rescued by clinicians in large teaching hospitals. In addition, objectives addressing the health care of indigenous peoples often illustrate dominant culture stereotypes. These biases can work at cross-purposes to the desired objectives from which they were drawn.

In addition to the biases that can creep into the cases themselves, it is difficult to ensure that all student groups achieve the objectives of the cases, particularly for cases that are relatively unstructured. The gain in student independence and development of self-directed learning skills with progressively less-structured cases must be balanced by the potential for students to miss dealing with some of the anticipated objectives of a case. Research on whether students achieve case objectives shows variable results.

Dolmans *et al.*(11) found that 62 per cent of faculty-generated objectives were definitely identified by the 12 tutorial groups they studied. Coulson and Osborne(12) analysed learning issues identified by students in PBL groups and compared them with learning objectives that faculty deemed essential. Groups identified an average of 61 per cent of the essential learning objectives.

One additional issue related to problems is their use in the clinical years. One would expect that a patient would be the best possible PBL problem. However, there has been an increasing trend towards introducing formal PBL tutorial groups into the clinical years. The merits of having such formal PBL tutorial groups in the clinical years are not altogether clear. Dornan *et al.*(13) conducted interviews with 14 general physicians after the University of Manchester extended PBL tutorial groups into the clinical years. The physician comments are poignant as they describe the loss of student excitement in clinical discovery that has accompanied the students' preoccupation with their PBL cases. From a non-physician perspective, it would seem a tragedy if PBL were to supplant readily available clinical mentoring by seasoned physicians. However, this type of instruction is becoming increasingly difficult to provide. Clinicians' comments about the wards included: 'falling numbers of beds, shorter lengths of stay, changing work patterns, pressure on staff and a narrower range of "material" were seen as constraints'(13, p. 167). The outpatient realm fared little better, with comments that dealt with space constraints, work pressure, productivity targets, patient expectations and the time-cost of teaching. As the clinical environment appears to be increasingly hostile to teaching, PBL may need to be the fallback to maintain clinical education at a reasonable level of quality. This may be especially true if medical education continues to progress towards competency-based education, and students will need to demonstrate core skills that may not be reliably obtained during the general course of clinical education.

Facilitators/tutors

Selection and training of facilitators

Selection

In the original McMaster PBL curriculum, Neville and Norman stated that tutors were not required to have any particular content expertise other than that contained in the tutorial guides. This was a conscious choice because it was believed that content experts would be unable to resist the temptation to lecture the students, thereby short-circuiting the students' opportunity to apply the knowledge that they might have to address the biomedical problems contained in the tutorial. Miflin(14) argues that given the norms of the time when PBL originated, tutors were expected to be physicians, and general medical expertise was an unstated assumption underlying the qualifications of tutors. In subsequent research, several studies found better learning outcomes if the facilitator/tutor had content expertise.(15,16) Zeitz and Paul(17) argue that these two studies were experiments in PBL in a larger, traditional curriculum and that the learners were novices regarding PBL. In their experience, when novices 'first attempt problem-based learning, the outcomes are better if the faculty facilitators are content *experts*' (17, p. 203). However, after one-to-two months, students enrolled in a PBL curriculum are so acculturated and so highly skilled in student-centred, self-directed learning that they are no longer so dependent on the facilitator. Zeitz and Paul further argue that in practice it is not feasible for facilitators to be content experts for all problems that they will facilitate. What they have found is that facilitators need to develop 'case expertness' by facilitating the case between three and five times. I have argued elsewhere that what we need to determine is not whether tutors need to be content experts, but what is the minimum content expertise and group facilitation expertise needed for tutors to be effective.(18) As far as what is needed regarding tutor expertise is concerned, I think the title of Miflin's(14) article summarises our current understanding: 'Problem-based learning: the confusion continues'.

Training

Facilitators need to be given specific guidelines about how they are to interact with students. Moving from content expert to facilitator is not necessarily natural for many faculty members, so practising the role during training will be helpful. The use of 'standardised' students, individuals who are trained to act like students, can make the practice closer to the real thing than it might otherwise be. However, it can be expensive and the fidelity of the simulation to real life may be difficult to maintain.

Facilitators should also be given all information about the case and any associated reading or materials that students will be given, as well as materials that will allow them to guide students in their search for knowledge. This includes the 'next steps' that students are expected to take. Anything that can help facilitators reach the case expertness described by Zeitz and Paul(17) more quickly is useful.

Facilitators also need to be prepared for students' reaction to the experience. If students are used to having faculty members serving as content deliverers, rather than facilitators, the transition to this type of relationship can be rocky. Initially, facilitators need to be prepared for students responding to their answering questions with questions by giving them a look that says, 'I pay X zillion dollars for this education, the least you can do is answer my question'. Over time, students learn that the facilitator is not there simply to answer their questions, but early on it can be a difficult adjustment for both students and facilitators.

Bowman and Hughes(19) use a clinical psychology framework and the similarity between PBL and small groups in clinical psychology to argue that PBL may be susceptible to the regressive and task-avoiding behaviours seen in clinical psychology groups. They cite four shared characteristics that can promote these problems: extended contact time (often more than six hours per week), non-directive role of tutor that facilitates uncertainty, the unpredictable nature of group process and the potential intimacy of PBL. While these characteristics may induce undesirable behaviour in students, Bowman and Hughes argue that the facilitator is also susceptible. To avoid tutor problems (wanting to be 'one of the gang', liked by students, in control, subverting the primary task with a new agenda, having a relationship with a student), training and follow-up should provide the following, according to Bowman and Hughes:(19)

- clear statements of the primary task of PBL tutors
- clear boundaries on the staff role and availability
- ongoing review and monitoring of tutor work
- social activities that are friendly but not intimate.

They argue for establishing monthly supervision, peer observation and mentoring for all PBL tutors.

How many facilitators per group?

The number of facilitators needed per group has not really been studied in a controlled manner, but there are practical considerations that lead to the conclusion that more than one will stretch facilitator resources pretty thin. There have been studies that examined the impact of having fewer than one facilitator per group. Farrell *et al.*(20) explored the use of a single facilitator who circulated among four groups, each of which had from three to four students in an ophthalmology section for second-year medical students. The authors found improvements in learning that were comparable to those made by students who had a more traditional ophthalmology experience, and high student satisfaction as well. Khaliq(21) reported substantial increases in student satisfaction ratings after introducing problem-solving exercises into lectures. In the problem-based course on public health for first-year medical students at the University of Wisconsin, we used two facilitators rotating among five groups (this was replicated with five different sets of facilitators and student groups). Each facilitator pair was composed of a methodologist and a clinical epidemiologist. The ability of the facilitators to discuss issues relative to their own experience base seemed to be synergistic, but there was substantial variability among the five different replications.

Small groups

Optimal size

Recommendations for optimal group size tend to be anecdotal. Dr David Matheson, a member of the PBL Best Practices Consortium (*see* Acknowledgements for details), offers the suggestion that 'groups should contain no more than seven members and no fewer than five. More than seven results in too many opportunities for reluctant members to hide. Fewer than five puts the spotlight on members permanently and removes much of the opportunity for "think" time'. Another member of the Consortium, Dr Gail Swarm, states, 'We have groups here that range from six to eight students. Having groups of seven students really seems to be a "magical" number'.

A search of PubMed using the terms 'PBL' and 'small-group size' yielded five hits, but none of them specifically examined small group size in relationship to PBL effectiveness. In 2009, my colleagues and I published an article detailing the development of the Integrated Systems

Model.(22) This model views students and the educational ecosystem as a type of complex adaptive system. As such, student behaviour in a small group will be difficult to predict, but there must be adequate time for each member to contribute to the group functioning, as well as the expectation that all members will make a contribution during each meeting. It makes the additional recommendation that there must be enough members in the group that the assignments will not deplete the reserves of members. This is a particular concern for the weaker members of the group, who may have to overcome weaknesses in their background preparation to be able to make a suitable contribution. A rule of thumb is that the groups should have at least four members but be small enough so that each student will have at least ten minutes each, assuming that speaking time is equally parsed to all members. So, if small groups meet for 90 minutes, no more than nine members should comprise the groups. From our earlier review, the additional recommendation can be made that group sizes over ten are no longer small.(6) Also, an even number of group members will make it more difficult to obtain a majority vote than will an odd number. Depending on whether or not one thinks that negotiating one's way out of tied votes is a skill worth promoting, this may or may not be desirable. There may be literature from business, counselling or psychiatry that could provide more insight into optimal small-group sizes for problem-solving exercises, but I will leave that to others.

Composition

The groups should be composed of students, of course, but what varieties? They come in many different shapes and sizes, so I would recommend randomisation, but stratified according to gender and particularly, academic ability. Also, students who are 'couples', especially if married, should be assigned to different groups to avoid problems in group dynamics.

Randomisation can do some unusual things, which is why statisticians acknowledge that error (usually 5 per cent) is a possibility in any given statistical test. So, for things that may impact on group functioning, such as the gender distribution, it is best to 'improve on chance' by having representation consistent with that of the larger group. If there are 50 per cent females in the class, a random assignment process should be used that results in approximately equal numbers of males and females in each group.

Stratifying groups by academic ability is also important and is particularly effective if linked to grading processes that reward the group for the co-operative success of the group as a whole. For example, in a co-operative learning PBL situation, any member of the group can be called upon to present their findings. The group member called upon could be the weakest member of the group, so it is in everyone's best interest to ensure that all members are adequately prepared to make their presentation. This approach values students teaching students and rewards those groups that are successful in doing so. It is also important to consider academic ability in group formation because it has been shown to have a lasting impact on physician careers. Gonnella *et al.*(23) followed graduates of Jefferson

Medical College who were in deciles based on first-year medical school grades into residency. They found a linear trend indicating that academically low performers were much less likely to thrive by various criteria. One approach to balancing ability would be to stratify so the groups are balanced in their representation by three levels of ability: bottom 25 per cent, middle 50 per cent and top 25 per cent. There are a number of challenges to stratifying by academic ability in a PBL curriculum. First, it may not be possible to determine who is in the bottom 25 per cent, let alone at other levels of performance, by the grading methods that are used in a PBL curriculum. For example, if a pass/fail grading system is used, it is almost impossible to determine who is in the bottom 25 per cent. In the absence of direct academic measures in medical school, admissions test performance can be used as a surrogate. In the USA, the Medical College Admissions Test (MCAT) has been shown to correlate relatively strongly with performance in medical school ($r = 0.60$).(24) Scores that average below 8 (the national mean of all who take the test and a point about one standard deviation below the mean of those who are admitted to medical school) on the primary subtests (biological and physical sciences and verbal reasoning) can serve as a reasonable substitute. For non-North American schools, admissions test performance that puts the students one or more standard deviations below the mean of admits can be used.

Structure and roles

It has become increasingly clear that just throwing a group of students together with a problem is not necessarily going to yield something useful. Guidelines and role assignments are often recommended to help students make a start on how to organise themselves to do productive work. Barrows (3, pp. 60, 61) recommends that students assume three separate administrative roles to make the process work smoothly, as follows:

- PBL module reader
- action master list handler
- recorder.

In the context Barrows was describing, students were working through what they called PBL modules. They were also instructed to formulate action lists. So, Barrows recommends having one student in the role of module reader, another handling the list of actions that need to be taken and a third who is a general recorder of activities.

David Matheson states,

> While it may be true that the world is run by those who turn up [Woody Allen], attendance at PBL sessions has to be mandatory to avoid group erosion and to underline the seriousness of the enterprise. Groups need rules and standards of acceptable behaviour. I have tried groups without rules, groups with minimal rules [such as be considerate of others] and all sorts of variations in between. In the end, each such group has decided to set out basic norms of acceptable behaviour comprising of, for example, when interruption is permitted, the attitudes towards latecomers, whether eating was allowed during a session, what to do if the tasks for the day were completed before time was out and so on. Importantly, these rules work best when generated by the group.

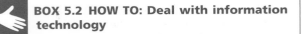

BOX 5.2 HOW TO: Deal with information technology

- Discussion is still supreme (as opposed to reading off a screen).
- Laptop work must be related to the group's tasks (no personal email, chat or other surfing/playing).
- System should be used for sharing information.
- Scribe should control the technology for the session.
- Wrap-up should include evaluation of how the technology is being used.
- Group agrees on what they believe is appropriate use.
- Give immediate feedback if technology is being used inappropriately.
- Agree that it is not appropriate to look up work that should have been prepared.
- Purpose of technology is to enhance group effectiveness.
- Quick look-ups allowed ~60 seconds.
- Single, group-only computer – no individual users.
- Add a spot for this in the facilitator evaluation of students (appropriate use of technology).

Source: http://oucom.ohiou.edu/fd/group_ground_rules.htm

Technology is also becoming a problem for small-group management and may interfere with problem-solving. Dr Stephen Davis, another member of the PBL Best Practices Consortium, provides a number of recommendations regarding ground rules for technology use, which are summarised in Box 5.2.

Time management

Dr Dennis Baker, another member of the Consortium, notes, 'It has been my experience that when students identify learning issues the learning issues are stated in very general terms which can lead to learning inefficiencies and additionally when the students come back together to discuss the learning issues the discussion of them can be lengthy and unfocused'. PBL adherents may not consider this type of situation to be necessarily bad, but simply the stage that students need to go through to become effective problem-solvers. It may also be that the facilitator should play a role in helping the students to see that their learning issues may not be sufficiently well delineated to yield productive searches. However, if it persists and students do not seem to be making progress in delineating clearer and more specific learning issues, the facilitator should take a more assertive role in pointing out the elements of the learning issues that are unclear before allowing students to go off on their independent assignments.

The facilitator should assist the groups by noting the time and pointing out how much progress needs to be made before they finish. This role should actually be taken over by the students themselves as they become more skilled in working in small groups. However, there may be some value in having a formally appointed timekeeper role, if it becomes apparent that discussion gets out of control and the group continually runs over the allotted time.

Resources

Space requirement

David Matheson recommends that rooms be dedicated to PBL and used only by an individual group. 'This helps create a sense of group cohesion and gives the group a place to call "home".' However, dedicated space in today's crowded health sciences learning centres can be hard to come by. As schools respond to the anticipated shortage of physicians by increasing class sizes, they will be even more hard-pressed to supply dedicated space for PBL groups. While it is not hard to see how dedicated space would be a desirable feature, it is not necessarily clear that the lack of dedicated space will have detrimental effects on student learning.

Computing resources

Matheson suggests that rooms need at least two networked computers to allow groups to access internet resources. He further recommends that the room should be wi-fi enabled so that anyone who wishes to can use the network via a laptop. However, the use of technology can have its drawbacks. Kerfoot *et al.*(25) noted that a large plasma screen monitor with internet access distracted students from engaging in problem-solving, as they searched the internet for answers to questions. Thus, care needs to be exercised so problem-solving exercises do not devolve into students using small-group time to look for answers on the Web.

Instructional resources

A well-stocked library is an important need for students in a PBL curriculum. Nolte(26) found that library use of reserve books increased 20-fold, after introducing a PBL course on neurobiology into the curriculum. With the more recent advent of the internet and online references, having internet access is essential. Literature search software such as PubMed is critical. Having general web-searching capability with software such as Google and Ask Jeeves will be useful for looking for non-library references, including policy statements and current events. However, as Kerfoot *et al.*(25) noted, there need to be guidelines for internet usage to avoid having the problem-solving process subverted by web searches.

Whiteboards and blackboards are also beneficial. Some schools have adopted electronic blackboards that enable electronic capturing of the material students write on the board.

Lectures can be an instructional resource, but Barrows recommends limiting them to 1–1.5 hours per day(3, p. 46). Barrows also recommends that basic science research staff should be a resource available to meet with students for 4–6 hours per week(3, p. 50).

With new learners, there is a danger of having too many resource options. Students can get bogged down looking for information and give too little attention to problem-solving, a problem similar to the one that Kerfoot *et al.* noted with plasma screen computer access to the Web.

Creature comforts

The instructional environment in the small group should be informal and as low-stress as possible. Lighting should be sufficient to see all types of educational resources that will be shared. The environment (chairs) should be comfortable, but not so comfortable as to make it difficult for students to stay awake. Students should be able to bring food and drink into the meeting room. Ready access to a refrigerator and even microwave helps make the room comfortable. David Matheson recommends having access to such things as a kettle, cups and teaspoons. If possible, it is desirable for each PBL group to have its own dedicated room where they can leave things out knowing that they will not be disturbed before the next time they meet.

Standardised patients

Barrows and Tamblyn(27) reported using standardised patients for both teaching and assessing students in PBL groups as early as 1973. Standardised patients can be particularly useful when students are learning communication skills and physical examination skills. Depending on the goals of the session, patients may need to be coached in the art of teaching and in the components of the examination that are being learnt. In cases where the goal is simply to give students an opportunity to work through the history and physical examination with a 'real' person, there may not be the need for such extensive training. However, it should be clear what the purpose of the session is in the determination of the training/skill needs of the standardised patients when the session is being scheduled. Generally, standardised patients are expensive to deploy and their use should be carefully considered in relation to the benefits derived. Patient involvement in medical education is discussed in detail in Chapter 17.

Organisation and grading

Administration and governance

Barrows(3) considers PBL to be most compatible with curricula that are organ-based. Such a curriculum aligns courses with different organs of the body. Thus, a course on the cardiovascular system would have the anatomy, physiology, biochemistry and so on, of the system all integrated. Because patient problems are often localised to a single organ system, it seems logical that PBL would be consistent with an organ-based curriculum.

However, organising staff for organ-system teaching and PBL can be difficult because most medical schools are organised around discipline-based departments (e.g. pathology, anatomy, surgery). Interdisciplinary collaboration can be difficult to sustain in a disciplinary-based medical school because it cuts across the organisational structure of the medical school, thereby requiring extra resources to sustain (effort to contact people who are at greater distances, travel to meetings outside the depart-

ment, more people to share academic credit with, less return on effort, etc.). Thus, while there is the excitement and energy of developing new organ-based curricula and PBL when a new dean arrives and marshals resources for the new curriculum, maintenance when the 'newness' wears off and resources are needed for other pressing matters is a challenge (this has been recognised as a problem for interdisciplinary research efforts).

Some newer medical schools in the USA are organising themselves differently from what has traditionally been the case. For example, Florida State University, a relatively recently opened medical school with a PBL curriculum, has organised itself around five departments that can be considered interdisciplinary: biomedical sciences; medical humanities and social sciences; clinical sciences; geriatrics; and family medicine and rural health. The University of New Mexico School of Medicine, another school with a PBL curriculum, has grouped its biological sciences into five departments: biochemistry and molecular biology; cell biology and physiology; molecular genetics/microbiology; neurosciences; and pathology. Organ-based curricula and PBL require interdisciplinary collaboration to be most effective. The interdisciplinary structure of these departments is more likely to sustain an organ system and PBL curriculum in the face of administrative changes and budget reductions because they require fewer resources to maintain than is the case in a medical school with discipline-based departments.

Programme evaluation

A combination of both formative and summative curricular evaluation processes is helpful. Formative evaluation is needed on an ongoing basis to identify and resolve small problems before they become big problems. Summative evaluations are designed to assess how effective the total learning experience has been, a critical element to inform stakeholders whether continual efforts to improve have had tangible benefits.

Barrows(3) recommends that the course co-ordinator meet weekly with groups for formative evaluation purposes. One of the advantages of modern technology is the ability of students to report issues as they occur through either email, posting to a website or any of the various social networking systems that instructors wish to employ. Students should be encouraged to report issues that are detracting from their learning experience as early as possible. Confidentiality should be assured because the PBL process is such a personal one that any criticisms can be misinterpreted or taken very personally. This becomes especially problematic with formative evaluation because it occurs while the PBL process is still in progress.

Summative evaluation relies on information that is generally collected after the completion of the learning experience. The goal is to determine the effectiveness of the experience. Student ratings are the most commonly used summative evaluation data. Students' success in achieving programme goals and objectives can also be a source of information. For PBL curricula in the preclinical years, ratings of preceptors in the clinical years have been useful. For entire curricula, the ratings of graduates and the residency supervisors of the graduates have also been useful. Performance on objective examinations, especially external ones such as the United States Medical Licensing Examination (USMLE) Step exams in the USA, can also serve as summative evidence. However, they have been criticised as being not very sensitive to the types of skills that PBL is attempting to develop. Progress tests, a long true/false or multiple choice test, administered repeatedly across the curriculum, have been used by some institutions such as McMaster and Maastricht for curriculum evaluation. Generally, one is better off using a range of different types of data to evaluate a programme and PBL is no different. Each type of data that one collects generally has its own weaknesses, but in aggregate the weaknesses can be mitigated. Over the past 15 years, the effectiveness of PBL has been the subject of at least eight separate literature reviews with somewhat controversial results. I will return to this in the final section when I deal with the impact of PBL.

Grading systems

Grading students in PBL offers challenges because there is the desire for collaborative and possibly co-operative learning among students. If the grading system is not properly designed, it can work at cross-purposes to this goal. In particular, if grading is competitive, with a fixed quota for the highest grades (e.g. reserve honours grades for the highest 16 per cent), students may be unwilling to help other students for fear that they would disadvantage themselves. As complex adaptive systems, students cannot be expected to do things that will diminish their prospects for success. Further, struggling students may be even less likely to help their colleagues if their survival in medical school is at risk, particularly if they see collaboration as taking time with no benefit. If collaboration and co-operation are desired, the value of doing so needs to be made clear to students and rewarded in the grading system.

There is also the component of PBL that has students working in groups and producing reports that are group work. Distinguishing individual performance in this type of activity is difficult and generally imprecise. A pass/fail grading system is most compatible with these elements of PBL. However, many staff and students believe that a pass/fail grading system does not provide the motivation for, or recognition of, achieving excellence. To recognise excellence, an honours grade beyond pass is sometimes added. The other concern is that staff appear to be loathe to award failing grades. To distinguish poorer performance in a way that staff appear to be more likely to use, a marginal or low pass grade is sometimes used as a buffer between fail and pass. Which system to use depends on the goals and aspirations of the school and the proclivities of its staff. The good thing is that if the grading system does not work, it can always be changed.

Student evaluation

Evaluating student performance in PBL is challenging; it would take an entire separate publication to treat it adequately. Here, I give a brief overview of selected methods that have been used. For each, I describe the method and briefly note its major strengths and weaknesses. For readers who are interested in more detailed descriptions of methods used to evaluate students in PBL, I refer you to Nendaz and Tekian,[28] and for an excellent reference on how to write test items and an analysis of the strengths and weaknesses of various approaches to student assessment, I recommend a free online manual.[29]

Multiple-choice exams

The use of multiple-choice examinations, including true/false and the extended matching variety, is common because of the ease of scoring. Writing multiple-choice questions that are appropriate for PBL, however, presents a formidable challenge and one that some would argue is not possible. Generally, there is no better way of covering a breadth of content more efficiently. Whether multiple-choice tests can assess the content at the level of problem-solving that PBL is designed to promote is an open question. There are those who believe that well-written multiple-choice questions are capable of assessing these problem-solving skills, and there are those who believe otherwise. At the very least, writing such sophisticated questions is a very complex skill, one that is unlikely to be particularly prevalent among the staff that are generally tasked to do this at the typical medical school.

That said, there is a form of multiple-choice examination that has been relatively widely used to assess PBL. The Progress Test has been used at the University of Maastricht since the early 1980s.[30] A version was adopted at McMaster University in 1992. A Progress Test reflects the end objectives of the curriculum and samples knowledge across all disciplines and content areas relevant for the medical degree. The Maastricht exam was composed of 250 true/false questions, while the McMaster exam contained 180 multiple-choice questions. At Maastricht the Progress Test is administered four times per year to all students in the medical school, while McMaster administers its test three times per year to all students. The Maastricht Progress Test has been found to have a strong correlation with a test on clinical reasoning ($r = 0.93$).[31] The McMaster version of the Progress Test was submitted to an extensive psychometric analysis and showed test–retest reliabilities over successive administrations ranging from 0.53 to 0.64, and predictive validity of the cumulative score was approximately 0.60.[32]

The main problem with a Progress Test is that it is inefficient. Neophyte examinees spend a lot of time answering questions the answers to which they can only hope to guess at (advanced clinical questions), and advanced examinees spend a lot of time answering questions that are too primitive for them (they answer them correctly with little thought needed). Measurement specialists prefer to administer relatively short tests that are appropriate for the learner's level and then scale the results to place the learner on an ability continuum. This, however, requires relatively advanced measurement methods (e.g. Item–Response Theory), lots of data and fairly sophisticated technical support. If the Progress Test is the only major knowledge evaluation taking up students' time in the curriculum, some inefficiency is probably acceptable.

Short-answer questions

Using a PBL scenario and then having students write their response at various stages of what would be the PBL process has the potential for being effective in assessing aspects of PBL, probably with less challenge than with the multiple-choice type question. Getting students to give answers to how they would respond in the first stage of the PBL process should be relatively easy to do in this format. After the first stage, however, it becomes more complicated. Should students' responses to the first stage be used in subsequent stages? If so, the answers will be idiosyncratic for each student and grading them objectively becomes exceedingly challenging. Also, if a student does poorly in an earlier stage, their later responses may be wrong, but correct given what they did earlier. Should they be given full credit, partial credit or no credit for these later answers? Generally, it is not good practice to have items that are linked in this manner. The answers to the questions are not independent and weighting them properly becomes problematic. A way around the linkage would be to provide a standard set of student choices for earlier stages, and ask the student to indicate what they would do now. This avoids the lack-of-independence problem but introduces an element of artificiality into the process. Some students would not have taken the earlier route through the case, and that makes it difficult for them to take the case from that point forward. Clearly, there are challenges in using short-answer questions to mirror the PBL process. Using short-answer as opposed to supplying the alternatives in a multiple-choice question solves the potential for students to get the answer correct by guessing, but does so with substantial added costs for grading.

Essay and modified essay questions

Essay questions provide the least structure and have the potential to offer insight into the thought processes underlying students' choices, when confronted with a patient problem. However, students who are not very skilled at writing essays could appear to be less accomplished than they are simply because they do not write well. Saunders *et al.*(33) describe what they call 'modified essay questions'. Each modified essay question covers nine areas of primarily internal medicine content. Each area is scored as fail, pass or good answer/above average. The advantage of the essay-type questions is in their relative ease of construction. The disadvantage is in their complexity and time necessary for scoring. Achieving reliable scores among graders is a major challenge, not to mention getting the essays graded in a timely manner.

Simulations

Simulations in medical education were first described by McGuire and Babbott in 1967.(34) At that time, technology involved the use of latent image pens that uncovered answers printed on paper that were only able to be disclosed by the use of the fluid contained in the pens. Unfortunately, such technology ended relatively abruptly in the late 1970s; urban rumour has it that the fluid was found to be a carcinogen. However, computers picked up where the 'carcinogen' left off, and today computer simulations are quite sophisticated. The USMLE Step 3 exam uses computer simulations as part of its assessment. In a PBL simulation, students are presented with a case and after giving it consideration, they indicate the next steps to be taken. The computer then shows the results of these actions. This proceeds until the designated end point of the simulation is reached. Some simulations end with the diagnosis, others end with management of the patient until the problem resolves itself or the virtual patient dies.

Computer simulations, the most likely ones to be encountered today, are complex and expensive to create. Grading student choices can also be complex if it must take into account every choice a student makes in working through what may be a complex process. Some simulations get around this problem by grading according to whether the desired end point is reached and not whether the desired route is taken to reach the end point. Other simulations are interested in the process that is taken as well as whether the end point is reached. These are the most complex simulations to grade.

Triple-jump exercise

The primary goal of a triple-jump exercise is to assess clinical problem-solving and self-directed learning skills.(35) In a triple-jump exercise, students discuss a written clinical scenario and identify the related learning goals, review the learning materials individually, and return to present their conclusions and judge their own performances. Students sometimes have three hours to complete their exercise, sometimes a week. This type of assessment is often used for formative evaluation purposes. It is less used for grading purposes because it is time-consuming, limiting the number of scenarios that can be evaluated, and as a result scores tend to be contextually bound to the specific problem assessed. I personally think the name choice is unfortunate because it is too close to the negative term 'jumping through hoops' – thrice.

Objective-Structured Clinical Exams

Objective-Structured Clinical Examinations (OSCE)s are performance-based examinations in which students rotate from station to station.(36) Stations often use standardised patients, computer simulations, literature search facilities, manikins and other types of 'hands-on' experience. The strengths of the OSCE are its face validity and standardised clinical experience for all examinees. There are relatively few other ways of assessing complex skills and abilities such as communication skills with the same degree of standardisation and reliability. The primary limitation of the OSCE pertains to its cost. It requires substantial infrastructure to administer: personnel to recruit, train and manage standardised patients and facilities. For a more detailed discussion of the OSCE, *see* Chapter 21.

Peer evaluations

Peer evaluation is what clinicians do on a daily basis in practice. As such, it has a certain natural appeal for use in

PBL, plus it relieves the facilitator from being the sole judge of student contributions. However, peer assessment should be used with caution. Because students are still learning what it means to be a professional, they do not have a solid basis for making peer judgments of knowledge. Further, because students may be competing with one another for grades, accolades and residency positions, peer evaluation can have a markedly disruptive effect on group dynamics. Complicating matters further, if a co-operative learning model is being used, students are expected to teach their peers. If they are expected to both teach and assess their peers, the two activities can be antagonistic. And, if after peer assessments, students are expected to come back and continue to work in their small groups, what might have been a functional group dynamic may no longer exist. If peer assessments are used for grading students, it may be best to use peer assessments of teaching contributions to colleagues than it would of learning accomplishment and group contributions. This aligns the students evaluative judgments with skills demonstrated by their peers that they are likely the very best judges, as well as reinforces to all students the importance of teaching one's peers.

Facilitator evaluations

Facilitator ratings of students are often used in PBL. Because the facilitator is present for the small-group meetings and can observe the interactions that occur, they can provide a unique perspective on each of the students' contributions. Several tools have been proposed to assess facilitator or tutor perceptions of student performance, but they vary markedly in their length and the frequency with which they are to be used. Hebert and Bravo[37] proposed Tutotest, an exhaustive 44-item instrument. Ladouceur et al.[38] developed a somewhat shorter instrument composed of 31 items, but this is still a formidable burden for facilitators. Several investigators have explored use of forms with five or fewer items.[39–41] The longer forms have been recommended for use at the end of a unit, while the shorter forms have been recommended for use at the end of each session. An instrument completed at the end of each unit will have one assessment completed every two-to-six weeks, while one completed at the end of each session will have from 4 to 18 assessments completed by the end of a unit. Scores from assessments completed at the end of each session have been found to have better psychometric properties. There is a problem, though, with facilitator evaluations as students – aware that their facilitator will be evaluating their performance – may behave differently in the facilitator's presence than they do in other group interactions. Inconsistency between facilitator and peer assessments in such a case may represent real differences and not psychometric weaknesses in either type of assessment.

Self-evaluations

One of the goals of PBL is to develop student's self-directed learning skills. The ability to accurately assess one's strengths and weaknesses and identify ways to address one's weaknesses are key components of achieving this goal. Accurate self-assessment is an important component of achieving self-directed learning skills. However, studies of self-assessment have demonstrated that poor performers tend to overestimate their performance and high performers tend to underestimate their performance.[42,43] Such tendencies cut across a wide variety of different skills. As a consequence, using self-assessments in grading may penalise the high performers and give undeserved increases in grades to the poorest performers (lowest 25 per cent). While self-assessment is a good activity for students to experience, it should be used with great care in assigning grades.

The theoretical basis for problem-based learning

The concept of contextual learning is often used to support PBL. The basic premise is that when we learn material in the context of how it will be used, it promotes learning and the ability to use the information. In PBL, the problem is usually portrayed in the real-life context of a patient coming to visit a doctor or some variation. Colliver[44] criticises the contextual learning argument on the grounds that it was drawn from a weak research finding and that almost all clinical education occurs in the contextually relevant process of patient care. However, other theories provide more compelling support.

Information-processing theory

Information-processing theory has been argued to underlie PBL.[45] This theory involves: prior-knowledge activation, encoding specificity and elaboration of knowledge. Prior-knowledge activation occurs when students use knowledge they already possess to understand and structure new information. Encoding specificity refers to transfer of learning being more likely to occur when the situation in which something is learnt more closely resembles the situation in which it will be applied. Elaboration of knowledge refers to information being better understood and remembered if there is opportunity for elaboration (discussion, answering questions, etc.). These three elements are commonly a part of PBL. They also have relatively strong documentation from the larger education and psychology literature. The single concept of encoding specificity incorporates most of the salient features of contextual learning theory suggesting that information processing theory provides a more comprehensive and parsimonious basis of support for PBL than does contextual learning theory alone.

Co-operative learning

Co-operative learning situations are those where individuals perceive that they can reach their goals if and only if the other group members also do so. The small-group format used in PBL often fits this definition. Qin et al.[46] conducted a meta-analysis of studies spanning the 20th century assessing the effect of co-operative versus competitive learning on problem-solving. Co-operation was operationally defined by the presence of joint goals, mutual rewards, shared resources and complementary roles among members of a group. Competitive learning situations were those where individuals perceived that they can reach their goals if and only if the other participants cannot attain their goals. Competition was operationally defined by the presence of a goal or reward that only one or a few group members could achieve by outperforming the others. Problem-solving was defined by situations that required participants to form a cognitive representation of a task, plan a procedure for solving it, execute the procedure and check the results. The authors concluded that overall, 'cooperative efforts produce higher quality problem-solving than do competitive efforts'.(46, p. 139) One possible reason for the success of co-operative learning is that it enables material to better mesh with students' level of cognitive development. In co-operative efforts, learners exchanged ideas and corrected each other's errors more frequently and effectively than did individuals competing with each other. It may be that students who are struggling to understand the material are more likely to be able to identify the sources of other students' misunderstandings than the expert instructor.

Self-determination theory

Self-determination theory distinguishes between two types of motivating conditions: controlled and autonomous.(47) Controlled motivators are termed maladaptive and include external demands and contingencies as well as 'introjected regulation', which are internalised contingencies about what they 'should' do. These are all accompanied by either explicit or implicit rewards or punishments, or in the case of the introjected regulation, what they term 'intrapsychic' or internal representations of rewards and punishments (self-aggrandisement and self-derogation). Under controlled forms of motivation, people act with a sense of pressure and anxiety. In educational situations, this takes the form of learning that is rote, short-lived and poorly integrated into students' long-term values and skills. It does not take much of a leap to infer that many traditional curricula are steeped in controlled forms of motivation. Autonomous motivators are those personally endorsed by the learner and reflect what the individual finds interesting and important. They include learners engaging in an activity simply because it is interesting and enjoyable, as well as situations in which the learner has identified with its value for functioning as a physician. In contrast to the external element of the rewards and punishments administered in controlled motivating conditions, autonomous motivation involves behaving with a sense of volition, agency and choice. Williams *et al.*(47) cite research which has demonstrated that, relative to controlled motivation, autonomous motivation for learning promotes greater conceptual understanding, better academic performance, higher academic achievement, stronger feelings of competence, enhanced creativity, a preference for optimal challenge over easy success, more positive feelings while learning, a tendency to cope more positively with failures and setbacks, greater persistence and better psychological adjustment.

A learning climate that promotes autonomous motivators includes one in which educators take the perspectives of students into account, provide relevant information and opportunities for choice, and encourage students to accept more responsibility for their own learning and behaviour. It also includes teachers being meaningfully involved in students' learning through dialogue, listening, asking students what they want, providing satisfying rather than superficial replies to student-generated questions, providing information and advice, and suspending judgement when soliciting the opinions and reactions of students. Such an environment minimises pressure and control, while encouraging a high level of performance. Clearly, autonomous motivators can be employed in either a PBL or a traditional curriculum. However, autonomous motivators would seem to be especially compatible with collaborative learning environments. Furthermore, PBL would seem to be an easier fit with autonomous motivators than would be the traditional curriculum.

Integrated System Model

While PBL began with no particular theory undergirding its design, over the intervening years, numerous theories have been advanced in its support and elsewhere, my colleagues and I have proposed an integrated model to explain behaviour in the relatively chaotic health care environment. The value of the model is its ability to incorporate a number of different models and theories into a cohesive unit. There are six major components to the Integrated System Model (ISM), as follows:
- superstructure
- change/adaptation
- feedback/regeneration
- environment/context and resources
- functional interactions
- complex adaptive system (CAS) behaviours.

In applying the ISM to medical students, the *learner* is represented as a form of complex adaptive system (CAS).(48) The CAS is built of interacting microsystems in which alignment of new material to be learned with the student's existing cognitive structure (also called 'scaffolding') is critical for learning to occur. Within the ISM, students are characterised as learning workers. Their mission is to learn the knowledge, skills, abilities and professional attributes that will prepare them for practice. The *superstructure* of the ISM is built upon Stufflebeam's Context, Inputs, Processes and Products (CIPP)(49) evaluation model and augmented by several models from human factors engineering.(50,51) The student is the sum of the Inputs, Processes and Products and an *upper change loop*. The upper change loop is critical to adapting to the world and enabling the learner to adapt to the demands of medical education. The *context* envelopes the student and provides the environment in which the student operates – the educational institution and larger community. The *inputs* for a student are what they bring with them to their latest learning job, including the sum of their genetics, education, life experiences, social supports and reserve capacity. The *process* is the means by which the student learns.

The *reserve* is the region that sits atop the inputs into which resources are sequestered for needs beyond the norm. The reserve powers the change loop, which enables the learner to do what it takes to succeed. The change loop is there to 'plug gaps'. The degree of alignment of new material with the existing cognitive structure and processes will determine the degree of energy needed to learn.

If the student's cognitive framework has a gap that leaves no way to absorb new material, the new material must be reduced to a level that the gap can be filled, and then the new material absorbed. Even if the cognitive structure has a fit for the new material and can absorb it, repetition is necessary to ensure that the fit endures.

Breaking sophisticated material down to a more basic level to fill a gap requires the expenditure of substantial time and energy. This engages the change loop and draws on reserves. Even if the instructor does the task of breaking the material down, the learners must fill the gap before they can absorb the material that is expected, essentially a double load. In terms of time, it is even more. The brain must be able to restructure in response to the new material. This requires downtime, when the learner is focusing on other things, such as sleeping, exercising or socialising. Without restructuring, there comes a point where to absorb new material, material that has already been absorbed needs to be expelled. This is counterproductive, and learning starts to shut down no matter how hard the learner tries. A learner cannot afford to have too much of their reserves devoted to filling gaps or they will fall behind.

Unlike previous applications of the ISM, where change was different from the norm, students are learning workers.(52) Their primary mission is to learn and evolve to become a more skilled individual who can assume professional roles and perform more complex tasks. For a learning-worker, learning itself generates resource return, as well as the reinforcement received from the system, such as grades or promotion. These things build back the reserves needed to keep the learner at work.

The ISM is a radical departure from models that typically describe undergraduate medical education because of: (i) the characterisation of students and teachers as CASs; (ii) the concept of resource reserves needed for learning; (iii) the need to align content complexity and structure of instruction with the existing level of cognitive development; and (iv) the need for alignment of the instructional operations with the research and service operations of the institution. Additionally, the integration of different models in one organism represents a clarification of the different types of change models and how they relate to one another. Despite its unique characteristics, the ISM melds well with findings from primary PBL research.

Effectiveness of PBL

The question that has dogged PBL since its inception has been to what degree it produces the types of change in learners that it was designed to produce. This includes self-directed learners who have a deeper knowledge of their discipline and who are better prepared to apply the science of medicine to patient care. Demonstrating these changes, however, has been a daunting challenge. Over the past 40 years, there have been hundreds of studies designed to test these differences, and at least 20 major reviews since 1990.(e.g., 5–7,29,53–56)

The attempts to do systematic reviews have either resorted to a very small set of controlled studies (*see* Vernon and Blake;(57) Newman;(58) Colliver(44)) or adopted a thematic approach (*see* Berkson(53)) or what might be called a 'best evidence approach', which used effect sizes when possible and a thematic approach when not (*see* Albanese and Mitchell(6)). For those who are certain that PBL is the best thing since sliced bread, these reviews have been disappointing. Newman summarised the earlier reviews as:

> Vernon and Blake (1993) concluded 'results generally support the superiority of the PBL approach over more traditional academic methods.' Albanese and Mitchell (1993) whilst acknowledging the weaknesses of the research literature concluded that PBL was more nurturing and enjoyable and that PBL graduates performed as well and sometimes better on clinical examinations and faculty evaluations. However, they also concluded that PBL graduates showed potentially important gaps in their cognitive knowledge base, did not demonstrate expert reasoning patterns, and that PBL was very costly. Berkson (1993) was unequivocal in her conclusion that 'the graduate of PBL is not distinguishable from his or her traditional counterpart'. She further argued that the experience of PBL can be stressful for the student and faculty and implementation may be unrealistically costly. The two more recent reviews also came to differing conclusions. Van den Bossche and colleagues (2000) concluded that PBL had a positive robust effect on the skills of students but a negative non-robust effect on knowledge. The review by Smits and colleagues (2002a) concluded that there was no consistent evidence that PBL is superior to other educational strategies in improving doctors knowledge and performance.((58, p. 13)

Newman's review was no more encouraging. Only for the outcome 'accumulation of knowledge' were there more than three studies that met the inclusion criteria. For this outcome, of 39 effect sizes computed, 16 favoured the PBL group and 23 the control. Generally, the state of the literature was not sufficient to make much out of it in his pilot review.

Dochy and colleagues(59) performed a meta-analysis of 43 studies, concluding that PBL had a negative effect on the knowledge base of students (effect size = −0.776) but a positive effect on their application of that knowledge (effect size = +0.658). Gijbels and colleagues(60) reported another meta-analysis of 40 studies in which they analysed the effects of PBL as a function of the type of cognitive skill assessed in the outcome: Concepts, Principles and Application. They found a slight negative effect size for concepts (−0.042) and positive effect sizes for Principles and Application (0.748 and 0.401, respectively).

However, I think the analysis of PBL must make a distinction between those studies conducted before and from 1993. The three reviews that came out that year apparently moved curricula towards what might be called 'hybrids' – a combination of structured activities directed at giving students the disciplinary conceptual frameworks (usually via lecture) combined with substantial time devoted to PBL. At the risk of 'cherry-picking' only the studies that have shown positive results, I will highlight what I think have been some of the findings of interest in that period. One of the more compelling studies comes from ten years

BOX 5.3 Effect sizes for MCAT and USMLE Steps 1 and 2 for pre-PBL, transition and post-PBL classes

Variable	1996 Pre-PBL	1997 Transition year	1998–2005/6 PBL years
MCAT	−0.23	−0.18	−0.06 (−0.17 to 0.07)
USMLE Step 1	−0.25	−0.10	0.30 (0.10 to 0.60)
USMLE Step 2	−0.50	0.00	0.38 (0.25 to 0.50)

of experience with PBL at the University of Missouri-Columbia. Hoffman *et al.*(61) present results for the USMLE Steps 1 and 2, and residency director perceptions of their graduate versus all other graduates for the period one year before implementation of PBL (1996 graduating year) and post-implementation (1997–2006 graduating years). The performances of the classes on the MCAT were also presented to demonstrate to what extent USMLE performance diverged from the pattern of MCAT scores. Hoffman *et al.* presented their results as effect sizes, with national means and standard deviations serving as comparison values for those from Missouri. Hoffman *et al.*'s results were presented in graph form; I estimated their values from the graphs to arrive at effect sizes for the year before PBL was implemented, the transition year (first year of PBL) and the mean effect size over the eight to nine years during which PBL was operating. The results are shown in Box 5.3.

Using MCAT effect sizes as an index for student entering academic ability, one would expect the Step 1 and Step 2 effect sizes to be comparable, unless the curriculum somehow affected the students' ability in a disproportionate way. In the pre-PBL year, the Step 1 effect size was almost identical to the MCAT effect size, which was approximately one-quarter of a standard deviation below the national mean. The Step 2 effect size was even more negative, approximately one-half standard deviation below the national mean. There was a relatively dramatic improvement in the transitional year that continued for the eight-to-nine years, since PBL was introduced into the curriculum. In that period, the MCAT effect sizes have risen from −0.23 to −0.06, but the changes in Step 1 and Step 2 have been stunning, rising to 0.30 and 0.38, respectively. Thus, during the PBL period, Step 1 and Step 2 performance exceeded, by over one-third of a standard deviation, that which would have been predicted from MCAT scores. Even more impressive is that the improvement in scores has been sustained over such a long period. The type of PBL used in the curriculum at Missouri would probably be termed 'hybrid'. They have about ten hours of lecture concurrent with an equal amount of time spent in PBL. This exceeds the limit on lectures that Barrows(3) recommended (1.5 hours per day; 7.5 hours per week). One other point is that concurrent with implementing PBL, they reduced the class size from 112 to 96 students. While the smaller class size may have

had some impact on the findings, it is hard to believe that this alone could have made such a large difference.

Examples of other recent findings include the survey responses Schmidt *et al.*(62) obtained from 820 of 2,081 (39 per cent) graduates of a PBL school and 621 of 3,268 (19 per cent) graduates of a traditional school in the Netherlands, regarding self-ratings of professional competence. For interpersonal competencies such as working in a team, interpersonal skills and skills required for running meetings, the PBL graduates rated themselves more skilled by an effect size of a whopping 1.30. For PBL-related competencies such as self-directed learning, problem-solving and information-gathering, the PBL graduates rated themselves as more highly skilled by an effect size of 0.78. For general academic competencies and task-supporting competencies, the differences were 0.14 and 031, respectively, which are small yet more positive for PBL graduates.

Schafer *et al.*(63) recently reported a randomised trial of PBL versus traditional curricula, regarding basic science and clinical knowledge. Students who had applied for the PBL track but due to limits on numbers were randomly assigned to the PBL track ($N = 122$) or to the traditional track ($N = 129$), and the remaining students in the traditional track ($N = 617$) were compared at three time points (beginning of first, third and fifth semester) using a 200-item progress test (1/3 basic science, 2/3 clinical). The results showed comparable gains by all groups on the basic science portion of the exam; however, by the third administration performance on the clinical section by the PBL students exceeded that of the other two groups by effect sizes greater than 1.17.

My colleagues and I have(64) examined the relationship of undergraduate science grade point averages (SGPA) to Step 1 failure rate for students in a PBL track and traditional track at one medical school and those at three other traditional medical schools. The relationship between the total MCAT score and Step 1 failure is shown in Figure 5.1.

The SGPA cutpoints represented in Figure 5.1 were obtained by 'cutting off' the group of examinees who fell below the cutpoint, and computing the percentage of those who failed Step 1. Thus, for 3.0, the examinees who had an SGPA below 3.0 were separated off and the percentage of those who failed Step 1 was determined and plotted on the graph. Although the overall failure rates for the three different groups were not different by a large margin (2 per cent), the pattern by which the three different groups reached the overall failure rate was strikingly different for the PBL track. While the traditional track and the three traditional medical schools had a relatively linear relationship between SGPA and Step 1 failure rate, the PBL school had almost no failures among those with SGPA values below 3.0. However, for SGPA values between 3.0 and 3.4, the PBL students had a much higher failure rate. Beyond an SGPA of 3.4, the failure rates of the different schools merged together.

These results raise the spectre that PBL may be better for some students, particularly those who have had relatively poor grades in prior course work (SGPA < 3.0), and worse for students who did relatively well, but not stellar, in prior course work (SGPA = 3.0–3.4). These results need to be

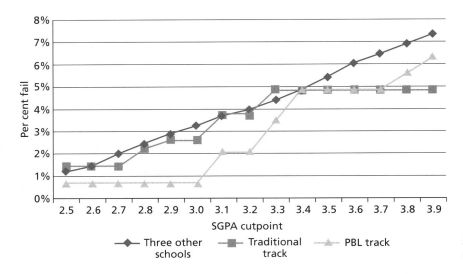

Figure 5.1 MCAT Step 1 failure rate vs. SGPA cutpoint.

confirmed with other schools but may explain why the results from studies of PBL have been so variable. If some students do better and others do worse, effects will be difficult to find as they will cancel each other out (*see* Box 5.4). Another factor that may affect studies of PBL is that Schmidt *et al.*(65) found the attrition rates of PBL schools in the Netherlands to be substantially below that of the conventional schools. Assuming academic problems are the main reason for attrition, the higher rate of elimination of poorer-performing students in the conventional schools may inflate their outcomes, masking the overall poorer performance of students in the conventional curricula.(66)

Summary

Beginning a PBL curriculum is not for the faint-hearted. There is much infrastructure that needs to be put into place, and there may be increased costs. While the effectiveness of PBL appears to be gaining better documentation, and we are gaining a better understanding of how to do PBL, there is still much we need to learn. In the meantime, it is important for anyone involved in implementing PBL to keep in mind what it is that one is trying to accomplish. Dolmans *et al.*(5) identified four important processes underlying PBL based on recent learning principles that provide a good synopsis of what one is trying to accomplish with PBL. These four processes are that learning should be a:
- constructive process
- self-directed process
- collaborative process
- contextual process.

By a constructive process, we mean that learning is an active process by which students 'construct or reconstruct their knowledge networks'. A self-directed process is one where learners are involved in planning, monitoring and evaluating the learning process. A collaborative learning process is one in which the social structure involves two or more students interacting, with a common goal, shared

BOX 5.4 WHERE'S THE EVIDENCE: For the effectiveness of PBL?

Reviews of PBL have generally been disappointing, showing at best that PBL is no worse than the traditional curriculum, but not consistently better. In recent years, more schools have moved to hybrid curricula, and there have been some notable successes and intriguing complexities identified.

Hoffman *et al.* present results for the United States Medical Licensing Examination (USMLE) Steps 1 and 2, and residency director perceptions of their graduates versus all other graduates that showed effect sizes over one-third of a standard deviation beyond what would be expected, based on the student's entering academic performance.

Schmidt *et al.*'s survey of graduates of a PBL school and traditional school in the Netherlands regarding self-ratings of professional competence found effect sizes from 0.78 to 1.3 for PBL-related competencies.

Schafer *et al.* reported a randomised trial of PBL versus traditional curricula regarding basic and clinical knowledge and found PBL students' performance on the clinical knowledge section exceeded that of the other groups by effect sizes greater than 1.17.

My colleagues and I examined the relationship of Medical College Admission Test (MCAT) and undergraduate science grade point averages (SGPA) to Step 1 failure rate for students in a PBL track and traditional track at one medical school and those at three other traditional medical schools. The relationship between the total MCAT score and SGPAs and Step 1 failure indicated that some students who do less well academically have lower-than-expected Step 1 failure rates and others who do better academically have higher-than-expected Step 1 failure rates in a PBL curriculum. This suggests that the problem demonstrating PBL effects may be due to differential effect for differing students.

BOX 5.5 FOCUS ON: The PBL Best Practices Consortium

PBL has been in existence for over 30 years. While there has been much research on it, there are elements that can best be described as relying on superstition and tradition. In establishing the PBL Best Practices Consortium, my goal was to develop a collection of individuals who were actively involved in conducting PBL, and tap their collective wisdom. I have defined a best practice as something that you wish someone had or did tell you before you started. Dues for enrolling in the group are the submission of one or more best practices that one wishes to share (although I have included some members who wanted to be involved in the e-conversations who were not actively involved in PBL). These enrolment dues were some of the sources of the recommendations in this paper (all attributed). I also plan to send monthly questions to the group, to collect a compendium of best practices. Through this means, I hope to dispel myths, or at least provide justification for their existence.

responsibilities, mutual dependency and a need to reach agreement through open interaction. A contextual process recognises that learning is context bound and that transfer to different contexts requires confronting cases or problems from multiple perspectives. No matter how someone decides to implement PBL ultimately, it is important that as they design their experience they keep clearly in mind what they are trying to accomplish and do not become distracted from their goal.

Acknowledgements

In addition to the literature cited I draw upon comments from selected members of the PBL Best Practices Consortium; Dennis Baker, Stephen Davis, David Matheson and Gail Swarm. Members of the Consortium offer best practices, things they wish someone had told them (or did tell them) about how to implement PBL, in response to monthly questions that I post to the group. Participation in the consortium is free and anyone can become a member by emailing me at: maalbane@wisc.edu (*see* Box 5.5) (details correct at the time of writing).

References

1 Neville AJ and Norman GR (2007) PBL in the undergraduate MD program at McMaster University: three iterations in three decades. *Academic Medicine*. **82**(4): 370–4.

2 Barrows HS (1986) A taxonomy of problem-based learning methods. *Medical Education*. **20**: 481–6.

3 Barrows HS (1985) *How to Design a Problem-based Curriculum for the Preclinical Years*. Springer, New York.

4 Wood DF (2003) ABC of learning and teaching in medicine: problem based learning. *British Medical Journal*. **326**: 328–30.

5 Dolmans DHJM, De Grave W, Wolfhagen IHAP and van der Vleuten CPM (2005) Problem-based learning: future challenges for educational practice and research. *Medical Education*. **39**: 732–41.

6 Albanese MA and Mitchell S (1993) Problem-based learning: a review of literature on its outcomes and implementation issues. *Academic Medicine*. **68**: 52–81.

7 Jones JW, Bieber LL, Echt R *et al.* (1984) A problem-based curriculum – ten years of experience. In: Schmidt HG and de Volder ML (eds) *Tutorials in Problem-based Learning*, pp. 181–98. Van Gorcum, Assen, Maastricht.

8 Wales CE and Stager R (1972) Design of an educational system. *Engineering Education*. **62**: 456–9.

9 Pawlak SM, Popovich NG, Blank JW and Russell JD (1989) Development and validation of guided design scenarios for problem-solving instruction. *American Journal of Pharmaceutical Education*. **53**: 7–16.

10 Hays R (2002) Problems with problems in problem-based curricula. *Medical Education*. **36**: 790.

11 Dolmans DHJM, Gijselaers WH and Schmidt HG (1992) Do students learn what their teachers intend they learn? Guiding processes in problem-based learning. Paper presented at the Annual Meeting of the American Educational Research Association, San Francisco, CA, April.

12 Coulson RL and Osborne CE (1984) Insuring curricular content in a student-directed problem-based learning program. In: Schmidt HG and de Volder ML (eds) *Tutorials in Problem-based Learning*, pp. 225–9. Van Gorcum, Assen, Maastricht.

13 Dornan T, Scherpbier A, King N and Boshuizen H (2005) Clinical teachers and problem-based learning: a phenomenological study. *Medical Education*. **39**: 163–70.

14 Miflin B (2004) Problem-based learning: the confusion continues. *Medical Education*. **38**: 921–6.

15 Eagle CJ, Harasym PH and Mandin H (1992) Effects of tutors with case expertise on problem-based learning issues. *Academic Medicine*. **67**: 465–9.

16 Davis WK, Nairn R, Paine ME *et al.* (1992) Effects of expert and non-expert facilitators on the small-group process and on student performance. *Academic Medicine*. **67**: 470–4.

17 Zeitz HJ and Paul H (1993) Facilitator expertise and problem-based learning in PBL and traditional curricula. *Academic Medicine*. **68**(3): 203–4.

18 Albanese M (2004) Treading tactfully on tutor turf: does PBL tutor content expertise make a difference? *Medical Education*. **38**: 916–20.

19 Bowman D and Hughes P (2005) Emotional responses of tutors and students in problem-based learning: lessons for staff development. *Medical Education*. **39**(2): 145–53.

20 Farrell T, Albanese MA and Pomrehn P (1999) Problem-based learning in ophthalmology: a pilot program for curricular renewal. *Archives of Ophthalmology*. **117**: 1223–6.

21 Khaliq F (2005) Introduction of problem-solving activities during conventional lectures. *Medical Education*. **39**: 1146–7.

22 Albanese M, Mejicano G, Xakellis G and Kokotailo P (2009) Physician practice change: a critical review and description of an integrated systems model. *Academic Medicine*. **84**(8): 1043–55.

23 Gonnella J, Erdmann J and Hojat M (2004) An empirical study of the predictive validity of number grades in medical school using three decades of longitudinal data: implications for a grading system. *Medical Education*. **38**: 425–34.

24 Julian ER (2005) Validity of the Medical College Admission Test for predicting medical school performance. *Academic Medicine*. **80**(10): 910–7.

25 Kerfoot BP, Masser BA and Hafler JP (2005) Influence of new educational technology on problem-based learning at Harvard Medical School. *Medical Education*. **39**(4): 380–7.

26 Nolte J, Eller P and Ringel SP (1988) Shifting toward problem-based learning in a medical school neurobiology course. In: *Research in Medical Education, 1988: Proceedings of the Twenty-Seventh Annual*

Conference, pp. 66–71. Association of American Medical Colleges, Washington, DC.

27 Barrows HS and Tamblyn RM (1976) An evaluation of problem-based learning in small groups utilizing a simulated patient. *Journal of Medical Education*. **51**: 52–4.

28 Nendaz MR and Tekian A (1999) Assessment in problem-based learning medical schools: a literature review. *Teaching and Learning in Medicine*. **11**(4): 232–43.

29 Case S and Swanson D (2001) *Constructing Written Test Questions for the Basic and Clinical Sciences* (3e). National Board of Medical Examiners, Philadelphia. (http://www.nbme.org/PDF/2001iwg.pdf; accessed 24 October 2006).

30 Van der Vleuten CPM, Verwijnen GM and Wijnen WHFW (1996) Fifteen years of experience with Progress Testing in a problem-based learning curriculum. *Medical Teacher*. **18**: 103–9.

31 Boshuizen HP, van der Vleuten CP, Schmidt HG and Machiels-Bongaerts M (1997) Measuring knowledge and clinical reasoning skills in a problem-based curriculum. *Medical Education*. **31**: 115–21.

32 Blake JM, Norman GR, Keane DR *et al.* (1996) Introducing progress testing in McMaster University's problem-based medical curriculum: psychometric properties and effect on learning. *Academic Medicine*. **71**: 1002–7.

33 Saunders NA, McIntosh J, McPherson J and Engel CE (1990) A comparison between University of Newcastle and University of Sydney final-year students: knowledge and competence. In: Nooman ZM, Schmidt HG and Ezzat ES (eds) *Innovation in Medical Education: An Evaluation of Its Present Status*, pp. 50–63, Springer, New York.

34 McGuire CH and Babbott D (1967) Simulation technique in the measurement of problem-solving skills. *Journal of Educational Measurement*. **4**(1): 1–10.

35 Painvin C, Neufeld V, Norman G, Walker I and Whelan G (1979) The 'triple jump' exercise–a structured measure of problem solving and self directed learning. *Annual Conference on Research in Medical Education*. **18**: 73–7.

36 Harden RM, Stevenson M, Downie WW and Wilson GM (1975) Assessment of clinical competence using objective structured examination. *British Medical Journal*. **1**: 447–51.

37 Hebert R and Bravo G (1996) Development and validation of an evaluation instrument for medical students in tutorials. *Academic Medicine*. **71**(5): 488–94.

38 Landouceur MG, Rideout DM, Black ME, Crooks DL, O'Mara LM and Schmuck ML (2004) Development of an instrument to assess individual student performance in small group tutorials. *Journal of Nursing Education*. **43**(10): 447–55.

39 Eva KW, Solomon P, Neville AJ *et al.* (2007) Using a sampling strategy to address psychometric challenges in tutorial-based assessments. *Advances in Health Sciences Education*. **12**(1): 19–33.

40 Chaves JF, Baker CM, Chaves JA and Fisher ML (2006) Self, peer and tutor assessments of MSN competencies using the PBL-evaluator. *Journal of Nursing Education*. **45**(1): 25–31.

41 Sim SM, Azila NM, Lian L, Tan CP and Tan NH (2006) A simple instrument for the assessment of student performance in problem-based learning tutorials. *Annals of the Academy of Medicine, Singapore*. **35**(9): 634–41.

42 Kruger J and Dunning D (1999) Unskilled and unaware of it: how difficulties in recognizing one's own incompetence lead to inflated self-assessments. *Journal of Personality and Social Psychology*. **77**(6): 1121–34.

43 Ward M, Gruppen L and Regehr G (2002) Measuring self-assessment: current state of the art. *Advances in Health Sciences Education*. **7**: 63–80.

44 Colliver J (2000) Effectiveness of problem based learning curricula. *Academic Medicine*. **75**: 259–66.

45 Schmidt HG (1983) Problem-based learning: rationale and description. *Medical Education*. **17**: 11–6.

46 Qin Z, Johnson DW and Johnson RT (1995) Cooperative versus competitive efforts and problem solving. *Review of Educational Research*. **65**(2): 129–43.

47 Williams GC, Saizow RB and Ryan RM (1999) The importance of self-determination theory for medical education. *Academic Medicine*. **74**(9): 992–5.

48 Plsek P (2001) Redesigning health care with insights from the science of complex adaptive systems. In: Committee on the Quality of Health Care in America (ed.) *Crossing the Quality Chasm: A New Health System for the 21st Century*, pp. 309–23. The National Academies Press, Washington, DC. (http://www.nap.edu/openbook.php?record_id=10027&page=309; accessed 22 March 2012).

49 Stufflebeam DL (2000) The CIPP model for evaluation. Chapter 16. In: Stufflebeam DL, Madaus GF and Kellaghan Y (eds) *Evaluation Models* (2e). Kluwer Academic Publishers, Boston, MA.

50 Carayon P, Schoofs Hundt A, Karsh B-T *et al.* (2006) Work system design for patient safety: the SEIPS model. *Quality and Safety in Health Care*. **15**: i50–8.

51 Karsh BT, Holden RJ, Alper SJ and Or CK (2006) A human factors engineering paradigm for patient safety: designing to support the performance of the healthcare professional. *Quality and Safety in Health Care*. **15**: 59–65.

52 Albanese MA (1999) Students are not customers: a new model for medical education. *Academic Medicine*. **74**(11): 1172–84.

53 Berkson L (1993) Problem-based learning: have the expectations been met? *Academic Medicine*. **68**(10): S79–88.

54 Norman GR and Schmidt HG (1992) The psychological basis of PBL. A review of the evidence. *Academic Medicine*. **67**(9): 557–65.

55 Smits P, Verbeek J and De Buisonje C (2002) Problem based learning in continuing medical education: a review of controlled evaluation studies. *British Medical Journal*. **324**: 153–6.

56 Van den Bossche P, Gijbels D and Dochy F (2000) Does problem based learning educate problem solvers? A meta-analysis on the effects of problem based learning. Paper presented at the VII EDINEB Conference, Newport Beach, CA, June 21–3, 2000.

57 Vernon DTA and Blake RL (1993) Does problem-based learning work? A meta-analysis of evaluative research. *Academic Medicine*. **68**: 550–63.

58 Newman M (2003) A Pilot Systematic Review and Meta-Analysis on the Effectiveness of Problem Based Learning. On behalf of the Campbell Collaboration Systematic Review Group on the effectiveness of problem based learning. Learning and Teaching Support Network, University of Newcastle, Newcastle.

59 Dochy F, Segers M, Van den Bossche P and Gijbels D (2003) Effects of problem-based learning: a meta-analysis. *Learning & Instruction*. **13**: 533–68.

60 Gijbels D, Dochy F, Van den Bossche P and Segers M (2005) Effects of problem-based learning: a meta-analysis from the angle of assessment. *Review of Educational Research*. **75**: 27–61.

61 Hoffman K, Hosokawa M, Blake R *et al.* (2006) Problem-based learning outcomes: ten years of experience at the University of Missouri-Columbia School of Medicine. *Academic Medicine*. **81**(7): 617–25.

62 Schmidt HG, Vermeulen L and van der Molen HT (2006) Long-term effects of problem-based learning on the attitudes of undergraduate health care students. *Medical Education*. **40**(6): 562–7.

63 Schafer T, Huenges B, Burger A and Rusche H (2006) A randomized controlled study on the progress in knowledge in a traditional versus problem-based curriculum. Proceedings of the 2006 Annual Meeting of the Association for Medical Education in Europe, Cotone Congressi, Genoa, Italy, 14–18 September. Abstract 10H2, . 208.

64 Albanese MA, Colliver J and Dottl SL (2006) Disrupting the tyranny of prior academic performance. Does PBL help or hinder. Proceedings of the 2006 Annual Meeting of the Association for Medical Education in Europe, Cotone Congressi, Genoa, Italy, 14–18 September. Abstract 10H1, . 208.

65 Schmidt HG, Cohen-Schotanus J and Arends LR (2009) Impact of problem-based, active learning on graduation rates for 10 generations of Dutch medical students. *Medical Education.* **43**: 211–8.

66 Albanese MA (2009) Life is tough for curriculum researchers. *Medical Education.* **43**: 199–201.

Further reading

Albanese M (2000) Problem based learning: why curricula are likely to show little effect on knowledge and clinical skills. *Medical Education.* **34**: 729–38.

Albanese MA and Mitchell S (1993) Problem-based learning: a review of literature on its outcomes and implementation issues. *Academic Medicine.* **68**: 52–81.

Barrows HS (1985) *How to Design a Problem-based Curriculum for the Preclinical Years.* Springer, New York.

Davis MH and Harden RM (1999) AMEE medical education guide number 15: problem-based learning: a practical guide. *Medical Teacher.* **21**: 130–40.

Norman GR and Schmidt HG (2000) Effectiveness of problem-based learning curricula: theory, practice and paper darts. *Medical Education.* **34**: 721–8.

6 Interprofessional education

Della Freeth

Centre for Medical Education, Queen Mary University of London, UK

> **ⓘ KEY MESSAGES**
>
> - Interprofessional education (IPE) is just a special case of professional education, so knowledge about good practice for learning and teaching in a wide range of contexts can be applied directly to IPE.
>
> - The uniqueness of IPE lies in deliberately creating heterogeneous groups. By bringing together participants from different professions around a particular task, it is anticipated that the increased diversity of knowledge and perspectives will enhance the learning of all.
>
> - The *raison d'être* for IPE is to enhance professional practice; uniprofessional as well as interprofessional.
>
> - Poorly planned or delivered IPE may be damaging if it generates a reluctance to engage in subsequent interprofessional collaboration or reinforces negative stereotypes.
>
> - IPE is not limited to formally planned and overtly labelled education. Whenever practitioners meet in multiprofessional groups to address complex needs or service evaluations and improvements, there is potential for interprofessional learning. This serendipitous IPE is a feature of daily practice.

Introduction

My starting position is that interprofessional education (IPE) is simply a special case of professional education, so all that we know about good practice in professional education applies to IPE too. What is different about IPE is a conscious decision to amplify the heterogeneity of learning groups.

Second, I view professional education as the range of formally planned and serendipitous experiences which, aided by reflection and a process of trying things out, form and continually modify our professional knowledge and practical wisdom.

I stress this broad view of education, a vibrant patchwork of experiences informing a lifelong project of development, because too much that is said about education portrays it narrowly as formal units of planned content. This view is often further restricted by the expectation of delivery by especially designated people in especially designated places using currently approved means of transmission and assessment. This is not to argue against formally planned and overtly labelled IPE delivered by university faculty and experienced health care professionals in a range of learning environments. Rather, it is a plea that in addition to valuing the important contributions of formal IPE, we should notice and value the contributions of *informal* interprofessional learning. *Both are inextricably linked to professional practice – (hopefully) high-quality interprofessional collaboration founded on complementary professional contributions to care.*Naturally, more will be said about formal IPE;

after all, serendipitous IPE happens spontaneously. But it is not quite that simple; geography, shared interests or problems, and organisational structures and cultures can promote or inhibit informal and serendipitous interprofessional learning. Some of these factors are amenable to re-engineering.

Defining interprofessional education

The most widely recognised and robustly debated definition of IPE was developed by the UK Centre for the Advancement of Interprofessional Education (CAIPE): 'Interprofessional education occurs when two or more professions learn with, from and about each other to improve collaboration and the quality of care'.[1,2] CAIPE elaborated this definition, stating that IPE includes: '. . . all such learning in academic and work-based settings before and after qualification, adopting an inclusive view of "professional" '.[2]

A number of key points can be drawn from the definition. Namely, that:
- education is defined by the occurrence of learning
- 'with, from and about' necessitates *active* learning and implies learning based on some type of exchange
- the main aims are to improve both collaboration and care.

IPE then is not just about a mixed group of people acquiring the *same* knowledge or developing the *same* clinical skill. This can be made clearer by oversimplifying for a

---

Understanding Medical Education: Evidence, Theory and Practice, Second Edition. Edited by Tim Swanwick.
© 2014 The Association for the Study of Medical Education. Published 2014 by John Wiley & Sons, Ltd.

BOX 6.1 Seven principles of interprofessional education

In 2006 the UK Centre for the Advancement of Interprofessional Education (CAIPE) published a vision of effective IPE,(1) summarised as seven principles. Namely that interprofessional education:

- works to improve the quality of care
- focuses on the needs of service users and carers
- involves service user and carers
- encourages professions to learn with, from and about each other
- respects the integrity and contribution of each profession
- enhances practice within professions
- increases personal satisfaction.

BOX 6.2 FOCUS ON: Competing terms

A proliferation of prefixes (such as inter-, multi- and trans-) and adjectives (such as shared, common, professional and disciplinary), combined with organisational and educational nouns (such as agency, sector and provider; learning, education and training) creates a confusing array of competing and inconsistently used phrases to describe IPE and related activities. For example, multidisciplinary education, shared learning, interagency training. People can mean the same or different things when they use these terms, necessitating clarification of what is meant and assumed. Provided below are simple descriptions of three commonly used terms in this area.

Interprofessional education
Learning with, from and about each other to improve collaboration and the quality of care.

Multiprofessional education
Learning side by side for whatever reason.

Uniprofessional education
The mainstay of pre-registration education and a substantial proportion of post-registration education. Consequently an important venue for the development of knowledge, skills and attitudes needed to underpin effective teamwork.

moment. During the exchanges of active IPE, representatives of profession X will learn about the expertise and perspectives of representatives of profession Y; meanwhile representatives of profession Y learn about the expertise and perspectives of representatives of profession X. Hopefully, all participants learn something about themselves and their own professional practice. In this way, everyone learns something different and can subsequently use that learning to enhance working as a particular type of professional within a multidisciplinary team.

CAIPE also developed seven principles(1) to guide provision, commissioning, development and evaluation of IPE (*see* Box 6.1). These have since been elaborated as values and principles for processes and outcomes.(3) The principles in Box 6.1 frame IPE as learning to practise in ways that are better for the people we serve, and better for ourselves and our colleagues because we focus on making a useful contribution to a collaborative effort. It is about trying to create a climate within which the different contributions of any pertinent people and organisations are valued, and, as far as is possible, well understood and well coordinated. IPE is not an instrument for creating generic health workers, smashing the power of professions or reducing funding.

Complementary forms of education

Interprofessional education is inextricably linked to multiprofessional education (MPE) and uniprofessional education (UPE). MPE is normally taken to be occasions when members or students of two or more professions learn side by side for whatever reason. Often this is because they have a common need to address particular content. Shared lectures and shared clinical skills sessions are examples of MPE. These only become IPE if active, exchange-based learning can be woven into the educational experience. MPE may provide some opportunities for interprofessional learning during relatively undirected time, for example, breaks or small group work. This is not meant to suggest that MPE is a good first step towards IPE: studies have

found that MPE can lead to resentment.(4) If the benefits of an interprofessional gathering are not realized, each group of participants can feel that their education is being 'diluted'. UPE will form the bulk of any pre-registration professional curriculum and may continue to form a substantial proportion of post-registration continuing education and workplace learning. Uniprofessional learning is, therefore, an extremely important venue for the development of knowledge, skills and attitudes that underpin interprofessional collaboration.

Competing terms

Unfortunately, from place to place, and author to author, there is inconsistency in the use of the terms IPE and MPE, and there is an unhelpful proliferation of terms used to describe IPE and MPE. There seems little point wading deeply into this 'semantic quagmire'.(5) It should be sufficient to remain mindful that when people use these competing and overlapping terms, they *may* do so inconsistently, with a vision that differs from your vision and without a clear conception of the defining features of this type of education. It will always be necessary to ascertain 'what exactly is being spoken of here?' *See* Box 6.2.

Some writers regard IPE as old-fashioned and inappropriately focused, preferring interprofessional *learning* (IPL). While the shift to focusing on learning is an important educational movement, the most widely adopted view of

IPE(1) defines education by the occurrence of learning, rendering the IPE/IPL debate redundant.

The recognition of competing terms and fashions is important because an unthinking rejection of differently labelled work could dislocate us from a rich heritage of valuable insights catalogued under terms that are not familiar or not currently in vogue. On the other hand, unthinking acceptance may have us working at cross-purposes with others.

The rationale for interprofessional education

The drivers for IPE have been well elaborated by a range of authors.(6–9) I do not intend to summarise all their arguments here. Instead, I will sketch out some key points that underpin the particular perspective I have taken in this chapter.

- Health care is delivered by multidisciplinary teams so interprofessional practice is inevitable. IPE may help to develop insights, shared knowledge and teamwork skills that promote effective collaboration to deliver high-quality care efficiently.
- The pace of change in the 21st century is very high, and there seems to be no end to increasing workloads. Perhaps these pressures and an attendant perception of fragmentation increase the felt need for formally identified IPE, while in gentler times less formal interprofessional learning opportunities might have been spotted and developed with little need for overt labelling and resource allocation.
- Concerns to monitor and promote equality of opportunity may also increase pressure to overtly label IPE and examine who is able to participate. Informality, while a great boon to creativity, can be susceptible to unintended and unexamined bias.
- In modern health care, traditional hierarchies, roles and boundaries are continually challenged because they have the potential to inhibit the efficient delivery of sound care. IPE can make a range of contributions to the ongoing challenge and renegotiation of established ways of thinking and being. For example, it can help participants to appreciate the contributions of different members of the team; it can promote shared examination of multifaceted problems and the formation of team plans, rather than a tangle of criss-crossing separate responses; it may promote healing and collaboration, when external pressures have damaged collaborative practice in a particular setting.
- When things go wrong in health care, subsequent investigations all too frequently identify failures in teamwork and failures in communication, often interprofessional or interagency teamwork and communication. IPE is often suggested as a contribution towards curing or immunising against poor collaboration. This has intuitive appeal and provides hints as to the nature of the required IPE.

Nevertheless, developing and sustaining good quality IPE takes significant effort. The following paragraphs may help you to focus your efforts efficiently and pragmatically.

By definition, IPE means bringing people from different groups together (physically or electronically). It is inevitable that this increases the complexity of agreeing mutually convenient times, finding a suitable venue and suitably skilled facilitators, identifying or creating learning resources that suit all participants; then negotiating responsibility for the associated costs and, where relevant, navigating the restrictions of multiple assessment schemes.

If the ideas and skills you wish to develop in a particular learning experience are not focused on improving both collaboration and the quality of care, there may be little gain in struggling to deliver that part of the overall curriculum on an interprofessional basis. This applies most strongly at the pre-registration level, where the number of potential participants can be huge and the assessment requirements of different professional curricula are least likely to match. Thus it is appropriate for most of each profession's curriculum to be delivered uniprofessionally. Nevertheless the pre-registration curriculum must address the nature of high-quality interprofessional collaboration for the effective delivery of high-quality care for many different needs in many different contexts. Within this, opportunities can be found to add value to the curriculum through interprofessional learning.

In post-qualification continuing professional development numbers are often smaller, assessment requirements may be more flexible and a higher proportion of educational activities will be concerned with improving the quality of collaboration and care for particular groups of people. Then the question 'Why do IPE?' becomes 'Why not do IPE?' Perhaps we should expect the majority of postgraduate education to be interprofessional.

Some aspects of improving interprofessional collaboration and improving care can be addressed quite well on a uniprofessional basis, reducing the need for IPE. For example, uniprofessional team-based activity, such as problem-based learning groups or action learning sets (*see* Chapters 5 and 9), may be a successful environment for facilitators to draw out learning about how teams function, the importance of diversity within team membership, the effects of people joining and leaving, and strategies for improving team functioning and individual contributions. These uniprofessional learning experiences may be sufficient in some circumstances; or they may be seen as having an important role in laying firm foundations for subsequent IPE that stretches learners a little further.

In addition to this pragmatic rationale for IPE, the evidence base is summarised in Box 6.3.

The diversity of interprofessional education

Elsewhere, colleagues and I have described a spectrum of IPE with two dimensions: first, variation in emphasis, and second, variation in the degree of planning and formalisation(49). It may be important for programme planners and course participants to be clear about where their IPE lies within this two-dimensional spectrum, since clarity

BOX 6.3 WHERE'S THE EVIDENCE: Interprofessional education

There are hundreds of peer-reviewed studies of interprofessional education (IPE), but their quality is variable and it is wise to pay most attention to the stronger studies. (10–12) Methodological approaches to researching IPE should be aligned with the aims, principles and processes of the particular IPE under investigation and pay heed to needs for improving practice, informing policy and increasing understanding.(13) Since IPE varies widely in its intentions, style and contexts, and studies vary in their purposes and intended audiences, wide variation should be expected in approaches to studying IPE.

Post-registration IPE

For post-registration learners there is evidence that IPE (mostly embedded in quality improvement initiatives) can improve the quality of care and the quality of working lives. To name just a few examples:

- progress with reducing infections and need for supplemental oxygen in neonatal intensive care(14) and reducing costs(15)
- improved preventative care, including increased screening or immunisation rates(16–21)
- improved teamwork and fewer errors observed in emergency departments(22)
- more regular briefing and better teamwork in operating theatres(23)
- reduced use of physical restraint in nursing homes,(24) without increasing risk of falls(25)
- better functional gains in stroke rehabilitation(26)
- increased interprofessional participation in planning and reviewing care(27–29)
- smoother work systems(20,30–32)
- more patient-centred communication(29,33)

There are also good studies of interprofessional teamwork that can inform thinking about informal and serendipitous IPE, or identify needs for post-registration IPE.(34,35)

Pre-registration IPE

Pre-registration education is always an investment in the future based on a professional consensus about desired content, policy drivers and economic realities. Viewed in isolation, most parts of any profession's curriculum will have a limited evidence base, and two questions serve to illustrate this: Do we know that the pharmacology content of medical education is

effectively integrated in subsequent professional practice? What do we know about the effectiveness of studying ethics at the pre-qualification level? So if we view IPE as content, we should not expect there to be an extensive evidence base.

On the other hand, if we view IPE as an educational method the evidence base we might expect would relate to its acceptability to learners and faculty; IPE's success in increasing knowledge of the topics addressed, changing attitudes and changed behaviour; studies of development and delivery; and models of integration with the wider curriculum, including assessment matters. In many ways the structure of the IPE evidence base would be similar to the structure of the evidence bases relating to, say, problem-based learning (*see* Chapter 5), simulation (*see* Chapter 13), or supervision and mentoring (*see* Chapter 8), while recognising these fields are all at different stages of development.

In fact, studies of pre-registration IPE have provided a wide range of insights. The list below is illustrative not exhaustive, and the examples referenced are just a small selection from an ever- increasing pool.

- Sustainable models of delivery that, over time, can accommodate large numbers of students.(36–40)
- Variable responses from students from different professions.(4,36,37,41,42)
- The pace and level of IPE needs to be closely matched to participants' prior experience.(36)
- IPE can develop more positive perceptions of members of other professions and constructive 'mutual inter-group differentiation' (*see* Box 6.5), and a more sophisticated understanding or roles within teams.(43–45)
- IPE can usefully extend (but is not a substitute for) uniprofessional learning, but students sometimes feel tension between profession-specific and interprofessional learning objectives.(38,43,46)
- Rehearsing interprofessional teamwork is valued.(38,43)
- An interprofessional clerkship in primary care increased the comprehensiveness of care and the number of patients seen by medical students.(38)
- IPE can increase interest in working in places or specialties where there are recruitment shortfalls.(47)
- Patients are pleased with care provided by interprofessional student teams.(38,48)
- Medical students sometimes feel less supported by clinical supervisors than other professions' students.(36,48)

will help everyone to set realistic learning goals and to make sound decisions about inclusion and exclusion.

The emphasis dimension runs from a primary focus on interprofessional collaboration as the subject matter for the IPE(50–52) to a secondary focus on interprofessional collaboration and a primary focus elsewhere (e.g. particular client group,(14,30,53–55) particular professional

skills,(43,56,57) policy innovation,(22,58) improving systems,(31,59) and responding to audit(16,32)). Many IPE initiatives seek to pay balanced attention to interprofessional collaboration and some other substantive content.(36,37,60)

The planning and formalisation dimension recognises that unplanned interprofessional learning is very influential and should be acknowledged. This often happens in daily practice when members of different professions review their work together, or encounter something slightly out of the ordinary, causing them to pause, more closely observe some aspect of overlapping concern, or seek out information from one another.

It is axiomatic that we cannot plan serendipitous learning, so we may think that it does not concern us in our roles as curriculum developers, tutors, facilitators or mentors, but we can pay more attention to creating the right conditions for positive unplanned learning. I stress conditions for *positive* learning because negative unplanned learning happens rather easily. Either way, these conditions form the 'hidden curriculum'.(61,62) I shall return to this later.

Beyond serendipitous interprofessional learning there is *informal* interprofessional learning that occurs more predictably because of work systems or the structure of educational programmes and events. Multidisciplinary team reviews of specific cases or processes can be good examples of informal IPE. These may be labelled as team meetings, action learning, audit, quality circles or external inspection, each with a different emphasis and potential for informal and formally recognised interprofessional learning. Many educational programmes and events provide opportunities for informal IPE simply by bringing people together; conferences and safety-related updates are common examples. The training and debate associated with introducing new equipment, processes or clinical guidelines provide further opportunities for informal interprofessional learning. Some of the examples cited at the beginning of this section to emphasise the diversity of IPE might be regarded as largely informal IPE.(14,31,32,56,59)

Students from different professions are often in the same clinical areas at the same time, providing opportunities for informal IPE even if the logistics of making this a formal part of the relevant professional curricula are too difficult to contemplate. The difficulties of converting informal IPE to formally recognised and structured IPE may relate to constant changes in the clinical area, the unpredictable availability of contributing practitioners, long time lags in curriculum change processes and a lack of funding for the formalisation process or to address sustainability. Nevertheless, if students and their supervising clinicians look out for opportunities for productive interprofessional exchange, valuable interprofessional learning can occur. Developing a habit of informal interprofessional learning can help students to mature into competent, collaborative professionals, confident with their own expertise and area of responsibility, willing to learn from and educate other professions.

The main dangers of promoting informal IPE and not paying attention to formal IPE include the following:
- the impossibility of monitoring equality of opportunity
- scope for duplication (although this should be limited if learners actively negotiate their learning with supervisors or colleagues)
- scope for individuals to avoid engaging with this important aspect of professional practice
- less motivation for engagement if the formal curriculum does not value interprofessional collaboration sufficiently to include appropriate interprofessional learning objectives, experiences and assessments.

Designing effective interprofessional education

There is growing understanding of the effectiveness of IPE (*see* Box 6.3). Effective IPE is simply good education with the added 'twist' of purposefully harnessing the knowledge, learning needs and dynamics of an interprofessional group. A large number of learning theorists and adult educators(63–77) have developed overlapping theories about adults' and professionals' learning. Key aspects include the following:
- the perceived relevance of the learning opportunity (which, due to the diversity of participants, may be a particular challenge for IPE)
- the perceived demands of the learning context
- the relationship of current learning to prior learning
- and learners' self-concepts.

These things are bound together by emotions evoked by learning experiences, including: excitement, admiration, motivation, satisfaction, empathy, ambivalence, anxiety, boredom, impatience, fatigue and disaffection. IPE developers and facilitators need to plan and manage interprofessional learning experiences in ways that create positive emotions and, if necessary, acknowledge and work with negative emotions (The role of the facilitator will be discussed later; *see also* Box 6.4.)

Poorly planned and delivered education of any type can waste resources and create ill-will. Poor-quality IPE may be particularly damaging if it creates increased reluctance to engage in subsequent interprofessional collaboration or reinforces negative stereotypes. We should try particularly hard to avoid delivering bruising or otherwise demotivating IPE.

Activities that do not allow each participating group to contribute and gain to more or less the same extent are unlikely to be a good foundation for sound IPE. The aim is for everyone to learn something productive through balanced exchanges, not for one group to plunder the expertise of another.

Learning theories highlight the motivational importance of the gap between what people think they know and what they think they need to know. Jarvis, in particular, highlighted this gap and used the term 'disjuncture'.(76) Disjuncture (providing it is not overwhelmingly large) stimulates learning. Generations of skilful educators have found ways to create or reveal constructive disjuncture. Slightly unfamiliar contexts, such as IPE, create disjuncture: revealing learning needs and motivating learners to close the gap. Furthermore, 'constructive friction' between a learning environment and learners' habitual approaches to learning can promote change and personal development.(78) IPE can be an excellent context for creating and harnessing appropriate levels of disjuncture and constructive friction.

The perceived relevance of the learning opportunity

Adult learners are life-centred and problem-centred, motivated to develop their knowledge and skills when they encounter an idea, a task or a problem that matters to them in their current context.(65,71,73,79) This may be something that is not going well at the moment or simply something new that they wish to explore. It is difficult to engage with things that do not interest us and seem to have little relevance.

IPE participants are likely to want to develop their knowledge and practice from multiple perspectives (as individuals, as members of a particular profession and as members of diverse teams). Furthermore, their primary focus will vary over time and in response to external demands. IPE normally addresses this personal, professional and team development by appealing to shared interest in delivering good care to *patients* (the 'object' of 'activity'(79)). This is most obvious within post-registration IPE: commonly labelled as *quality improvement* (some examples are provided in Box 6.3). People may not even notice they are engaged in IPE: learning with, from and about each other to improve collaboration and the quality of care. Participants from diverse backgrounds are focused on and motivated by their shared practice-based problem.

In other circumstances, establishing relevance and authenticity requires active attention from curriculum developers and facilitators. They will try to ensure that learning opportunities (in clinical practice, university and staff development settings) are well aligned with the anticipated participants' concerns, interests and levels of expertise. This can be particularly challenging for IPE because the diversity of concerns, interests and expertise is normally greater within an interprofessional group. Students have been shown to engage more fully with IPE when they perceive it as supportive of their own, profession-specific, development.(80)

For practice-based interprofessional learning, it may be easier for an interested organisational 'insider' to create alignment and convince participants of the relevance of the interprofessional learning.(81) If such 'insiders' work in partnership with experienced 'outsiders' who bring particular expertise in interprofessional learning, professional development or service development (and sufficient distance from practitioners' immediate concerns to be better placed to reframe and challenge local understandings), the development and delivery of IPE harness the complementary strengths of 'insiders' and 'outsiders' and also 'walks the talk' of interprofessional or inter-organisational collaboration.

While diversity can stimulate learning and enjoyment, it can also overstretch the skills of the facilitators or the ingenuity of the curriculum developers who provide trigger material and structure for interprofessional learning. It is wise to work with a manageable level of diversity and select a theme that is fairly easily recognised as relevant to all participants.

The perceived demands of the learning context

Learners' *perceptions* of the learning environment and what is expected from them (more than any objective reality) affect what and how they learn(82,83) – for example, whether they mainly seek to absorb and reproduce knowledge or behaviours from facilitators or learning materials;

focus on understanding and generating new knowledge; hope to transform their professional lives; or seek to please important gatekeepers. Overloading learners is known to encourage a reproducing (surface) approach to learning, faulty learning, disengagement or a strategic approach to studying.(84) Thus, for example, it is not helpful to place an optional, experiential interprofessional learning opportunity shortly before a high-stakes summative assessment (usually examinations for individuals or external inspections, audits or reviews for service delivery teams). While this may seem too obvious to mention, it is surprisingly easy to overlook important conflicting demands faced by one or more of the groups from whom participation is desired. This will constrain their participation and alter the overall dynamics of the interprofessional learning. Such oversights are more easily avoided when care is taken to include a member of each participating group in the planning process.

Learners' perceptions are shaped by explicit and implicit messages. Explicit messages include the following:

- the course description (as published and as spoken by facilitators)
- perhaps a handbook containing aims or intended learning outcomes
- the learning materials and assessment requirements.

These all convey the 'target understanding'(85) that curriculum developers, tutors and examiners have in mind (and any lack of alignment can create confusion).

Implicit messages, the 'hidden curriculum', include the following:

- perceptions of the importance of a particular learning opportunity based on, for example, who chooses to attend or otherwise contribute and the attitudes they display
- any attendance or assessment requirements
- whether the event is allocated a bright and airy room with access to adequate technology and refreshments
- whether the event is pushed to the fringes of the timetable such as late on Friday afternoon
- many other subtle ways of reinforcing or undermining the official explicit messages.

IPE can be enhanced or undermined by the explicit and implicit messages delivered and (more importantly) perceived about its relationship to the (properly) dominant activities of uniprofessional education and practice.

The self-concept of the learner

Professional and interprofessional education address learners who wish mainly to see themselves as competent, self-directed, appropriately self-evaluative and exercising choice(46,65,67) – in short, skilfully self-regulating.(86) Any education that attacks these aspects of self-concept will produce resistance and possibly rejection. Of course, it is perfectly reasonable to dislike coercion and to try to avoid embarrassment or failure. Successful education will challenge learners (cognitively and affectively) but will monitor and adjust the degree of challenge to maintain productive learning. IPE participants bring along their constantly evolving professional persona and expertise. Skilful curriculum planning and facilitation are needed to ensure that their expertise and values are acknowledged and that challenge is supportive. This is most easily achieved when levels of expertise are appropriate for the task at hand. A practical response in post-registration interprofessional practice development is to ensure that participants are drawn from the correct levels within their particular profession or specialisation: those who really know about the processes under scrutiny and those who have the ability to effect change in the relevant environments. For pre-registration IPE we may sometimes match participants to learning activities, but more often we will match learning activities to available participants. This means that IPE curriculum developers must take time to examine the anticipated participants' prior learning and competing learning needs.

Adults' need for self-direction coexists with a need for structure, particularly in unfamiliar learning milieu.(87,88) IPE will be less familiar than UPE, so at the beginning, participants may feel quite strongly that the programme details and facilitators' actions should structure the learning experience for them. As confidence grows, the participants will have less need for this 'scaffolding',(89,90) so it is sensible to focus on supporting learners in the early stages of a learning encounter and then shift in the direction of measured challenge.

Links to prior learning

Prior learning influences subsequent learning, and this has many dimensions. Learning proceeds more quickly and is better retained if it relates to earlier experience and learning.(91) The accuracy or otherwise of earlier learning, particularly the understanding of key concepts, lays firm or shaky foundations for later learning. This has been shown to be especially important in scientific fields.(92,93) Learning from prior experiences may support or inhibit new learning by providing relevant or distracting procedural and technical knowledge, and supportive or undermining emotional associations.(63,71,94) Prior learning will also influence the approaches to learning with which IPE participants feel comfortable. Facilitators and curriculum developers should try to maintain an up-to-date understanding of the probable prior learning (curricula and extent of practice experience) for the learners to whom each IPE initiative is addressed. A recent study reports some effects of mismatched prior learning (compounded by differing perceptions of relevance).(95)

Some learners develop unhelpful approaches to learning,(96,97) and it may be very difficult for them to change these.(98) Skilful facilitators will not underestimate the degree of personal challenge that IPE might present to some learners as a result of their prior learning, and will work more closely with these learners to provide additional scaffolding.

Interprofessional education and the curriculum

Curriculum design is not about identifying *the right way* to do things, but a matter of making value-laden choices that are fit for purpose within a particular context. This chapter argues that there is no ideal or essential location for IPE within a curriculum, rather that there are many opportunities for enhancing learning through IPE. Those selected will depend on the preferences of the curriculum developers and local opportunities. The choices made also reflect developers' conceptions of the purposes of IPE.

Some people think that IPE must occur as early as possible in pre-registration education to avoid the development of negative stereotypes and a preference for uniprofessional working over collaborative practice. But our students are not blank pages on which we write, or empty vessels that we fill: they arrive with life-based and media-based stereotypes and a strong commitment to their chosen profession. Nevertheless, early IPE can work well, provided it is appropriate to learners' current knowledge, experience and learning needs.(99–101) It is worth remembering that junior students may be more biddable than their seniors, so absenteeism is less likely to be a problem at this stage. Well-received early IPE might encourage later engagement within a spiral curriculum (*see* Chapter 3), which revisits interprofessional collaboration with increasing levels of sophistication and challenge. It is important that each return to IPE builds on rather than repeats earlier interprofessional and uniprofessional learning; otherwise, disengagement and resistance are highly likely.

If local constraints make early IPE difficult, it may be more efficient to ensure that pre-registration curricula across the professions have elements that *systematically* and *explicitly* work towards developing skills and insights that will aid later engagement with IPE and collaborative practice. Later engagement might occur during the middle years when students have begun to build a reasonably secure technical knowledge base relating to their own profession. By this stage they have some experience of professional practice, they have begun to appreciate the complexities of communication skills, teamwork, decision-making, working in partnership with patients and carers, ethical practice, professionalism and patient safety. They may also be developing understanding of the limits of medical knowledge and resources. At this stage students have some useful profession-specific knowledge and experiences that they can share, and they tend to be hungry for new experiences.(47,102)

If engagement with formal IPE is delayed until the final years of pre-qualification curricula, it will be particularly important to recognise the competing priorities of high-stakes examinations and securing a job for the following year. It is also important to remember that students will by now have experienced informal and serendipitous IPE while engaging with other things, particularly while gaining experience in various clinical areas. They would not want to feel that a new block in the curriculum, formally labelled as IPE, is repeating ground they have already covered. It must be clear that any revisiting is raising the level of thinking and skills; this is what a spiral curriculum demands.(103) But interprofessional learning can be a logical pinnacle within a spiral curriculum and there are studies of IPE used this way.(43,104) In the closing months of pre-qualification curricula, students are naturally preoccupied with the impending responsibilities and realities of professional practice. IPE that speaks to these strongly felt learning needs is likely to be well received.

As mentioned earlier, interprofessional continuing professional development is often more natural than uniprofessional development in improving certain clinical practices and developing services. IPE at this level can help ensure that resources are used wisely, that effective and patient-centred care are the main priorities and, importantly, that attention is given to the quality of working lives.

Overtly labelling particular learning experiences as interprofessional offers the advantage of visibility for an important aspect of professional practice, but creating isolated interprofessional elements within the curriculum can make IPE vulnerable to attack and easy to cut when times are hard. My (probably controversial) suggestion is that sustainability may be more easily achieved if interprofessional learning is embedded as a taken-for-granted part of certain other strands of activity. There are many possibilities, but obvious choices include the following:

- clinical and service-based quality improvement initiatives where the embedded model is already well developed at the post-qualification level
- multiprofessional student teams shadowing real teams or providing supervised care (see next section for further discussion)
- curriculum strands that address patient groups whose needs can only be met through interprofessional or inter-agency collaboration
- patient-safety initiatives.

It has to be recognised that IPE will always present logistical challenges that are not so strongly felt in UPE. It may also present political and financial challenges.

Delivering effective interprofessional education

Most modes of educational delivery could potentially have some application in IPE, but some are more naturally suited to the task. I shall consider four here.

Case-based learning

Many IPE experiences trigger learning by using real cases and incidents, or authored scenarios drawn from a synthesis of past experience. This is a natural format, because all the participating professions are likely to be familiar with learning in this way and because relevance to the concerns of participants should be achievable. Well-selected or well-crafted triggers ensure that each profession can make a valued contribution. One randomised study showed that augmenting case triggers with an Interprofessional Team Reasoning Framework and video examples of interprofessional interactions improved students' perceptions of team skills and their case presentations.(105)

I have avoided using the term problem-based learning (PBL) and should explain why. In IPE it is often the problem focus that matters; it may not be necessary or appropriate to conduct the IPE as a PBL experience in manner described

in Chapter 5. A second reason is that different groups of participants may have different conceptions of PBL, which have grown up within their uniprofessional experiences to suit their profession-specific needs. It is the same as with the earlier warning to be alert to whether everyone in the group you are working with means the same thing when they talk about IPE. It can be an unnecessary distraction for IPE participants to be told that they will engage in PBL and then find things do not proceed according to the formula that they associate with the term.

Simulation

The term simulation covers everything from table-top exercises and simple role play (e.g. a telephone call) to medium-fidelity simulation in clinical skills centres and on to high-fidelity clinical simulations supported by sophisticated technology or highly skilled simulated patients (*see* Chapter 13). The purposes of simulation include the following:

- providing a safe learning environment that protects patients and learners, where mistakes can be allowed to occur as learning opportunities
- providing learning opportunities that do not disrupt the normal delivery of care
- speeding up or slowing the passage of time to enhance learning
- allowing repeated practice, preferably after feedback or self-assessment
- providing managed formative exposure to things not yet experienced or only rarely experienced
- creating appropriate levels of disjuncture to stimulate learning.

It is worth remembering that the fidelity of any simulation only needs to be as high as is necessary to achieve the intended learning. Costs can be contained by examining which aspects of a situation need to be simulated and looking for the simplest way to do this.

Naturally, people fear failure and embarrassment. Some types of simulation offer scope for public humiliation and thus require particularly careful planning and skilful facilitation to avoid creating 'miseducative experiences'.(106)

Since professional practice is interprofessional, it makes sense for some simulation-based education to be interprofessional. Examples include extending earlier uniprofessional learning through the development of interprofessional scenarios for rehearsing aspects of communication with simulated patients(43) and rehearsing case and workload management.(100,107)

Shadowing

Reciprocated shadowing, with associated discussion and reflection, can make an excellent contribution to interprofessional understanding of roles, responsibilities, constraints, expertise and models of practice. Passive observation tends not to be integrated with earlier learning and is soon forgotten. Thus a shadowing experience needs structure and follow-up activities that promote active learning. This increases the chance that learning will become integrated in subsequent professional practice. Some wider IPE initiatives include shadowing elements.(37,108–110)

Clinical work in interprofessional student teams

Several IPE initiatives, in a variety of clinical contexts, have involved interprofessional student teams providing care under the supervision of qualified practitioners.(36,38,40, 48,108,111) These models show how a rolling programme of IPE in a particular service delivery setting can, over time, allow large numbers of students to rehearse and reflect on interprofessional teamwork. Patients tend to be highly satisfied with care provided by interprofessional student teams,(38,48) and follow-up studies show that students retain strong and largely positive memories of this type of IPE.(112,113) However, these models can be vulnerable to sudden changes in the clinical area, resulting in loss of staff to provide the level of supervision students require, or a change in the caseload rendering a clinical area too demanding for student teams. Studies have also noted that supervising student teams and facilitating effortful reflection can be a draining role for clinicians and faculty.(112,114)

A model that stops short of providing care involves interprofessional student team members assessing patients with complex needs and conducting an interdisciplinary case conference to integrate their findings and develop a care plan.(37) (This can be considered a form of shadowing.) The students' care plan is then presented to members of the client's actual care team for discussion and (formative) assessment; *see* The assessment of interprofessional education section, below.

The role of facilitation

To enable *active* learning *with*, *from* and *about* members of other professions, IPE normally adopts some form of small group learning. Advice on facilitating small group learning has been ably addressed by a wide range of authors (115–117) and *see also* Chapters 5 and 9. Their insights are directly applicable to IPE. The added dimensions of facilitating interprofessional small group work are, first, that IPE groups are deliberately heterogeneous; and second, that the aim of IPE is to harness the different perspectives, skills and insights of participants from different professions.

Uniprofessional groups contain learners from different cultures, of different ages, with different abilities, varying prior experiences and different levels of interest in the topic under consideration. Consequently, faculty and practice-based supervisors are already skilled in playing to the strengths of different learners and supporting everyone to make a valued contribution; providing tailored feedback and sufficient (but not too much) challenge; also managing group dynamics, including conflict. Thus, experienced teachers already have most of the skills they will need to facilitate IPE. Nevertheless, the greater diversity within an interprofessional learning group may stretch these skills. More effort is involved in finding out about the expertise and prior experience of participants, necessitating greater advance preparation to ensure that learning materials and activities are pitched at the correct level and allow all groups to contribute. It can be harder to draw out a valued contribution from a quiet learner if you are unsure of the relevant profession's contribution yourself, again pointing to the need for advance preparation. On the other hand, the diversity of the group can make for a rich variety of contributions that enthuses everyone; then the facilitator's main roles may be to keep an eye on the time and to help summarise learning and plans before everyone disperses.

Interprofessional co-tutoring is one way to mitigate tutors' inadequate knowledge of all participating professions and their usual approaches to learning and teaching, but there are costs to be balanced. The extra cost of additional facilitators would need to be offset by larger groups or reduced contact time. In addition, co-facilitators can feel that their own professional expertise is under the spotlight to a greater extent than in their routine work; this can be experienced as enjoyable or nerve-wracking. It is also important that co-tutors role-model high-quality interprofessional collaboration, otherwise the credibility of the learning experience may be damaged.

For a comfortable learning experience, the content and pace of the IPE need to feel appropriate to all participants (this links to the importance of perceived relevance and perceived demands, discussed earlier). Indicative content, and by implication pace, will be set when the IPE is planned. But any exchange-based learning relies on participants' contributions and, therefore, the facilitator must continually evaluate contributions and learners' engagement to judge when to expand themes or deepen thinking, and when to move the group on to something new. The diversity of interprofessional groups might make this task more challenging. IPE researchers have reported that gender balance and the balance of professional membership can affect group dynamics.(104) There may be opportunities for facilitators to allocate group membership in ways that maintain sufficient balance to safeguard productive interprofessional discussion.

Tutors grow accustomed to working with learners from particular professions (often the tutor's own profession) and, with varying degrees of awareness, may adopt profession-based norms for learning and teaching encounters. Translating their consequent facilitation style and expectations directly into IPE can cause alarm and discomfort to some participants, particularly those from other professions. IPE facilitators should try to remain vigilant for signs of discomfort or resistance. These might indicate that the facilitation style needs some modification. On the other hand, unfamiliar educational approaches may be causing the anxiety, suggesting that certain participants need extra support to begin to feel at ease with the IPE activities (see earlier discussion of learners' self-concepts and links to prior learning). For example, some IPE participants may find reflective practice a natural state, while others are rather uncomfortable with such self-examination. Succinct displays of certainty may be the carefully developed cultural norm for one group, but this could be seen as arrogant and narrow-minded by another group. In addition, similar terms may be used by different professions to mean rather different things. It is best not to assume that everyone means the same thing when they say problem-based learning, self-directed learning, OSCE, clinical skills and many other terms.

Discomfort generated by lack of familiarity with IPE or with particular approaches to teaching and learning may cause some participants to try to change the nature of the learning experience so that it becomes more familiar. The conflicting expectations of different groups mean it is possible facilitators will have to contend with participants trying to tug the learning experience in different directions. It may become necessary to reflect this process back to the group and ask them to suspend resistance for a while, or to negotiate an acceptable compromise with respect to the learning activities.

Conflict may be more likely in a group where firmly held professional positions are being exposed to scrutiny. Facilitators need to develop skills to productively harness the energy of conflict and set clear limits on acceptable behaviour. The Contact Hypothesis (*see* Box 6.4) suggests how prejudice and its associated conflict might be reduced. It highlights the importance of facilitators drawing out both similarities and differences between participating groups.

 BOX 6.4 FOCUS ON: The Contact Hypothesis

The Contact Hypothesis(118–120) was developed from studies of religious and racial tension. It suggests that hostility between social groups would be reduced, if members experienced greater contact, provided a set of 'conditions' is met, as follows:(121)

- each group should have equal status
- interaction should be conducted in a cooperative atmosphere
- participants should be working towards common goal and experience successful joint working
- 'the authorities' should support the initiative – for IPE this would mean professional bodies, health care providers, senior managers, clinicians, universities and faculty.
- participants should be made aware of group similarities and group differences – members of one group compare their group's characteristics (in-group) with the characteristics of other groups (out-group) in an effort to establish positively valued distinctiveness.(122) IPE can usefully encourage mutual inter-group differentiation so that there can be shared acknowledgement of valued aspects of each group's identity(123)
- participants should have positive expectations
- participants from different groups should perceive one another as typical members of their group.

Listed thus, it sounds like a tall order for any educational initiative. Nevertheless, people have found the Contact Hypothesis a useful framework for developing or evaluating IPE that seeks to address unhelpful stereotypes and expectations.(4,44,81,123–126) The list of conditions provides useful guidance for curriculum developers and facilitators. It is in harmony with discussion within four earlier subsections focused on Designing Effective IPE (relevance, perceived demands, self-concept and prior learning).

Most IPE facilitators find that conflict remains productive and manageable if there is a central focus on patients and improving the quality of services. Improving the quality of working lives by improving team communication and local processes is also an effective focus at post-qualification level.

Facilitators new to IPE may bring concerns,(127) which sensitive faculty development can address.

Facilitating online IPE

Is e-moderation for interprofessional e-learning the same as uniprofessional e-moderation? In most respects the answer should be yes, so general e-moderation advice will be sound.(124) Predictable differences for e-IPE might include an unbalanced dynamic if members of each profession already know fellow e-learners from their own profession but are just 'meeting' the other professions' learners in their e-IPE set. This is most likely to happen at the pre-qualification level when learners from different disciplines, possibly attending courses at different campuses, 'meet' to undertake e-IPE. Blending this with initial face-to-face IPE can help even out the degree to which learners feel they know one another.

Continuing with the case of pre-registration e-IPE, the ebb and flow of different professions' courses mean that any e-IPE group designed to run over an extended period will encounter times when one or other group leaves campus to gain experience in clinical settings. Even if faculty have planned continuing e-IPE, learners' access to the relevant network platform may be curtailed and, furthermore, students' attention may be almost completely diverted to their clinical experiences. This can lead to a profession unofficially dropping out for a while, changing the experience for those who remain (particularly in the extreme case of only two participating professions when the e-IPE comes to an unscheduled halt).

On their return, the temporarily absent learners will find themselves behind with the wider group's learning and need to catch up. Learners from other professions may have become irritated by the disengagement, so e-moderators may have to help the group to reintegrate . . . and then another profession goes out for a month's clinical experience. Happily, the downside of disengagement and re-entry is counterbalanced because re-entering learners often invigorate the e-IPE with insights and questions drawn from their recent clinical experience. E-moderators can help to initiate this process by welcoming people back and asking questions that help learners to link their recent experience with the e-IPE themes. Similar fluctuations in engagement with e-IPE can be seen when each participating profession approaches important summative assessments.

For a refreshingly candid description of delivering e-IPE, *see* Bluteau and Jackson.(128)

The assessment of interprofessional education

Should we assess IPE at all? It might be argued that immersion in the process of IPE is more important than assessment. However, most people perceive value in including some formative or summative assessment. But how should we approach this? I would argue that the key concept is 'constructive alignment',(129) that is, assessment that by its nature reinforces the intended outcomes of the IPE. Since IPE is extremely varied, we should expect assessment associated with IPE to be equally varied.

Beginning with the most straightforward form of IPE, interprofessional quality improvement initiatives, the most appropriate form of assessment will be indicators drawn from the process of service delivery, and there are several good examples in Box 6.3. Within these team-based initiatives it is not usually felt to be necessary to assess the outcomes of IPE at the level of individual practitioners.

Individual practitioners will be assessed while they are undertaking specialist training or an award-bearing course. Formative assessment may well comprise feedback from colleagues and supervisors. Some of this will be informal, as needs and opportunities arise, but increasingly this is complemented by more structured feedback – perhaps from a range of colleagues from different professions: i.e. multi-source feedback.(130,131) Structured feedback is based on expected competences and can span formative and summative assessment. Summative assessments must have clearly defined criteria, and this is quite a complex undertaking for competences associated with interprofessional collaboration, but surely no more complex than trying to assess many other aspects of professionalism.

Pre-registration IPE and award-bearing post-registration IPE have to contend with the assessment requirements of all the participating professions and university departments, and practicalities too. This can feel like a problem without a solution and it is common for no summative assessment to be attached to IPE. The risk is that curriculum strands without assessment are interpreted as less valued, making disengagement and absenteeism more likely. Consequently, the most basic form of assessment for pre-registration IPE can be meeting an attendance or participation requirement. Attendance and participation are reasonable demands if interprofessional collaboration is viewed as a core facet of professionalism. Nevertheless, many initiatives prefer to offer opt-in IPE to avoid the necessity of managing recalcitrant learners.

Some IPE is assessed formatively or summatively through knowledge tests, essays, reflective journals and group presentations in various media (e.g. posters, patchwork texts, film, drama or through the ubiquitous presentation of software slide shows). Presentations may be delivered to peers, tutors, relevant practitioners or service users, providing different emphases within any resultant feedback or discussion. Whatever the format, learners gain most from active engagement with the activities that are assessed; this may need to be pointed out to group members who appear to be aiming for minimal participation. Encouraging self-assessment and including peer-assessment can be helpful here.

Faculty need to decide whether to assess teams or individuals, but current assessment regulations may limit options. This may signal a need for longer term work to align assessments with the principles of IPE, perhaps

beginning with securing permission to pilot innovative assessments.

There are many who feel that assessment of interprofessional leaning, and even the development of interprofessional curricula, require much more attention to defining interprofessional competencies. This has spawned considerable efforts to develop and agree interprofessional competencies.(132–134) Some professional accreditation frameworks now incorporate interprofessional competencies.(135)

Tidal flows in interprofessional education

Whichever beach you are sitting on, it is likely to feel as if interest in IPE comes and goes like the tide. This applies to areas of practice as well as geographical locations, and beaches differ with respect to the amount of variation between high and low tide.

IPE matching the description at the beginning of this chapter has been recorded since the 1960s. While there was national variation, early foci often included interprofessional teamwork in mental health and learning disabilities services, community and primary care. The 1970s saw increased attention to child protection and palliative care, while the 1980s brought IPE relating to HIV/AIDS. By the end of the 20th century interest had broadened considerably and IPE had developed for maternity care, rehabilitation, chronic illnesses, ethics, management; to address the needs of ageing populations, increasingly dispersed families, cost containment and workforce shortages. Most of these foci have endured, although relatively little is now written about some of the early foci. Hopefully, interprofessional collaboration and learning are too well embedded to be remarkable. Most early IPE occurred between qualified practitioners.

So far, 21st century IPE foci have continued to include chronic illnesses, responding to social and demographic changes, improving the quality and efficiency of services, and care for vulnerable groups with complex needs (such as children, older people, people with mental health challenges, people at risk from domestic violence and people with inadequate (or no) housing – IPE centred on supporting people with learning disabilities is much less common and, arguably, much needed). Newer foci include patient safety, disaster planning spurred on by heightened fears of terrorism, professionalism and new health care roles. The major health professions now mandate or strongly advise the inclusion of interprofessional learning opportunities within pre-registration education. For several years a significant strand of IPE development in Australasia and North America focused on meeting the needs of underserved populations, particularly rural communities and indigenous peoples. Catching this tide and the tides of cost-containment and workforce shortages, in 2010 two major reports (136,137) declared IPE central to addressing global health and global health workforce challenges, see Boxes 6.5 and 6.6. In 2012 the US Department of Health and Human Services announced a large investment in a co-ordinating centre to promote interprofessional education and collaborative practice.(138)

BOX 6.5 FOCUS ON: WHO Framework for Action

The authors of the WHO Framework for Action on Interprofessional Education and Collaborative Practice(136) argued that collaborative practice strengthens health systems and improves health outcomes. It positioned IPE as preparation for collaborative practice and contributing to the achievement of global health goals in the context of global health workforce shortages, fragmented services and unmet need. They stressed the importance of health and education systems working together and highlighted local and regional variation in mechanisms underpinning effective IPE and collaborative practice. Therefore the Framework for Action aimed to provide policy-makers with strategies and ideas to support context-sensitive implementation of IPE and collaborative practice. The Framework divides mechanisms

supporting IPE into educator mechanisms and curricular mechanisms and divides mechanisms supporting collaborative practice into three themes: institutional support, working culture and environment. The Framework also examines mechanisms through which health services are delivered and patients are protected.

The Framework is a call to action to improve health outcomes through embedding IPE in the education of the health workforce and advancing collaborative practice within and beyond health services. Examples and suggested actions are provided at provider and system levels. Leaders at all levels are asked to 'contextualise, commit and champion'.

BOX 6.6 FOCUS ON: A global independent commission

Spurred on by the centenary of the Flexner Report(139) – which shaped a significant science-based shift in health professions' education at the beginning of the 20th century – *The Lancet* established a group to consider the education of health professionals for the 21st century and in doing so, explore contemporary concerns about gaps and inequalities in health and 21st century health needs and expectations. The Commission's report, *Health Professionals for a New Century: Transforming Education to Strengthen Health Systems in an Interdependent World*,(137) highlights that the global health workforce is highly mobile, which exacerbates gaps and inequality. The ambitious report advocates wide-ranging and fundamental changes in professional education, and in the relationships between health care providers, educational institutions and the populations they serve.

Of interest in this chapter, the report is concerned about 'professional tribalism' and 'silos'. It advocates: '. . . interprofessional and transprofessional education that breaks down professional silos while enhancing collaborative and non-hierarchical relationships in effective teams . . .'((137), p.1924)

The report describes 'transprofessional' education as preparation for teamwork with basic and ancillary health workers, administrators, managers, policy-makers and local community leaders. As discussed at the beginning of the chapter and in Box 6.2, the CAIPE definition of IPE and vision of interprofessional collaboration encompasses the Commission's view of transprofessional education, so introducing the additional term may serve to confuse rather than illuminate (not least because it is also used rather differently elsewhere,(140) to mean something closer to transcending the limited perspective of one's profession to adopt a more holistic patient-centred integrated-service view). However, this report usefully highlights the breadth of collaborative practice in which 21st century professionals must engage and the growing importance to health care of basic and ancillary workers, community leaders and volunteers. Health professions' education, through IPE and other aspects of the curriculum, must support 21st century practitioners to develop expertise for less-hierarchal collaboration with a wider range of contributors.

Interest and innovation in IPE in Europe (particularly the Nordic countries and the UK, but also elsewhere), Canada, the USA, Australia, New Zealand and, more recently Japan, is significant and likely to endure, although levels of interest and funding tend to fluctuate. If you sit on any beach long enough the tide will ebb and flow.

References

1 CAIPE (2006) CAIPE re-issues its statement on the definition and principles of interprofessional education. *CAIPE Bulletin.* **26**: 3.

2 CAIPE (2012) Home page. (http://caipe.org.uk/; accessed 17 September 2012).

3 Barr H and Low H (2011) Principles for interprofessional education.(http://caipe.org.uk/resources/principles-of-interprofessional-education/; accessed 17 September 2012).

4 Carpenter J and Hewstone M (1996) Shared learning for doctors and social workers: evaluation of a programme. *British Journal of Social Work.* **26**(2): 239–57.

5 Leathard A (1994) Interprofessional developments in Britain: an overview. In: Leathard A (ed.) *Going Inter-Professional: Working Together for Health and Welfare,* pp. 3–37. Routledge, London.

6 Barr H (2005) Interprofessional education: today, yesterday and tomorrow (revised). LTSN for Health Sciences and Practice,

London. (http://repos.hsap.kcl.ac.uk/content/m10122/latest/occp1_revised2005.pdf; accessed 17 September 2012).

7 Leathard A (2003) *Interprofessional Collaboration: From Policy to Practice in Health and Social Care*. Brunner-Routledge, Hove.

8 Irvine R, Kerridge I, McPhee J and Freeman S (2002) Interprofessionalism and ethics: consensus or clash of cultures? *Journal of Interprofessional Care*. **16**(3): 199–210.

9 Øvretveit J, Mattias P and Thompson T (eds) (1997) *Interprofessional Working in Health and Social Care*. Palgrave Macmillan, London.

10 Freeth D, Hammick M, Koppel I, Reeves S and Barr H (2002) A critical review of evaluations of interprofessional education. Learning and Teaching Support Network Health Sciences and Practice, London. (http://repos.hsap.kcl.ac.uk/content/m10123/latest/occp2.pdf; accessed 5 November 2012).

11 Hammick M, Freeth D, Koppel I, Reeves S and Barr H (2007) A best evidence systematic review of interprofessional education: BEME Guide No. 9. *Medical Teacher*. **29**(8): 735–51.

12 Reeves S, Perrier L, Goldman J, Freeth D, Zwarenstein M (2013) Interprofessional education: effects on professional practice and healthcare outcomes (update). *Cochrane Database of Systematic Reviews*. Issue 3. Art. No.: CD002213

13 De Bere SR (2003) Evaluating the implications of complex interprofessional education for improvements in collaborative practice: a multidimensional model. *British Educational Research Journal*. **29**(1): 105–24.

14 Horbar JD, Rogowski J, Plsek PE *et al*. (2001) Collaborative quality improvement for neonatal intensive care. *Pediatrics*. **107**(1): 14–22.

15 Rogowski JA, Horbar JD, Plsek PE *et al*. (2001) Economic implications of neonatal intensive care unit collaborative quality improvement. *Pediatrics*. **107**(1): 23–9.

16 Fraser S, Wilson T, Burch K, Osborne M-A and Knightley M (2002) Using collaborative improvement in a single organisation: improving anti-coagulant care. *International Journal of Health Care Quality Assurance*. **15**(4): 152–8.

17 Shafer MB, Tebb KB, Pantell RH *et al*. (2002) Effect of a clinical practice improvement intervention on chlamydial screening among adolescent girls. *JAMA: The Journal of the American Medical Association*. **288**(22): 2846–52.

18 Thomas P (1994) The Liverpool Primary Health Care Facilitation Project 1989–94. Liverpool FHSA, Liverpool.

19 Janson SL, Cooke M, McGrath KW, Kroon LA, Robinson S and Baron RB (2009) Improving chronic care of type 2 diabetes using teams of interprofessional learners. *Academic Medicine*. **84**(11): 1540–8.

20 Taylor CR, Hepworth JT, Buerhaus PI, Dittus R and Speroff T (2007) Effect of crew resource management on diabetes care and patient outcomes in an inner-city primary care clinic. *Quality and Safety in Health Care*. **16**(4): 244–7.

21 Thompson RS, Rivara FP, Thompson DC *et al*. (2000) Identification and management of domestic violence: a randomized trial. *American Journal of Preventive Medicine*. **19**(4): 253–63.

22 Stein J and Brown H (1995) 'All in this together': an evaluation of joint training on the abuse of adults with learning disabilities. *Health and Social Care in the Community*. **3**(4): 205–14.

23 Weaver SJ, Rosen MA, DiazGranados D *et al*. (2010) Does teamwork improve performance in the operating room? A multilevel evaluation. *Joint Commission Journal on Quality and Patient Safety*. **36**(3): 133–42.

24 Dunbar JM, Neufeld RR, White HC and Libow LS (1996) Retrain, don't restrain: the educational intervention of the national nursing home restraint removal project. *The Gerontologist*. **36**(4): 539–42.

25 Rask K, Parmelee PA, Taylor JA *et al*. (2007) Implementation and evaluation of a nursing home fall management program. *Journal of the American Geriatrics Society*. **55**(3): 342–9.

26 Strasser DC, Falconer JA, Stevens AB *et al*. (2008) Team training and stroke rehabilitation outcomes: a cluster randomized trial. *Archives of Physical Medicine and Rehabilitation*. **89**(1): 10–5.

27 Berman S, Miller AC, Rosen C and Bicchieri S (2000) Assessment training and team functioning for treating children with disabilities. *Archives of Physical Medicine and Rehabilitation*. **81**(5): 628–33.

28 Walsh PL, Garbs CA, Goodwin M and Wolff EM (1995) An impact evaluation of a VA geriatric team development program. *Gerontology and Geriatrics Education*. **15**(3): 19–35.

29 Cameron KA, Engel KG, McCarthy DM *et al*. (2010) Examining emergency department communication through a staff-based participatory research method: identifying barriers and solutions to meaningful change. *Annals of Emergency Medicine*. **56**(6): 614–22.

30 Nash A and Hoy A (1993) Terminal care in the community- an evaluation of residential workshops for general practitioner/district nurse teams. *Palliative Medicine*. **7**(1): 5–17.

31 Cox S, Wilcock P and Young J (1999) Improving the repeat prescribing process in a busy general practice. A study using continuous quality improvement methodology. *Quality in Health Care*. **8**(2): 119–25.

32 Ketola E, Sipilä R, Mäkelä M and Klockars M (2000) Quality improvement programme for cardiovascular disease risk factor recording in primary care. *Quality in Health Care*. **9**(3): 175–80.

33 Helitzer DL, Lanoue M, Wilson B, de Hernandez BU, Warner T and Roter D (2011) A randomized controlled trial of communication training with primary care providers to improve patient-centeredness and health risk communication. *Patient Education and Counseling*. **82**(1): 21–9.

34 Robinson M and Cottrell D (2005) Health professionals in multi-disciplinary and multi-agency teams: changing professional practice. *Journal of Interprofessional Care*. **19**(6): 547–60.

35 White S and Featherstone B (2005) Communicating misunderstandings: multi-agency work as social practice. *Child and Family Social Work*. **10**(3): 207–16.

36 Ponzer S, Hylin U, Kusoffsky A *et al*. (2004) Interprofessional training in the context of clinical practice: goals and students' perceptions on clinical education wards. *Medical Education*. **38**(7): 727–36.

37 Barber G, Borders K, Holland B and Roberts K (1997) Life span forum. *Gerontology & Geriatrics Education*. **18**(1): 47–59.

38 Dienst E and Byl N (1981) Evaluation of an educational program in health care teams. *Journal of Community Health*. **6**(4): 282–98.

39 Lennox A and Anderson ED (2007) Leicester Medical School: the Leicester model of interprofessional education: a practical guide for implementation in health and social care. Higher Education Academy, Newcastle upon Tyne. (http://www.medev.ac.uk/static/uploads/resources/SR9_Leicester_Model.pdf; accessed 5 November 2012).

40 Pelling S, Kalen A, Hammar M and Wahlström O (2011) Preparation for becoming members of health care teams: findings from a 5-year evaluation of a student interprofessional training ward. *Journal of Interprofessional Care*. **25**(5): 328–32.

41 McFadyen AK, Webster VS, Maclaren WM and O'Neill MA (2010) Interprofessional attitudes and perceptions: results from a longitudinal controlled trial of pre-registration health and social care students in Scotland. *Journal of Interprofessional Care*. **24**(5): 549–64.

42 Buckley S, Hensman M, Thomas S, Dudley R, Nevin G and Coleman J (2012) Developing interprofessional simulation in the undergraduate setting: experience with five different professional groups. *Journal of Interprofessional Care*. **26**(5): 362–9.

43 Cooke S, Chew G, Boggis C and Wakefield A (2003) 'I never realised that doctors were into feelings too': changing student perceptions though interprofessonal education. *Learning in Health and Social Care*. **2**(2): 137–46.

44 Carpenter J (1995) Interprofessional education for medical and nursing students: evaluation of a programme. *Medical Education*. **29**(4): 265–72.

45 Mires G, Williams F, Harden R and Howie P (2001) The benefits of a multiprofessional education programme can be sustained. *Medical Teacher.* **23**(3): 300–4.

46 Wijma MB and Fallsberg K (1999) Student attitudes towards the goals of an inter-professional training ward. *Medical Teacher.* **21**(6): 576–81.

47 Mu K, Chao CC, Jensen GM and Royeen CB (2004) Effects of interprofessional rural training on students' perceptions of inter-professional health care services. *Journal of Allied Health.* **33**(2): 125–31.

48 Reeves S, Freeth D, McCrorie P and Perry D (2002) 'It teaches you what to expect in future . . .': interprofessional learning on a training ward for medical, nursing, occupational therapy and physiotherapy students. *Medical Education.* **36**(4): 337–44.

49 Freeth D, Hammick M, Reeves S, Koppel I and Barr H (2005) *Effective Interprofessional Education: Development, Delivery and Evaluation.* Blackwell, Oxford.

50 Gilbert J, Camp R, Cole C, Bruce C, Fielding D and Stanton S (2003) Preparing students for interprofessional teamwork in health care. *Journal of Interprofessional Care.* **14**(3): 223–35.

51 Cooper H, Spencer-Dawe E and Mclean E (2005) Beginning the process of teamwork: design, implementation and evaluation of an inter-professional education intervention for first year undergraduate students. *Journal of Interprofessional Care.* **19**(5): 492–508.

52 van Staa AL, Visser A and van der Zouwe N (2000) Caring for caregivers: experiences and evaluation of interventions for a palliative care team. *Patient Education and Counseling.* **41**(1): 93–105.

53 Tepper M (1997) Providing comprehensive sexual health care in a spinal cord injury rehabilitation: implementation and evaluation of a new curriculum for health care professionals. *Sexuality and Disability.* **15**(3): 131–65.

54 Mann K, Weld-Viscount P, Cogdon A, Davidson K, Langille D and MacCara M (1996) Multidisciplinary learning in continuing professional education: the Heart health Nova Scotia experience. *The Journal of Continuing Education in the Health Professions.* **16**(1): 50–60.

55 Adamowski K, Dickinson G, Weitzman B, Roessler C and Carter-Snell C (1993) Sudden unexpected death in the emergency department: caring for the survivors. *Canadian Medical Association Journal.* **149**(10): 1445–51.

56 Treadwell M, Frank L and Vichinsky E (2002) Using quality improvement strategies to enhance pediatric pain assessment. *International Journal for Quality in Health Care.* **14**(1): 39–47.

57 Crawford M, Turnbull G and Wessely S (1998) Deliberate self harm assessment by accident and emergency staff an intervention study. *Journal of Accident and Emergency Medicine.* **15**(1): 18–22.

58 Morey J, Simon R, Gregory D *et al.* (2002) Error reduction and performance improvement in the emergency department through formal teamwork training: evaluation results of the MedTeams project. *Health Services Research.* **37**(6): 1553–61.

59 Allison M and Toy P (1996) A quality improvement team on autologous and directed-donor blood availability. *The Joint Commission Journal on Quality Improvement.* **22**(12): 801–10.

60 Sully P (2002) Commitment to partnership: interdisciplinary initiatives in developing expert practice in the care of survivors of violence. *Nurse Education in Practice.* **2**(2): 92–8.

61 Snyder B (1973) *The Hidden Curriculum.* MIT Press, Boston.

62 Margolis E (ed.) (2001) *The Hidden Curriculum in Higher Education.* Routledge, New York.

63 Kolb DA (1984) *Experiential Learning: Experience as the Source of Learning and Development.* Prentice Hall, Englewood Cliffs, NJ.

64 Brookfield S (1986) *Understanding and Facilitating Adult Learning: A Comprehensive Analysis of Principles and Effective Practices.* Open University Press, Milton Keynes.

65 Schön DA (1983) *The Reflective Practitioner: How Professionals Think in Action.* Basic Books, New York.

66 Entwistle N (1998) Approaches to learning and forms of understanding. In: Dart B and Boulton-Lewis G (eds) *Teaching and Learning in Higher Eduction,* pp. 72–101. Australian Council for Educational Research, Melbourne.

67 Rogers CR and Freiberg HJ (1994) *Freedom to Learn* (3e). Merrill, New York.

68 Eraut M (1994) *Developing Professional Knowledge and Competence.* Falmer, London.

69 Engeström Y, Engeström R and Kärkkäinen M (1995) Polycontextuality and boundary crossing in expert cognition: learning and problem solving in complex work activities. *Learning and Instruction.* **5**(4): 319–36.

70 Marton F and Booth S (1997) *Learning and Awareness.* L. Erlbaum Associates, Mahwah, NJ.

71 Knowles MS, Holton EF and Swanson RA (2011) *The Adult Learner: The Definitive Classic in Adult Education and Human Resource Development* (7e). Butterworth-Heinemann, Oxford.

72 Wenger E (1998) *Communities of Practice: Learning, Meaning, and Identity.* Cambridge University Press, Cambridge.

73 Mezirow J (2000) *Learning as Transformation: Critical Perspectives on a Theory in Progress.* Jossey-Bass, San Francisco, CA.

74 Eraut M (2000) Non-formal learning, implicit learning and tacit knowledge in professional work. In: Coffield F (ed.) *The Necessity of Informal Learning,* pp. 12–31. Policy Press, Bristol.

75 Engestrom Y (2001) Expansive learning at work: toward an activity theoretical reconceptualization. *Journal of Education and Work.* **14**(1): 133–56.

76 Jarvis P (2006) *Towards a Comprehensive Theory of Human Learning.* Routledge, London.

77 Illeris K (2007) *How We Learn: Learning and Non-Learning in School and Beyond.* Routledge, London.

78 Vermunt JD and Verloop N (1999) Congruence and friction between learning and teaching. *LearningF and Instruction.* **9**(3): 257–80.

79 Engestrom Y (1999) Expansive visibilization of work: an activity-theoretical perspective. *Computer Supported Cooperative Work.* **8**(1–2): 63–93.

80 Green C (2012) Relative distancing: a grounded theory of how learners negotiate the interprofessional. *Journal of Interprofessional Care.* **27**(1): 34–42.

81 Furness PJ, Armitage HR and Pitt R (2012) Qualitative evaluation of interprofessional learning initiatives in practice: application of the contact hypothesis. *International Journal of Medical Education.* **3**: 83–91.

82 Marton F and Saljo R (1976) On qualitative differences in learning: II outcomes as a function of the learner's conception of the task. *The British Journal of Educational Psychology.* **46**(2): 115–27.

83 Prosser M and Trigwell K (1999) *Understanding Learning and Teaching: The Experience in Higher Education.* Society for Research into Higher Education and Open University Press, Buckingham.

84 Entwistle NJ (2009) *Teaching for Understanding at University: Deep Approaches and Distinctive Ways of Thinking.* Palgrave Macmillan, Basingstoke.

85 Entwistle N and Smith C (2002) Personal understanding and target understanding: mapping influences on the outcomes of learning. *The British Journal of Educational Psychology.* **72**(3): 321–42.

86 Zimmerman B (1998) Developing self-fulfilling cycles of academic regulation: an analysis of exemplary instructional models. In: Schunk D and Zimmerman B (eds) *Self-Regulated Learning: From Teaching to Self-Regulated Practice,* pp. 1–19. Guildford Press, New York.

87 Kahl TN and Cropley AJ (1986) Face-to-face versus distance learning: psychological consequences and practical implications. *Distance Education.* **7**(1): 38–48.

88 Laurillard D (2012) *Teaching as a Design Science: Building Pedagogical Patterns for Learning and Technology.* Routledge, New York.

89 Jaramillo J (1996) Vygotsky's sociocultural theory and contributions to the development of constructivist curricula. *Education.* **117**(1): 133–40.

90 Hogan K and Pressley M (1997) *Scaffolding Student Learning: Instructional Approaches and Issues.* Brookline Books, Cambridge, MA.

91 Healy A, King C, Clawson D *et al.* (1995) Optimizing the long-term retention of skills. In: Healy A and Bourne L (eds) *Learning and Memory of Knowledge and Skills,* pp. 1–29. Sage, Thousand Oaks, CA.

92 Laurillard D (2002) *Rethinking University Teaching: A Framework for the Effective Use of Learning Technologies* (2e). Routledge Falmer, London.

93 Prosser M (1987) The effects of cognitive structure and learning strategy on student achievement. In: Richardson J, Eysenck M and Piper D (eds) *Student Learning: Research in Education and Cognitive Psychology,* pp. 29–38. SRHE/Open University Press, Milton Keynes.

94 Bandura A (1986) *Social Foundations of Thought and Action: A Social Cognitive Theory.* Prentice Hall, Englewood Cliffs, NJ.

95 Flynn L, Michalska B, Han H and Gupta S (2012) Teaching and learning interprofessionally: family medicine residents differ from other healthcare learners. *Journal of Research in Interprofessional Practice and Education* [online]. **2**(2): 205–18. (http://www.jripe.org/index.php/journal/article/view/32; accessed 5 November 2012).

96 Pask G and Scott B (1972) Learning strategies and individual competence. *International Journal of Man-Machine Studies.* **4**: 217–53.

97 Perry WG (1970) *Forms of Intellectual and Ethical Development in the College Years: A Scheme.* Holt, Rinehart and Winston, San Francisco, CA.

98 Perry WG (1981) Cognitive and ethical growth: the making of meaning. In: Chickering A (ed.) *The Modern American College,* pp. 76–116. Jossey-Bass, San Francisco, CA.

99 Areskog N-H (1995) Multiprofessional education at the undergraduate level. In: Soothill K, Mackay L and Webb C (eds) *Interprofessional Relations in Health Care,* pp. 125–39. Edward Arnold, London.

100 Ker J, Mole L and Bradley P (2003) Early introduction to interprofessional learning: a simulated ward environment. *Medical Education.* **37**(3): 248–55.

101 Miller C, Woolf C and Mackintosh N (2006) National Evaluation of Common Learning and AHP First Wave Sites. Final Report (Department of Health Commission 0160050). University of Brighton, Brighton. (http://www.ihse.qmul.ac.uk/medicaleducation/Documents/29271.doc; accessed 8 October 2012).

102 Itano JK, Williams J, Deaton MD and Oishi N (1991) Impact of a student interdisciplinary oncology team project. *Journal of Cancer Education.* **6**(4): 219–26.

103 Bruner JS (1977) *The Process of Education.* Harvard University Press, Cambridge, MA.

104 Kilminster S, Hale C, Lascelles M *et al.* (2004) Learning for real life: patient-focused interprofessional workshops offer added value. *Medical Education.* **38**(7): 717–26.

105 Packard K, Chelal H, Maio A *et al.* (2012) Interprofessional team reasoning framework as a tool for case study analysis with health professions students: a randomized study. *Journal of Research in Interprofessional Practice and Education* [online]. **2**(3): 250–263. (http://www.jripe.org/index.php/journal/article/view/96; accessed 5 November 2012).

106 Dewey J (1998/1938) *Experience and Education* (*60th anniversary edition*). Kappa Delta Phi., West Lafayette, IA.

107 Freeth D and Chaput de Saintonge M (2000) Helping medical students become good house officers: interprofessional learning in a skills centre. *Medical Teacher.* **22**(4): 392–8.

108 Madsen M, Gresh A, Petterson B and Taugher M (1988) An interdisciplinary clinic for neurologically impaired adults: a pilot project for educating students. *Journal of Allied Health.* **17**: 135–41.

109 Steven A, Dickinson C and Pearson P (2007) Practice-based interprofessional education: looking into the black box. *Journal of Interprofessional Care.* **21**(3): 251–64.

110 Wright A, Hawkes G, Baker B and Lindqvist SM (2012) Reflections and unprompted observations by healthcare students of an interprofessional shadowing visit. *Journal of Interprofessional Care.* **26**(4): 305–11.

111 Hayward KS (2005) Facilitating interdisciplinary practice through mobile service provision to the rural older adult. *Geriatric Nursing.* **26**(1): 29–33.

112 Reeves S and Freeth D (2002) The London training ward: an innovative interprofessional learning initiative. *Journal of Interprofessional Care.* **16**(1): 41–52.

113 Hylin U, Nyholm H, Mattiasson A-C and Ponzer S (2007) Interprofessional training in clinical practice on a training ward for healthcare students: a two-year follow-up. *Journal of Interprofessional Care.* **21**(3): 277–88.

114 Wahlstrom O and Sanden I (1988) Multiprofessional training at Linkoping University: early experience. *Education for Health.* **11**: 225–31.

115 Jaques D and Salmon G (2007) *Learning in Groups: A Handbook for Face-to-Face and Online Environments* (4e). Routledge, London.

116 Light G, Cox R and Calkins S (2009) *Learning and Teaching in Higher Education: The Reflective Professional* (2e). Sage, London.

117 Savin-Baden M (2003) *Facilitating Problem-Based Learning: Illuminating Perspectives.* Society for Research into Higher Education, Maidenhead.

118 Allport GW (1975) *The Nature of Prejudice* (*25th anniversary edition*). Addison-Wesley, Reading, MA.

119 Hean S and Dickinson C (2005) The contact hypothesis: an exploration of its further potential in interprofessional education. *Journal of Interprofessional Care.* **19**(5): 480–91.

120 Amir Y (1969) Contact hypothesis in ethnic relations. *Psychological Bulletin.* **71**(5): 319–42.

121 Hewstone M and Brown R (1986) Contact is not enough: an intergroup perspective on the 'contact hypothesis'. In: Hewstone M and Brown R (eds) *Contact and Conflit in Intergroup Encounters,* pp. 1–44. Blackwell, Oxford.

122 Tajfel H (1981) *Human Groups and Social Categories: Studies in Social Psychology.* Cambridge University Press, Cambridge.

123 Barnes D, Carpenter J and Dickinson C (2000) Interprofessional education for community mental health: attitudes to community care and professional stereotypes. *Social Work Education.* **19**(6): 565–83.

124 Hewstone M, Carpenter J, Routh D and Franklyn-Stokes A (1994) Intergroup contact between professional groups: two evaluation studies. *Journal of Community and Applied Social Psychology.* **4**(5): 347–63.

125 Carpenter J (1995) Doctors and nurses: stereotypes and stereotype change in interprofessional education. *Journal of Interprofessional Care.* **9**(2): 151–61.

126 Mohaupt J, van Soeren M, Andrusyszyn M-A, MacMillan K, Devlin-Cop S and Reeves S (2012) Understanding interprofessional relationships by the use of contact theory. *Journal of Interprofessional Care.* **26**(5): 370–5.

127 Anderson ES, Thorpe LN and Hammick M (2011) Interprofessional staff development: changing attitudes and winning hearts and minds. *Journal of Interprofessional Care.* **25**(1): 11–7.

128 Bluteau P and Jackson A (2009) An e learning model of interprofessional education. In: Bluteau P and Jackson A (eds) *Interprofessional Education: Making It Happen,* pp. 107–21. Palgrave Macmillan, Basingstoke.

129 Biggs JB and Tang CS-K (2011) *Teaching for Quality Learning at University: What the Student Does* (4e). McGraw-Hill/Society for Research into Higher Education/Open University Press, Maidenhead.

130 Multisource Feedback Work Group of the Academy of Medical Royal Colleges (2009) Multisource feedback, patient surveys and revalidation: report and recommendations. Academy of Medical Royal Colleges, London. (http://www.gmc-uk.org/Item_6e___Annex_C_AoMRC_MSF_and_PF_Report.pdf_28987521.pdf; accessed 8 October 2012).

131 Wood L, Hassell A, Whitehouse A, Bullock A and Wall D (2006) A literature review of multi-source feedback systems within and without health services, leading to 10 tips for their successful design. *Medical Teacher*. **28**(7): e185–91.

132 Wood V, Flavell A, Vanstolk D, Bainbridge L and Nasmith L (2009) The road to collaboration: developing an interprofessional competency framework. *Journal of Interprofessional Care*. **23**(6): 621–9.

133 Canadian Interprofessional Health Collaborative (2010) A National Interprofessional Competency Framework. Canadian Interprofessional Health Collaborative, Vancouver, BC. (http://www.cihc.ca/files/CIHC_IPCompetencies_Feb1210r.pdf; accessed 8 October 2012).

134 Tashiro J, Byrne C, Kitchen L, Vogel E and Bianco C (2011) The development of competencies in interprofessional health care for use in health science educational programs. *Journal of Research in Interprofessional Practice and Education* [online]. **2**(1): 63–82. (http://www.jripe.org/index.php/journal/article/view/64%3C/div%3E; accessed 17 October 2012).

135 Zorek J and Raehl C (2012) Interprofessional education accreditation standards in the USA: a comparative analysis. *Journal of Interprofessional Care*. **27**(2): 123–30.

136 WHO Study Group on Interprofessional Education and Collaborative Practice (2010) Framework for action on interprofessional education and collaborative practice. World Health Organization, Geneva. (http://www.who.int/hrh/resources/framework_action/en/index.html; accessed 8 October 2012).

137 Frenk J, Chen L, Bhutta ZA *et al.* (2010) Health professionals for a new century: transforming education to strengthen health systems in an interdependent world. *The Lancet*. **376**(9756): 1923–58.

138 National Center for Interprofessional Practice and Education (2012) Frequently asked questions http://www.ahceducation.umn.edu/prod/groups/ahc/@pub/@ahc/@educ/documents/article/ahc_article_425404.pdf; accessed 15 June 2013. (http://www.hrsa.gov/about/news/pressreleases/120914interprofessional.html; accessed 8 October 2012).

139 Flexner A (1910) *Medical Education in the United States and Canada: A Report to the Carnegie Foundation for the Advancement of Teaching*. The Carnegie Foundation for the Advancement of Teaching, New York.

140 Thylefors I, Persson O and Hellström D (2005) Team types, perceived efficiency and team climate in Swedish cross-professional teamwork. *Journal of Interprofessional Care*. **19**(2): 102–14.

141 Bluteau P and Jackson A (2009) *Interprofessional Education: Making It Happen*. Palgrave Macmillan, Basingstoke.

142 Howkins E and Bray J (2008) *Preparing for Interprofessional Teaching: Theory and Practice*. Radcliffe, Oxford.

143 Hammick M, Freeth D, Copperman J and Goodsman D (2009) *Being Interprofessional*. Polity Press, Cambridge.

144 Littlechild B and Smith R (eds) (2013) *A Handbook for Interprofessional Practice in the Human Services: Learning to Work Together*. Pearson, Harlow.

145 Day J (2013) *Interprofessional Working: An Essential Guide for Health and Social Care Professionals*. Cengage Learning EMEA, Andover.

Further reading

Many of the other chapters in this book are valuable sources of additional reading to inform the development and delivery of IPE.

Good studies of IPE are dispersed across many journals, their location often reflecting the clinical setting for the IPE or the professional backgrounds of the authors. However, the most extensive single collection of papers about IPE – descriptions, evaluations and theoretical debate – can be found in the *Journal of Interprofessional Care* (www.informa healthcare.com/jic).

This chapter has not discussed the evaluation of IPE, although many of the cited studies ably demonstrate varied approaches to evaluating IPE, selected according to context and the nature of the research questions. I have contributed to an extended discussion of evaluating IPE in Part III of Freeth D, Hammick M, Reeves S, Koppel and Barr H (2005) *Effective Interprofessional Education: development, delivery and evaluation*. Blackwell, Oxford.

The UK Centre for the Advancement of Interprofessional Education maintains a website with important content and useful links to organisations, projects and freely available learning and teaching resources (www.caipe.org.uk).

The Canadian Interprofessional Health Collaborative will keep you up to date with the burgeoning activity in Canada (www.cihc.ca).

In 2009 the Social Care Institute for Excellence (SCIE) published an e-learning resource on interprofessional and interagency collaboration (www.scie.org.uk/publications/elearning/ipiac)

Several recent books focus on developing, delivering and evaluating IPE,(49,141,142) or on interprofessional and interagency collaboration.(143–145)

7 Work-based learning

Clare Morris[1] and David Blaney[2]
[1] Clinical Education and Leadership, University of Bedfordshire, UK
[2] Medical Protection Society, UK; University of York, UK

KEY MESSAGES

- The workplace is a fundamentally important site for learning in both undergraduate and postgraduate medical education.

- The erosion of time-served methods of apprenticeship creates challenges for those tasked with ensuring that health care professionals are appropriately trained to deliver safe, efficient and effective patient care.

- Insight into the theoretical concepts underpinning work-based learning reveals a range of tools and approaches that can be employed to 'revive' apprenticeship and support work-based learning.

- Faculty development for clinical teachers drawing on social theories of learning provides a way forward to enhance work-based learning in medical settings.

Introduction

Work is where we spend a considerable amount of our life and expend a great deal of physical and emotional energy. Work is how many people define themselves, be it in relation to their role – 'I am a doctor' – or to their place of work – 'I work for the University of. . .'. For doctors, work and the workplace is where their professional learning is made real, where knowledge and skills are acquired, crafted and developed. We all have different experiences of work and workplaces. We influence our workplace, and it influences and shapes us. The workplace can be a nurturing environment where knowledge and skills are fostered, extended and developed through work activity and interactions with others. Equally, it can be a dysfunctional environment that stifles creativity, dampens professional motivation and leads to psychological and physical ill health.(1,2)

In this chapter we explore the value of work-based learning in an ever-changing landscape, outline current conceptions of work-based learning and their underpinning theoretical perspectives, and propose strategies to enhance work-based learning for medical students and trainees. Whilst medical education is the chosen exemplar, we recognise the challenges faced by other health care professionals involved in supporting work-based learning in clinical contexts.

The changing landscape of medical education and training

Health care professionals' education is dependent upon the interplay between two complex systems, the higher education institution and the health 'service'.(3) Changes in one will impact upon the other, whether intended or otherwise. For example, a call for early patient contact in the curriculum has resource implications for those supporting such placements in practice settings. Changes in clinical service organisation and delivery have resulted in patients spending less time in hospitals, traditionally the main provider of work-based experiences. In medical education, concerns have been raised that 'healthcare as a business may threaten medicine as a calling', with clinical teachers being challenged to provide opportunities for learning through experience and practice.(4) Others argue that teaching and patient care have become subordinate to research, with the increased demand for productivity eroding teaching time.(5) Responses to working time directives lead to concerns about the availability of supervised work-based learning experiences,(6,7) with some evidence emerging that trainees are experiencing significant reductions in work-based learning opportunities.(8)

Both the higher education and health sectors have undergone periods of unprecedented, rapid and ongoing change in the past decade. Tensions arise between liberal ambitions of universities, seeking to promote academic excellence and produce world-class graduates, and the more instrumental ambitions of employers wishing to recruit staff who are able to deliver care efficiently and effectively.(5) One exemplar is the reform of postgraduate medical training in the UK, with a move away from costly time-served models of apprenticeship to more closely regulated time-measured, outcomes based, competency assessed training models(9) leading to debates about whether 'competence' or 'excellence' should be the benchmark for training.(8) The UK is certainly not unique in facing such challenges or engaging in such debates.(10,11) Recent calls for reform of medical

Understanding Medical Education: Evidence, Theory and Practice, Second Edition. Edited by Tim Swanwick.
© 2014 The Association for the Study of Medical Education. Published 2014 by John Wiley & Sons, Ltd.

education in the USA, for example, seek the standardisation of learning outcomes and competency based assessment.(12) Across Europe, commentators question the value and meaning of competence and argue for training based upon professional judgement embedded in the concept of 'entrustable professional activity'.(13) An analysis of the relative merits of such models is beyond the scope of this chapter; but the ways in which medical training is framed, however, will shape and skew the types of work activity that are deemed to have learning value.

Whilst work-based learning is recognised as a fundamental aspect of education and training, its perceived status has been challenged by the privileges afforded to formal teaching. This is evidenced in protected teaching time, investment in formal teaching spaces and simulation resources within clinical environments, and investment in off-site development opportunities for trainees and their trainers. The danger of this is that work-based learning is marginalised and undervalued. Yet, as we argue in the next section, the curriculum of the workplace is fundamentally important to the development of future doctors.

The current state of work-based learning in medical education

Irrespective of the continual reshaping of health care provision, clinical workplaces continue to be a significant site for learning at all stages of a medical career. Students undertake work-based placements throughout their undergraduate education. Trainees/residents rotate through a range of clinical specialties and contexts in their postgraduate years, whilst more senior medical staff continue to develop, adapt and innovate in their practice. Workplace-based learning is clearly important but inherently problematic. Alongside the debates about curriculum models and trainees' ability to access to sufficient work-based learning opportunities, other concerns emerge.

Holmboe and colleagues(14) adopt a critical stance to the deeply entrenched approach to medical rotations for students and trainees, noting that very little empirical evidence exists on the optimal timing and duration of rotations, and how transitions should be supported. They question an approach based on multiple, short rotations, noting that from a sociological perspective this undermines the capacity to understand and engage in different cultures of teams, contexts and specialties. They argue that 'the lack of ongoing supervision and longitudinal relationships with faculty profoundly conflict with growing evidence from the literature on the development of expertise'.(14, p. 76)

Longer, integrated clinical attachments offer a range of potential benefits, including enhanced professionalism, more holistic appreciation of the course of illnesses and greater patient-centredness.(15,16) A recent study showed that students undertaking these types of clerkships were more actively engaged in independent patient care activity at the end of a year, than those undertaking more traditional block rotations.(16)

The issue of graduate preparedness has attracted considerable interest in the UK. There is evidence to suggest that a significant proportion of medical graduates do not feel suitably prepared for clinical practice and have concerns about dealing with the day-to-day realities of working life, be it dealing with acutely ill patients, prescribing, managing their workload or being on call.(17–21) Significantly, additional challenges, such as understanding their role and boundaries, may only become evident in their first posts.(18) The reasons why some graduates feel unprepared are complex and span individual and organisational dimensions. However, the amount and nature of work-based experience undergraduates have and their opportunity to shadow first posts before commencing employment appears to increase their preparedness. Early experiences of the workplace were noted to have an impact on intended career pathways for half of those in the British Medical Association cohort study, with working conditions and work hours the main reasons cited for planned changes.(19)

Others have moved the emphasis on graduate preparedness, turning attention to issues of transition throughout a medical career.(22,23) They argue that transition is an underresearched area in medicine, yet other high-risk occupations have documented that it is at periods of transition that performance is compromised, linking this to adverse outcomes. Researching periods when trainees assume greater levels of medical responsibility, they argue that doctors can never be fully prepared because 'performance occurs in the interface between the doctor and the work itself in a specific setting'.(22, p.1013) Others might understand these issues in terms of the capacity of learners to put their knowledge to work in new situations or contexts.(24)

Regular access to high-quality supervision is fundamental to successful work-based learning experiences, whatever stage of a medical career. The fragmentation of supervisory relationships underpins many of the issues highlighted above. It is perhaps unsurprising, therefore, that attention is turning to the selection, preparation and recognition and approval of clinical faculty undertaking supervisory responsibilities.(12,25,26) *See* also Box 7.1.

There is little doubt that doctors in training value work-based learning experiences and seek opportunities to engage in work-based learning. They want a structured environment where work-based learning is valued, protected and appropriately supervised and supported. However, reform of health care, education and training, and threats to the time-served nature of training are placing significant challenges on those in training and those who are charged with supporting and fostering their development in the workplace. Access to a range of theoretical tools and conceptions of work-based learning may be the key to overcoming such challenges.(27)

Learning and work

In this section we provide an overview of the ways working and learning relationships are conceptualised; this inevitably leads to a review of theories of learning, some of which have already been covered in detail in Chapter 2. Sfard(28) argues that the views we hold about learning are significant, shaping the ways in which we engage with learners and the pedagogic practices we adopt. Scott(29) provides a thoughtful critique of curriculum theories, and drawing on Bernstein's model of curriculum as performance,(30) he identifies the following predominant elements in mainstream education:

- the strong focus on traditional forms of knowledge (discipline-based)
- distinctions between lower and higher domains of knowledge
- differentiation of learners and the curriculum (selection, differentiation)
- the teacher's role being to impart knowledge.(29)

While his critique focuses on schooling, there are parallels with professional education. In medicine, as with other health professions, the curriculum has been based on a model of technical rationality, where knowledge (in the mind of the learner) is 'applied' to the world of practice. Although this model has been challenged,(31) it persists in the minds of many as the 'best' way to educate, leading to a continued focus on imitation and instruction as the primary tools of the teacher. However, several commentators(32–34) have argued that the tendency to compare work-based learning with formal learning, or to draw on formal models of learning in the workplace, is unhelpful. Responding to this, we examine existing and emerging notions of work-based learning and the potential to develop new approaches to professional education and training.

Informal and non-formal learning

Medical education has tended to draw a distinction between 'formal' learning (medical school) and 'informal' learning (in the clinical work environment). Formal learning is typically characterised by timetables, aims and objectives, a defined curriculum and often, progressive, linear teaching and examinations. In contrast, informal learning, usually in the workplace, has traditionally been less valued by teachers and students, viewed as haphazard, opportunistic and lacking any formal educational rigour, process or structure. As noted previously, these criticisms arise in part because work-based learning is compared with the process and pedagogy of formal learning, rather than being viewed as having a pedagogy and process of its own.

Eraut(35) proposes a move away from the use of the term 'informal learning' to that of 'non-formal learning'. In so doing he proposes a typology of *non-formal* learning, focusing on the learner's intention to learn. *Implicit learning* is characterised by learning that takes place without any prior intention to learn by the learner, with the learner being unaware of the learning at the time. He contrasts this with *deliberative learning*, where the learner sets time aside to learn and approaches learning in a planned and purposeful way. Between these two points, Eraut describes *reactive learning*, which happens almost spontaneously as a result of situation and circumstance. Whilst the learning is not consciously planned, learners recognise learning opportunities, are prepared for emergent learning opportunities and are likely to engage in brief, almost spontaneous reflection on learning events or experiences. This distinction is helpful when we consider ways to promote work-based learning, suggesting the possibility of explicitly recognising, responding to and valuing the learning that arises during everyday practice, and encouraging students and trainees to do the same.

Work-based learning

Work-based learning spans all stages of medical education and training, from early undergraduate years, through specialist training and, increasingly, continuing medical education. Boud and Solomon have explored the place of work-based learning in professional education, noting that undergraduate courses now: 'Acknowledge the workplace as a site of learning and as a source for making the curriculum more relevant. As such they are a signal of the blurring distinctions between the university and the workplace'.(36, p. 34)

They go on to note that this 'blurring' signals the increasing legitimisation of learning outside formal academic contexts and argue that this creates both opportunities and challenges for students and trainees: 'Learning tasks are influenced by the nature of work and, in turn, work is influenced by the nature of the learning that occurs. The two are complementary. Learners are workers; workers are learners. They need to be able to manage both their roles'.(36, p. 34)

This dual role is particularly striking in postgraduate training, where trainees are also employees and therefore have service as well as learning commitments. Seagraves and Boyd(37) distinguishes three 'links' between work and learning, as follows:

- learning *for* work
- learning *at* work
- learning *from* work.

These semantic distinctions are important, signalling, albeit implicitly, different relationships between working and learning, and the intended purposes of that learning. The question that arises is whether, for example, the medical curriculum is designed or intended to enhance working practice or professional practice. In other words, is the learning undertaken for the benefit of the employer or the individual? To some extent, this depends on the perspective from which work is viewed.

Evans *et al.*(38) provide the following three perspectives, which are of value in viewing work-based learning:

- industrial relations
- sociological
- social learning theory.

Viewed from the *industrial relations* perspective, work is a contested activity, with constant tension between employee and employer over rights, obligations and the prevention or misuse of employee skills and labour. Work-based learning is driven by the needs of the workplace, rather than those within it, with access to further training and development opportunities being driven by desires to promote innovation or efficiency. Work-based learning is something employers control (e.g. study leave). For medical students and trainees this is visible in issues such as access to study leave, hours of work and rotas, and the emphasis on statutory training.

Viewed from the *sociological* perspective, however, work is more of a place of and for social interaction, socialisation and identity formation. Clearly, this is of influence in the development of professional roles and identities, where interpersonal relationships, power, authority and status are all part of the dynamic of the workplace. In this context, how an individual trainee or student relates to others and how they are perceived by others may have a bearing on the types of learning experiences they are offered, the training they receive and the professional identity they ultimately develop.(39,40) How work is perceived will have an effect on how an individual views and approaches work-based learning. Work involves professional activity, but also demands of doctors, trainees and students additional duties, roles and responsibilities. Understanding this is central to work-based learning and, as we will argue later, is important if students and trainees wish to maximise their learning at work. The difficulty is that the privileging of, and overemphasis on, formal learning in undergraduate years may influence student and trainee ability to recognise the learning that is embedded in working activity.(41) The value of social learning theory in helping make sense of medical education is specifically explored below.

Theorising work-based learning

Theories of learning can be seen to sit within different educational schools of thought, distinctions between them drawn in a range of ways. One broad distinction is between those that focus on individual learning (behavioural and cognitive theories) and those that focus on shared or distributed learning (social learning theories).(33,34) Others differentiate on the basis of psychological, sociological or socio-cultural origins.(42) Sfard(28) differentiates on the basis of the underpinning metaphors, contrasting learning-as-acquisition with learning-as-participation. In the former, the goal of learning is the acquisition and accumulation of knowledge and skills – i.e. cognitive and behavioural theories. This metaphor allows us to consider issues of transfer of knowledge from one situation or context to another (seen, for example, in concerns about preparedness). In the latter, the goal of learning is to become a full participant of a community of learners or workers – i.e. socio-cultural theories. This metaphor captures processes of professional identity formation and enculturation (seen in concerns about transitions). Chapter 2 summarises a broad range of learning theory, and helpful critiques of workplace learning theories can be found in the wider learning literatures.(43) In this chapter however, we have endeavoured to highlight some helpful explanatory and analytical ways of thinking specifically about work-based learning, as it relates to medicine, notably behavioural, cognitive and social orientations to learning.

Behavioural conceptions of learning
Behavioural orientations to learning have their traditions in psychology, tending to focus on skill acquisition of individual learners, with the influence of context relatively 'silent'. Broadly speaking, behaviourism contests that learning is manifested by changes in behaviour, these changes being the result of stimuli that are external to the individual, that is, environmental factors. Hartley argues that the learning principles arising from the behaviourist

school are focused on the importance of the following components:
- learning by doing
- frequent practice in varied contexts
- reinforcement as a prime motivator
- the need to have clearly defined behavioural objectives that are communicated to the learner.(44)

These learning principles are readily observed in popular models of skills-based teaching in medicine and the rise of competency-based education. But however desirable the models may seem, they belie the complexity of work-based and professional learning. As Hager cautions, 'The notion that job performance can be fully specifiable in advance remains a seductively attractive one. This false hope has underpinned much of the support that competency-based training has garnered in recent times'.(43, p.18)

Cognitive conceptions of learning
The cognitive orientation to learning can be seen as a shift from the behaviourist's focus on the external world to one that focuses on the internal world of the learner and changes in their thinking. Here, the focus is on the acquisition of knowledge and skills, be it as a result of input from a more able 'other' (through processes of transmission) or through engagement with one's own experiences (constructivism). Referred to as the 'standard'(44) and 'dominant'(28,33) paradigm, it is where learning is understood as:
- residing in individual minds
- being propositional in nature
- expressible verbally or in writing
- transparent to the mind.(45)

Constructivism, within the cognitive school and closely linked to the work of Jean Piaget, posits that meaning (or learning) is generated through human engagement with experience. As Scott and Palinscar note: 'Constructivists argue there is no such thing as ready-made knowledge; regardless of what a teacher does, learners construct their own knowledge. All learning . . . requires reinterpreting the information to be learnt or used in light of one's existing understandings and abilities'.(46, p. 31)

Cognitive views on learning are readily found in medical education research and practice. As Swanwick notes, the contested concepts of *andragogy*,(47) *experiential learning* (48) and *reflection* (49,50) have led to the almost wholesale adoption of portfolios, appraisal and personal development planning in all walks of medical education and training.(34) What is important to note here, however, is that these models present learning as essentially unmediated activity, which happens as a result of learner engagement with their own experiences. For example, Kolb's learning cycle of concrete experience, reflection, conceptualisation and experimentation(48) is abstracted from a social context and tells us little about the types of experience that may foster this cyclical process or the role of more expert practitioners in encouraging or supervising subsequent reflection, conceptualisation and experimentation. The 'cognitive apprenticeship' model(51,52) is a helpful supplement here. *See* Box 7.1.

Lee *et al.* note this emphasis on rational and cognitive aspects leads to work performance being 'conceived as

BOX 7.1 FOCUS ON: Cognitive apprenticeship

The cognitive apprenticeship model derives from traditional craft apprenticeship, but makes 'thinking visible'.(52) Collins *et al.*(51) identified the following six stages to their model, which can be readily adopted in work-based teaching and is particularly useful in teaching decision making, ethics, communication skills and other cognitively complex areas of professional practice.

Modelling: allow the learner to observe your practice in order to build up a conceptualisation of that practice.

Coaching: watch the learner practise, offering them guidance, critique and feedback.

Scaffolding: offer the learner more opportunities to practise, gradually and purposefully increasing complexity of the work undertaken while slowly fading out your input.

Articulation: use questioning and supervision time to encourage the learner to talk you through what they are doing, why and how, providing a rationale for the approaches taken.

Reflection: encourage the learner to consider his or her performance analytically and to compare it with that of the expert to identify ways to further enhance his or her own performance.

Exploration: provide opportunities for the learner to undertake new tasks and activities, prompting the learner to become independent in his or her activity and his or her thinking.

thinking or reflection followed by application of the thinking or reflection'.(53, p. 7) Central to these models is the individual learner's capacity to engage with an experience, reflect critically on it and deduce the lessons learnt that need to be applied to future activity. Cognitive perspectives of learning will tend to lead to an emphasis on instructional methods, with the importance of structure being stressed. The importance of building on prior knowledge is key, and so distinctions between individual learners are important when planning teaching or supervision. Cognitive feedback (successes and failures) is an important dimension, providing learners with new information to assimilate and accommodate. However, cognitive models of learning are increasingly being called into question as the dominant model for work-based learning in medicine.(14,22,33,34,54)

Social-contextual conceptions of learning

Theories of learning that recognise and explicitly emphasise the social, participatory and context specific nature of learning are argued to be of greater relevance to complex practice that happens in teams and communities of workers and learners. Three of these – *social cognitive theory*, *social constructivism* and *socio-cultural theories* – are considered in this section.

Social theories of learning pay attention to both the inner and external worlds of learners, and the interaction between individuals and those around them is central to the process of meaning making. Each of the theoretical perspectives explored in the following section places different levels of emphasis on this interaction and the impact of the social elements on learning and practice. All offer valuable insights into the potential nature of work-based learning in medicine and suggest ways of working with students and trainees to foster learning.

Social cognitive theory

Social cognitive theory can be seen as a coming together or a bridging of the behaviourists' concern with external, environmental stimuli and the cognitive theorists' concern with the internal mind. Bandura(55) proposed a model of learning to capture what he saw as the dynamic interplay between the personal, the cognitive and the environmental, which, combined, determine an individual's behaviour (*see* Figure 2.1). He described this as *reciprocal determinism*.

Social cognitive theory is discussed in more detail in Chapter 2, but to summarise here, Bandura identified five fundamental human capabilities, as follows:

- *symbolising* (in order to give structure, meaning and continuity to their lives)
- *forethought* (planning for action, considering potential consequence of actions)
- *self-regulation* (through the positive and negative consequences that their behaviour produces)
- *self-reflection* (in relation to own functioning and self-efficacy)
- *vicarious learning* (through close observation of others).

It can be argued, therefore, that what people think, feel and believe will influence how they behave, with self-belief (also described as self-efficacy(56)) being an important determinant of motivation and achievement (*see* Box 2.3). The capability for vicarious learning has been argued to be an important element of role-modelling in medicine and a powerful means of transmitting values, attitudes and patterns of behaviour, be it through imitation or identification.(57)

Role-modelling is foregrounded in the medical education literature as a key process in professional development and enculturation,(58,59) and Box 7.2 summarises some

BOX 7.2 HOW TO: Be a good role model(57–60)

- Be positive about what you do
- Be enthusiastic, compassionate and open
- Analyse your own performance as a role model
- Model reflection and facilitate the reflections of others
- Articulate and discuss values
- Make the implicit more explicit
- Be learner-centred in your teaching
- Allow time for discussion and debrief
- Engage in personal and professional development activity
- Show respect to colleagues
- Work to improve workplace culture and values.

of the characteristics that 'good' role models are said to display. A review of the literature pertaining to 'good clinical teaching' notes the dominance of non-cognitive characteristics based on personal and relationship-based attributes.(60) It is unsurprising, therefore, that concerns have been raised about the erosion of role-modelling through the demise of apprenticeship and the commercialisation of health care.(5,61) Despite the central importance ascribed to role-modelling, its basis remains largely unexamined and considerable assumptions are made of its effectiveness.(57)

Social constructivism

In constructivist models the emphasis is on how the individual learner 'constructs' knowledge, that is, how the learner makes sense of new information and experiences provided by the teacher, the environment and their wider experience. Social constructivism goes one step further, emphasising the importance of social engagement in the learning process. In other words, learners make sense of new ideas and information by engaging with others, be it their teachers, their fellow students or others around them. An example of social constructivism influences to medical education would be problem-based learning (in its purest form).

Vygotsky,(62) who developed his theories of learning from observational studies of children interacting with adults, was a key contributor to social constructivism. He noted that children were more successful in learning tasks when they engaged with adults (a more knowledgeable 'other') than when they worked independently, arguing that learning awakens developmental processes that are able to operate only when the child is interacting with their peers and others in their environment. This is significantly different from models of experiential learning explored above, which suggest that the provision of a learning experience itself leads to learning. Vygotsky drew attention to the concepts and tools teachers use to mediate the learning of another, stressing the importance of language (or shared talk) in the developmental process. Importantly, he introduced what has been described as a fundamentally new approach to the need to match learning to the learner's developmental stage, through the construct of the *zone of proximal development*.(46) This refers to what a learner can do with the support of a more knowledgeable other (be it their teacher or their peers) and is contrasted with their *zone of actual development*, or what they can do independently. Box 7.3 illustrates the ways in which Vygotsky's work can shape approaches to clinical teaching.

Social cognitive theory and constructivist approaches help us understand ways in which we might support student or trainee learning. However, even these models are limited in helping us better understand the complexity of work-based learning. It is here that socio-cultural theories of learning have the greatest potential utility.(54)

Socio-cultural learning

It has been argued that junior doctors learn by 'situated learning in communities of practice',(63) explicitly referring to the work of socio-cultural theorists and, in particu-

---

 BOX 7.3 FOCUS ON: Vygotsky

Consider the mediated nature of learning activity
Vygotsky drew attention to the 'tools' that we use to 'mediate' a learning experience, be it the language we use to explain or guide, or the tools we use to exemplify, such as handouts, paper cases, X-rays and patients-as-cases. This can help us look more purposefully at informal learning encounters, and recognise and make explicit the everyday tools and learning resources we use.

Identify learners' needs and learning potential
Vygotsky drew a distinction between what he termed the *zone of actual development* (what the learner can actually do unassisted) and the *zone of proximal development* (what the learner can do with some assistance or guidance). Learning is what takes place in the zone of proximal development, where we guide, assist, support and coach our learners. In working with students and trainees, therefore, it is important to recognise what they can do independently and then to work out how we can *scaffold* their learning so that they can move forward.

Engage 'more knowledgeable others' in the learning process
Vygotsky saw engagement with peers and others in the environment as an essential prerequisite for learning to take place. Recognising and valuing the contributions made by all members of the care team and the learners' peer group are essential to effective learning in the workplace.

---

lar, the work of Lave and Wenger.(64) The evidence base supporting this assertion is explored in Box 7.4. Socio-cultural theories of learning have broad disciplinary origins and embrace a wide range of theoretical perspectives. However, it has been argued that they share some core tenets, these being that learning is:

- situated (shaped by the context in which it occurs)
- mediated (by a range of symbolic and conceptual tools)
- historically and culturally influenced.

Social-cultural theories have undoubtedly been influenced by Vygotsky's work (and others from the social-constructivism school), but they draw even greater attention to the wider context in which learning takes place, and the role of the wider community in which learners learn. They emphasise the historical context of practice, in other words they argue that in order for a student to understand workplace practices, they need to have a sense of the history of those practices and how they have evolved over time. This gives support to the idea that it is important to recognise what has been successful in work-based learning in medicine and to find ways to ensure that these historically successful strategies can evolve to be equally successful in new times and contexts.

BOX 7.4 WHERE'S THE EVIDENCE: For situated learning

Lave and Wenger(64) developed their viewpoints on learning through ethnographic studies of traditional 'apprenticeships' as diverse as the apprenticeships of Yucatec midwives, Vai and Gola tailors, butchers, quartermasters and members of Alcoholics Anonymous. From this work they developed ideas around situated learning and communities of practice, both of which have been influential on thinking about informal and work-based learning generally and, increasingly, in medical education specifically. Claims have been made for the value of drawing on their viewpoints, when looking at work-based learning in medicine;(3,14,33,34,54,65–69) however, few studies have been undertaken to explicitly explore the extent to which their claims are true of medical education.

A qualitative study of medical student learning on clinical attachments supported the idea that attachments could be seen as times spent in communities of practice, albeit in a descriptive sense. The limits placed on student engagement in authentic work-based activity, the extent to which students and their teachers identify the learning resources embedded in this day-to-day activity and the hierarchical (and sometimes authoritarian) stance towards teaching and learning limited the extent to which this claim could be supported.(70) Likewise, a qualitative study of general practice training revealed that registrars may not be able to become full participants in the practices of a community, nor may they be able to access and engage with all of the community members to develop shared understandings of practice.(68) The work around preparedness of graduates for practice(18,19) and the limited nature of student engagement in authentic clinical activity(69) also question the extent to which they are able to become full participants through legitimate peripheral participatory practices.

Socio-cultural theorists see the distinction between learning and working (or practice) as being artificial. They start from the assumption that learning is part and parcel of our everyday experience and practice. So, for example, when we talk to our colleagues about patients we are having difficulty with, or we 'think aloud' management options on the ward round, we are engaged in both a working activity and a learning activity. Our understanding of each other, our patients and their illnesses is influenced by the conversations we have, and this becomes part of the learning in the workplace. When we encounter a complex patient or a complex situation, we draw on the 'learning resources' around us (our peers, our seniors, other members of the health care team) to consider how to move forward. We might consult other types of resource, such as internet search engines, but seldom do we immediately 'rush off to be taught' to address these issues. As students develop their practice, they are learning at the same time. Learning is therefore an everyday activity and is developed by joint participation. In other words, learning is 'situated' and collective, with a shift in emphasis from a focus on the individual learner or teacher, to one that focuses on the 'team' or 'community'.

In recent years, the term 'community of practice' has been adopted by those in professional education and used, often uncritically, to capture a desire to foster collaborative working, be it face-to-face or online. *See* Chapter 22. However, its original use was much more specific and was to capture examples of situated learning in a range of 'apprenticeship systems' observed ethnographically by Lave and Wenger.(64) Their seminal text identifies a defining feature of learning in these contexts, that of legitimate peripheral participation, described as: 'A way to speak about the relations between newcomers and old-timers, and about activities, identities, artefacts and communities of knowledge and practice. It concerns the process by which newcomers become part of a community of practice. A person's intentions to learn are engaged and the meaning of learning is configured through the process of becoming a full participant in a socio-cultural practice'.(64, p. 29)

Four key ideas emerge from Lave and Wenger's work, which have particular relevance to work-based learning in medicine and newly emerging models of apprenticeship, as follows:

- learning is part of social practice
- learning takes place in communities of practice
- learning takes place through legitimate peripheral participation
- language is a central part of practice.

Let's explore these ideas in more depth. First, *learning is part of social practice*. Every day at work we encounter new situations, new patients, new colleagues, trainees or students that lead us to question what we know, what we do, and how and why we do it. This is clearly a 'learning' situation, although we might not always label it as such. Second, *learning takes place in communities of practice*,(71) which can be identified and defined by common expertise. The practice of a surgical team or the psychiatric outreach team demonstrates this in that their practice is effective because of the shared endeavour, the collective 'team think' that leads to successful outcomes. If we compare these two 'teams', while each contains doctors, nurses and health care professionals, they are clearly distinct in terms of the specialist work they do, the ways they do this and the 'cultures' of their practice (how they dress, how they talk to each other and their patients, etc.). Clearly, within medicine there are many distinct communities of practice, and students and trainees need to learn how to participate within them and indeed, across them.(70) Third, *learning has a central defining process, that of 'legitimate peripheral participation'*, a process that enables the student to develop the expertise necessary to permit full access and participation in a community. When we delegate work to students and trainees, we need to ensure it allows increasing engagement in 'real' work activity, from the periphery (e.g. scrubbing up to observe the surgical procedure) to more central core activity (e.g. leading the surgical procedure). It is important to note that the relationships described between 'newcomers' and 'old-timers' here are very different from the traditional hierarchical educational models of novice to expert. This is an important distinction as it recognises the valuable contributions students and trainees can make to shaping and developing practice and the impact they can have on the workplace. Finally, *language is a central part of practice*, not only in terms of learning from talk, but rather in terms of learning to talk – a process of talking one's way into the expertise. For example, when students and trainees 'present cases', with implicit structures and cultures of doing so – 'Mrs Smith is a 55-year-old woman, who presented to A and E with a three-day history of. . .' – they are learning 'to talk' medicine and therefore learning medicine itself.

Socio-cultural perspectives on work-based learning clearly offer some theoretical and conceptual tools to allow researchers and practitioners to analyse important aspects of work-based learning. The emphasis on learning as being something that encompasses the processes of 'belonging, becoming and identity', as well as meaning making,(71) encourages closer attention to what others have termed the 'hidden curriculum' of medical education and training. However, Lave and Wenger's work has been criticised for its lack of attention to a number of important issues, namely:

- individual variations in accessing learning in the workplace(72)
- the ways in which 'old timers' continue to learn in the workplace(73)
- emotional dimensions of work-based learning(2)
- the role of formal learning opportunities for workers,(73,74)

Billett, in particular, argues the need to pay attention to the *invitational qualities* of the workplace, in terms of the ways in which the workplace provides and allows access to learning activities.(32,72) A concrete example can be seen in obstetrics and gynaecology attachments for medical students, where male students are likely to access fewer hands-on learning experiences than female students, due to patient preferences.(75) More subtle variations of opportunity may exist on the basis of 'qualities' attributed to students by staff. For example, more able students who express high levels of confidence, enthusiasm and interest in a specialty may access more learning opportunities than a shy or struggling student or one perceived to have limited insight into their own performance. In this latter case it may be that those who most need experience to develop confidence and competence are denied these experiences.(65) Despite these criticisms, social perspectives on learning can be seen as a way forward to understanding and therefore more effectively shaping the work-based learning opportunities offered to students and trainees.

Any single theory of learning will have its limitations. Cognitive and behavioural orientations help explain the ways in which knowledge and skills are acquired and provide a language to talk about transfer, yet fail to offer a way to explain learning within and across teams. Traditional understandings of medical apprenticeship have been shaped by this thinking, focused on the instruction and development of the apprentice in the workplace. The focus is very much on the development of the individual, through engagement with the supervising expert. It does not accommodate the idea that the expert may learn from the apprentice and that the apprentice may in fact shape the practice in which they both engage. Contemporary views of apprenticeship, building on socio-cultural theories of learning, accommodate not only the reciprocal nature of learning between 'apprentice and master', but also the contributions made by others in the professional community. New formulations of apprenticeship are emerging that enable us to look beyond the novice–expert dualism and consider a social apprenticeship that much more actively recognises the contributions made by the wider community of the workplace.(73) Whilst social-cultural orientations offer contextual ways to analyse and re-think medical apprenticeship, including processes of professional formation and practice, they too have their limits. They downplay the role of cognition, restrict thinking about transfer and are most valuable in understanding stable working practices. However, medical education is undergoing periods of significant reform, traditional approaches to apprenticeship are being eroded and working teams being fragmented by system reform. More expansive orientations, with the potential to explain complex medical learning and practice are starting to emerge, drawing on activity theory and actor-network theory.(66,76,77)

Curriculum and work-based learning: a complex relationship

In describing these different theoretical schools of thought, we have drawn out the ways in which work-based learning can be conceptualised in its own right. The distinctiveness of work-based learning can also be highlighted in relation to the curriculum.

Traditional approaches to curriculum design,(78,79) based on formal education, focus on the curriculum as transmission of a body of knowledge (e.g. paediatrics) or on the definition of desired end points and outcomes (e.g. a competent doctor). The emphasis is on the clear delineation of specific knowledge, skills and attitudes, which are seen as measurable outputs of learning.

The risk with this model as a framework for work-based learning is that it assumes that all worthwhile attainments are visible and quantifiable,(29,43,45) that those external to the learner are best placed to identify what it is the learner needs and that learning itself is devalued with the emphasis on outcomes (to be signed off) rather than processes of learning,(80,81) The emphasis on competence, as opposed to excellence, has also been questioned – for instance, in the UK following the wholesale introduction of work-based curriculum and assessment tools in postgraduate medical education.(8)

When we turn to social theories of learning, however, additional understandings of the work-based curriculum become available. The 'process curriculum', drawing on a social constructivist perspective, focuses on the construction of meaning and collaborative engagement. As Stenhouse argues: 'The superficialities of the disciplines may be taught by pure instruction, but the capacity to think within the disciplines can only be taught by inquiry'.(82, p. 38)

A process-based curriculum places importance on the relationships between trainer and trainee and the outcome of their interaction. It is grounded in the individual experience of the trainee, resulting from their clinical and professional experiences. A process curriculum assumes that trainers have experience and knowledge, that they understand their role and have a mature and internalised concept of what they are trying to achieve with the trainee. The content of the trainee's learning is to a great extent built on and derived from their experiences and is developed by promoting critical dialogue and thinking, reflecting both in and on outcomes and activity. In the process curriculum, both trainer and trainee seek to critically test knowledge, and the learning is continually adapted by both trainer and trainee. The consequence of such an approach is that learning outcomes can vary between trainees and are negotiable depending on the trainee's capability. However, the purpose of the curriculum is to extend the trainee and to seek to maximise their potential, rather than simply achieve competence. The learner is actively involved and manages the process of learning with the trainer, and the interaction and relationship with the trainer is central to this process.

The contrast between 'product' and 'process' models of curriculum lead us to consider the appropriateness of each *for* the workplace. However, socio-cultural theories of learning focus on the workplace and work *as* the curriculum; in other words, there is little separation between participation in working life and learning.(64,83) If the workplace is the curriculum, the challenge for those with educational roles in the workplace is to make the learning that can arise from working more explicit, and to ensure that learners are engaged in the process of seeking and accepting these opportunities to learn.

This is underlined by studies exploring the nature of work-based learning in clinical settings, which have emphasised the importance of:

- initiation processes to engage learners as part of the team (69)
- active involvement in patient care(65–69)
- access to conversations, coaching and feedback in order to foster professional thinking and skill development.(84)

Constraints may arise in terms of the number of 'learners' attached to a particular setting, and the nature and scope of work activity undertaken by the team.(66) It is important to emphasise that if the workplace is the curriculum, the learning relationships to be developed must extend beyond those between individual learner and teacher to encompass the whole team.(33) More recent framings of apprenticeship(73) adopt these broader perspectives on learning and curriculum and identify the ways in which the workplace can both expand and restrict opportunities for learning.

Implications for the clinical teacher

The question reasonably arises: What does this all mean for an individual clinical teacher, trainer or supervisor? The direct implications can be summarised as follows.

1 Learning is part of everyday social practice(64)

Implication: We need to make learning opportunities explicit to our learners. We also need to make explicit specific workplace cultures and practices to help students and trainees 'make sense' of what they see, hear, sense and do.

2 Teams can be seen as 'communities of practice', which are identified and defined by their shared expertise(71)
Implication: We need to involve the whole team (community) in supporting student/trainee learning.

3 Novices become experts through participation in communities of practice(64)
Implication: We need to consider the ways in which we can meaningfully involve our students/trainees in workplace activity.

4 Workplaces do not always readily invite learners in and do not always offer equal opportunities to all learners(72)
Implication: We need to consider how we can create the right conditions for learning to take place in our workplace and to ensure certain students or groups of students/trainees are not inadvertently disadvantaged.

5 Horizontal learning is as important as vertical learning in the workplace(85)
Implication: We need to understand what our students/trainees already know (where they are coming from) and help them to use it to make sense of what they see, hear and do in the workplace.

6 'Talk' is a central part of practice – learners need to 'learn to talk their way into expertise', rather than just learn from the talk of an expert(64)
Implication: We need to find strategies to help our students and trainees talk themselves into the expertise, by using techniques such as 'thinking aloud' and case-based discussion.

7 Students and trainees learn from their entire setting (72,73)
Implication: We need to be aware of the workplace climate and the effect this will have on trainees. This includes how staff relate to them and to each other, how staff are valued, and how they value their work and workplace.

8 Students require multiple learning experiences and learning methods
Implication: A balance needs to be found between the duration of attachments – sufficient to allow students to become immersed in the workplace – and providing enough attachments to give exposure to other workplaces and specialties.

9 Feedback to students and a sense of belonging are important in allowing them to feel confident and become active participants in the workplace
Implication: Regular feedback is important, and we need to provide trainees with increasing exposure to and involvement in workplace activities.

10 Learning in the workplace is an iterative process, and trainees are active participants and can influence the workplace
Implication: We need to allow and value feedback from students and give them the opportunity to feed back their views and impressions of the workplace.

Challenges to work-based learning in medical education

As we hope we have illuminated, the workplace has the potential to be the central site for professional learning and development in both undergraduate and postgraduate years. However, it is important not to underestimate the potential barriers to effective work-based learning. Clearly, there is an ongoing tension between working and learning, and the intensity of work for both trainers and trainees has a significant bearing on this. Trainees need opportunities to learn through working, but they also need to be released to access the formal aspects of their training and to have time to consider and discuss the learning that arises through engagement in work activity. The sheer number of learners in the workplace is also significant, and those with responsibility for organising training need to consider how to avoid the creation of learner hierarchies, which are at risk of favouring issues of seniority, power or status over learning need. The importance of organisational and work dynamics should not be overlooked.

The shortening and fragmentation of training has eroded time-served traditional apprenticeship models. However, the importance of the relationship between trainer and trainee continues to feature highly in studies of work-based learning in medicine. Developing safe and effective supervision strategies will be key, as will be the need to draw on new models of apprenticeship that value the relationships between and contributions of other members of the team. Finally, the rise of competency-based models of education, training and assessment brings a risk of a 'tick-box' mentality to training that must be challenged. The focus on process aspects of the curriculum will be fundamental to the ongoing development of trainees.

Throughout this chapter we have drawn attention to the ways in which conceptions of work-based learning can shape our practice, and the importance of a critical engagement with theoretical perspectives on learning, which can illuminate ways in which we can best support work-based learning in medicine. We have argued that social theories of learning, in particular, which emphasise the social, participatory, mediated and context-specific aspects of learning, are best placed to support our activity. In the final section we will summarise the implications for those who organise, manage and deliver education and training in the medical workplace.

Developing and promoting work-based learning

Implications for clinical teachers

In addition to the suggestions above, reviving apprenticeship demands a change of mindset from one that focuses on 'sitting at the master's feet' to one that focuses on the community, that is, a collective model of newcomers and old-timers working and learning together.(64,85) Clinical supervisors can assist this process by ensuring appropriate orientation to patient care and teamworking, and by highlighting opportunities to work and learn with all members of the team, including patients, carers and peers. Effective

BOX 7.5 HOW TO: Make the implicit 'explicit'

- Label the learning opportunities that arise spontaneously in day-to-day work.
- Signal expectations in terms of culture (dress code, ways of addressing members of the team and patients), practices (preferred ways of doing things and why) and participation.
- Encourage learners to articulate and discuss observed differences in culture and practice in different settings or specialties, and consider why these may occur.(39,40)
- Be clear about the importance given to learning from work and set aside time to consider lessons learned (brief and debrief).
- Prime learners for observation and shadowing (using advanced organisers), making clear what it is possible to learn.
- Adopt the principles of 'articulation and reflection' in your approaches to clinical teaching cognitive apprenticeship.
- Talk about what you are role-modelling and why.

clinical teaching will involve planning for learning, which includes making sure that learners are open to the learning opportunities that arise through work.(35) The need to make the implicit 'explicit' arises as a key factor here (*see* Box 7.5).

A second shift of mindset may be from that of 'teacher' to 'facilitator of learning' to ensure that precious protected teaching time is not wasted. This will mean ensuring that you have a clear sense of the starting points of individual learners and that you have identified what they can do with the assistance of a more knowledgeable other, who may be one of their peers or another team member, rather than the named supervisor. Kilminster *et al.*'s(86) guidance on effective supervision is particularly helpful here.

The effective use of authentic, work-based assessments can be invaluable. Learners provided with appropriate support are able to access a broader range of working, and therefore learning, experiences. The emphasis on learning through participation with other team members allows the supervisor to be more targeted and effective with time set aside for teaching. Conceptualising this as time set aside for developmental conversations may help this process. The importance of shared talk, learning to talk and to articulate reasoning, cannot be overemphasised here. Launer's model of narrative-based supervision is flexible enough to encompass formal and informal supervision sessions, as well as the skills needed to conduct case-based discussion more effectively.(87)

Implications for educational leaders and managers

Those charged with responsibility for overseeing the training of individuals (e.g. educational supervisors) or groups of trainees (e.g. directors of medical education, training programme organisers) can build on the strategies for clinical teachers highlighted above. Re-conceptualising training as an opportunity for an 'expansive apprenticeship'(73) leads to a closer consideration of the value of time spent in a range of clinical settings (albeit for relatively short periods compared with old) and the need to balance this with time 'out' for formal training and thinking time. Seeing induction as an opportunity to orientate learners to ways in which to make the most of the learning that happens in the workplace will be key. This will include the following:

- making explicit the value of learning through working
- supervision as an opportunity for developmental conversations
- work-based assessment as the key tool to identify learning needs and ensure regular and targeted feedback
- the cultural expectation of learning through teamwork.

Peer learning should be emphasised and explicitly valued, with the positive impact of mentoring relationships being explored. Interprofessional induction helps strengthen the value placed on working and learning in teams that go across professional boundaries.

Implications for faculty developers

Swanwick argues that the professionalisation of medical education, increased accountability and aspirations to excellence have heightened the attention being placed on faculty development in medicine.(88) There is a growing expectation that all doctors who teach will undertake suitable training and be willing to demonstrate their competence to carry out their roles.(12,25,26) However, attention has been drawn to the organisational deterrents to engagement in faculty development,(89) and it is worth noting that historically this activity has been based within medical schools (with the resulting emphasis on formal teaching), rather than the clinical workplace. If, as we have argued, a revival of medical apprenticeship requires shifts in mindset as well as practice, faculty development has the potential to be invaluable. Clearly, there are some areas where developing teaching and assessing skills will be necessary. Norcini,(90) for example, argues that faculty development is key to the successful use of assessment methods based on observation of routine encounters. Faculty development that moves beyond a focus on teacher competence to a concern with the need to foster a critical dialogue between those who share responsibility for medical education and training is vital.(91) Faculty developers working with clinical teachers should be tasked with sharing insights into work-based learning that draw on social and participatory schools of thought, rather than the cognitive models that dominate the formal educational arena. Approaches to faculty development that recognise the value of coaching, mentoring and peer observation of teaching will model the social and participatory aspects of learning through work and can be balanced with more traditional workshop-based activity focusing on skill rehearsal, dialogue and feedback.

Conclusion

The value and importance of work-based learning has never been clearer, nor the challenges faced greater. Reform of health care, medical education and training are eroding time-served approaches to training and demand a revival and creation of new models of apprenticeship. Conceptions of work-based learning, alongside a closer examination of educational theories and perspectives, may provide us with the tools to do this. Whilst it will be important to hold on firmly to the time-honoured features of apprenticeship, rooted in a developmental relationship between trainer and trainee, there are opportunities to embrace opportunities for learning as active participants in patient care, supported by peers and colleagues within the communities in which we work and learn.

References

1 Firth-Cozens J (2006) A perspective on stress and depression. In: Cox J, King J, Hutchinson A and McAvoy P (eds) *Understanding Doctors' Performance*, pp. 22–37. Radcliffe Publishing, Oxford.

2 Turnbull S (ed.) (2000) The role of emotional in situated learning and communities of practice. Productive learning at work. Working Paper 59. Lancaster University Management School, University of Technology, Sydney, NSW.

3 Morris C (2009) Developing pedagogy for doctors-as-teachers: the role of activity theory. In: Daniels H, Lauder H and Porter J (eds) *Knowledge, Values and Educational Policy. A Critical Perspective*, pp. 273–81. Routledge, Oxford.

4 Department of Health (2004) Modernising Medical Careers – the next steps. The Future of Foundation, Specialist and General Practice Training Programmes. Department of Health, London.

5 Cooke M, Irby D, Sullivan W and Ludmerer K (2006) American medical education 100 years after the Flexner Report. *New England Journal of Medicine*. **355**: 1339–45.

6 Temple J (2010) Time for Training. A review of the impact of the European Working Time Directive on the quality of training. Medical Education England, London. (http://www.mee.nhs.uk/PDF/14274%20Bookmark%20Web%20Version.pdf; accessed 5 January 2013).

7 Wilson I (2009). Maintaining quality of training in a reduced training opportunity environment. Medical Education England, London. (http://www.mee.nhs.uk/PDF/Quality%20of%20Training%20FINAL.pdf; accessed 5 January 2013).

8 Tooke J (2008) *Aspiring to Excellence: findings and recommendations of the Independent Inquiry into Modernising Medical Careers*. MMC Inquiry, London.

9 Morris C (2011) From time-served apprenticeship to time-measured training: new challenges for postgraduate medical education. Thesis submitted in partial fulfilment of Doctor of Education (EdD), Institute of Education, University of London.

10 Whitcomb M (2003) Editorial. The most serious challenge facing academic medicine's institutions. *Academic Medicine*. **78**: 1201–2.

11 Gwee M (2011) Commentary. Medical and health care professional education in the 21st century: institutional, national and global perspectives. *Medical Education*. **45**: 25–8.

12 Cook M, Irby D and O'Brien B (2010) *Educating Physicians: A Call for Reform of Medical School and Residency*. Jossey Bass, San Francisco, CA.

13 Ten Cate O (2005) Commentary. Entrustability of professional activities and competency-based training. *Medical Education*. **39**: 1176–7.

14 Holmboe E, Ginsburg S and Bernabeo E (2011) The rotational approach to medical education: time to confront our assumptions? *Medical Education*. **45**: 69–80.

15 Walters L, Greenhill J, Richards J et al. (2012) Outcomes of longitudinal integrated clinical placements for students, clinicians and society. *Medical Education*. **46**: 1028–41.

16 O'Brien B, Poncelet A, Hansen L *et al.* (2012) Students' workplace learning in two clerkship models: a multi-site observational study. *Medical Education.* **46**: 613–24.

17 Goldacre M, Lambert T, Evans J and Turner J (2003) Preregistration house officers' views on whether their experience at medical school prepared them well for their jobs: national questionnaire survey. *British Medical Journal.* **328**: 1011–2.

18 Illing J, Davies C and Baldauf B (2008) *How Prepared Are Medical Graduates to Begin Practice. A Comparison of Three Diverse Medical Schools.* Report to Education Committee. General Medical Council, London.

19 British Medical Association Health Policy and Economic Research Unit (2008) First report of the BMA cohort study of 2006 medical graduates. British Medical Association, London. (http://bma .org.uk/working-for-change/negotiating-for-the-profession/ workforce/cohort-study; accessed 9 January 2012).

20 Cave J, Goldacre M, Lambert T *et al.* (2007) Newly qualified doctors' views about whether their medical school had trained them well: questionnaire surveys. *BMC Medical Education.* **7**: 38.

21 Tallentire V, Smith SE, Skinner J and Cameron HS (2011) Understanding the behaviour of newly qualified doctors in acute care contexts. *Medical Education.* **45**: 995–1005.

22 Kilminster S, Zukas M, Quinton N and Roberts T (2011) Preparedness is not enough: understanding transitions as critically intensive learning periods. *Medical Education.* **45**: 1006–15.

23 Roberts T (2009) *Learning responsibility? Exploring Doctors' Transitions to New Levels of Medical Responsibilty: Full Research Report ESRC End of Award Report (RES 153-25-0084).* Swindon: Economic and Social Research Council.

24 Evans K, Guile D, Harris J and Allan H (2010) Putting Knowledge to Work. *Nurse Education Today.* **30**: 245–51.

25 Academy of Medical Educators (2010) A framework for the professional development of postgraduate medical supervisors. London: Academy of Medical Eductors. (http://www.medicaleducators.org; accessed 13 June 2013).

26 General Medical Council (2012) *Recognising and approving trainers: the implementation plan.* General Medical Council, London.

27 Reeves S and Hean S (2013) Editorial. Why we need theory to help us better understand the nature of interprofessional education, practice and care. *Journal of Interprofessional Care.* **27**: 1–3.

28 Sfard A (1998) On two metaphors for learning and the dangers of chosing just one. *Educational Researcher.* **27**: 4–13.

29 Scott D (2008) *Critical Essays on Major Curriculum Theorists.* Routledge, London.

30 Bernstein B (1996) *Pedagogy, Symbolic Control and Identity: Theory, Research and Critique.* Taylor and Francis, London.

31 Schon D (1983) *The Reflective Practitioner: How Professionals Think in Action.* Basic Books, New York.

32 Billett S (2001) *Learning in the Workplace. Strategies for Effective Practice.* Allen and Unwin, Crows Nest, NSW.

33 Bleakley A (2006) Broadening conceptions of learning in medical education: the message from teamworking. *Medical Education.* **40**: 150–7.

34 Swanwick T (2005) Informal learning in postgraduate medical education: from cognitivism to 'culturism'. *Medical Education.* **39**: 859–65.

35 Eraut M (2000) Non-formal learning, implicit learning and tacit knowledge in professional work. In: Coffield F (ed.) *The Necessity of Informal Learning*, pp. 12–21. The Policy Press, Bristol.

36 Boud D and Solomon N (2003) *Work-based Learning. A New Higher Education?* The Society for Research into Higher Education, Open University Press, Buckingham.

37 Seagraves L and Boyd A (1996) *Supporting Learners in the Workplace: Guidelines for Learning Advisers in Small and Medium Sized Companies.* University of Stirling, Stirling.

38 Evans K, Hodkinson P, Rainbird H and Unwin L (2006) *Improving Workplace Learning.* Routledge, Oxford.

39 Monrouxe L, Rees C and Hu W (2011) Differences in medical students' explicit discourses of professionalism: acting, representing, becoming. *Medical Education.* **45**: 585–602.

40 Gordon J, Markham P, Lipworth W, Kerridge I and Little M (2012) The dual nature of medical enculturation in postgraduate medical training and practice. *Medical Education.* **46**: 894–902.

41 Swanwick T and Morris C (2010) Shifting conceptions of learning in the workplace. *Medical Education.* **44**: 538–9.

42 Mann K, Dornan T and Teunissen P (2011) Perspectives on learning. In: Dornan T, Mann K, Scherpbier A and Spencer J (eds) *Medical Education. Theory and Practice.* Churchill Livingstone, Edinburgh.

43 Hager P (2011) Theories of workplace learning. In: Malloch M, Cairns L, Evans K and O'Connor B (eds) *The Sage Handbook of Workplace Learning.* Sage, London.

44 Hartley J (1998) *Learning and Studying. A Research Perspective.* Routledge, London.

45 Hager P (2004) The conceptualization and measurement of learning at work. In: Rainbird H, Fuller A and Munro A (eds) *Workplace Learning in Context*, pp. 242–58. Routledge, London.

46 Scott S and Palinscar A (2009) The influence of constructivism on teaching and learning in classrooms. In: Daniels H, Lauder H and Porter J (eds) *Knowledge, Values and Educational Policy: A Critical Perspective*, pp. 29–43. Routledge, London.

47 Knowles M (1973) *The Adult Learner. A Neglected Species.* Gulf Publishing, Houston, TX.

48 Kolb D (1984) *Experiential Learning.* Prentice Hall, Englewood Cliffs, NJ.

49 Schon D (1983) *The Reflective Practitioner: How Professionals Think in Action.* Basic Books, New York.

50 Schon D (1987) *Educating the Reflective Practitioner: Towards a New Design for Teaching and Learning in the Professions.* Jossey-Bass, San Fransisco, CA.

51 Collins A, Brown J and Newman S (1989) Cognitive apprenticeship: teaching the crafts of reading, writing and mathematics. In: Resnick L (ed.) *Knowing, Learning, and Instruction: Essays in Honour of Robert Glaser*, pp. 453–94. Lawrence Erlbaum Associates, Hillsdale, NJ.

52 Wooley N and Jarvis Y (2007) Situated cognition and cognitive apprenticeship: a model for teaching and learning clinical skills in a technologically rich and authentic learning environment. *Nurse Education Today.* **27**: 73–9.

53 Lee T, Fuller A, Ashton D *et al.* (2004) Workplace learning: main themes and perspectives. Learning as work. Research Paper 2. University of Leicester, Centre for Labour Market Studies, Leicester.

54 Cook V, Daly C and Newman M (2012) *Work-based learning in Clinical Settings – Insights from Socio-Cultural Perspectives.* Radcliffe, Oxford.

55 Bandura A (1977) *Social Learning Theory.* Prentice-Hall, Englewood Cliffs, NJ.

56 Bandura A (1997) *Self-Efficacy: The Exercise of Control.* WH Freeman, New York.

57 Kenny N, Mann K and MacLeod H (2003) Role modeling in physicians' professional formation: reconsidering an essential but untapped educational strategy. *Academic Medicine.* **78**: 1203–10.

58 Cruess SR, Cruess RL and Steinert Y (2008) Role Modelling – making the most of a powerful teaching strategy. *British Medical Journal.* **336**: 718–21.

59 Paice E, Heard S and Moss F (2002) How important are role models in making good doctors? *British Medical Journal.* **325**: 707–10.

60 Sutkin G, Wagner E, Harris I and Schiffer R (2008) What makes a good clinical teacher in medicine? A review of the literature. *Academic Medicine.* **83**: 452–66.

61 Dornan T (2005) Osler, Flexner, apprenticeship and 'the new medical education'. *Journal of the Royal Society of Medicine.* **96**: 91–6.

62 Vygotsky L (1978) Interaction between learning and development. In: Cole M, John-Steiner V, Scribner S and Souberman S (eds) *Mind*

in Society: The Development of Higher Psychological Processes. Harvard University Press, Cambridge, MA, pp. 79–91.

63 Postgraduate Medical Education and Training Board (2008) *Educating Tomorrow's Doctors: future models of medical training; medical workforce shape and trainee expectations.* PMETB, London.

64 Lave J and Wenger E (1991) *Situated Learning: Legitimate Peripheral Participation.* Cambridge University Press, Cambridge.

65 Sheehan D, Wilkinson T and Billett S (2005) Interns' participation and learning in clinical environments in a New Zealand hospital. *Academic Medicine.* **80**: 302–8.

66 Morris C (2012) From classroom to clinic: an activity theory perspective. In: Cook V, Daly C and Newman M (eds) *Work-Based Learning in Clinical Settings – Insights from Socio-Cultural Perspectives.* Radcliffe, Oxford.

67 Bleakley A (2002) Pre-registration house officers and ward-based learning: a 'new apprenticeship' model. *Medical Education.* **36**: 9–15.

68 Cornford C and Carrington B (2006) A qualitative study of the experiences of training in general practice: a community of practice? *Journal of Education for Teaching.* **32**: 269–82.

69 Lyon P (2004) A model of teaching and learning in the operating theatre. *Medical Education.* **38**: 1278–87.

70 Morris C (2012) Re-imagining 'the firm': clinical attachments as time spent in communities of practice. In: Cook V, Daly C and Newman M (eds) *Work-Based Learning in Clinical Settings – Insights from Socio-Cultural Perspectives.* Radcliffe, Oxford.

71 Wenger E (1999) *Communities of Practice. Learning, Meaning and Identity.* Cambridge University Press, Cambridge.

72 Billett S (2002) Toward a workplace pedagogy: guidance, participation and engagement. *Adult Education Quarterly.* **53**: 27–43.

73 Fuller A and Unwin L (2006) Expansive and restrictive learning environments. In: Evans K, Hodkinson P, Rainbird H and Unwin L (eds) *Improving Workplace Learning*, pp. 27–48. Routledge, London.

74 Solomon N (1999) Culture and difference in workplace learning. In: Boud D and Garrick J (eds) *Understanding Learning at Work*, pp. 119–31. Routledge, London.

75 Higham J and Steer PJ (2004) Gender. gap in undergraduate experience and performance in obstetrics and gynaecology: analysis of clinical experience logs. *British Medical Journal.* **328**: 142–3.

76 Bleakley A (2012) Establishing patient safety nets: how Actor-Network-Theory can inform clinical education research. In: Cook V, Daly C and Newman M (eds) *Work-Based Learning in Clinical Settings – Insights from Socio-Cultural Perspectives.* Radcliffe, Oxford.

77 Bleakley A (2013) Working in "teams" in an era of "liquid" healthcare: what is the use of theory? *Journal of Interprofessional Care.* **27**: 18–26.

78 Bobbitt F (1918) *The Curriculum.* Houghton Miflin, Boston, MA.

79 Tyler R (1950) *Basic Principles of Curriculum and Instruction.* University of Chicago Press, Chicago, IL.

80 Prideaux D (2004) Clarity of outcomes in medical education: do we know if it really makes a difference? *Medical Education.* **38**: 580–1.

81 Talbot M (2004) Outcomes-based teaching: 'monkey see, monkey do': a critique of the competency model in graduate medical education. *Medical Education.* **38**: 587–92.

82 Stenhouse L (1975) *An Introduction to Curriculum Research and Development.* Heinemann, London.

83 Billett S (2004) Learning through work. Workplace participatory practices. In: Rainbird H, Fuller A and Munro A (eds) *Workplace Learning in Context*, pp. 119–31. Routledge, London.

84 Dornan T, Boshuizen H, King N and Sherpbier A (2007) Experience-based learning: a model linking the processes and outcomes of medical students' workplace learning. *Medical Education.* **41**: 84–91.

85 Griffiths T and Guile D (2003) A connective model of learning: the implications for work process knowledge. *European Educational Research Journal.* **2**: 56–73.

86 Kilminster S, Cottrell D, Grant J and Jolly B (2007) AMEE guide no. 27: effective educational and clinical supervision. *Medical Teacher.* **29**: 2–19.

87 Launer J (2006) *Supervision, Mentoring and Coaching: One-to-One Learning Encounters in Medical Education.* Association for the Study of Medical Education, Edinburgh.

88 Swanwick T (2008) See one, do one, then what? Faculty development in postgraduate medical education. *Postgraduate Medical Journal.* **84**: 339–43.

89 Steinert Y, McLeod P, Boillat M *et al.* (2009) Faculty Development: a 'field of dreams'? *Medical Education.* **43**: 42–9.

90 Norcini J (2007) *Workplace-Based Assessment in Clinical Training.* Association for the Study of Medical Education, Edinburgh.

91 D'Eon M, Overgaard V and Harding S (2000) Teaching as a social practice: implications for faculty development. *Advances in Health Sciences Education: Theory and Practice.* **5**: 151–62.

Further reading

Cook V, Daly C and Newman M (2012) *Work-Based Learning in Clinical Settings – Insights from Socio-Cultural Perspectives.* Radcliffe, Oxford.

Dornan T, Mann K, Scherpbier A and Spencer J (2011) *Medical Education. Theory and Practice.* Churchill Livingstone, Edinburgh.

Lave J and Wenger E (1991) *Situated Learning: Legitimate Peripheral Participation.* Cambridge University Press, Cambridge.

Malloch M, Cairns L, Evans K and O'Connor B (2011) *The Sage Handbook of Workplace Learning.* Sage, London.

Rainbird H, Fuller A and Munro A (2004) *Workplace Learning in Context.* Routledge, London.

8 Supervision, mentoring and coaching

John Launer
Professional Development, Health Education South London, UK

KEY MESSAGES

- Supervision and one-to-one support occur throughout medical education and the medical career cycle. They often form the most important part of professional learning and act as the foundation of reflective practice. They may play an essential part in motivating and retaining practitioners, and in preventing stress and burnout.

- One-to-one supervision can take a variety of forms and names, including clinical supervision, educational supervision, mentoring and coaching. The boundaries between these activities are often unclear. Terminology can be confusing, but definitions are probably less important than understanding the context and purpose of any encounter.

- All one-to-one supervision contains an element of professional development and an element of performance monitoring or standard setting. These elements may be present either implicitly or explicitly. The emphasis on one or the other will vary greatly, depending on the circumstances.

- There are three principal types of focus for supervision: clinical cases, the wider contexts of these cases (e.g. professional networks) and career choices. Sometimes the focus will move around between these.

- One-to-one supervision can occur formally or informally; on an obligatory basis or a voluntary one; and in a hierarchical relationship or between peers. It can take place as part of management, training, remediation or routine professional work.

- Whatever its form or context, good supervision depends on the same set of skills. These include affirmation, emotional attunement, awareness of external requirements and standards, and ability to question and challenge people appropriately.

- Skills for supervision can be taught and learned. These include the use of questions designed to help learners extend their understanding without raising excessive anxiety.

Introduction

Traditionally, medicine has been an area where the emphasis has been on didactic training, rather than facilitated learning. The reasons for this are fairly obvious. Doctors need to acquire, and to keep acquiring, tremendous amounts of factual knowledge and practical skills. In social terms, medicine has always had a hierarchical structure, alongside a high social status. As a reflection of this, the chief mode of medical school teaching has traditionally been the ward round: a senior male doctor in a suit addressing and interrogating a group of medical students in short white coats, in the presence of a silent and supine patient.

In spite of this, most doctors can probably remember one-to-one encounters and relationships from every stage of their undergraduate and postgraduate careers that helped or influenced them. Such supervision, coaching or mentorship – whether or not it was formally named as such – may have been the most important part of their learning. For those who have always provided it, particularly junior hospital doctors in the case of teaching medical students, it may have been one of the most gratifying parts of their work.

Approaches to teaching and learning in medical careers are now undergoing a transformation in many places. This is bringing one-to-one activities such as supervision and mentoring to the fore in two ways. First, the kinds of encounter that are taking place within medicine and medical education are often different from how they might have been in the past. They are likely to be more informal and dialogical in style, and perhaps more tentative as well. They may also go beyond informational input, and involve discursive and wide-ranging consideration of cases and work issues. They are therefore coming closer to the notion of 'bringing forth' understanding. Second, the structures within which such one-to-one support takes place are likely to be less 'ad hoc' and more organised or rigorous. Thus, in an increasing number of settings, one-to-one support is being placed at the centre of professional learning. In the UK, for example, this now include the following:
- tutorials for trainee general practitioners (GPs)(1)
- educational supervision for newly qualified doctors and those in speciality training(2,3)
- appraisal of doctors(4)
- mentoring for hospital specialists or GPs(5)

Understanding Medical Education: Evidence, Theory and Practice, Second Edition. Edited by Tim Swanwick.
© 2014 The Association for the Study of Medical Education. Published 2014 by John Wiley & Sons, Ltd.

- executive coaching for senior doctors(6)
- remedial work done under the aegis of departments of postgraduate medical education.(7)

The factors that have led to such changes are many, but the following are probably the most significant:

- Education in many professional fields has undergone widespread change, with an emphasis on adult learning as opposed to traditional pedagogy, and on reflective practice rather than on the acquisition of facts.(8–10)
- Social developments have made both patients and learners less deferent in many societies and therefore less likely to accept authoritative or directive instruction without question or challenge; 'patient-centred' and 'learner-centred' styles are becoming the norm.(11)
- Doctors now work more closely with other professionals such as nurses, social workers, psychologists and psychotherapists, who have all established one-to-one supervision as the mainstay of their basic training and continuing professional development.(12–16)
- There is an increasing need for lifelong learning in medicine, and this has led to some loss of the boundary between initial training and continuous professional development, including work-based learning.(17–19)
- Many doctors have a greater awareness of medical ethics and new areas of exploration, such as complexity,(20) social constructionism,(21) whole-systems approaches (22) and narrative.(23) They are therefore aware that any clinical case may be amenable to multiple interpretations and possible solutions.
- Political influences in many countries have put quality, performance, clinical governance and patient-centred care permanently on the medical agenda, and these in turn have all required doctors to be more open about their failings and uncertainties, and more amenable to discussion of their competencies.(24)

Although there is still far less of a tradition of organised, regular, one-to-one pedagogy within medicine than in some other professions, the situation is changing rapidly. It is now possible that one-to-one support may become the mainstay of basic training and lifelong learning in the medical profession, although much still needs to be done for this to happen.

What does supervision mean?

There are many definitions of one-to-one learning activities such as supervision, mentoring and coaching. Different authors take different approaches, largely according to their own professional backgrounds, experience and agendas. Some use the terms supervision and clinical supervision interchangeably. Others introduce phrases or hybrid terms of their own such as 'learning support'(25) or 'coach-mentoring'.(26) It is easy to get bogged down in semantics and lose sight of the important principles. This section attempts to cut through the jargon and focus on what matters in one-to-one support.

The term 'supervision' originated in professions outside medicine. It has been used for many years in the mental health world and nursing to mean regular, structured, extended encounters aimed at reflecting on casework.(27) Over time, people in these professions and more widely have come to take a far wider view of its meaning, suggesting that it should cover any encounter that provides support in a clinical context, whether this is formal or informal, hierarchical or non-hierarchical, and part of a training programme or outside one. Butterworth, for example, offers this very inclusive definition from a nursing perspective: 'An exchange between professionals to enable the development of professional skills'.(28) Burton and Launer, looking at primary care, define it as 'facilitated learning in relation to live practical issues'.(29) Clark *et al.* have suggested that supervision should be considered an umbrella term, covering all one-to-one professional encounters and thus including mentoring and coaching, as well as activities that include an element of management, training, assessment or remediation.(30)

In this chapter, the term 'supervision' is used in this wider sense to cover all one-to-one encounters aimed at promoting competence and reflective practice, including mentoring and coaching. Box 8.1 outlines the argument in favour of doctors adopting the term in this way, to cover the entire range of one-to-one encounters.

One cause for controversy is whether supervision is principally about professional development or about monitoring and standard-setting. This may arise from the inherent ambiguity in the English word 'supervision' itself; some people automatically assume it to mean 'looking after someone', while others understand it to mean 'looking over someone's shoulder'. As the word is used in both senses, both colloquially and within education, it is probably best to acknowledge that the word can carry either meaning, or both, depending on the speaker and the context. Again, that is the approach adopted in this chapter.

In practical terms, it may be useful to think of supervision in terms of two overlapping circles labelled 'develop-

---

BOX 8.1 Should doctors use the word supervision?

Within medicine, people often cannot hear the words 'clinical supervision' or 'supervision' without feeling it involves mainly instruction. Many doctors say they would sometimes prefer an alternative term for conversations aimed at promoting reflective practice: for example, 'case discussion', 'clinical case analysis' and so on. In spite of this, there are good reasons to promote both the word and the concept of supervision in the wide sense that is now understood in other fields. This usage connects doctors with the richness of thinking about supervision that has gone on in these fields, especially in nursing and the mental health professions. It also enables people to identify the many encounters in medicine that have an element of supervision in them, although they may not be named as such. Over time, this may help to promote an enhanced culture of supervision within medicine, not just within training, but throughout professional life.

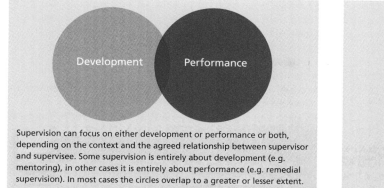

Supervision can focus on either development or performance or both, depending on the context and the agreed relationship between supervisor and supervisee. Some supervision is entirely about development (e.g. mentoring), in other cases it is entirely about performance (e.g. remedial supervision). In most cases the circles overlap to a greater or lesser extent.

Figure 8.1 The two faces of supervision.

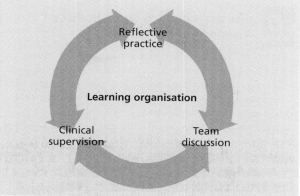

Figure 8.2 The learning organisation.

ment' and 'performance' (*see* Figure 8.1). On some occasions, the focus will be entirely on personal and professional development. The supervisor will be more or less able to take performance standards for granted. This occurs, for example, where a doctor is helping an experienced and proficient colleague to think through a highly complex case and consider a range of different management options. On other occasions, supervision has to move almost entirely towards directive teaching. This may happen, for example, when a supervisee presents a case for discussion but exposes a huge ignorance of basic knowledge in doing so.

In both these extremes, however, it is clear that supervision will always pay attention to both development and performance to some extent. Even when two experienced peers are discussing a case, both colleagues will assume certain norms that define the options that are worth considering – even if the norms remain unspoken during the supervision itself. Similarly, the supervisor who pulls up a poor trainee on the facts is still working within a framework of development and aiming to foster a relationship where standards can be assumed.

What is supervision for?

It is generally helpful to make a distinction between supervision on the one hand, and straightforward didactic training on the other. While training addresses the high ground of facts, figures, rules and guidelines, supervision in all its forms addresses the 'swampy lowlands' of everyday practice:(9) the uncomfortable, inconvenient realities that professionals face all the time. They are realities for which the textbook never quite seems to have the answer, and which never exactly correspond to any case that the practitioner has seen before. For students, such cases may initially seem rare. As professionals advance in their careers, they may become more frequent rather than less; curiosity and courage have increased with experience; and problems that were previously disguised or withheld appear.

There is an inseparable connection between supervision and reflective practice. One way of looking at this is to regard supervision as an intelligent conversation with a colleague about a case or issue, and reflective practice as

an intelligent conversation with oneself.(31) Supervision nurtures reflective practice, while reflective practice in turn leads to a thirst for supervision in all its forms. The same can be said in connection with team discussion, which may or may not be present in the workplace as a regular activity and as an attitude of mind.

Not surprisingly, the same transferable skills operate in relation to consultations with patients, good supervision with colleagues and effective team discussion. These include careful listening, the formation of credible hypotheses, and the construction of helpful and challenging questions. All these skills enhance critical thinking and, as such, generate a vision in the workplace that is 'open and malleable, not closed and fixed'.(8)

The relationship between reflective practice, supervision, team discussion and the learning workplace is symbolised in Figure 8.2.

One useful set of concepts to help understand the different purposes of supervision is the one provided by Proctor.(32) She regards supervision as having three aspects: 'normative', 'formative' and 'restorative'. The normative aspect is what links supervision to the 'world out there', where there are standards to meet and rules to be followed. The formative aspect is what helps supervisees to develop. The restorative aspect is what sustains colleagues in their jobs. Each of these aspects may come to the fore or remain in the background, according to the context and the circumstances.

Looking specifically at formal professional supervision, Morton-Cooper and Palmer list its purposes as follows:(25)

- as a defence against feelings of disorientation, disillusionment and burnout
- as a framework for clarifying human values
- as a way of recovering meaning in our social relationships
- as a means of providing skill rehearsal and access to appropriate role models in the workplace (both personally and collegially)
- as a device for evaluating and disseminating best practice in health care
- as a way of acquiring 'emotional literacy to deal constructively with our emotions in a mutually beneficial way'.

BOX 8.2 WHERE'S THE EVIDENCE: is supervision effective?

In terms of effectiveness, there are several studies from professions such as nursing showing that recipients place a high value on supervision, mentoring and coaching for what they bring about in terms of general well-being, knowledge, confidence, morale, understanding, self-awareness, job satisfaction and professional endurance.(33–37) There are also studies showing benefits to those who offer mentoring to their organisations.(38) However, there are few, if any, studies showing a direct relationship between the presence of supervision, or its quality, and its effects on patient satisfaction or patient outcome. There are a number of reasons for this, including the difficulty of assessing the clinical efficacy of any complex educational intervention with may variables involved.(39) There is clearly a need to develop methodologies that will allow researchers to establish what difference it makes to patients for clinicians to have regular supervision or other forms of one-to-one support, and which approaches to supervision seem to make the most difference.(40) In this connection, some writers have questioned the assumption that supervision automatically enhances good practice, and they have suggested that it can also sometimes lead to collusion and complacency.(5,41) It can also be limited by poor supervision skills, bad matching, intrusive management or other obstacles.

Although supervision is generally understood as a very different concept from clinical governance, there is an argument for regarding supervision as an important means of putting governance into action. While guidelines, protocols, audits and other tools may provide an external framework for acceptable practice, supervision can be thought of as a collective activity through which professionals refine and develop their own personal practice. In other words, it is a literally a regulatory activity, but one of continual mutual regulation.

One aspect of supervision that is vital but often understated is that of imagination. As with research supervision in an academic context, supervision in a clinical setting can at times (and in some hands) be a very dull affair, but it also has the potential to inspire people to perform at their best, and to go to places clinically and professionally that they may never have been able to reach otherwise.

Box 8.2 covers the issue of evidence and evaluation in relation to supervision, mentoring and coaching.

Cases, contexts, careers: the three domains of supervision

Cases

Most supervision takes place mainly in order to address cases, namely the everyday work that professionals undertake. These cases may be approached from the point of view of straightforward technical case management, for example, what is good practice or best practice. Far more commonly, however, cases needing supervision raise issues far broader than this, such as the following:

- when there is no one easy answer
- ethical issues
- complex co-morbidity
- when it is unclear when to stop investigations or treatment
- 'grey area' cases, for example, somatisation, frequent attenders, chronic fatigue, irritable bowel
- complaints, distressed families, angry patients, unlikeable patients.

In all cases like these, discussion of the technical or pragmatic options that may be available is inseparable from what has been called 'emotional work', that is, the processing of difficult emotions attached to the case. This may involve a simple discharge of negative feelings, or it may require something more complex and skilled, depending on the capacities of both supervisor and supervisee: a careful analysis of why particular feelings have arisen and what information this provides in respect of the dynamics of the case and the doctor–patient relationship.

Contexts

Most supervision in medicine relates to the content of cases only, because the working context is itself quite unproblematic. However, sometimes this is not the case. Even at the best of times, careful case management can depend on thinking about the work setting as much as the clinical issues involved. In postgraduate medical education, it is rare to have an intelligent discussion about any case without at some point having to consider how the professional network is functioning, and whether it is supporting or hindering practitioners in their work. Similarly, formal or informal case discussions among experienced hospital doctors will regularly address issues such as professional or inter-professional rivalries and problems concerning communication, money, politics or power. In addition, much supervision addresses difficulties in relation to roles and boundaries, for example, the extent and limits of what patients can legitimately expect from clinicians and what colleagues or team members can legitimately expect from each other. Supervision may also need to address other relevant contexts, including how best to conduct interactions with the patient's family, as well as cultural or faith issues that may be appropriate to the patient's care.

Careers

While specific discussions aimed at clarifying the client's career goals and choices do sometimes take place, it is probably more common for these to be addressed incidentally in the course of discussions about cases or network issues. For example, a clinical case may well bring certain learning needs to light and raise issues about whether the client should undertake further training to improve their level of skill. Similarly, supervision in relation to a difficulty in the workplace may lead to the question, 'Is this any longer the right workplace for the supervisee?' The case of professional appraisal is interesting in this respect. Although it is not often considered a form of supervision or mentoring,

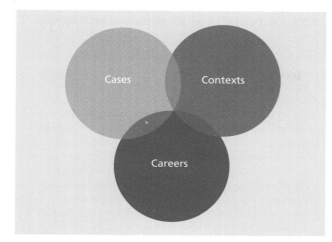

Figure 8.3 The three domains of supervision.

professional appraisal does offer similar opportunities by creating a space where clients can reflect on their competencies, learning needs and future aspirations.(42) However, there are clearly conflicts when appraisal is linked with professional revalidation or re-accreditation and some have argued that supervision and mentoring cannot be combined with anything that has regulatory implications.(43) Figure 8.3 highlights the inter-relationship of these three supervisory 'domains'.

Types of supervision

This section describes some of the commonest types of supervision, with examples of each type. The typology used here is adapted from Clark *et al.*(30)

Informal supervision

Informal supervision takes the form of opportunistic exchanges that are generally short and arise spontaneously in the context of everyday work. Typical examples are chats over coffee, in the corridor or in the operating theatre changing room. While formal supervision is usually given by someone more experienced, informal supervision can come from all sorts of people, including juniors, clerical staff and even spouses. In many circumstances, such supervision 'on the hoof' provides the mainstay of much postgraduate learning and support, whether or not this is explicitly noticed or acknowledged. Colleagues who work well together and respect each other may be able to provide excellent and challenging supervision, even in brief moments snatched from the hurly-burly of everyday work. However, the commonest risk in informal supervision is that it takes the form of swapping anecdotes or reinforces banal or stereotypical practice. This is especially the case if it takes place in the absence of any regular or reflective supervision, or as a substitute for it.

Sometimes the most imaginative supervision that doctors ever receive comes spontaneously and unexpectedly from people outside the medical profession – for example, from

BOX 8.3 Informal supervision: an example

Dr K was working late one evening in her family practice, when a new patient arrived without an advance appointment. The patient had a complicated and long-standing problem of back pain. He demanded a full clinical assessment and immediate referral to an orthopaedic surgeon. Dr K felt pressurised. She responded by telling the patient very firmly about the appointment system in the practice and by insisting that he must return for a booked appointment with full details of all his previous tests and medication. Later, before locking up her office, Dr K talked to her receptionist and expressed her frustration at patients like this, and how she hated having to behave 'like a police officer'. The receptionist remarked that Dr K would probably have handled the patient more carefully if he had come in the morning, when she was less tired. The comment led Dr K to realise that she had probably been too harsh with the man, who may have been pressurising her because his pain was so bad. She also felt she should have carried out at least a basic examination to rule out any serious pathology.

lay people commenting on their own medical experiences in social encounters.(29) Some have argued that other personal experiences, including reading novels and poetry, seeing films and operas, or walks in the countryside, are among opportunities for 'self-supervision', since they may provide the conditions for processing the thoughts and emotions that arise from everyday work (*see* Box 8.3).

Clinical supervision

Clinical supervision is the commonest form of supervision in most medical settings. It consists of the day-to-day discussion of clinical cases and their management, and any issues arising from this. It may take a variety of forms, from very brief discussions on ward rounds or in clinics, to more extended and reflective discussions of complex cases or options for clinical management. In a training context, clinical supervision may overlap with didactic training, particularly where case discussions reveal gaps in knowledge or skills. Even here, however, a conversational approach based on questioning is often more effective than giving advice since this will help to establish the supervisee's existing ideas and promote independent thinking. It will also ensure that any advice that is needed is pitched at the right level.

Doctors do not generally use the term 'clinical supervision' for case discussions taking place beyond the training years. Nevertheless, much clinical supervision does take place between peers or within teams, although it may not necessarily be labelled as such. Typical forms of this include case review meetings, primary care team meetings and phone calls to colleagues to seek expert advice or an independent view of a problem. Many established doctors, particularly those working in isolation, express a wish for more regular or systematic opportunities to discuss cases than their work patterns may allow.(44,45)

Educational supervision

Educational supervision is regular supervision taking place in the context of a recognised training in order to establish learning needs and review progress. It is most common in the early years of postgraduate training. Arguably, this is the most complex and challenging form of supervision, since the educational supervisor has to fulfil many overlapping and (in some situations) conflicting roles. As well as facilitating learning, the supervisor has a responsibility to assess the supervisee's performance, while the supervision is taking place, or by formal means at a later date.

The concept and practice of educational supervision has come to the fore in the UK, with the introduction of national curricula for all doctors in training grades. Educational supervisors play a key role in the delivery of such curricula (46) and their tasks include the following:

- setting learning objectives
- establishing a learning contract
- assisting the supervisee in maintaining a learning portfolio
- coordinating the supervisee's educational experience and graded exposure to casework
- offering opportunities for case-based discussion
- offering career guidance
- undertaking appraisal
- carrying out assessment
- producing reports.

Educational supervisors are also more likely to have to offer pastoral care at times, particularly for students and trainees who are going through crises in their personal lives or careers.

An educational supervisor may or may not take on the task of day-to-day clinical supervision. In general practice, for example, it is likely that one and the same person will do both jobs. On a programme of hospital training, by contrast, it may be preferable to have a single skilled and trained educator assigned to a trainee as an educational supervisor for the duration of the programme, while the day-to-day clinical supervision is carried out by clinicians working with the trainee at any given time. This is especially the case when trainees rotate through a number of different specialties and where an educational supervisor could not possibly have the skills to offer case-based discussion across the whole range of work. When this kind of arrangement is in place, it is essential to have close coordination between all the people involved, to prevent people working at cross-purposes or giving conflicting messages to the trainee. It also makes sense to link the approval of training placements to the quality of the supervision arrangements on offer. This is particularly important because research has shown that the quality of the supervisory relationship is the key to effective supervision in medical settings.(47)

In all educational supervision, there is a tension between assessment and supervision. Trainees may feel that their performance is being judged covertly under the guise of a supportive discussion or that their qualifications and careers may depend on what they say in apparently innocent discussions. Equally, it is hard for educators to stop themselves from being influenced by how trainees present

> **BOX 8.4 Educational supervision: an example**
>
> Dr P is the educational supervisor for Alan T, a doctor who qualified 18 months ago. As a paediatrician, Dr P is also the clinical supervisor while Alan is working on the children's ward. Over the past few weeks, there have been several children on the ward who are possible victims of physical abuse by their parents. Dr P has been concerned about Alan's apparently simplistic and judgemental attitude towards the problem: he seems to believe that the only desirable solution in every case is adoption outside the family. Dr P arranges for Alan to spend some time with the child and the family mental health team, seeing them do therapeutic work with parents who have abused their children but have also (in many cases) themselves been victims of abuse in the past. He also fixes up for Alan to attend a case conference, in which some of the complexities of a particular case are examined. He uses their regular education supervision sessions to review what Alan has learnt and to discuss how he might record this in a reflective piece of writing for his learning portfolio.

themselves in the course of day-to-day exchanges about casework. Because of this, it is important to remain aware of the two different contexts and be willing to address this difference transparently. When real concerns arise about a trainee's competence, it is fairer and more effective to say so, to set explicit targets, with a clear timetable and (if necessary) an explanation of possible sanctions (*see* Box 8.4).

Remedial supervision

Remedial supervision occurs when a regulatory agency has formally determined that there are concerns about someone's performance. This can only happen if the agency has the authority to assess performance and prescribe the supervision as a proposed remedy.

Remedial supervision takes place within a framework of assessments and reports. Essentially, remedial supervision is a type of educational supervision where the context is one of prescribed retraining, rather than basic training undertaken on a voluntary basis (*see* Box 8.5). Although the term 'remedial supervision' is not widely used, partly because of the stigma attached, it is useful for those practising it to be aware of its difference from other forms of supervision.

Professional supervision

Professional supervision consists of regular, extended one-to-one meetings between established practitioners, mainly to discuss specific cases. It is particularly common in professions such as counselling and psychotherapy, where it is generally a requirement of continuing professional practice. Such supervision is often devoted to reflection on the emotions provoked by these cases, and on the information that these emotions represent.(48) In the context of medicine (with the exception of psychiatry and a small number of GPs) such supervision is uncommon. Professional super-

BOX 8.5 Remedial supervision: an example

Dr L has had a considerable number of complaints from patients. His local health board has referred him to an agency that specialises in assessing and helping doctors whose performance is causing concern. The agency has carried out an occupational psychology assessment, some tests of Dr L's knowledge and skills, and a review of selected case notes. On the basis of this, they have found that Dr L has particular difficulty managing 'grey area' cases that involve vague somatic symptoms with low-grade depression. He tends to dismiss such patients, putting them on antidepressants straightaway without first doing adequate investigations. The agency has now assigned Dr L a remedial supervisor who has sat in on some of his surgeries and reviewed some video records of his consultations. The supervisor has now held a series of meetings with Dr L to go through some cases systematically and challenge him on his approach and attitude, in order to help him attain an acceptable level of practice.

BOX 8.6 Professional supervision: an example

Dr J, a psychiatrist, goes to an experienced psychotherapist colleague once a month to discuss cases that are causing him concern. His last supervision session was taken up with an account of a patient he is seeing regularly, who has made several suicide attempts. This session was spent examining Dr J's feelings of helplessness in relation to his patient's behaviour, and also his sense of personal responsibility for her. His supervisor helped him to understand how he was picking up the patient's own feelings of helplessness, and touched on memories of a family member who had committed suicide some years previously in spite of psychological help. They also looked at how Dr J could help the patient understand that others did feel responsible for her and care for her, in spite of her fixed belief that nobody ever did.

BOX 8.7 Managerial supervision: an example

Ms B, a community nurse, was seeing a woman who caused her concern because of how depressed she seemed. The woman came from Thailand, had been married only a year and had just had twins. She seemed cowed by her European husband, who clearly expected her to keep the house immaculate in spite of having two new babies. Ms B had never come across a family situation like this and she felt insufficiently trained to know what to do. She took the case to her regular meeting with her nurse manager. The manager spent nearly an hour with her exploring all the different issues in the case. These included the risk of serious puerperal depression, the demands of twins, the cultural and age differences between the parents, homesickness and isolation, and the difference in perception between the nurse and the husband. Through the meeting with her manager, Ms B came to realise that she could make things worse by trying to 'rescue' the woman from her husband and that she needed to build up his trust instead. She also came away from the discussion with a range of options in her mind. These included a joint visit with the doctor, putting the mother in touch with the local twins' club and exploring to see if there were any other Thai mothers in the locality who might be willing to make contact with the woman.

vision is usually, although not always, delivered by experienced members of the same profession. However, it is reasonably common for senior mental health professionals such as psychologists to offer supervision to members of other professions, including doctors and nurses. Depending on the cases being discussed, and their context, the supervisor's lack of specific technical knowledge may or may not matter (*see* Box 8.6).

Managerial supervision

Managerial supervision is supervision carried out by someone with direct management responsibility for the supervisee. This may or may not take place within an educational framework (e.g. nurse training) and may or may not involve explicit assessment. In some of the non-medical literature, anything involving clinical line management or direct accountability in employment terms is explicitly disqualified as a form of supervision. By contrast, it is often the norm within the nursing profession. It probably makes sense to regard managerial supervision as an inevitability in some circumstances (*see* Box 8.7).

Mentoring

Mentoring is usually understood as guidance and support offered by a more experienced colleague,(47,49,50) although there are also descriptions of peer mentoring or co-mentoring.(51) Mentoring may be either informal or formal. Where it is informal, it may have arisen naturally between colleagues and may not even be described as mentoring except in retrospect. Where offered as part of a formal scheme, mentoring is often wide-ranging, covering not just clinical work but professional relationships and career plans as well. Although it should not be confused with counselling, life-cycle issues such as family events will quite often come into the picture. It is often an entirely private encounter, with total confidentiality given and expected on both sides. Virtually all the literature concerning mentoring includes the assumption, implicitly or explicitly, that the arrangement is both voluntary and confidential, although agencies funding mentors may want to know in general terms that their clients are finding it useful (*see* Box 8.8).

Coaching

Coaching is a form of supervision that has been defined as 'unlocking a person's potential to maximise their own

BOX 8.8 Mentoring: an example

Since attaining her first hospital consultant post three years ago, Dr M has had meetings every few months with an experienced doctor she met when she was in training. She has used these meetings to discuss the inevitable difficulties she has had in adjusting to life not just as a newly qualified radiologist, but also as a team leader, a manager and (most recently) a new mother. Over the past two or three mentoring sessions, the same theme has come up repeatedly: the feeling that her male colleagues are paternalistic and sexist. At her most recent session her mentor simply asked her, 'Are you really just asking my permission to get out?' Dr M felt enormous relief at being asked the question. She realised that she did indeed want to move on, but had feared her mentor would be critical of her for leaving her first senior post so soon.

BOX 8.9 Coaching: an example

Dr T, a gastroenterologist, was recently promoted from medical director of his hospital to chief executive. As a result, he has decided to give up most of his clinical work, except for a small private endoscopy practice, and to concentrate on his management role. He is paying to see a coach from a private consultancy organisation to help him develop his new professional identity. Quite a few of his fortnightly coaching sessions have been spent examining how he can keep his trusting relationships with his medical colleagues at the hospital (some of whom have been his friends for many years), while also behaving equitably and responsibly in relation to all the other staff groups at the hospital, including nurses, technicians, non-clinical staff and manual workers.

performance'.(52) The coaching relationship, like mentoring, is a voluntary and confidential one. A useful analogy here is with sports coaching, where the client already has an advanced degree of proficiency and the coach, who may or may not be an exponent of the sport, helps the client to work towards further excellence. However, even the word 'coaching' can be somewhat confusing, since it is also used colloquially when someone needs extra help (e.g. 'She needs specific coaching in how to talk to patients'). Recently, the term has come more into vogue within medicine, either within the context of 'life coaching'(53) to help people achieve personal and career fulfilment, or in a more general sense to describe any one-to-one learning relationship that does not involve management or assessment. Some writers use the terms 'mentoring' and 'coaching' interchangeably, or have abandoned one term in favour of the other. It is too early to say which terminology will catch on or whether in time people will be happy to use the umbrella term 'supervision' as used in a broad sense in this chapter (*see* Box 8.9).

The types of supervision listed here are not exhaustive or mutually exclusive. Among the huge variety of learning encounters that occur in medicine, there will be many that only loosely fit any of the categories described here, while other encounters may include aspects of several types of supervision, or shift between supervision and training from moment to moment. Clark *et al.* have suggested that it is less important to achieve consensus on terms than to ask the following questions in relation to any supervision activity.(30)

- Who is asking for this to be done?
- What do they want, and why?
- Do they know what the supervisor does and does not offer?
- Will the client be attending voluntarily?
- Is anyone expecting specific outcomes, should they be and, if so, what?
- Who is paying whom, and do all the parties know this?
- Who is reporting to whom, about what, exactly when, and do all the parties know this?
- Is everyone agreed on the terms being used, and on their meaning?

Similarly, Proctor has proposed that 'What the role relationship is called is probably unimportant in practice . . . The roles, responsibilities and rights need to be identified from the beginning, and to be discussed, made real and reviewed.'(54)

Conceptual frameworks for supervision

There is no single conceptual framework that is universally recognised within the world of supervision and mentorship. Different writers use – or assume – frameworks that draw on various fields, including psychoanalysis,(55–57) systemic psychotherapy,(58–60) Rogerian counselling,(61) neuro-linguistic programming(62) and learning theory, with a particular emphasis on authorities such as Schon (10) and Kolb.(63) Some explicitly address learning styles or personality types.(64,65) Many writers have adapted the work of educational theorists in order to construct models that fit the professional context of supervision. One useful model based on learning theory comes from Proctor,(32) drawing on Wackman *et al.*(66) This suggests that learners move continually through a cycle from 'unconscious incompetence' through 'conscious incompetence' to 'conscious competence' and finally 'unconscious competence'. In other words, supervision invites people to consider how they may be avoiding more adventurous areas of practice, and to explore these – at first tentatively, then as a matter of course – until they are ready to extend themselves even further (*see* Figure 8.4).

Certain themes arise again and again in the supervision literature, suggesting that there is a consensus about particular ideas that cross theoretical boundaries. These themes include the following.

- Supervision should be about enabling, empowerment and sustaining human values.
- Supervisors may need at different times to take on a variety of roles, including guide, advisor, role model, sponsor, teacher and facilitator.
- Supervision needs to pay attention to the personal, professional and relational aspects of the work.

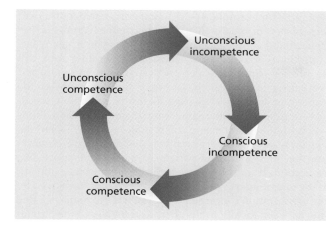

Figure 8.4 The supervision cycle.

- Supervisors always have to bear in mind three separate 'clients': the supervisee, the patient and the organisation or agency.
- Supervision needs to address the complexity and unique-ness of the problems brought, in order to generate solutions or options that are the best fit.
- Supervision is an interactional process. To be effective, it depends on emotional attunement, mutual trust and usually an evolving relationship between supervisor and supervisee.

In keeping with the modern emphasis on narratives and their importance, a number of writers have suggested that supervision is inherently a narrative-making activity.(67,68) The role of the supervisor is therefore to elicit an existing narrative of 'the problem' as it is currently understood, and to question the supervisee in such a way that a new under-standing emerges, in the form of a different narrative in which 'the problem' is either lessened or has dissolved. One advantage of using this approach in a medical context is that it places less emphasis on eliciting emotion and more on 'bringing forth new stories'. Many doctors without spe-cific training in psychotherapy or counselling find it more comfortable and more appropriate to take such a narrative-based approach, rather than adopting a technique that is centred on the direct examination of emotions or on learn-ing theory. In addition, a narrative-based technique allows the technical and factual content of cases to be integrated into the evolving story that the supervisee brings (*see* Box 8.10).

A set of operational 'rules' for effective supervision, based on this narrative approach, appears in Box 8.11. The rules are generic: they can be used or adapted for a wide range and variety of supervision encounters, both formal and informal. They can also be used in the context of con-sultations; indeed, it has been suggested that consultations are really just about providing supervision for the patient. Self-evidently, guidelines such as these cannot be trans-ferred simplistically from the written page to everyday practice. They are the starting points for a spiral learning process that may involve both formal and informal train-ing, as well as sustained reflective practice in conversa-tional skills.

BOX 8.10 FOCUS ON: Narrative-based supervision

In the context of training doctors to carry out effective supervision, I have developed a simple theoretical framework for a narrative-based approach, summarised as 'the seven Cs'.(23)

1 *Conversation.* Wherever possible, supervision should aim to resolve problems through the conversation itself rather then through giving advice.

2 *Curiosity.* The best stance for the supervisor is one of curiosity: establishing what the supervisees already know and what options they have already thought of, or want to explore further.

3 *Contexts.* It is often more important to discover the contexts for a problem rather than focusing on the content. These contexts include the patient's and the supervisee's beliefs, values and preference, and the needs and pressures of the organisation.

4 *Complexity.* Most problems brought to supervision are inherently complex, involving many levels of difficulty or intersecting difficulties. Supervision mainly offers opportunities for supervisees to enrich their understanding of what is going on, in order to find a way forward. It rarely helps by finding a 'quick fix'.

5 *Challenge.* Supervision requires frankness and risk taking on both sides.

6 *Caution.* It also requires respect and circumspection: operating within the limits of the supervisee's capacity to tolerate anxiety, while not avoiding the challenge within those limits.

7 *Care.* Most of all, supervision requires attentiveness and positive regard.

Common tensions in supervision

As with any human relationship, supervision and related activities are subject to particular tensions. The ones most commonly experienced by practitioners and cited in the literature are:

- facilitation versus training
- the needs of the client versus the needs of the organisation
- affirmation versus challenge.

This section addresses each of these tensions in turn.

Facilitation versus training

In a technical specialty such as medicine, supervisors may have an overriding wish to bring out the best in their super-visees, and yet at the same time will be aware of the need for a secure basis of knowledge and skills. There are certain facts that any practitioner needs to know. These may be scientific facts that are fairly solid and indisputable (such as how to tell the difference between herpes simplex and shingles), or they may be pragmatic facts because there is

BOX 8.11 HOW TO: Do effective supervision(72)

- The supervisor is not considered to be in a position of authority over the supervisee, except where this is clearly required by the context (e.g. in training contexts).
- Wherever possible, the supervisor's role is to help the supervisee reflect and expand the problem they are presenting in a non-judgemental way.
- The supervisor should offer advice only when this is specifically requested by the supervisee.
- The supervisor needs to pay close attention to the words used by the supervisee and to pursue their meaning.
- Wherever possible, the supervisor should ask questions rather than offer interpretations.
- Each question should, wherever possible, be based on the response to the previous question.
- The supervisor should note non-verbal cues and body language and use this to help frame subsequent questions at the right level of challenge.
- The supervisor will necessarily base their questions on their own knowledge and experience but needs to be wary of making assumptions and imposing these on the supervisee, unless this is necessary for medical safety.
- The conversation does not at first set out to explore the supervisee's feelings, although their emotional response may become an important factor to consider.
- The skill of the supervisor often involves working 'on the cusp', offering enough challenge to the supervisee to help in the exploration of new ideas, but not so much that the supervisee becomes excessively defensive or anxious.
- It is not necessarily expected that the conversation will lead directly to any solution, but may simply help shift the dilemma or case narrative in a more helpful way for the supervisee.

a professional of political consensus about them (such as guidelines on smoking cessation). There is little point in trying to 'bring forth' such knowledge where it is absent. On the other hand, there is always the risk that supervisors will be tempted to remain in a didactic, knowledge-imparting mode, even when this is unhelpful. For example, teaching about the safe use of antidepressants can easily slide into direct advice about prescribing them in a case where it might be more helpful to widen the discussion into areas such as the patient's social circumstances. Supervisees can put pressure on their supervisors, consciously or unconsciously, to offer a quick fix. Supervisors therefore need to offer clear signposting for areas of professional certainty (e.g. the correct doses of drugs) and areas of considerable uncertainty (e.g. the wider contexts of case management).

The client versus the organisation

In some circumstances the tension between the client's needs and those of the organisation can be almost entirely ignored – for example, in a voluntary arrangement for peer supervision or mentorship undertaken between two experienced and competent colleagues. However, in many circumstances organisational needs, spoken or unspoken, will be present. From one perspective, the organisation and regulatory bodies can be a proxy for the needs of the patient, in so far as they exist to ensure acceptable standards of practice. At the same time, there may be situations where the reverse tension exists – for example, where the person receiving supervision believes that they are pursuing the interests of the patient in the face of oppressive restrictions from the agency, including financial or bureaucratic ones. Supervisors and mentors who are employed by the organisation concerned therefore have to manage a fine line between loyalty to the client and loyalty to the organisation. Trust and transparency are needed to negotiate this kind of tension.

Affirmation and challenge

The core tension in any form of supervision is the extent to which the supervisor sets out to support or challenge the client. Every supervisor or mentor wants their clients to feel good about themselves. Equally, every supervisor wants (or should want) clients to be capable of change and to develop as far as their potential will allow. Much of the skill of supervision depends on a capacity to go just beyond the 'comfort zone'. This involves offering enough challenge to the supervisee to help in the exploration of new ideas and new possibilities, but not so much that the supervisee becomes excessively anxious, defensive or deskilled. It may also involve fine judgement as to whether the context permits some careful exploration of personal issues that may be impeding professional performance. Like the skill of consulting with patients who may be anxious or fearful, this is not something that can be learned from books or articles. It depends on a gradual, sometimes lifelong, acquisition of the capacity to calibrate every utterance with the exact circumstances and with the wishes and needs of the client.

Raising the profile of supervision: changing the culture of medicine

Regulatory changes play a part in making sure that supervision happens on a regular basis, but they cannot necessarily ensure its quality. There are no simple prescriptions for promoting a culture change within medicine involving greater emphasis on supervision as a way of bringing about reflective practice. Proctor in particular has emphasised the great importance of every profession and discipline discovering its own approach to supervision; while general principles can be transferred from one profession to another, each will also have its own demands, its own established ways of working and its own supervision needs.(32) Readers will no doubt be able to call to mind some imaginative and creative examples of incremental change in this direction within a variety of medical settings and specialties, including medical schools.(69) Such examples will often involve individual doctors taking the initiative to move from traditional forms of learning (such as lectures, conventional ward rounds or team meetings mainly devoted to administrative matters) towards more enlightened and engaging types of learning approach involving one-to-one reflection.

Conclusions

Medical work is not just about scientific facts. It requires practitioners to apply scientific knowledge in the context of individual lives and complex human systems. It crosses many domains of knowledge, including the social and interpersonal. Doctors are exposed constantly to risks, including stress, alienation, over-involvement, automatic behaviour and burnout. Other professions have rightly recognised that they need organised support as professional oxygen in order to sustain reflective practice in the face of such risks. The medical profession has until now been in the paradoxical position of needing as much of this oxygen as any other group of clinicians (if not more) but generally getting less.

To practise reflectively, doctors need emotional and intellectual trust, so that they can reflect frankly on their own work and learn continually without feeling overexposed or under excessive scrutiny. Activities such as supervision, mentoring and coaching provide opportunities for them to examine their own work safely and effectively, based on their everyday professional experience, and in a way that complements other forms of education and training.

Doctors are always pulled in two directions. On the one hand, there is a clear need for concrete facts, explicit guidelines and consistent policies – in other words, for certainty. On the other hand, there is also the need for practitioners to gain in confidence and in wisdom, and to be able to grapple with the complex, multidimensional problems that they encounter with an ever-increasing level of understanding, sophistication and adventurousness – in other words, for the management of uncertainty. Supervision, mentoring and coaching have the capacity to ensure that medical practice rises consistently above the uninspired, the routine and the automatic. They are often what is needed in order to transform excellence in theory into excellence in action.

There are compelling reasons why the profile of supervision and related activities in medicine should now be raised greatly. These include the increasing complexity of the work, and of the demands placed on practitioners. They also include the pressures placed on doctors by patients, governments and society, and the need to maintain a medical workforce that is well motivated. The challenge of promoting effective methods of supervision, mentoring and coaching among doctors, and of training a generation of competent supervisors, may be one of the most important and exciting projects now facing medical educators.(70–72)

Acknowledgements

Many colleagues made helpful comments on an earlier draft of this work. I particularly want to thank Dr Jonathan Burton, Dr Julie Draper, Dr Anat Gaver (Tel Aviv, Israel), Dr Helen Halpern, Dr Gareth Holsgrove, Dr Tim Swanwick, Prof. Frank Smith and Dr Per Stensland (Bergen, Norway).

References

1 Gray R (2001) A framework for looking at the trainer/registrar tutorial in general practice. *Education for General Practice.* **12**: 153–62.

2 NHS Modernising Medical Careers (2005) *Curriculum for the Foundation Years in Postgraduate Education and Training.* Department of Health, London.

3 NHS Modernising Medical Careers (2008) *A Reference Guide for Postgraduate Speciality Training in the UK: The Gold Guide* (2e). Department of Health, London. (http://www.mmc.nhs.uk/pdf/Gold%20 Guide%202008%20-%20FINAL.pdf; accessed 13 February 2009).

4 School of Health and Related Research (ScHARR) (2001) Appraisal for GPs. (http://www.dh.gov.uk/assetRoot/04/03/47/75/04034775 .pdf; accessed 13 February 2009).

5 Garrett-Harris R and Garvey B (2005) *Towards a Framework for Mentoring in the NHS.* Mentoring and Coaching Research Unit, Faculty of Organisation and Management, Sheffield Hallam University, Sheffield.

6 Beecham B, Dammers J and van Zwanenberg T (2004) Leadership coaching for general practitioners. *Education for Primary Care.* **15**: 579–83.

7 Bowden R and Schofield J (2004) Work based learning and poor performance. In: Burton J and Jackson N (eds) *Work Based Learning in Primary Care.* Radcliffe Publishing, Oxford.

8 Brookfield S (1987) *Developing Critical Thinkers: Challenging Adults to Explore Alternative Ways of Thinking and Acting.* Open University Press, Milton Keynes.

9 Schon D (1983) *The Reflective Practitioner: How Professionals Think in Action.* Temple Smith, London.

10 Schon D (1987) *Educating the Reflective Practitioner: Towards a New Design for Teaching and Learning in the Professions.* Basic Books, New York.

11 Stewart M, Brown J, Weston W *et al.* (2004) *Patient-Centred Medicine: Transforming the Clinical Method* (2e). Radcliffe Publishing, Oxford.

12 Bishop V (ed.) (1988) *Clinical Supervision in Practice, Some Questions, Answers and Guidelines.* Macmillan, London.

13 Bond M and Holland S (1998) *Skills of Clinical Supervision for Nurses.* Open University Press, Buckingham.

14 Cutcliffe J, Butterworth T and Proctor B (2001) *Fundamental Themes in Clinical Supervision.* Routledge, London.

15 Hawkins P and Shohet R (eds) (1989) *Supervision in the Helping Professions.* Open University Press, Milton Keynes.

16 RCN Institute (2000) *Realising Clinical Effectiveness and Clinical Governance through Clinical Supervision.* Radcliffe Medical Press, Oxford.

17 Boud D and Solomon N (eds) (2001) *Work-based Learning: A New Higher Education.* Open University Press, Buckingham.

18 Department of Health (2001) *Working Together, Learning Together: a framework for lifelong learning.* Department of Health, London.

19 Burton J and Jackson N (eds) (2004) *Work Based Learning in Primary Care.* Radcliffe Publishing, Oxford.

20 Steinberg D (2005) *Complexity in Healthcare and the Language of Consultation.* Radcliffe Publishing, Oxford.

21 Lupton D (1994) *Medicine as Culture: Illness, Disease and the Body in Western Societies.* Sage, London.

22 Thomas P (2006) *Integrating Primary Care: Leading, Managing, Facilitating.* Radcliffe Publishing, Oxford.

23 Launer J (2002) *Narrative-Based Primary Care: A Practical Guide.* Radcliffe Medical Press, Oxford.

24 Department of Health (2004) *Modernising Medical Careers: the next steps: the future shape of foundation specialist and general practice training programmes.* Department of Health, London.

25 Morton-Cooper A and Palmer A (eds) (2000) *Mentorship, Preceptorship and Clinical Supervision: A Guide to Professional Support Roles in Clinical Practice* (2e). Blackwell, Oxford.

26 Foster-Turner J (2006) *Coaching and Mentoring in Health and Social Care.* Radcliffe Publishing, Oxford.

27 Scaife J (2001) *Supervision in Mental Health Professions: A Practitioner's Guide.* Brunner Routledge, Hove.

28 Butterworth T (1992) Clinical supervision as an emerging idea in nursing. In: Butterworth T and Faugier J (eds) *Clinical Supervision and Mentorship in Nursing.* Stanley Thornes, Cheltenham.

29 Burton J and Launer J (eds) (2003) *Supervision and Support in Primary Care.* Radcliffe Medical Press, Oxford.

30 Clark P, Jamieson A, Launer J *et al.* (2006) Intending to be a supervisor, mentor or coach: which, what for and why? *Education for Primary Care.* **17**: 109–16.

31 Launer J (2003) Practice, supervision, consultancy and appraisal: a continuum of learning. *British Journal of General Practice.* **53**: 662–5.

32 Proctor B (2001) Training for the supervision attitude, skills and intention. In: Cutcliffe J, Butterworth T and Proctor B (eds) *Fundamental Themes in Clinical Supervision.* Routledge, London.

33 Begat I, Severinsson E and Berggren I (1997) Implementation of clinical supervision in a medical department: nurses' views of the effects. *Journal of Clinical Nursing.* **6**: 389–94.

34 Butterworth T, Bishop V and Carson J (1996) First steps towards evaluating clinical supervision in nursing and health visiting. I. Theory, policy and practice development: a review. *Journal of Clinical Nursing.* **5**: 127–32.

35 Hallberg I, Hansson U and Axelsson K (1994) Satisfaction with nursing care and work during a year of clinical supervision and individualised care: comparison between two wards for the care of severely demented patients. *Journal of Nursing Management.* **1**: 296–307.

36 Kelly B, Long A and McKenna H (2001) Clinical supervision: personal and professional development or the nursing novelty of the 1990s? In: Cutcliffe J, Butterworth T and Proctor B (eds) *Fundamental Themes in Clinical Supervision.* Routledge, London.

37 Winstanley J (2001) Developing methods for evaluating clinical supervision. In: Cutcliffe J, Butterworth T and Proctor B (eds) *Fundamental Themes in Clinical Supervision.* Routledge, London.

38 Garvey B and Garrett-Harris R (2005) *The Benefits of Mentoring: a literature review.* Sheffield Hallam University, Mentoring and Coaching Research Unit, Sheffield.

39 Feltham C (2000) Counselling supervision: baselines, problems and possibilities. In: Lawton B and Feltham C (eds) *Taking Supervision Forward: Enquiries and Trends in Counselling and Psychotherapy.* Sage, London.

40 Kilminster SM and Jolly BC (2000) Effective supervision in clinical practice settings: a literature review. *Medical Education.* **24**: 827–40.

41 Kirkpatrick D (1967) Evaluation of training. In: Craig R and Bittel I (eds) *Training and Development Handbook.* McGraw-Hill, New York.

42 Pringle M (2003) Re-evaluating revalidation and appraisal. *British Journal of General Practice.* **53**: 437–8.

43 Bulstrode C and Hunt V (2000) What is mentoring? *Lancet.* **356**: 178–8.

44 Owen D and Shohet R (eds) (2012) *Clinical Supervision in the Medical Profession: Structured Reflective Practice.* Open University Press, Milton Keynes.

45 Sommers L and Launer J (eds) (2013) *Clinical Uncertainty in Primary Care: The Challenge of Engagement.* Springer, New York.

46 General Medical Council (2012) *Recognising and Approving Trainers: the Implementation Plan.* General Medical Council, London.

47 Cottrell D, Kilminster S, Jolly B and Grant J (2002) What is effective supervision and how does it happen? A critical incident study. *Medical Education.* **36**: 1042–9.

48 Shipton G (ed.) (1997) *Supervision of Psychotherapy and Counselling: Making a Place to Think.* Open University Press, Buckingham.

49 Gupta R and Lingam S (2000) *Mentoring for Doctors and Dentists.* Blackwell, Oxford.

50 Department of Health (2004) *Mentoring for Doctors: signposts to current practice for career grade doctors.* Department of Health, Doctors' Forum, London.

51 Sackin P, Barnett M, Eastaugh A and Paxton P (1997) Peer supported learning. *British Journal of General Practice.* **47**: 67–8.

52 Whitmore J (1996) *Coaching for Performance.* Nicholas Brierley, London.

53 Kersley S (2006) *Prescription for Change: For Doctors Who Want a Life* (2e). Radcliffe Publishing, Oxford.

54 Proctor B (2000) Postscript. In: Morton-Cooper A and Palmer A (eds) *Mentorship, Preceptorship and Clinical Supervision: A Guide to Professional Support Roles in Clinical Practice* (2e). Blackwell, Oxford, p. 221.

55 Casement P (1988) *On Learning from the Patient.* Routledge, London.

56 Obholzer A and Roberts V (eds) (1994) *The Unconscious at Work: Individual and Organisational Stress in the Human Services.* Routledge, London.

57 Salinsky J and Sackin P (eds) (2000) *What are You Feeling Doctor? Identifying and Avoiding Defensive Patterns in the Consultation.* Radcliffe Medical Press, Oxford.

58 Burnham J (1993) Systemic supervision. The evolution of reflexivity in the context of the supervising relationship. *Human Systems.* **4**: 349–81.

59 Todd T and Storm C (eds) (1997) *The Complete Systemic Supervisor: Contexts, Philosophy and Pragmatics.* Allyn and Bacon, London.

60 Campbell B and Mason B (2002) *Perspectives on Supervision.* Karnac, London.

61 Patterson C (1997) Client centred supervision. In: Watkins C (ed.) *Handbook of Psychotherapy Supervision.* John Wiley, New York.

62 Claridge M-T and Lewis T (2005) *Coaching for Effective Learning.* Radcliffe Publishing, Oxford.

63 Kolb D (1984) *Experiential Learning.* Prentice Hall, Englewood Cliffs, NJ.

64 Honey P and Mumford A (1992) *Manual of Learning Styles.* Honey, Maidenhead.

65 Houghton A and Allen J (2005) Understanding personality type: doctor–patient communication. *BMJ Career Focus.* **330**: 36–7.

66 Wackman DB, Miller S and Nunnally EW (1976) *Student Workbook: Increasing Awareness and Communication Skills.* Interpersonal Communication Programmes, Minneapolis, MN.

67 Benner P, Tanner C and Chesla C (1986) *Expertise in Nursing Practice – Caring, Clinical Judgment and Ethics.* Springer, New York.

68 Launer J (2003) A narrative based approach to primary care supervision. In: Burton J and Launer J (eds) *Supervision and Support in Primary Care.* Radcliffe Medical Press, Oxford.

69 Driessen E, van Tartwijk J, Overeem K *et al.* (2005) Student learning: conditions for successful reflective use of portfolios in undergraduate education. *Medical Education.* **39**: 1230–5.

70 Bennett J, Gardener B and James F (2001) Implementing clinical supervision in an NHS community trust: sharing the vision. In: Cutcliffe J, Butterworth T and Proctor B (eds) *Fundamental Themes in Clinical Supervision.* Routledge, London.

71 Launer J (2004) Training GP educators in clinical supervision. *Work based Learning in Primary Care.* **2**: 366–9.

72 Launer J and Halpern H (2006) Reflective practice in clinical supervision: an approach to promoting clinical supervision amongst general practitioners. *Work based Learning in Primary Care.* **4**: 629–32.

9 Teaching and leading small groups

Peter McCrorie
St George's University of London, UK

🔑 KEY MESSAGES

- Always consider whether a session can better be run in small groups.
- Plan the session carefully in plenty of time.
- Vary the session plan according to the size of the group and the venue.
- For large groups (~ 30) run the session in workshop format, by splitting the group into four or five smaller groups.
- Consider which format is most appropriate for the group task.
- Include a range of formats in any one session, recognising that active learning is likely to be more successful than passive learning.

- Consider your own role in the group process; remember that being the group leader is only one of several options.
- Remember the importance of maintaining good group dynamics.
- Deal with issues as and when they arise, bearing in mind that it is often better to let the group address the issues themselves.
- Take care not to overstep boundaries and destroy good working relationships.

Introduction

Two people give a lecture on a medical topic. One is charismatic and inspirational. He holds the audience in his hands – they are on the edge of their seats throughout the lecture. He does not use notes, illustrates his talk with a few well-chosen photos and uses the traditional 'talk and chalk' approach. He regularly wins the 'best lecturer' prize. Contrast this with the second lecturer – a very dry and serious speaker, who has carefully prepared every word he intends to use, uses a myriad of PowerPoint slides, each laden with detailed information, and who whips each slide away before his audience has had a chance to get down the half of what he says. Now imagine that each sets an examination question based on his lecture. Which question do you think the students would perform better in?

In fact, they would get higher marks in the second, less charismatic, lecturer's question. Why? Because in order to make any sense of his lecture, the students would have made a beeline for their textbooks and this self-directed learning would have enabled them to learn and retain the information more effectively. While the first lecture was stunning at the time, the students would have assumed they would remember every word of it several weeks later and therefore would not have bothered reading around the subject – an approach that would let them down on the day.

The conclusion from the above is that an active, self-directed approach is likely to have a much greater impact on a student's learning than passive, lecture-based learn-

ing. Lectures should be used sparingly and for broad overviews, summaries and difficult topics. Sadly, only about 5 per cent of what is taught in lectures is actually retained, and too many people use lectures for imparting large quantities of detailed information that could easily be picked up, and more effectively, by reading a textbook. (*See* Chapter 10 for more on lectures and lecturing.)

Learning in small groups is a sort of halfway house, involving active learning, or more precisely *interactive* learning. But here the direction of learning is determined by the group as a whole, rather than the individual. Group learning can be a most rewarding and effective experience at all stages in a medical career – undergraduate, postgraduate and throughout years of continuing professional development. Too many people still consider that unless material is passed on from professor to student or consultant to trainee in a formal lecture, it would not be learnt properly. This chapter aims to challenge that assumption and to provide some ideas and suggestions, backed up by theory and the available evidence, for getting the most out of the small group learning experience.

The learner experience

If you were to ask a group of medical graduates to relate their personal experiences of small group work in their undergraduate course or postgraduate training, their responses would vary considerably. But the two factors

---

Understanding Medical Education: Evidence, Theory and Practice, Second Edition. Edited by Tim Swanwick.
© 2014 The Association for the Study of Medical Education. Published 2014 by John Wiley & Sons, Ltd.

most likely to underpin their accounts would probably relate to *tutor variability* and *curriculum philosophy*.

A *tutor* who creates a relaxed atmosphere, who keeps the group focused on the task in hand, who deals effectively with group dynamics, who allows the learners to take ownership of their learning and who helps make the process an effective, yet enjoyable, experience will produce strongly positive and enthusiastic responses. On the other hand, a tutor who talks all the time, who does not encourage group participation, who belittles learners who answer questions incorrectly, who has clear favourites in the group and who creates an atmosphere where one is frightened to open one's mouth does an extreme disservice to education.

A traditional *curriculum*, heavily dependent on imparting information through lectures, where students or trainees are seen as an inconvenience and a hindrance to research and their clinical practice, rather than as a benefit and an opportunity to mould and influence the future medical workforce, and where time spent by large numbers of tutors on small group teaching is perceived as an ineffective use of staff time, is likely to be received unfavourably. A progressive university or postgraduate team that values its students, believes in active learning, encourages small group teaching and trains its staff in the art of facilitation of learning will undoubtedly invoke a positive response.

At the postgraduate level, lectures are of even less value than at the undergraduate level, yet they are used just as frequently. Trainees gain far more from small group teaching sessions and on-the-job training than from, for instance, revision courses for passing membership exams. In the UK, primary care has tended to lead the way with its long-established one-to-one training relationship and regular group-based release courses, but effective education and training are also possible in secondary care. Bulstrode and Hunt, in their training manual *Educating Consultants*,(1) offer a number of constructive suggestions for running on-the-job training that allow consultants to carry out effective education, while at the same time maintaining their clinical practice load. And the training need not be one to one. It is common practice to train senior doctors, junior doctors and medical students at the same time. Bedside teaching is an example of this, but sadly such sessions are often still run in an inappropriate and humiliating way. The effectiveness of bedside teaching is discussed by Jolly in his book entitled *Bedside Manners*.(2)

De Villiers *et al.*,(3) in a report of an evaluation of a continuing professional development programme for primary care medical practitioners in South Africa, suggest that the following aspects should be incorporated into the design of small group activities to make them effective. Namely that they should:

- build on prior knowledge and experience
- relate to the perceived learning needs of the participants
- involve active learning
- be focused on problems
- be immediately applicable to practice
- involve cycles of action–reflection
- allow the acquisition of technical skills.

Steinert(4) researched medical students' perceptions of small group teaching in a Canadian medical school. Her conclusions at the undergraduate level were not a million miles away from de Villiers' findings at the postgraduate level, that is that positive student perceptions of small group teaching were related to:

- effective small group facilitation
- a positive group atmosphere
- active student participation and group interaction
- adherence to small group goals
- clinical relevance and integration
- cases that promote thinking and problem solving.

The inefficiency argument is often used by those opposed to small group teaching. Twenty-five tutors spending two-to-three hours working with students in small groups of eight is clearly less efficient than one lecturer talking to 200 students all at once – but only in terms of delivery of material. Efficiency does not just take account of the delivery of *teaching*; what the students *learn* is what matters. I return to the point made earlier, that the taught curriculum is not the same as the learnt curriculum. Through small group discussion, much more is retained, especially if the learning is contextualised, for example, in case scenarios. In terms of efficiency of learning, small group work wins hands down. More particularly, small group work encourages critical thinking, which, although not impossible, is less common in lectures. *See* Box 9.1.

What constitutes a small group?

The ideal size of a small group is probably around seven or eight. If the group is smaller, it becomes too threatening,

---

BOX 9.1 WHERE'S THE EVIDENCE: Does small group work encourage critical thinking?

Most of the research around small group work relates specifically to problem-based learning (PBL) – a specialised form of small group learning discussed in detail in Chapter 5. The nature of courses structured around PBL is such that small group work, and the subsequent self-directed learning, is the main vehicle by which students gain information, with lectures contributing relatively little to students' knowledge acquisition. This is in contrast to courses where lectures and other forms of didactic teaching provide the main source of information for students, and where small group teaching is really an adjunct to their learning. Tiwari *et al.*(5) have compared the effects of these two course styles on the development of students' critical thinking. They found that PBL students had significantly higher levels of critical thinking (measured using the California Critical Thinking Disposition Inventory(6)) compared with students on a predominantly lecture-based course. Furthermore, they continued to have higher scores for two years afterwards. Similar conclusions have emerged from a variety of other sources.(7–9) the synergistic effect – the collective knowledge of the group being greater than the sum of the knowledge of each member of the group – is reduced and the interaction is less successful. If the number increases above eight, some learners can get by without fully participating, or without joining in at all, and others are less able to get their voice heard, because the size of the group deters them from expressing their point of view. For problem-based learning (PBL), the size of the tutorial group rarely exceeds eight – the process would simply fall apart were there any more in the group. Norman(10) recently carried out an email survey of a cross-section of medical schools around the world using PBL, asking about the size of group they felt was appropriate, and eight turned out to be the norm. Peters(11) cites academic evidence that supports his own findings that the optimum size of a group is somewhere between five and ten.

Some medical schools are so short of willing and able teachers that they operate small groups of 20 or more. This can still be successful, however, if the larger group is run in workshop format, where the whole group is given a task to carry out in smaller subgroups of seven or eight. Here, one facilitator handles several groups. Many postgraduate training courses are run this way.

Group size is probably less important than what the group actually does. The purist view of small group teaching is that it must be learner-centred, with all students joining in free discussion of a particular topic. Some teaching may indeed take place in small groups but sits outside this definition. The seminar is a case in point, where invited speakers present on a topic about which they are passionate. The seminar has its place in a university – particularly at the Bachelor of Science or Master's level – but is invariably teacher-centred, with any discussion taking the form of questions and answers.

Even within the confines of our working definition, a wide range of styles of small group work exists, and many of these are discussed later.

Housekeeping

Before embarking on small group teaching, some thought needs to be given to the environmental arrangements. It seems obvious to say it, but the first requirement is to hold the session in an appropriately sized room. What is appropriate depends on the number of learners participating. Consideration should also be given to heating, lighting and temperature control in the room, all of which are the unique responsibility of the group leader.

For a group of eight or so undertaking PBL or some similar activity, a room with a table in it, preferably round- or oval-shaped and big enough for all to sit around it comfortably – including the tutor, who should be part of the group and not outside it – is ideal (*see* Figure 9.1). The walls of the room should be lined with whiteboards or flipcharts for students to write and draw on.

For a session where argument is more important than capturing information, for example, an ethical debate, then a circle of chairs is all that is required (*see* Figure 9.2).

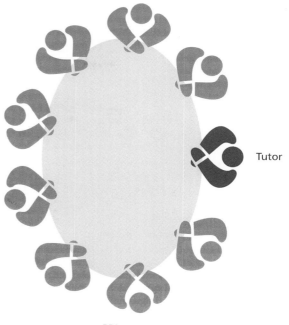

PBL group

Figure 9.1 Seating arrangement for a problem-based learning (PBL) tutorial.

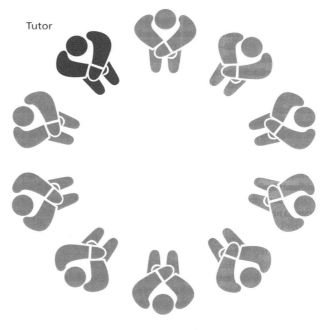

Discussion circle

Figure 9.2 Seating arrangement for a group discussion.

The positioning of the tutor is important. To maximise the effectiveness of the process, the tutor should be *in* the group, rather than *separate* from it. Sitting in a circle has two advantages:
• everyone in the circle is equal
• everyone has eye contact with each other.

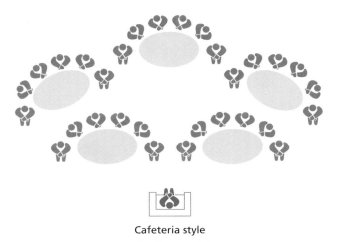

Cafeteria style

Figure 9.3 Seating arrangement for a workshop.

This arrangement also suits the role of the tutor as *facilitator*.

For larger groups, the workshop format is the method of choice, and hence the room has to be larger and laid out in cafeteria style (several round tables with chairs round them, laid out like a cafeteria; *see* Figure 9.3). There needs to be space at the front of the room for the tutor, PowerPoint and/or overhead projector facilities (including an accessible power source), and whiteboard(s) that everyone can see. Ideally, each group should have a flipchart as well. Again, if there is no requirement for a table, then several circles of chairs will suffice.

Positioning of the tutor is different for a workshop. Plenary sessions are commonly part of a workshop, usually at the beginning to introduce the topic or task, and at the end to take feedback from the groups and summarise what has been achieved. Since the tutor needs to be able to engage everyone together, he or she needs to stand or be seated at the front of the class for these plenaries. However, for the rest of the session, the tutor's job is to go round the groups to check how they are getting on.

The role of the tutor

The tutor can adopt a range of roles depending on the nature of the small group session. Rudduck(12) suggests that tutors can have four differing roles:
- the *instructor*, who is there to impart information to the students
- the *devil's advocate*, who intentionally adopts a controversial view in order to stimulate discussion
- the *neutral chair*, who literally chairs the discussion but expresses no strong opinions
- the *consultant*, who is not part of the group, but is there for the students to ask questions.

To these roles, I would add a fifth:
- the *facilitator*, similar to the neutral chair, but with more of a guiding role, for example, asking the group open-ended questions to facilitate their progress with the

task in hand. The facilitator need not be the chair of the group – this role might fall to a student.

Tutors may adopt any or all of the above roles during the course of a small group teaching session. They may begin the session in instructor mode, defining the task for the students. During the rest of the session, they may adopt a more facilitatory role, at times prompting discussion by playing the role of the devil's advocate or taking up a chairing role. If the students get stuck, they may even take on the role of expert to allow them to move on (not in PBL, of course, where the tutor must reflect any questions back to the group and encourage them to research the answers for themselves).

Richmond(13) defines more specific roles for tutors, which he refers to as 'strategic interventions':
- to start and finish group discussion by outlining the group task, summarising the group's or groups' achievements and conclusions, and setting further learning activities
- to maintain the flow of content, for example, by preventing sidetracking and keeping the group(s) focused on the task
- to manage group dynamics by encouraging the shy or bored student(s) and by handling the dominant, aggressive, offensive or nuisance student(s)
- to facilitate goal achievement through open questioning, making suggestions and checking group understanding
- to manage the group environment by keeping an eye on the time and dealing with any distractions (e.g. noise, insufficient flipchart paper, pens running dry, heating).

According to Brown,(14) tutors need a range of skills in order to make a success of small group teaching. These include questioning, listening, reinforcing, reacting, summarising and leadership. But the real skill, one that Brown refers to as a *super skill*, is the skill of knowing when to use which skill.

Getting started

The first time the tutor meets with a new group of students or trainees is always exciting. Is it going to be the group from heaven or the group from hell? Often, the first encounter is the defining moment for the group. How the tutor handles the opening small group teaching session may establish the atmosphere for the sessions that follow.

The group members may or may not know each other. At the start of the course they almost certainly would not; but even later on, particularly in undergraduate curricula, because of the trend to have large numbers of students on courses, group members may still not know every other person on the course. Ice-breakers have a useful role here – ways of introducing strangers, trying to relax the group and getting group members to interact with each other.

There are many ice-breakers in common use – some simple, some elaborate. A standard technique is to ask the group members to pair up and talk to someone they do not know. Their task is to learn something about their partners and report it back to the group. This exercise works better if the task is fairly specific, and in addition to their partners'

BOX 9.2 Examples of ground rules for small groups

- Turn up punctually
- Finish on time
- Do not talk over each other
- Do not interrupt
- Value each person's contribution
- Respect each other's viewpoint
- Turn off mobile phone
- Turn up prepared
- Join in the discussion
- Keep personal issues outside
- Maintain confidentiality within the group

---

student and discuss their thoughts with each other. After another five minutes, the pairs are invited to join with another pair, and all four students continue their discussion. Two sets of fours then compare notes, and so on. The process is called 'snowballing' because of its resemblance to a snowball rolling down a hill, gathering more and more snow and getting bigger and bigger in size. The big advantage of this technique is that everyone has to participate, even the most reticent of students. By allowing time for them to gather their own thoughts and then share these thoughts with one other, it gives even the shyest student confidence to speak. A variation on snowballing is called *jigsaw groups*, where the participants divide into small groups and discuss an issue. After a period, the groups re-form into new groups, with each of the new groups containing one member of each of the old groups, thereby maximising the mix of participants (*see* Figure 9.4).

names and brief biographical details, participants may be asked to report back on the most interesting place their partners have visited, something unusual that they have done in their life or something they have done of which they are proud. Participants could also be asked to imagine themselves as a musical instrument or a vehicle or a colour, and to describe which most closely matches their character – all of which can be quite revealing!

An example of a more complex ice-breaker, which needs a bit of time, is to divide the group into two teams which have to compete with each other to build a bridge of specific dimensions and requirements out of Lego bricks in a specified time. The dimensions and rules they have to adhere to make this a hard task, but it enables the tutor to observe how each member of the team behaves under pressure. It also provides an opportunity for discussing people's behaviours at the end of the exercise, and seeing how each team worked. Such exercises or games are common on off-campus postgraduate training courses.

Having got the group talking, the next thing to do is set the ground rules. This is a really important activity and should never be omitted. It is essential that the group itself comes up with the ground rules – they must not be imposed by the tutor. Box 9.2 shows examples of ground rules that my own undergraduate students have come up with. Probably the most important ground rule is to do with valuing each other's contribution. That way a relaxed atmosphere is created where no one is embarrassed about saying something stupid. Humiliation must be avoided at all costs.

Techniques to use in small groups

Following on from the ice-breaker, a good technique to get a group engaged in the topic under discussion is known as *snowballing*. The students are given a question, for example, 'How might cystic fibrosis affect the life of a 15-year-old young man?', and asked to think about it individually, without conferring with anyone else. After five minutes, the students are asked to pair up with another

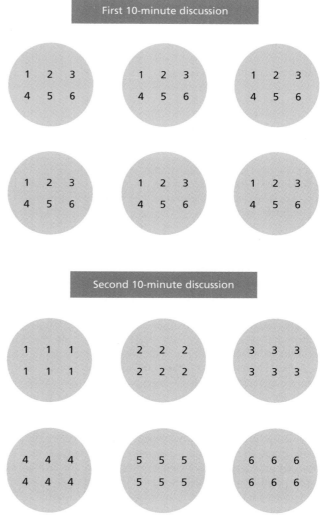

Figure 9.4 How jigsaw groups work.

Brainstorming is another widely used technique. Again, learners are given something to think about (e.g. possible diagnoses for a patient who presents with lower back pain). One group member acts as scribe and writes all the suggestions from the group – in this case possible diagnoses – on a whiteboard. Absolutely everything is written up, no matter how unlikely the suggestion may be. No one is allowed to make any value judgements on the suggestions at this stage. A reflective analysis of what has been written up follows, where items are prioritised, grouped together or removed altogether.

A third introductory technique involves the use of *buzz groups*. This technique is more generally used in lectures, but can also be used in small groups, if the group becomes stuck in its thinking. The tutor who senses an impasse can interrupt the discussion and throw in a question for the group to ponder in pairs or threes, to help the members get back on track. If students are struggling to understand respiratory acidosis, for instance, the tutor might ask them to discuss in pairs what the role of the kidney is in maintaining pH or what blood buffers exist. When this technique is used in lectures, there is a loud 'buzz', as members of the audience start talking with their neighbours – hence the name.

Further on in the life of the learning group, a number of other techniques may be used.

Simply *chairing a discussion* – or, better still, getting one of the group members to do so – works well when there is more than one perspective about an issue, such as a genuine ethical dilemma like abortion, animal experimentation or euthanasia. Occasionally with moral and ethical arguments, the tutor may need to step in to clarify matters of fact, such as primary legislation, case law or professional guidelines – an example of the tutor acting as a consultant or expert. A more imaginative and hands-off approach to such issues would be to get the students to set up a *formal debate*, with students primed to speak for or against a particular motion, such as 'This house believes that patients with coronary artery disease, who continue to smoke after they have been repeatedly counselled about the dangers of smoking, should be refused heart bypass surgery'. The advantage here is that the relevant factual elements to the discussion are prepared in advance.

A variation of the discussion group is called *line-ups*. The tutor makes a controversial statement, such as 'Doctors should be allowed to hasten the death of old people who have a terminal illness'. The tutor identifies a point in one corner of the room where everyone who strongly agrees with the statement should stand. Another point is identified, as far away as possible, where those who strongly disagree should stand. The rest of the group members have to line up somewhere between the two points, according to how much they agree or disagree with the statement. The participants have to talk to the others in the line and argue their point of view. The tutors, and indeed the participants, get an immediate view of the spread of participants' opinions on the topic. If the line-up is carried out at the beginning and the end of a session, the tutor can gauge if there has been a change of opinion after the session has been run and the participants are better informed.

There are a number of variations on the discussion approach to small group teaching. Some of these are less than satisfactory, however. One approach used frequently in postgraduate medical education is the *journal club*. Staff are asked to present their comments on recent papers in the medical literature. This works well, provided the topic is of direct relevance to everyone and there is plenty of opportunity for discussion. It is less successful at the undergraduate level, where it is more usual to run the session along the lines of a syndicate presentation, where a topic such as diabetes is subdivided into several subtopics (e.g. mechanism of action of insulin, diabetic ketoacidosis, clinical presentation of diabetes, treatment of diabetes) and each of these subtopics is given to a student or pair of students to research. They then all report back at the next tutorial. The problem with both of these methods is that the presentations become mini-lectures, are frequently delivered in an uninspiring manner and, frankly, bore the pants off everyone. Discussion is limited because only the chosen few have researched the topic, and then only the subtopic they were allocated. Unless everyone researches everything, the only people who join in the discussion are those who researched the topic and the tutor!

Another old favourite at the undergraduate level is the *post-lecture tutorial*. This is another disaster site. Most students come unprepared and have not read up around the lecture topic (indeed, they may not even have attended the lecture or may be blissfully unaware what lecture topic is being discussed). Many students see it as an opportunity to listen to a rerun of the original lecture, which is what it often turns into, particularly if the tutor gets monosyllabic responses to the questions they ask to try to stimulate the students. There is really only one solution to this – ensure that students are given a self-directed learning exercise to prepare *before* the tutorial. A good example would be to give them a detailed case study to read up, with some questions attached for them to research, for example, a case history of a patient with a peptic ulcer, followed by a series of questions on, for instance, medical imaging, regulation of intestinal pH, *Helicobacter pylori*, drug treatment and dietary advice. In this way, the students know what the topic of the tutorial is, have done their homework, and therefore feel able to join in the discussion and get a lot more out of the whole exercise.

The *use of triggers* provides an ideal springboard for a tutorial. The tutor can design a whole session around one or more of these. They are commonly used when running sessions in the workshop format. At the beginning of the session, after a brief introduction, the tutor hands out a trigger. A trigger is simply a tool to get the discussion started. They might take various forms, such as the following:

• an electrocardiogram (ECG) strip from a patient with ventricular fibrillation – to stimulate a discussion about cardiac muscle, the sinoatrial node, ECGs, arrythmias, defibrillation
• a photomicrograph showing neoplastic growth changes to stimulate discussion about the appearance of cancerous tissue, the characteristics of cancer cells, metastasis

- a chest X-ray showing a pneumothorax to stimulate discussion about X-rays, pleura of the lungs, pneumothorax – its causes, presentation and treatment
- an audiogram from a patient with age- and noise-related hearing loss to stimulate discussion about the anatomy of the ear, the hearing mechanism, sensorineural hearing loss, audiometry, Rinne and Weber's tests
- a copy of *Good Medical Practice* to stimulate discussion on what constitutes a good standard of practice and patient care, professionalism, working with colleagues and probity
- an anonymised or mock-up of a patient record for students to discuss record-keeping in the context of a particular case
- a photograph of a patient with an obvious goitre and exophthalmos to stimulate discussion around the thyroid gland and thyroid disorders, including clinical signs, symptoms and treatment
- a photograph of a man in a wheelchair playing with a young child to stimulate discussion around disability, psychosocial sequelae of chronic illness, social care, child care, single-parent families
- a family pedigree, showing the distribution of a genetic disorder such as haemophilia to trigger a discussion on genes and patterns of inheritance
- a video showing, for example, a doctor explaining to a couple that their baby has Down syndrome
- a paper, or excerpts from a paper, showing some statistical data, in order to get the students talking about *P*-values or odds ratios or randomised controlled trials.

In PBL, a paper-based case scenario would normally act as the trigger, and there are two main variants of this: one where the case is presented in the form of a short summary; the other where the case is much longer and is released in stages by the tutor (presentation, history, examination findings, investigations, treatment, patient progress and outcome). The former is generally used for school leavers, the latter for graduates. The tutor has rather different roles in the two versions. In short-case PBL tutorials, the students take turns at being chair of the group and the tutor is passive, intervening only to ask the odd question to stimulate discussion or to keep the group on track. In the long, progressive-release version of PBL, the tutor acts as the chair, moves the group along when their discussion has come to a halt and occasionally asks specific, programmed questions. Both styles of PBL are student-centred and produce deep and high-level discussions, particularly with graduate students. PBL is covered in more detail in Chapter 5.

Role play also uses a trigger. Students are given a scenario to act out, for example, taking a headache history, explaining a medication regime for eczema or breaking bad news about a cervical smear result. Professional actors are often employed to simulate real patients, and students can try out their clinical communication skills in a safe environment. If the students are video-recorded as well, they can study their communication attempts in their own time and work on improving their technique before encountering the real thing. This technique works well at the postgraduate level too, especially with doctors who have been identified as having a communication problem. Watching your own performance can be very revealing and informative. Discussing your performance, captured on videotape, with a trained communication skills expert is invaluable and always leads to improvement. The secret is to have enough insight and be brave enough to do it in the first place.

Clinical skills are also taught in small groups, but rather than using a trigger, the clinician will demonstrate the skill to the group before letting them have a go. One commonly used technique(15) takes place in four stages:

- the tutor demonstrates the skill in silence
- the tutor runs through it again, but explains the rationale behind the technique at the same time
- the students then talk the tutor through the technique
- finally, a volunteer student runs through the technique without tutor intervention.

The *Balint group*(16,17) is a special kind of group activity undertaken mainly by general practitioners (GPs), although increasingly patients, and even students, are becoming involved. Michael Balint was a Hungarian psychoanalyst who worked extensively with UK GPs in helping them to understand the psychology behind the doctor–patient relationship. He set up discussion groups with GPs to allow them to share their personal experiences of specific problems or dilemmas that had arisen in their practice. A modern-day Balint group consists of a handful of GPs, who meet on a regular basis, often with a psychoanalyst and sometimes with one or more patients, to discuss specific issues concerning patients arising from their daily practice. The presenting clinician brings to the group cases that have given cause for thought. The purpose of the group is to increase understanding of the doctor–patient relationship, not to find solutions to the patient's problem. Discomfort or distress in the doctor are not ignored, but are worked through in the context of the needs and problems of the patient rather than of the doctor. Balint group members find that the benefit gained by sharing their experiences far outweighs any pain they may feel as a result of the experience. Balint groups are not for everyone and should not to be entered into lightly.

Another type of group activity used in the postgraduate arena is the *action learning set*. An action learning set is a group of six-to-eight people who meet regularly to help each other learn from their experiences. The set is not a team, since its focus is on the actions of the individuals within it, rather than on a shared set of work objectives. Sets are usually facilitated by a set adviser whose responsibility is to create a suitable learning environment by encouraging, challenging and focusing on learning. Action learning is based on the concept of learning by reflection on experience. It is underpinned by the cycle of experiential learning,(18) as shown in Figure 9.5, where the stages of reflection and generalisation are worked through with the members of the set.

The action learning approach was first developed by Revans.(19) Each participant works on a project or task over the life of the set (which may be a few weeks, or spread over several months). The set decides on its own way of working, but usually a meeting involves participants taking turns to present their project to the set. This will normally involve the following:

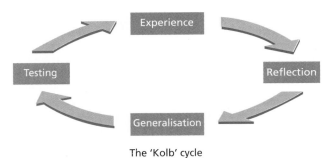

The 'Kolb' cycle

Figure 9.5 The 'Kolb' cycle.

- an update of progress on actions from the last meeting
- a discussion about current issues or problems
- an agreement on actions for the future.

Participants work with the presenter, by listening and questioning, to help them decide what actions to take. This kind of group is useful for individuals working on an educational or research project largely on their own.

Group dynamics

Before considering the role of the tutor in addressing issues of poor group dynamics, it is worthwhile taking a look at how a group evolves during its lifetime. Tuckman[20] has summarised it into four stages, which have been further interpreted by Walton[21] and Mulholland.[22]

Forming

The participants get to know each other, form alliances and establish themselves. The tutor must ensure they are introduced to each other.

Norming

The participants set the ground rules for working as a group. Being unfamiliar with what is expected of them can lead to some uncertainty and insecurity at this point. The tutor may need to explain the way the tutorials are to be run to alleviate anxiety at this point.

Storming

The group begins to function. Individuals adopt the roles with which they feel comfortable. One might be a leader; another good at initiating conversation; a third might be skilled at asking probing questions; a fourth might be good at clarifying and explaining; another might be good at keeping the team together, coming to the rescue of anyone who appears lost, frustrated or angry; one or two may simply be good listeners and may only contribute to the process when they have something to say. There is the potential for a good deal of friction during this stage, while the group is sorting itself out. The tutor needs to keep a careful watch on the group members, identifying problems and trying to relieve tensions. If the participants are mature enough, they may be able to address their own issues as a group. This is to be encouraged. The less the tutor gets involved, the better. Such a group skill takes time to develop

and the tutor will undoubtedly need to facilitate the process initially.

Performing

This is the position every group should aim for. Essentially the group has settled down and is functioning well. The group members are comfortable with their roles. There is a good atmosphere within the group and the goals of each tutorial are generally accomplished through successful collaboration. The tutor can now relax.

Unfortunately, some groups never achieve this state. This is usually due to one or two personality clashes and the odd difficult student. If the group cannot sort itself out, the tutor must act. Otherwise participants and tutor will dread meeting up for tutorials and attendance will fall off.

Adjourning

Also called *mourning,* this is the final stage of working in groups. The lifetime of the group has run out, and members move on to join new groups. This phase is a mixture of celebration and sadness (or relief, in the case of an unsuccessful group). A good group will look back over its achievements and reflect on each other's contribution, on lessons learnt, on what worked well and what could have been done better.

This process of reflection can be formalized, and the tutor can help the group debrief itself in a structured way. One process that works quite well is carried out in two stages. First, the group rates itself as a whole against set criteria. The criteria depend on the nature and purpose of the small group work, but might include attendance and punctuality, preparedness for the sessions, adequacy of input into the sessions and behaviour towards each other within each session. Having established a group rating for each criterion, the members of the group then rate themselves against the group rating. Everyone shares their scores and a discussion ensues. A good group will recognise individuals' strengths and weaknesses, will be constructively critical, and will try to be supportive and encouraging to the more self-effacing members of the group. A good group will also not shirk its responsibility to address issues arising from individuals who are lacking in insight as to their own behaviour. Often, as a result of this kind of caring, inward reflection, change does take place when these members move on to their next groups (*see* Box 9.3).

The interprofessional group

Interprofessional learning is considered important at both the undergraduate and the postgraduate levels (*see* Chapter 6 for a full discussion).[25] Health care is all about working in teams, and it is sensible therefore to have regular joint educational training throughout the continuum of learning. The key to interprofessional education is that it should relate to real practice and should not be contrived just so that the box can be ticked for the next accreditation visit. Furthermore, interprofessional education does not require the participation of *all* the professions at each session – only those for whom it is appropriate.

BOX 9.3 FOCUS ON: Discussion in small groups

Visschers-Pleijers *et al.*(23) have carried out an analysis of verbal interactions in tutorial groups. They have subdivided these interactions into five types:

- exploratory questioning – exchanging ideas, critical exchange of ideas
- cumulative reasoning – uncritical accumulation of information
- handling conflicts about knowledge – discussion of contradictory information; arguments and counter-arguments
- procedural interactions – conversations relating to process matters
- off task/irrelevant interactions – general asides; discussion about the weather

Most of the interactions (about 80 per cent) were learning-oriented, demonstrating the high task involvement of the group and confirming the findings of De Grave *et al.*(24)

Interprofessional team meetings are common at the postgraduate level, interprofessional training less so, although both acute and primary care trusts provide programmes of training sessions for their staff. Quite a few of these are interprofessional, although they tend to be for large numbers, rather than small groups. Training in leadership and management for senior staff is less likely to be profession-specific and often follows the workshop format.

At the undergraduate level, certainly in the UK, there is only a small amount of useful interprofessional education taking place. What there is takes a variety of forms, ranging from a common foundation term with shared PBL, lectures and anatomy sessions,(26) shared clinical skills training,(27,28) a simulated ward environment for junior medical and nursing students,(29) and an interprofessional training ward(30–32) to regular joint interprofessional sessions spread over a number of years.(33) Apart from the lectures and the anatomy sessions, most of this involves small group work.

The skills training described,(27,28) involved final-year medical students with newly qualified staff nurses and took place in an interprofessional clinical skills centre. The programme was based around a developing patient scenario, which was pertinent to the participants' area of practice. Each session was led by an experienced nurse lecturer and doctor, supported by specialist contributors. The style of learning was participative, with small interprofessional groups addressing a range of patient management issues. In this way, relevant clinical and communication skills were integrated within the context of holistic patient care. This short exposure to interprofessional learning appears to have been highly effective.

The interprofessional training ward takes small group learning in the context of simulation even further. Here, final-year nurses, physiotherapists, occupational therapists and medical students look after a small ward.(30–32) They work shifts, carry out all ward duties, work extensively with each other and learn about each other's professions, while at the same time building up their uniprofessional skills. Handover from one shift to another is key to the learning process. This provides students with an excellent preparation for working on the wards when they graduate, and is again popular with most students.

Undergraduate or postgraduate, the issues around interprofessional learning are the same and revolve around group relations (*see* Bion in the 'Further Reading' section). There is a strong hierarchical culture, which pervades all areas of the health service. When people from different professions find themselves being trained together, there is a tendency to adopt these hierarchical roles. Even at the undergraduate level, medical students, physiotherapists, occupational therapists and nurses all have different entry requirements, and immediately a barrier exists. Of course, one of the aims of interprofessional education is to break down such barriers. Another aim is for the members of one profession to have a clear understanding of the roles of the other health care professionals. Putting these two aims together leads to the third, overarching, aim – to learn how to work in teams, thereby leading to a more efficient and effective health service. Small group learning in interprofessional groups is one way to help achieve this last aim.

For an inter-professional group, good facilitation is essential. If the guidance described for any small group work activity is followed, the majority of problems will soon disappear. Setting clear ground rules and ensuring that the group adheres to them is vital – particularly the rule about valuing everyone's input. In addition, the topic or activity needs to be inclusive, that is appropriate for all professions present. The learning needs of the students or trainees must be taken into account, as they will not be the same for all professions. Where they *are* the same, then joint interprofessional learning is more likely to succeed.

Dealing with difficult group members

Dealing with difficult group members is a key role of the tutor running small group teaching sessions. Box 9.4 features a list of common problems encountered, and regular group leaders will recognise them all. It is not the purpose of this chapter to provide suggestions for dealing with *each* form of aberrant behaviour – for a full discussion of this topic read Tiberius's excellent book *Small Group Teaching: a trouble shooters guide*.(34) One general point though is worth emphasising, that is wherever possible, the group should sort out its own problems. This is liable to be much more effective in the long term than the tutor taking control, which often leads to resentment. The tutor's role here is to raise the group's awareness of the issue. One way of doing this is to say, 'Let's take time out for a minute. Is everyone happy the way the group is working? Does anyone want to make a comment about the group process?' Then stand back and watch the sparks fly!

Of course, this is not always appropriate, nor does it always work. In such circumstances, the group leader has

BOX 9.4 Challenging learners

- The dominant learner
- The arrogant learner – the know it all
- The learner who wants to be the centre of attention all the time
- The aggressive or argumentative learner
- The offensive and rude learner
- The politically incorrect learner
- The flirtatious learner
- The joke-a-minute learner
- The garrulous learner
- The disengaged learner
- The bored learner
- The learner who relies on everyone else to do the work
- The lazy learner
- The shy learner
- The delicate, tearful learner
- The over-dependent learner
- The constantly late learner
- The frequently ill learner
- The mentally disturbed learner

to step in. Sometimes issues have to be addressed in the presence of the group; at other times the leader needs to address the issue outside the group – for example, in the case of a learner who is clearly upset, or one who has failed to respond to everything the tutor has tried in the session. Failure to address group dynamics by one means or another can be very harmful, not just for that particular group, but for future groups. The issue will rarely go away of its own accord and often gets worse and worse if nothing is done about it. No matter how difficult or painful it is, the tutor has a responsibility to sort matters out.

Here are some ideas.

The dominant group member

People can dominate discussions for a number of reasons:
- they simply know a lot
- they think they know a lot – but are frequently wrong
- they like to be the centre of attention and are showing off
- they want to impress the tutor, or their girlfriend/boyfriend
- they enjoy teaching others and are keen to share their knowledge
- they feel that someone has to start the ball rolling, as no one else seems to want to.

If dominating group members are allowed to continue, the group will get really angry, the shy group members will disappear into their shells, and people will either switch off or drop out. Often the dominant member can contribute successfully to a group and does actually have some really

useful information to bring. The secret is to reduce their input, while not causing offence.

Sometimes group members realise that they have a tendency to dominate and readily accept being told to keep quiet. Not many have such insight, though, and one suggestion for dealing with those who do not is to give them a specific task to do, for example, acting as scribe for the rest of the group. Make sure, however, that they do put up the group's ideas on the whiteboard, and not just their own interpretation. Another technique is to ask them to discuss a particular point and let them have their say, but next time invite someone else to start the ball rolling. Seating can also play a key role. If the tutor sits opposite the dominant student, then that student has the eye of the tutor for the whole session. On the other hand, if the dominant student sits *beside* the tutor, interaction is significantly reduced and the tutor's eye catches other students much more readily. The use of the sweeping hand gesture directed at the dominant student can sometimes be effective – the held-up hand is saying, 'Hang on a minute. I want to hear contributions from other students.' Indeed, sometimes the tutor has to speak these very words aloud. If none of this works, then a word outside the session is necessary, explaining how valuable the individual's contribution is, but how it is important to give *everyone* a chance to be heard.

The reticent group member

The converse of the above is reticent group members. Again there are many reasons for this, including the following:
- they *are* innately shy
- they are upset or worried about something going on in their lives
- they are in a bad mood
- they are upset with someone in the group
- they have not done any work for the session
- they do not know anything about the topic
- they are completely out of their depth
- they are very tired
- they are very bored
- they have lost their motivation to be a doctor
- they are ill or depressed.

Some of these issues are most definitely not in the group tutor's remit to deal with, particularly the last one. Ill or depressed group members need to be seen by qualified practitioners – GPs, occupational health physicians or student counsellors. Under no circumstances should the small group learning tutor attempt to address such issues. Other issues may need to be taken up with the learner's personal tutor, trainer or educational supervisor. The group leader's role is to encourage the individual concerned to seek help from the appropriate person, and to help identify who that person might be.

However, dealing with a genuinely shy, or work-shy, learner is down to the tutor of the small group session. The former needs to be subtly encouraged to join in. Snowballing and buzz groups work quite well, since the learner does not have to speak in front of the whole group. Like the dominant group member, giving the shy individual a task to do, such as being scribe, works well. They are responding to the rest of the group's ideas, a role they are comfortable with. Pointing a finger at them and asking them a direct question is likely to send them deeper into their shell. Humiliating them in any way, for instance by laughing at their answers, is hugely counterproductive. Getting them to comment on something that they are almost certain to know might work, but sometimes the shy person simply needs to be left alone for a while, particularly if the reason for their non-involvement is transitory.

As to the work-shy, usually peer pressure takes care of this, but if not, then a quiet word outside the group is the solution. If a student is really out of his or her depth, this is a more serious situation and needs reporting to the appropriate member of staff responsible for academic progress, so that they can consider whether some form of remediation would help.

The flirtatious, 'jokey' or offensive group member

These are definitely examples of situations when the tutor should get the *group* to deal with the issue. One way is to get the group to take time out from the session and ask them if everyone is comfortable with the atmosphere in the group, or with the behaviour of everyone in the group. Usually someone is heartily sick of it and says so. If this does not do the trick, the tutor should speak to the student out of hearing of the group. The tutor should be very firm with them.

The late or absent group member

Groups can get really angry with perpetually late or absent group members and usually make their feelings on the matter quite clear. Starting the group later to accommodate the perpetually late learner is not an option. The only possible exception to this is the person who has *genuine* problems getting in for, say, a 9 a.m. start – perhaps for child care reasons or finishing off a ward round. If they really are unable to change their arrangements, then the issue should be taken up with the group right at the beginning, when forming the ground rules.

Persistent absence is a course or programme attendance issue, even if this is due to illness. The learner may, as a result, be held back, and the school or postgraduate dean may refuse to sign them off or award credits. These are issues of professionalism, and unprofessional behaviour must be addressed when it first appears, not left to smoulder until it is too late to help learners amend their behaviour.

And there is one other essential ground rule, particularly at the undergraduate level: if a person is unable to attend a session for whatever reason – planned or last-minute – they must inform the tutor prior to their absence, or as soon after as is possible. If the tutor is unavailable, then they must inform someone in the group. In the era of mobile phones, there really is no excuse for not adhering to this policy.

The over-dependent group member

Here, the tutor has to learn to keep a distance from that individual and must take great care not to overindulge him or her. Some people are good at manipulating vulnerable

members of staff for their own ends – another instance when the person concerned should be seated out of the sightline of the tutor.

Exploring boundaries

Before taking charge of a small group, it is essential to be trained in the art of facilitation. Usually such training will itself take the form of a workshop in which an experienced facilitator demonstrates how to facilitate a small group by example. The facilitator is likely to cover the issues described in this chapter. The training session is likely to include some consideration about handling difficult group members and may also include some consideration about interpersonal boundaries – boundaries for the students, and boundaries for the staff. Boxes 9.5–9.8 depict four scenarios that illustrate some situations that may arise for group leaders. There are no comments on these scenarios. They are presented for the reader to think about whether the tutor's response was appropriate.

BOX 9.5 Case A

Stephen is tutor to a group in which Tom and Sarah are students. Tom is a likeable but dominant member of the group, who has strong knowledge that he likes to demonstrate to the group. Sarah is a student who comes from an arts background and is not confident about her ability. During a session, Tom begins (as always) to tell the group about his understanding of the learning issues. Stephen stops Tom briefly, and asks everyone if they understand what Tom is describing. The group nods, apart from Sarah, who replies, 'This is all over my head, but don't worry about me. I just don't have the basic knowledge to join in this conversation. I'll catch up one day I'm sure.' Tom continues his feedback, and Sarah immerses herself in a textbook. Stephen is sympathetic to Sarah but does not want the group to get behind. He believes that it is important that the group finishes its work in the time allocated and never allows the session to run over. Anyway, he has a lecture to give immediately after the session.

BOX 9.6 Case B

Hannah is a student in Rebecca's group. Hannah is a lively and strong character, who has said quite openly that she 'wears her heart on her sleeve'. During a tutorial that focuses on lung cancer, Hannah spends a lot of time describing very emotionally how her grandmother died from lung cancer last year. As learning issues are written up on the board, Hannah says that she does not think she will 'be able to do many of these as it's all too close to home for me'. Later in the tutorial, Hannah suddenly begins to cry and says, 'It,s all too much for me', and runs out of the tutorial in tears. Rebecca follows her and is out of the room for about 20 minutes.

BOX 9.7 Case C

Claire has been a student in Maria's group for several weeks. She is known to be struggling with the course and is open about a number of personal problems that she says are 'affecting her work'. Maria is concerned about Claire and has become something of a confidante to her. At various points in tutorials, Maria has mouthed the words, 'Are you okay?' to Claire. Maria has offered to talk to Claire 'any time' about her difficulties, and Claire has taken to staying behind after teaching sessions to chat to Maria.

BOX 9.8 Case D

Mike is a student in Hardeep's group. Mike is an extremely confident and able student, who is a lively and enthusiastic contributor to the group. At the start of the tutorial Hardeep asks the group how their week has been. Most members of the group make comments about how useful they have found the lectures so far and how they have enjoyed their GP visits. Mike adds, looking at Hardeep, 'The content of that Asian guy's session was crap. I could hardly make out one word he said'. Later, when the students are presented with the first page of a new problem, Hardeep asks them to identify its key features. The front cover to the week's problem shows a picture of a young woman in some distress. Mike says, 'Well, she's blonde, about 20 and far too skinny. Not my type at all. She's probably gay, anyway!' The group dissolve into laughter. Hardeep joins in.

Frequently asked questions

How long should a small group teaching session last?

There is no simple answer to this. Everyone's attention span is limited. The key is to vary the activities on a regular basis. This is easy in a workshop format, but in, for instance, a PBL session, students may be incarcerated in a windowless room, engaged in more or less the same activity for up to three hours. In any lengthy session, it is essential to build in a reasonable break for rest and refreshment. In summary, a session should last between 45 minutes and 3 hours, depending on the activity. The less the students are engaged in active learning, the shorter the session has to be.

Many postgraduate workshops last all day, sometimes they are spread over two or three days, or even a week – for example, for residential training courses. All-day workshops must be split into manageable chunks, separated by frequent refreshment breaks. Week-long courses should include at least a half day of relaxation.

How often should group membership be changed?

In undergraduate education, a group should generally remain together for something between a term and a year.

It is important for students to learn to mix and establish new teams. Groups that function well never want to change; groups that function poorly cannot wait to change. A term is probably a good compromise.

In postgraduate education, for example, day-release courses in vocational GP training schemes or Balint groups, it is important to maintain as much continuity as possible, and groups should stay together for their natural lifetime (welcoming newcomers as appropriate).

Should learners who do not get on be swapped into other groups?

As far as medical students are concerned, absolutely not – under any circumstances! Doctors have to work in teams for the rest of their lives. These teams may not always function ideally. There may be personality clashes, jealousy, rivalry – but they still have to work as a team. The sooner they learn to find a way to get on with people they do not like, the better they will function when it really matters.

In postgraduate education, doctors know their own needs (unfortunately, not always) and are free to attend whatever courses they feel they will gain the most from. Continuing professional development is a requirement for all health care professionals, but apart from essential updating of skills (for example, resuscitation and life-support courses), few courses are compulsory and most are one-offs. Apart from GPs and psychiatrists, doctors therefore do not tend to attend regular workshops with the same people, although they do meet together as teams all the time. Instead, doctors tend to create their own 'clubs' and meet up frequently at conferences. Rarely, these national or international meetings involve small group work, consisting mainly of hundreds of usually fairly dire presentations.

Do I need to be a subject expert to run a small group?

It depends. For PBL, there is some evidence that the best tutors are those who are expert facilitators, but that it helps to have knowledge expertise as well.(35,36) Knowledge experts who have no skills of facilitation and who turn each PBL session into a question-and-answer session, or worse still, a mini-lecture, make poor tutors, as do those who do not even have the excuse of being knowledge experts and who are unable to grasp the principles of PBL (and indeed scorn the whole approach to learning). But for other small group activities, such as a seminar or workshop, and for most postgraduate teaching, where the tutor has more input, knowledge expertise is indeed necessary, again alongside the skills of small group facilitation.

Can a group survive with a series of different facilitators?

Generally, continuity of group leader is important, although rarely is an undergraduate tutor available to take every session in a term because of other commitments. One solution to this is to have paired tutors, so that when one is absent, the other can take over.

In the case of, say, a series of small group sessions covering a range of specialist topics, such as in day-release workshops for junior doctors, it is actually desirable to have different tutors because specialist medical expertise is required. The problem then is that the group never really has the time to develop a meaningful relationship with each tutor, because they are with them for such a short time. The group may get beyond the forming stage, but the tutor rarely does. There are two solutions to this: reduce the number of guest tutors, or maintain continuity through the use of a regular co-facilitator.

Is there such a thing as a floating facilitator?

In fact, that is exactly what a workshop facilitator does. But the question is more to do with a single facilitator looking after more than one group simultaneously, where the groups are not located in the same space but, for example, in nearby rooms. This is rather like the consultant surgeon keeping an eye on his trainees in adjacent operating theatres – common enough practice, but is it *good* practice? Usually this kind of multi-group facilitation only happens because of tutor shortages, and is aimed at making economies. The economies are really perceived economies rather than actual economies, because they only take into account savings in staff time and not quality of student learning. The learning experience is unlikely to be beneficial to the student (although sharing one good tutor is undoubtedly better than being tutored by two separate bad tutors). For multi-group facilitation to work, the activities being undertaken by each group must be task-based, with the tutor popping in now and again to check on group progress. Again, in the postgraduate arena, where the learners are often more committed and motivated, groups can be left to get on with the task by themselves for a while, which leads in nicely to the next frequently asked question.

Do groups need a facilitator at all?

Again, the answer is that it depends. Students in the early stages of their course undoubtedly need a facilitator around. Partly, this is simply because they do not know what to do, and partly, for reassurance that they are learning what they are supposed to be learning. 'Will it come up in the exam?' is a question frequently asked of tutors. As students develop and become more mature, the need for a tutor is reduced. Such students can facilitate their own groups. Once they are let loose on the wards, students revert to Stage One again and need a bit of mollycoddling and guidance.

Postgraduate groups can survive without a tutor if the purpose of the small group session is clear. They may then appoint a chair from within the group and get on with the task in hand.

Summary

Learning in small groups can be very productive, if at times challenging. Not everyone enjoys the process, particularly if the group is dysfunctional. Here, the skills of the facilitator are put to the greatest test, although there are guidelines for handling difficult group members, which are touched on here and elsewhere. A poor facilitator can jeopardise the success of even the best of groups, however – through bul-

lying, humiliating, patronising, prejudicial or over-didactic behaviour. A good facilitator can help the group to achieve a high standard of learning, by encouraging active learning and reflective thinking, by questioning and challenging, and by setting a good example. The most successful groups are tutored by people who are good at facilitation, and not necessarily those who have subject expertise.

Small group learning is particularly successful if the facilitator adopts a variety of techniques during sessions. Workshops, which often last a morning or afternoon, must be split up into a range of activities – discussion, role play, debate, exercises using triggers, watching videos, practising skills, observing demonstrations, problem solving, question-and-answer sessions, presentations – the list is endless.

Facilitation expertise does not grow on trees. People who are brilliant teachers do not necessarily make good facilitators, because they may find it hard to get out of the information-giving mode in which they excel. Group facilitation should never be forced on such people. It is more sensible to recognise their skills and make use of them in the more didactic elements of a course, leaving facilitation to those who are good at it. Would that life were that simple . . .

References

1 Bulstrode CJK and Hunt VL (1997) *Educating Consultants*. SUMIT, Oxford.

2 Jolly BC (1994) *Bedside Manners: teaching in the hospital setting*. Universitaire Pers Maastricht, Maastricht.

3 De Villiers M, Bresick G and Mash B (2003) The value of small group learning: an evaluation of an innovative CPD programme for primary care medical practitioners. *Medical Education*. 37: 815–21.

4 Steinert Y (2004) Student perceptions of effective small group teaching. *Medical Education*. 38: 286–93.

5 Tiwari A, Lai P, So M and Yuen K (2006) A comparison of the effects of problem-based learning and lecturing on the development of students' critical thinking. *Medical Education*. 40: 547–54.

6 Facione NC, Facione PA and Sanchez CA (1994) Critical thinking disposition as a measure of competent clinical judgement: the development of the Californian Critical Thinking Disposition Inventory. *Journal of Nursing Education*. 33: 345–50.

7 Barrows HS (1986) A taxonomy of problem-based learning methods. *Medical Education*. 20: 481–6.

8 Engel CE (1997) Not just a method but a way of learning. In: Boud D and Feletti G (eds) *The Challenge of Problem-Based Learning* (2e), pp. 17–27. Kogan Page, London.

9 Kamin CS, O'Sullivan PS, Younger M and Deterding R (2001) Measuring critical thinking in problem-based learning discourse. *Teaching and Learning in Medicine*. 13: 27–35.

10 Norman GR (2006) Personal communication.

11 Peters T (1995) *In Search of Excellence: Lessons from America's Best-Run Companies*. Harper Collins Business, London.

12 Rudduck J (1979) Learning to teach through discussion. Centre for Applied Research in Education occasional publications no. 8. University of East Anglia, Norwich.

13 Richmond DE (1984) Improving the effectiveness of small-group learning with strategic intervention. *Medical Teacher*. 6: 138–45.

14 Brown G (1982) How to improve small group teaching in medicine. In: Cox KR and Ewan CE (eds) *The Medical Teacher*, pp. 70–8. Churchill Livingstone, Edinburgh.

15 Peyton JWR (1998) *Teaching and Learning in Medical Practice*. Manticore Europe, Rickmansworth.

16 Balint M (1957) *The Doctor, His Patient and the Illness*. Churchill Livingstone, Edinburgh. [1964, reprinted 1986].

17 Balint E and Norell J (eds) (1983) *Six Minutes for the Patient: Interaction in General Practice Consultations*. Tavistock Publications, London.

18 Kolb DA (1984) *Experiential Learning: Experience as the Source of Learning and Development*. Prentice Hall, Englewood Cliffs, NJ.

19 Revans R (1982) *The Origins and Growth of Action Learning*. Chartwell Bratt, Bromley.

20 Tuckman BW (1965) Development sequence in small groups. *Psychological Bulletin*. **63**: 384–99.

21 Walton HJ (1997) *Small Group Methods in Medical Teaching*. ASME medical education booklet no. 1. Association for the Study of Medical Education, Edinburgh.

22 Mulholland H (1994) Teaching small groups: facilitating learning. *Hospital Update*. **20**: 382–4.

23 Visschers-Pleijers AJSF, Dolmans DHJ, de Lang BA *et al.* (2006) Analysis of verbal interactions in tutorial groups: a process study. *Medical Education*. **40**: 129–37.

24 De Grave WS, Boshuizen HPA and Schmidt HG (1996) Problem-based learning: cognitive and metacognitive processes during problem analysis. *Instructional Science*. **24**: 321–41.

25 Molyneaux J (2001) Interprofessional teamworking: what makes teams work well? *Journal of Interprofessional Care*. **15**: 29–35.

26 Mitchell BS, McCrorie P and Sedgwick P (2004) Student attitudes towards anatomy teaching and learning in a multiprofessional context. *Medical Education*. **38**: 737–48.

27 Freeth D and Nicol M (1998) Learning clinical skills: an interprofessional approach. *Nurse Education Today*. **18**: 455–61.

28 Tucker K, Wakefield A, Boggis C *et al.* (2003) Learning together: clinical skills teaching for medical and nursing students. *Medical Education*. **37**: 630–7.

29 Ker J, Mole L and Bradley P (2003) Early introduction to interprofessional learning: a simulated ward environment. *Medical Education*. **37**: 248–55.

30 Areskog N (1994) Multiprofessional education at the undergraduate level – the Linköping model. *Journal of Interprofessional Care*. **8**: 279–82.

31 Reeves S, Freeth D, McCrorie P and Perry D (2002) 'It teaches you what to expect in future . . .': interprofessional learning on a training ward for medical, nursing, occupational therapy and physiotherapy students. *Medical Education*. **36**: 337–44.

32 Kirk A, Parish K and Buckingham I (2006) Interprofessional education – the benefits and drawbacks of an interprofessional training ward. Paper presented at the 12th International Ottawa Conference on Clinical Competence, New York, 20–24 May.

33 O'Halloran C, Hean S, Humphris D and Macleod-Clark J (2006) Developing common learning: the New Generation Project under-graduate curriculum model. *Journal of Interprofessional Care*. **20**: 12–28.

34 Tiberius RG (1990) *Small Group Teaching: A Trouble-Shooting Guide*. Ontario Institute for Studies in Education Press, Toronto.

35 Barrows HS (1988) *The Tutorial Process* (2e). Southern Illinois University School of Medicine, Springfield, IL.

36 Schmidt HG, van der Arend A, Moust JHC *et al.* (1993) Influence of tutors' subject-matter expertise on student effort and achievement in problem based learning. *Academic Medicine*. **68**: 784–91.

Further reading

Bion WR (1952) Group dynamics: a review. *The International Journal of Psycho-Analysis*. **33**: 235–47. [Reprinted in: Klein M, Heimann P and Money-Kyrle R (eds) (1955) *New Directions in Psychoanalysis*, pp. 440–77. Tavistock Publications, London; Bion (1961), pp. 141–91].

Bion WR (1961) *Experiences in Groups*. Tavistock Publications, London.

Campkin M (1986) Is there a place for Balint in vocational training? *Journal of the Association of Course Organizers*. **1**: 100–4.

Dennick R and Exley K (2004) *Small Group Teaching: Tutorials, Seminars and Beyond*. Routledge, Abingdon.

Edmunds S and Brown G (2010) Effective small group learning: AMEE Guide No. 48. *Medical Teacher*. **32**(9): 715–26.

Habeshaw S, Habeshaw T and Gibbs G (1988) *53 Interesting Things to Do in Your Seminars and Tutorials*. Technical & Educational Services, Bristol.

Jacques D (2000) *Learning in Groups: A Handbook for Improving Group Work* (3e). Kogan Page, London.

Jacques D (2003) Teaching small groups. *British Medical Journal*. **326**: 492–4.

Lee A and Higgs J (1988) How to help students learn in small groups. In: Cox KR and Ewan CE (eds) *The Medical Teacher* (2e), pp. 37–47. Churchill Livingstone, Edinburgh.

McGill I and Beaty L (1995) *Action Learning, a Guide for Professional, Management & Educational Development* (2e). Kogan Page, London.

Newble D and Cannon R (2001) Chapter 3: teaching in small groups. In: *A Handbook for Medical Teachers* (4e), pp. 39–54. Kluwer Academic Publishers, Dordrecht.

Norman GR and Schmidt HG (2000) Effectiveness of problem-based learning curricula: theory, practice and paper darts. *Medical Education*. **34**: 721–8.

Weinstein K (1995) *Action Learning: A Journey in Discovery and Development*. Harper Collins, London.

Westberg J and Jason H (1996) *Fostering Learning in Small Groups*. Springer Publishing Company, New York.

10 Lectures and large groups

Andrew Long[1] and Bridget Lock[2]
[1]Royal College of Paediatrics and Child Health, UK; University College London, UK; Great Ormond Street Hospital, UK
[2]South London Healthcare NHS Trust, UK

 KEY MESSAGES

- Lectures continue to be one of the main methods of knowledge transmission in both undergraduate and postgraduate education, despite evidence to suggest that they have little impact on 'deep' learning.

- A better understanding by lecturers of the limitations of the human memory, and the ability of the learner to be able to concentrate over an extended period of time, could lead to lectures becoming more effective learning opportunities.

- A well-structured lecture with explicit learning objectives, defined contextual relationships and linkage of theory to experience is more likely to maximise the learning opportunity for those attending the lecture.

- Preparation by those attending the lecture as well as those organising and speaking will enhance the educational experience.

- Lectures provide a focus for the 'community of learners', offering opportunities for extended learning and professional conversations that can serve to widen debate and offer knowledge-sharing opportunities for all participants.

- Interactivity during lectures is an important adjunct to allow questioning and engagement of the learners, which is likely to improve the learning experience.

- A range of different techniques may be employed to engage larger groups in constructive learning processes that lead to better concentration and sustained enjoyment for all participants.

- Visual aids, used wisely, enhance the quality of the spoken word and improve the experience for most learners.

Some people talk in their sleep. Lecturers talk while other people sleep.

Albert Camus

Introduction

Traditional lectures, during which information is imparted to a passively receptive audience, have been the mainstay of undergraduate and postgraduate education for centuries, but there is an increasing body of evidence questioning the place of this style of learning in medical education. Only a small percentage of the information delivered during a lecture is retained, and often what is told does not equate to what is learnt.(1) Despite this widely recognised fact, most undergraduate courses continue to have a significant lecture component within their curricula and practising clinicians continue to choose to attend lecture-based meetings at the local, national and international level as part of their professional development. This suggests that even in the information-rich 21st century lectures still have a place.(2) The challenge is to reconcile the inherent educational problems of the lecture format with the expressed need of the professional community for this activity and to use valuable professional time productively.

This chapter explores the difficulties of the lecture format from both theoretical and educational perspectives and aims to offer practical solutions on how the organisation and delivery of lectures can be adapted to effectively meet the educational needs of clinicians of both current and future generations. As with much of this volume, although the focus for this chapter is on medical education, the messages within it apply equally well across the health care professions.

Clinical knowledge

Clinicians require what has been termed *propositional* knowledge to inform their practice.(3) Such knowledge is available in the public domain and provides a shared theoretical and practical base for the profession's activities. Propositional knowledge is available from published sources – journals, textbooks, the Internet – or educational programmes, examinations and courses, and an experienced doctor can easily find and acquire the necessary facts. But the complex professional activity of clinical practice cannot be described by a simple algorithmic processing of data alone, as it requires an amalgam of propositional, practical, situational, technical and *personal* experiential

---

knowledge applied to each new situation to make a justifiable, informed clinical judgement.(4) Each new piece of knowledge that comes the clinician's way is judged in relation to its applicability to the context of everyday practice.(5)

Professional frameworks such as the UK General Medical Council's *Good Medical Practice*(6) emphasise that developing knowledge that is useful to practice is a professional duty. Knowledge to inform clinical decision making is derived from a number of sources, including reflection on the variance of actual to expected outcome.(7) But it is the unexpected that can yield the most benefit to an individual's fund of experiential knowledge, and the capacity to manage uncertainty and the unexpected is a hallmark of a professional.(8) Solitary reflection is important in developing practice but in itself is not sufficient.

Like medicine itself, professional learning is a social activity. If lectures, for instance, are to be of any worth, they need to be valued by the community of learners, and they also need to offer an insight into the context in which the knowledge was generated,(9) its place within accepted wisdom and how it fits into or serves to modify current practice. The presentation must be delivered in a manner that can be readily assimilated by clinicians and drawn on when required for clinical practice.(10)

Communities of practice

Deeply embedded in the medical profession is the concept of specialisation and the development of expertise for both a broad aspect of practice and the opportunity to sub-specialise into smaller divisions. Each of the subspecialties may be viewed as communities of practice, united by a professional activity, focusing on a particular area of expertise.(11) Each member of the community holds a professional duty to engage in continuing professional development. This includes both learning and teaching of specialist professional knowledge in its widest sense, and assessment of the value of new information for patients through questioning of, and deliberation on, emerging research knowledge within a 'safe' professional grouping. By engaging in debate about practice, the scale of importance of new and current research can be determined.

New entrants to the community have to learn the tradition and knowledge of the profession for its continuity. Working within the professional community and engaging in conversation about the work of the community enables situated learning and allows limited participation of newcomers.(12) A professional works in dialogue with a patient but develops the expertise that professionals need to draw on for practice within their professional community, with all the multiple interrelationships and opportunities for learning that membership implies. Through these 'professional' conversations, the professional then learns to 'walk-the-walk' and 'talk-the-talk' of professional practice.(13)

Communities of practice have cognitive benefits too. By researching a case alone, a doctor can only have a unique view of a piece of information attained in whatever form. However, this may not be a sufficient depth of knowledge to practise safely. It is too limited in its range of viewpoints to gauge its value when the doctor is required to make a clinical judgement. A critical collaborative review of research knowledge or an overview of a subject will reveal the flaws in an argument and allow the identification of strengths or weaknesses of new research and due interpretation in the context of accepted practice. In-depth enquiry and group discussion through questioning can bring fallacies to light. The larger the number and variety of experiences among discussants, the better the insight into the value of a piece of information.

In order to deliberate, communities have to meet, and although teleconferencing and web-based discussion forums are now readily available, the interaction and opportunities for learning can be rather one-dimensional. However, if the community is to assemble, then learning needs to be facilitated, and this requires some structure and planning. A lecture or large group can provide this opportunity.

Lectures and learning

Within a community of practice a range of educational activity can occur, with the method of learning varying according to the nature of the subject matter. A balance of all types of educational activity is needed as one style of learning does not suit all.(14) Bligh has usefully summarised the evidence that provides the basis for the continuance of lectures as a useful instructional method.(15) It is suggested that lectures are at least as effective as any other method for transmitting information. However, while lectures can provide a new insight into a difficult subject matter, and provoke thought and debate, there is little evidence to suggest that they have any role in modifying behaviour or values, or in inspiring interest. On the contrary, lectures have the potential to induce a sense of complacency in the recipient – even if they take notes in the ill-founded belief that this information can be recalled from memory when needed. Alternatively, and perhaps even more dangerously, lectures may engender a sense of inadequacy and impotence as listeners are overwhelmed by the volume of information for which they have no context and can develop no new understanding. In this instance, they will have no opportunity to situate the initial information with present knowledge before more complex ideas are delivered, and may be left disheartened and disengaged.

If the purpose of a given learning event is the presentation of new information, a review of new developments in an area of study, or merely to highlight some key issues, then a lecture format may be appropriate. If this is the case then the manner of presentation should aid learning, and how this task is approached depends on an understanding of how learning occurs from a psychological and physiological perspective.

Memory, learning and performance

Theories of how memory is laid down and knowledge retrieved for later use offer some insight into how a presenter might support his or her audience in their learning.

**BOX 10.1 WHERE'S THE EVIDENCE:
Attention and recall**

During the course of an hour-long lecture:

- attention is at its height during the first 10–20 minutes and the final five minutes(18)
- the most note-taking occurs during the first 10 minutes(19)
- only 42 per cent of the key points of a lecture can be recalled immediately afterwards
- this drops to 20 per cent within one week

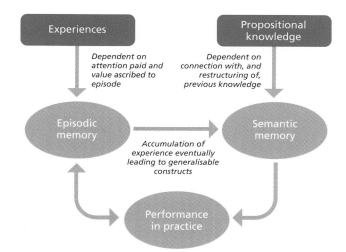

Figure 10.1 Memory, learning and performance.
Source: Eraut.(21)

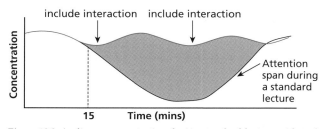

Figure 10.2 Audience concentration during standard lecture with and without interaction.
Source: Higher Education Academy Engineering Subject Centre.(24)

As words are heard and understood they are assimilated into working or short-term memory through the recognition of patterns and context. Without context, the information is forgotten if not learnt through immediate repetition. To secure the information into long-term memory, coding must occur.(16) Two forms of long-term memory have been identified; procedural or non-declarative (implicit) memory is related to learning 'unconscious' skills (e.g. riding a bicycle), whereas declarative (or explicit) memory refers to memories which can be consciously recalled (e.g. facts or knowledge). Declarative memory is thought to have two inter-dependent components; an *episodic* memory, which stores personal experiences and events and a *semantic* memory, which stores factual knowledge that does not rely on personal experience.(17) Episodic memory makes multiple associations or links with events, sequences, sounds, smells or sights over time. Recall is dependent on the importance of the event and on developed connections to other pieces of retained knowledge in its many forms (*see* Box 10.1). Something heard or seen may 'strike a chord' in relation to a patient seen previously or an event experienced. Filing, or coding, episodes into long-term memory is personal, dependent on the attention paid and the value ascribed to the episode by the individual, as well as how it connects with other previously retained knowledge.(20) Semantic memory refers to the development of concept-based knowledge built from individual components of factual information which give meaning in the context of previous experience. This interpretation takes time, and without adequate time to construct links and formulate code, information will not be assimilated into long-term memory and is subsequently discarded from short-term memory. The relationship between learning memory and professional performance is summarised in Figure 10.1.

Limits to learning

Key to understanding the importance of this is the recognition that there is both a physiological *rate limit* to the system (too fast a delivery and the mechanism of retention is overwhelmed) and a physiological *capacity* to the system (overload of information will lead to a lack of capacity for retention). The capacity of the system relies on a full engagement of concentration generated by motivation for the learning task in hand.

The presenter should heed these physical limitations and take care not to swamp the memory with too much information delivered too fast or exceed reasonable concentration limits. Some tactics can be adopted to enhance memory retention – for example, providing the description of an event, setting memorable context or assisting in the development of relevant connections or anchors.(22) Lecturers must offer an opportunity for questioning at reasonable time intervals, enabling listeners to check their construction of knowledge and reveal and correct misunderstandings. As little is recalled after 20 minutes of uninterrupted concentration,(23) introducing variety in presentation every 15–20 minutes will aid learning (Figure 10.2). A listener needs an opportunity to participate or question to avoid misinterpretation and thus incorrect integration into existing knowledge. The marked decline in attention after 15 minutes might offer the opportunity for a brief anecdote illustrating the principles described by the lecture. This will act to embed the delivered ideas in the narrative component of the listener's long-term memory, complementing information previously stored in conceptual or semantic memory.(25)

Of even greater concern, Bligh describes processes that may result in memory *loss*: those of *retroactive* and *proactive* interference.(15) The former relates to when there is a requirement to learn a new series of facts shortly after committing the first set to short-term memory, such as in successive lectures. The latter occurs where memorising the first set of facts interferes with remembering the second set. Presenters therefore need to take account of both the volume and the concordance of the subject matter presented. It is also relevant to note that there is a beneficial effect in repetition, which has the opposite effect of interference and tends to consolidate learning, although if learning has not taken place the first time (i.e. the listener did not understand), then repetition has no additional benefit.

This has necessarily been a simplified description of a dynamic and complex process, but viewing a presentation from the perspective of the learner's capability to assimilate new information may assist lecturers in structuring their presentation to facilitate, rather than inhibit, learning. Useful learning occurs when the learner makes connections with pre-existing knowledge and can anchor new knowledge to previous concepts.(22) A context for information is also needed both for understanding and for recall. The level of understanding will depend on the listener's level of expertise; those that already have core knowledge will find their knowledge base enhanced in a different way to a naive listener. Similarly, a generalist in a field may enlarge his or her range of knowledge and understanding of *specialist* expertise. Each listener will have personal levels of depth and breadth of understanding related to past experience and motivation for learning. What is learnt depends on knowledge of the range of the subject; old information may become obsolete or be viewed with different importance, and new information develops and finds a place. But this will only be of use in patient care, if the learner has the internal connections to draw out the information when needed and put it into practice (Box 10.1).

Lecturing and listening

Lecturing, then, offers an opportunity for a student or a practitioner to establish where the new information sits in relation to his or her present knowledge. The resultant new knowledge will be unique to the learner as it is the result of selective attention and engaged interest, and the product of the learner's active efforts to relate new knowledge to pre-existing concepts.

The listener has social responsibilities as a participant and needs to be more than a passive recipient of information. The lecturer has offered his or her view, but the use remains the prerogative and responsibility of the recipients as they integrate what they hear into their established knowledge and in doing so have the opportunity to reshape it.(26) Before a lecture is delivered, the listeners should take a little time to prepare, even if it is only to ask himself or herself, 'What do I know of this subject?' and call to the front of his or her consciousness their present knowledge and understanding. It is not unreasonable for the listeners to challenge themselves, or the arguments of the lecturer, as this level of mental engagement facilitates the active process of learning, develops additional connections and aids coding into long-term memory. The role of active listening also involves noting problems of understanding for questioning at an appropriate opportunity.

Until this point, it has been implied that the deliverer is always 'the expert' and that the recipient is generally a relative novice to the subject. This is not necessarily the case. In most national and international settings, clinicians and research workers with expertise in a localised area of knowledge will present their ideas to an audience with profound experience in their field for adjudication of its value to present knowledge. In contrast, at the local level, a young doctor may present a difficult case for debate by a group of experienced doctors to advance his own clinical judgement through public deliberation on practice. An experienced teacher may lay out the framework of a topic for first-year undergraduate medical students in the morning and listen to a visiting professor discourse on a specialist subject in the afternoon. These are examples of a community of professional educational practice where the roles taken by participants vary, depending on the educational purpose of the activity. What is learnt by listeners and deliverers will vary with circumstance, but the teachers may learn as much or more than the learners.

In some roles, what is learnt may demonstrate an individual's need for help in developing clinical understanding. This is a different purpose from the transmission of information in a didactic fashion. The organisers of the meeting and the presenters need to take heed of underpinning theory to enable effective learning to occur, especially the time for discussion. And it is to the organisation and delivery of effective lectures that we now turn our attention.

Putting theory into practice

Organisational aspects

Lectures have the advantage of economy of scale, but to be cost-effective they must succeed in their primary purpose. At all levels of education the number of individuals that can be 'taught' by a single lecturer is increased by the use of this format. The more 'students' that can be taught by a single 'teacher', the better the return on investment, and as academic staff are relatively expensive and in short supply, this seems to make good economic sense. It is not often the case that those responsible for managing the budgets within organisations are charged with considering the value of the intervention for the recipient.

Organisers of educational events that include lectures and large groups need to make sure that there is clear guidance for chair, speakers and listeners well in advance of the event. Electronic support for dialogue must be efficient and enabling of debate. A chairman must facilitate intelligently. At large gatherings, participants need time and information about the presentations on offer to enable choice of learning. Résumés of the presentation help memory recall at a later date and enable concentration during a delivery, as listeners are not distracted by the need to take copious notes and can listen for understanding, annotating as they wish.

Since lectures form the backbone of most major conferences at the postgraduate level, often attended by thousands of delegates, many of whom have attained high levels of educational qualifications, it must be perceived by those attending that the lectures are of personal value. It would appear that those who attend voluntarily, as part of an educational plan, expect to be educated and are therefore prepared to engage with the educational process. There are, of course, a multitude of reasons why delegates choose to attend conferences, and there will be differences for each of them.

If we assume that most people who attend lectures are motivated to do so, then it offers an opportunity to enhance learning. The critical need is to ensure that those who attend remain engaged during the lecture, as there is evidence to suggest that not all who attend are equal in terms of their ability to learn in a primarily auditory fashion;(27) their ability to work at the same pace; their high-volume memory capacity; their basic knowledge required for the lecture; and their note-taking ability.(28) At least part of the solution is to ensure that lecture techniques are optimised to accommodate the principles of learning discussed previously.

The public role of each participant should be clear for each educational activity. The lecturer should present and the audience should have the opportunity to inquire for understanding. It is entirely inappropriate for a member of the audience to stand and offer a discourse of their own or interrogate the presenter. In some circumstances, however, the audience may become the teachers as they are invited to give a view of the weighting of the value of information. Explicit guidance must be offered to audience and presenters before the event, and signals for role changes must be made clear by the nominated chair to ensure the rules of the game are understood and observed. Without guidance, the event becomes a meaningless shambles to everybody's dissatisfaction because the activity will not fulfil its purpose.

Building the community

Delivering the content is not the only purpose of a lecture. A secondary function can be viewed as the essential creation of community links and exchange of clinical knowledge. The essential 'informal space' created by refreshment breaks offers the opportunity for attendees to engage in networking and community building. Collaborative learning is at the centre of developing communities of practice and credit needs to be given to the discussion that takes place between engaged learners united by a common goal and establishing virtual relationships where the focus is on the exchange of ideas and information.(11)

Providing adequate time, space and comfortable surroundings aids reflection on what has been heard. This can be offered within an informal setting or as more formal groups. The latter may benefit from a facilitator and a published summary, but the spontaneity of the former may be of considerable benefit to an individual's understanding. The development of extensive memory connections is enhanced by early revisiting of the material covered during dialogue with other participants. The provision of an unthreatening and intellectually stimulating learning environment is key to the success of both the formal and the informal educational event.

Developments in information technology and the ability to engage in a number of different modes of online learning have been challenges to the existing lecture format. A move towards transforming lectures and similar large-group settings to make them more academically and socially interactive is a welcome development. If teachers truly understand the limitations and potential of this teaching methodology, then there is an opportunity to significantly enhance learning.

Preparation

The most important part of any successful lecture is the preparation. The audience to whom the talk is to be given should be taken into account, and the lecturer should ask the course leader or conference organiser about the context and type of talk expected. Poor preparation may compromise whole teaching programmes and has led to many courses being poorly valued by either the recipient or the deliverer. If the assumption is made that each episode offers a unique educational event that will never be repeated and that its value will be enhanced by the contribution of the lecturer and the audience, then it is likely to be successful, enjoyable and well received. It is a fundamental principle of educational and professional practice that all participants should treat one another with respect and courtesy. To do other than prepare for an educational event is discourteous.

Most lecturers who are asked to present on undergraduate courses or at international and national meetings are informed many months in advance, and it is common practice to start preparation of thought processes and development of ideas in debate with others a long time before the presentation. There is often a temptation to 'rehash' a previous lecture that has been well received. However, if the talk is not tailored to the specific context, it will be discordant and uncomfortable for both the recipients and the deliverer. This should be avoided as it does not show due regard for the new audience that will be receiving the talk for the first time, nor for the organisers of the meeting who have invited the lecturer. There are a number of valuable texts on how to present at meetings (*see* 'Further Reading' section), and many offer a wide range of 'hints and tips' for use by anyone, from novice to expert.

Brown and Manogue(29) outline a model that demonstrates the method by which the recipients of a lecture learn from the event. It is based on work from Baddeley,(30) which identified modes of information processing and their effect on human memory, and confirmed much of previous observational work undertaken by previous authors.(31) It suggests that there is a dynamic relationship between the lecturer and his or her audience that has a direct effect on the way the lecture is delivered. Four components seem to contribute to making lectures more effective, as follows:

- *intentions* of the lecturer *and* the recipient
- *transmission*, including both verbal and non-verbal messages
- *receipt* of key messages by the learner
- *output*, in terms of both the immediate response of the recipient and the ability of the learner to store

information in short-term memory, transfer to long-term memory and effect changes in attitudes and behaviour.

The authors suggest that it is this reciprocity that makes it so difficult to convert lectures entirely to an electronic medium. Encouraging interaction is then essential to good learning, but this opportunity may be denied to a 'live' audience when programmers curtail discussion time in order to provide more speakers; or a lecturer, desperate to impart more facts, overruns into question time so denying the audience the opportunity to fully understand the speaker's reasoning through debate.

The principle of 'more is not always better' is useful to consider. As we have established, this simply overloads the long-term memory. Getting value from the activity in terms of its contribution to understanding and learning is more useful than delivering large volumes of talks. Professionals may travel long distances to meet since they perceive the value of debate to professional practice and the ability to understand the information proffered.

There is a strong association between subject knowledge and competence in teaching.(29) But the most effective teaching is also underpinned by an insight into the knowledge and level of understanding of the audience. It is essential to successful lecturing to prepare the talk by taking into account the diversity of the stages of learning of the audience, and to structure the talk accordingly. The enthusiasm of the lecturer for their subject matter is a prime motivator in the interest level generated in the listeners, promoting engagement with the topic and encouraging a positive approach to learning. Therefore an in-depth knowledge and extended level of interest on behalf of the lecturer is much more likely to have a beneficial outcome for the student wrestling with understanding new facts and concepts, because they are much more likely to be explained in relatively simple terms.

One of the cardinal rules of lecturing is the requirement to set objectives. These should be stated early on in the presentation and repeated as often as necessary to optimise learning. It may also be necessary for the lecturer to try to understand what the student is feeling and how this affects their belief in the subject matter that the lecturer inspires. The outcome from the learning event should be the product of the understanding and feeling, which should aid interpretation and the ability to process information and store it in memory. This is helped by visual and auditory imagery, which aids recall from deeply stored memories. Too much detail and content within lectures blunts learning(15) – detail can be learnt from texts. Students most value explanation supported by a structure and framework on which to build concepts of learning.

It is therefore apparent that a lecturer needs to prepare an outline that fits the purpose before adding the content. If the lecturer can identify a clear path through the duration of their talk, it is highly likely they will convey that structure to the listener. A sense of order in the presentation of facts will aid learning as it will prevent the audience from having to make cognitive leaps in order to follow the train of thought – another possible source of interference in learning (*see* Box 10.2).

 BOX 10.2 HOW TO: Structure a lecture

Approximate timing of the performance is important to ensure understanding and maximum recall of the lecture content. Understanding of the human mind and memory offers a rationale for action about which a more detailed discussion is to be found in the text. Here is some guidance (and a rationale) for structuring a traditional hour-long lecture:

- 5 minutes: Introduction and scoping
  sets minds
- 5 minutes: Ascertain knowledge base question
  engages mind and memory
- 15 minutes: Delivery
  just enough new information – at just the right speed
- 10 minutes: Question and discussion
  set connections in long-term memory
- 15 minutes: Delivery
  check volume and speed of delivery
- 5 minutes: Questions
  consolidate connections
- 5 minutes: Summary and close
  pull it together

Content

The main danger for the lecturer is to try to cover too much in a single presentation. Too much information can cause a number of serious problems that may adversely affect learning. First, there is a temptation to increase the pace of delivery in order to include all the subject matter. Audio-visual aids become either too crowded or too numerous, and there is inadequate time for the learner to grasp the essential facts, add some context and transfer to note form. To compensate for the last factor, many lecturers produce printouts of the slides from their talk. This may lead to students attending, collecting the handout and leaving before the talk starts (or even more cynically, getting someone else to collect the paperwork). These actions deny the participants the most useful portion of the lecture: the interaction with the lecturer and the learning community.

It therefore makes sense for the lecturer to identify the key messages they wish to deliver, ensure this material is covered and fits into a logical structure and then enhance it with information that cannot be gleaned from written sources, such as practical examples, personal experience and expert insight. All participants, at any stage of learning, gain added value from examples that demonstrate theory worked out in practice, harnessing episodic memory and encouraging contextual understanding.(32) It is often useful to introduce controversial or challenging components at key points during the presentation to excite (possibly flagging) interest and engage the attention of the participants. Experienced and skilful lecturers might allow (or even plan) some deviation from their 'script', if they feel it is likely to enhance understanding, and it might be worth identifying in advance such detours and possible variance in reaching the desired endpoint.

The content should be put into a structure that allows the learner to follow clearly the thought trains that underpin the delivery. This generally includes the following:

- an *introduction*, which should be designed to capture the interest of even the most disaffected participant and provide some explanation of the context and importance of the subject matter
- the *body* of the presentation, which contains the facts that are to be presented
- the *conclusion*, where the main points should be emphasised and summarised.

Style

The style of lecturing relates in part to the experience, level of confidence and comfort of the lecturer, and in part to the type of presentation, the audience and the subject matter being covered. It also appears that there is considerable variation in lecturing style across cultures and academic disciplines,(33) which may reflect the different volume of material being delivered and affect the speed of delivery. Lecture styles do seem to have generational differences, perhaps reflecting learners' needs, or possibly because lecturers and institutions are becoming more aware of the limitations of their medium and adjusting style to match the evidence relating to effectiveness of lectures in general. Certainly, a move to a more participatory style has introduced a cultural shift – from a lecturer-centred to a learner-centred teaching event.

Dudley-Evans and Johns(34) identified three distinct lecturing styles that seem to be contributory to, or inhibitive of, interactivity during the lecture. The traditional *reading* style, where the lecturer sticks closely to a script, which is often pre-rehearsed, offers the least opportunity for interaction, is least conducive to learning and is probably obsolete in 21st century informed society, as the knowledge conveyed is best read from source. This style is often adopted by lecturers who lack confidence, either in themselves or in their material. It has been observed that this style offers the greatest opportunity of being 'the process whereby a lecturer's notes are transferred to a student notebook without the need for mental effort on anybody's part'.(35) This type of lecture is more likely to be delivered in a monotonous fashion and may be less well understood by those for whom the language in which it is delivered is not their first language. This style also encourages more monologues and less dialogue.

The second style of lecturing described is the *conversational* style, where the lecturer speaks more informally, either without notes or from a notation format rather than a script. It is helpful if the lecturer encourages discussion at regular intervals to check that learning is taking place. This more informal style encourages interaction and offers a more explanatory approach within lectures, and the tonal expression tends to have a more beneficial effect in engaging the learner. The additive effect of engagement facilitates learning by pacing to encourage physiological retention.

The lecturer is generally more relaxed and less rigid in the lecture content. This style seems to be the most predominant in all areas of higher education.

The third lecturing style involves the lecturer taking a role as a performer. The *rhetorical* style is characterised by frequent digressions and asides. It is much more akin to daily conversation and implies a much greater sense of informality between the lecturer and the listener. The style is very interactive; the structure is less rigid and requires a great deal of confidence on the part of the speaker. The tempo of the lecture is much more upbeat, with a wide range of tonal variance, and it is often the style that is entertained when lectures are being video-taped, emphasising the function of the lecturer as a performer. It is, of course, the case that during a single lecture or study course, combinations of styles might be employed and use of audiovisual aids might well predetermine the style and content of the lecture.

Brown and Bakhtar(36) have taken a different approach to describing lecturing styles based on the characteristics of the individual lecturers. They describe that *oral presenters*, who tend to use no visual aids, are less likely to rely on notes and tend not to provide lecture notes. The *visual presenter*, on the other hand, tends to make full use of all media to aid explanation and uses diagrams and structures to help the student to understand. They are likely to use full notes and will offer more time to students during the lecture. The *exemplary performer* uses a wide range of techniques and is generally very confident in their presentation, offering students a highly structured approach and setting clear learning objectives. *Eclectic performers* also use a variety of techniques, including humour, but lack confidence and tend to be more disorganised, often digressing from the main content of the lecture, whereas the *amorphous talker* is very confident but ill-prepared, vague and less likely to consider the structure or objectives of their lecture.

Understanding the strengths and weaknesses of these lecturing styles is essential for the lecturer wishing to complement the learning process for the recipient and develop their own style. Careful thought in planning and preparing each lecture with due regard for the knowledge base of the audience, the agreed learning objectives and the time frame for presentation will avoid the novice lecturer falling into a style that fails to meet the needs of the audience.

Aids to lecturing

Visual aids can significantly enhance lecturing and add an extra dimension when explaining or describing difficult or complex inter-relationships. However, they can also be an unnecessary distraction, illegible and incomprehensible, and serve no purpose in aiding learning.(37) Therefore, if aids are used, they should complement the subject and the context being taught, add rather than subtract from the aural presentation, be instantly understandable and used appropriately.

The chalkboard and chalk as a teaching methodology, although still used in some parts of the world, has now been largely superseded by the whiteboard or flipchart and coloured marker pens. This ancient technology has been updated in recent times by adding functionality, such as the ability to electronically project, record and print written scripts, together with the use of magnetic strips and other highlighting techniques. When used appropriately, it can be an extremely effective teaching aid, although it is generally more appropriate for smaller rather than large groups. However, its use requires careful thought and preparation to maximise its potential, as it is easy to produce a messy and even more confusing display if the contents are produced in an unstructured fashion. Its use is generally more suited to the conversational or rhetorical style of presentation, as there is more informality, and it can be used in a fashion where ideas are built up throughout the duration of the lecture. It requires the lecturer to turn away from their audience, which results in some loss of interaction and the ability to gauge audience response. However, this medium can be used to encourage learner participation and engagement with the subject matter.

Thought should be given to both the colours and nature of the medium being used. The lecturer's handwriting is key to effective delivery, and complex diagrams should be planned well in advance. It is always best to start and finish with a clean board, and care should be taken that the marker pens used on whiteboards are water-soluble.

The overhead projector (OHP) became the medium that initially threatened the chalkboard as the premier teaching medium. The ability for the lecturer to face the audience while writing, the 'build' capacity where layered overheads could be interlaced to provide a structured diagram and the potential to prepare 'acetates' in advance were significant advantages in favour of the OHP. Once again this medium can prove to be as fallible as other media with their reliance on intact power supply, functioning bulbs and transparencies with colours that are visible and text that does not smudge. The OHP also offers the temptation to photocopy small text and complex diagrams onto transparencies in the hope that they will be comprehensible. There is continuing debate about the benefits of displaying each part of the screen sequentially or whether the whole screen should be displayed at the same time so that the observer is not constantly trying to guess what will be revealed next. Like all use of audiovisual media, in the hands of an expert they will enhance a good presentation, and for novice lecturers they provide the opportunity for additional clarity of presentation with relatively few technical demands, provided the medium is used wisely.

The major change in the use of audiovisual aids for lecturing came with the Microsoft dominance of the world of personal computing and the introduction of 'bundled' Office software, which included PowerPoint. Before this, the 35-mm slide dominated significant educational events and was the recommended media for important talks prepared at any level, from local presentations to international meetings. Slides were generally difficult to prepare, expensive to produce and inflexible to change. The advent of widespread use of PowerPoint brought its own challenges, as it became the accepted standard; however, the ability to transport talks easily was limited by disk capacity. Now the increased availability and relative cheapness of USB memory sticks has meant that almost any size of talk can be accommodated, and changes can be made easily at any time before the start of the presentation; however, renewed concerns about computer virus transfer has resulted in increasing dependence on 'encrypted' sticks which do not always translate into easily compatible software transfer.

The full functionality of PowerPoint is rarely utilised. However, it now dominates the audiovisual league table and is largely accepted as the international standard. There are many texts that offer sound advice on the best use of this media (*see* 'Further Reading' section), and it is not intended to replicate the information here. However, it is reasonable to review some of the strengths and weaknesses of this technology. The ability of PowerPoint to produce a full range of slides, outlines, lecture notes and handouts makes producing lecture material relatively easy, and talks can be translated from computer-projected slides to transparencies for projection on an OHP or even into web-based annotated presentations as part of a virtual learning environment. Nearly all lecture theatres, classrooms and auditoriums now have PC projection equipment installed, and the relatively low cost of portable projectors and laptop computers has made this an increasingly affordable and transportable means of providing highly professional presentations in almost any venue.

All types of audiovisual aid have the ability to be abused, and generally the higher the degree of technological dependence, the higher the risk for the presenter. While the 'hardware' technology has become increasingly reliable, although is still subject to power loss and bulb failure, the temptation for the lecturer to extend the limits of safety to achieve dazzling effects has sometimes overshadowed the message that is being promoted. PowerPoint comes with a range of colourful backgrounds, artistic fonts and highly sophisticated 'build' and 'transition' effects, complete with sound. There is the ability to add in video clips to enhance and extend the range of demonstrable material, and sometimes the technology becomes overwhelmed almost as much as the audience. Evidence suggests that increasing volume of images and competing inputs might challenge the ability of the learner to store the information being transmitted in their short-term memory.(38) It has also been clearly demonstrated(39) that students' perception of the images they are shown is highly variable, and it is often necessary for the lecturer to pause a presentation to emphasise a point or check that there is consensus on the material presented at that time.

There is little doubt that emerging technologies will make audiovisual media even more exciting in the future. The ability to provide images of 'virtual reality', the ability to video-conference across large distances and the possibility of widely distributed networks with interactive functionality introduces opportunities that are restricted only by the imagination of the presenter. However, it should always be remembered that the key objective is the imparting of information and any medium that clouds the message being presented is harmful, both for the learner and for the reputation of the speaker (*see* Box 10.3).

Delivery

The final and perhaps the most important aspect of lecturing is the presentation itself. Once the talk has been pre-

BOX 10.3 HOW TO: Design a PowerPoint presentation

- Ensure that PowerPoint is the best format for the type of talk you are giving and the audience you are addressing.
- Use background colours and contrasting text that will be seen well – white or yellow on a blue background project well under most circumstances.
- Try to use the same font throughout and a type size that will be easily visible.
- Using bold type or text 'shadowing' can improve the legibility, and the use of bold, italics or underlining may serve to enhance key points.
- Don't overcrowd the slides – as a general rule there should be no more than seven words per line and seven lines of text per slide.
- Use 'exciting' slide transition and slide 'build' with caution – listeners might become more interested in the action on the slide rather than the message you wish to convey, although a dynamic build sequence can enhance the message.
- Break up blocks of solid text with pictures, cartoons or photographs. Visual images can serve to embed messages into long-term memory.
- Exercise caution with the use of graphics – try to use only simple graphs and tables that do not have too much information or require too much explanation.
- Running video clips from within presentations can produce spectacular results but is fraught with technical risks.
- It is best not to read the text from the slide but allow the audience to read the slide contents and talk around the key points raised.
- As a general rule allow one minute per slide – too many slides might lead to your talk overrunning, which will not be popular with the chairman or audience.
- Use an introduction slide to explain the structure of your talk and a summary slide of your conclusions – 'tell them what you are going to tell them; tell them; tell them what you have told them'.
- Practise your talks with a friendly audience so you can judge timing, content and presentation style.

pared, taking into account aspects of style, content and audiovisual aids, it is the lecturer's responsibility to convey his or her message clearly. This in itself requires some forethought and preparation no matter how experienced or skilled the lecturer. Much depends on the familiarity of the presenter with the group and the venue for the talk, but it is all too easy to become complacent, which in itself may prejudice an excellent presentation.

It is essential that the lecturer arrives at the venue in plenty of time to prepare themselves and (if appropriate) the group to whom they are presenting. Depending on the media being used, it will be necessary to check equip-

ment, both for correct functionality and for ease of use, to gain familiarity with the mode of operation and to enable the presenter to feel comfortable. It may offer an opportunity to start a process of engagement with the learners, to check assumed knowledge levels and to demonstrate appropriate intent to ensure that learning opportunities are maximised.

When the presentation starts, the expert lecturer will take clues from the audience to judge the pace of the talk and the degree of detail required. The importance of maintaining eye contact with the recipients cannot be overemphasised, and interpretation of body language and non-verbal clues about their well-being and receptivity is learned over a period of time. The novice lecturer might wish to gauge audience response by asking questions or inviting responses. Timing is very important, and the risk of preparing and expecting too much has already been emphasised. All the evidence suggests that the more enthusiastic the presenter, the better prepared the presentation and the simpler the message, the more likely it is to be understood and to have a positive impact. The use of handouts as an aid to both clarity and retention is discussed in Box 10.4.

Beyond lecturing

Learning in all environments can be improved if learners are actively involved in the process, are expected to develop knowledge and understanding, receive feedback on their work and feel part of a community of learning. The organisation of a lecture can be adapted to increase its effectiveness in the light of new concepts of effective learning. Provided lecturers understand the context of the lecture and are prepared to try to establish the baseline knowledge of the audience, agree and set objectives from the lecture, and retain the interest of the listener by using interactive elements, they can be very useful educational events. Furthermore, the organisers should ensure that topics presented are current (and perhaps controversial) and that lecturers are selected for their presentation abilities, including their ability to engage with the audience, as well as their knowledge and experience. Structuring the programme to allow frequent breaks at roughly 20-minute intervals and encouraging participants to take notes, ask relevant questions and interact with other learners all helps build the community of practice facilitating the development of collaborative professional working and learning.

A range of other techniques may be used to engage learners and create an environment of 'active learning' during the lecture. The 'Further Reading' section includes a book entitled *53 Interesting Things to Do in Your Lectures*, which presents a wide range of hints and tips designed to stimulate the interest of students and increase the enjoyment and effectiveness of lectures. *Cinemeducation. A comprehensive guide to using film in medical education* also includes a number of ideas on how commercial film clips may be used to liven up an otherwise dull subject and aid learning by providing a contextual basis for the subject of the lecture through the provision of examples. A range of other relatively simple techniques may also be used to break up a lecture and ensure audience participation.

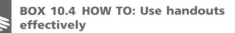

BOX 10.4 HOW TO: Use handouts effectively

- Think clearly about the purpose of the handout – simple regurgitation of the PowerPoint presentation is easy to do but does not necessarily aid learning.

- Handouts may be the most effective way of conveying key, complex information and diagrammatic representations that need detailed explanation.

- Consider the audience to which you are talking and design the handout to suit the learning needs of those attending.

- An 'outline' handout may be just a one-page summary of the contents of the lecture with key references.

- Providing electronic 'hot links' and references within handouts will offer the opportunity for those attending the talk to undertake further reading at a later date.

- 'Skeletal notes', which contain a set of the lecture notes with pieces of information missing, might be valuable in maintaining attention, adding some interaction to the lecture and thereby enhancing learning.

- If you choose to provide printouts of a PowerPoint presentation, remove unnecessary slides and use the format that best conveys the information required with minimum wasted paper (three slides or six slides per sheet).

- Consider whether you wish to provide handouts before the talk so participants can use them for note taking or distribute them after the talk so attention is not distracted during the presentation.

- Using a handout to set tasks or raise controversial issue for discussion may facilitate small group work within the lecture or provide material for 'break-out' groups following the talk.

- Handouts might be used to provide personal background information before a lecture to ensure commonality of knowledge across a whole group.

- It might be easier to make handouts available electronically after a talk, thereby reducing paper wastage and maximising the capability to provide electronic links for further information.

Source: Bligh.(15, p. 148)

Questioning

This is the simplest of interactive lecturing techniques, but often the most valuable. Individuals within large groups might potentially feel threatened, and this often leads to migration to the back row if there is a fear that questions will be asked and knowledge gaps identified. The wise lecturer, however, will judge the 'educational climate' and introduce this technique in a fashion that is non-threatening, such as through the use of humour to lighten the inevitable tension when questions are introduced. A simple 'show of hands' might provide the answer, and anonymised 'audience response' keypads are becoming ever more affordable. As a general rule, questions should be 'open' rather than

'closed' (yes/no answers), and used wisely, this technique will identify the level of group knowledge, enable planning of future direction and offer the opportunity for fears and concerns to be addressed. Allow plenty of time for responses, giving the audience time to think; if responses are poor, try rephrasing the question rather than offering an answer.

Buzz groups

While most traditional lecturers try to discourage talking between students attending lectures, an alternative approach is to recognise that this is likely to happen anyway and will encourage interchange of ideas at appropriate intervals. The concept is to set a task for groups of two or more students to discuss at regular intervals. The task can be related to the preceding section of the lecture or a controversial issue raised, or (perhaps even braver) it can provide the opportunity for the learners to 'shape' the next section of the lecture. The challenge is always to regain the interest of the students, but the task should include a requirement for selected feedback to the rest of the audience to maximise group learning.

Brainstorming

This is a method widely used in commerce and can be used by teachers to test group knowledge or discuss areas where there are likely to be a range of viewpoints. The lecturer invites answers to a question or problem from the audience, and it is important to emphasise that each contribution will be treated with equal importance and should be written down without further comment. The list of answers will then form the basis for a discussion with the audience and should lead naturally to the next part of the talk.

Snowballing

This aptly describes a process where each individual member of the audience is invited to work alone on a problem or issue for a couple of minutes, then share with their neighbour for a similar length of time, the two of them generating a discussion which they then share with another pair, and so on. This process can be time-consuming, so it generally suits smaller groups, and enough time should be included to get useful feedback from all the groups before the lecture continues or comes to an end.

Nominal group technique

For some groups and suitable subject material, it may prove desirable to divide the audience into smaller groups with a set task. This particular technique gives all group members the right to express any opinion without challenge. All the group contributions are written down by a nominated group leader and time is then given for elucidation, explanation and challenge to the ideas raised. At this point similar items can either be aggregated if they are very similar, or disaggregated if a group's members feel they are materially different. After this period of discussion the group members are invited to vote for the issues raised, identifying their perceived importance, and the key issues are then fed back to the wider audience.

Evidence suggests that interactive lectures promote understanding in the audience rather than simply encouraging fact retention.(40) Interactivity also offers the opportunity for lecturers to check assumptions and participants to feel included, engenders collective learning and aids retention of learning through facilitating different learning styles and empowering the audience in the learning process.

Conclusion

Lectures will continue to hold a useful place among the methods of learning that may be included in the educational toolbox of medical educators. They will remain the bedrock for most professional and interprofessional educational meetings at the local, national and international level. However, to be effective, they must be employed judiciously with a clearly thought-through purpose for the presenter and the audience. The manner of delivery and the aids used must be carefully tailored to facilitate effective learning, giving due responsibility equally to the organisers, the lecturer and the audience, recognising the limitations of human physiology and taking heed of the capabilities and needs of the audience. Preparation for each unique learning event is essential and due regard should be given to the opportunity for those attending to continue discussion during refreshment breaks, sharing knowledge and good practice and continuing to build the community of learning. Due consideration should be given to the place of interactive learning, and lecturers might learn a great deal if they are required to sit through their own lectures, a learning opportunity that is now freely available through the use of modern digital recording techniques.

References

1 Dunkin MJ (1983) A review of research on lecturing. *Higher Education Research and Development.* **2**: 63–78.

2 Charlton BG (2006) Lectures are an effective learning method because they exploit human nature to improve learning. *Medical Hypotheses.* **67**: 1261–5.

3 Fish D and de Cossart L (2003) *Cultivating a Thinking Surgeon: New Perspectives on Clinical Teaching, Learning and Assessment.* tfm Publishing, Shifnal, Shropshire.

4 Ashcroft RE (2004) Current epistemological problems in evidence based medicine. *Journal of Medical Ethics.* **30**: 131–5.

5 Dewey J (1938) *Experience and Education.* Macmillan, New York.

6 General Medical Council (2013) *Good Medical Practice.* GMC, London.

7 Schön DA (1983) *The Reflective Practitioner: How Professionals Think in Action.* Basic Books, New York.

8 Schön DA (1987) *Educating the Reflective Practitioner: Towards a New Design for Teaching and Learning in the Professions.* Jossey-Bass, San Francisco, CA.

9 Eraut M (1994) *Developing Professional Knowledge and Competence.* Routledge Falmer, London.

10 Benner P (1984) *From Novice to Expert: Excellence and Power in Clinical Nursing Practice.* Addison-Wesley, London.

11 Wenger E (1998) Communities of practice: learning as a social system. *Systems Thinker.* (http://www.co-i-l.com/coil/knowledge-garden/cop/lss.shtml; accessed 15 November 2012).

12 Lave J and Wenger E (1991) *Situated Learning: Legitimate Peripheral Participation.* Cambridge University Press, Cambridge.

13 Swanwick T (2005) Informal learning in postgraduate medical education: from cognitivism to 'culturism'. *Medical Education.* **39**: 859–65.

14 Stenhouse L (1975) *An Introduction to Curriculum Research and Development.* Heinemann, London.

15 Bligh DA (2000) *What's the Use of Lectures?* Jossey-Bass, San Francisco, CA.

16 Entwistle NJ (1988) *Styles of Learning and Teaching.* David Fulton, London.

17 Tulving E (1972) Episodic and semantic memory. In: Tulving E and Donaldson W (eds) *Organisation of Memory*, pp. 381–403. Academic Press, London.

18 Verner C and Dickinson G (1967) The lecture: an analysis and review of research. *Adult Education.* **17**: 85–100.

19 Gardiner L (1994) *Redesigning Higher Education: Producing Dramatic Gains in Student Learning.* George Washington University, Washington, DC. ASHE-ERIC Higher Education Report No. 7. (http://bern.library.nenu.edu.cn/upload/soft/0-article/021/21052.pdf; accessed 15 November 2012).

20 Neisser U (1976) *Cognition and Reality.* Freeman, San Francisco, CA.

21 Eraut M (2000) Non-formal learning and tacit knowledge in professional work. *British Journal of Educational Psychology.* **70**: 113–36.

22 Ausubel DP (1968) *Educational Psychology: A Cognitive View.* Holt, Reinehart and Winston, Austin, TX.

23 Stuart J and Rutherford RJD (1978) Medical student concentration during lectures. *Lancet.* **2**: 514–6.

24 Higher Education Academy Engineering Subject Centre (2005) Guide to Lecturing. (http://www.heacademy.ac.uk/assets/documents/subjects/engineering/guide-to-lecturing.pdf; accessed 16 June 2013).

25 Ellis AW and Young AW (1988) *Human Cognitive Neuropsychology.* Erlbaum, Hillsdale, NJ.

26 Biggs J (1999) *Teaching for Quality Learning at University.* Open University Press, Buckingham.

27 Baddeley A (1992) Working memory. *Science.* **255**: 556–9.

28 Kiewra K (1988) Cognitive aspects of autonomous note taking: control processes, learning strategies, and prior knowledge. *Educational Psychologist.* **3**: 39–56.

29 Brown G and Manogue M (2001) AMEE Medical Education Guide No. 22: refreshing lecturing: a guide for lecturers. *Medical Teacher.* **23**: 231–44.

30 Baddeley A (1996) *Your Memory: A User's Guide.* Penguin, Harmondsworth.

31 Strodt-Lopez B (1991) Tying it all in: asides in university lectures. *Applied Linguistics.* **12**: 117–40.

32 Tulving E (2002) Episodic memory: from mind to brain. *Annual Review of Psychology.* **53**: 1–25.

33 Nesi H (2001) A corpus-based analysis of academic lectures across disciplines. In: Cotterill J and Ife A (eds) *Language across Boundaries*, pp. 201–18. BAAL in Association with Continuum Press, London.

34 Dudley-Evans A and Johns T (1981) A team teaching approach to lecture comprehension for overseas students. In: *The Teaching of Listening Comprehension*, pp. 30–46. ELT Documents Special. The British Council, London.

35 Chaudron C and Richards JC (1986) The effect of discourse markers on the comprehension of lectures. *Applied Linguistics.* **7**: 113–27.

36 Brown GA and Bakhtar M (1987) Styles of lecturing: a study and its implications. *Research Papers in Education.* **3**: 131–53.

37 Norvig P (2003) PowerPoint: shot with its own bullets. *Lancet.* **362**: 343–4.

38 Baddeley A (1996) *Human Memory: Theory and Practice.* Erlbaum, Hillsdale, NJ.

39 Abercrombie MLJ (1960) *The Anatomy of Judgment: Concerning the Processes of Perception, Communication, and Reasoning.* Hutchinson, London.

40 Social Policy and Social Work Subject Centre. Activities to try in lectures. The Higher Education Academy Social Policy and Social Work (SWAP) website. (http://www.swap.ac.uk/resources/publs/digests.html; accessed 1 August 2013).

Further reading

Alexander M, Lenahan P and Pavlov A (eds) (2005) *Cinemeducation. A Comprehensive Guide to Using Film in Medical Education.* Radcliffe, Oxford.

Bligh DA (2000) *What's the Use of Lectures?* Jossey-Bass, San Francisco, CA.

Brown G and Manogue M (2001) AMEE Medical Education Guide No. 22: refreshing lecturing: a guide for lecturers. *Medical Teacher.* **23**: 231–44.

Cantillon P, Hutchinson L and Wood D (eds) (2003) *ABC of Learning and Teaching in Medicine.* BMJ Publishing, London.

Gibbs G, Habeshaw S and Habeshaw T (2000) *53 Interesting Things to Do in Your Lectures.* Cromwell Press, Trowbridge.

Hall G (ed.) (2007) *How to Present at Meetings.* Blackwell, Oxford.

Carpenter S, Simons F (eds). (2005) Guide to Lecturing. Higher Education Academy Engineering Subject Centre. (http://www.heacademy.ac.uk/assets/documents/subjects/engineering/guide-to-lecturing.pdf; accessed 1 August 2013).

Midmer D (2003) Presentation magic. *BMJ Careers.* **326**: S120.

Newble D and Cannon R (1983) *A Handbook for Clinical Teachers.* MTP Press, London.

Social Policy and Social Work Subject Centre. (2008) SWAP digest 4a. Maximising student learning in lectures. Social Policy and Social Work Subject Centre, Higher Education Academy. (http://www.swap.ac.uk/docs/digests/swapdigest_4a.pdf; accessed 1 August 2013).

Social Policy and Social Work Subject Centre. (2008) SWAP digest 4b. What makes a good lecturer? The student perspective. Social Policy and Social Work Subject Centre, Higher Education Academy. (http://www.swap.ac.uk/docs/digests/swapdigest_4b.pdf; accessed 1 August 2013).

11 Technology-enhanced learning

Alison Bullock[1] and Peter GM de Jong[2]

[1]Cardiff University School of Social Sciences, UK
[2]Center for Innovation in Medical Education, Leiden University Medical Center, The Netherlands

KEY MESSAGES

- Technology has the potential to enhance learning but needs to be integrated into educational processes, related to learning aims and outcomes, connected to reflective practice and linked to learner needs and preferences. The technology itself, should not be viewed in isolation.

- Both knowledge acquisition and participation in social practice are essential elements of learning; there is an intimate connection between knowledge and activity in a community of practice; the motivations and experiences of adult learners also need to be given consideration.

- Uptake by educators of technological innovations to support learning is affected by the individual, by the skills,

knowledge and motivations of teachers, and by organisational factors such as resources and infrastructure.

- A number of frameworks are available to help structure the evaluation of the potential of technology to enhance learning. These underscore the importance of not only looking at the technology/tools but also to other factors such as the learners, the task, the physical environment and organisational characteristics. This makes the job of assessing the impact of technology on learning a complex one.

- Further research is needed to address gaps in our understanding of TEL use and impact.

Introduction

This book carries chapters on e-learning and simulation (*see* Chapters 12 and 13) so why a chapter on technology enhanced learning (TEL) as well? There is overlap between the terms certainly, but notably 'TEL' as a term underscores how technology should be used to *enhance* learning, that technology should not merely be used to replace traditional learning, but rather it should add something to the learning process. So putting lecture notes and PowerPoint presentations into a virtual learning environment (VLE) is *not* TEL. Although it might enable remote 'any place, any time' access to material, such an activity does not improve the learning process. As Robin and colleagues argue, 'just converting . . . lecture notes to digital format is not enough'.(1) On the other hand, including self-assessments and feedback, incorporating synchronised or asynchronised peer-to-peer discussion and using varied modes of presentation (e.g. video clips) exploits technology in ways which have potential to enhance the learning process. Technology has the power to 'help students become active participants not just in their own learning, but in creating knowledge'.(2)

The technologies discussed in this chapter are not additional to those referred to in the e-learning or simulation chapters, and beyond offering some examples time will not be spent rehearsing their diversity. Rather, we seek to outline some relevant theories of learning and set out examples which show ways in which technology has been

used to enhance learning. We will talk a little about the importance of reflection and note some of the main criteria or questions to think about as an educator planning to use technology to enhance learning. The e-learning chapter highlights the importance of structure in both computer-aided learning (CAL) and simulation, as well as technology used to support more unstructured learning in the workplace by providing just-in-time information. Emphasis is given to time for reflection which is needed for knowledge assimilation. This chapter develops those ideas and underscores the importance of viewing technology as a *tool* that can be used to enhance learning; viewing it not in isolation, but as an integral part of the educational process. *See* Box 11.1.

Examples of learning technology

There is a wealth of potential ways to enhance learning through using technology and this diversity is ever-changing and developing (*see* Chapter 12). We say 'potential' because the use of technology should never be assumed to enhance the learning but certainly if computers, the internet and mobile technology are used in a correct way, enhancement is possible. Technology offers ways to supplement or in some cases, replace traditional learning methods.

Jenkins *et al.* define technology enhanced learning as 'any online facility or system that directly supports learning and

Understanding Medical Education: Evidence, Theory and Practice, Second Edition. Edited by Tim Swanwick.
© 2014 The Association for the Study of Medical Education. Published 2014 by John Wiley & Sons, Ltd.

Box 11.1 FOCUS ON: Some fundamental questions in technology enhanced learning

What is the purpose of the educational intervention?

Technology should support and serve learning rather than drive the learning experience. However, technology also creates new possibilities, and as educators we should think about how it can develop learning and help us to achieve worthwhile educational goals.

What is the right tool for the job?

An important question for educators to consider is the fit between the learning mode and the desired outcomes.

Does the technology support the active engagement of the learner?

Different uses of technology have implications for the role of the learner and their position vis-a-vis the learning content.

How do the learners like to learn?

Learner preferences are important and need to be factored into the instructional design.

Has the technology supported the achievement of the learning outcomes?

This can be difficult to assess as it is dependent on such things as learner attitude, learner aptitude, context and the course design rather than just the technology. And even the best designed resources are not always used as intended.

Box 11.2 Examples of technology potentially enhancing learning

e-Learning

Online learning materials, sometimes 'blended' with face-to-face events, providing an individualised approach to learning.

Web 2.0 tools

Enhancing the active engagement of the learner through the generation of material (e.g. blogs, and wikis), and/or communication via social networking software (e.g. Facebook, Twitter).

Mobile devices and apps

Specific, downloadable software programmes supporting learning in the workplace by providing ready access to information.

Simulation

Including mannequins, case scenarios and computerised environments that imitate the real world offering structured expose and enabling skills practice in a safe environment.

MOOCs

Non-award-bearing, free structured courses, offering the potential to free up class time for deeper learning.

---

teaching'.(3) An obvious type of system is **e-learning**, which is defined as learning that is facilitated, supported or made possible through technology. It may be entirely online or **blended.** A blended approach is one in which a mix of approaches is adopted – for example, e-learning and face-to-face small group work. E-learning has been demonstrated to be as equally as effective in achieving learning outcomes as traditional approaches, especially when used in a blended environment.(4)

TEL also includes **Web 2.0** tools. These are tools that support communication and sharing where users generate content and develop web-based communities (through social networking software such as Facebook or Twitter, for example) or use blogs or wikis for course updates, reference sharing, or for recording immediate reflections. Such tools may be accessed from **mobile devices**.(5) A mobile computing device is a hand-held, multi-function device. It is a personal computer – with internet and email capability – a mobile phone, a camera, a notepad, radio, gaming device and many other things. Its functions can be extended through the use of **apps**. Apps are software programmes which can be downloaded onto the device. Hun-

dreds of thousands of apps are available, some with specific use in medical fields (such as steps in specific clinical procedures).

In the last few years, simulations have become increasingly prevalent and a preferred part of the learning process. **Simulations** are diverse and include actors taking the role of patients (standardised patients), computerised mannequins, case scenarios and computerised environments that imitate the real world.(6) Computer-based simulations of highly interactive, dynamic environments employ aspects of **gaming**.(7) These scenario-based games allow players to interact, experiment and manipulate variables.(8) An example might mimic a real-world spread of a virus across a population where players see the effects of their treatments. By making use of technology, education providers can capitalise on the gaming experience of younger generations. However, although the virtual world of 'Second Life' has been seen as a future environment for online medical simulations, the idea never really took off.

A recent development is the emergence of **MOOCs** (massive open online courses). These are non-award-bearing, free academic courses run on platforms operated by companies such as Udacity, Coursera or edX. The structured courses, devised by academics from some of the world's best universities, provide feedback to the many thousands of students they attract. (*See* Box 11.2.)

Why use technology to enhance learning?

Offering new opportunities

Using technology as part of the learning process has become widespread.(9) Jenkins *et al.*(3) found the departments within higher education institutions (HEIs) making most use of TEL were medicine, nursing and health and that the most important driver was a general concern to enhance the quality of teaching and learning. Fundamental to the use of TEL are questions about the purpose of education – what is it for? Technology should support, serve and develop learning, rather than drive the learning experience. Technology is a means to an end, rather than an end in itself. In medical education, those ends should relate to good patient care – for example, developing and maintaining the knowledge and skills that lie behind good clinical decision-making. As Olson(10) remarks 'we need to decide our purpose, and then choose the right tools for the job', and different uses of TEL will have implications for the role of the learner. Dror *et al.*(11) remind us that we need to be mindful of the role for the learner that the technology assumes. For example, watching a video is a passive activity for the learner but videos can be made interactive and so engage and challenge the learner, providing a more cognitively effective activity.

E-learning programmes that provide help when needed and are responsive to learners' developing knowledge and skills offer dynamic scaffolding. Simulations allow learners to practise in a safe environment, decreasing risk to patients and can deliver structured exposure to the workplace environment and patient treatments. Simulation gaming offers opportunities for users to control variables and learn from the consequences of their decisions. Mobile devices are used to support learning in the workplace through providing ready access to information. A recent study indicated that 82 per cent of UK doctors own a smartphone,(12) with 300,000 apps developed between 2007 and 2010.(13) Wallace *et al.*(5) report that over 85 per cent of the medical students, residents and faculty in the large Canadian medical school in their study used a mobile-computing device. These smartphone or tablet devices allowed users to check information 'on the go' and the great majority regularly used at least one medical app. In the UK, the MoMEd (Mobile Medical Education) project with final year medical students(14) and the iDoc project with trainee doctors(15) both use 'Dr Companion' software (Medhand International AB, UK), which provides a search tool and core medical textbooks including the *British National Formulary*. In both projects, this use of the smartphone supported learners by providing access to just-in-time information and was used to complement rather than replace other forms of learning.

Olson also recognises that technology brings 'new possibilities for collaboration' and suggests we should also think about 'what worthwhile ends can we achieve' given these new developments.(10) E-learning can facilitate an individualised approach to learning(16) and with the introduction of Web 2.0 technologies, it has potential to become more participative, social and mobile.(17) George and Dellasega provide an example of a tool which allows students to 'use mobile devices to contribute to discussions, ask and answer questions and respond directly to teacher prompts in real-time through multiple social networking platforms, including Facebook and Twitter'.(18) They also report how 'tweets' are displayed on big screens in classroom settings to encourage communication across groups. Using social media can change the position of the learner vis-a-vis the learning content. Learners can directly create and contribute to content, a role which, some have argued,(18) makes the learning process more egalitarian and can develop engagement with a social community of learners. Synchronous interaction via web or video-conferencing can help build collaboration skills and offers 'far greater opportunities for education than taking satellite courses or streaming lectures through the internet'.(19) The use of MOOCs may also create benefits by freeing up class time for more interactive, deeper learning activities, although Corbyn comments that there is little that is 'pedagogically adventurous about the instructional model commonly used'(20) within MOOCs and reports dropout rates in excess of 90 percent.

Changing the nature of work

Seminal work by Zuboff(21) raises our awareness of the significant effects of technology on the nature of labour, on the transparency of information and on workplace learning. She explains how technology has changed how many of us work – from activities with people and things, to working in computer-mediated environments – and how this increasing 'abstraction' of work challenges the meaningfulness of the traditional distinction between white and blue collar workers. She introduces the concept of 'informating', a process whereby technology takes information and translates it into action. Through informating, technology makes systems and processes explicit, and such symbolic representation (abstraction) of events and organisational processes makes them transparent and visible, thus enabling them to be known by others and shared. Zuboff writes: 'Activities, events, and objects are translated into and made visible by information when a technology *informates* as well as *automates*', and explains these processes with the example of a programmer not only telling the machine 'what to do' but also telling 'what the machine has done – translating the production process and making it visible'. In the education context, this brings to mind the quantity of data produced by programme analytics that report records not only of users' responses to assessment questions in an online learning programme, but also the different pages visited, the duration of time spent on each page and from what which machine etc. According to Zuboff, in the 'informated organization . . . learning is no longer a separate activity that occurs either before one enters the workplace or in remote classroom settings . . . learning is the heart of productive activity . . . To put it simply, learning is the new form of labor'.((21), p. 395)

Drawing on the work of Eraut,(22) we might ask how technology contributes to workplace learning activities such as getting information, listening and observing, reflecting, learning from mistakes and giving and receiving feedback. As Zuboff(21) points out, the effects of technology on the workplace are not neutral: it allows and enables some experiences and closes off others. Nor is our interaction neutral – we shape the future by choosing to use technology in some ways but not others. And we operate within social, political and cultural norms and expectations which shape further developments. The three combined – the technology itself, the individual and the social context – result in both intended and unintended consequences. Thus technology has the capacity to create learning environments that develop deeper learning through greater learner access to knowledge and participation in knowledge creation, which challenges traditional hierarchies, or it can be used unimaginatively to serve the needs of the teacher in ways which do not warrant the label 'technology *enhanced* learning', or used by learners to plagiarise the work and ideas of others and to access inappropriate material which fails to treat others with dignity.

Evidence of effect

In a meta-analysis of the effectiveness of internet-based educational interventions for health care professionals, Cook *et al.*(4) report studies that clearly revealed gains from e-learning interventions. However, there was no single message from a comparison between e-learning and more traditional approaches: studies showed varying results in terms of relative effectiveness.(23–25) Cook, Levinson and Garside(26) in their systematic review of the literature on time and efficiency in internet-based learning found little difference between e-learning and traditional methods. However, they noted that efficiency can only be examined within a given course and context and that efficiency is dependent on learner aptitude and course design rather than computer technology per se.

An important question for educators to consider is the fit between the learning mode and the desired outcomes. A study by Genischen and colleagues(27) suggested e-learning was particularly suited to virtual clinical case studies and for updating medical knowledge. They found that by combining different modes of teaching, a mixed learning approach can facilitate learning preferences and offer new training opportunities. Learner preferences are also important. In research on problem-based learning (PBL), Robson(28) showed that an online interaction was an acceptable alternative to more traditional group learning. In some contrast, Stewart and colleagues(19) reported that although about 25 per cent of higher education students in the USA had enrolled on one or more online courses in 2008, they still wanted face-to-face contact. Dror *et al.*(11) suggest that if the material is intended for face-to-face presentation, then converting it to electronic format can even be detrimental to the learning experience.

Simulations have been shown to enhance teamwork and technical skills.(26) Following a systematic review, Rosen *et al.*(29) conclude that 'in situ simulation', an approach that blends simulation in a real workplace environment, helps with learning transfer. Some argue that this transfer to real world performance should be the primary outcome measure when judging the efficacy of the training.(6)

Box 11.3 WHERE'S THE EVIDENCE: Can technology enhance learning?

E-learning is at least as efficient and effective as traditional lecture-based learning,(4,30–32,36,37) but efficiency depends on learner aptitude and course design,(26) and mode of 'delivery' needs to suit purpose.(11)

A blended approach can facilitate learning preferences and face-to-face contact is important.(19,27)

Simulation can enhance teamwork and technical skills and simulation blended in a real workplace environment, helps with learning transfer.(29)

For further evidence *see*:

http://repository.alt.ac.uk/839/2/ALT_TEL_evidence_document_for_BIS_low-res.pdf

Given evidence leading to a conclusion that e-learning is not *less* efficient or effective than traditional lecture-based learning,(26,27,30–32) it could be a more *cost*-effective alternative, creating savings in terms of travel costs, institutional infrastructure and instructor training time.(27,33) However, cost-effectiveness is affected by the use of technology in combination with other teaching modes, notably in combination with face-to-face teaching and there are strong educational reasons for adopting a blended approach. Sandars(34) refers to 'nagging doubts' about how e-learning can be used to best effect and even the best designed resources may not be used as intended and learners make variable use of resources.(35) In all this we need to keep asking how the technology is *enhancing* the educational experience. (*See* Box 11.3.)

Theoretical groundings for TEL

In this section we explore the nature of knowledge and learning in order to better understand the significance technology has for educational processes. In this, we adopt a broad conception of learning which includes informal learning in the workplace.

Learning processes
In Chapter 7 Morris and Blaney discuss the ideas of Anna Sfard(38) who describes two 'metaphors' for learning, which she labels 'acquisition' and 'participation'. The two models are contrasted; in the acquisition model, emphasis is given to an individual's attainment of knowledge whereas the participation model of learning focuses on the bonds between individuals, where learning is seen more as an ongoing process of belonging and not separable from context. Importantly, Sfard(38) argues that learners need both to acquire knowledge and participate in learning processes, that it is neither desirable nor possible to ignore

the place of acquisition in learning development. In relation to participation, we note here the notion of 'communities of practice' from the work of Lave and Wenger.(39) Their ideas are pertinent to trainee doctors' learning in the workplace. They contend that to become a member of the community involves much more than the technical, explicit knowledge or skills associated with undertaking certain tasks. Members of the community engage in a set of relationships over time which gives rise to a shared sense of enterprise and identity. Initially the trainee joins the community and learns at the periphery, engaging in 'legitimate peripheral participation'. As they become more competent, they move towards the 'centre' of the community. Learning is thus both about the acquisition of knowledge and also a process of social participation.

Forms of knowledge and knowledge conversion

The capacity of technology to enhance learning is influenced by the nature of the knowledge. Here we draw attention to the distinction between two main forms of knowledge – explicit and tacit. Explicit knowledge is codified (arranged in an organised system) and can be expressed in formal, declarative statements (as in textbooks, for example). Tacit knowledge, on the other hand, is hard to formalise and communicate in words and is expressed in action and experience. Tacit knowledge is developed or learnt through observation, imitation and practice. The medical practitioner needs both. Nonaka(40) described the interactions between the different forms of knowledge, identifying four distinct processes of 'knowledge conversion' and represented these in a four-quadrant diagram. According to this model, 'combination' is the process of creating new explicit knowledge. This can be done through classifying or reconfiguring existing explicit knowledge. 'Internalisation' is the word used by Nonaka(40) to describe the process by which explicit knowledge is shared and converted (internalised) into tacit knowledge. This, he argues, occurs through action and experimentation. The process which converts tacit knowledge to new tacit knowledge is 'socialisation' where, by spending time together, experiences are shared. The conversion of tacit knowledge to explicit knowledge is described as a process of 'externalisation', whereby the tacit knowledge is articulated in a way that enables it to be shared by others. This is a difficult process but one which is helped by the use of stories and metaphors and by repeated and extended dialogue and discussion.

How does this relate to TEL? Knowledge creation, sharing and conversion are central learning processes, and understanding the place of both explicit and tacit knowledge in medical education can assist educators in determining their use of technology to enhance learning. A students' or trainees' knowledge of a workplace, a context, a situation is determined by a mix of explicit and tacit knowledge.(22) A library of texts on a smartphone, for example, provides ready access to explicit knowledge and, as explicit and tacit knowledge are complementary, development of

one can help in knowledge conversion processes. Timely access to explicit information may support internalisation and the development of tacit knowledge. Another illustration can be drawn from the use of Web 2.0 technologies in supporting learning communities and assisting processes of externalisation. And if, as has been argued, much of doctors' knowledge is implicit or tacit,(41) this becomes an important process in medical education.

Adult learning and reflective practice

Malcolm Knowles(42) developed a set of principles for adult learning based on his identification of the motivations and learning preferences of adults. The characteristics of adult learners and the implications they present for teaching and learning have been set out in an earlier chapter (*see* Chapter 2) and will not be rehearsed here; nor will theory of reflective practice. Suffice to say, the capacity of technology to enhance learning should not be viewed in isolation from educational theory. Reflection has many facets – short/long, group/individual, focused/spontaneous(43) – and is an essential part of the learning process. It is through reflection that learners can make sense of their educational experience, be that attendance at a traditional lecture, an experience in a simulation lab or a workplace placement in a clinical setting. It enables learners to digest, convert and embed knowledge. Kolb(44) and Moon(45) view reflection as an iterative process that allows new knowledge to be assimilated and acted upon. Morris and Blaney (*see* Chapter 7) writing specifically about work-based learning, warn that Kolb presents an essentially cognitive view of learning. This leads to an emphasis on individuals, their engagement with learning and their prior knowledge and experience, which underplays the complexity of learning processes and the importance of the social and participatory workplace context. Eraut (43) developed a three-dimensional framework for considering reflection. These dimensions relate to purpose, focus and context. We emphasise the importance of context and community but make the point here that when looking at technology and how it supports learning, we need also to consider the place of reflection, albeit at the level of the individual learner.(46)

Knowledge and innovation transfer

There is a whole body of literature on the transfer of knowledge and innovation which seeks to address the gap between the creation of new knowledge and innovative developments (some forms of TEL would be an example) and what happens in practice. The UK's National Institute for Health Research (NIHR) and similar bodies internationally are concerned with the lack of knowledge transfer from universities into health care delivery.(47) Such concern dates back over 30 years,(48) but research has failed to reveal major breakthroughs in how to improve it. A recent UK review led by Sir Ian Carruthers, *Innovation, Health and Wealth: Accelerating Adoption and Diffusion in the NHS*(49) placed innovation at the top of the service agenda and set out ambitious recommendations to encourage quicker transfer of new practices. Focused on technology, Schifferdecker *et al.* summarise aspects that need to be considered when seeking to enhance the adoption of innovations, as follows:

- the needs of potential adopters
- perceived and real benefits of change for adopters
- the computer- or technology-related knowledge and skills of the potential adopters
- the resources (e.g. time, money, support) required to make the change
- features (e.g. complexity, compatibility) of the technology, item or programme to be adopted.(50)

The authors(50) report how these factors apply to the adoption of the computer-assisted learning in paediatrics programme (CLIPP) centred on virtual patients. The needs of potential adopters related to a number of aspects including gaps in experience, licensing requirements and desire to improve teaching and learning. These also related to the perceived (improved learning) and real (licensure) benefits. In addition, motivations were important. Regarding the required technology skills, the authors(50) found that their users had sufficient skills and commented that they thought this aspect would become less important as successive generations become increasingly skilled (although here we note that technological developments require ever-changing skills). As for resources, the authors(50) comment that either the innovation should require little additional time or adopters should be given sufficient time. However they add that for educators the ease of adoption 'may be at odds with the time required to appropriately integrate' the technology into the programme. In the conclusion they point to the need for adequate staff training. Finally, regarding the technological features, CLIPP was described as relatively simple and followed a national curriculum.

Planning to use TEL: Evaluation frameworks

In considering the impact of technology on learning, it can be useful to borrow ideas from systems engineering(29) and consider the learners, the technology/tools, the task, the physical environment and organisational characteristics.(51) Carroll and colleagues(52) developed a framework for reviewing e-learning programmes and suggest that the learning experience is enhanced if all five areas are addressed. These are:

- presentation and course design (applicability, attractiveness, usability)
- flexibility (off-line working, asynchronous engagement)
- peer communication (asynchronous engagement, learner interaction, peer support)
- support (moderated learning, formal and peer support)
- knowledge validation (assessment and formal support).

To enhance the experience of e-learning, Carroll *et al.*(33) reason that courses need to address these areas. To this we can also add some assessment of the quality of the content of the educational material. At the University of Leeds, Asarbakah and Sandars(53) have devised a usability checklist for e-learning which comprises three aspects: the learner and context, the technological aspects of design, and the content of interventions. Wallace *et al.*(5) raise concern about users' failure to apply quality checks and distinguish good learning resources and material. Participants in their study made uncritical use of Wikipedia and apps, for example. Shortt *et al.* argue for 'the need to define quality criteria for accredited online modules'.(54) Although they found no list of quality criteria from their review of literature, they identified a number of key themes, as follows.

- **The fit with the way physicians prefer to learn** Doctors, as adult learners, prefer to learn at their own pace. They reflect on change and implications for practice and like the online modules to accommodate needs-based, goal-directed learning.
- **The fit with content preferences** Doctors prefer a systematic approach to the presentation of content, with the inclusion of clinical cases or problems. They like to interact with the content and with experts and peers. And the content should be seen by the doctor as facilitating change and practice improvement.
- **Technical aspects** The e-learning modules should be user-friendly, make effective use of multi-media and include links to other resources.
- **Evaluation component** This theme relates to the inclusion of learner self-assessments and the evaluation of the course itself and its outcomes.

We have experience of using Kirkpatrick's model of programme evaluation to guide the gathering of evidence of effectiveness.(55,56) The original framework comprises four levels. *Level 1* is concerned with assessing the participants 'reaction' or satisfaction with the programme: for example, do the learners think that the course met their expectations? Such responses can be collected from end-of-course, online questionnaires, for example. *Level 2* is about 'learning' (knowledge and skills): for example, do the participants report gains in knowledge and skills development? There are different ways to collect evidence of learning and these include pre and post-testing, review of the content of discussion boards or associated assignments or through the submission of reflective diaries. *Level 3* focuses on behaviour change (performance) and the extent to which new learning is applied to practice: for example, as a result of the course, do participants narrate a change in their clinical practice? Direct evidence may be collected from observation, or indirectly through self reports recorded in audio diaries or from interviews, for example. *Level 4* looks at outcomes, exploring whether organisational performance (and ultimately patient outcomes) improves. Evidence to demonstrate effect at each level is progressively difficult. An example of level 4 evidence might be from a pre- and post-course audit of prescribing practice following an educational intervention. However, disentangling the contextual factors related to the educational input and teacher affect, makes evaluation of impact particularly challenging. (*See* Box 11.4.)

Box 11.4 A framework for evaluating effectiveness (adapted from Kirkpatrick(55))

Level 4 *Outcomes*: tangible results of the programme in terms of health care outcomes

Level 3 *Performance*: changes in practice resulting from the learning

Level 2 *Learning or knowledge*: principles, facts and techniques learned

Level 1 *Reaction*: participants' reaction to the programme

Implementation issues

Assumptions about learners

The 'net generation'(57) and 'digital natives'(58) are terms that have been used to describe a generation of students who have grown up with technology and have developed sophisticated technical skills and learning preferences. Although it is expected that health care professionals are computer and information literate when they register, there are difficulties in appraising learners' attitudes to e-learning and their skills,(59) not least because measures have not been updated in line with technological advances. The educator needs to exercise some caution in making assumptions about their learners' ability to make best use of some forms to technological learning tools, particularly the more recent developments.

Learner access to technology should also not be assumed. For example, the prevalence of smartphones and tablet devices (e.g. iPads) is undeniable. But this does not mean either that all learners have access to such kit or that all learners have sufficient technological skills to use it well to support their learning. Watson and Pecchioni argue that it is a 'dangerous assumption' to think that 'students living in new media environments automatically comprehend how to use the new technologies'.(2)

Politics and practicalities

In practice, how technology is used to support learning processes is affected not only by pedagogical concerns but also by politics and practicalities. Jenkins *et al.*(3) report that TEL needs committed local champions, a factor found to be more important than the availability of external funding. Writing specifically about the use of simulation technology in education and training, Curtis *et al.*(6) provide the following four guidelines:

- know who you are training (so that training can be appropriately tailored)
- clearly identify training objectives
- understand budget constraints
- treat simulation fidelity as a multidimensional concept. This means being aware of not just the high-low dimension but also the physical, functional and psychological aspects of fidelity.

An implication of such guidelines is the need for staff training. Challenges for the future include the development of staff skills particularly in the light of recent and prospective developments.(3)

Learning contexts

Learning context can be differentiated in a number of ways, four of the most obvious being: *level* – undergraduate, postgraduate and continuing; *place* – classroom, simulation lab, workplace, home; *mode* – on-line/off-line; and *extent of specification of intended learning outcomes*. For example, using a smartphone to support learning in the workplace will be more informal in approach than following a structured e-learning package as part of an award-bearing programme of study. And although there are specialty differences (such as the use of simulation technology in anaesthetics, surgery and emergency medicine), in general the use of technology in continuing education has lagged behind TEL in undergraduate and postgraduate education.(12)

We need to be mindful of the learning setting as the application of technology to support and enhance learning in one setting may not be fitting in other contexts, or there may be practical impediments to use. Take for example the use of internet-based online learning packages by busy doctors in their hospital workplace. Time, space and internet access all work against this as a useful learning mode. Blanket internet suppression in some hospitals means that learners are unable to access resources and Prince *et al.*(60) for example, found that podcasts were often difficult to view and lacked sound. They argue that without taking account of logistical considerations, learners who are enthusiastic at the outset can quickly become disenchanted. In developing online courses, educators have to overcome a range of cognitive, pedagogical, motivational and social challenges.(61) Context, access and content are all important.

Work undertaken at the London Knowledge Lab in the UK has focused on technology, learning and context.(62) Although the learner operates in one local context at a time, context is complex and 'reflects their interactions with multiple resources: people, artefacts and environments'.(62) The team there have devised an 'Ecology of Resources' model to represent how learners interact with resources and build meaning through internalisation.(63)

Superficial learning

A number of debates about learning are raised by TEL. One concern is that it may support (indeed, encourage) superficial rather than deep learning. Wallace *et al.* argue that rapid access to information 'may inhibit the internalisation of knowledge . . . leading to the potential for "superficial learning"'(5) and offer some illustrative quotations from participants in their study to back this up. These extracts suggest that users develop a tendency to rely on the devices for information rather than commit it to their own memory. However, there is no indication that this in itself is a bad thing educationally, as it can be argued that knowing where to find information is as important as having that information in your own memory, particularly where that information is subject to regular update and change as in the case of medical drug prescribing, for example.

Wallace *et al.* also point to how smartphones can be a distraction – in both the classroom and the clinical workplace; rather than giving their full attention to the teaching or experience in hand, individuals were 'more globally connected but less locally present'. They conclude that 'this new technology offers the potential to enhance learning and patient care, but also has potential problems associated with its use'.(5)

Netiquette and mobiquette

Rice and McKendree in Chapter 12 draw our attention to the need for agreed principles regarding how users speak to each other in forums which relate to the use of courteous language and not writing excessive amounts. A study by Chretien *et al.*(64) found that 60 per cent of US medical schools had incidents of students posting unprofessional content online. These incidents included profane and discriminatory language, sexually suggestive material and violations of patient confidentiality. The concluded that medical schools should look to include a digital media component in the professionalism curriculum and review their policies about online behaviour.

We would extend the notion of etiquette to the use of mobile devices in the workplace and classroom (so called 'mobiquette'). In the workplace, it is important that colleagues know what the device is being used for. Some places specifically state that doctors will face disciplinary action if they use mobile phones in the clinical setting. The iDoc project(15) advises all participants to:

- Inform all relevant colleagues (such as the ward nursing and administrative staff, consultants, seniors, peers and teams) that you are participating in the iDoc project, which means that you will be using your smartphone to search for information across medical textbooks.
- Reassure colleagues that you will not be 'playing' or making inappropriate use of your smartphone in work time.
- When using the mobile device in front to patients and their families (if present), inform them that you are accessing information quickly from reliable sources (textbooks). Show them the results of your searches if appropriate and explain how the information may help in their care. It may not be appropriate to do this and you may need to look up the information away from the patient. Exercise careful judgement with each patient.
- Only use your smartphone device for medical purposes.

In the classroom, to avoid inappropriate use of mobile devices during teaching sessions, some lecturers specifically build in breaks for text and email checking, for example.

The need for rigorous research

Gaps in the literature have been highlighted. For example, the use of mobile technology providing immediate access to electronic resources has undergone limited evaluation in workplace settings in health care.(65) Others – Stewart *et al.*,(19) for example – identify the lack of 'a theoretically-guided and empirically-grounded study of practice', or, put simply, 'what students and teachers are actually doing with technology'. Ellaway(66) argues that e-learning is sufficiently mature now to focus research effort on understanding how technology enhances learning. The importance of a critical approach to researching and evaluating the use of TEL cannot be over-emphasised(12) and writers point to the need for more rigorous research.(29) An evangelical approach, extolling the prevalence, power and potential of some new technology, heralded as the panacea to untold ills, is associated with atheoretical, sloppy 'research' with no appreciation of the technology's limitations. To illustrate this point, Selwyn(67) warns of hyperbole arising from the distorted position of 'ed-tech' experts' enthusiastic use of the latest technology which leaves them out-of-touch with realities 'on the ground'. Elsewhere he describes education and technology as a not 'especially coherent' area of study that attracts a 'ragbag of individuals' and goes on to make ten suggestions for improving academic research in education and technology.(68) These are summarised in Box 11.5.

These suggestions draw attention to the importance of social science aspects that need highlighting in studying and researching the use of technology in education. Picking up on the last of Selwyn's(68) suggestions, the goal of improved efficiency is usually not an educator's single

---

Box 11.5 HOW TO: Improve research into TEL (adapted from Selwyn(68))

1. Have nothing to sell.
2. Be certain only of the uncertainty of it all – 'technologies are subjected continually to complex interactions and negotiations with the social, economic, political cultural contexts into which they are situated.'
3. Be close (but not *too* close) to the digital technologies that are being researched.
4. Always ask, 'What is new here?' Be aware of 'old wine in new bottles'.
5. Retain a sense of history – to work against over-estimating the short term and under-estimating long-term impacts.
6. Be aware of global, national *and* local contexts of education and technology. Notably, 'show sensitivity towards the importance of local contexts, cultures and circumstances'.
7. Engage with the politics of education and technology – recognising issues of 'power, control, conflict and resistance'.
8. Make good use of theory when and where it is helpful.
9. Be open-minded and curious when it comes to methodology-- be rigorous and appropriate when it comes to methods.
10. Always consider how education, technology and society might be made fairer. 'The best academic research is pursued with the intention of making education *fairer* as well as merely more 'effective' or 'efficient'.

focus. Although concerned to make best use of learners' effort, educators may be seeking to offer, for example, opportunities for the co-creation and sharing of knowledge and may be more concerned with matters of equity and power than just with learning efficiency or effectiveness.

Practical applications: Three case studies

Little is known about the influence of TEL on the organisation of learning. But that there is some influence is obvious. Take for example the use of audience response systems: this allows the teacher to be much better informed about the students' level of knowledge and understanding. This in turn enables the teacher to adapt the lecture to fill knowledge gaps. And because of the new ways of easy communication between students, information can be shared much more quickly than before and this has the potential to affect the organisation of teaching. With the rise of mobile devices and new developments in TEL, the learning environment has for many changed dramatically over the last five years. As teachers it is timely to review and adapt our teaching methods. In this final section we provide three evidenced case studies of innovation and practice points.

Clickers in the classroom
A simple to use but effective and popular technology-based learning tool is the audience response system (ARS).(69) These devices, also known as 'clickers', have enhanced the interactivity in large scale lectures. The old way of provoking discussion by asking questions and showing hands, could be disappointing. Students are not easily willing to show their differing opinion, or risk being wrong in front of the class. When personal or ethical topics are under discussion it is especially hard to get feedback from a large group.(70)

When using clickers students are much more willing to respond to the questions posed. Their willingness relates to anonymity. Neither participants nor the teacher will know who were the ones providing the wrong answer. The technique shows the participants the distribution of answers or opinions. This has educational benefit, as it provides feedback to the audience as well as indicating to the teacher how many need further explanation. Presenters that use ARS questions in their lecture, can better gauge their audience and from the feedback they gain new insights and ideas for improvement for future lectures.(71)

Another benefit of the technology is the way it can be used to chunk the lecture into smaller parts. It is known that attention span decreases rapidly, which causes students to remember less from the second part of lecture. By asking one or more questions during the lecture, students and their memories are activated, resulting in greater long-term retention;(72) indirectly it also causes an increase in motivation.(73)

Clickers can be applied in several scenarios. The first example is about knowledge measurement. The teacher can measure the level of understanding of the group, and based on that outcome, adjust the lecture. When using questions at the start and at the end of a lecture or series of lectures, the teacher can measure gains in knowledge. A second example relates to opinions. As people may be unwilling to show their personal preference in public, the use of clickers to respond anonymously can lead to richer discussions.(73) A third example is the lecture on demand. By asking the audience if they want to learn more about topic A or topic B, the learners can change the course of the lecture. This approach requires the teacher to prepare both topics but can better meet the needs of a majority of the audience. Finally, the clinical reasoning and problem-solving scenario is very effective in medical education.(74) By using interactive cases, classes can decide which steps in the clinical treatment process need to be taken. This approach helps students engage more actively with the case presented and confronts them with possible wrong actions based on class majority.

Mobile devices for learning
Arguably one of the biggest steps in TEL of the last decade is that learners do not need to be in a specific location in order to connect to their educational materials. Before the introduction of mobile wireless devices, you needed to go to a computer which was wired to the network. Despite the claim that one of the greatest advantages of computer-based learning was 'place independence', this was not true. Computer rooms were situated in specific locations, and the learner needed to be there. And those places were not usually available 24/7. This has now changed dramatically. The introduction of small wireless devices with internet access such as laptops, tablet computers and smartphones really opened the opportunity to access learning material anywhere. While before theory and practice were generally separated in time and place, these two now can easily be blended. Students use mobile devices to search for information and critique the quality (accuracy, reliability, credibility).(75) Whilst on the ward, the physician can demonstrate a procedure to a patient. Trainees can instantaneously access relevant information. The use of first PDAs (personal digital assistants) and later smartphones in clerkships is a good example of the revolution in the capacity of technology to support learning in the workplace. What began with a few doctors using such mobile devices, quickly turned to widespread prevalence.(10)

As almost every medical trainee and student has a smartphone, tablet or iPad, the step to using these devices in education is a small one. Projects like the MoMEd with final year medical students(14) and the iDoc project(15) both provide a library of texts on smartphones to support learning through access to just-in-time, reliable information. Even the traditional clickers (ARS) are being replaced by online voting through smartphones.

There are issues related to the use of mobile devices. Firstly, there are equity issues. We should not assume that every student or trainee has an operational device. Another issue is the use of mobile devices in the presence of others, notably patients. Many would currently assume that the smartphone use was personal rather than for learning and it is important that the educational use is communicated appropriately. Using mobile devices requires communication skills. Finally, the use of mobile devices for patient records risks data security. Accessing personal data, of patients or students, on a mobile device makes it more easily available to others. These issues urge us to use mobile devices prudently in our teaching.

Web 2.0 tools to enhance collaboration

New web technologies offer unique opportunities in the field of collaboration and can help students develop learning communities. By using a computer or a mobile device, students can stay connected to each other independently of their physical location. And once connected, they can work together on assignments or research projects. Simple communication tools such as Skype are used for virtual meetings, replacing the much more complex systems of institutional video conferencing. Other tools, such as wikis and blogs, are more focused on content sharing in order to support document development by different people from different places.(76) Besides the option to share a document, these technologies support collaboration and knowledge construction skills. Twitter can be used between teacher and students, but also among students themselves.(77) Some of the Web 2.0 tools specifically focus on social relationships, like Facebook. However, we now see groups of students organising themselves in Facebook groups to discuss learning materials in a safe and readily accessible environment.

Several schools use a combination of social media in education. Pen State College of Medicine applied Twitter, YouTube, Flickr, blogging and Skype in elective courses for fourth year students to improve their skills in problem-solving, networking and collaboration.(18) In this school George and Dellasega provide an example of a tool which allows students to 'use mobile devices to contribute to discussions, ask and answer questions and respond directly to teacher prompts in real-time through multiple social networking platforms, including Facebook and Twitter'.(18) Bahner and colleagues(78) at The Ohio State University used Twitter and Facebook simultaneously to deliver content to students directly to their mobile devices.

Conclusions

Education is a complex, context-dependent experience which *can* be enhanced by technological devices and programmes but we should take care to make sure that the technology serves the educational experience rather than drives it. Having said that, technology also presents new opportunities to facilitate the sharing and creation of educational material and the more active engagement of learners. Mobile technology, for example, profoundly effects the place and context of learning. In turn, it may start to make non-formal learning a core component of student and trainee development. Eraut suggests that 'person-to-person networking may yet prove to be [technology's] biggest impact'.(22) To enhance the adoption of technological advances in the support of education, educators should understand not only how the technology may address their needs and bring benefits, but also the implications for the learners and for resources, which may include time for

educator training. There is a need also to be aware of organisational politics and practicalities and, despite the prevalence of technological devices, it remains important for educators to avoid making assumptions either about learners' capacity to use technology or their access to it.

The importance of seeing technology as *a part* of the educational process cannot be over emphasised. Technology should not distract from the need for learners to reflect on their educational experiences so that their knowledge and learning can be embedded and applied to practice.

The availability of technology raises a number of issues for educators and currently, use of technology appears 'to be running ahead of leaders, policy-makers and educators'.(5) Educators have a role in supporting a more critical approach to learners' use of technology such as apps, Web 2.0 tools and the internet. Issues around etiquette point to the need for professionalism education to be built into TEL. Leaders of medical education need to play a key role in guiding the use of technology so that it *enhances* learning and in promoting rigorous research into what works, in what contexts and for whom.

References

1 Robin BR, Cook DA and McNeil SG (2012) Letter to the Editor. More about technology-enhanced learning in medical education: in reply. *Academic Medicine.* **87**(3): 256.

2 Watson JA and Pecchioni LL (2011) Digital natives and digital media in the college classroom: assignment design and impacts on student learning. *Educational Media International.* **48**(4): 307–20.

3 Jenkins M, Browne T, Walker R and Hewitt R (2011) The development of technology enhanced learning: findings from a 2008 survey of UK higher education institutions. *Interactive Learning Environments.* **19**(5): 447–65.

4 Cook DA, Levinson AJ, Garside S, Dupras DM, Erwin PJ and Montori VM (2008) Internet-based learning in the health professions: a meta-analysis. *Journal of the American Medical Association.* **300**: 1181–96.

5 Wallace S, Clark M and White J (2012) 'It's on my iPhone': attitudes to the use of mobile computing devices in medical education, a mixed-methods study. *BMJ Open.* **2**(4): e001099.

6 Curtis MT, Diaz Granados D and Feldman M (2012) Judicious use of simulation technology in continuing medical education. *Journal of Continuing Education in the Health Professions.* **32**(4): 255–60.

7 Westera W, Nadolski RJ, Hummel HGK and Wopereis IGJH (2008) Serious games for higher education: a framework for reducing design complexity. *Journal of Computer Assisted Learning.* **24**(5): 420–32.

8 Prensky M (2001) *Digital Game-Based Learning.* McGraw Hill, New York.

9 Harris JM, Sklar BM, Amend RW and Novalis-Marine C (2010) The growth, characteristics and future of online CME. *Journal of Continuing Education in the Health Professions.* **30**(1): 3–10.

10 Olson CA (2012) Editorial. CME congress, simulation technology, and the relationship between means and ends. *Journal of Continuing Education in the Health Professions.* **32**(4): 227–9.

11 Dror I, Schmidt P and O'Connor L (2011) A cognitive perspective on technology enhanced learning in medical training: great opportunities, pitfalls and challenges. *Medical Teacher.* **33**(4): 291–6.

12 Nolan T (2011) A smarter way to practise. *British Medical Journal.* **342**: d1124.

13 Gill P, Kamath A and Gill T (2012) Distraction: an assessment of smartphone usage in health care work settings. *Risk Management and Healthcare Policy.* **5**: 105–14.

14 Davies BS, Rafique J, Vincent TR *et al.* (2012) Mobile Medical Education (MoMEd) – how mobile information resources contribute to learning for undergraduate clinical students – a mixed methods study. *BMC Medical Education.* **12**: 1.

15 Hardyman W, Bullock AD, Brown A, Carter-Ingram S and Stacey M (2013) Mobile technology supporting trainee doctors' workplace learning and patient care: an evaluation. *BMC Medical Education.* **13**(6): 1–10. (http://www.biomedcentral.com/1472-6920/13/6; accessed 23 February 2013).

16 Yalcinalp S and Gulbahar Y (2010) Ontology and taxonomy design and development for personalised web-based learning systems. *British Journal of Educational Technology.* **41**: 883–96.

17 Fuad A and Hsu C-Y (2012) Letter to the Editor. E-learning=inequity in learning? *Medical Teacher.* **34**: 1087.

18 George DR and Dellasega C (2011) Use if social media in graduate-level medical humanities education: two pilot studies from Penn State College of Medicine. *Medical Teacher.* **33**: e429–34.

19 Stewart AR, Harlow DB and DeBacco K (2011) Students' experience of synchronous learning in distributed environments. *Distance Education.* **32**(3): 357–81.

20 Corbyn Z (2012) This could be huge. *Times Higher Education.* 6/12/12: 34–9.

21 Zuboff S (1988) *In the Age of the Smart Machine: The Future of Work and Power.* Basic, New York.

22 Eraut M and Hirsh W (2007) The significance of workplace learning for individuals, groups and organisations. SKOPE. (http://www.skope.ox.ac.uk/sites/default/files/Monogrpah%209.pdf; accessed 23 February 2013).

23 Meckfessel S, Stühmer C, Bormann KH *et al.* (2010) Introduction of e-learning in dental radiology reveals significantly improved results in final examination. *Journal of Cranio-Maxillo-Facial Surgery.* **39**(1): 40–8.

24 Raza A, Coomarasamy A and Khan KS (2009) Best Evidence continuous medical education. *Archives of Gynecology and Obstetrics.* **280**(4): 683–7.

25 Mazzoleni MC, Rognoni C, Finozzi E *et al.* (2009) Usage and effectiveness of e-learning curses for continuous medical education. *Studies in Health Technology and Informatics.* **150**: 921–5.

26 Cook DA, Levinson AJ and Garside S (2010) Time and learning efficiency in Internet-based learning: a systematic review and meta-analysis. *Advances in Health Sciences Education: Theory and Practice.* **15**: 755–70.

27 Gensichen J, Vollmar HC, Sönnichsen A, Waldmann U-M and Sandars J (2009) E-learning for education in primary healthcare – turning the hype into reality: a Delphi study. *European Journal of General Practice.* **15**: 11–4.

28 Robson J (2009) Web-based learning strategies in combination with published guidelines to change practice of primary care professionals. *British Journal of General Practice.* **59**(559): 104–9.

29 Rosen MA, Hunt EA, Pronovost PJ, Federowicz MA and Weaver SJ (2012) In situ simulation in continuing education for the health care professions: a systematic review. *Journal of Continuing Education in the Health Professions.* **32**(4): 243–54.

30 Kulier R, Coppus S, Zamora J *et al.* (2009) The effectiveness of a clinically integrated e-learning course in evidence-based medicine: a cluster randomised controlled trial. *BMC Medical Education.* **9**: 21.

31 Hugenholtz NI, de Croon EM, Smits PB, van Dijk FJ and Nieuwenhuijsen K (2008) Effectiveness of e-learning in continuing medical education for occupational physicians. *Occupational Medicine.* **58**(5): 370–2.

32 Wutoh R, Boren SA and Balas EA (2004) E-learning: a review of internet-based continuing medical education. *Journal of Continuing Education in the Health Professions.* **24**(1): 20–30.

33 Carroll C, Booth A, Papaioannou D, Sutton A and Wong R (2009) UK health-care professionals' experience of online learning techniques: a systematic review of qualitative data. *Journal of Continuing Education in the Health Professions.* **29**(4): 235–41.

34 Sandars J (2011) It appeared to be a good idea at the time but . . . A few steps closer to understanding how technology can enhance teaching and learning in medical education. *Medical Teacher.* **33**: 265–7.

35 Khogali SEO, Davies DA, Donnan PT *et al.* (2011) Integration of e-learning resources into a medical school curriculum. *Medical Teacher.* **33**: 311–8.

36 Hadley J, Kulier R, Zaomra J *et al.* (2010) Effectiveness of an e-learning course in evidence-based medicine for foundation (internship) training. *Journal of the Royal Society of Medicine.* **103**(7): 288–94.

37 Garland KV (2010) E-learning vs. classroom instruction in infection control in a dental hygiene program. *Journal of Dental Education.* **74**(6): 637–43.

38 Sfard A (1998) On two metaphors for learning and the dangers of choosing just one. *Educational Researcher.* **27**(2): 4–13.

39 Lave J and Wenger E (1991) *Situated Learning: Legitimate Peripheral Participation.* Cambridge University Press, Cambridge, UK.

40 Nonaka I (1994) A dynamic theory of organizational knowledge creation. *Organization Science.* **5**(1): 14–37.

41 Fish D and de Cossart L (2007) *Developing the Wise Doctor.* Royal Society of Medicine Press, London.

42 Knowles MS (1973) *The Adult Learner: A Neglected Species.* Gulf Publishing, Houston, TX.

43 Eraut M (2004) The practice of reflection. *Learning in Health and Social Care.* **3**(2): 47–52.

44 Kolb D (1984) *Experiential Learning.* Prentice-Hall, Englewood Cliffs, NJ.

45 Moon J (1999) *A Handbook of Reflective and Experiential Learning.* Routledge, London.

46 Delany C and Molloy E (2009) Critical reflection in clinical education: beyond the 'swampy lowlands'. In: Delany C and Molloy E (eds) *Clinical Education in the Health Professions,* pp. 3–24. Elsevier, Melbourne, Australia.

47 Cooksey D (2006) *A Review of UK Health Research Funding.* HM Treasury, London.

48 Mitton C, Adair C, McKenzie E, Patten S and Perry B (2007) Knowledge transfer and exchange: review and synthesis of the literature. *Milbank Quarterly.* **85**: 729–68.

49 Department of Health (2011) Innovation Health and Wealth: accelerating adoption and diffusion in the NHS. Department of Health, London.

50 Schifferdecker KE, Berman NB, Fall LH and Fischer MR (2012) Adoption of computer-assisted learning in medical education: the educators' perspective. *Medical Education.* **46**: 1063–73.

51 Carayon P, Hundt AS, Karsh B-T *et al.* (2006) Work system design for patient safety: the SEIPS model. *Quality and Safety in Health Care.* **15**(Suppl I): 50–5.

52 Naidr JP, Adla T, Janda A, Feberová J, Kassal P and Hladiková M (2004) Long-term retention of knowledge after a distance course in medical informatics at Charles University Prague. *Teaching and Learning in Medicine.* **16**(3): 255–9.

53 Asarbakhsh M and Sandars J (2013) E-learning: the essential usability perspective. *The Clinical Teacher.* **10**: 47–50.

54 Shortt SED, Guillemette J-M, Duncan AM and Kirby F (2010) Defining quality criteria for online continuing medical education modules using modified nominal group technique. *Journal of Continuing Education in the Health Professions.* **30**(4): 246–25.

55 Kirkpatrick D (1979) Techniques for evaluating training programs. *Training and Development.* **33**(6): 78–92.

56 Kirkpatrick D (1996) Great ideas revisited. Techniques for evaluating training programs. Revisiting Kirkpatrick's four-level model. *Training and Development.* **50**(1): 54–9.

57 Tapscott D (1998) *Growing Up Digital: The Rise of the Net Generation.* McGraw-Hill, New York.

58 Prensky M (2001) Digital natives, digital immigrants part 2: do they really think differently? *On the Horizon*. **9**(6): 1–6.

59 Wilkinson A, While AE and Roberts J (2009) Measurement of information and communication technology experience and attitudes to e-learning of students in the healthcare professions: integrative review. *Journal of Advanced Nursing*. **65**: 755–72.

60 Prince MJ, Cass HD and Klaber RE (2010) Accessing e-learning and e-resources. *Medical Education*. **44**: 436–7.

61 Schlager M (2004) Enabling new forms of online engagement: challenges for e-learning design and research. In: Duffy TM and Kirkley JR (eds) *Learner-Centered Theory and Practice in Distance Education: Cases from Higher Education*, pp. 91–104. Lawrence Erlbaum Associates Publishers, Mahwah, NJ.

62 London Knowledge Lab. The SCARLET – Scaffolding Rich Learning Experiences through Technology – project. (http://www.lkl.ac.uk/cms/index.php?option=com_content&task=view&id=419&Itemid=91; accessed 8 March 2013).

63 Luckin R (2008) The learner centric ecology of resources: a framework for using technology to scaffold learning. *Computers and Education*. **50**: 449–62.

64 Chretien KC, Greysen SR, Chretien JP and Kind T (2009) Online posting of unprofessional content by medical students. *Journal of the American Medical Association*. **302**(12): 1309–15.

65 Prgomet M, Georgiou A and Westbrook JI (2009) The impact of mobile handheld technology on hospital physicians' work practices and patient care: a systematic review. *Journal of the American Medical Informatics Association*. **16**(6): 792–801.

66 Ellaway R (2011) E-learning: is the revolution over? *Medical Teacher*. **33**: 297–302.

67 Selwyn N (2012) Editorial. Bursting out of the 'ed-tech' bubble. *Learning Media and Technology*. **37**(4): 331–4.

68 Selwyn N (2012) Editorial. Ten suggestions for improving academic research in education and technology. *Learning Media and Technology*. **37**(3): 213–9.

69 Bruff D (2009) *Teaching with Classroom Response Systems. Creating Active Learning Environments*. Jossey-Bass, San Francisco.

70 Premkumar K and Coupal C (2008) Rules of engagement – 12 tips for successful use of 'clickers' in the classroom. *Medical Teacher*. **30**: 146–9.

71 Nayak L and Erinjeri JP (2008) Audience response systems in medical student education benefit learner and presenters. *Academic Radiology*. **15**: 383–9.

72 Rubio EI, Bassignani MJ, White MA and Brant WE (2008) Effect of an audience response system on resident learning and retention of lecture material. *AJR. American Journal of Roentgenology*. **190**(6): W319–22.

73 Doucet M, Vrins A and Harvey D (2009) Effect of using an audience response system on learning environment, motivation and long term retention, during case-discussions in a large group of undergraduate veterinary clinical pharmacology students. *Medical Teacher*. **32**: e570–9.

74 Russel JS, McWilliams M, Chasen L and Faley J (2011) Using clickers for clinical reasoning and problem solving. *Nurse Educator*. **36**(1): 13–5.

75 Smith CM (2012) Harnessing mobile devices in the classroom. *Journal of Continuing Education in Nursing*. **43**(12): 539–40.

76 Rasmussen A, Lewis M and White J (2013) The application of wiki technology in medical education. *Medical Teacher*. **35**(2): 109–14.

77 Forgie SE, Duff JP and Ross S (2013) Twelve tips for using Twitter as a learning tool in medical education. *Medical Teacher*. **35**: 8–14.

78 Bahner DP, Adkins E, Patel N, Donley C, Nagel R and Kman NE (2012) How we use social media to supplement a novel curriculum in medical education. *Medical Teacher*. **34**: 439–44.

Further reading and resources

Department of Business Innovation and Skills (2010) Technology in learning. (http://repository.alt.ac.uk/839/2/ALT_TEL_evidence_document_for_BIS_low-res.pdf; accessed 9 March 2013).

http://edutechwiki.unige.ch/en/Main_Page
EduTechWiki from the University of Geneva is a resource kit for educational technology teaching and research. It contains over 1,200 articles.

http://www.qotfc.edu.au/resource/index.html
A module aimed at the occupational therapy practitioner considering educating a student on placement. It includes a range of reference documents, worksheets and resource templates.

http://resources4adultlearning.excellencegateway.org.uk/default.htm
Resources provided by the UK Quality Improvement Agency for improving adult learning.

http://www.lkl.ac.uk/cms/index.php
The London Knowledge lab of the Institute of Education, London. 'Exploring the future of learning with digital technologies'.

http://www.leeds.ac.uk/medicine/prof_dev/free.html
A link to free learning materials from the University of Leeds School of Medicine. Includes access to a checklist for designers of educational e-learning material.

12 e-Learning

Scott Rice[1] and Jean McKendree[2]
[1] University College London, UK
[2] Hull York Medical School, UK

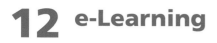

> **KEY MESSAGES**
>
> - Effective e-learning, or learning by using computer-based technology should be viewed as a curriculum design issue; technologies are tools, not teachers.
> - Blended learning, combining online and face-to-face teaching, is the most common approach to e-learning in undergraduate medical education.
> - Informal, opportunistic learning linked to the use of e-portfolios is increasingly prevalent in postgraduate settings and continuing professional development.
>
> - The bottom-up development of web 2.0 technologies and digital social networking is resulting in new communities of practice.
> - Using computer-based technologies effectively requires knowledge of how people learn, how to design interactions with the tools and how to evaluate best use given the desired learning outcomes.

Introduction

Claims about the ability of technology to transform teaching and learning are not new. The latest emerging technology is invariably heralded as the 'killer' invention that will make learning effortless. Most recently, claims have been made that using computers and the internet, an educational strategy often called e-learning, will lead us to reconceptualise learning and make teachers, schools and formal education obsolete:

> . . . the computer, and particularly, its future development, will change 'children's relationship with knowledge' producing a revolution comparable to that of the 'advent of printing and writing'.(1)
>
> In the new economy, where mindcraft replaces handicraft as the main form of work, HL [hyperlearning] makes obsolete the teaching, testing, and failure on which academic credentialism rests.(2)

Such effusive pronouncements are usually followed by a period of backlash and criticism attacking the enthusiasts and calling for a return to basic, traditional teaching, whatever that is conceived to be at the time. The aim of this chapter is to steer a course through this sea of hyperbole to find a safe harbour for those who are interested in using e-learning, but would like to anchor it on the rocks of research evidence and shared best practice.

Technologies on their own will not alter the fundamental fact that learning a discipline such as medicine will always require considerable effort on the part of students and teachers. However, there is evidence that technology can enhance teaching and learning, when used thoughtfully and appropriately.

This chapter outlines such approaches based on available research on using new (and not so new) technologies effectively. There are some references to examples and web resources in the text, and at the end of the chapter, but these have been kept brief deliberately, as there is no guarantee that the links will be there when you look for them – one pitfall of the internet as a learning resource. For a broader examination of the relationship between technology, and learning, *see* Chapter 11.

Computers and learning

The term 'electronic learning' or 'e-learning' is currently used in a variety of ways. Sometimes it refers to learning in which content or activity is delivered via computers in any way, sometimes to learning content from the worldwide web (www) and sometimes to the use of a virtual learning environment (VLE) or digital social network (DSN). For the purposes of this chapter, we use the term 'e-learning' to refer to any computer-aided approaches, although this use of the term is waning and web-based and VLE meanings are becoming more common. However, as many of the concepts apply to the wider scope, we will first cover non-internet-based learning approaches, as much of the fundamental research on effective learning with computers has been done in these areas.

Understanding Medical Education: Evidence, Theory and Practice, Second Edition. Edited by Tim Swanwick.
© 2014 The Association for the Study of Medical Education. Published 2014 by John Wiley & Sons, Ltd.

So, does computer-based learning 'work'? There are so many different types of and approaches to e-learning that it is almost impossible to give a simple 'yes or no' answer to this question. Instead, we will break it down into its component parts and examine some of the key research evidence.

Hypertext and read-only websites (web 1.0)

Over the last 15 years the worldwide web has developed as an information space with more than a billion users. It is a vast network of widely dispersed individuals, both in time and place, connecting to form virtual networks and communities. The original version of the web (web 1.0) is widely regarded as a medium in which a relatively small number of people published and most browsed.(3) Most of this publishing is founded in hypertext, or electronically linked, non-linear text. This established widespread use in late 1980s when HyperCard became available on the Macintosh computer, although the basic concept was outlined by Vannevar Bush in 1945,(4) and the term 'hypertext' was coined by Ted Nelson in 1963.(5) Prior to web-based delivery, early hypertexts tended to be tightly constructed, stand-alone programmes, rather like electronic textbooks. With the advent of the Internet, this type of resource varies now from online books, to packages of organised and inter-related materials, to random collections of text studded with links to pages all over the world.

Here we shall look only at the hypertext resources that have been designed primarily for teaching and consist mostly of text, with images, animations and videos. Do these facilitate learning? Does a textbook? The answer to both is, of course, 'yes', but only if the person reading the material pays attention and engages at a deep level. A great deal of research has shown that people who read material actively, that is, asking questions as they go, stopping to summarise points, taking notes, anticipating what the author will write next, can learn effectively from either online or paper texts.(6)

Such learning depends not only on the learner, but also on the quality of the resource. Just as some books are not very good, some web pages are not very useful. What is *not* effective is to put up a large amount of poorly structured, fragmented material with no guidance about what is intended to be learnt from it or how to approach learning.(7) Studies of hypertexts show that comprehension from large, complex, hyperlinked materials is generally poorer than from a well-structured book with the same information, and that readers tend not to see all the available information – in effect they get lost in hyperspace.(8)

However, well-designed hypertext can be useful for learning, when it makes explicit the connections between chunks of information in the domain (*see* Box 12.1). Navigating hypertext links can give the learner a clearer idea of the way that the information fits together in the domain to form a coherent whole. Some possible ways this can be accomplished is to design hypertexts around goal-oriented tasks, such as answering questions as they read, or by constructing a *concept map*(9) which explicitly displays the

BOX 12.1 HOW TO: Use online hypertext

- If putting up large amounts of text electronically, make sure there is a clear index or navigation structure and consider breaking it into sensible chunks in case students prefer to print it out and read it.

- If such a text is intended to be used with other, more interactive electronic resources, consider removing it to a separate 'user manual' or introduction selection, rather than including it with the interactive resources.

- Consider using graphical navigation and a suggested set of activities for hypertexts that are intended to be read in their entirety.

- Often the most useful online hypertexts are reference books that are easily searchable and not intended to be read fully (e.g. http://www.statsoft.com/textbook).

relationships between different sections of a hypertext. A good example of such an approach is the Visual Thesaurus at http://www.visualthesaurus.com.

Computer-aided learning

These are increasingly web-based e-learning software packages that have not only textual and pictorial information, but interactive exercises as well. This type of package is referred to as, variously, computer-aided learning, computer-based tutorials or training, computer-assisted instruction, or simply courseware. The NHS has invested heavily in this approach using a web-based e-learning software platform as a base to its e-learning for Healthcare platform http://www.e-lfh.org.uk to support, among other areas, speciality training.

Many such packages have self-assessment questions included as students work through the software. Given equivalent amounts of time, students using these types of package that more or less reproduce a coursebook – with perhaps some animations and assessment questions – generally learn at a very similar level to the level they would learn at if they were using a textbook, and they often enjoy using the software packages more than they enjoy using textbooks. A screenshot of a typical computer-aided learning package is shown in Figure 12.1.

In some computer-aided learning packages, the student is presented with structured exercises emphasising repeated practice of an increasing skill, often until a certain criterion is met. This was the fundamental idea behind BF Skinner's *Teaching Machines* in the late 1950s,(10) and more recently in *Integrated Learning Systems* used in many UK schools. A typical example would be software that lets children practise addition and subtraction skills. Such programmes have also been used to help students in the health professions become proficient at dosage calculations, radiograph interpretation, electrocardiogram lead placement and other

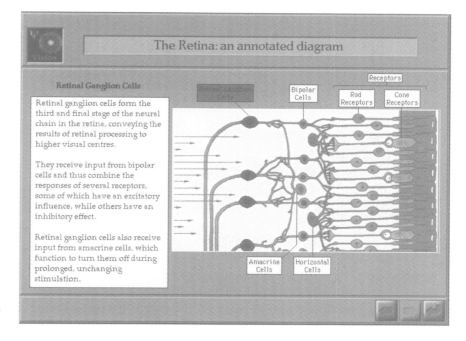

Figure 12.1 Example of a computer-assisted learning software screen.
Source: From PsyCLE © University of York for the TLTP PsyCLE consortium; used with permission.

skills that benefit from extended practice. This type of 'drill-and-practice' software is sometimes maligned as being proscriptive, unimaginative and old-fashioned. However, when used appropriately, it can teach fundamental skills very effectively.

Using technology to practise basic skills can be highly effective according to a large body of data and a long history of use.(11) Students usually learn more, and learn more rapidly, in courses that use computer-assisted instruction (CAI). This has been shown to be the case across all subject areas, from pre-school to higher education, and in both regular and special education classes. Fletcher *et al.*(12) report that in the military, where emphasis is on short and efficient training time, the use of CAI can cut training time by one-third. CAI can also be more cost-effective than additional tutoring, reduced class size or increased instruction time to attain equivalent educational gains.(13)

While this kind of e-learning can indeed lead to better mastery of procedures that lend themselves to repeated practice, research has shown that spaced exposure is very important – ten minutes per day three-to-four times a week is more effective than 30–40 minutes at one go.(14) This is a finding backed up by decades of psychological research on learning in general – and which dictates against cramming for exams, too.

Again, exercises need to be well designed. This crucial issue of instructional design is important in all forms of teaching, of course, and is one that is all too frequently ignored. Another reason for the effective learning seen in these systems is the delivery of instantaneous feedback. Feedback is critical for all learning, but immediate feedback is especially effective when basic skills are involved, where

practising incorrectly can cause a wrong method to become engrained and difficult to change.(15)

Simulation

A giant step up in complexity from these practical exercise-based systems is simulation. In simulation, a student must work through an exercise of some sort, but one that exemplifies much of the complexity of a real-world situation. Simulations may or may not involve instructional feedback; the problems may be highly complex or relatively simple; they may be high or low fidelity. In all of these, the goal is for the student to actually *apply* knowledge in order to solve a problem or resolve the situation in an environment that attempts to capture at least some of the important features of the real world.

These types of programme can lead to very effective learning, if they capture the critical characteristics of the situation the student is intended to be learning. It is fairly obvious, and there is plenty of supporting evidence, that high-fidelity (and highly expensive) simulators such as those used for teaching airplane pilots or surgeons can be effective. Less high-fidelity e-learning simulations can also teach students effectively, when they emphasise the reasoning and knowledge underlying the concepts being taught. However, with all simulation teaching, other factors such as feedback and integration into the larger curriculum are critical for effective learning.(16)

However, with such simulations there can be a problem with students becoming proficient at playing the 'game' without learning the underlying lessons. It is critical to combine relatively unstructured simulations with

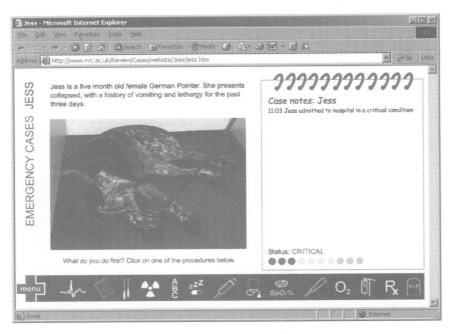

Figure 12.2 Example simulation: Jess the dog.
Source: Emergency Case Simulator © Royal Veterinary College 2006; used with permission.

discussions of the concepts students are intended to illustrate and specific tasks or assessments in order to best promote learning. Any exercise using concrete examples, electronic or not, can benefit from being explicitly framed in the larger domain to promote a grasp of abstract concepts.(17) Indeed, to be effective, the e-learning approaches discussed in this chapter should always be embedded and framed in an educational environment that includes activities, discussion and reflection – this 'learning conversation' is designed to be conducive to promoting effective learning (Figure 12.2).

The range of available simulation equipment and the effective design and use of simulation is covered in detail in Chapter 13.

Learning styles and e-Learning

There is an intuitive appeal to the popular idea that e-learning may be effective because it caters to different learning styles. While this may be true, evidence is very mixed and the area is controversial. One difficulty is that there are many different meanings of 'learning style' and many different instruments to measure it. A systematic review of learning style studies(18) found over 70 different measures being used in the literature, only a handful of which had been researched sufficiently to make sound judgements about reliability or predictive validity.

There is also variation in the underlying assumptions about where learning style differences might originate. The measures found in the review suggested three sources of learning style variation: constitutional and ability measures, and instructional preferences.

The *constitutional measures*, implying an innate or fixed trait, tend to be tied either to sensory modality (e.g. visual, kinaesthetic or auditory) or to a stable personality measure. The review concluded that there was no reliable evidence that matching teaching either to adult learners' measured sensory preference or to their personality measure aided learning. In fact, some studies cited suggested that pictorial materials helped *all* learners, no matter what their self-reported preference, and may have had the biggest benefit for those labelled as 'verbal' by the learning style instruments.

Nevertheless, there is evidence that presenting information in more than one modality may help all learners, no matter what their particular score on any given measure.(19) The 'dual-code' theory(20) that originated in the 1970s indicates that presenting information in multiple ways allows learners to integrate knowledge by having multiple representations and links, so that assimilation with existing knowledge is stronger, and therefore recall is improved.

Ability measures of learning style are those that consider that learners have relatively stable, if not fixed, abilities that direct their learning preferences and are not likely to change (e.g. convergent-divergent thinking, focusing-scanning). Again, there is inconclusive evidence that matching teaching and learning styles promotes better learning, but another confounding factor is that these measures tend to be correlated with various measures of aptitude,(18) and thus may simply be reflecting variations in general intelligence, rather than a 'learning style' in the usual sense of equally effective but different approaches to learning. There is much debate here whether instruction should match the students' abilities or should create a mismatch in order to encourage adoption of a wider range of approaches to learning.

The final category of learning style addresses *instructional preferences* or approaches to study. These tend to emphasise that students have preferences about approaches to learning, but these may be flexible depending on context and motivation. In fact, the evidence is that good learners are 'versatile': able to adapt their approach to what needs to be learnt and the amount of time available to do so. Probably one of the best known researchers in this area currently is Noel Entwistle, who has evolved the Approaches to Study Skills Inventory for Students (ASSIST) over the past 30 years.(21) The ASSIST instrument gives an indication of whether students tend to be deep, strategic or shallow learners. Entwistle discusses the difference between a student's *style*, which is the preferred approach to learning, and *strategy*, which is the approach adopted at any given time according to the perceived demands of the task at hand.

Briefly, surface learners have an extrinsic motivation for learning: earning a high mark, fear of failure. Typically, this results in an emphasis on rote learning and a focus on getting through assessments. Deep learners have more intrinsic motivations: curiosity, commitment to the subject. They will make more of an attempt to analyse new knowledge, derive general principles and seek understanding, rather than learning just enough to pass exams. Strategic learners use a combination of strategies. They become adept at choosing study methods based on the cues they have picked up as to what type of work will result in the best outcomes for the given curriculum. Some studies have shown that medical students, often the very good ones, tend to start out as deep learners, but may move towards being strategic, probably due to the heavy demands of a typical course, plus the traditional emphasis on summative, knowledge-based assessments. In fact, strategic learning has a significant positive correlation with final marks,(22) so in the current climate, this may be the best strategy for students to adopt.

In the end, students will adopt what is suggested by the teaching – surface learning will emerge under time pressure and examinations that stress factual learning; deep learning emerges via extended activities, student–student interaction, learning conversations and problem-based learning.(23)

So what can we conclude about the relationship between these various style measures and e-learning? The lack of strong evidence for matching preferred style to presentation of learning content does not necessarily mean it is not useful, but this is a complex and contested area. While the debate rumbles on, it is best to design materials using as many of the modes of presentation as are appropriate to the domain, which may also tend to allow more flexibility in use, according to student needs.

It is also the case that learning style measures can be useful as tools to generate a discussion with students about their own learning processes. Students often find these scales very interesting and can learn important lessons by working through one (it does not really matter which one) and then comparing their results with those of other students. This often demonstrates that people do not all choose to approach learning in the same way, which can be a useful insight for students and may help smooth tensions – for instance, in a problem-based learning group or an online discussion in which people prefer to approach the learning along different paths.

Workplace-based learning and continuing professional development

In the previous sections, the emphasis has been on *e-learning* in a formal course of instruction, particularly in an undergraduate medical curriculum. Of course, doctors are learning informally and formally throughout their careers, in the workplace and through a process of continuing professional development (CPD). Increasingly, these established practitioners depend on technology for supporting this learning.

Some online resources offer easily accessible and quickly updated sources of information, such as the electronic *British National Formulary* (http://www.bnf.org) or point of care decision-making aids such as DynaMed (https://dynamed.ebscohost.com/). Moreover, the explosion in advanced mobile technologies such as smart-phones and tablet-computers has seen a proliferation in 'apps' or mobile applications that are downloaded from the internet and used as a mobile reference. While these are not e-learning tools per se, such resources begin to blur the lines between reference books and professional development tools. For instance, all general practitioners (GPs) in the UK now use computers in consultations, and many will regularly consult systems such as GP Notebook (http://www.gpnotebook.co.uk), an online reference database that also offers a tracking service that records the information that the doctor has looked up and collates it for use as evidence of educational activity during the year. The GP can then add personal notes and record their learning needs in the electronic record.

This 'just-in-time' learning, what Eraut(24) refers to as 'opportunistic' or 'reactive' learning, is where much new knowledge is encountered once doctors are practising. The danger with this approach is that such knowledge may remain tacit or disconnected from other knowledge and perhaps difficult to recall or apply in future. To be most fruitful, such informally encountered knowledge must be integrated with other experiences and eventually become more generalised so that it is not tied to a single context or incident. Time for reflection is needed to assimilate and clarify information, and turn such reactive learning encounters into more usable knowledge. Portfolio-based tools, such as the NHS e-Portfolio developed by NHS Education for Scotland (http://www.nhseportfolios.org) are intended to promote this type of reflection on experience in a professional context.

Online CPD, a more formal approach to work-based learning, is becoming more commonplace. Some courses involve timetabled modules with online tutor support such as those leading to university-accredited postgraduate awards. Some can be started at any time, but offer interactions with other students and tutors during a specified time period. Some offer modules that can be worked through at any time, with self-assessment questions at the end, which carry CPD credit, a good example of which is the extensive suite of offerings from BMJ Learning http://n3.learning.bmj.com/learning/home.html

Virtual learning environments

The term 'e-learning' is often used to refer to the use of a *virtual* or *managed* learning environment. These systems are not actually learning technologies themselves, in terms of being the content to be learned, but they provide a framework or infrastructure into which materials are placed and in which activities take place. They are part of a larger learning environment, in the way that classrooms, computers networks and libraries are in a university. Just as these physical facilities need to be planned to be effective for students, so the choice and use of a virtual learning environment need planning and support to be usefully implemented.

In general, although the terminology is still evolving, a VLE refers to the teaching and administrative tools available in a system, while a managed learning environment also includes tools such as those for admissions, finance and enrolment at an institutional level. You may also find these called 'enterprise systems', which generally refers to very large, commercial VLEs intended to manage and integrate data from many institutional information sources. This section will refer to VLEs, because it concentrates on those tools that directly affect the tutors and students in a medical course. It does not go into any great detail about specific VLEs, since they are evolving constantly. The example screenshots are from the system used at Hull York Medical School, which happens to be Blackboard™, but this is not intended to be an endorsement, simply a convenience.

Blended learning

There is a common misunderstanding that e-learning via a VLE implies that the course is a distance-learning course, that is, one in which the learner is at a location geographically distant from the tutors and never sees them face to face. There are some courses like this delivered using VLEs, such as those from the Open University (www.open.ac.uk), but VLEs are actually predominantly used as one aspect of a course in which students meet regularly with tutors and other students, sometimes in an otherwise relatively traditional course. This use of VLEs combined with face-to-face teaching is called *blended learning*.

The crucial aspect of blended learning is to think very hard about which aspects of a course are well supported by a VLE and which are best supported face to face, or in other ways. The next section reviews some of the current uses for VLEs in medical schools.

Content delivery

In the early days of the web and VLEs, many course instructors simply put up all their lecture notes and PowerPoint presentations electronically and did nothing more. The VLE certainly can be a useful repository for *content* such as presentations, especially those with colour images that may best be viewed on a screen rather than on a small, black-and-white printout. Such content areas can be very useful for student revision by gathering the resources from each year into a single, readily accessible area, and they can help to manage content in the curriculum by timing the release of items, providing rapid updates of documents and allowing access to commonly used items such as student forms. The screenshot in Figure 12.3 shows a content area in which a radiograph appears as part of a consultation with a 'virtual patient', and the VLE has posted an announcement for the students to review it for the next problem-based learning session.

There are an increasing number of repositories of useful electronic teaching resources being shared among institutions. They contain a variety of types of content, such as images, videos, short interactive exercises and self-assessment questions. These content items are often called *reusable learning objects*. The concept behind this growing area is that objects can be designed to be downloaded and used flexibly in the local VLE by tutors in the context of their own curriculum, rather than having a large amount of fixed content such as most of the computer-aided learning packages discussed previously.

Assessment

Another very common use of VLEs is to deliver assessment, either formative (that does not feed into an official assessment for the course) or summative (that is part of the official assessment). Most VLEs come with tools to write common types of questions such as multiple choice, extended matching, fill in the blank and true/false. Testing tools allow flexible administration, such as having tests appear and disappear either at a specified time or when a student has completed another activity satisfactorily, allowing students to have one or multiple attempts, presenting randomised questions, and marking automatically and entering the marks into an online gradebook. Also, many VLEs allow seamless integration of external online assessment packages such as Questionmark Perception™ (https://www.questionmark.com/uk/perception), which is widely used for both formative and summative exams (Box 12.2).

E-portfolios

A more recent VLE development is the *e-portfolio*. While these tools are still developing, most allow students and other learners to organise and annotate any materials they have online, including essays, personal statements, feedback collected from tutors, images, or any other item that might feed into a portfolio and is available electronically. Students can submit material to a specified tutor for marking and feedback, and the tutor mark will automatically be recorded in the online gradebook in the VLE. Some

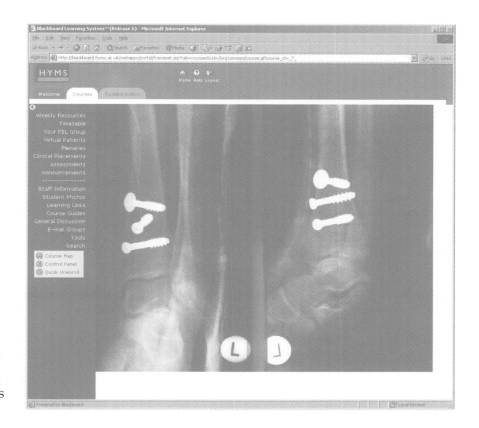

Figure 12.3 Example of content in a virtual learning environment.
Source: Screenshot from Hull York Medical School Blackboard™ VLE, copyright HYMS 2006.

BOX 12.2 FOCUS ON: Computer-based assessment

Computer-based assessment is a major area that in increasing in sophistication and use. Chapter 18 covers this in greater detail, but a few of the possibilities and advantages will be mentioned here.

Of course, one major reason for using computer-based testing is the opportunity for automated scoring and immediate feedback to students. In the past, test items have been limited to easily scored question types such as multiple choice, true-false and matching. Recently, however, researchers have made progress in automated scoring of essays using Latent Semantic Analysis.(25)

Because computers can monitor a students' performance in real time, it is possible for a system to adapt the test to the ability and level of the individual student. In sequential testing, a

short test is given to all candidates. If the calculated confidence interval shows that a student has clearly passed or clearly failed, those students do not have to continue. For those students for whom there is still uncertainty, more test items can be presented, until a judgement can be made or the system runs out of test items.

Computer-adaptive testing is similar in concept, but here the system begins by presenting all candidates with a test item that has been judged to be moderately difficult. If the student answers correctly, a more difficult item is presented; if the candidate answers incorrectly, an easier one is given. Using this method, the relative competence of the candidate can be gauged, and the system can suggest areas where further study should be considered.

---

portfolio tools also allow students to sign up for tutorial sessions and record the agreed outcomes of such meetings, keep learning diaries, link evidence to specific learning outcomes for personal development planning or reaccreditation, or build an online curriculum vitae. The student can manage the content, so that material can be kept private, made public or permission granted to specified people

only. E-portfolios are also in common use in postgraduate training and continuing professional development where evidence is collected to form the basis of periodic reviews of progression or fitness for continuance of practice. The University of Newcastle (UK) provides a useful resource for those interested in e-portfolios and personal development planning (PDP) at http://www.eportfolios.ac.uk.

Communication

Perhaps most interestingly, VLEs are widely used to facilitate different types of communication. Email, of course, is used widely by students and tutors, and discussion lists and chat rooms were around long before the appearance of VLEs. But a VLE can pull together different methods and allow students and tutors to choose the most appropriate methods for the moment. Probably the most widely used communication tool in most VLEs is the *asynchronous threaded discussion forum*. These tools allow learners or tutors to log in at any time, read contributions by others and respond without the need for anyone else to be using the tool at the same time. Figure 12.4 is a screenshot showing an example of one such forum. In this example, a student posted a question about confidence intervals, and a list of the headings of responses by other students appears at the bottom of the screen. In this case, the students themselves answered the question satisfactorily, possibly more quickly than a tutor would have done. Tutors should monitor the discussions regularly to make sure that the information is correct, but often it is the case that students are perfectly capable of answering the questions. This can be a very important factor in promoting the acceptance by students of their peers as a 'learning resource' and can reduce the attitude that only lecturers are acceptable as sources of help.

Discussion forums

Discussion forums can be useful for allowing tutors or students to post and discuss questions and debate issues. An important aspect of using these forums, however, is to establish rules for using the forum, sometimes called 'netiquette'. Generally, these are commonsense guidelines, such as keeping to the topic, being courteous, using appropriate language and not writing huge amounts. It is a good idea for somebody with some authority to monitor forums in case something gets out of hand or posts need to be removed for whatever reason.

An important factor in using discussion forums effectively, particularly if you want to include student discussion as an official component of the course, is defining specific tasks to get students started. It is seldom sufficient to simply say, 'Discuss the course here'. Often, the first task in a course is for students to post a short introduction about themselves in order to learn how to use the forum. The tutor may then post a specific question for discussion or may assign students to summarise a reading and post a question. Such discussion areas can be very effective as learning tools, if used as an integral part of the course, just as face-to-face discussion can be a very useful pedagogical intervention.(17)

Administration and management

And finally, while perhaps not as pedagogically interesting, VLEs can be very useful for administration and management functions, such as submitting and time-stamping assignments, signing up for student electives, sending group emails and posting reminders or urgent announcements. Many now integrate anti-plagiarism software within the uploading platform, and some have been used to release official exam results: after authenticating via their system login, students are allowed to see final marks in the gradebook.

Figure 12.5 shows the results from a survey of 51 UK medical, dental and veterinary schools summarising the

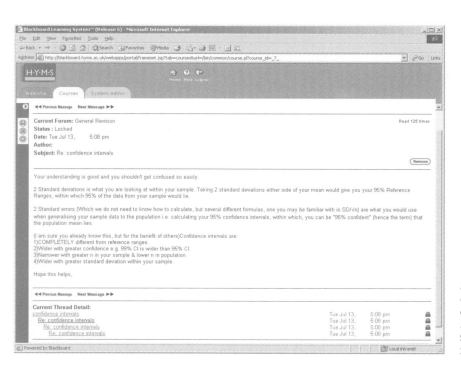

Figure 12.4 Example of an asynchronous discussion forum in a virtual learning environment.
Source: Screenshot from Hull York Medical School Blackboard™ VLE, copyright HYMS 2006.

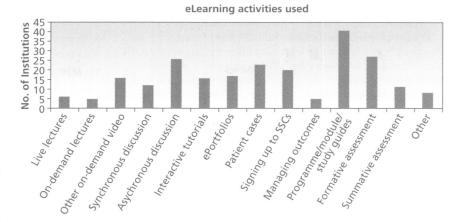

Figure 12.5 Use of virtual learning environments in UK medical schools. *Source*: ©University of Bristol, as appeared in the Subject Centre for Medicine, Dentistry and Veterinary Medicine Newsletter, Spring 2006.

different uses of their VLEs.(26) It is apparent that schools choose to use these tools in different ways, adapting and selecting them based on their own curriculum needs.

Web 2.0 technologies

Web 2.0 technology or 'participatory web' refers to a new set of internet applications allowing users to generate content, comment and evaluate others users' actions, and belong to various virtual communities.(27) The term is used to describe a second generation of web-based communities that have emerged following the development and implementation of a wide range of social networking software. This key feature of web 2.0 technologies is the requirement of minimal technical expertise to develop content and interact with others, thus enhancing individuals' ability to manage their virtual environment. It is user-driven and directed and may be seen as 'bottom up' delivery system of content, in contrast with the original structure of the internet, which required specialist skills and little interaction.

In medical education there are now a range of approaches that allow individuals to produce content and to develop and manage their virtual networks. The advent of web 2.0 has enabled more users to connect and collaborate through digital social networks and a new generation of VLEs. Web 2.0 services are not really technologies as such, but services (or user processes) created using the building blocks of the technologies and open standards that underpin the internet and the web.(3) As with many e-learning tools, some of the newly emerging technologies emphasise communication among learners and there are several web 2.0 applications used in medical education.

Instant messaging

This allows synchronous communication between learners and/or teachers individually or in groups. Examples include Facebook™ Messenger (http://www.facebook.com), Twitter™ (https://twitter.com) and Yahoo!™ Messenger

(www.yahoo.com). Additionally, applications such as Skype™ enable group communication with video-conferencing and voice through the internet. Skype has been used as a powerful tool to support learning, where students are based remotely from campus. It enables face-to-face communication with the personal tutor to discuss progress and any problems that have been encountered in real time. It requires relatively low technology (a workstation with appropriate software and/or a 3G phone) and is of low or no cost to the student.

Blogs

The weblog is a more recent use of online communication. These are websites where new pages or entries can be entered easily without knowing HTML or web page authoring software. However, contributions to blogs are generally restricted to the owner or a chosen group of members. They are similar to a discussion forum, but are generally organised as pages of text, rather than threads or hierarchies, as is typical of a discussion forum. Many VLEs now supply blog tools, and the weblog has been adopted in some institutions as a personal online journal accessible by all web users, including fellow students.

A particularly powerful example of the flexibility of web 2.0 applications and the spectrum of stand-alone versions is demonstrated in the BMJ blog (http://blogs.bmj.com). This site provides numerous different blogs in topics, ranging from childhood disease to the thoughts of those currently training. There is a comments feature built in within the blog, where readers are able to give 'rapid responses'. It is also is supported by Real Simple Syndication (RSS feeds), which keeps users up-to-date when comments are made or the blog is updated.

Wikis

These are similar to blogs but allow the text on the website to be edited by others, with the creation of a common document that can be shared between individuals. Wikis are thus collaborative web applications. Probably one of the best-known examples of a wiki is *Wikipedia* (http://

www.wikipedia.org), a shared and constantly evolving encyclopaedia to which anyone can contribute.

Wikipedia's definition of a wiki is: 'A **wiki** ("wee-kee" or "wick-ey") is a type of website that allows anyone visiting the site to add, to remove, or otherwise to edit all content, very quickly and easily . . . This ease of interaction and operation makes a wiki an effective tool for collaborative writing'.

There has been some debate about the academic accuracy of material on a wiki, *Wikipedia* in particular. A major criticism is there is little quality assurance and some, if not a majority, of the information is unreliable with no source author. Clearly, within clinical education the focus must therefore be on teaching and developing of critical appraisal skills and challenging the reliability of all information, including that on web 2.0 applications.

Social bookmarking

An individual's favourite websites, including blogs, can be 'bookmarked' and stored on a website or mobile internet device. Examples include del.icio.us (http://del.icio.us/) and digg (www.digg.com). These bookmarks can be shared with others. Whilst not a primary learning resource, these applications are a useful adjunct to online learning and may be incorporated into individual students VLEs or social networks to share information and pages of interest.

Media sharing

Visual media can be uploaded and stored on a website, such as Flickr (www.flickr.com) for photographs and You Tube (www.youtube.com) for videos. These media can then be shared with others. This may be particularly powerful in medical education, as practical procedures or clinical photographs may be recorded and uploaded by the teacher and accessed by learners remotely. The use of hand-held devices such as the iPad or iPhone enables students to review practical procedures in a clinical area.

Digital social networking

Digital social networking (DSN) is no longer a niche phenomenon and is quickly becoming ubiquitous online as a key feature of web 2.0 technology, with the most popular networks including Facebook™ (www.facebook.com) and Twitter™ (www.twitter.com). Box 12.3 provides a more comprehensive list. DSNs enable individuals to: construct a public or semi-public profile within a system; articulate a list of other users with whom they share a connection; and view and traverse their list of connections and those made by others within the system.(28) The unique feature of DSNs is their ability to be mobile and 'always on'.

The use of DSNs in education is accelerating and some medical education institutions themselves are beginning to apply this technology to develop online student identities and e-communities. An example of this is the development of Community@Brighton.(29) This is currently believed to be the world's largest higher education-based social network with some 36,000 registered users, comprising students, staff and associates of the medical school and university.

Challenges of participatory web, and DSNs in particular, are predominantly based around privacy, intellectual prop-

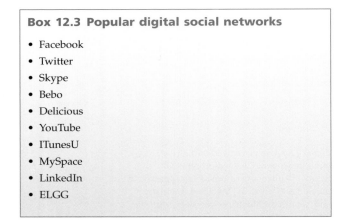

Box 12.3 Popular digital social networks

- Facebook
- Twitter
- Skype
- Bebo
- Delicious
- YouTube
- ITunesU
- MySpace
- LinkedIn
- ELGG

erty and the longevity of digital information. Although DSNs offer novel opportunities for interaction among their users, they also attract non-users' attention, particularly within medical education, because of the privacy concerns they raise.(30) Such concerns may be well placed; each post, message or 'conversation' may be recorded indefinitely and can be searched, replicated and altered, and even accessed by others without the knowledge of the individual making the initial post. Crucially, all activities within DSNs are underpinned by a public domain approach to issues of intellectual property rights, where concerns over propriety do not hinder the distribution and use of online content.(31) Thus, content may remain linked with an individual long after the user's attitudes and behaviours have changed.

Massive open online courses

A recent development are online courses aimed at large-scale participation and open access via the internet. Originating in Canada, the aim is to 'provide all who want to learn with access to available resources at any time in their lives; empower all who want to share what they know to find those who want to learn it from them; and, finally furnish all who want to present an issue to the public with the opportunity to make their challenge known'.(32) Course content is often aggregated via RSS feeds and made available via web pages or email, and learners could participate with their choice of tools: threaded discussions in Moodle, blog posts, Second Life and synchronous online meetings.(33)

The key aspect of Massive Open Online Courses (MOOC) are platforms that enable the operations involved to be done effectively. There are now two types of MOOC. One is cMOOC, a model that encourages knowledge creation, creativity, autonomy and learning via social networking. The other is xMOOC, a system that focuses on knowledge duplication and skill acquisition.(32) There has been a surge of interest recently in MOOCs. Universities around the world have been combining to place course material online and make it available for free or for nominal fees. The most established courses are offered by Udacity (www.udacity.com), Coursera (www.coursera.org), which now has 33 partner universities, and edX (https://www.edx.org), which has content from several major US institutions.

Pedagogical aspects of web 2.0-mediated learning

The participatory web (web 2.0) provides potential to develop new approaches to curriculum development. With abundant content and sources, educators can draw from a pool of open educational resources and provide students with better and more varied teaching than individual teachers could develop alone.(32) This new 'learning territory' presents new opportunities in medical education and incorporates aspects of formal teaching, the hidden curriculum and role modelling.

The basic approach of much of web 2.0-based teaching remains based on traditional pedagogy, relying primarily on information transmission, computer-marked assignments and sometimes peer assessment. Most xMOOCs use approaches that are already well known in distance learning, such as structured texts, videos or PowerPoint presentations, followed by exercises to apply what has been presented, ideally followed by immediate feedback. More participatory technologies such as blogs and RSS feeds may personalise learning but this, in reality, is often simply an alternative route through material. A true pedagogical challenge therefore is to stimulate an online community of practice where discussion, motivation and an understanding of an individual student's needs are addressed through extended engagement with experts and fellow students to foster deep understanding and personal ownership of learning.

In medical education one of the most powerful ways of learning professional behaviour and values is through experience of positive role models, both formally and informally. In role-modelling, students observe behaviours of others, and a teacher will traditionally guide a group to make sense of these observed behaviours. With participatory web-based learning and the development of MOOCs and an e-curriculum, learning of some areas of knowledge, skills and attitudes in virtual spaces (e.g. through gaming) may not need to replicate the real world. DSNs therefore constitute an extended social context where role-modelling occurs within a wider 'learning territory' with multiple communities of practice.

Emerging approaches and technologies

New technologies that could be integrated into e-learning frameworks are constantly being introduced. This section mentions just a few such new developments with pointers to some examples of use. However, the basic principle is still the same: why are you using these in the context of your curriculum? Do not feel the need to cave in to students demanding the latest 'whizzy' technology unless there is a good reason to do so and adequate expertise and support are available. Having said that, often the students themselves may be a source of such expertise and may help schools develop innovative uses of these new tools.

The flipped classroom
A blended learning approach is one in which podcasts of lectures are distributed to be watched by students before coming to the scheduled classroom session. That meeting then becomes a time for facilitated discussion around the questions or issues raised by students and activities applying the content of the recorded lectures, such as analysis of clinical scenarios or other real problems in the domain. This promotes self-regulated learning in the students and fosters a more personalised experience for the group, allowing the time with the expert to be used for active experimentation, exploration and dialogue. Stanford University Medical School is considering replacing all lectures with this approach.(34)

Mobile learning
Sometimes called M-learning or nomadic learning, it refers to learning in which the student is using a mobile device such as a phone, hand-held personal computer (PC), or tablet computer. While this is very similar to e-learning with VLEs, the primary difference is the ability to 'carry the learning' so that resources are at hand wherever they might be needed. Also, information can be 'beamed' to a device when it is detected, to deliver information at the most appropriate time and place. This type of mobile resource is also becoming common in schools and hospitals for accessing information such as formularies, filling in common forms and recording other information, as well as for learning purposes.

Haptic technologies
These are high-fidelity, web 2.0-based technologies that integrate tactile sensation applying force, vibration or motion to a user. Their use in medicine is being translated from the gaming industry and is being developed in surgery to allow surgical trainees to practise procedures. Haptic technology aids simulation by creating a realistic environment of touch.

Web 3.0
Web 3.0 is much talked about but poorly defined. Some consider the next generation of web technologies to be the convergence of the virtual and physical world, with a platform capability layer that includes TV-quality open video, 3D simulation, augmented reality and pervasive broadband or wireless capabilities. Web 3.0's most defining characteristic will be the mass diffusion of high-definition quality video to TVs, laptops, tablets and mobile devices, along with intuitive searching, automatic location recognition and person-specific search results. According to some internet experts, web 3.0 will allow the user to sit back and let the internet do all of the work for them.

Conclusions

So what is e-learning? Currently, the term tends to be used in a very techno-centric way, with definitions built around descriptions of the types of hardware and software used in teaching and learning. However, views are changing and conceptualisations of e-learning are becoming less about delivery and more about the more interaction with the learner. A recent research review proposes a new definition: 'e-Learning is the capability required of a learner/user in order that they can manage their own learning . . .

using technology as appropriate to context, sector and task'.(35)

In essence, this captures the main argument of this chapter – e-learning technologies by themselves are tools, not teachers. Too often, e-learning resources are left isolated from the rest of the educational experience. Decades of research on technology-supported learning has shown that this approach is not the most effective means for using these tools, and the key is to use these tools when and if appropriate, with thought given as to how to integrate them into the curriculum and help students and tutors become proficient and discerning users. Factors that are important for design of effective e-learning, adapted from Issenberg *et al.*, include the following:

• *curriculum integration*: integration of [e-learning]-based exercises into the standard medical school or postgradu-

ate educational curriculum is an essential feature of their effective use

• *providing feedback*: educational feedback is the most important feature of [e-learning]-based medical education

• *individualised learning*: the importance of having . . . educational experiences where learners are active participants, not passive bystanders

• *defined outcomes*: clearly stated goals with tangible outcome[s] . . . will more likely lead to [effective learning].(16)

Figure 12.6 encapsulates some of these principles and summarises a framework for designing and using VLEs and associated computer-based learning resources in a blended model of e-learning. The key is to create a resource that is useful to the students and to keep it relevant and current in order to make the most effective use of your educational environment.

Phase 1: preparation of the course (design phase)	Establish your rationale for using computer-based learning resources, and identify what links there will be between computer-based and other activities. Present students with a clear need to work online, i.e. demonstrate how the virtual component is relevant and adds value. Devise an assessment scheme that promotes learning in both eLearning and other activities.
Phase 2: Socialising learners and tutors (start of the course)	Orientate tutors and students to the aims and objectives of the module, along with your approach and what they're likely to gain from it. Induct participants to your selected tools. Set expectations regarding their participation and 'netiquette'. Build in preparatory exercises that encourage knowledge sharing and discussion, and a sense of collective ownership over the site by welcoming and responding to feedback.
Phase 3: Supporting participation online and maintaining activity	Provide ongoing support to minimise any user anxiety and build confidence. Actively guide and facilitate online; model targeted learning; provide feedback; encourage students to discuss and share. Maintain currency of site, e.g. introduce new resources, and stage new activities. Recognise online contribution and make connections to other activities. Consider periodic assessment, formative or summative, covering eLearning materials.
Phase 4: Summing up the learning outcomes for the course	Provide feedback on students' online activities, e.g. knowledge sharing, research tasks or collaboration, and request feedback from participants on eLearning activities in the context of the entire curriculum. Re-emphasise links between online process and other activities. Highlight key learning outcomes for the module and comment on issues that arose in the blended approach. Address outstanding issues online in final class sessions.

Figure 12.6 A framework for designing and delivering blended e-learning.
Source: Adapted from Planning Your Blended Module, eLearning Development Team, Univ of York © 2005; with permission.

References

1 Murphy E (1996) Book Review: Seymour Papert (1993) The children's machine: rethinking school in the age of the computer. (http://www.ucs.mun.ca/~emurphy/stemnet/papert.html; accessed 15 August 2013).

2 Perelman LJ (1993) School's Out: The hyperlearning revolution will replace public education. Wired, p. 3. (http://www.wired.com/wired/archive/1.01/hyperlearning.html; accessed 12 July 2013).

3 Anderson P (2007) What is Web 2.0? Ideas, technologies and implications for Education. JISC Report. (http://www.jisc.ac.uk/media/documents/techwatch/tsw0701b.pdf; accessed 15 August 2013).

4 Bush V (1945) As we may think. *Atlantic Monthly.* **176**(1): 101–8. (http://www.theatlantic.com/magazine/archive/1969/12/as-we-may-think/3881/; accessed 15 August 2013).

5 Nelson TH (1965) Complex information processing: a file structure for the complex, the changing and the indeterminate. Proceedings of the Association for Computing Machinery 20th Annual Conference, pp. 84–100. Available from the ACM Digital Library (http://portal.acm.org/dl.cfm; accessed 15 August 2013).

6 Kintsch W (1998) *Comprehension: A Paradigm for Cognition.* Cambridge University Press, Cambridge, UK.

7 McKendree J, Reader W and Hammond N (1995) The homeopathic fallacy in learning from hypertext. *Interactions.* **2**(3): 74–82.

8 Charney D (1994) The impact of hypertext on processes of reading and writing. In: Hillgoss S and Selfe C (eds) *Literacy and Computers*, pp. 238–63. Modern Language Association, New York.

9 Novak J (1998) *Learning, Creating, and Using Knowledge: Concept Maps as Facilitative Tools in Schools and Corporations.* Lawrence Erlbaum Associates, Mahwah, NJ.

10 Skinner BF (1958) Teaching machines. *Science.* **128**: 969–77.

11 Kulik JA (1994) Meta-analytic studies of findings on computer-based instruction. In: Baker EL and O'Neil HF Jr (eds) *Technology Assessment in Education and Training.* Lawrence Erlbaum Associates, Mahwah, NJ.

12 Fletcher JD, Hawley DE and Piele PK (1990) Costs, effects, and utility of microcomputer assisted instruction in the classroom. *American Educational Research Journal.* **27**: 783–806.

13 Kosakowski J (1998) The benefits of information technology. ERIC Digest, Report ED420302 1998-06-00, Washington, DC. (http://eric.ed.gov/?id=ED420302; accessed 15 August 2013).

14 Underwood J, Cavendish S, Dowling S, Fogelman K and Lawson T (1996) Are integrated learning systems effective learning support tools? *Computers and Education.* **26**(1–3): 33–40.

15 McKendree J (1990) Effective feedback content for tutoring complex skills. *Human-Computer Interaction.* **5**: 381–413.

16 Issenberg SB, McGaghie WC, Petrusa ER, Gordon DL and Scalese RJ (2005) Features and uses of high-fidelity medical simulations that lead to effective learning: a BEME systematic review. *Medical Teacher.* **27**(1): 10–28.

17 McKendree J (2002) The role of discussion in learning. Paper presented at Association for Medical Education in Europe conference, 29th August to 1st September 2002, Lisbon, Portugal. Full paper available from the author.

18 Coffield F, Moseley D, Hall E and Ecclestone K (2004) Learning styles and pedagogy in post-16 learning: a systematic and critical review. Report for Learning and Skills Research Centre. (http://www.voced.edu.au/content/ngv13692; accessed 15 August 2013).

19 Mayer RE and Sims VK (1994) For whom is a picture worth a thousand words? Extensions of a dual-coding theory of multimedia learning. *Journal of Educational Psychology.* **86**(3): 389–401.

20 Paivio A (1971) *Imagery and Verbal Processes.* Holt, Rinehart and Winston, New York.

21 Entwistle N (2005) Contrasting perspectives on learning. In: Marton F, Hounsell D and Entwistle N (eds) *The Experience of Learning: Implications for Teaching and Studying in Higher Education* (3e), pp. 3–22. University of Edinburgh, Centre for Teaching, Learning and Assessment, Edinburgh.

22 Ferguson E, James D and Madeley L (2002) Factors associated with success in medical school: systematic review of the literature. *British Medical Journal.* **324**: 952–7.

23 Dochy F, Segers M, Van den Bossche P and Gijbels D (2003) Effects of problem-based learning: a meta-analysis. *Learning and Instruction.* **13**(5): 533–68.

24 Eraut M (2000) Non-formal learning and tacit knowledge in professional work. *British Journal of Educational Psychology.* **70**: 113–36.

25 Landauer TK, Laham D and Foltz P (2003) Automatic essay assessment. *Assessment in Education: Principles, Policy and Practice.* **10**(3): 295–308.

26 Cook J (2005) Review of virtual learning environments in UK medical, dental and veterinary education. Newcastle: Subject Centre For Medicine, Dentistry And Veterinary Medicine. Report 6.

27 Moubarak G, Guiot A, Benhamou Y *et al.* (2011) Global medical ethics: Facebook activity of residents and fellows and its impact on the doctor–patient relationship. *Journal of Medical Ethics.* **37**: 101–4.

28 Boyd D and Ellison N (2007) Social network sites: definition, history, and scholarship. In: Boyd D and Ellison N (eds). Special Issue of JCMC on Social Network Sites. London.

29 Stanner S (2010) Community@Brighton – the development of an institutional Shared Learning Environment. In: O'Donoghue J (ed.) *Technology-Supported Environments for Personalized Learning: Methods and Case Studies.* Information Science, London.

30 Cain J (2008) Online social networking issues within academia and pharmacy education. *American Journal of Pharmaceutical Education.* **72**: 10.

31 Selwyn N (2007) Web 2.0 applications as alternative environments for informal learning: A critical review. In: Alternative learning environments in practice: Using ICT to change impact and outcomes. Presentation and paper for the OECD-KERIS expert meeting, Korea. (http://www.oecd.org/dataoecd/32/3/39458556.pdf; accessed 15 August 2013).

32 Daniel J (2012) Making sense of MOOCs: musings in a maze of myth, paradox and possibility. Seoul: Korean National Open University. (http://www.academicpartnerships.com/research/white-paper-making-sense-of-moocs; accessed 15 August 2013).

33 Masters K (2011) A brief guide to understanding MOOCs. *Internet Journal of Medical Education.* **1**(2). (http://archive.ispub.com/journal/theinternet-journal-of-medical-education/volume-1-number-2/a-brief-guide-to-understanding-moocs.html#sthash.nkwWRR2w.dpbs; accessed 15 August 2013).

34 Prober CG and Heath C (2012) Lecture halls without lectures – a proposal for medical education. *The New England Journal of Medicine.* **366**: 1657–9.

35 Coultas J, Luckin R and du Boulay B (2004) How compelling is the evidence for the effectiveness of e-Learning in the post-16 sector? Consultation Paper. Eduserv Expert Seminar. (http://www.reveel.sussex.ac.uk/files/ConsultES204.pdf; accessed 15 August 2013).

Further reading

Approaches and Study Skills Inventory for Students (ASSIT): http://www.etl.tla.ed.ac.uk//questionnaires/ASSIST.pdf

Summary of concept mapping theory and tools: http://www.cocon.com/observetory/conceptmappingvs1.htm

JISC report on Innovative practice with e-learning: http://www.jisc.ac.uk/eli_practice.html

Higher Education Academy e-learning Resources: http://www.heacademy.ac.uk/resources

13 Simulation in medical education

Jean Ker[1] and Paul Bradley[2]
[1] College of Medicine, Dentistry and Nursing, University of Dundee, UK
[2] Institute of Medical Education, University of Swansea, UK

 KEY MESSAGES

- Simulation is a powerful learning tool, when learning outcomes are clearly defined
- Simulation is a safe, learner-centred educational method
- Simulation should be integrated within the curriculum, not stand-alone
- Debriefing and feedback are essential in assisting transfer of learning into practice
- The authenticity of the simulation should relate to the learning outcomes

- The development of procedural expertise requires 'deliberate' practice
- Simulation research should focus on instructional design, outcomes and translation into practice
- Simulation cannot replace clinical experience, but is a valuable technique in preparing clinicians for safe and effective practice

Introduction

This is an exciting time to become involved in the use of simulation in health care education. The increasing emphasis on patient safety,(1,2) and the evidence of the impact of simulation from other high-reliability organizations, such as aviation, has led to a realisation that it needs to become integrated in health care professional education.(3–5)

This chapter introduces the reader to the potential of simulation in medical education and in doing so covers four key areas, as follows:
- definitions and classifications
- application of educational theories
- the role of debriefing and feedback
- practical applications.

Research into the use of simulation has until recently focused on its effectiveness(6) and efficiency, which were often limited to descriptive, low-level evaluations.(7) There is an increasing shift to explore simulation from the perspective of conceptual generalisability – what can we learn about theory and the social context of learning.(8–10)

Historical perspective

Simulation has been around for centuries in many areas of human endeavour.(11) Simulators in health care learning date back as far as 18th century France, when Madame Du Coudray used her fetal model and pelvis to train midwives.(12) The modern movement in simulation training coincided with developments of the part-task trainer.

Resusci Anne led the way in standardising resuscitation training by making available a simple, low-cost, practical and effective manikin.(13) *Sim-One*, a higher-fidelity human patient simulator, was developed by Abrahamson at the University of Southern California School of Medicine to help novice anaesthetists develop skills in inserting endotracheal tubes.(14,15) Since then anaesthesia has been at the forefront of simulator development. The 1980s saw the development of *Gainesville Anaesthetic Simulator*(16) and the *Comprehensive Anaesthesia Simulation Environment* (CASE).(17) The CASE group linked the simulator to a programme on anaesthesia crisis resource management,(18,19) which was the start of many disciplines using simulation for learning both in technical and in non-technical skills.(20,21) Barrows introduced simulated patients, providing learners with a controlled, staged experience of simulated practice.(22) Following recent technological developments, computer-assisted simulation, virtual reality and the use of haptics (tactile sensations) have been added to the simulation armamentarium.

What is simulation?

Simulation is a technique which can be used to facilitate any learning, whether in the cognitive, psychomotor or affective domains. It may involve a wide range of activities and approaches and is applicable to learners, from novice to expert – one of the major underlying drivers being to develop and maintain safe health care practitioners (*see* Figure 13.1).

Understanding Medical Education: Evidence, Theory and Practice, Second Edition. Edited by Tim Swanwick.
© 2014 The Association for the Study of Medical Education. Published 2014 by John Wiley & Sons, Ltd.

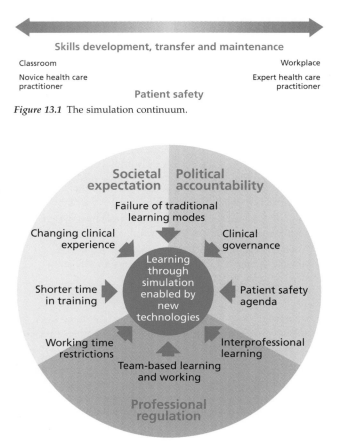

Skills development, transfer and maintenance

Classroom

Novice health care
practitioner

Workplace

Expert health care
practitioner

Patient safety

Figure 13.1 The simulation continuum.

Societal
expectation

Political
accountability

Failure of traditional
learning modes

Changing clinical
experience

Clinical
governance

Learning
through
simulation
enabled by
new
technologies

Shorter time
in training

Patient safety
agenda

Working time
restrictions

Interprofessional
learning

Team-based learning
and working

Professional
regulation

Figure 13.2 Drivers for the development of simulation.

Simulation is not defined in terms of either high (or low) technology, nor is it confined to interactions with people or models, physical or virtual; it could just as easily be a paper-based activity. It can be used effectively in the classroom, in a specialist facility or centre, or in the health care environment. What drives any simulation event is the learning that is expected to be achieved.

Why use simulation?

A number of societal, political, clinical and educational influences have driven the development of simulation over the past 40 years (*see* Figure 13.2).

Patients remain important participants in health care education and increasingly question the process of their care and share in the decisions made about their management.(23,24) There is now an expectation that learners and health care practitioners will be prepared to an acceptable level, for their sphere of clinical practice before caring for patients.(25,26) An additional challenge over the past ten years has been the enormous changes in health care delivery, which have resulted in fewer opportunities for students to learn from the breadth of patients in the clinical area.(27) This has been exacerbated by the changing roles of other health care professionals, which has reduced learning opportunities in practice.(28–30)

Reports such as *To Err Is Human*(31) and *An Organisation with a Memory*(32) increased awareness of adverse events and their underlying causes. This has been recognised at policy-making level in terms of the role simulation can have in addressing these concerns. Scotland is the first country in the world to have a national clinical skills strategy,(33) and the Department of Health in England has recognised the essential role simulation can play in the development of a safe culture in its health service.(34) The development by the World Health Organization (WHO) of a curriculum on patient safety for undergraduate medical education highlights the recognition of the central role simulation can play.(35)

Simulation can specifically help address the patient safety agenda and clinical governance requirements for standards of practice by preparing health care practitioners for rare and unexpected events.(36) It can also help educate staff in defined processes in a realistic health care context with defined and assessed outcomes. Simulation can improve patient care through team-based approaches,(37–45) and aid the development of non-technical skills.(2–4,46–49) Safe technical skills can also be enhanced and standardised using simulation.(50–52) New diagnostic and therapeutic technologies, for example, endoscopy and minimally invasive surgery, have revolutionised clinical practice, but they have also imposed a requirement for safe, effective training for both trainee and established practitioners.(53–59) New interventional techniques can be pioneered through simulation.

Worldwide, there have been major changes in medical education, both undergraduate and postgraduate, which recognise the need to incorporate all aspects of a doctor's practice, including knowledge, skills and expected attitudes, within an outcomes-based framework.(60–66) The defined outcomes of competency-based curricula lend themselves to using a simulation approach. With more emphasis on the cost-effectiveness of clinical care and a reduction in working times, clinical teaching has been squeezed, with learners receiving less time on direct bedside teaching.(67–69) There has also been significant evidence of the failure of traditional serendipitous approaches to skills acquisition across a wide range of core skills.(70–78) The traditional apprenticeship model in this context is no longer effective and simulation offers a feasible alternative to learning procedural skills,(79) and the opportunity to rehearse performance in complex integrated scenarios in a safe, protected, learner-centred simulated clinical setting.(38,80–83)

Assessment and monitoring of both non-technical and technical skills can also be delivered in educationally supportive clinical skills and simulation centres.(84–91) Behaviours observed in a simulated environment can provide a prediction of how professionals will behave in the reality of practice.(92) A more extensive list of potential applications is listed in Box 13.1.

Simulation fidelity

How well a learning event using simulation replicates reality is a key question in designing simulation-based edu-

BOX 13.1 Potential applications of simulation(11)

- Routine learning and rehearsal of clinical and communication skills at all levels
- Routine basic training of individuals and teams
- Practice of complex clinical situations
- Training of teams in crisis resource management
- Rehearsal of serious and/or rare events
- Rehearsal of planned, novel or infrequent interventions
- Induction into new clinical environments and use of equipment
- Design and testing of new clinical equipment
- Performance assessment of staff at all levels
- Refresher training of staff at all levels

BOX 13.2 Fidelity

Miller(97)
- Psychological fidelity – degree to which the skills or skill in real task are captured in the simulated task.
- Physical or engineering fidelity – degree to which the device or environment replicates the physical characteristics of the real environment.

Rehmann(98)
- Equipment fidelity – degree to which the simulator duplicates reality.
- Environmental fidelity – degree to which the simulator duplicates the visual and other sensory clues.
- Psychological fidelity – degree of reality perceived by the trainee or student.

cation. There is a widespread assumption that the quality of a simulation experience equates to its level of replication of reality.(93) This assumption has been repeatedly criticised.(94,95) Simulation fidelity needs to be related to the goals or learning outcomes of the simulation learning event.

Uwe Laucken(96) describes three modes of thinking in relation to fidelity or realism which can be applied to the simulation context, as follows:

- *Physical* mode of thinking relates to entities that can be measured in terms of physical dimensions such as weight height and physical characteristics of the simulator.
- *Semantical* mode of thinking relates to interpretation of relationships and acceptance of these by agreements, such as a box representing an ECG machine.
- *Phenomenological* mode of thinking relates to the participant's own self-awareness and emotions, and in the case of simulation is the reality for the person immersed in the learning. They can relate the relevant experience of the simulation event to their clinical practice.

This approach to the different modes of thinking in relation to reality can provide guidance on the development of scenarios using simulation to ensure learning outcomes are achieved. Other approaches to classifying fidelity are shared below.

Meller(97) developed a classification scheme for a medical simulation with the following four components to explain his concept of fidelity:

- the patient and/or disease process
- the procedure, test or equipment
- the physician or other practitioners (learner)
- the expert practitioner (teacher).

However, an analysis that looks at the fidelity of the simulation, the simulator and the component parts is probably more meaningful. Simulation can be viewed as a continuum that runs from low to high levels of fidelity and from low to high levels of authenticity, dependent on the learners and learning context (*see* Box 13.2).

Fidelity can be described as the extent to which the appearance or/and behaviour of the simulation or simulator matches the appearance and behaviour of the real system.(99) Miller(97) made the distinction between two different types of fidelity: psychological and physical. Rehmann(98) further expanded physical fidelity to incorporate equipment and environmental fidelity. This typology is, of course, based on the trainer's perspective. The required overall fidelity configuration is best determined by intended learning outcomes.(100)

Simulation has also been classified as high (hi) or low (lo) fidelity, traditionally related to the level of technical sophistication. However, hi- or lo-fidelity relates to more than advanced technology, and simulation authenticity should be considered in relation to the real world and community of practice.

Such classifications of fidelity do not fully embrace all the determinants of realism relating to a defined simulation event. The fidelity of simulation required for teaching a novice the technique of venepuncture is very different from that needed to recreate a multi-professional team in the throes of an operating theatre-based crisis. Contextual fidelity, which has both clinical and temporal components, is a very important consideration. Our own model, which describes simulation not as a task, but as an event influenced by a number of factors relating to fidelity, is shown in Figure 13.3.

Classification of simulators

A range of simulators and types of simulation event are available to medical education (*see* Box 13.3), and in this section we will review those in common use.(31,101) An extensive list of available simulators is available at: http://www.pennstatehershey.org/web/simlab/home.

Part-task trainers

Part-task trainers (PTTs) are often used to teach and learn psychomotor, procedural and technical skills. They are

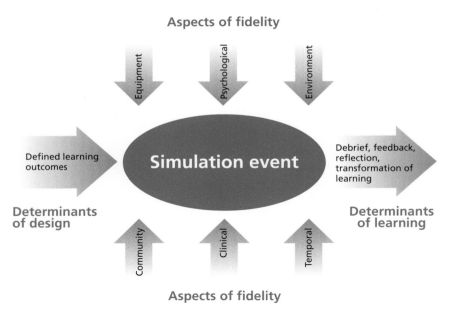

Figure 13.3 Factors influencing simulation fidelity.

BOX 13.3 Classification of simulators

Simulator type	Examples
Part-task trainers	Venepuncture arms, arterial arms Male and female pelvic models Skin and tissue jigs for injection and suture practice
Computer-based systems	Emergency medicine (*Microsim*, Laerdal) *Anesoft* – range of modules including anaesthesia simulator, haemodynamic simulator, critical care and bioterrorism
Virtual reality and haptic systems	
Precision placement	Venepuncture trainer IV cannulation
Simple manipulation	Endoscopy trainer Ultrasound trainer
Complex manipulation	Minimally invasive surgery Complex surgical procedures
Integrated simulators	
Instructor-driven simulators	*SimMan*
Model-driven simulators	*METI* (Medical Education Technologies Inc. adult and paediatric simulators)
Simulated patients	
Simulated environments	Wards, operating rooms, intensive care suites, etc.

Source: Kneebone (101) and Maran and Glavin (43)

---

used to develop mastery of these skills in an educational setting. As well as lo-fidelity trainers, for example, venepuncture arms, PTTs also include highly sophisticated computerised human patient simulators such as *Harvey* and *Simulator K.*(102,103)

Taking venepuncture as an example, with a PTT (and a little imagination) the tutor can incorporate clear demonstration of communication skills, health and safety issues (including patient identification, clinical hygiene, handwashing, safe disposal of sharps and clinical waste, and use of universal precautions), completion of documentation, labelling of specimens, safe handling of specimens, and proper handling and despatch to ensure the best-quality specimens arrive at the laboratory. Therefore, even for this relatively low level of skill, a fairly sophisticated set-up and performance may be required, placing the learning in the context in which it will eventually be applied.(38,104)

Computer-based systems

There have been significant developments in computer-based simulations. Learners are provided with interfaces that allow them to interact with materials relating to basic sciences, which can be staged and can progress at the student's own pace. These programmes ensure learners receive relevant feedback to reinforce their learning.

A number of programmes have been produced that include sophisticated physiological models. Some also provide feedback on the decision-making ability and performance of the user; in the case of Laerdal's *MicroSim* suite, it can be used to reinforce an emergency care curriculum.

Virtual reality and haptic systems

Virtual reality generates images representative of objects or environments with which the user interacts and which respond to those actions. Haptic systems provide the kinaesthetic and tactile sensation. These two approaches may be combined to provide training in basic skills such as venepuncture, and more sophisticated skills such as endoscopic, laparoscopic and endovascular procedures. Such simulation systems can also generate user data, which can be presented subsequently as detailed feedback on performance and maintained as an ongoing record.

Integrated simulator models

Integrated simulators combine a whole- or part-body manikin with a computer that controls the model's physiology and the output to monitors showing graphic displays. The observed clinical vital signs and the electrical readouts can be controlled and altered in response to interventions and therapies initiated by the users interacting with the manikin. The capabilities of modern integrated simulators are extensive, encompassing the life-like representation of body parts and functions, to generating realistic monitoring data such as electrocardiography and pulse oximetry, and providing a hi-fidelity means of rehearsing a range of procedures such as the insertion of a chest drain or urinary catheters.

Integrated simulators are divided into two subgroups: model and instructor driven. **Model-driven** simulators – also known as hi-fidelity simulators — are physiological and pharmacological models that directly control the manikin's responses to intervention and treatments. Examples include the highly sophisticated METI (Medical Education Technologies Inc.) adult and paediatric simulators, which have up to 100 changeable physiological parameters to recreate accurate patient responses to illness and therapies. Such hi-fidelity simulators usually require dedicated facilities, faculty and specialised technical support. **Instructor-driven** – or intermediate fidelity simulators – respond to instructor intervention, either directly via the computer keyboard or via a pre-written computer algorithm. They are less resource-intensive than hi-fidelity simulators and are widely used by skills and simulation centres.

Simulated patients

The terms 'standardised patient' and 'simulated patient' are often used interchangeably. Barrows defined a simulated patient as 'a well person trained to simulate a patient's illness in a standardized way'.(22) They are used for both learning and assessment.(105,106) Simulated patients may be usefully involved in the teaching of a number of domains, including communication and consultation skills, physical examination, non-invasive procedural skills and the assessment of professionalism. There is also a special group that provides learners with opportunities to undertake male and female genital and digital rectal examination, and female breast examination. These people are trained and give the learners feedback on all aspects of their performance.(107–109)

Simulated patients need training and considerable organisation in relation to matching simulated patient training needs to scripts and in timetabling simulated patients for both training sessions and student/learner training programmes and needs. This can be even more complex, when simulated patients are required to provide feedback to students or to participate in assessment or

---

BOX 13.4 FOCUS ON: 'Patients' in simulation

Standardised patient

A person with a particular history and/or physical signs, trained to present them in a consistent manner for the purposes of teaching or assessment.

Simulated patient

A person without a history or physical signs who is trained to portray a role and/or mimic particular physical signs for the purposes of teaching or assessment.

Real patient

A person with minimal training who consents to present his or her history and findings for the purposes of teaching or assessment.

Lay educator/patient teacher/expert patient/patient instructor

A patient with a particular condition who has been trained to provide facilitation, feedback and assessment about their condition and its history and findings.

Role-play patient

The recreation of a patient role or event by a learner or teacher.

---

complex health care scenarios, when simulated patient training may require more than one session. The impact of being involved in education has been reported in the literature with increased stress, although only mild symptoms reported in more challenging roles.(110) A database can be used to manage the bank of simulated patients effectively.(80) There will also need to be considerable investment in time and resources, and the financial costs may be high, particularly if your simulated patients are professional actors.

Script development for simulated patient exercises can be used to support wider learning outcomes beyond the simulation and immediate learning goals. Inevitably, however, there are some physical signs and situations that cannot be simulated and such patients can in no way substitute for direct clinical experience (*see* Box 13.4).

Simulated environments

The development of clinical skills and simulation centres provides varying degrees of recreation of the clinical setting in a protected environment.(85,111–113) Within these venues, application of contextual fidelity enables the suspension of disbelief and facilitates transfer to the real world. It might be argued that real clinical settings are better places for learning and increasingly simulation scenarios are being recreated in the workplace.(114) However, the disruption of normal clinical activity and the distraction of peripheral

BOX 13.5 The range of simulated settings

- Generic teaching and learning rooms
- Consultation rooms
- Simulated ward
- Operating theatre, including anaesthetic room, scrub area and recovery room
- Emergency department cubicles and resuscitation area
- High dependency and intensive care areas
- Domestic settings
- Roadside and motor vehicle
- How about pharmacy setting

BOX 13.6 HOW TO: Design a simulation event

Gaba analysed simulation events in 11 dimensions.(115) These provide a way of approaching the design and delivery, ensuring all aspects are aligned for maximum benefit. We have adapted his approach and condensed these considerations under three 'Ps': purpose, process and participants.

Purpose is an essential consideration for any learning programme, as identification of intended outcomes ensures that the learning is integral to the overall curricular programme.

Process relates to the reality factor; whether this is computer, real patients (RP), part-task trainers (PTT), simulated patients (SP), virtual reality (VR), replicated clinical environment (RCE) or the actual clinical environment (ACE). The reality factor is crucial to the process and needs to be judged in relation to both the purpose and the participants. Often the focus is on too much realism, which can distract from the purpose of the event in the first place.

Participants should be considered carefully. Are the right people present and is the simulation at the right level for the healthcare professional concerned? Simulation can provide excellent inter-professional learning opportunities.

events may prevent the required learning. One advantage of a dedicated facility is access to additional educational and audio-visual resources (*see* Boxes 13.5 and 13.6).

The theoretical basis of simulation

A number of theories of learning and instruction underpin the design and delivery of the simulated clinical experience, and these can be used not only to affirm educational credibility, but also to develop appropriate research questions. What follows is a short description of the major rel-

evant educational theories, with examples of their relevance to simulation. For a more detailed exposition of some of the educational theories described, readers are directed to Chapter 2.

Some additional theoretical considerations will also be mentioned, as they specifically impact on the construction of learning events using simulation. These include the concepts of expertise, skill decay, unlearning,(116) deliberate practice and suspension of disbelief. There has also been some concern over the use of the term 'skills' in relation to simulation. 'Skill' here is used in its broadest sense and may refer to cognitive, psychomotor or affective skills as composite requirements in professional development. This recognises the complexity of the domains of practice that can be influenced and enhanced by simulation.

Behaviourism

Behaviourism(117,118) ignores the 'black box' of the mind and describes a model in which a stimulus is used to produce a response that may be 'rewarded' or 'punished' to reinforce or weaken the response through a process known as 'conditioning'. Knowledge is therefore seen as a repertoire of behaviours. Neo-behaviourists, such as Bandura,(119) also point out that a reciprocal determinism exists between the behaviour, the environment and a number of personal factors, such as personality, affect and knowledge.

In simulation training, feedback is used extensively to bring about new behaviours. Simulation also permits 'over-learning' as a means of making such behaviours automatic. An example of such a behaviourist approach in simulation is the 'skills and drills' of resuscitation training to which we are all exposed throughout our undergraduate and postgraduate career.(120,121)

Cognitivism

Cognitivism, as expounded by Piaget(122) and Bruner,(123) posits that learners develop new ideas, constructs, hypotheses and decisions based on their interaction with the world and their own prior knowledge as an internal mental process. Learning is assimilated (the experience fits into the existing structure and adds to the body of examples) or accommodated (the experience does not fit the existing structure, which must be changed to incorporate the new knowledge) into a cognitive structure that gives meaning and organisation to the knowledge.

In the context of simulation, the tutor can help facilitate the learners' learning by establishing their preconceptions, presenting a cognitive conflict, drawing attention to the discrepancy between learners' expectation and experience of the event, asking questions and engaging in dialogue to prepare the learners to be receptive to new ideas, teaching the new ideas and drawing attention to the way in which they are better than the learners' previous knowledge structures. Simulation also enables the learner to move from the lower levels of Bloom's cognitive taxonomy,(124) such as comprehension, to higher, more complex, levels, such as the application, analysis and even synthesis of knowledge.(125)

Social constructivism

Rooted in the work of Vygovsky,(126) social constructivism emphasises social interaction as the means of learning. Language and culture are considered central to human intellectual development and how the world is perceived. Knowledge is co-constructed as a social phenomenon. The tutor can work collaboratively to support ('scaffold') the learner's development and in time remove such support to encourage independence. Through, for example, discussion of salient points and problems arising, the tutor mediates social interactions. Constructivism requires the learning environment to be safe, where ridicule or embarrassment will not follow mistakes and, by extrapolation, patients would not be at risk.

Situated learning and cognitive apprenticeship

Lave and Wegner(127) introduced the term 'legitimate peripheral participation', describing the position of learners within a community of practice. The learning is described as a product of the activity, culture and context (the social interaction within the workplace). As a learner moves from the periphery towards the centre, they become more actively involved and socialised (accepting beliefs and behaviours) and take on more senior and expert roles. This process is often not deliberate but evolutionary.

In a related model, Collins *et al.*(128) developed the concept of the cognitive apprenticeship, where the processes of the task are identified and made visible; abstract tasks are situated in the context of authentic settings; situations are varied to emphasise commonalities; and transfer of learning is promoted, that is, through a process of:

* modelling
* coaching
* scaffolding
* articulation
* reflection
* exploration/transferability.

The cognitive apprenticeship approach can be used in the teaching of a practical skill prior to its integration, application and transfer to the clinical environment, whereas situated learning is the more appropriate paradigm in the workplace environment where a junior learner would increasingly become part of the team during a clinical attachment and their learning would benefit from that socialisation.(129)

Experiential learning

Although criticised as an oversimplification with a weak theoretical basis, experiential learning, as defined by Kolb,(130) provides a useful model for simulation training (*see* Figure 2.2 in Chapter 2). Experience provides the main motivation for learning and new knowledge is established from reflection. The model of learning from experience includes concrete experience (apprehension) and abstract conceptualisation (comprehension) as means of perceiving experience, and critical reflection (intension) and active experimentation (extension) as means of transforming the experience.

Engaging learners in a health care exercise using simulation provides both the realism relevant to the learner's experience and the time in which to analyse and interpret different potential scenarios and their outcomes. The experiential learning process using simulation techniques allows learners to reflect critically on how they felt during the exercise. They can then begin to formulate concepts and hypotheses concerning the experience through discussion and individual reflection. Further experimentation with newly formed concepts and experiences can then lead to further reflection on experimentation. In this way, simulation provides a safe opportunity to experience health care, again without compromising patients.(131,132)

Reflective and transformative learning

Reflection-in-action (thinking on your feet) and reflection-on-action (evaluating after the event) are key concepts in the work of Schön.(133,134) Reflection-in-action occurs during an event; little time is given or available and recall of reflection might be limited, but prior experiences and knowledge are drawn upon and applied (almost experimentally) within the content of an unfolding situation, adding to the wealth of experiences already in place. Reflection-on-action is more indirect and formalised; writings, recording and other recall may be used to analyse an event, actions and outcomes.

Transformative learning(135) involves the reconfiguration of ideas, knowledge and meaning stimulated by a process of critical reflection. Learners are empowered to identify and incorporate new learning as their own. The use of video recordings in the learning of communication skills is an example of these educational approaches. Video can result in reflection both in- and on-action, and through facilitated discussion after the event it can result in a transformative restructuring and the development of an action plan and new learning goals.(136–139)

Activity theory

Engeström and other activity theorists(140–142) posit that conscious learning comes from human activity; forms of behaviour that are socially formed and conscious, structured, dynamic and self-regulating and motivated by needs and objects. Activities create motor and mental actions directed by conscious goals. Actions themselves are implemented through operations, which are dependent on conditions in the (external and internal) system.(143)

This seemingly complex interaction illustrates the underlying principle that learning, knowledge and activity are intrinsically interlinked and that learning is a socially mediated activity. Relationships between one activity system and another – for example, the simulated environment and the clinical setting might help us understand issues surrounding the transfer of skills and how clinical education might best be engineered. A crisis resource management or interprofessional exercise would find this educational approach most beneficial in a simulated setting. This would enable teams to rehearse their skills using hi-fidelity simulation and to transfer the skills into clinical practice.(144–146)

Unlearning and skill decay

One of the challenges which simulation can support in health care education is unlearning.(147) The evidence based for health care practices is continuously changing and can require routine or deep unlearning. This refers to the loss or decay of trained or acquired skills, and there is evidence of what influences this process in terms of retention and decay. These factors include the length of the retention interval; the degree of over-learning aspect of the characteristics of the task – whether closed or open looped tasks; the methods used in testing; the conditions for retrieval of the skill and instructional strategies. Although all these aspects are influential, the most influential appears to be the degree of over-learning.(148)

Deliberate practice

Ericsson(149) introduced the term deliberate practice to explain the large variation in individual performance despite experience. He suggests a framework to explain how the acquisition of expert performance requires engagement in deliberate practice. He describes the theories of skills acquisition(150,151) with the development of a mastery level of proficiency. In any area of skill, however, he quotes the work by Simon and Chase, which suggests that attaining an expert of performance in whatever skill requires over ten years' involvement. Deliberate practice enables consistent high levels of performance. The key challenge for facilitators and learners is to stop developing the skill, when reaching a level of automaticity and to develop cognitive skills to continue to improve. This requires the learner to seek out different situations in which to exceed their current level of competence.

'As if' and the suspension of disbelief

When learner participate in a simulation event, they need to behave towards the part-task trainer, the manikin or the simulated patient as if they were in the clinical workplace. The 'as if' concept enables the participants to rehearse modes of thinking in relation to both their own self-awareness and immersion in the simulation event. This enables the facilitator to present relevant information about the scenario in a timely and learner-centred way so that it almost becomes more real. It is about suspending disbelief and can facilitate learning from a simulation scenario.(8)

Models of expertise

In considering all the educational approaches above, it is also important to recognise the development of expertise and its impact on any simulated exercise. Expertise may be considered as the end point in a stepwise development of cognitive, psychomotor and affective skills. The Dreyfus brothers(152,153) describe five levels of development of expertise from novice to expert. Experiences in simulation should be modelled in accordance with the levels of expertise expected of the learner.

Debriefing and feedback

Health care practitioners like most people want to know how well they are doing and how they can improve their performance. Debriefing and feedback are essential in simulation – closing the learning loop. Feedback may be intrinsic or extrinsic. Intrinsic feedback, as described by Laurillard,(154) refers to a conversational framework embedded within the teaching and learning experience. Extrinsic feedback, by contrast, is usually available only after the event has taken place.

In an ideal world, learners should be able to compare their own performance with a standard, and be able to diagnose their own strengths and weaknesses. A simulated learning environment should permit such self-criticism, providing an atmosphere of trust and encouraging excellence. Most learners welcome the opportunity to discuss their strengths and areas for self-improvement, and in maximising the impact of learning from a simulation episode, extrinsic feedback is crucial. But when, how often and how well it is done is often disappointing.(155)

Who should give feedback?

In recent years, there has been a move towards the widespread use of multisource feedback, particularly as evidence of performance in the workplace.(156,157) Such a tool can also be useful in the simulated context where the event has involved a team.(158) Peer-group feedback can give learners a realistic perspective on standards of performance.

The simulators can provide instant feedback by collecting data of events and interactions and from attached monitors. Video-recording a simulated learning event, whether a hi-fidelity scenario(137) or other simulated encounters,(159) may also provide the learner with an opportunity for later reflection;(160) although it may be no more superior for immediate feedback than oral feedback alone.(139) Tutors and facilitators can provide feedback where the main focus is on striving for better professional practice, and trained simulated patients can also offer a unique perspective on the learning episode.(161,162)

The purpose of feedback

Feedback ensures that learners are clear about the learning outcome expected, can have areas of performance clarified, are given time and space to make connections with what they already know and can generalise to what training might be required in the future.(163) Feedback also raises the learner's self-awareness. It can reinforce good practice and be corrective by encouraging modifications of behaviour. Feedback should be an integral component of the learning process and is analogous to the reflective thinking process needed for safe clinical practice.

The feedback process

There are approaches on how to debrief and provide feedback following a simulation learning event.

The terms are often used inter-changeably and often reflect the facilitator's own professional background. The term 'debriefing' or 'after-action review' originated in the military to identify lessons from one mission that could enhance the next.(164) Feedback emerged in the education arena as a way of identifying how curricular or learning could be improved and also how learners could enhance their knowledge and knowledge application.(165) There are different approaches as to when it is best to provide feedback but more experienced learners prefer to complete the simulation learning event, rather than being interrupted.(166)

We describe the following four-stage approach in which feedback is integral to the simulation learning event.

1. *Preparation for feedback:* This is important and should be addressed prior to the simulation exercise. Learners can be asked to complete a questionnaire or to discuss in small groups the intended learning outcomes for the simulation exercise. This process helps to assess prior knowledge or similar experiences, to explore awareness of the learners' own competence and confidence, and to identify previous concerns or difficulties.

2. *Coming out of role:* During a simulation a learner takes on a health professional role caring for a 'patient' (simulator) in a situation of 'suspended disbelief'. Giving time to come out of role is important to allow the emotional responses of the learner to be addressed. This should not diminish the consequences of inappropriate action but helps promote conditions for deep learning. A learner has to acknowledge himself or herself as a student in learning, not a doctor or a health care professional responsible for the safety of the patient's life.(167) Concern for emotional impact must also be considered in relation to the experiences of simulated patients.(110,168,169)

3. *Constructive feedback:* Several models for constructive feedback exist which are relevant to learning from simulation. Most of these share a common goal of constructing what learning from performance has occurred. Examples include Pendleton's Rules(170) and the Cambridge–Calgary SETGO method,(171,172) both of which are widely used in consultation skills training; CORBS,(173) from the supervision literature; and GREAT,(174) a simple checklist developed specifically to debrief after an advocacy inquiry approach.(175) The 3D model of debriefing identifies three phases – defusing, discovering and deepening – as a way to enhance daily practice and patient outcomes simulator-based training.(176)

4. *Contemplation:* In this final stage the facilitator encourages the student to link up what has happened in the simulator with prior relevant learning experiences and to think about transfer of learning to the workplace – to generalise their learning so that it is accessible in different contexts. A subsequent post-encounter meeting can further support this process.

Feedback and its role in formative assessment and development are covered in more detail in Chapter 23.

Practical approaches to teaching, learning and assessment using simulation

To illustrate some of the theoretical concepts already highlighted in this chapter, this section explores the practical applications for simulation in the teaching and learning of technical and non-technical skills, and how the influence of the environment on practice can be analysed by recreating health care settings.

Teaching and learning a practical skill

Whether teaching components of a practical skill or learning more complex professional skills using simulation, knowledge is required to underpin practice. However, in medicine, as in other complex areas of professional work, it is not just necessary to recall facts, but it also necessary to be able to use knowledge.(177) Eraut(178) categorises knowledge as propositional, procedural and personal; the latter two being gained only through experience and reflection, whether simulated or real practice. Gagne(179) lists the following three phases in instructional design when contemplating the teaching of a technical skill:

- early or cognitive phase (consciously developing a routine with cues from a facilitator)
- intermediate or associative phase (component parts becoming integrated)
- final or autonomous phase (skill becomes automatic).

Studies have shown that rest periods interspersed with periods of practice are more effective than continuous practice. A practical application of the above is found in the Advanced Trauma Life Support and Advanced Life Support courses, and this approach can be further adopted and adapted.(180)

Joyce and Showers(181) stressed the importance of learning in context, modelling through real-time demonstration, repeat demonstration with explanation of actions, supervised practice and feedback to guide further development through further repeated practice. Their work also emphasised the importance of feedback and further coaching in ensuring effective implementation of new learning (*see* Box 13.7).

This standardised approach to skills teaching and learning is less easily transferable to a setting where there may be large cohorts of learners and smaller teaching faculties. However, it is possible to build on the model, as Joyce and Showers(181) also identified, that while feedback and coaching are essential in skills training, they do not necessarily have to be done by the trainers or in the initial training session. Therefore, a modified approach may be adopted in which initial teaching is delivered to groups and learning is consolidated through deliberate practice and peer review (*see* Box 13.8).

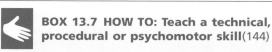

BOX 13.7 HOW TO: Teach a technical, procedural or psychomotor skill(144)

- Demonstrate the skill in real time without discussing with the learners.
- Repeat the demonstration but with explanation of what is being done and why.
- Allow a learner to lead the tutor through another run of the demonstration.
- The learner performs a demonstration.
- All learners practise.

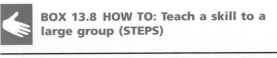

BOX 13.8 HOW TO: Teach a skill to a large group (STEPS)

S   Set the foundation of prior learning, the importance of the skill and the context in which it will be learned and applied.

T   Tutor demonstration in real time without commentary.

E   Explanation with repeat demonstration.

P   Practise under supervision with feedback from peer and tutor.

S   Subsequent deliberate practice encouraged through self-directed learning and with peer assessment and feedback.

BOX 13.9 Guide to effective simulation-based training(183)

- Understand the learner – the needs and the requirements.
- Embed measurements of performance both technical and non-technical for both individuals and teams.
- Ensure feedback is facilitated (e.g. video) and provided.
- Create scenarios based on learning outcomes.
- Guide the practice, including mistakes, and provide resources and support to seek improvement.
- Create synergy between content experts (clinicians) and process experts (educationalists).
- Evaluate the programme at all levels of the Kirkpatrick hierarchy.

In learning communication skills a more immersive approach can be utilised in facilitating skills development.(182) The 'SISFR' approach involves the following steps:

S – setting the context and identifying roles and outcomes expected

I – immersing in roles to practise using simulation for an agreed time frame

S – summary by participant of progress with simulation event

F – feedback from self, peers and tutor

R – refine by further immersion in practice building on feedback

Learning using patient scenarios

Planning and structuring are essential to developing successful patient-based scenarios, and here it is important to avoid the lure of the 'bells and whistles' of the technological capabilities of simulators. They are a means to an end. Patient scenarios can form a useful teaching aid in a variety of settings at all levels of simulation complexity. Salas *et al.* (183) provide a simple but effective blueprint for such an approach (*see* Box 13.9).

In patient scenario teaching, particularly when using hi-fidelity simulators, the feedback component is often referred to as 'the debrief'. This has two elements: the clinical/technical aspects of the exercise and the non-technical professional skills. Useful frameworks have been validated to support non-technical skills debriefing, such as the Anaesthetic Non Technical Skills (ANTS) framework (184) and others.(185) Again, feedback to learners is absolutely essential,(186) and the stages of feedback described above should be followed.

Learning using different health care settings

Simulations incorporating the health care environment are increasingly being used to develop and rehearse non-technical skills, such as prioritisation, decision-making and situational awareness. Examples include simulated out-patient and ward environments,(38,187,188) anaesthetic settings(17) and complete operating theatres.(145) In a

simulated health care environment significant events in practice can be recreated with errors and adverse events built in to test systems.(189)

Learning using team scenarios

There are several examples of simulation used to explore the functioning of the health care teams. In Basel, Switzerland, an operating theatre has been the venue in which the whole team are presented with an emergency situation; video-recording facilitates analysis of team performance, leadership and follower roles, delegation of tasks, effective communication and feedback.(190) It also tests the safety procedures and organisational systems.(191) This can lead to better understanding of how teams can work better together and why errors arise.(192,193) At Imperial College, London, simulated operating theatres have been used to explore the technical and non-technical differences between grades of surgeons.(194)

Other examples include: emergency medicine,(42) obstetrics,(120) the management of acutely ill patients,(195) advanced cardiac life support, trauma team training and neonatal resuscitation,(41) as well as in many other disciplines.(196) Team and interprofessional simulation-based learning is also used in the undergraduate years – for example, in clinical skills,(197,198) communication skills,(199) resuscitation (200) and in addressing patient safety issues (146) – although these bring challenges of their own.(201)

Assessment

The use of simulation in assessment usually focuses on the assessment of competence; therefore, the simulation needs to be as authentic as possible, if the assessment is to offer a reasonable indication of whether a person is able to perform in the reality of practice. Miller's(202) pyramid is often used as a model for the assessment of clinical competence, with four tiers representing 'knows', 'knows how', 'shows how' and 'does'. Simulation sits at the top of the third level and is able to provide an environment for testing the 'shows how' of clinical ability. Formative assessment through debriefing and feedback should form an integral part of clinically oriented simulated-assessment events. In more high-stakes summative assessment, the full range of simulators may be used, often in the format of an Objective Structured Clinical Examinations(203) or structured clinical skills assessment (*see* Chapter 21). In the classical format of this exam, candidates would typically rotate through a number of stations where they might encounter simulated patients, part-task simulators (e.g. venepuncture arm), simulated patient charts and results, resuscitation manikins, computer-based simulations and even whole-patient simulators, and will usually be tested on a range of psychomotor and communication skills. High levels of reliability and validity can be achieved in these exams,(204) where, interestingly, checklists and global scales show almost equal reliability.(205)

Hi-fidelity simulators offer the potential to examine higher levels of expertise among clinicians, testing knowledge, procedural and psychomotor skills, decision-making, team working, communication and professional behaviour. Of key importance is that the testing process must be rigorously assessed itself for reliability and validity, if the assessment is going to be used in a high-stakes setting.(87,206,207) It should be noted that there is currently limited evidence to support the use of hi-fidelity simulators and complex clinical scenarios in high-stakes assessments.

The apex of Miller's pyramid – 'does' – can be assessed using simulation, but in the real practice environment, an example being incognito simulated patients who are trained to visit a practitioner in their practice and then score their performance.(208)

Transferability

Throughout this chapter we have tried to highlight how simulations may be designed and delivered to most effectively promote transfer of learning to the workplace. These 'transferability factors' are summarised in Box 13.10. It should be noted that transferability is affected not only by the teaching regime, but also the characteristics of the individual learner.(209)

Limitations to simulation

Simulation is not, and can never be, a replacement for authentic experiential learning in the real world of clinical practice. It can, however, prepare practitioners for the real world, providing a structure for deliberate practice analogous to the hours put in by a professional golfer on a golf range or a concert pianist working their way through books of technical studies.(210) Simulation is not a tool to replace other modes of learning, but a powerful adjunct, and at its most useful when fully integrated into the curriculum.(211) Simulation should not be viewed as limited to training but as enhancing all aspects of professional education, particularly in relation to clinical reasoning and professional judgement.

There is a question over the transferability of learning from the simulated to the clinical environment. Recently, there have been concerns expressed about a disparity

BOX 13.10 HOW TO: Enhance transferability

- The role of the facilitator or tutor in a learning episode involving simulation is crucial in ensuring integration and transfer through a reflective action.
- Place the learning in context.
- Stage the simulation in a progressive and staged manner.
- A haptic component of a simulator in a simulated learning episode can add value to transfer of learning to context.
- The non-verbal skills of simulated patients, more than the content of their script, promote engagement with the learner. The resulting deep learning creates transferability potential.
- Recreation of the real clinical environment facilitates 'suspension of disbelief' and aids transfer of competence to performance.
- Structuring the learning to move from the specific to the general at the end of a learning session using simulation promotes transfer.
- Giving inexperienced learners specific relevant tasks in the workplace can reinforce learning in the simulated setting.
- Build a time into the learning session to encourage generalisability to the workplace.
- Feedback is crucial in enabling learners to generalise their learning for future practice.
- Ensure learning facilities using simulation are located close to or in the context of the workplace.
- Link the timing of the simulation to workplace experience.

between confidence and assessed competence of new graduates, and calls for the improved and systematic teaching of clinical skills.(212,213) However, it is still not clear how well these transfer into practice,(214) and it may be that simulation, while providing varying degrees of fidelity, does not attend to the noisy, messy and emotional reality of clinical practice. An approach exposing learners to this milieu may have more relevance,(79,104) and it has also been suggested that close geographical location of workplace and simulation facilities – where learners can more readily avail themselves of learning opportunities as their needs are identified – is helpful for transfer. As a general rule, training should be more aligned to fulfilling capability and less to time-limited competency end points.(215)

Planning of learning needs to support the development of skills through a process that stages acquisition linked to increasing authenticity.(129) It should be realised that learning in the simulated environment is not an end in itself. It is unrealistic to expect that one or two episodes of teaching and learning using simulation are sufficient to produce competence or proficiency. Learners still need to apply their learning in the real world, under supervision, and to receive feedback so that their skills base may become consolidated, refined and adaptable. In terms of unintended learning, there may be the danger of abnormal risk-taking behaviours being adopted by learners if their simulated experience, which is risk and harm free, is not tempered with the need for them to recognise their own limitations and to call for senior help in difficult circumstances.

Some learners may form a comfort zone within the simulated environment and might retreat to this in the face of a challenging clinical workplace – 'simulation-seeking behaviour'; these learners require encouragement and support to put the lessons from simulation into practice in the workplace, with suitable supervision and feedback, akin to Vygotsky's 'zone of proximal development'.(216)

The workplace may also be the source of contradictory practice and negative role modelling that causes dissonance for the learner, who needs to be prepared for this eventuality.

There is no doubt that there are significant costs associated with establishing simulation-based learning, whether this is in clinical skills facilities or simulation centres.(217) The costs relate not only to the technological aspects but also to the physical infrastructure, the personnel and the ongoing costs associated with a programme of this sort. This needs to be offset against the potential gain in terms of patient safety, potential reduced litigation and the satisfaction of a better-prepared health care workforce. However, it is important to ensure the most cost-effective approach is used for learning and to recognise that simulation may not always be appropriate.

The future of simulation

Simulation needs more supportive evidence; both in relation to its effectiveness and its efficiency in medical education (*see* Box 13.11). Simulation is resource-intensive, both

---

BOX 13.11 WHERE'S THE EVIDENCE?

There is an increasing literature regarding the use of simulation in medical education (*see* Figure 13.4), but most studies have been at the lower levels of Kirkpatrick's evaluation hierarchy.(7) Some research has looked beyond learner satisfaction and has reported on impact on learning. For example, analysis of performance data from virtual reality simulators has shown that simulator training is associated with a reduction in performance time and enhanced proficiency(218) and, more importantly, that this gain transfers to the real world.(219)

Simulation is increasingly being used to investigate performance-shaping behaviours, such as fatigue(220) or the introduction of new equipment, techniques and facilities for trial and rehearsal prior to being implemented in the workplace.(221–225) The use of simulation may also improve cognitive ability, as suggested by Rogers *et al.*(226) in a study of fourth-year medical students' thinking and application of skills for managing critically ill patients, and similarly by Steadman *et al.*(227) There have also been reports of simulators used to teach basic sciences with the aim of bridging the

theory–practice gap.(228,229) That said, there are also several studies that indicate lack of impact of simulation.(230–232) In a recent systematic review, Issenberg *et al.*(211) identified that although much of the primary literature was weak, certain features of hi-fidelity simulation were consistently reported as facilitating learning. These were:

- providing feedback
- allowing repetitive practice
- integrating within curriculum
- providing a range of difficulties
- being adaptable; allowing multiple learning strategies
- providing a range of clinical scenarios
- providing a safe, educationally supportive learning environment
- active learning based on individualised needs
- defining outcomes
- ensuring simulator validity as a realistic recreation of complex clinical situations.

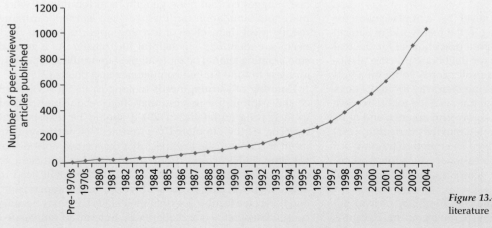

Figure 13.4 The growth in 'simulation' literature pre-1970s–2004.

financially and in human resources costs,(217) and therefore has to justify its role in terms of both outcomes and deliverables. Despite an almost exponential boom in the simulation literature (*see* Figure 3.4), more robust studies are required that link educational theory with the demands of service, studies which demonstrate changes in workplace behaviour that impact on patient outcomes, occurring as a direct result of simulated interventions. More specifically, there is also a need for an explicit understanding of clinical thinking; rehearsal of decision-making processes through simulation may help to avoid errors and increase physician awareness.(233) McGaghie *et al.*'s(234) critical review of simulation-based medical education research has identified the 12 features and best practices of simulation-based medical education. These include: feedback, deliberate practice, curriculum integration, outcome measurement, simulation fidelity, skills acquisition and maintenance, mastery learning, transfer to practice, team training, high-stakes testing, instructor training and education and professional context. In addition, Okuda *et al.*(235) published a useful review of the evidence of the utility of simulation in medical education. This highlighted that doctors trained on simulators were more likely to adhere to life support protocols than those not trained in this way.(236,237) In other areas there is evidence that the use of simulation has led to improvements in knowledge, in confidence and in practical procedures,(238) and can be reliable in testing learners and teaching teamwork.(239)

The research agenda derived from the simulation-based health care education Utstein meeting has begun to develop an international consensus about what needs to be done.(9) The need to agree terminology will ensure that clinical skills researchers and simulation-based researchers work together on international collaborations related to the research agenda.

For the moment though, with an increasing professional and societal emphasis on patient safety, it looks like simulation is not only here to stay, but will become even bigger business over the next few years, particularly with increased understanding of human factors training. Greater public accountability will require that doctors rehearse and practise their skills away from the bedside, consulting room or operating theatre before putting patients in the firing line. The challenge for simulation is to prove that it can make a difference.

References

1 Leape LL (1994) Error in medicine. *JAMA*. **272**: 1851–7.

2 Helmreich RL (2000) On error management: lessons from aviation. *BMJ*. **320**: 781–5.

3 Reason J (2000) Human error: models and management. *BMJ*. **320**: 768–70.

4 Burke CS, Salas E, Wilson-Donnelly K and Priest H (2004) How to turn a team of experts into an expert medical team: guidance from the aviation and military communities. *Quality and Safety in Health Care*. **13**: i96–104.

5 Anon (2007) 'Out of this nettle, danger, we pluck this flower, safety': healthcare vs. aviation and other high-hazard industries. *Simulation in Healthcare*. **2**: 213–7.

6 Ker J, Hogg G and Maran N (2010) Cost effective simulation. In: Walsh K (ed.) *Cost Effectiveness in Medical Education*, pp. 61–71. Radcliffe, Abingdon.

7 Kirkpatrick DL (1994) *Evaluating Training Programs: The Four Levels*. Berrett-Koehler Publishers, San Francisco, CA.

8 Dieckmann P, Gaba D and Rall M (2007) Deepening the theoretical foundations of patient simulation as social practice. *Simulation in Healthcare*. **2**: 183–93.

9 Issenberg S, Ringsted C, Ostergaard D and Dieckmann P (2011) Setting a research agenda for simulation-based healthcare education. A synthesis of the outcome from an Utstein style meeting. *Simulation in Healthcare*. **6**: 155–67.

10 Reeves S, Albert M, Kuper A and Hodges BD (2008) Why use theories in qualitative research? *BMJ*. **337**: a949.

11 Bradley P (2006) History of simulation in medical education and possible future directions. *Medical Education*. **40**: 254–62.

12 Le Boursier du Coudray A (1759) *Abrégé de l'art des accouchements*. Vve. Delaguette, Paris; cited in van Meurs WL (2006) Evolution of acute care simulation: a european perspective. Medisch Journaal. 35: 116.

13 Tjomsland N and Baskett P (2002) Resuscitation greats: Armund S Laerdal. *Resuscitation*. **53**: 115–9.

14 Abrahamson S, Denson JS and Wolf RM (2004) Effectiveness of a simulator in training anesthesiology residents. *Quality and Safety in Health Care*. **13**: 395–7.

15 Good ML (2003) Patient simulation for training basic and advanced clinical skills. *Medical Education*. **37**: 14–21.

16 Good ML and Gravenstein JS (1989) Anaesthesia simulators and training devices. *International Anesthesiology Clinics*. **27**: 161–6.

17 Gaba DM and DeAnda A (1988) A comprehensive anaesthesia simulation environment: re-creating the operating room for research and training. *Anaesthesiology*. **69**: 387–94.

18 Howard SK, Gaba DM, Fish KJ, Yang G and Sarnquist FH (1992) Anesthesia crisis resource management training: teaching anesthesiologists to handle critical incidents. *Aviation, Space, and Environmental Medicine*. **63**: 763–70.

19 Gaba DM, Fish KJ and Howard SK (1994) *Crisis Management in Anesthesiology*. Churchill Livingstone, New York.

20 Flin R and Maran NJ (2004) Identifying and training non-technical skills for teams in acute medicine. *Quality and Safety in Health Care*. **13**(1): 80–4.

21 Glavin RJ and Maran NJ (2003) Integrating human factors into the medical curriculum. *Medical Education*. **37**: 59–64.

22 Barrows HS (1993) An overview of the uses of standardized patients for teaching and evaluating clinical skills. *Academic Medicine*. **68**: 443–51.

23 Santen S, Hemphill R, McDonald M and Jo C (2004) Patients' willingness to allow residents to learn to practice medical procedures. *Academic Medicine*. **79**: 144–7.

24 Santen SA, Hemphill RR, Spanier CM and Fletcher ND (2005) 'Sorry, it's my first time!' Will patients consent to medical students learning procedures? *Medical Education*. **39**: 365–9.

25 Sedlack RE and Kolars JC (2004) Computer simulator training enhances the competency of gastroenterology fellows at colonoscopy: results of a pilot study. *The American Journal of Gastroenterology*. **99**: 33–7.

26 Sedlack RE, Kolars JC and Alexander JA (2004) Computer simulation training enhances patient comfort during endoscopy. *Clinical Gastroenterology and Hepatology*. **2**: 348–52.

27 McManus I, Richards P and Winder B (1998) Clinical experience of UK medical students. *Lancet*. **351**: 802–3.

28 Hunt G and Wainwright P (eds) (1994) *Expanding the Role of the Nurse*. Blackwell Scientific Publications, Oxford.

29 Department of Health (2002) *Developing Key Roles for Nurses and Midwives – A Guide for Managers*. Department of Health, London.

30 Department of Health (2003) The Chief health professions officer's ten key roles for allied health professionals. Department of Health. (http://www.acprc.org.uk/dmdocuments/10_key_roles.pdf; accessed 12 June 2013).

31 Kohn LT, Corrigan JM and Donaldson MS (2000) *To Err is Human: Building a Safer Health System*. National Academy Press, Washington, DC.

32 Department of Health (2000) *An Organisation with a Memory*. HMSO, London.

33 NHS Education for Scotland (2007) Partnerships for care – taking forward the Scottish Clinical Skills strategy. Executive Summary. (http://www.csmen.scot.nhs.uk/media/1867/scottish_clinical_skills_strategy_exec_summary.pdf; accessed 18 December 2012).

34 Donaldson L (2009) CMO Annual Report: Safer Medical Practice: machines, manikins and polo mints. Department of Health, London.

35 Walton M, Woodward H, Van Staalduinen S et al. (2010) The WHO patient safety curriculum guide for medical schools. *Quality and Safety in Health Care*. **19**: 542–6.

36 Blike G, Cravero J, Andeweg S, Jensen J and Christoffersen K (2005) Standardized simulated events for provocative testing of medical care system rescue capabilities. In: Henricksen K, Battles JB (eds) *Advances in Patient Safety: From Research to Implementation*, pp. 193–207. Agency for Healthcare Research and Quality, Rockville, MD.

37 Donovan T, Hutchison T and Kelly A (2003) Using simulated patients in a multiprofessional communications skills programme: reflections from the programme facilitators. *European Journal of Cancer Care*. **12**: 123–8.

38 Ker J, Mole L and Bradley P (2003) Early introduction to interprofessional learning: a simulated ward environment. *Medical Education*. **37**: 248–55.

39 Macedonia CR, Gherman RB and Satin AJ (2003) Simulation laboratories for training in obstetrics and gynecology. *Obstetrics and Gynecology*. **102**: 388–92.

40 Beaubien JM and Baker DP (2004) The use of simulation for training teamwork skills in health care: how low can you go? *Quality and Safety in Health Care*. **13**: i51–6.

41 Ostergaard HT, Ostergaard D and Lippert A (2004) Implementation of team training in medical education in Denmark. *Quality and Safety in Health Care*. **13**: i91–5.

42 Shapiro MJ, Morey JC, Small SD et al. (2004) Simulation based teamwork training for emergency department staff: does it improve clinical team performance when added to an existing didactic teamwork curriculum? *Quality and Safety in Health Care*. **13**: 417–21.

43 Maran NJ and Glavin RJ (2003) Low- to high-fidelity simulation – a continuum of medical education? *Medical Education*. **37**: 22–8.

44 Watterson L, Flanagan B, Donovan B and Robinson B (2000) Anaesthetic simulators: training for the broader health-care profession. *ANZ Journal of Surgery*. **70**: 735–7.

45 Rosen MA, Salas E, Wilson KA et al. (2008) Measuring team performance in simulation-based training: adopting best practices for healthcare. *Simulation in Healthcare*. **3**: 33–41.

46 Shapiro MJ and Jay GD (2003) High reliability organizational change for hospitals: translating tenets for medical professionals. *Quality and Safety in Health Care*. **12**: 238–9.

47 Sexton J, Thomas E and Helmreich R (2000) Error, stress, and teamwork in medicine and aviation: cross sectional surveys. *BMJ*. **320**: 745–9.

48 Leonard M, Graham S, Bonacum D (2004) The human factor: the critical importance of effective teamwork and communication in providing safe care. *Quality and Safety in Health Care*. **13**: i85–90.

49 Wayne DB, Didwania A, Feinglass J, Fudala MJ, Barsuk JH and McGaghie WC (2008) Simulation-based education improves quality of care during cardiac arrest team responses at an academic teaching hospital: a case-control study. *Chest*. **133**: 56–61.

50 Wulf G, Shea C, Lewthwaite R (2010) Motor skill learning and performance: a review of influential factors. *Medical Education*. **44**: 75–84.

51 Draycott T, Sibanda T, Owen L et al. (2006) Does training in obstetric emergencies improve neonatal outcome? *BJOG: An International Journal of Obstetrics and Gynaecology*. **113**: 177–82.

52 Kneebone RL (2009) Practice, rehearsal, and performance: an approach for simulation-based surgical and procedure training. *JAMA*. **302**: 1336–8.

53 Ecke U, Klimek L, Müller W, Ziegler R and Mann W (1998) Virtual reality: preparation and execution of sinus surgery. *Computer Aided Surgery*. **3**: 45–50.

54 Ladas SD, Malfertheiner P and Axon A (2002) An introductory course for training in endoscopy. *Digestive Diseases*. **20**: 242–5.

55 Letterie GS (2002) How virtual reality may enhance training in obstetrics and gynecology. *American Journal of Obstetrics and Gynecology*. **187**: s37–40.

56 Reznek M, Harter P and Krummel T (2002) Virtual reality and simulation: training the future emergency physician. *Academic Emergency Medicine*. **9**: 78–87.

57 Adrales GL, Chu UB, Witzke DB et al. (2003) Evaluating minimally invasive surgery training using low-cost mechanical simulations. *Surgical Endoscopy*. **17**: 580–5.

58 Fichera A, Prachand V, Kives S, Levine R and Hasson H (2005) Physical reality simulation for training of laparoscopists in the 21st century. A multispecialty, multi-institutional study. *JSLS*. **9**: 125–9.

59 Aggarwal R, Grantcharov T, Moorthy K, Hance J and Darzi A (2006) A competency-based virtual reality training curriculum for the acquisition of laparoscopic psychomotor skill. *American Journal of Surgery*. **191**: 128–33.

60 Education Committee of the General Medical Council (2002) *Tomorrow's Doctors: Recommendations on Undergraduate Medical Education*. General Medical Council, London.

61 General Medical Council Education Committee (2005) *The New Doctor: Recommendations on General Clinical Training*. General Medical Council, London.

62 General Medical Council (2013) *Good Medical Practice*. General Medical Council, London.

63 Accreditation Council for Graduate Medical Education (1999) ACGME outcome project. Accreditation Council for Graduate Medical Education. (http://www.acgme.org; accessed 25 July 2013).

64 Association of American Medical Colleges (1998) *Report on Learning Objectives for Medical Student Education: Guidelines for Medical Schools*. Medical School Objectives Project. Washington, DC.

65 Frank JR (ed.) (2005) *The CanMEDS 2005 Physician Competency Framework. Better Standards. Better Physicians. Better Care*. The Royal College of Physicians and Surgeons of Canada, Ottawa, ON.

66 Department of Health (2004) *Modernising Medical Careers – The Next Steps*. UK Health Departments, London.

67 Richards P and Gumpel M (1997) Save our service. *BMJ*. **314**: 1756–8.

68 Rahman A (2005) Teaching students – whose job is it anyway? *BMJ*. **330**: 153.

69 Richards T (1997) Disillusioned doctors. *BMJ*. **314**: 1705.

70 Skinner DV, Camm AJ and Miles S (1985) Cardiopulmonary resuscitation skills of preregistration house officers. *BMJ*. **290**: 1549–50.

71 Carter R, Aitchison M, Mufti G and Scott R (1990) Catheterisation: your urethra in their hands. *BMJ*. **301**: 905.

72 Feher M, Harris-St John K and Lant A (1992) Blood pressure measurement by junior hospital doctors – a gap in medical education? *Health Trends*. **24**: 59–61.

73 Taylor DM (1997) Undergraduate procedural skills training in Victoria: is it adequate? *Medical Journal of Australia.* **166**: 1–3.

74 Fox RA, Ingham Clark CL, Scotland AD and Dacre JE (2000) A study of pre-registration house officers' clinical skills. *Medical Education.* **34**: 1007–12.

75 Turner KJ and Brewster SF (2000) Rectal examination and urethral catheterization by medical students and house officers: taught but not used. *BJU International.* **86**: 422–6.

76 Goodfellow PB and Claydon P (2001) Students sitting medical finals – ready to be house officers? *Journal of the Royal Society of Medicine.* **94**: 516–20.

77 Boltri J, Hash R and, Vogel R (2003) Are family practice residents able to interpret electrocardiograms? *Advances in Health Sciences Education: Theory and Practice.* **8**: 149–53.

78 Cartwright MS, Reynolds PS, Rodriguez ZM, Breyer WA and Cruz JM (2005) Lumbar puncture experience among medical school graduates: the need for formal procedural skills training. *Medical Education.* **39**: 437.

79 Kneebone R, Nestel D, Yadollahi F *et al.* (2006) Assessing procedural skills in context: exploring the feasibility of an Integrated Procedural Performance Instrument (IPPI). *Medical Education.* **40**: 1105–14.

80 Ker JS, Dowie A, Dowell J *et al.* (2005) Twelve tips for developing and maintaining a simulated patient bank. *Medical Teacher.* **27**: 4–9.

81 Ker J, Hesketh A, Anderson F and Johnston D (2005) PRHO views on the usefulness of a pilot ward simulation exercise. *Hospital Medicine.* **66**: 168–70.

82 Wayne DB, Siddall VJ, Butter J *et al.* (2006) A longitudinal study of internal medicine residents' retention of advanced cardiac life support skills. *Academic Medicine.* **81**: S9–12.

83 Barsuk J, Cohen E, McGaghie W and Wayne D (2010) Long-term retention of central venous catheter insertion skills after simulation-based mastery learning. *Academic Medicine.* **85**: S9–12.

84 Morgan PJ and Cleave-Hogg D (2000) A Canadian simulation experience: faculty and student opinions of a performance evaluation study. *British Journal of Anaesthesia.* **85**: 779–81.

85 Bradley P and Postlethwaite K (2003) Setting up a clinical skills learning facility. *Medical Education.* **37**: 6–13.

86 McLaughlin SA, Doezema D and Sklar DP (2002) Human simulation in emergency medicine training: a model curriculum. *Academic Emergency Medicine.* **9**: 1310–8.

87 Devitt JH, Kurrek MM, Cohen MM and Cleave-Hogg D (2001) The validity of performance assessments using simulation. *Anesthesiology.* **95**: 36–42.

88 Forrest FC, Taylor MA, Postlethwaite K and Aspinall R (2002) Use of a high-fidelity simulator to develop testing of the technical performance of novice anaesthetists. *British Journal of Anaesthesia.* **88**: 338–44.

89 Edler AA, Fanning RG, Chen MI *et al.* (2009) Patient simulation: a literary synthesis of assessment tools in anesthesiology. *Journal of Educational Evaluation for Health Professions.* **6**: 3.

90 Boursicot K, Etheridge L, Setna Z *et al.* (2011) Performance in assessment: consensus statement and recommendations from the Ottawa conference. *Medical Teacher.* **33**: 370–83.

91 Stirling K, Smith G and Hogg G (2012) The benefits of a ward simulation exercise as a learning experience. *British Journal of Nursing.* **21**: 116–8.

92 Weller J, Wilson L and Robinson B (2003) Survey of change in practice following simulation-based training in crisis management. *Anaesthesia.* **58**: 471–3.

93 Salas E and Burke CS (2002) Simulation for training is effective when. . . . *Quality and Safety in Health Care.* **11**: 119–20.

94 Hays RT and Singer MJ (1989) *Simulation Fidelity in Training System Design: Bridging the Gap between Reality and Training.* Springer-Verlag, New York.

95 Salas E, Bowers CA and Rhodenizer L (1998) It is not how much you have but how you use it: toward a rational use of simulation to support aviation training. *The International Journal of Aviation Psychology.* **8**: 197–208.

96 Laucken U (2003) [*Theoretical Psychology. Forms of Thought and Social Practices*]. Bibliotheks- und Informationssystem der Universität Oldenburg, Oldenburg.

97 Miller RB (1953) *Handbook on Training and Training Equipment Design.* Air Research and Development Command, United States Air Force, Dayton, OH.

98 Rehmann AJ, Mitman RD and Reynolds MC (1995) *A Handbook of Flight Simulation Fidelity Requirements for Human Factors Research.* Crew System Ergonomics Information Analysis Center, Wright-Patterson Airforce Base, Dayton, OH.

99 Farmer E, van Rooij J, Riemersma J, Joma P and Morall J (1999) *Handbook of Simulator Based Training.* Ashgate, Aldershot.

100 Oser RL, Cannon-Bowers JA, Salas E and Dwyer DJ (1999) Enhancing human performance in technology-rich environments: guidelines for scenario-based training. In: Salas E (ed.) *Human/Technology Interaction in Complex Systems*, pp. 175–202. JAI Press Inc, Greenwich, CT.

101 Kneebone R (2003) Simulation in surgical training: educational issues and practical implications. *Medical Education.* **37**: 267–77.

102 Gordon MS, Ewy GA, Felner JM *et al.* (1980) Teaching bedside cardiologic examination skills using 'Harvey', the cardiology patient simulator. *The Medical Clinics of North America.* **64**: 305–13.

103 Takashina T, Shimizu M and Katayama H (1997) A new cardiology simulator. *Cardiology.* **88**: 408–13.

104 Kneebone R, Kidd J, Nestel D, Asvall S, Paraskeva P and Darzi A (2002) An innovative model for teaching and learning clinical procedures. *Medical Education.* **36**: 628–34.

105 Stillman PL, Regan MB, Philbin M and Haley HL (1990) Results of a survey on the use of standardized patients to teach and evaluate clinical skills. *Academic Medicine.* **65**: 288–92.

106 Cantillon P, Stewart B, Haeck K, Bills J, Ker J and Rethans J-J (2010) Simulated patient programmes in Europe: collegiality or separate development? *Medical Teacher.* **32**: e106–10.

107 Pickard S, Baraitser P, Rymer J and Piper J (2003) Can gynaecology teaching associates provide high quality effective training for medical students in the United Kingdom? Comparative study. *BMJ.* **327**: 1389–92.

108 Rochelson B, Baker D, Mann W, Monheit A and Stone M (1985) Use of male and female professional patient teams in teaching physical examination of the genitalia. *Journal of Reproductive Medicine.* **30**: 864–6.

109 Wånggren K, Pettersson G, Csemiczky G and Gemzell-Danielsson K (2005) Teaching medical students gynaecological examination using professional patients—evaluation of students' skills and feelings. *Medical Teacher.* **27**: 130–5.

110 Bokken L, Van Dalen J and Rethans J-J (2004) Performance-related stress symptoms in simulated patients. *Medical Education.* **38**: 1089–94.

111 Dacre J, Nicol M, Holroyd D and Ingram D (1996) The development of a clinical skills centre. *Journal of the Royal College of Physicians of London.* **30**: 318–24.

112 du Boulay C and Medway C (1999) The clinical skills resource: a review of current practice. *Medical Education.* **33**: 185–91.

113 Bradley P and Bligh J (1999) One year's experience with a clinical skills resource centre. *Medical Education.* **33**: 114–20.

114 Miller KK, Riley W, Davis S and Hansen HE (2008) In situ simulation: a method of experiential learning to promote safety and team behavior. *The Journal of Perinatal and Neonatal Nursing.* **22**: 105–13.

115 Gaba DM (2004) The future vision of simulation in health care. *Quality & Safety in Health Care.* **13**(s1): i2–i10.

116 Glavin RJ (2011) Skills, training, and education. *Simulation in Healthcare.* **6**: 4–7.

117 Skinner B (1978) *Reflections on Behaviorism and Society.* Prentice-Hall, Englewood Cliffs, NJ.

118 Watson JB (1924) *Behaviorism.* Norton, New York.

119 Bandura A (2001) Social cognitive theory: an agentic perspective. *Annual Review of Psychology.* **52**: 1–26.

120 Thompson S, Neal S and Clark V (2004) Clinical risk management in obstetrics: eclampsia drills. *BMJ.* **328**: 269–71.

121 Douglas JDM and Laird C (2004) Clinical fire drills and skill decay: can we develop an evidence base for policy and a language for training? *Medical Education.* **38**: 14–6.

122 McCarthy GJ and Reid DK (1981) *The Learning Theory of Piaget and Inhelder.* Brooks/Cole Pub. Co., Monterey, CA.

123 Bruner J (1966) *Toward a Theory of Instruction.* Harvard University Press, Cambridge, MA.

124 Bloom B (1956) *Taxonomy of Educational Objectives, the Classification of Educational Goals – Handbook I: Cognitive Domain.* McKay, New York.

125 Zigmont JJ, Kappus LJ and Sudikoff SN (2011) Theoretical foundations of learning through simulation. *Seminars in Perinatology.* **35**: 47–51.

126 Jarvis P, Holford J and Griffin C (2004) *The Theory and Practice of Learning.* RoutledgeFalmer, London.

127 Lave J and Wegner E (1991) *Situated Learning: Legitimate Peripheral Partcipation.* Cambridge University Press, Cambridge, UK.

128 Collins A, Brown JS and Newman SE (1986) *Cognitive Apprenticeship: Teaching the Craft of Reading, Writing, and Mathematics.* BBN Labs., Inc., Cambridge, MA.

129 Gott SP, Kane RS and Lesgold A (1995) *Tutoring Transfer of Technical Competence.* Armstrong Lab., Brooks AFB, TX.

130 Kolb D (1984) *Experiential Learning.* Prentice Hall Inc., Englewood Cliffs, NJ.

131 Reeves S, Freeth D, McCrorie P and Perry D (2002) 'It teaches you what to expect in future': interprofessional learning on a training ward for medical, nursing, occupational therapy and physiotherapy students. *Medical Education.* **36**: 337–44.

132 Wahlstrom O, Sanden I and Hammar M (1997) Multiprofessional education in the medical curriculum. *Medical Education.* **31**: 425–9.

133 Schön D (1983) *The Reflective Practitioner.* Basic Books, New York.

134 Schön D (1987) *Educating the Reflective Practitioner.* Jossey-Bass, San Francisco, CA.

135 Mezirow J (1991) *Transformative Dimensions of Adult Learning.* Jossey-Bass, San Francisco, CA.

136 Seropian M (2003) General concepts in full scale simulation: getting started. *Anesthesia and Analgesia.* **97**: 1695–705.

137 Byrne AJ, Sellen AJ, Jones JG *et al.* (2002) Effect of videotape feedback on anaesthetists' performance while managing simulated anaesthetic crises: a multicentre study. *Anaesthesia.* **57**: 176–9.

138 Roter DL, Larson S, Shinitzky H *et al.* (2004) Use of an innovative video feedback technique to enhance communication skills training. *Medical Education.* **38**: 145–57.

139 Savoldelli GL, Naik VN, Park J, Joo HS, Chow R and Hamstra SJ (2006) Value of debriefing during simulated crisis management: oral versusvideo-assisted oral feedback. *Anesthesiology.* **105**: 279–85.

140 Bedny GZ, Seglin MH and Meister D (2000) Activity theory: history, research and application. *Theoretical Issues in Ergonomics Science.* **1**: 168–206.

141 Engeström Y, Miettinen R and Punamäki R (1999) Activity theory and individual and social transformation. In: Engestrom Y, Miettinen R, Punamaki R *et al.* (eds) *Perspectives on Activity Theory.* Cambridge University Press, Cambridge, UK.

142 Brown K and Cole M (1999) Cultural historical activity theory and the expansion of opportunities for learning after school. (http://lchc.ucsd.edu/People/MCole/browncole.html; accessed 27 July 2013).

143 Engestrom Y (1987) *Learning by Expanding: An Activity-Theoretical Approach to Developmental Research.* Orienta-Konsultit, Helsinki.

144 Small S, Wuerz R, Simon R, Shapiro N, Conn A and Setnik G (1999) Demonstration of high-fidelity simulation team training for emergency medicine. *Academic Emergency Medicine.* **6**: 312–23.

145 Aggarwal R, Undre S, Moorthy K, Vincent C and Darzi A (2004) The simulated operating theatre: comprehensive training for surgical teams. *Quality and Safety in Health Care.* **13**: i27–32.

146 Kyrkjebø JM, Brattebø G and Smith-Strøm H (2006) Improving patient safety by using interprofessional simulation training in health professional education. *Journal of Interprofessional Care.* **20**: 507–16.

147 Rushmer R and Davies HTO (2004) Unlearning in health care. *Quality and Safety in Health Care.* **13**: ii10–5.

148 Arthur Jr W, Bennett Jr W, Stanush PL and McNelly TL (1998) Factors that influence skill decay and retention: a quantitative review and analysis. *Human Performance.* **11**: 57–101.

149 Ericsson KA (2004) Deliberate practice and the acquisition and maintenance of expert performance in medicine and related domains. *Academic Medicine.* **79**: S70–81.

150 Fitts PM and Posner MI (1967) *Human Performance.* Brooks and Cole, elmont, CA.

151 Anderson JR (1982) Acquisition of cognitive skill. *Psychological Review.* **89**: 369.

152 Dreyfus H and Dreyfus S (1986) *Mind over Machine: The Power of Human Intuition and Expertise in the Era of the Computer.* Basil Blackwell, Oxford.

153 Dreyfus HL and Dreyfus SE (2005) Expertise in real world contexts. *Organization Studies.* **26**: 779–92.

154 Laurillard D (1997) Learning formal representation through multimedia. In: Marton F, Hounsell D, Entwhistle NF (eds) *The Experience of Learning* (2e), pp. 172–83. Scottish Academic Press, Edinburgh.

155 Cowan G (ed.) (2001) *Assessment and Appraisal of Doctors in Training. Principles and Practice.* Royal College of Physicians of London, Salisbury.

156 Lockyer J (2003) Multisource feedback in the assessment of physician competencies. *Journal of Continuing Education in the Health Professions.* **23**: 4–12.

157 Archer JC, Norcini J and Davies HA (2005) Use of SPRAT for peer review of paediatricians in training. *BMJ.* **330**: 1251–3.

158 Beaubien J and Baker D (2003) Post-training feedback: the relative effectiveness of team- versus instructor-led debriefings. In *47th Annual Meeting of the Human Factors and Ergonomics Society*, pp. 2033–6. Human Factors and Ergonomics Society, Santa Monica, CA. Cited in Beaubien JM and Baker DP (2004) The use of simulation for training teamwork skills in health care: how low can you go? Quality and Safety in Health Care. 2013(S2031): i2051–6.

159 Fuller G and Smith P (2001) Rediscovering the wheel: teaching communication skills using video taped clinical consultations in specialist training. *Clinical Medicine.* **1**: 203–4.

160 Festa LM, Baliko B, Mangiafico T and Jarosinski J (2000) Maximizing learning outcomes by videotaping nursing students' interactions with a standardized patient. *Journal of Psychosocial Nursing and Mental Health Services.* **38**: 37–44.

161 McGraw RC and O'Connor HM (1999) Standardized patients in the early acquisition of clinical skills. *Medical Education.* **33**: 572–8.

162 Howley L and Martindale J (2004) The efficacy of standardized patient feedback in clinical teaching: a mixed methods analysis. *Medical Education Online.* **9**: 18. (http://www.med-ed-online.org/res00104.htm; accessed 25 July 2013).

163 Rogers J (2001) *Adults Learning.* Open University Press, Maidenhead, UK.

164 Fanning RM and Gaba DM (2007) The role of debriefing in simulation-based learning. *Simulation in Healthcare.* 2: 115–25.

165 Rudolph JW, Simon R, Raemer DB and Eppich WJ (2008) Debriefing as formative assessment: closing performance gaps in medical education. *Academic Emergency Medicine.* 15: 1010–6.

166 Van Heukelom JN, Begaz T and Treat R (2010) Comparison of postsimulation debriefing versus in-simulation debriefing in medical simulation. *Simulation in Healthcare.* 5: 91.

167 Stafford F (2005) The significance of de-roling and debriefing in training medical students using simulation to train medical students. *Medical Education.* 39: 1083–5.

168 Spencer J and Dales J (2006) Meeting the needs of simulated patients and caring for the person behind them? *Medical Education.* 40: 3–5.

169 Bokken L, van Dalen J and Rethans J-J (2006) The impact of simulation on people who act as simulated patients: a focus group study. *Medical Education.* 40: 781–6.

170 Pendleton D, Schofield T, Tate P and Havelock P (1984) *The Consultation: An Approach to Learning and Teaching.* Oxford University Press, Oxford.

171 Silverman J, Draper J and Kurtz SM (1996) The Calgary-Cambridge approach to communication skills teaching 1: agenda-led outcome-based analysis of the consultation. *Education for General Practice.* 7: 279–378.

172 Kurtz S, Silverman J and Draper J (1998) *Teaching and Learning Communication Skills in Medicine.* Radcliffe Medical Press, Oxford.

173 Hawkins P and Shohet R (2000) *Supervision in the Helping Professions: An Individual, Group and Organizational Approach.* Open University Press, Milton Keynes, UK.

174 Owen H and Follows V (2006) GREAT simulation debriefing. *Medical Education.* 40: 488–9.

175 Rudolph JW, Simon R, Rivard P, Dufresne RL and Raemer DB (2007) Debriefing with good judgment: combining rigorous feedback with genuine inquiry. *Anesthesiology Clinics.* 25: 361–76.

176 Zigmont JJ, Kappus LJ and Sudikoff SN (2011) The 3D model of debriefing: defusing, discovering, and deepening. *Seminars in Perinatology.* 35: 52–8, Elsevier.

177 Bloom BS (1956) *Taxonomy of Educational Objectives: The Classification of Educational Goals. Handbook I: Cognitive Domain.* Longmans, New York.

178 Eraut M (1994) *Developing Professional Knowledge and Competence.* Falmer Press, London.

179 Gagne RM (1985) *The Conditions of Learning and Theory of Instruction.* Holt, Rinehart and Winston, New York.

180 Advanced Life Support Group (1998) *Pocket Guide to Teaching for Medical Instructors.* BMJ Books, London.

181 Joyce BR and Showers B (1980) Improving in-service training: the messages of research. *Educational Leadership.* 37: 379–85.

182 Ker J and Ambrose L (2008) How to make the most of your CSC teaching session. Getting started in the clinical skills centre, pp. 2–12. University of Dundee, Centre for Medical Education.

183 Salas E, Wilson KA, Burke CS and Priest HA (2005) Using simulation-based training to improve patient safety: what does it take? *Joint Commission Journal on Quality and Patient Safety.* 37: 363–71.

184 Fletcher G, Flin R, McGeorge P, Glavin R, Maran N and Patey R (2003) Anaesthetists' non-technical skills (ANTS): evaluation of a behavioural marker system. *British Journal of Anaesthesia.* 90: 580–8.

185 Rudolph J, Raemer D, Simpson R and Dufresne R (2004) Debriefing in a simulation environment: An introduction and immersion. In Institute for Medical Simulation Comprehensive Workshop, Center for Medical Simulation, Boston, MA.

186 Gaba DM, Howard SK, Flanagan B, Smith BE, Fish KJ and Botney R (1998) Assessment of clinical performance during simulated crises using both technical and behavioral ratings. *Anesthesiology.* 89: 8–18.

187 Ker JS, Hesketh EA, Anderson F and Johnston DA (2006) Can a ward simulation exercise achieve the realism that reflects the complexity of everyday practice junior doctors encounter? *Medical Teacher.* 28: 330–4.

188 Hogg G, Stewart F and Ker J (2011) Over the counter clinical skills for pharmacists. *The Clinical Teacher.* 8: 109–13.

189 Crosskerry P (2003) The importance of cognitive errors in diagnosis and strategies to try and minimise them. *Academic Medicine.* 78: 1–6.

190 Helmreich RL and Schaefer H (1994) Team performance in the operating room. In: Bogner M (ed.) *Human Error in Medicine*, pp. 225–53. Lawrence Erlbaum Associates, Hillsdale, NJ.

191 Watling C, Driessen E, van der Vleuten CPM and Lingard L (2012) Learning from clinical work: the roles of learning cues and credibility judgements. *Medical Education.* 46: 192–200.

192 Helmreich RL and Davies JM (1996) Human factors in the operating room: interpersonal determinants of safety, efficiency, and morale. In: Aitkenhead AR (ed.) *Ballièrés Clinical Anaesthesiology: Safety and Risk Management in Anaesthesia*, pp. 277–96. Ballière Tindall, London.

193 Salas E, DiazGranados D, Weaver SJ and King H (2008) Does team training work? Principles for health care. *Academic Emergency Medicine.* 15: 1002–9.

194 Moorthy K, Munz Y, Adams S, Pandey V and Darzi A (2005) A human factors analysis of technical and team skills among surgical trainees during procedural simulations in a simulated operating theatre. *Annals of Surgery.* 242: 631–9.

195 Smith GB, Osgood VM and Crane S (2002) ALERT(TM)–a multiprofessional training course in the care of the acutely ill adult patient. *Resuscitation.* 52: 281–6.

196 Baker DP, Gustafson S, Beaubien JM, Salas E and Barach P (2005) Medical team training programs in health care. In: Henricksen K, Battles JB (eds) *Advances in Patient Safety: From Research to Implementation*, pp. 253–67. Agency for Healthcare Research and Quality, Rockville, MD.

197 Freeth D and Nicol M (1998) Learning clinical skills: an interprofessional approach. *Nurse Education Today.* 18: 455–61.

198 Tucker K, Wakefield A, Boggis C, Lawson M, Roberts T and Gooch J (2003) Learning together: clinical skills teaching for medical and nursing students. *Medical Education.* 37: 630–7.

199 Ross F and Southgate L (2000) Learning together in medical and nursing training: aspirations and activity. *Medical Education.* 34: 739–43.

200 Pirrie A, Wilson V, Harden RM and Elsegood J (1998) AMEE Guide No. 12: multiprofessional education: part 2 – promoting cohesive practice in health care. *Medical Teacher.* 20: 409–16.

201 Lorente M, Hogg G and Ker J (2006) The challenges of initiating a multi-professional clinical skills project. *Journal of Interprofessional Care.* 20: 290–301.

202 Miller GE (1990) The assessment of clinical skills/competence/performance. *Academic Medicine.* 65: S63–7.

203 Harden R, Stevenson M, Downie W and Wilson G (1975) Assessment of clinical competence using objective structured examination. *BMJ.* 1: 447–51.

204 Newble D (2004) Techniques for measuring clinical competence: objective structured clinical examinations. *Medical Education.* 38: 199–203.

205 Regehr G, MacRae H, Reznick RK and Szalay D (1998) Comparing the psychometric properties of checklists and global rating scales for assessing performance on an OSCE-format examination. *Academic Medicine.* 73: 993–7.

206 Byrne AJ and Greaves JD (2001) Assessment instruments used during anaesthetic simulation: review of published studies. *British Journal of Anaesthesia.* 86: 445–50.

207 Devitt J, Kurrek M, Cohen M *et al.* (1998) Testing internal consistency and construct validity during evaluation of performance in a patient simulator. *Anesthesia and Analgesia.* **86**: 1160–4.

208 Rethans JJ, Sturmans F, Drop R and van der Vleuten C (1991) Assessment of the performance of general practitioners by the use of standardized (simulated) patients. [see comment]. *British Journal of General Practice.* **41**: 97–9.

209 Barnett SM and Ceci SJ (2002) When and where do we apply what we learn? A taxonomy for far transfer. *Psychological Bulletin.* **128**: 612–37.

210 Ericsson KA, Krampe RT and Tesch Roemer C (1993) The role of deliberate practice in the acquisition of expert performance. *Psychological Review.* **100**: 363–406.

211 Issenberg SB, McGaghie WC, Petrusa ER, Gordon DL and Scalese RJ (2005) Features and uses of high-fidelity medical simulations that lead to effective learning: a BEME systematic review. *Medical Teacher.* **27**: 10–28.

212 Barnsley L, Lyon PM, Ralston SJ *et al.* (2004) Clinical skills in junior medical officers: a comparison of self-reported confidence and observed competence. *Medical Education.* **38**: 358–67.

213 Evans DE, Wood DF and Roberts CM (2004) The effect of an extended hospital induction on perceived confidence and assessed clinical skills of newly qualified pre-registration house officers. *Medical Education.* **38**: 998–1001.

214 Silverman J and Wood DF (2004) New approaches to learning clinical skills. *Medical Education.* **38**: 1021–3.

215 Kneebone RL, Scott W, Darzi A and Horrocks M (2004) Simulation and clinical practice: strengthening the relationship. *Medical Education.* **38**: 1095–102.

216 Bockarie A (2002) The potential of Vygotsky's contributions to our understanding of cognitive apprenticeship as a process of development in adult vocational and technical education. *Journal of Career and Technical Education.* **19**: 47–66.

217 Kurrek MM and Devitt JH (1997) The cost for construction and operation of a simulation centre. *Canadian Journal of Anaesthesia.* **44**: 1191–5.

218 Kneebone RL, Nestel D, Moorthy K *et al.* (2003) Learning the skills of flexible sigmoidoscopy – the wider perspective. *Medical Education.* **37**: 50–8.

219 Grantcharov TP, Kristiansen VB, Bendix J, Bardram L, Rosenberg J and Funch-Jensen P (2004) Randomized clinical trial of virtual reality simulation for laparoscopic skills training. *British Journal of Surgery.* **91**: 146–50.

220 Howard SK, Gaba DM, Smith BE *et al.* (2003) Simulation study of rested versus sleep-deprived anesthesiologists. *Anesthesiology.* **98**: 1345–55.

221 Kobayashi L, Shapiro MJ, Sucov A *et al.* (2006) Portable advanced medical simulation for new emergency department testing and orientation. *Academic Emergency Medicine.* **13**: 691–5.

222 Vadodaria BS, Gandhi SD and McIndoe AK (2004) Comparison of four different emergency airway access equipment sets on a human patient simulator. *Anaesthesia.* **59**: 73–9.

223 Sanders J, Haas RE, Geisler M and Lupien AE (1998) Using the human patient simulator to test the efficacy of an experimental emergency percutaneous transtracheal airway. *Military Medicine.* **163**: 544–51.

224 Lim TJ, Lim Y and Liu EHC (2005) Evaluation of ease of intubation with the GlideScope or Macintosh laryngoscope by anaesthetists in simulated easy and difficult laryngoscopy. *Anaesthesia.* **60**: 180–3.

225 Anderson K, Gambhir S, Glavin R and Kinsella J (2006) The use of an anaesthetic simulator to assess single-use laryngoscopy equipment. *International Journal for Quality in Health Care.* **18**: 17–22.

226 Rogers PL, Jacob H, Thomas EA, Harwell M, Willenkin RL and Pinsky MR (2000) Medical students can learn the basic application, analytic, evaluative, and psychomotor skills of critical care medicine. *Critical Care Medicine.* **28**: 550–4.

227 Steadman RH (2010) Improving on reality: can simulation facilitate practice change? *Anesthesiology.* **112**: 775–6.

228 Morgan PJ, Cleave-Hogg D, Desousa S and Lam-McCulloch J (2006) Applying theory to practice in undergraduate education using high fidelity simulation. *Medical Teacher.* **28**: e10–e15.

229 Tan GM, Ti LK, Suresh S, Ho BS and Lee TL (2002) Teaching first-year medical students physiology: does the human patient simulator allow for more effective teaching? *Singapore Medical Journal.* **43**: 238–42.

230 Gordon J, Shaffer D, Raemer D, Pawlowski J, Hurford W and Cooper J (2006) A randomized controlled trial of simulation-based teaching versus traditional instruction in medicine: a pilot study among clinical medical students. *Advances in Health Sciences Education: Theory and Practice.* **11**: 33–9.

231 Morgan PJ, Cleave-Hogg D, McIlroy J and Devitt JH (2002) Simulation technology: a comparison of experiential and visual learning for undergraduate medical students. *Anesthesiology.* **96**: 10–6.

232 Engum SA, Jeffries P and Fisher L (2003) Intravenous catheter training system: computer-based education versus traditional learning methods. *American Journal of Surgery.* **186**: 67–74.

233 Eva KW and Norman GR (2005) Heuristics and biases; a biased perspective on clinical reasoning. *Medical Education.* **39**: 870–2.

234 McGaghie WC, Issenberg SB, Petrusa ER and Scalese RJ (2010) A critical review of simulation-based medical education research: 2003–2009. *Medical Education.* **44**: 50–63.

235 Okuda Y, Bryson EO, DeMaria S *et al.* (2009) The utility of simulation in medical education: what is the evidence? *Mount Sinai Journal of Medicine, New York.* **76**: 330–43.

236 Wayne DB, Butter J, Siddall VJ *et al.* (2006) Mastery learning of advanced cardiac life support skills by internal medicine residents using simulation technology and deliberate practice. *Journal of General Internal Medicine.* **21**: 251–6.

237 Eppich WJ, Adler MD and McGaghie WC (2006) Emergency and critical care pediatrics: use of medical simulation for training in acute pediatric emergencies. *Current Opinion in Pediatrics.* **18**: 266–71.

238 McLeod R, Mires G and Ker J (2012) Direct observed procedural skills assessment in the undergraduate setting. *The Clinical Teacher.* **9**: 228–32.

239 Chakraborti C, Boonyasai RT, Wright SM and Kern DE (2008) A systematic review of teamwork training interventions in medical student and resident education. *Journal of General Internal Medicine.* **23**: 846–53.

14 Portfolios in personal and professional development

Erik Driessen[1] and Jan van Tartwijk[2]
[1] Maastricht University, The Netherlands
[2] Utrecht University, The Netherlands

 KEY MESSAGES

- Portfolios are a useful vehicle for supporting and assessing learning in the clinical workplace.
- In medical education portfolios serve three main goals: monitoring and planning learner development, assessment and stimulating reflection.

- Depending on their purpose, portfolios may differ significantly in scope, structure and content.
- The assessment of portfolios requires a qualitative interpretative approach.
- Mentors are a crucial factor in portfolio effectiveness.

Introduction

In 1990, Miller described the challenges of assessing 'clinical skills/competence/performance'. At that time, he signalled that in medical education instruments were available for assessing knowledge, skills and competence, but not for assessing what a graduate does when functioning independently in a clinical practice.(1) Because of their ability to fill this gap in assessment, in recent decades portfolios have gained a prominent position in medical education.(2,3)

The portfolio concept is borrowed from the arts and architecture, where work samples and evidence of quality were traditionally kept in a portable case, a portfolio. Today's educational portfolios may be digital or paper-based. Content may be prescribed or left to the discretion of individual learners, and the portfolio can report on work done, feedback received, progress made, plans for improving competence, and reflections on performance and development.(4,5) What makes the portfolio eminently suitable for supporting and assessing learning in the clinical workplace is its ability to accommodate non-standardised information about performance, and thereby do justice to the characteristics and challenges of individual learners and specific workplaces.(6) As a result, the portfolio is in perfect alignment with recent developments in education with a strong focus on learning in practice, such as outcomes-based education and competency-based learning.

This chapter focuses on the following topics:
- diversity of portfolios
- the use of portfolios for the monitoring and planning of competency development
- portfolio assessment
- the use of portfolios to stimulate reflection.

The evidence base for portfolios in medical education is summarised in Box 14.1.(5,7,8) For the rest of this chapter we will use the term 'student' to refer to any learner in undergraduate or postgraduate medical education or practitioners undertaking continuing professional development.

Diversity of portfolios

Scope
Portfolios can differ substantially in scope.(9) They may vary from being very limited (such as a portfolio for presentation skills only) focused on one single skill, competency domain, or curricular component, to being very broad, covering the learner's development across all relevant competency domains over a prolonged period of time.

Open or closed
Learners composing a portfolio can be offered different degrees of structuring or guidance, with clear consequences for the content and structure of the portfolio. A 'closed' portfolio with detailed guidelines and strict regulations allows learners relatively little freedom to determine the format and content of their own portfolios. Closed portfolios are easy to compare and navigate, which is an advantage for large-scale portfolio assessment. The downside is that the portfolio cannot really do justice to

---

BOX 14.1 WHERE'S THE EVIDENCE?
Factors promoting portfolio success

Factor	Recommendation
Goals	Clearly explain the goals of working with the portfolio.
	Combine goals (learning and assessment).
Introducing the portfolio	Provide clear guidelines about the procedure, the format and the content of the portfolio.
	Be on guard against problems with information technology.
	Use a hands-on introduction with a briefing on the objective of the portfolio and the procedures used.
Mentoring/ interaction	Arrange for mentoring by teachers, trainers, supervisors, or peers.
Assessment	Incorporate safeguards in the assessment procedure, like intermittent feedback cycles, involvement of relevant resource persons (including the student), a sequential judgement procedure.
	Use assessment panels of two to three assessors depending on the stakes of the assessment.
	Train assessors.
	Use holistic scoring rubrics (global performance descriptors).
Portfolio format	Keep the portfolio format flexible.
	Avoid being overly prescriptive with regard to portfolio content.
	Avoid excessive paper work.
Position in the curriculum	Integrate the portfolio with other educational activities in the curriculum.
	Be moderately ambitious with regard to early-undergraduate portfolio use.

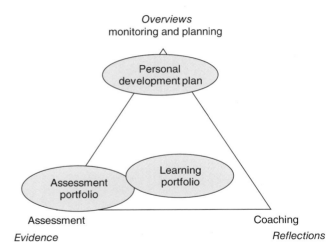

Figure 14.1 Purposes and content of portfolios.

BOX 14.2 Structural models of portfolios(10)

Shopping trolley
The portfolio is used to collect anything that could be seen as a vehicle to learning, and the choice is limited only by what the student considers to be appropriate. There are rarely any linking strategies between components.

Toast rack
The portfolio contains a number of pre-determined 'slots' that must be filled for each module of a programme (e.g. action plans, reflective accounts of significant events, skills checklists). Each component is formally assessed in isolation.

Cake mix
The parts of the portfolio are blended in that students are expected to provide evidence that they have achieved specified learning outcomes whilst on placement. The 'mixing' is provided by reflective commentaries addressing analytical criteria.

Spinal column
A series of competency statements form the central column of the portfolio and evidence is collected by students to demonstrate their achievement. One piece of evidence may be used against multiple statements.

---

the characteristics of individual learners and specific workplaces. A more 'open' portfolio results when directions are rather loose and general, allowing learners considerable freedom with respect to portfolio content and format. As a consequence, learners can provide richer descriptions of their individual learning processes and pay attention to specific characteristics of the workplaces in which they have worked.

Goals and their relation to portfolio design

In medical education, portfolios serve three main goals: assessment, reflection and learner development. Which goal or goals predominate drives the structure and content of the portfolio, as summarised in Figure 14.1.(2) In portfolios used for *assessment*, the evidence of competency attainment takes centre stage. In portfolios primarily aimed at

stimulating reflection, the core of the portfolio consists of written evaluations and performance analyses to direct performance improvement. In portfolios that are used to *monitor and plan development*, the main features are overviews of achievements and targets. In practice, most portfolios combine all or some of these goals, and the goal mix determines what the portfolio looks like (*see* Box 14.2). There is no 'one size fits all' and in the next part of this chapter we focus on the three main goals of portfolio use:

monitoring and planning development, assessment and stimulating reflection.

Portfolios for monitoring and planning development

From an educational perspective, workplaces are not the most suitable environment to enable learners to comply with the demands of a structured curriculum. For while learning outcomes and competencies can be determined in advance, whether the workplace offers opportunities to achieve them depends on the presence of patients with different pathologies and the presence of clinical teachers to supervise students. To put it differently, learning in the workplace depends on the availability of learning opportunities, and this inevitably varies from learner to learner.(11) On top of this, it is rare in undergraduate education (perhaps less so in postgraduate training) for students to have the same supervisor for more than one or two weeks.(12) The clinical workplace is thus by nature an erratic environment in which it is difficult for students to direct their own learning. While being immersed in clinical practice, students have a hard time perceiving exactly how their experiences can contribute to the overarching learning objectives and competency achievements required by the curriculum. Moreover, lack of continuity of supervision and limited observation of student activities stand in the way of effective monitoring of learner development. These problems can be solved by including in the portfolio a systematic overview of tasks undertaken to obtain specific competencies, the competency levels achieved, and areas where more work is needed.(13) (*see* Box 14.3).

Setting learning goals

For such a portfolio to be effective, it is essential that well-defined learning goals are set for a specific period. Purposeful activities are one of the pillars of workplace-based learning.(16) Learning goals are often incorporated in personal development plans which are included in the portfolio and used to guide progress interviews. Learning goals can be determined based on the following:(17)

- the programme requirements and the availability of a placement for the upcoming period
- the analysis of the portfolio and the progress interview – defining aspects that require special attention
- the learner's personal learning objectives – elective subjects, special interests, etc.

For learning goals to be effective, it is important that both learner and teacher are committed to achieving them. The teacher should see to it that objectives are concrete and that a feasible plan is drawn up to achieve them. A useful aid for this is the SMART model: objectives should be Specific, Measurable, Acceptable, Realistic and Time-bound, for only if these criteria are met is there a real chance that objectives will actually be achieved.(18)

Box 14.3 FOCUS ON: Entrustable professional activities (Figure 14.2)

Educational frameworks to structure workplace-based learning are often constructed using competencies and/or intended learning outcomes. Competencies and outcomes emphasise that the focus is not exclusively on medical knowledge and skills but on general competencies as well, while additionally they are used to guide learning and assessment. Learning activities – varying from simulations, formal teaching and participation in patient care – can be linked to competencies. However, in practice, linking abstract competencies to clinical work can be problematic, and the danger of bureaucratisation looms large. While records of student performance may suggest adherence to the formal curriculum, in reality the connection between the formal curriculum and what students actually learn in the workplace may be paper-thin. To bridge the gap between abstract competencies and clinical practice, Ten Cate and Scheele(14) have introduced the concept of 'entrustable professional activities' (EPA), tasks that are considered to be crucial to a certain profession and which every student must have mastered at the end of the course or curriculum. Given their importance, the EPAs are given special attention during the programme. Scheele *et al.*(15) developed three criteria to define EPAs: a task of high importance for daily practice; a high-risk or error-prone task; and a task that is exemplary of specific competencies.

In the portfolio the learner can collect materials in evidence of attainment of competency in one of the EPAs. Figure 14.2 shows an example of an EPA for postgraduate training in obstetrics and gynaecology in the Netherlands.

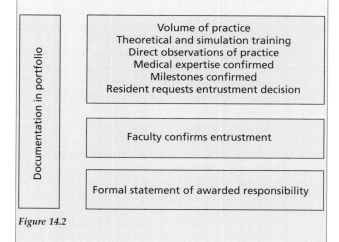

Figure 14.2

Portfolio structure and content

In portfolios that are used as instruments to promote and monitor development, overviews of what has been mastered and what remains to be achieved are important. Many portfolios provide overviews to be completed by learners to show what they have done, where they have done it, what they have learned as a result, and how they are planning to proceed.(13)

Such overviews could contain the following information:

- Procedures or patient cases
  Which procedures? What was the level of supervision? Which types of patients? What was learned? Were the activities assessed? Plans?
- Prior work experience
  Where? When? Which tasks? Strengths and weaknesses? Which competencies or skills were developed? Evaluation by the learner?
- Prior education and training
  Which courses or programmes? Where? When? What was learned? Completed successfully? Evaluation by the learner?
- Experiences within and outside the course/programme
  Where? When? Which tasks? What was done? Strengths and weaknesses? Which competencies or skills were developed? Evaluation by the learner? Plans?
- Components of the course/programme
  Which components have been attended so far? Which remain to be attended? When? What was learned? Completed successfully? Evaluation by the learner? Plans?
- Competencies or skills
  Where addressed? Level of proficiency? Plans? Preferences?

Portfolios for assessment

In recent years, there has been a marked change in the thinking about ways of assessing portfolios. The traditional psychometric approach, characterised by a focus on objective judgement based on standardisation and analytical assessment criteria has been found to be incompatible with the essentially non-standardised nature of many portfolios centred around the individual characteristics and challenges of individual learners and specific workplaces.(19,20) The psychometric quantitative approach does not quite fit with portfolios containing a variety of qualitative information, in addition to numerical information (scores).(6,21) Portfolios are not used to assess technical skills only: they are especially suited to assess non-technical skills, including professionalism.(22) This kind of assessment task cannot be translated into an analytical procedure with a standardised checklist and a list of strictly defined criteria.(23) Consequently, due to the presence of diverse qualitative information, assessors in weighing the information in a portfolio to assess competency inevitably have to rely on their personal judgement.(20,24,25)

To achieve a match between portfolio assessment and portfolio characteristics, we advocate an approach that leans heavily on the methodology of qualitative research.(19,20) As is the case with most portfolios, qualitative research requires interpretation of different kinds of qualitative information to arrive at meaningful statements about ill-defined problems. The strategies listed below can be useful when assessing portfolios.(2,19)

Strategies in portfolio assessment

Arrange for feedback cycles

Conduct periodical feedback cycles to ensure that learners are not taken by surprise when the final judgement arrives. Since portfolio contents are usually compiled over a longer period of time, it is ill advised to wait until the end of the period to make pronouncements about the quality of the portfolio. Intermediate formative assessments, such as feedback from a mentor,[1] are useful to allow learners to adapt and improve their portfolio. Regular feedback at different stages of portfolio development is advisable not only from an assessment perspective but from a learning perspective as well.(13,26)

Involve multiple informants

In addition to the assessors who judge the completed portfolio at the end of the period, different people who are in some way involved in the portfolio process can also make a valuable contribution to the assessment. The mentor is usually the first to comment on the quality of the portfolio.(27) He or she often knows the learner best, is in a position to ascertain the authenticity of the materials, and is familiar with the learner's work habits.(28) Peers are another group that can contribute to the assessment. The advantages of peer assessment are two-fold: peers know from experience what it means to produce a portfolio and by engaging in peer assessment they can familiarise themselves with the portfolio's assessment standards. Finally, learners can also self-assess the quality of their portfolios – for instance, by responding to the mentor's comments and/or by self-assessing their competencies. The literature shows that self-assessments tend to be biased.(29) To mitigate this bias, Eva and Regehr(30) recommended that learners should be encouraged to actively seek external information about their performance to arrive at well-validated self-assessments. In a similar vein, learners' self-assessments of their portfolios could be supported by mentor judgements to arrive at valid self-assessments.(31)

Train assessors

Organise a meeting (before the final assessment round and at an intermediate stage during the portfolio period) in which assessors can calibrate their judgements and discuss the assessment procedure and its results. Assessing vast amounts of highly diverse information in personalised portfolios requires professional judgement. Assessors inev-

---

[1] We use the term 'mentor' for a teacher or peer that supports the learner's development over a certain period of time. Other terms that could be used are tutor, coach, (clinical) teacher or supervisor.

itably use assessment criteria idiosyncratically, with judgement depending, for instance, on prior experiences and individual notions and beliefs about education and the competencies to be judged.(32) Differences between assessors can be reduced by engaging them in a discussion of the judgement process.(33) After discussing a benchmark portfolio, for example, assessors' interpretations of assessment criteria may converge and a joint understanding of the procedure to be followed can be built. Such discussions should preferably be scheduled not only immediately before an assessment round but also at an intermediate stage of the portfolio period when assessors can compare their own portfolio judgements with those of their colleagues and discuss differences of interpretation.(34) After the final assessment, information about all the assessments should be communicated to assessors to help improve their understanding of the entire process.

Develop sequential assessment

At Maastricht Medical School a procedure has been developed to optimise efficient use of the time available for assessment in which conflicting information triggers gathering more information.(19) Mentors make a recommendation for the assessment of the portfolios of the students under their guidance. Individual students and an assessor decide whether they agree with the mentor's recommendation. Agreement signals the completion of the assessment procedure. In cases where there is no agreement, the portfolio is submitted to a larger group of assessors. In this way it is ensured that portfolios causing doubt are judged more carefully than portfolios where judgement is unanimous. As more judges are consulted, the trustworthiness of the assessment increases. Additionally, the discussions between the assessors will enhance clarity with respect to the application of the criteria (*see* also under 'Train assessors').

Include narrative information.

Incorporate in the portfolio requests for qualitative, narrative feedback and give this information substantial weight in the assessment procedure. Narrative comments offer learners and assessors much richer information than quantitative, numerical feedback.(16) A score of seven on a ten-point scale gives little insight into what a learner has and has not done well. Only when strengths and weaknesses of performance are explicated in narrative feedback does assessment become truly informative. A related problem in workplace assessment is rater's leniency. For various reasons low scores are a rarity in practice, and consequently scores generally do not discriminate very well.(35) Narrative feedback, however, often provides more detailed and discriminative information about learner performance. Assessors can be encouraged to give narrative feedback by providing dedicated spaces in the assessment form.

Use clear rubrics or descriptors

Education institutions often put a great deal of energy into generating competency profiles. The important thing is to strike a balance between very long lists of concrete criteria detailing everything a learner must be able to do ('can do-statements') on the one hand and on the other hand global descriptions offering a general outline but little practical guidance for assessors. In other words, the trick is to strike the right balance between analytical and global criteria. To achieve this one might give learners and assessors an idea of the level to be attained for each global competency. A very useful instrument for this is rubrics or descriptors, which typically contain descriptions of each competency at different levels, such as the levels to be expected from a novice, a competent professional and an expert.(36)

Portfolio structure and content

Portfolios were first introduced into education for assessment purposes. These portfolios were basically nothing more than containers for storing various types of evidence of quality of performance. However, experiments with portfolios revealed that for evidence in a portfolio to be meaningful to assessors, it should be organised to reflect the competencies learners wish to demonstrate or the tasks they wish to illustrate.(37) To this end captions should be attached to the evidence in the portfolio, explaining what the evidence is supposed to show. The nature and diversity of the materials determine the richness of the picture the portfolio paints of the learner's activities and achievements. Although it may be tempting for learners to include a vast amount of materials leaving it up to the assessor to determine their value, this strategy is to be discouraged. For not only does it increase the assessors' workload, it can also cause confusion by preventing assessors from seeing the wood for the trees. It is therefore important for learners to be selective, and an excellent selection criterion is that materials should provide insight into the learner's development and progress. The variety of materials that may be included in a portfolio is huge. We distinguish the following three types.(2)

- Products – reports, papers, patient management plans, letters of discharge, critical appraisals of a topic
- Impressions – photographs, videos, observation reports
- Evaluations – test scores, feedback forms (e.g. mini-CEX, multisource feedback), letters from patients or colleagues expressing appreciation, certificates.

Portfolios to stimulate reflection

Cycles of reflection

Elsewhere we have defined 'reflection' as 'letting future behaviour be guided by a systematic and critical analysis of past actions and their consequences'.(38) Learning from participating in the workplace is the process of transforming experiences into knowledge, skills, attitudes and values, a process that can be represented graphically by experiential learning cycles, such as those proposed by Korthagen and colleagues and Kolb and Fry.(39,40) Concrete experiences, evaluation, analysis, formulation of abstract concepts and generalisations, and testing the implications in new situations are the stations of these cyclical models. At several of these stages, portfolios have a contribution to make. We will illustrate this using Korthagen's ALACT model (*see* Figure 14.3).(31,39)

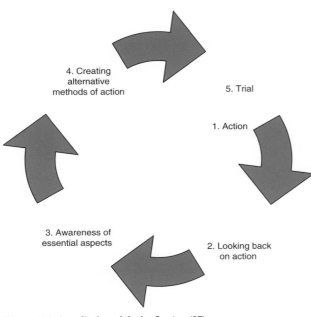

Figure 14.3 A cyclical model of reflection.(37)

Action

The cycle kicks off with action. To enable learners to improve their existing competencies while concurrently acquiring new ones, it is important to pre-select a task mix covering all the competencies required.

Looking back on action: Evaluation

Because unguided self-assessment is generally of (quite) poor quality, Eva and Regehr(30) proposed 'self-directed assessment seeking' as an alternative for this stage in professional development cycles. Following Boud,(41) they describe self-directed assessment seeking as a process of taking personal responsibility for looking outward by explicitly seeking feedback and information from external sources. At this stage, the portfolio would be the 'folder' in which the information is stored and organised in line with the competencies to be attained and with captions indicating what the evidence shows and the conclusions to be drawn about the level of performance.

Awareness of essential aspects: Analysis

In the next step, the analysis, data are examined, patterns detected, and cause and effect associations identified. At this stage, theory can be helpful to identify patterns and causal associations. Research shows that it is not self-evident that learners are able to analyse their own performance appropriately.(42) In view of this, Korthagen *et al.*(39) recommend that mentors should ask questions to stimulate learners to discover and explicate the reasons underlying their own and others' actions and to pinpoint any inconsistencies in the analysis.

Creating or identifying alternative methods of action: Change

Following and based on the analysis, alternative methods of action should be selected. It is the role of the mentor to encourage the learner to consider alternative courses of action, decide which one to use, and justify that choice. A SMART (specific, measurable, acceptable, realistic, time-bound) action plan initiates the next cycle of reflective learning.

For more on reflection and reflective practice, *see* Chapters 2 and 23.

Portfolio structure and content

In portfolios aimed at stimulating reflection, written contributions feature prominently. These reflections can relate to the competencies the learner wishes to acquire, and the learner will generally also evaluate performance, analyse what has already been mastered, and determine which competencies need further development.(31) The reflections can also pertain to the learner's motivation for attending the programme, and/or how the learner views his self as a doctor/professional. These reflections can serve as a long-term agenda for learners.

In portfolios that are specifically aimed at stimulating reflection, the reflections are central in the portfolio structure, with learners supporting their reflections by referring to materials and overviews in the portfolio.(43) This helps to focus the reflections, because learners are likely to aim for consistency of reflections and evidential materials. The requirement that reflections be supported by evidence helps to make reflections less non-committal. It is, for instance, not acceptable for learners to simply state that they have learned how to give a clinical presentation: they have to substantiate this statement by evidential materials and overviews demonstrating why and how they have done this.

Conclusions

The portfolio approach has theoretical as well as practical merits. It can capture performance and development in the workplace using qualitative information that can take into account unique characteristics of specific workplaces. In this way the portfolio closes the assessment gap by enabling assessment at Miller's 'does' level. Portfolios that include reflective writing require learners to engage in a 'conversation with self', which can be enhanced by reflective discussions with another person and by aiming for consistency with the evidence in the portfolio. Reflection provides learners and teachers a means to keep an overview of what has already been achieved and what still remains to be done.

Portfolios do not work of and by themselves. For a portfolio to be effective, certain conditions must be fulfilled. Probably the most crucial factor is the mentor: a person with whom the learner discusses the content of his/her portfolio (see Box 14.4).

Acknowledgement

We would like to thank Mereke Gorsira for revising the language of this article and to acknowledge John Pitts, whose chapter in the first edition of this book informed our writing of this one.

BOX 14.4 HOW TO: Combine the role of mentor and assessor

Teachers commonly fulfil the combined role of coach and assessor for their students. It has been argued, however, that combining these roles threatens the safety of the learning environment.(44) Elsewhere we have described alternative scenarios for the role of the mentor in assessment.(2)

The PhD supervisor

In some scenarios the role of the mentor in the assessment procedure of the portfolio resembles that of supervisors of PhD students. In many countries, dissertations are formally assessed by a committee. When the supervisor considers the dissertation to be up to standard, he/she invites peers with relevant expertise to sit on the assessment committee, of which the supervisor is not a member. As a negative assessment would be harmful to the supervisor's reputation, supervisors are highly unlikely to convene a committee unless they are convinced the dissertation meets the criteria. In this type of procedure, mentors and learners have a shared interest: to produce a dissertation or portfolio that merits a positive judgement.

The driving instructor

In this model the roles of the mentor and the assessor are strictly separate. The mentor/driving instructor coaches the learner in achieving the required competencies, shown in the portfolio. When the mentor thinks the learner is sufficiently competent, he or she invites an assessor from the relevant professional body (i.e. the Driver and Vehicle Licensing Agency) to assess the competencies of the learner. It is also possible for learners to take the initiative to approach the licensing agency.

The coach

In this model, the learners take the initiative. They may ask a senior colleague to coach them until they have achieved the required level of competence. This scenario is appropriate for instance when a professional wants to obtain an additional qualification. The assessor would be someone from an external body.

References

1 Miller GE (1990) The assessment of clinical skills/competence/performance. *Academic Medicine.* **65**(9 Suppl): S63–7.

2 Van Tartwijk J and Driessen EW (2009) Portfolios for assessment and learning: AMEE Guide no. 45. *Medical Teacher.* **31**(9): 790–801.

3 Davis MH, Friedman Ben-David M, Harden RM *et al.* (2001) Portfolio assessment in medical students' final examinations. *Medical Teacher.* **23**(4): 357–66.

4 Paulson FL, Paulson PR and Meyer CA (1991) What makes a portfolio a portfolio. *Educational Leadership.* **48**(5): 60–3.

5 Driessen E, van Tartwijk J, van der Vleuten C and Wass V (2007) Portfolios in medical education: why do they meet with mixed success? A systematic review. *Medical Education.* **41**(12): 1224–33.

6 Snadden D (1999) Portfolios – attempting to measure the unmeasurable? *Medical Education.* **33**(7): 478–9.

7 Buckley S, Coleman J, Davison I *et al.* (2009) The educational effects of portfolios on undergraduate student learning: a Best Evidence Medical Education (BEME) systematic review. BEME Guide No. 11. *Medical Teacher.* **31**(4): 282–98.

8 Tochel C, Haig A, Hesketh A *et al.* (2009) The effectiveness of portfolios for post-graduate assessment and education: BEME Guide No. 12. *Medical Teacher.* **31**(4): 299–318.

9 Van Tartwijk T, Driessen E, Hoeberigs B *et al.* (2003) *Werken met een elektronisch portfolio (To Work with an Electronic Portfolio).* Wolters-Noordhoff, Groningen.

10 Webb C (2002) Models of portfolios. *Medical Education.* **36**: 897–8.

11 Billet S (2006) Constituting the workplace curriuclum. *Journal of Curriculum Studies.* **38**(1): 31–48.

12 Jones MD Jr, Rosenberg AA, Gilhooly JT and Carraccio CL (2011) Perspective: competencies, outcomes, and controversy–linking professional activities to competencies to improve resident education and practice. *Academic Medicine.* **86**(2): 161–5.

13 Driessen EW, van Tartwijk J, Govaerts M, Teunissen P and van der Vleuten CP (2012) The use of programmatic assessment in the clinical workplace: a Maastricht case report. *Medical Teacher.* **34**(3): 226–31.

14 ten Cate O and Scheele F (2007) Competency-based postgraduate training: can we bridge the gap between theory and clinical practice? *Academic Medicine.* **82**(6): 542–7.

15 Scheele F, Teunissen P, Van Luijk S *et al.* (2008) Introducing competency-based postgraduate medical education in the Netherlands. *Medical Teacher.* **30**(3): 248–53.

16 Overeem K, Wollersheim H, Driessen E *et al.* (2009) Doctors' perceptions of why 360-degree feedback does (not) work: a qualitative study. *Medical Education.* **43**(9): 874–82.

17 Driessen E, Kenter G, de Leede B *et al.* (2011) Richtlijn voortgangsgesprek in de medische vervolgopleiding. *Tijdschrift voor Medisch Onderwijs.* **30**(6 Suppl 3): 51–62.

18 Overeem K, Driessen EW, Arah OA, Lombarts KM, Wollersheim HC and Grol RP (2010) Peer mentoring in doctor performance assessment: strategies, obstacles and benefits. *Medical Education.* **44**(2): 140–7.

19 Driessen E, van der Vleuten C, Schuwirth L, van Tartwijk J and Vermunt J (2005) The use of qualitative research criteria for portfolio assessment as an alternative to reliability evaluation: a case study. *Medical Education.* **39**(2): 214–20.

20 Van der Vleuten CP, Schuwirth LW, Scheele F, Driessen EW and Hodges B (2010) The assessment of professional competence: building blocks for theory development. *Best Practice and Research. Clinical Obstetrics and Gynaecology.* **24**(6): 703–19.

21 Pitts J and Coles C (2003) The challenge of non-standardised asessment of professionals-the need for a paradigm shift. *Education for Primary Care.* **14**: 397–405.

22 Driessen E (2009) Portfolio critics: do they have a point? *Medical Teacher.* **31**(4): 279–81.

23 Kuper A, Reeves S, Albert M and Hodges BD (2007) Assessment: do we need to broaden our methodological horizons? *Medical Education.* **41**(12): 1121–3.

24 van der Vleuten CP, Schuwirth LW, Driessen EW *et al.* (2012) A model for programmatic assessment fit for purpose. *Medical Teacher.* **34**(3): 205–14.

25 Eva KW and Hodges BD (2012) Scylla or Charybdis? Can we navigate between objectification and judgement in assessment? *Medical Education.* **46**(9): 914–9.

26 Altahawi F, Sisk B, Poloskey S, Hicks C and Dannefer EF (2012) Student perspectives on assessment: experience in a competency-based portfolio system. *Medical Teacher.* **34**(3): 221–5.

27 Dekker H, Driessen E, Ter Braak E *et al.* (2009) Mentoring portfolio use in undergraduate and postgraduate medical education. *Medical Teacher.* **31**(10): 903–9.

28 Driessen E, van Tartwijk J, Vermunt JD and van der Vleuten CP (2003) Use of portfolios in early undergraduate medical training. *Medical Teacher.* **25**(1): 18–23.

29 Davis DA, Mazmanian PE, Fordis M, Van Harrison R, Thorpe KE and Perrier L (2006) Accuracy of physician self-assessment compared with observed measures of competence: a systematic review. *Journal of the American Medical Association.* **296**(9): 1094–102.

30 Eva KW and Regehr G (2008) 'I'll never play professional football' and other fallacies of self-assessment. *Journal of Continuing Education in the Health Professions.* **28**(1): 14–9.

31 Driessen E, Overeem K and Van Tartwijk J (2010) Learning from practice: mentoring, feedback, and porfolios. In: Dornan T, Mann K, Scherpbier A and Spencer J (eds) *Medical Education: Theory and Practice*, pp. 211–27. Churchill Livingstone Elsevier, Edinburgh.

32 Govaerts MJ, Van de Wiel MW, Schuwirth LW, Van der Vleuten CP and Muijtjens AM (2013) Workplace-based assessment: raters' performance theories and constructs. *Advances in Health Sciences Education.* **18**(3): 375–96.

33 Pitts J, Coles C, Thomas P and Smith F (2002) Enhancing reliability in portfolio assessment: discussions between assessors. *Medical Teacher.* **24**(2): 197–201.

34 Rees CE and Sheard CE (2004) The reliability of assessment criteria for undergraduate medical students' communication skills portfolios: the Nottingham experience. *Medical Education.* **38**(2): 138–44.

35 Williams RG and Dunnington G (2004) Prognostic value of resident clinical performance ratings. *Journal of the American College of Surgeons.* **199**(4): 620–7.

36 Meade LB, Borden SH, Mcardle P, Rosenblum MJ, Picchioni MS and Hinchey KT (2012) From theory to actual practice: creation and application of milestones in an internal medicine residency program, 2004–2010. *Medical Teacher.* **34**(9): 717–23.

37 Bird T (1990) The schoolteacher's portfolio: an essay on possibilities. In: Millman J and Darling-Hammond L (eds) *The New Handbook of Teacher Evaluation: Assessing Elementary and Secondary School Teachers*, pp. 241–56. Corwin Press Inc., Newbury Park, CA.

38 Driessen E, van Tartwijk J and Dornan T (2008) The self critical doctor: helping students become more reflective. *BMJ (Clinical Research Ed.).* **336**(7648): 827–30.

39 Korthagen FAJ, Kessels J, Koster B, Lagerwerf B and Wubbels T (2001) *Linking Theory and Practice: The Pedagogy of Realistic Teacher Education.* Lawrence Erlbaum Associates, Mahwah, NY.

40 Kolb DA (1984) *Experiential Learning: Experience as the Source of Learning and Development.* Prentice Hall, Englewood Cliffs, NJ.

41 Boud D (1999) Avoiding the traps: seeking good practice in the use of self assessment and reflection in professional courses. *Social Work in Education.* **18**: 121–32.

42 Mansvelder-Longayroux DD, Beijaard D and Verloop N (2007) The portfolio as a tool for stimulating reflection by student teachers. *Teaching and Teacher Education.* **23**(1): 47–62.

43 Van Tartwijk J, Van Rijswijk M, Tuithof H and Driessen EW (2008) Using an analogy in the introduction of a portfolio. *Teaching and Teacher Education.* **24**: 927–38.

44 Tigelaar D, Dolmans D, Wolfhagen H and Van der Vleuten C (2004) Using a conceptual framework and the opinion of portfolio experts to develop a teaching portfolio prototype. *Studies in Educational Evaluation.* **30**: 305–21.

Further reading

Driessen E, van der Vleuten C, Schuwirth L, van Tartwijk J and Vermunt J (2005) The use of qualitative research criteria for portfolio assessment as an alternative to reliability evaluation: a case study. *Medical Education* **39**(2): 214–20.

Holmboe E and Hawkins R (eds) (2008) *Practical Guide to the Evaluation of Clinical Competence.* Mosby Elsevier, Philadelphia.

Klenowski V (2002) *Developing Portfolios for Learning and Assessment. Processes and Principles.* RoutledgeFalmer, London.

15 Self-regulated learning in medical education

Casey B White[1], Larry D Gruppen[2] and Joseph C Fantone[3]
[1] University of Virginia School of Medicine, USA
[2] Department of Medical Education, University of Michigan Medical School, USA
[3] University of Florida College of Medicine, USA

KEY MESSAGES

- Self-regulated learning is vital for continuing professional development.

- There is little evidence to suggest that medical schools and postgraduate institutions are successfully helping students become effective self-regulated learners.

- Researchers in medical education have most often studied self-regulated learning in the narrower context of self-assessment.

- Self-regulated learning involves four steps: *planning, learning, assessment* and *adjustment*.

- Self-regulated learning skills can be learnt – and therefore taught.

Introduction

The need for physicians to engage in effective self-regulated learning (SRL) is well documented and pressing, given the links between continuing medical education and the quality of health care.(1,2) However, there is little published evidence that medical schools and postgraduate institutions are successfully helping students become effective self-regulated learners. This is in spite of formal goals for 'life-long learning' prevalent among medical schools and residency programmes, and the availability of research findings to guide efforts to integrate SRL into education and training programmes.

Since the 1980s, educators and psychologists outside medicine have conducted extensive research into SRL. Characteristics and habits of identified self-regulated learners have been compiled and explored, and specific strategies have been identified and tested. Psychological dimensions, task conditions, attributes and processes have been categorised under constructs bounded by the scientific questions of why, how, what and where learners engage in SRL. Models have been presented characterising the complex and intersecting networks that underlie SRL and that include personality, cognition and development. Outcomes of this research provide evidence that SRL comprises a set of skills that *can* be learnt.

Undergraduate and graduate medical programmes have yet to grapple with this concept in a systematic and uniform way. This has been attributed in part to different interpretations of SRL among teachers and students,(3) and to the inconsistency with which it is defined and studied by medical educators and academics. In a 2005 review of the medical education literature reporting on SRL, Ainoda

et al.(4) found that only five out of 63 articles (8%) identified actually defined SRL, and those definitions were not consistent with one another.

In medical education, among the studies conducted on self-assessment and self-regulation, agreement on and evidence of a systematic, feedback-driven programme of SRL appears to be highly variable.(5–7) In fact, researchers in medical education have most often studied SRL in the narrower context of self-assessment, based on the notion that self-assessment is the first step in a two-step process: (a) self-assessment of knowledge and skills, followed by (b) self-regulated education to address areas of concern or weakness.(8) Yet there is evidence that physicians have limited ability to self-assess their strengths and weaknesses,(9) and that those physicians who are the least skilled are also the most confident and the weakest self-assessors.(10) This is perhaps why we have focused our research efforts on self-assessment and its accuracy – if one cannot self-assess accurately, one cannot focus self-education where it is most needed. While this is in fact correct, where does our limited success in predicting factors that are key to effective self-assessment leave us in terms of helping learners become effective self-assessors? Perhaps the problem in achieving this very important outcome lies in our perception of SRL and self-assessment.

Educational psychologists view SRL as a complex cycle comprising intermingling elements such as psychological characteristics (e.g. self-efficacy, motivation, beliefs and learning style), personal choices (effort expended, learning strategies), judgements (self-assessment, attributions) and personal actions (e.g. goal setting, adjustment).(6) They recommend a systematic integration of SRL into educational

Understanding Medical Education: Evidence, Theory and Practice, Second Edition. Edited by Tim Swanwick.
© 2014 The Association for the Study of Medical Education. Published 2014 by John Wiley & Sons, Ltd.

programmes, with monitoring and feedback to assure effective skills are acquired.

This chapter is meant to assure medical educators that SRL *can* be taught and that educators play a pivotal role in helping learners to develop the relevant skills.(11) The chapter provides theoretical and practical information about a broader and more complex cycle of SRL, and proposes a model for its integration into medical curricula. The model, adapted from research in educational psychology, reflects four steps that comprise the cycle of SRL (planning, learning, feedback/assessment and adjustment), and the underlying elements within each. Adoption of a consistent, evidence-based model within and across the continuum of medical education (i.e. undergraduate to postgraduate) and across programmes (i.e. around the country or around the world) will help us explore the effectiveness of this approach in helping learners set personal goals, consider how what they bring to their learning as unique individuals influences their learning, monitor (i.e. self-assess) their learning and make adjustments to assure that they meet their goals. Such a model can also help medical educators meet their own goals of training physicians who are prepared for self-regulated, lifelong learning.

A model for self-regulated learning

Medical educators are understandably eager to help students and physicians become capable of effective SRL. However, even medical programmes with clear expectations and requirements for their learners to engage in SRL do not necessarily have programmes in place to monitor the quality or effectiveness of SRL strategies used by students.(12)

Zimmerman reported that learners can be described as self-regulating to the extent that they are 'metacognitively, motivationally, and behaviourally active participants in their own learning process'.(13) Much of the research focused specifically on SRL has been grounded in elementary or middle school educational contexts, with some studies at more advanced educational levels. However, this work can be adapted and used as a framework for integrating SRL into medical education. The framework in Figure 15.1 adapts this research and models SRL as a cycle of four phases: planning, learning, assessment and adjustment.

Educators can contemplate different contexts (lecture hall, classroom, clinic, hospital) for applying elements of the model. Although it is important for learners to understand that ultimately the principles must apply across learning contexts, the elements can be introduced at earlier stages and then reinforced at later stages. In the next section of this chapter, each phase and element of the model is explicated, followed by an example of how the model may be applied (*see* Box 15.1).

Planning
To self-regulate effectively, learners must set personal goals. Goals guide the decisions we make related to learning (e.g. value, strategies), and they are the specific measure against which we self-assess learning and performance. Motivation

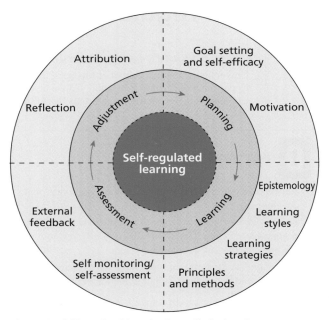

Figure 15.1 Self-regulated learning in medical education.

BOX 15.1 Case study

The extended example used in this chapter relates to the 'longitudinal cases' in use at the University of Michigan Medical School. These robust paper- and video-based cases developed from real patients are designed to help students recognise and grapple with the existence and complexity of psychosocial issues in patient care. Clinical topics in the cases align with what students are learning in concurrent organ-based courses. Each case is presented in two or three two-hour small group sessions; specific intended learning outcomes and questions or problems are provided for students to work through and respond to in a small group, facilitated setting.

Each small group leader participates in a number of development sessions to learn how to facilitate student-led discussions effectively and to assess student development. Midway through the Autumn term of the first year, all students participate in a teaching and learning workshop. Here they are introduced to developmental theory, (active) learning theory and methods, learning strategies and learning styles. They also learn how to write intended learning outcomes.

Assessment is Pass/Fail and is scaled on advancing levels of cognitive development in specific dimensions (e.g. quality of teaching, critical thinking and problem-solving, quality of participation), not on case content.

---

is a goal-guided process through which individuals instigate and sustain activities directly linked to goal achievement.(14) In the cycle of SRL, achievement of learning goals influences self-efficacy, which in turn reinforces motivation (*see* Box 15.2).

BOX 15.2 FOCUS ON: Factors that influence goal choice and commitment(16)

Personal factors

Previous performance	Individuals are most likely to attempt goals with which they have had previous success
Skill level	It is unlikely that individuals will attempt to achieve goals that are far beyond their level to achieve
Value	Individuals have personal beliefs about the importance or value in achieving a specific goal
Attributions	Attributing failure to unstable (controllable) causes such as low effort can lead to setting higher goals on subsequent tasks
Self-efficacy*	There is a positive correlation between high self-efficacy (personal belief that a goal is achievable) and strong commitment to goals

Social-environmental factors

Normative environment	Higher group norms encourage individuals to set higher personal goals
Group and peers	A peer or group can exert pressure in support of a group goal that encourages group members (or partner)
Role-modelling	Positive role modelling of goal setting by others encourages individuals to set higher personal goals
Feedback*	Feedback that stresses challenge, mastery, self-improvement and achievement towards goal has the most positive effect

*key factor

Goal-setting and self-efficacy

Goal-setting is the establishment of specific standards of performance or resulting outcomes. The motivational benefits of goals are dependent not just on goal-setting, but on learner commitment to achieving them.(15)

Personal and social-environmental factors influence goal choice and goal commitment. Personal factors include skill level, previous performance, beliefs about goal value and attribution of performance. However, self-efficacy is the most important influence on personal goal-setting.(15) Self-efficacy is an individual's belief in his or her ability to achieve specific goals.(16) A strong, positive sense of self-efficacy is critical to setting and achieving challenging yet attainable goals, which translate into personal successes that support setting more difficult goals.

Social-environmental factors include group norms (higher norms lead to higher personal goals), group and

peer goals, and role-modelling by peers. Feedback from others is an essential influence, especially when it comprises positive self-efficacy information that emphasises challenge, mastery, self-improvement and achieved progress towards goal (*see* Box 15.2).(15)

Motivation

It is useful to distinguish between intrinsic motivation, doing something because it is inherently interesting and enjoyable, and extrinsic motivation, doing something to obtain an outcome separate from the activity. Although intrinsic motivation results in high-quality learning, educators cannot depend on all learners to be intrinsically motivated across all learning tasks.

Self-determination theory emphasises that learners who are intrinsically motivated embrace learning as a valued activity in and of itself, regardless of rewards or outcomes.(17) Although this would seem to be an ideal orientation to learning, frankly, many of the tasks learners need to engage in to reach their learning goals are not inherently enjoyable.

Categories of extrinsic motivation range from the learner feeling the task(s) is controlled by external forces that produce rewards or punishments, to the learner feeling some sense of control over the task(s). Within this extrinsic framework, learner attitudes can range from resentment or disinterest to willingness.

The least autonomous form of extrinsic motivation is *external regulation*, in which individuals perform to satisfy an external demand or to reap an external reward. Next is *introjection*, in which individuals still feel external control, but perform to maintain self-esteem or a feeling of self-value. *Identification* is a more autonomous form of motivation in which an individual finds personal importance in an action and internalises it as a means to a broader personal goal. The most autonomous form of extrinsic motivation is *integration*, in which individuals internalise reasons for an action and assimilate them totally into themselves. Although identification and integration share important qualities with intrinsic motivation, these are still extrinsic motivation because individuals are motivated to achieve a goal that they see as separate from their behaviour.

Although all learners bring some level of motivation to their learning,(18) educators can create environments that support development of intrinsic motivation and autonomy. Such environments offer optimal challenges, interpersonal involvement in learning, acknowledgement of feelings, opportunities to make choices about learning, and also opportunities for learners to evaluate their own and others' learning.(19)

Medical students and junior doctors are certainly, at least generally, viewed as highly motivated learners. While this might be true within the boundaries and 'safety' of a formal educational programme, autonomy is key to lifelong learning, and intrinsic motivation is key to the development of autonomy. Also, extrinsically motivated learners who no longer have a strong reward system or direct oversight/feedback might not be effective self-regulated learners. If our goal is to help students and trainees become self-regulated learners who will pursue excellence throughout their professional careers, research relevant to motivation needs to become a greater focus in medical education (*see* Box 15.3).

Learning

Learning can be defined as 'a persisting change in performance or performance potential that results from experience and interaction with the world'.(21) Individuals perceive and interact with the environment in personal and unique ways based on characteristics such as intelligence, personality, beliefs, experiences and culture. Because of this, there is no single idea, principle, paradigm or belief that defines how individuals learn most effectively. Furthermore, educators should be aware of how their own and their learners' beliefs about learning influence learning, as well as the presence of learning styles and their potential to influence the effectiveness of learning.

Epistemology

Personal epistemology is an individual's beliefs about knowledge and knowing. There is growing interest in how epistemology influences knowledge acquisition, cognition (i.e. thinking and reasoning), and decisions educators and learners make about learning.(22)

Research provides evidence that individuals traverse through a patterned sequence of development in their beliefs about knowledge and knowing, becoming more complex as they advance through college.(23) One schema proposes four distinct categories and transition stages along a continuum ranging from a simplistic belief that knowledge exists as a fixed entity to be transmitted from knower to learner, to a more complex belief that knowledge is fluid, changing and contextual, and must be individually discovered (*see* Figure 15.2). This journey tends to be reinitiated when new areas of knowledge are first addressed.

In their progress towards self-regulation, learners should be aware of their own beliefs and how they influence their efforts to reach their academic goals. Using a number of methods, educators can help learners understand where they are along the epistemological (i.e. developmental) continuum and how they can move forward.

BOX 15.3 Self-regulated learning in practice: Planning

At the first meeting of the longitudinal case (LC) small groups, early in the first year, students are introduced to the format of the cases and the nature of the problems/questions, as well as the expectations for their performance and participation. Personal responsibility for ensuring self-learning (with guidance and resources as needed/requested) and peer learning is emphasised to foster and support appropriate motivation for learning.

At this first meeting, students are asked to set personal learning goals for the LCs. Goals should address all domains, not just knowledge, and they should be articulated at an appropriate level (Bloom's *Taxonomy*(20) is used as a guide). Students discuss their goals with their facilitator (briefly) in an early small group. They may adjust their goals/learning outcomes and re-submit them at any time, and they are encouraged to do so at the start of each term (if detailed, these can also serve as a learning plan for the next stage of the cycle).

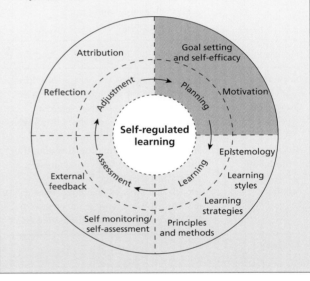

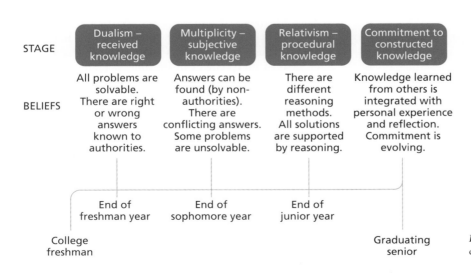

Figure 15.2 Intellectual development in the college years.(23)

Most college students have advanced beyond viewing knowledge as concrete and static; they are moving towards seeing it as dynamic and changing, and see themselves as active constructors of their own knowledge. Autonomous learning, including accurate and effective self-assessment, requires the ability to look at one's self objectively, something that is only possible at the higher levels of the developmental continuum.(24)

Given this evidence, it makes sense for medical students and trainees to be challenged to learn and practise these skills in increasingly complex contexts, if only because physicians use self-assessment skills in complex contexts in their professional lives. Based on evidence of strong correlations between epistemological beliefs and cognitive strategies that students use for learning, both educators and learners should have a solid understanding of their own beliefs about the acquisition of knowledge and how these can influence decisions related to teaching and to learning.

Learning styles

Learning styles can be thought of as innate characteristics possessed by learners that underlie and influence their learning, as opposed to learning strategies, which are the techniques learners choose. Although there is skepticism about the validity of learning styles as a construct, researchers continue to propose and categorise individual styles; one example of many is Kolb's 'cycle of experiential learning'.(25)

There is increasing evidence that many learners have multimodal preferences for learning, depending on time, circumstance and context.(26) In medical education a study of first year medical students using the VARK (visual, audio, read/write, kinaesthetic) inventory revealed that the majority of students preferred multiple modes.(27)

What is most important is that teachers and learners recognise that individuals can and do have different preferences for learning, just as they have different personalities. Knowledge about how they learn most effectively can help learners strategise and choose techniques, as they approach their learning, and also help them assess more effectively their progress towards learning goals. Both learning styles and learning strategies are critical to effective SRL because of their key and personal connections to achieving learning outcomes or goals.

Learning strategies

Learning strategies are important in self-regulation because they are one area in which learners, in formal educational programmes, can exercise direct control or autonomy. Making decisions about strategies is a dynamic process that requires attention to different learning elements: individual learner needs (e.g. high aptitude for particular content versus low aptitude); styles (e.g. visual learner versus auditory); contexts (e.g. studying biochemistry versus studying the cardiac examination); and other factors such as environment and time of day.(28)

The effectiveness of strategies will also change as learners advance or change contexts in a particular discipline or domain. A strategy for learning the very basics of the cardiac examination (e.g. how to place a stethoscope) will not be effective for more advanced skills (e.g. detecting/recognising a cardiac abnormality). Learners need to be attentive to this and to self-monitoring outcomes that indicate the success or failure of specific strategies in helping them to achieve learning goals.

Finally, learners can encounter problems choosing and deploying the most appropriate strategies. They might not effectively match strategies with study/learning conditions, they might not be proficient in strategies they choose, or they might even lack the motivation necessary to employ certain strategies.(29) Such problems can be mitigated with effective monitoring and formative feedback.(30)

Principles and methods

Connecting principles with methods enables the building of a bridge of understanding between teachers and learners. As epistemological beliefs evolve – that is, as learners begin to see they have a personal role in their acquisition of knowledge and see knowledge as more dynamic – problem-solving skills improve. This suggests that educators should consider their own epistemological beliefs in light of the pedagogical decisions they make based on those beliefs, and how those decisions affect the beliefs, knowledge acquisition and cognitive development of their learners.

It is important for educators to articulate specific principles underlying expectations and approaches, if they are to help individuals become autonomous, self-regulating learners; it is equally important that learners understand these principles, so that they are prepared to meet these expectations. For example, in a course or programme one underlying principle might be to help individuals become self-directed learners. This should be stated explicitly, and learners should be given specific information about what is expected of them. For instance, as self-directed learners 'in training' they will be expected to set their own goals, use experts and resources to help them achieve their goals, be willing to take responsibility for their own learning and productivity, be able to manage their own time and projects, and assess themselves and their peers.(31) The 'Zone of Proximal Development' (ZPD) – the space between what learners cannot do at all and what they can do independently – provides an excellent foundation for helping students to develop learning autonomy.(32) In the ZPD, learners are guided and encouraged by instructors and more knowledgeable peers; guidance is provided at the starting point, and then increasingly diminished until it becomes unnecessary. Active learning exercises designed for collaborative work are based on the premise that peers (as well as instructors) can provide scaffolding for each other's learning.

Teachers can conceptualise, construct and model specific learning activities that encourage ongoing cognitive growth and acquisition of increasingly complex reasoning skills. Approaches that foster development and provide logical opportunities for self-regulation include pedagogies with progressively increased emphasis on learners' participation and responsibility for their own and their peers' learning. Active learning methods such as collaboration

BOX 15.4 Self-regulated learning in practice: Learning

Expectations for student performance are presented and discussed in the first meeting. There is not an explicit assessment of learning styles or strategies; rather, students choose their own strategies for personal learning, and they are given the control and autonomy to choose the methods by which they will teach in the longitudinal cases.

Questions/problems related to the cases are presented in a provocative manner to challenge students to grapple with complex and uncomfortable issues, to help them develop appropriate problem-solving skills, to encourage introspection and reflection, and to foster integration of personal experiences into new learning. The processes and heuristics students use to tackle these problems – thinking through potential and alternate solutions, applying values, and considering and weighing evidence and opinions – provide essential information about developmental level and cognitive and professional characteristics. Peers and facilitator provide feedback.

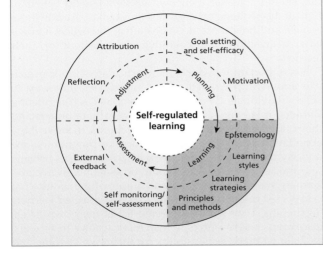

and opportunities for learners to discuss and analyse ill-structured problems and controversial issues help foster the advanced cognitive skills that are inherent in higher levels of development (*see* Box 15.4).(33,34)

A concept nicknamed the 'flipped classroom' is gaining momentum across education. Students learn lower-order principles and concepts outside the classroom, before coming to class, allowing instructors to engage students in higher-order approaches to learning inside the classroom, where students can collaborate and instructors can guide. In higher order activities, students are at the very least *applying* the information they have learned in more authentic contexts, which sparks curiosity and interest, and fosters contextual recall (i.e. 'stickiness').(35)

Feedback and assessment

Feedback is a key component of SRL.(30) In a perfect world, self-regulated learners generate criteria against which to monitor their progress, as they create their own goals for

achievement. They then systematically monitor and interpret their progress against goals and adjust, as needed. However, their interpretation of their progress might vary in accuracy because learners hold differing beliefs about learning and about their own self-efficacy, and they might also have knowledge or learning deficits of which they are not aware (i.e. 'you don't know what you don't know'). Thus, it is critical that learners receive timely, targeted and systematic feedback to help improve learning and to help them develop skills for effective self-monitoring and SRL.

Internal monitoring/self-assessment

Educational psychologists study the impact of feedback on the self-monitoring process as a means of exploring links between self-monitoring and self-regulated learning.(36) Engaging in SRL activities improves academic performance within formal educational structures where it is fostered and where feedback is part of the SRL cycle.(37,38) In fact, SRL and feedback are inextricably linked in school, where learners begin to understand, practise and then ultimately master SRL. Formative assessment includes both feedback and self-monitoring. The goal of many instructional systems is to facilitate the transition from feedback to self-monitoring.(39)

Internal monitoring is a conscious, pivotal element of learning that guides SRL. Learners identify goals, choose strategies and apply those strategies to a task(s) that yields a specific (learning) product or outcome. Self-monitoring during this process produces internal feedback (self-assessment) that compares the evolving state of the task to the goal. This provides the basis for further action(s) on the part of the learner, such as adjustment of strategies or even adjustment of goals.

Research on self-monitoring suggests that most learners do not inherently possess optimal skills.(40) When left to regulate on their own, learners will often monitor their progress incorrectly (e.g. believing they have mastered what they intended to) and terminate learning activities before achieving goals. Reasons for this vary, and some are linked with learners' choice of learning strategies. If the strategy chosen is not linked effectively with what the learner needs to accomplish in the task at hand, the same faulty thinking that led to that choice might contribute to incorrectly judging progress towards goals.(36) Also, during self-monitoring, learners might misperceive cues (specific criteria representing their progress) and thus misperceive progress, or they might be overwhelmed by cognitive demands that skew internal feedback on progress.

Studies of self-assessment across undergraduate and postgraduate medical education have tended to focus on assessment of outcomes, rather than internal formative feedback that guides learning and sharpens self-regulated learning actions. Many of these studies ask medical students or trainees to estimate their performance in a small group setting, an examination or essay, or a clinical performance (e.g. Objective Structured Clinical Examination station with a standardised patient), treating self-assessment as a separate and distinct entity. These studies focus on learner accuracy, usually as a comparison of a self-estimated performance measured against an 'actual' performance

BOX 15.5 WHERE'S THE EVIDENCE: Self-assessment(47)

There is a lack of published research to answer the important questions:

• Does self-assessment help identify learning needs?

• Does self-assessment bring about change in learner activity or clinical practice?

Most research focuses on the accuracy of self-assessment.

Some studies have looked at the impact of gender. The evidence is inconclusive, although a very large study (*n* = 1152) indicates men overestimate their ability more than women do.

Poor performers tend to overestimate their ability, while competent individuals are more likely to be accurate.

Students are more accurate at self-assessing practice skills than knowledge.

Feedback in the form of video, benchmarking and instruction can improve self-assessment accuracy.

Research on self-assessment has been fraught with methodological problems.

There is need for further research in this area to examine the impact of self-assessment.

as scored or judged by an expert. Such 'accuracy studies' have provided evidence that even medical practitioners are poor self-assessors, when their self-assessments are compared with others' assessments of their knowledge and skills.(10,41)

The medical education literature on self-assessment (*see* Box 15.5) reports at least one finding that is similar to the educational psychology literature on self-monitoring: while some learners are accurate self-assessors, many or even most are not.(42–44) Self-assessment accuracy is task- and context-specific (as are SRL strategies), but when the context changes, the better self-assessors remain better than the poorer self-assessors.(45) Attempts to identify characteristics of good self-assessors (i.e. reasons why some learners are more accurate than others) have provided limited useful information.(46)

There are those who blame the lack of enlightening findings on the methodologies used for the various studies on medical student self-assessment.(47) While this might certainly be true, another basic problem might be how medical education perceives and conceptualises the role of self-assessment. Educators believe self-assessment is a critical element in the process or cycle of SRL.(48,49) However, few medical educators or medical education programmes focus on the process of self-monitoring to achieve personal and external learning outcomes, or on how formative feedback can influence both performance and self-monitoring of performance. Rather, medical education is focused on the outcome of self-assessment – whether students self-assess their grade/score accurately. This means our assessment

systems are focused more on providing summative information than formative feedback, and without formative feedback, attempts to integrate self-regulation are likely to have only limited success.

External formative feedback

Formative feedback occurs when teachers provide information to learners designed to enable them to learn better, improve performance, and enhance their self-reflective and self-monitoring processes. Effective formative feedback focuses learners' attention on their progress towards achieving goals, provides specific information that helps them to recognise and close gaps, and integrates review, reflection and self-assessment components. In its purest form, formative feedback does not involve scoring or grading.

Educators can serve as guides, as learners develop their goals and choose learning strategies, but learners must self-monitor their own progress; faculty can then provide formative feedback that confirms or rectifies internal feedback. Both roles must be integrated into the curriculum and into expectations for learners and faculty.

Unfortunately, we know that the paucity of formative feedback in medical education is a critical issue and stems from two major causes: infrequent faculty observation of trainees/students; and discomfort among preceptors in giving feedback. Both lead to general and non-specific feedback (student to preceptor: 'How am I doing?'; preceptor to student: 'Fine') that fails to give students sufficiently specific information to reflect on their performance in the context of progress towards goals, and to adjust personal goals, strategies or techniques.

Problems with sufficient time to give formative feedback are exacerbated by regulations restricting the number of hours juniors can work; such legislation has influenced the availability of preceptors to provide feedback to learners in many clinical disciplines.(50) Experienced educators have proposed teaching models such as the 'One-minute Preceptor' that incorporate timely formative feedback.(51,52) Another model is the Clinical Encounter Card, which incorporates specific, timely feedback to students. At one institution medical students used the feedback to improve their performance and were encouraged by faculty using the cards to develop their own learning objectives on the rotation.(53)

Faculty development workshops designed to help preceptors sharpen feedback skills and improve comfort levels with giving feedback have been well received.(54) At the very least, specific guidelines for what constitutes formative feedback can help improve the timing and quality of formative feedback, which in turn provides learners with the information they need to reflect on their performance and make necessary adjustments.(55) Formative feedback is covered in more detail in Chapter 23 (*see* Box 15.6).

Adjustment

Self-regulated learners must synthesise self- and externally generated feedback related to progress towards learning goals and take action such as adjustments to goals or strategies. Reflection (as a foundation for synthesis) and

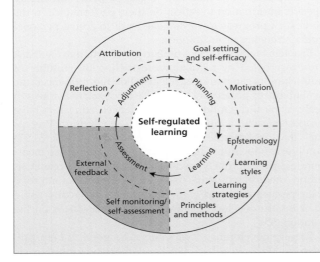
attribution (as a foundation for action) are central issues to consider in this part of the cycle.

Affect plays a key role in this phase. Preceptors are cautioned to keep their own personal feelings separate from the feedback they provide to learners. However, learners are bound to have feelings related to what they hear about their performance. In the process of reflection, learners can acknowledge their feelings and then learn to put them to productive use. Positive feedback and successful progress can boost feelings of self-efficacy and motivation and thus begin another round through the cycle. Negative feedback can diminish self-efficacy and motivation, especially if learners let their emotions interfere with understanding where and how they can adjust. Placing the blame for disappointing or frustrating performance on poor choices of goals (perhaps too ambitious) or strategies (perhaps not aligned well with goals) will help learners make the changes they need to make and to continue effectively through the SRL cycle. Placing the blame on self (not smart enough) or others (the resident did not like me) can get learners 'stuck' in the cycle and unable to move forward. Insufficient feedback leaves learners with insufficient information to move forward as well.

It is important for learners to acknowledge feelings (particularly where learning is focused on attitudes), but it is just as important for them to have a sense of control over their learning – a sense that if efforts are not entirely successful, they can adjust as needed and achieve success.

Reflection

Reflection is an advanced cognitive skill that requires individuals to examine new information/material, weigh its validity and relevance, and draw conclusions that they either incorporate into existing cognitive structures, or use to construct new structures with links to existing ones.(56) Reflection, an essential element of learning, is just as essential for developing SRL competency in learners.(57) In the context of SRL, reflection encourages individuals to consider themselves as learners with personal goals, beliefs and styles, to evaluate the processes or strategies they have chosen, and then to weigh the level of success these have contributed towards achievement of goals. Reflection provides important information as learners approach learning in the future (i.e. continue once again through the cycle).

Schön(58) conceptualised the reflective practitioner, who possesses certain tacit expertise that is revealed through skilful performance. Reflection-*on*-action is a process individuals use to ponder their performance after a task has been completed, reflecting on what worked well and what would they have done differently. Reflection-*in*-action is a process individuals use, as they are working on a task and encounter situations in which their knowledge-in-action does not work in some new or changed context; in this circumstance reflection allows the learner to adjust an activity or task 'on the fly', that is, while it is ongoing.

Reflection-in-action can also be conceptualised as reflection-in-learning, where reflection during the learning process is encouraged and enhanced by self-monitoring and external, formative feedback. Guidance or feedback on the reflection process might be in order because some learners do not naturally engage in reflection and others can become more productive in their reflective activities. However, there is evidence that due in part to insufficient training, faculty charged with helping students become reflective are not prepared to do so. Faculty development should address appropriate training and expectations.(59)

Educators can employ different methods to help learners become comfortable with reflection, such as portfolios or writing in journals. As development advances, reflection can also be integrated as a key step in solving complex or ill-structured problems. Reflective practice is discussed in more depth in Chapter 2.

Attribution

Learners make causal attributions about whether specific performances are the result of ability or effort extended. Poor performance attributed to insufficient ability can discourage efforts to improve, while poor performance attributed to learning strategies can encourage efforts to experiment with different strategies in order to improve.(28)

Attribution theory provides a useful contemporary framework for thinking about specific factors to which learners attribute their academic successes or failures.(60) There are three types of explanation that individuals tend to make about success or failure.

- The cause of success or failure might be *internal* or *external* (factors within us or factors within the environment).
- The cause of success or failure might be *stable* or *unstable* (stable if we believe the outcome will be the same if we perform the same behaviour again, unstable if we believe the outcome might be different).
- The cause of success or failure might be *controllable* or *uncontrollable* (we can alter controllable factors if we wish, we cannot easily alter uncontrollable factors).

Learners will be most successful at achieving learning goals and outcomes, when they attribute poor academic performance to internal, unstable factors over which they have control (i.e. effort). However, a key assumption of attribution theory is that learners will want to attribute academic success or failure in ways that maintain a positive self-image. Thus, when they achieve intended outcomes, learners will tend to attribute success to their own effort or ability, but when they do *not* achieve intended outcomes, they will tend to attribute failure to poor teaching or bad luck – factors over which they have no control. The ideal attribution for academic success is ability plus effort, and in practical terms effort can be defined as devoting effective learning time and strategies to academic tasks.

Learners who engage in the strategic, step-by-step learning that characterises SRL will tend to attribute success or failure on learning tasks to the presence or absence of sufficient strategic approaches, and they will blame failed efforts on their approaches, rather than on their innate ability or on others. They can adjust their approaches to assure better outcomes, that is, they are in control of this process and thus they are in control of the outcomes.(61)

Outcomes of successfully employed SRL include learners' positive feelings about their accomplishments and the responsibility and self-control they engaged to accomplish what they did, which cyclically provides motivation to progress to the next step of learning (*see* Box 15.7).(62)

Conclusion

This chapter has described a model for SRL that was synthesised from existing theory and evidence, most of which was undertaken and reported by educational psychologists. Scholars and educators involved in this research believe that effective SRL habits can be learnt, and that

---

BOX 15.7 Self-regulated learning in practice: Adjustment

Given the nature of the psychosocial issues in the longitudinal cases and the presence of attitudinal intended learning outcomes, students are provided with opportunities for reflection about issues. These opportunities for practising reflection are meant to prepare them for reflection on personal issues such as beliefs, goals and performance.

Students are provided with a variety of resources, but they are free to make decisions about strategies they use to study and methods they use to learn and to help their classmates learn. With that freedom comes responsibility for assuring that learning is occurring and progress is made towards goals or learning outcomes. If progress is slower than expected or off-target, reflection about what might be wrong and how to adjust is encouraged.

Each (end-of-term) assessment period, facilitators submit their assessments of students and then review and discuss with each student faculty assessment, self-assessment and progress towards course and personal goals. Because the assessment instrument is scaled on distal learning outcomes, proximal goals are encouraged. In their one-on-one meetings with students (formal meeting times are scheduled twice each year), facilitators make explicit connections between personal goals and personal responsibility for learning (attributing performance appropriately). Students are reminded of the expectations for them in the context of the course, and are encouraged to discuss areas where they believe more or different goals and effort are required.

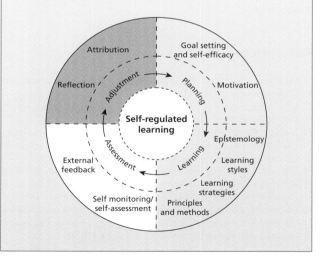

---

educators play a key role – through intentional practice – in helping learners understand and master these habits.

Medical educators believe self-assessment is a vital skill in professional practice – particularly in light of its links to the quality of medical care; researchers connected with medical education have investigated this phenomenon inside and outside the classroom and clinic. They have, however, thus far been stymied in attempts to draw evidence-based conclusions that guide educators in how to help learners master the ability to self-assess themselves effectively. Perhaps this is because these efforts have been focused solely on self-assessment, and on measuring self-assessment accuracy.

In fact, practising professionals are not *just* self-assessing. They are self-regulating their learning through the decisions they make related to what to learn (goals), how to learn it (epistemology, styles, strategies, methods), whether or not they have learnt what they intended to learn (assessment) and what to do if they have not learnt what they intended to learn (adjustment). They are self-regulating, but perhaps not as effectively as they might if they had been trained to think about each of those steps consciously with the intent that they become habit.

The model proposed here takes a broader look at the self in the context of learning, beyond self-assessment as the 'driving force' in lifelong learning. Such a model gives us, as educators, a broader focus for helping our learners to become intentional self-regulators; within this context self-assessment remains key, but as a process interlinked with personal goals, actions and outcomes that reciprocally reinforce each other. It is within this broader context that learners can see and understand the importance of self-assessment in the process of learning, and the importance of assuming greater and greater responsibility for their own learning.

Acknowledgement

With thanks to Professor Jan Illing at the University of Durham for her contribution to this chapter on self-assessment.

References

1 Westberg J and Jason H (1994) Fostering learners' reflection and self-assessment. *Family Medicine*. **26**: 278–82.

2 Lowenthal W (1981) Continuing education for professionals: voluntary or mandatory? *Journal of Higher Education*. **52**: 519–38.

3 Miflin B, Campbell CB and Price DA (1999) A lesson from the introduction of a problem-based, graduate entry course: the effects of different view of self-direction. *Medical Education*. **33**: 801–7.

4 Ainoda N, Onishi H and Yasuda Y (2005) Definitions and goals of self-directed learning in contemporary medical education literature. *Annals of the Academy of Medicine, Singapore*. **34**: 515–9.

5 Dornan H, Hadfield J, Brown M *et al.* (2005) How can medical students learn in a self-directed way in the clinical environment? Design-based research. *Medical Education*. **39**: 356–64.

6 White CB (2007) Smoothing out transitions: how pedagogy influences medical students' achievement of self-regulated learning goals. *Advances in Health Sciences Education: Theory and Practice*. **12**: 279–97.

7 Harvey BJ, Rothman AI and Frecker RC (2003) Effect of an undergraduate medical curriculum on students' self-directed learning. *Academic Medicine*. **78**: 1259–65.

8 Regehr G, Hodges B, Tiberius R and Lofchy J (1996) Measuring self-assessment skills: an innovative relative ranking model. *Academic Medicine*. **71**(10): S52–4.

9 Eva KW and Regehr G (2005) Self-assessment in the health professions: reformulation and research agenda. *Academic Medicine*. **80**(10): S46–54.

10 Davis DA, Mazmanian PE, Fordis M *et al.* (2006) Accuracy of physician self-assessment compared with observed measures of competence. *Journal of the American Medical Association*. **296**: 1094–103.

11 Pintrich PR (1995) *Understanding Self-Regulated Learning. New Directions for Teaching and Learning*, no. 63. Jossey-Bass, San Francisco, CA.

12 Evensen DH, Salisbury-Glennon JD and Glenn J (2001) A qualitative study of six medical students in a problem-based curriculum: toward a situated model of self-regulation. *Journal of Educational Psychology*. **93**: 659–76.

13 Zimmerman BJ (1989) A social cognitive view of self-regulated learning. *Journal of Educational Psychology*. **81**: 329–39.

14 Pintrich PR and Schunck DH (2002) *Motivation in Education: Theory, Research and Applications* (2e). Merrill Prentice Hall, Upper Saddle River, NJ.

15 Locke EA and Latham GP (1990) *A Theory of Goal Setting and Task Performance*. Prentice Hall, Englewood Cliffs, NJ.

16 Bandura A (1994) Self-efficacy. In: Ramachaudran VS (ed.) *Encyclopedia of Human Behavior* (vol. 4), pp. 71–81. Academic Press, New York.

17 Ryan RM and Deci EL (2000) Intrinsic and extrinsic motivations: classic definitions and new directions. *Contemporary Educational Psychology*. **25**: 54–67.

18 Winne PH (1997) Experimenting to bootstrap self-regulated learning. *Journal of Educational Psychology*. **89**: 397–410.

19 Deci EL, Vallerand RJ, Pelletier LG and Ryan RM (1991) Motivation and education: the self-determination perspective. *Educational Psychologist*. **26**: 325–46.

20 Bloom B, Englehart M, Furst E *et al.* (1956) *Taxonomy of Educational Objectives: The Classification of Educational Goals. Handbook I: Cognitive Domain*. Longmans, Green, New York and Toronto.

21 Driscoll MP (1999) *Psychology of Learning for Instruction*. Allyn and Bacon, Boston, MA.

22 Hofer BK (2006) Domain specificity of personal epistemology: resolved questions, persistent issues, new models. *International Journal of Educational Research*. **45**: 85–95.

23 Perry WG (1970) *Forms of Intellectual and Ethical Development in the College Years: A Scheme*. Holt, Rinehart, and Winston, New York.

24 Kegan R (1994) *In Over Our Heads: The Mental Demands of Modern Life*. Cambridge University Press, Cambridge, MA.

25 Kolb DA (1984) *Experiential Learning*. Prentice Hall, Upper Saddle River, NJ.

26 Gurpinar E, Bati H and Tetik C (2011) Learning styles of medical students in relation to time. *Advances in Physiology Education*. **35**: 307–11.

27 Lujan HL and Di Carlo SE (2006) First-year medical students prefer multiple learning styles. *Advances in Physiology Education*. **30**: 13–6.

28 Zimmerman BJ (2000) Attaining self-regulation: a social-cognitive perspectives. In: Boekaerts M, Pintrich PR and Zeidner MH (eds) *Handbook of Self-Regulation*, pp. 13–39. Academic Press, San Diego, CA.

29 Winne PH (1982) Minimizing the black box problem to enhance the validity of theories about instructional effects. *Instructional Science*. **11**: 13–28.

30 Butler DL and Winne PH (1995) Feedback and self-regulated learning: a theoretical synthesis. *Review of Educational Research*. **65**: 245–81.

31 Grow G (1991) Teaching learners to be self-directed. *Adult Education Quarterly*. **41**: 125–49.

32 Vygotsky LS (1978) *Mind in Society: The Development of Higher Psychological Processes*. Harvard University Press, Cambridge, MA.

33 Baxter Magolda MB (1999) *Creating Contexts for Learning and Self-authorship: Constructive-Developmental Pedagogy*. Vanderbilt University Press, Nashville, TN.

34 King P and Kitchener KS (1994) *Developing Reflective Judgment: Understanding and Promoting Intellectual Growth and Critical Thinking in Adolescents and Adults*. Jossey-Bass, San Francisco, CA.

35 Prober C and Heath C (2012) Lecture halls without lectures: a proposal for medical education. *New England Journal of Medicine.* **366**(18): 1657–9.

36 Balzer WK, Doherty ME and O'Connor R (1989) Effects of cognitive feedback on performance. *Psychological Bulletin.* **106**: 410–33.

37 Shokar GS, Shokar NK, Romero CM and Bulik RJ (2002) Self-directed learning: looking at outcomes with medical students. *Family Medicine.* **34**: 197–200.

38 Andrews GR and Debus RL (1978) Persistence and the causal perception of failure: modifying cognitive attributions. *Journal of Educational Psychology.* **70**: 154–66.

39 Sadler DR (1989) Formative assessment and the design of instructional systems. *Instructional Science.* **18**: 119–44.

40 Baker L (1984) Children's effective use of multiple standards for evaluating their comprehension. *Journal of Educational Psychology.* **76**: 588–97.

41 Boerebach BC, Arah QA, Busch OR and Lombarts KM (2012) Reliable and valid tools for measuring surgeons' performance: residents' vs. self evaluation. *Journal of Surgical Education.* **69**(4): 511–20.

42 Rezler AG (1989) Self-assessment in problem-based groups. *Medical Teacher.* **11**: 151–6.

43 Das M and Mpofu D (1998) Self and tutor evaluations in problem-based learning tutorials: is there a relationship? *Medical Education.* **32**: 411–8.

44 Tousignant M and DesMarchais JE (2002) Accuracy of student self-assessment ability compared to their own performance in a problem-based learning medical program: a correlation study. *Advances in Health Sciences Education: Theory and Practice.* **7**: 19–27.

45 Fitzgerald JT, White CB and Gruppen LD (2003) A longitudinal study of self-assessment accuracy. *Medical Education.* **37**: 645–9.

46 Baliga S, Gruppen LD, Fitzgerald JT *et al.* (1998) Do personal characteristics and background influence self-assessment accuracy? Paper presented at the Eight Ottawa Conference on Medical Education, Philadelphia, PA, June.

47 Colthart I, Bagnall, Evans A et al.(2008) The effectiveness of self-assessment on the identification of learner needs, learner activity, and impact on clinical practice: BEME Guide no. 10. *Medical Teacher.* **30**(2): 124–45.

48 Engel CE (1991) Not just a method but a way of learning. In: Boud B and Geletti G (eds) *The Challenge of Problem-Based Learning,* pp. 23–33. Kogan Page, London.

49 Berkson L (1993) Problem-based learning: have the expectations been met? *Academic Medicine.* **68**(10): S79–88.

50 White CB, Haftel HM, Purkiss JA *et al.* (2006) Multi-dimensional effects of the 80-hour work week. *Academic Medicine.* **81**: 57–62.

51 Irby DM, Aagaard E and Teherani A (2004) Teaching points identified by preceptors observing one-minute preceptor and traditional preceptor encounters. *Academic Medicine.* **79**: 50–5.

52 Aagaard E, Teherani A and Irby D (2004) The effectiveness of the one-minute preceptor model for diagnosing the patient and the learner. *Academic Medicine.* **79**: 42–9.

53 Greenberg LW (2004) Medical students' perceptions of feedback in a busy ambulatory setting: a descriptive study using a clinical encounter card. *Southern Medical Journal.* **97**: 1174–8.

54 McIlwrick J, Nair B and Montgomery G (2006) 'How am I doing?' Man problems but few solutions related to feedback delivery in undergraduate psychiatry education. *Academic Psychiatry.* **30**: 130–5.

55 Ende J (1983) Feedback in clinical medical education. *JAMA.* **250**: 777–81.

56 Meyers C and Jones TB (1993) *Promoting Active Learning: Strategies for the College Classroom.* Jossey-Bass, San Francisco, CA.

57 Chi MTH (1996) Constructing self-explanations and scaffolded explanations in tutoring. *Applied Cognitive Psychology.* **10**: 1–17.

58 Schön DA (1987) Teaching artistry through reflection-in-action. In: Schon DA (ed.) *Educating the Reflective Practitioner,* pp. 22–40. Jossey-Bass, San Francisco, CA.

59 McGrath D and Higgins A (2006) Implementing and evaluative reflective practice group sessions. *Nurse Education in Practice.* **6**: 175–81.

60 Wiener B (1972) Attribution theory, achievement motivation, and the educational process. *Review of Educational Research.* **42**: 203–15.

61 Prawat RS (1998) Current self-regulation views of learning and motivation viewed through a Deweyan lens: the problems with dualism. *American Educational Research Journal.* **35**: 199–224.

62 Paris SG and Paris AH (2001) Classroom applications of research on self-regulated learning. *Educational Psychologist.* **36**: 89–101.

Further reading

There is a substantial body of research and relevant literature on self-regulated learning. Although a fair amount of the work was done in kindergarten to 12th grade contexts, there is some evidence reported at the college level. As with any body of scholarly work in an academic field, some of this work is theoretical, some is quite complex, written in disciplinary vernacular and designed to inform researchers about the work that has been done and the evidence it has yielded, and some is practical, written in terms that help educators understand how theory has been applied effectively in classroom contexts. The reference list includes a lot of this work, across these various domains.

16 Learning medicine from the humanities

J Jill Gordon[1] and H Martyn Evans[2]
[1]University of Sydney, Australia
[2]School of Medicine and Health, Durham University, UK

 KEY MESSAGES

- Professional competence is enhanced when students are broadly educated; the humanities can foster personal and professional maturation by providing insights into the human experience of illness, disability and medical interventions.

- Despite the importance of the arts and humanities, their position within medical curricula tends to be precarious; educators need a clear and defensible view on teaching and learning medicine from the humanities.

- Philosophy, history and literature are key humanities disciplines, and their relationship with medicine should be part of the core curriculum; students should also have access

to self-selected study modules suited to their particular interests.

- The processes involved in learning medicine from the humanities are as important as the course content.

- The humanities can often blend with other elements of the medical curriculum, rather than being in direct competition. Teaching, assessment and evaluation should be aligned with each other and reflect the core values of the programme more generally.

- A rich supply of resources for teaching and learning is available.

Felix, qui potuit rerum cognoscere causas
Happy are they who are able to understand the cause of things.

Virgil, *Georgics: Book 2*, Line 490.

Introduction

In developed societies, medical practice relies heavily on science and technology, and doctors are often accused of losing sight of some fundamental elements of good doctoring, including an empathic understanding of the other. Technological dominance has been harmful for both patients and the profession. Perhaps, it is suggested, doctors more versed in the medical humanities would help to redress the balance between the science and the art of medical care.

Medical students usually enter medical school with the desire, as Virgil puts it, 'to understand the cause of things' in the world of biomedicine. They also want to use this knowledge to help others. At the outset, students generally acknowledge that 'helping others' means more than simply solving medical problems, and that curing is not equivalent to healing. (When students are not immediately clear on the difference, the analogy of a burglary can be helpful. The police may track down the burglar and recover your possessions. This may 'cure' your material loss, but that will not guarantee your emotional recovery.) Understanding the many causes of human behaviour is just as important as understanding the cause of 'things', but in medical

school, students quickly discover that teaching and assessment both focus on the medical sciences, rather than the social sciences. To understand the cause of things is to reduce everything to its smallest component, as defined by each biomedical discipline.

Students also observe that the doctors who deal with the broad philosophical and social challenges posed in primary care, mental health, rehabilitation, ageing and end-of-life care generally occupy the lower rungs of the medical hierarchy, whilst those who avoid the complex issues in medical care and focus on the technological specialties tend to occupy the higher rungs.

In short, biomedicine values 'objective' science, whilst the medical humanities are distinguished by their concern with recording and interpreting human experiences in relation to illness, disability and medical intervention. Students experience the medical humanities at the most basic level, whenever they attend to patients' stories, rather than simply extracting 'medically relevant' information and whenever they themselves reflect on, and give expression to, their own and others' experiences of health, illness and care-giving. In addition to these immediate experiences of the doctor–patient relationship, students can also access representations of illness, disability and medical intervention portrayed by others – writers, historians, philosophers, artists and musicians.

These opportunities are particularly important for students from relatively narrow cultural backgrounds with limited experience of the values, attitudes, needs and concerns of the majority of people. Although many medical

Understanding Medical Education: Evidence, Theory and Practice, Second Edition. Edited by Tim Swanwick.
© 2014 The Association for the Study of Medical Education. Published 2014 by John Wiley & Sons, Ltd.

schools now try to select students from a wide range of backgrounds, many students are still disadvantaged by their material advantages, when it comes to understanding other people's lives. The humanities can help such students to venture out into a less controlled and ordered world.

The term 'medical humanities' was coined by an Australian surgeon, Anthony Moore, in 1976. He described his approach to using literature in teaching undergraduate medical students at the University of Melbourne,(1) as a way of understanding the experience of health and illness and as a way of exploring ethical issues in clinical practice.(2) At the same time, the University of La Plata in the Argentine Republic, among others, was making a specific commitment to teaching and learning in the medical humanities.(3) Over the past 20 years, other educational initiatives in medical humanities have flourished, albeit with more theoretical than empirical support. In 1984 the Hastings Center commissioned Eric Cassell to write a paper on *The Place of the Humanities in Medicine*.(4) Cassell argued that in medicine there is 'an entire spectrum of functions that can be provided only by the humanities'. (4, p. 54) In the same year, Edmund Pellegrino outlined three particular uses for the humanities in medical education: 'They are vehicles for teaching the liberal arts, they convey a special kind of knowledge that liberates the imagination and they are sources of delectation for the human spirit'. (5, p. 254)

Self(6) also talks about three goals for the medical humanities: 'cultural transmission', 'affective development' and cognitive development, with an emphasis on reasoning around scientific, social and moral issues.

In a similar vein, Grant at the University of Auckland in New Zealand(7) has set out four main roles for medical humanities, as follows:

- to increase understanding of the human condition
- to expose students to the critical analysis of ideas
- to make more allowance for individual differences
- to provide pockets of expertise and lifelong interests.

Finally, Brody(8) has defined 'medical humanities' via three complementary conceptions – as a list of disciplines, as a programme of moral development and as a supportive friend.

We agree with all of these perspectives and would summarise them as: first, to introduce the idea that the arts and humanities can contribute to health care; second, to extend the range of future doctors' sensitivities and insights regarding human experience in all its variety; and third, to deepen our understanding beyond merely biomedical interpretations of health and illness (*see* Box 16.1).

Helping students to learn from the humanities

Whether you are involved at undergraduate, postgraduate or continuing professional development level, your role may encompass one or more of the following:

- the design of all or part of a curriculum (whether it is integrated or discipline-based, hospital- or community-oriented)

BOX 16.1 What can the humanities do for medical education?

- Help learners (including medical students, junior doctors, more advanced trainees and established practitioners) to develop skills in interpreting their own experiences and the experiences of others
- Provide a wide range of opportunities for students to encounter and appreciate human diversity
- Help students to develop their own personal values
- Encourage medical students to take experience and subjectivity seriously
- Enable medical education to move from a technical training to a genuine university education
- Nourish a sense of wonder at embodied human nature and embodied consciousness, leading to medical education that is, in its essence, reverential
- Helps students to appreciate the dangers of ignoring the lessons of history
- Help students to develop communication skills

- organising a large- or small-group learning activity
- providing curriculum content, perhaps in relation to your own particular discipline
- offering specific interest and expertise in one or more of the medical humanities.

Your background may be in medicine, other health sciences, the arts, humanities or social sciences, or a combination of these. Many doctors are amateurs in the best sense of the word. We maintain a deep love of the humanities, because they take us beyond the dogmatic world of 'single best answers'. Whilst as doctors we are motivated to share this love of learning, our opportunities for deep scholarship in the humanities tend to be limited by the demands of a medical career. All too often the result is a limited approach that takes the form of stories about medicine's achievements, the discoveries and breakthrough moments. But this is only one side of the story.

A medical humanities programme needs to engage scholars from other disciplines, but if you are a professional humanities scholar invited to teach in a medical school, you may be accused of having insufficient 'street cred', because you are too far removed from the realities of medical practice. If you make the mistake of offering too pointed a critique of biomedicine or of doctors, you may lose goodwill and end up talking to an empty room.(9) Then again, if you are deferential and apologetic, you may find yourself largely ignored. Even the least gifted lecturer in physiology or pathology will command a certain amount of respect, if there are to be questions in the exam, but the professional humanities scholar may have no such pulling power.

In 1976, whilst writing about vocational education in general, Scally made a plea to humanities teachers to enter the world of the student, and not to simply stand outside and reject technology: 'A student should gain . . . a vision of personal and social alternatives . . . encouraging the awareness that there are other ways of living, other value structures, other social constructs besides the familiar'.(10, p. 225)

Finding the balance between the science and the art

In 2006, in the journal *Medical Education*, Weatherall wrote on science in the 20th-century medical curriculum. He concluded the article with these words:

> as this essay was restricted to the role of science in medical education, it has not been possible to enlarge on how its teaching can be accommodated with the numerous other skills that have been introduced into the curriculum, including an over-liberal dose of the humanities, with the aim of humanising our doctors of the future. But when I see a surgeon poised over my abdomen with a knife, all that I ask is that he or she is a humble, self-critical professional whose biological and technical training has prepared their mind to cope with the infinite possibilities that lie beneath the skin, and that, when finished, they can communicate what they have done to my relatives in simple, kindly language; at that moment their skills at deciphering the arcane meanings of multiple-choice questions or their acquaintance, or lack of, with the late string quartets of Beethoven will not bother me too much.(11, p. 201)

The arguments are important, since they are ones that you are likely to encounter. They can be summarised as follows:

- science and the humanities must compete for curriculum time.
- I doubt that studying the humanities 'humanises' doctors.
- I would prefer a kind and competent surgeon to a highly sophisticated but incompetent one.

How to respond? You might wish to acknowledge that you would all share the same anxious desire, should the need arise, for access to a competent surgeon who is also humble and self-critical. Those qualities are fundamental, if one is to avoid putting one's life into the care of someone who is insufficiently capable on the one hand and insufficiently risk-averse on the other. In relation to the medical curriculum, the more helpful question to ask might be how to achieve the best educational outcomes in the time available, using the most relevant academic resources.

The argument that surgeons should always communicate in simple, kind language may evoke in you slightly uncomfortable memories of rather more paternalistic days. Better perhaps to wish for a surgeon with the insight into making an accurate judgement of individual needs and to respond appropriately.(12) You might mention that many doctors fail to elicit patients' complaints and concerns, and comprehend little of the emotional and social impact of the illness. Even worse, they fail to appreciate the adverse effects of their own well-intentioned behaviour on their patients.(13)

Perhaps you would also take the time to defend multiple-choice questions and poor Beethoven; there is, after all,

evidence that well-constructed multiple-choice questions can indeed discriminate between candidates who know their science and those who do not,(14,15) and a shared love of the late string quartets of Beethoven may be deeply relevant for doctors who work in places such as the palliative care ward.(16) Finally, of course, you might wish to point out that competent surgeons do not need to be cultural philistines.

A medical school that offered an 'over-liberal dose of the humanities' would be bound to raise antibodies with some academic staff as well as with students. Do such curricula exist? What, we might wonder, is the right 'dose' of humanities? Is it wise to think of the humanities in the currency of teaching hours, with the implication that the humanities are taught in a discrete disciplinary 'slot'? If this were the case, would an average of an hour per week be too much, too little or just right? A review of 41 humanities programmes in North America, and some international schools was provided by the journal *Academic Medicine* in 2003.(17) With only a few exceptions, most of the medical schools reported on modest, often elective programmes, with very limited hours of study. Few, if any, would offer as much as the equivalent of one hour per week.

We labour all of these points because you will face such challenges, even when the medical humanities component of your curriculum seems well embedded. Describing the position of the medical humanities as 'precarious', Friedman(18) argues that the humanities must be protected so that they can offer students different ways of analysing information, viewing the world and confronting dilemmas. The humanities raise issues that can help students confront questions about both their chosen field and their particular places within it. They do not need to compete with the biomedical sciences; each part of the curriculum needs to be assessed in terms of its intrinsic worth and its utility in the lives of students and graduates. However, if your curriculum does not currently provide any opportunities for students to learn medicine from the humanities, you may face the problem familiar to any who have tried it: 'It is easier to win a war than to change the medical curriculum by even one half hour'.(19, p. 227)

Meeting curricula requirements

The UK General Medical Council's publication *Tomorrow's Doctors*(20) emphasises points of particular relevance to learning medicine from the humanities. The document deals with the following:

- qualities that are appropriate to future responsibilities
- a core curriculum supported by student-selected components
- skills of exploration, evaluation, integration and critical appraisal of evidence
- experience in a variety of clinical settings with early clinical experience
- up-to-date teaching and learning systems.

Let us examine these curricula requirements, and how the humanities can support their delivery.

Qualities appropriate to future responsibilities

'A number of concepts from history, the social sciences and the humanities are central to understanding and internalizing professionalism'.(21) It has been argued that 'humanism' and 'professionalism' are qualities that must be taught and learnt,(22–24) but less acknowledged is the role of the learning environment.(25–27) There is ample evidence of the negative effects of inhumane environments in relation to the socialisation of medical students and junior doctors.(28) It is hard to imagine an educational or a working environment within which careful and genuine attention to the humanities would not help students and doctors avoid crossing over to the 'dark side' – the dehumanised working environment that causes the cynicism and despair portrayed in novels such as *The House of God* (29) and *Bodies*.(30) Contrast these examples with the enormously popular American television series *M*A*S*H*,(31) in which a supportive work environment is shown to help doctors to cope with even the most challenging medical situations. The difference is clearly due to the sympathy and humour with which *M*A*S*H* portrayed the human experiences of illness and injury through the eyes of the subversive medical draftees.

However, any attempt to force-feed professionalism using the humanities will serve only to discredit this approach, especially when it is done by non-medical teachers. Even students from humanities backgrounds who are trying to come to grips with the sheer volume of material to cover, in an undergraduate programme or during their specialty training, find themselves driven to ask, 'What's likely to be in the exams?' They will have little patience with 'irrelevant' subjects or topics that are seen as digressions from the 'core' of the programme. For this reason, many educators have aimed to 'embed' the humanities(32) and to more clearly demonstrate their relevance,(33) as more likely to appeal to learners. Poetry may not make 'better' doctors,(34) and it may not be a predictable way to teach ethics,(35) but if the resources drawn from the arts, humanities and social sciences are of high quality, they cannot help but 'liberate the imagination' and provide 'delectation for the human spirit', both of which support the qualities that in turn support professional practice.

A core curriculum supported by student-selected components

'Student-selected components' have provided one way of challenging the rigidity of the traditional curriculum. Limiting the reach of a potentially inexhaustible core curriculum is a way of reducing rote learning and promoting deep understanding. Over the past ten years, many accounts of humanities special study modules (in other countries, often called 'options' or 'electives') have been published.(36–41) Whilst these are generally received with enthusiasm by the students who volunteer, they have led to the understandable concern that the humanities might be relegated to parts of the curriculum that will be taken up only by this small subgroup. A compromise can be reached by identifying a medical humanities 'core' (defined in terms of intellectual skills, rather than content) complemented by self-selected components, recognising that not all students will take the latter.

Emphasis on the skills of exploration, evaluation, integration and critical appraisal of evidence

If humanities students were required to undertake a course of study defined in terms of content alone, they would probably miss the benefits of a university education. What unites scholars across the arts and humanities is not the content of their studies, but the acquisition of intellectual skills. Whether graduating with a major in philosophy, history, literature, languages or a social science, humanities students are expected to be capable of rigorous and independent thought, to account for their decisions, and to be creative, imaginative and tolerant of ambiguity.

Unlike humanities students, who demonstrate these qualities through essay writing, medical students tend not to be required to write many essays; the introduction of reflective writing is a relatively new approach.(42) However, medical students and graduates do tend to participate in small-group tutorials, especially if a course of study is problem or case based. Tutorials provide an ideal opportunity for students to share their experiences and refine their ideas and values; this is often overlooked as an example of learning medicine from the humanities. Deep learning(43) occurs when students learn to see things from different perspectives, discuss their ideas with others and apply knowledge in the real world.(39,44) These approaches respond directly to the General Medical Council's requirement for students to 'explore knowledge, and evaluate and integrate (bring together) evidence critically. The curriculum can motivate students to develop the skills for self-directed learning'.(20, p. 3) If you have responsibility for organising teaching and learning, then small-group tutorials, appropriately facilitated, are the ideal way to achieve many of these goals. Small-group discussions should help students to reflect on experience and to extend their insights by drawing on the humanities and social sciences. Many different ways of achieving the goal of reflective practice have been identified,(45–48) and some of these may work well in your own situation.

Learning in a variety of settings and early clinical experience

Learning in a variety of settings has generally meant that, in addition to hospital-based experience, students now learn in general practices, community health facilities and patients' homes. These naturally introduce some of the complexities of context and relationships that are so often lost, when patients are seen out of context, in a hospital bed. The humanities and social sciences can provide invaluable insights into the human experience of illness, disability and medical intervention in the patient's own setting. In addition, students can explore the roles of a broader range of health professionals, consider the operation of power structures and even participate in (or at the very least observe) inter-professional care. 'Poetry on rounds' was found to have a levelling effect(49) between attending physicians, house staff and medical students: 'Rounds became a time when the team shared not only medical knowledge but also life and emotional experiences'.(50, p. 449)

Instead of feeling that they have little to offer, students can be encouraged to consider unfamiliarity as a gift, embodied in the Polish proverb, 'The guest sees in one hour what the owner of the house does not see in a lifetime'. Seeing with a fresh eye is essential to remaining clinically alert over a professional lifetime, and students need explicit encouragement to do that, so that they are less likely to be socialised into accepting some of the less desirable aspects of the health care environment. Professional historians use this approach when they try to 'make the familiar strange' – to take nothing for granted.

Social history resources and fictional depictions of families can help medical students prepare for clinical attachments in patients' homes, hospitals, clinics and GP surgeries. Historical, philosophical, literary and artistic representations can be chosen to pique their interest without adding a large burden of additional study. You might invite beginning students to reflect on the difference between their way of seeing patients and the way an experienced clinician might see them.

Cultural competence is a relatively recent goal in medical education. It addresses the provision of appropriate health care, when there are ethnic and cultural differences between patients, families and caregivers to consider. Kleinman and Benson,(51) who work at the interface between medicine and anthropology, have proposed an 'explanatory models' approach, which provides practical help for students. They aim 'to open clinicians to human communication and set their expert knowledge alongside (not over and above) the patient's own explanation and viewpoint'. They have outlined six steps that simultaneously illustrate the relevance of the humanities. Students should be able to:

- find out about [how] the patient's ethnicity relates to how she or he sees herself or himself and place within family, work and social networks
- evaluate what is at stake in terms of close relationships, material resources, religious commitments and even life itself
- reconstruct the patient's narrative in order to understand the meaning of the illness
- consider ongoing stresses and social supports
- examine culture in terms of its influence on clinical relationships, using critical self-reflection to explore, for example, the culture of biomedicine, 'including bias, inappropriate and excessive use of advanced technology interventions, and of course stereotyping'(51, p. 1675)
- reflect on the effects of attending to cultural difference – is it relevant and helpful for this patient in these circumstances?

Learners at all levels will find themselves revisiting these quite subtle and complex skills. In *The Spirit Catches You and You Fall Down*,(49) Anne Fadiman provides a powerful example of how well-intentioned care can go wrong. Her storied account of the health care system is a great educational resource. Greenhalgh(52) also gives examples of the power of stories to reduce the barrier of ethnic difference.

Narrative accounts of illness by real patients offer important learning opportunities.(53) Suitable patients are likely to have chronic conditions such as cystic fibrosis, diabetes, epilepsy or mental illnesses. They have an advantage over 'book learning', because students see and talk to them in a particular clinical context (whether at home, in a hospital ward, tutorial room or lecture theatre). Contextual factors make these experiences memorable; anyone who has organised such opportunities for students will be aware of the deep impression they can create. Most medical graduates can remember certain patients many decades after graduation, and one patient who describes the impact of a less-than-perfect encounter with the health care system may sometimes have a greater effect than statistical analyses of medical error.

Up-to-date learning and teaching systems: Integration and problem-based learning

The humanities can make sense of a medical curriculum by integrating all aspects of a patient's problem, avoiding the 'silo effect' that is typical of a traditional curriculum. Integration needs to be both vertical (preclinical and clinical) and horizontal (dealing with all aspects from the human perspective).

The approach is not new; in 1992, Almy *et al.*(54) reported on a course for fourth-year students which used a problem-based approach that demonstrated the relevance of the social sciences and humanities to clinical decision-making. The course culminated in an assessment of individual students using a simulated patient with a complex management problem. Kirklin(39) describes the way in which the arts and humanities can be used to teach around a specific medical problem, such as genetic disorders and therapies. If your curriculum uses problem-based learning (PBL), you may wish to identify resources that complement the cases your students study. Such resources bring convincingly drawn 'patients' to life and remind students that every real-life case occurs within a context from which the human experience of illness proceeds. If your medical school has created PBL cases using comic-book characters with demeaning nicknames, object and then have them changed. Stereotypes are neither harmless nor amusing; they simply perpetuate the idea that patients are mere vehicles for interesting diseases. Students need to learn that the humanity they share with their patients(55) is just as important as the knowledge they bring to their service.

The *Journal of the American Medical Association* provides beautiful annotated examples from art, as well as from the other humanities disciplines (*see Poetry and Medicine* and *A Piece of My Mind*). The Medical Humanities pages at the New York University School of Medicine (http://medhum.med.nyu.edu) provide resources and also links to other sites. In 2003, New York University published *Editor's Choices from the Literature, Arts and Medicine Database*(56) to celebrate its tenth anniversary. The Association of American Medical Colleges has produced selections from the journal *Academic Medicine* to commemorate ten years of medicine and the arts.(57) The University of Pennsylvania has produced a CD-ROM on literature and medicine.(58) Radcliffe Publishing has produced a number of medical humanities titles (*see* 'Further Reading' section). Last but not least, students will respond to invitations to write and post their own compositions and book reviews, tasks that provide opportunities for their broader professional development.

A curriculum for the medical humanities?

Macnaughton(59) has described some of the ways in which students can learn medicine from the humanities. Evans and Mcnaughton have asked, 'Is there, or could (should) there be, an agreed and coherent core curriculum for the study of medical humanities as such?'(60, p. 65). They suggest that the core curriculum should be guided by four principles, as follows:
- disciplinary openness
- humility in enquiry
- respect for subjectivity
- openness to a sense of wonder at embodied human nature.

The first three are, of course, applicable to all scholarship. The last one is especially important in medicine; wonder can often disappear under the weight of anxiety, sadness and the frustration that a doctor's life entails.

Not only is this a useful template against which to judge your own initiatives in medical humanities, it is also a prescription for the learning environment itself.(61) Philosophy, history and literature clearly provide a disciplinary core that meets all of these criteria, whilst social sciences (especially sociology and anthropology), art and music provide a 'second string' that meets some of them, to some extent. Your own decision-making about what to include will obviously take advantage of the local expertise available and the opportunities that arise. Not infrequently will you find other academics in a clinical, para-clinical or preclinical discipline, such as palliative care or infectious diseases, who will be enthusiastic collaborators (*see* Box 16.2).

Philosophy

There is a tendency to assume that bioethics, now a distinct component of many medical curricula, is all that is required to 'cover' philosophy in a medical degree programme. However, philosophy of medicine, as an organised disciplinary strand, is much broader; its job is to ask questions about the questions that medicine asks.(62) It examines, for example, the phenomena of health and illness, the nature of the clinical encounter and many of the assumptions of modern medical practice. Because we are focusing on educating doctors and not humanities scholars, it is particularly important for students to see the point of 'studying philosophically', rather than 'studying philosophy'. Philosophy promotes logic and reasoning, and encourages the understanding of multiple perspectives.(63)

In the course of their studies, medical students learn to consider the human body of daily experience as a medical body, the object of scientific enquiry, standardised rather than individuated. The sense of mystery and the symbolic significance of the body can be lost quite easily, if students come to consider it as merely a source of data on the physical status of a patient, and to consider it in terms of function alone.(62) However, the study of clinical medicine combines both universal and existential knowledge and can give concrete form to many of philosophy's traditional questions.

Louhiala(64) has described four different ways of approaching philosophy within a medical curriculum, only two of which he recommends, as follows:
- traditional lectures on philosophy without connection to medicine
- an academic philosophy of medicine course, as for philosophy students
- philosophy of medicine teaching related to the students' experiences
- full integration into the curriculum using, for example, PBL.

Traditional lectures, unconnected to medicine and with their content suited to philosophy, rather than to medical courses, are unlikely to appeal to students. We know that the teaching needs to be related to students' experiences and that it is most effective when fully integrated.

History of medicine

George Santayana famously warned that those who cannot learn from history are doomed to repeat it. This is particularly important for medicine. In the course of history, countless patients have suffered unnecessarily from inappropriate and even dangerous medical interventions.

Dufflin, author of *History of Medicine: a scandalously short introduction*,(65) argues that the study of history in relation to medicine can be used to:
- foster critical thinking, or to instil scepticism about the content and durability of everything else students are taught in their professional training
- demonstrate that history is a research discipline, built on fascinating questions, rigorous methods and a wide variety of raw materials – a research discipline not unlike those in the clinical and basic sciences.

Dufflin(66) has also provided useful advice on the 'why', 'who', 'how' and 'what' of teaching medical students. Confronted with a choice of physician historians or professional historians, her advice is to prefer expertise and to take whatever opportunities present themselves with respect to timing: with Year 1 students, whilst medicine is still fresh; with Year 4, when it is less daunting. With respect to scheduling, 'Friday afternoons are suicidal. Instructors who agree to schedule their lessons in such a slot have

---

BOX 16.2 A curriculum for the medical humanities

Philosophy

History of medicine

Literature

Narrative

Art and music

Spirituality

participated in their own demise'.(66, p. 159) The content is the least important consideration: 'As long as the information is accurate and relevant, the "what" does not matter as much as the "why," the "who" and the "how"'.

There are abundant resources for teaching in the history of medicine. Some are listed in the 'Further Reading' section. Porter's legacy alone is substantial.(67–69)

Literature

Evan(70) suggests four medical educational 'goods' that literature supports, as follows:

- an education (as opposed to mere training)
- ethics and communication skills
- the development of personal values
- a sense of wonder at embodied human nature.

Medical curricula that include the arts and humanities often begin with literature. This is not surprising, given the range of forms: novels, poems, plays and non-fiction accounts of the experience of illness (so-called 'pathography'(71)), plus health providers' narratives, including reflective writing. To this list we can add film, as an increasingly popular way of accessing the humanities.(72,73) Others have promoted 'narrative medicine',(74) which is said to offer a way of understanding the medical history as the patient's story; 'narrative therapy' has grown out of this perspective.

William Osler often advised students and young doctors to intersperse their studies with reading in the humanities. One hundred years ago his recommended reading list included *The Bible*, Plutarch, Marcus Aurelius, Epictetus, Shakespeare, Montaigne, Miguel de Cervantes, Ralph Waldo Emerson and Oliver Wendell Holmes. Given the choice, students are unlikely to select from this sample today and will often select films or modern novels and poetry that may be less familiar to an older generation. If you find yourself unable to outrun the avalanche of modern literature, it can be helpful to take advantage of students' choices to build your own collection.

In *The Moral of the Story: An anthology of ethics through literature*,(75) Singer and Singer provide excerpts from literary works that are both enjoyable and thought-provoking. Twenty-nine of their 79 authors were born in the 20th century. The book uses excerpts that question the nature of ethics, values and duties, racism and sexism, war and suicide, and so on. Literature used as a stimulus for teaching ethics raises particular issues. As pointed out earlier, Wear and Aultman(9) found that some of their students were uncomfortable with literature that dealt with challenging social issues such as domestic violence, and Pickering(35) has pointed out that using poetry, for instance to teach ethics, can have unpredictable results. The underlying purpose of the exercise is to foster critical thinking, rather than inculcating a point of view, even in the well-intentioned goal of achieving 'professionalism'. Students are quick to react to perceived criticism of the profession, whilst they are taking their first tentative steps towards acquiring a professional identity. This is one reason why team teaching, with a supportive humanities scholar and a clinician working together, is an important philosophical and practical consideration.

Special study modules remain the most popular means of including literature in the curriculum. Other approaches include the use of short excerpts that relate to clinical conditions being studied in a PBL or case-based curriculum. These can be used to provide a change of pace, for example, towards the end of a small-group discussion. Shapiro *et al.*(76) introduced medicine-related poetry and prose to a Year 3 family medicine clerkship, using clinical notes in the 'SOAP' (Subjective, Objective, Assessment, Plan) format and into an end-of-clerkship Objective Structured Clinical Examination. Students were moderately interested and felt that the experience had been positive in terms of encouraging empathic responses to patients.

Louis-Courvoisier and Wenger(48) have argued that the study of literature can help students to realise the extent to which their view of the world is context-dependent and culturally shaped. 'Distancing' enables students to become aware that their point of view is only one of many alternative ways of seeing. They suggest that team teaching can overcome many of the difficulties that occur when literature is taught by medical teachers who lack the professional expertise of the literary scholar, or by literary scholars who lack a deep understanding of the context of medical care. 'Team teaching entails numerous discussions and negotiations. It is a time-consuming process, but quite exciting because it is the result of a dynamic process and of a constructive confrontation rather than a mere juxtaposition of expertise'.(48, p. 54) Because of the importance of role models in medicine, the admired clinician who gives critical endorsement to this approach and who can describe why they enjoy particular writers and films is likely to encourage students to read or view films with a discerning eye.

Narrative medicine

'Narrative medicine' has recently laid claim to a greater role in medical education(74) for the purpose of helping doctors to understand the different perspectives of doctors and patients.(77) Students are said to move towards narrative competence, as they demonstrate 'the set of skills required to recognize, absorb, interpret and be moved by the stories one hears or reads. This competence requires a combination of textual skills (identifying a story's structure, adopting its multiple perspectives, recognising metaphors and allusions), creative skills (imagining many interpretations, building curiosity, inventing multiple endings), and affective skills (tolerating uncertainty as a story unfolds, entering the story's mood)'.(78) Greenhalgh and Hurwitz(79) describe the illness experience as a narrative embedded within a broader life narrative.

Is this really new or different? Are not these skills the 'bread and butter' of many communication skills training programmes? In a systematic review of such programmes, Gysels *et al.*(80) found that not all of them included all the components of narrative medicine training. They concluded that 'learner-centred (communication training) programmes using several methods, combining a didactic component focusing on theoretical knowledge with practical rehearsal and constructive feedback from peers and skilled facilitators, proved to be very effective. Small groups encouraged more intensive participation'.(80, p. 366)

Clark and Mishler(81) have provided evidence of the practical utility of an approach that could be seen as related to narrative medicine. They present a comparative analysis of two clinical consultations and compare the successful story-telling exemplified by one with the constantly interrupted narrative in the other. The authors point out how focusing on the patient's attempts to tell a story can illuminate the exercise of authority in clinical encounters. The results from this research provide a powerful teaching tool. Many educators will be familiar with the use of video- and/or audio-recording to teach communication skills, but these authors offer a detailed account of how stories are developed or suppressed. 'Attending to the patient's authorship of her/his story highlights the vicissitudes of authority in clinical encounters and the social transformation of illness in clinical relationships'.(81, p. 368)

Equally useful for teaching communication is the rhetorical approach outlined by Lingard and Haber(82). She points out that rhetoric is a science that can deepen understanding of communication and improve teaching, rather than relying on implicit, ad hoc teaching without a theoretical base. Books such as these are useful for staff development; clinical teachers will recognise the authentic contexts within which the research has taken place and see more clearly the benefits of the humanities in teaching and learning.

Your own curriculum may approach the skills described above using a range of teaching methods, without ever mentioning 'narrative competence'. What is important is that the teachers have a model or models to enable them to understand what they are trying to achieve when they teach communication skills.

Art and music

Some claims have been made for the role of the visual arts in learning and teaching. From an essentialist point of view, art education can be justified for the aesthetic experience alone, whilst from an instrumentalist perspective, art education can be justified as a means of achieving curriculum goals, by sharpening students' powers of observation, for example.(83,84,85) Tapajos(86) points out the advantages of viewing a medical condition such as HIV/AIDS through a humanities lens; artistic representations of cancer have been a focal point for other initiatives, such as special study modules.(87)

There have been some published evaluations of the use of art and music to achieve curriculum goals; not surprisingly, these are all positive, since positive outcome bias is probably just as applicable in medical humanities research as it is in clinical medicine.(88) Whilst the evaluations themselves tend to be methodologically weak and/or to involve small numbers, the fact that such initiatives are part of a medical school curriculum contains an implicit message about what is valued in the curriculum, including student well-being. A more rigorous evaluation was carried out by Shapiro *et al*.(89) in comparing the observation skills of a medical student group trained with clinical photographs and paper cases, and a group trained with art plus dance. Pattern recognition probably improved as a result of the first group's experience, but the second group thought that

their emotional recognition, empathy, identification of story and narrative, and awareness of multiple perspectives had improved. Dolev *et al*.(90) randomised first-year students to a control or intervention group in which the students attended the Yale Center for British Art for visual training as part of the general curriculum. The researchers found a modest, statistically significant improvement in observations skills in the intervention group and commented that this could be used as the basis for a continuing curriculum applicable to all physicians.

Family physicians participated in a workshop in Israel in which they discussed and wrote about artistic representations of suffering. Participants commented that this type of experience is rare.(91) At the University of California, San Francisco, interns are given the opportunity to use artistic expression through drawing, collage and mask-making, which encourages reflection, and like other initiatives it has been well received.(86) These examples all provide ideas for educators looking for opportunities for the humanities. Kirklin *et al*.(87) identified seven 'keys to success' based on their experience of a special study module that included art at University College London.

They include the following:
- dedicated course co-ordinator
- enthusiastic tutors
- identification of students needing extra support
- flexibility to modify the course
- supportive environment
- opportunities for reflection and feedback
- individual feedback to students.

Whilst educators claim a place for philosophy, bioethics, history, literature, art and so on, music has fewer advocates for a place in the core curriculum. However, at medical schools such as Dalhousie University in Canada,(92) strong advocacy at the highest levels has resulted in a programme that not only includes medical humanities in the curriculum, but also brings faculty together for musical performances as a means of strengthening the sense of belonging to a community of scholars (http://humanities.medicine.dal.ca).

Spirituality

The acceptance that good medical care requires a biopsychosocial or, perhaps more accurately, an 'existential' approach can lead to a discussion of the spiritual qualities that doctors need, if they are to be able to respond to a range of different needs in their patients. Evans suggests that doctors need to draw on 'a type of spiritual confidence that does not arise merely from a narrow scientific training; a spirit perhaps more dependent on ways of thinking, rather than content of thought; genuine education rather than training; development of personal qualities rather than acquired techniques; a completeness or fullness of human being'.(93, p. 13) This type of 'spiritual confidence' should be distinguished from religious faith, but refers rather to the 'human spirit.'.

In the USA, the Medical School Objectives Project(94) has defined learning objectives for spirituality. The American Association of Medical Colleges reported in a survey carried out in 2000 that approximately 70 medical schools were addressing spirituality in their curricula. By 2004, that number had reached 84.(95) Berlinger(96) from the Hastings Center has discussed the ethical implications of such courses, some of which are linked to developments in 'integrative' and 'complementary' medicine.(97,98) She points out some of the pitfalls of incorporating spirituality into the curriculum – for example, the fact that the research evidence linking spiritual and religious beliefs and practices to health and healing is very poor, that the practice of taking a 'spiritual history' from a patient is potentially intrusive and coercive, and that doctors who see themselves as healers may become overly impressed with their own mystique and regress to a less patient-centred and more paternalistic model of patient care.

Individual medical schools or training programmes should consider the extent to which spirituality needs to be singled out for special attention, as opposed to being incorporated into a programme that emphasises respectful care and sensitivity to difference. Kleinman's(51) work on the skills required to manage cultural difference, outlined above, is equally relevant when applied to the different faiths and non-faiths that doctors and their patients hold.

Course design and assessment

Whether the medical humanities component of a curriculum is stand-alone or embedded, compulsory or voluntary, there are similar design questions to be addressed. By beginning with your curriculum goals in mind, you can try to ensure congruence between whatever type of programme you run and the assessment methods used (*see* Box 16.3).(44)

Consider assessment early. Do you have the resources and time to carry out both the learning activities and the related assessments? How practical are they? Will they survive the initial wave of enthusiasm?

If we are dealing with biomedical topics, it is relatively easy to ask, 'How can we ensure that students have adequate knowledge of anatomy/physiology/pathology, etc., to progress safely to the next stage of learning?' This is not a question that can be applied to the humanities, and it is important for students to know that we are not trying to turn them into humanities scholars, but into more broadly educated doctors. We are therefore forced to acknowledge that humanities assessment cannot sample knowledge in a statistically defensible way, especially given the fact that both the cognitive and affective components of the humanities curriculum are important. However, when students are required to prepare a reflective essay, for example, not only does it challenge their higher-order skills, but it also indicates the value that the faculty places on this skill.

Take every opportunity to integrate the assessment into formats that are already being used for other parts of the curriculum. However, because of the different cognitive and affective requirements of assessments in biomedicine and the humanities, you may need to use a different approach, but keep it as simple as you can.

Essays and reflective diaries work well for many humanities subjects, because they take time to draft, review and

---

BOX 16.3 HOW TO: Implement a medical humanities curriculum

Questions for programme designers

- Does our programme provide opportunities for students to reflect on their experiences? Do they have opportunities to explore the works of significant thinkers? Can our students interpret messages in different forms – literary, historical, artistic, musical, etc.? Can we ensure that they use language precisely, and that they can develop and defend a logical argument?

- How and when does our programme ensure that students encounter other sets of values and other experience of the world? How do we ensure that students can demonstrate their understanding of the subjective experiences of others? How are they required to provide evidence of, for example, 'cultural competence'?

- Does our programme foster independent thinking? Can our students articulate and defend their personal values? Can they describe their view of a morally good life? Can they use the resources of literature, philosophy, history, etc. in achieving these goals?

- How do we ensure that students understand the respective contributions of the natural and human sciences to our understanding of the world? To what extent do we enable them to see that objective and subjective 'cures' need not be the same? Can they distinguish between disease and illness?

- How do we nourish, test for and demonstrate that students have acquired the generic skills associated with a university education – high-level reasoning, tolerance of ambiguity, creativity and imagination?

- How are students challenged to consider the 'why' versus the 'how'? Are they encouraged to tap onto their own aesthetic and emotional responses to human nature and its representation in the arts and humanities? Do they have opportunities to learn about the intellectual traditions of the range of cultures that they are likely to encounter? Do they have opportunities to see how patients and doctors share an awareness of our vulnerability, mortality and transcendence?

- Does our curriculum provide examples of the pitfalls of treating other human beings as means rather than as ends in themselves? What can we learn from the history of medical error both past and present? Do we equip students to understand how mistakes might be avoided in the future?

- How does my programme utilise insights, approaches and techniques derived from the humanities to help students to become more competent in communication? As well as demonstrating oral communication skills, are they required to demonstrate clear written communication? Is there a focus on the progressive development of these skills, using examples from the humanities?

BOX 16.4 HOW TO: Implement a medical humanities curriculum

Barriers and how to overcome them

Barriers	Possible solutions
Power: Influential faculty, from the dean downwards, tend to be trained in the biomedical model that has both defined and served their careers; a different approach may engender anxiety and resistance.	Ensure that the dean and other influential people have been adequately briefed. Identify other potential supporters; form a faculty interest group. Describe how learning from the humanities will enrich both students and faculty; trial innovative approaches on a small scale and if the students feedback is positive, use it to help you to move forward.
Expertise: Faculties typically employ hundreds of biomedical scientists and very few scholars in the humanities and social sciences, and the latter group tends not to be in positions of leadership.	Foster faculty expertise by encouraging contributions to teaching. Make links with humanities departments and identify potential teaching exchanges. Scour research teams for humanities scholars engaged in interdisciplinary research: are they willing to contribute to the teaching programme?
Language: The language of the humanities is often unfamiliar and obscure; it can appear dismissive and derogatory in discussions of science and scientists.	Take account of the learning needs of the least humanities-oriented students. Use texts that take science seriously; avoid obscure language and hyper-critical humanities academicians. Use literary texts that show how the language of biomedicine can also be used to exclude others.
Objectivity: Medical science is concerned with reducing variables, achieving detachment and emphasising generalisability.	Highlight the limits of a purely scientific approach in the real world, especially with, for example, chronic illnesses. Use literature to illustrate the complexity of human experience. Distinguish the challenges of diagnosis from those of management.
Overcoming the problems of 'two cultures': Medicine focuses on health improvement and progress, minimising error and doubt, whilst the humanities investigate and celebrate uncertainty and ambiguity.	Demonstrate the utility of both approaches. Help students to see why scientific knowledge is always provisional; invite students to identify the inherent weaknesses and biases of scholarly activity. Communicate some of the lessons of history. Discuss the need for an 'illness service' and a 'health service'.
Competition for time in the curriculum: Medical curricula are typically crowded (and there is also competition between 'old' and 'new' biomedical subjects).	Look for opportunities for synergy: integrate the humanities with biomedical teaching, learning and assessment wherever possible. Look for opportunities to collaborate when new topics or courses are being developed. Stress the benefits for learning of a 'change of pace' between science and the humanities.
Values: Concerns are expressed about the status of personal and values.	Demonstrate to students that no human activity is value-neutral. Articulate the values of your medical school without forcing them onto students. Encourage open-minded debate.

---

prepare for presentation, which are important skills for students to acquire and polish. Another approach that can work well is to assign topics for a group presentation and/or group poster. The process of preparing such a product requires students to consider other viewpoints around the topic. You might like to consider selecting a different theme each year, so students can compare their efforts and learn from one another. Your students should also be required to make a statement about the relative contribution of each group member, similar to that required of scholars submitting a paper to an academic journal (*see* Box 16.4).

Programme evaluation and research opportunities

Whilst attempts have been made to evaluate individual modules or complete strands or themes, evaluations are generally limited to feedback from surveys, questionnaires, individual interviews and focus groups to assess student satisfaction. Reports of feedback on special study modules usually acknowledge that students self-select into areas in which they have a particular interest, and only occasionally into areas in which they feel deficient.

Student feedback is essential for course correction and continuous quality improvement, which are dear to the hearts of educators who care about their courses. However, most enthusiastic teachers will elicit positive feedback, and this can lull one into a false sense of security concerning the impact of a course of study. It is important to remember that such evaluations do not test the commonly proffered argument that the humanities make students and doctors more humane. This argument is often made in terms of questions that are presented rhetorically as, 'How could one fail to respond to the lessons of history, or the magnificence of great literature or the insights of art or the cogency of the philosophical reasoning?', and so on. In reply, one could point out that our medical schools still graduate, year after year, a tiny number of students who are at risk for unprofessional behaviour. They may have participated in excellent programmes that incorporate the medical humanities, or they may not. However excellent their educational experience, it will not have been enough to change the values, beliefs, attitudes and behaviour of the psychopath or sociopath.

Leaving aside the minute number in this category, a more appropriate question would be whether the medical humanities are likely to provide fundamentally humane students with additional insights that are of value to themselves and of potential value to their patients. Theoretically, this question could be answered by a randomised controlled trial of sufficient size (a multi-centre trial perhaps), but one can imagine the practical challenges of randomisation within medical schools and the philosophical challenges of choosing outcome measures. In addition, such a trial would not answer two key questions concerning opportunity cost. The first can be formulated as the question, 'Does any specific educational experience within a medical humanities course yield better outcomes than another?' (e.g. is a course on the history of medicine of greater value than a course on medicine and literature?). The second question is the one posed earlier by Weatherall(11) concerning the relative importance of the humanities and the biomedical sciences for individual practitioners. Are insights into the history of medicine more important than knowing the detailed structure of, for example, cytokine receptors? The answer is, of course, 'It depends'. Because graduates follow so many different career paths, we can only look at individual students, and then only with the benefit of hindsight, after they have chosen their particular career paths. We are left, as is so often the case in medical education, with innumerable variables intertwined. This is not, however, a counsel of despair. Excellent research is being done on a small scale, and the researchers deserve full credit for sourcing funds and carrying out interesting and innovative research projects on teaching, learning and assessment involving the humanities.

Creating the right environment

Through the biomedical sciences, students learn about how bodies function and malfunction. Through the humanities disciplines, students learn about how and why we think, feel and behave as we do; the humanities invite us to make sense of Socrates' observation that the unexamined life is not worth living. Much of the students' humanities-based knowledge is acquired in the same way that their non-medical fellows acquire it – through reading, reflecting, debating, discussing, listening and looking, as a part of everyday life. Without reflection we all live in a state of relative philosophical confusion and disorder.(99,100) In addition to the knowledge acquired as part of a broad education, doctors acquire insights through their privileged relationships with patients and families, and with society at large. The humanities can encourage students to

trust their own aesthetic perceptions and judgements – a process that happens most readily when there is space for students to make personally relevant connections.

Medical teachers have the capacity to foster or neglect their students' personal and professional development alongside learning in the biomedical sciences.(61) Whether in primary, secondary, tertiary or post-tertiary learning, certain institutional factors consistently help students to achieve the twin goals of mastering the art and science of medicine. Here are just some of the characteristics of successful medical schools, against which you might like to compare your own organisation.

- To what extent do you have strong and effective leaders who value teaching and learning in both science and the humanities?
- Do you have competent teachers with respect to both humanities content and process?
- Do your courses encourage high levels of critical thinking, creativity, problem-solving and teamwork?
- Does engagement with medical humanities foster a sense of belonging and pride and emphasise respect, tolerance, inclusion and diversity of views?
- Are all students required to master foundational knowledge and skills, acknowledging that some will go further with elective experiences?
- Is humanities teaching adequately resourced?
- Are assessment processes defensible?
- Are there good evaluation and monitoring systems in place?

Resources

There are now so many schools with interesting programmes running that it is impossible to describe them all. Once you access a website for one of the schools that have committed to the medical humanities, you will find yourself in a rich maze of resources. At medical schools such as Dalhousie, strong advocacy at the highest levels has resulted in a programme that not only includes medical humanities in the curriculum, but uses the arts and humanities to bring students and faculty together for musical performances, art competitions and to promote humanistic engagement: http://humanities.medicine.dal.ca.

Examples in the USA can be found at:
- http://litmed.med.nyu.edu Literature, Arts, and Medicine Database at NYU School of Medicine
- http://medhum.med.nyu.edu/syllabi.html Medical humanities syllabi listing
- http://www.meded.uci.edu/Medhum/index.html UC Irvine School of Medicine, Medical Humanities and Arts
- http://www.utmb.edu/imh University of Texas Medical Branch, Institute for Medical Humanities
- http://www.stonybrook.edu/bioethics/ Center for Medical Humanities, Compassionate Care, and Bioethics at Stony Brook University

Examples in the UK can be found at:
- http://www.dur.ac.uk/cmh/ Centre for Medical Humanities, Durham University

- http://www.kcl.ac.uk/research/groups/chh/ Centre for the Humanities and Health, King's College London

Students can also be directed to web-based discussions and blogs:

- http://medhum.blogspot.com
- http://www.medhumanities.org
- http://blogs.bmj.com/medical-humanities/
- http://medhum.med.nyu.edu/blog/
- http://humanitiesandhealth.wordpress.com/

Whilst it is not possible to acknowledge all of the resources available for teaching and learning in the humanities, it is even more daunting to try to list the philosophical, literary, historical, anthropological, sociological, artistic and musical resources that have the potential to open doors to the recording and interpreting of human experience in relation to illness, disability and medical care. We have not attempted to do so! You and your colleagues will find your own favourites, especially those with local relevance.

Conclusion

When Virgil wrote the words with which we began our chapter, he was concerned with the science of agriculture. Small land owners in the second century BCE were being taken over by large farming 'companies' with access to slave labour – shades of the globalisation to come. Virgil was trying to restore a sense of balance – a sense that farming is not just about the 'bottom line', but also about the wise, scientifically based use of limited resources. All over the world, profit-driven agriculture is depleting vital food stocks on land and in the sea. The science of agriculture was, and is, potentially life-saving, just as medicine is. Little wonder that the deep understanding of 'the cause of things' in any of the natural sciences gives rise to a particular kind of satisfaction, one that is distinctively different from the satisfaction derived from the study of the social sciences and humanities.

It is sometimes tempting for medical students, selected to a large degree for their scientific ability, to focus on those areas of understanding over which they have the fullest mastery – physiology, pathology and so on. However, when biomedicine fails, as it must, they may be ill prepared to respond. The social sciences and humanities defy reduction to formulae. They demand that we learn to live in a 'polysemic' world – a complex world of multiple meanings. It is not simply a question of how to learn medicine from the humanities; rather, it might be said that without the humanities medicine can never be truly learnt. The educator's task is to help students see how much wisdom, insight, support and comfort the humanities can provide for them and for their patients.

References

1 Moore A (1976) Medical humanities – a new medical adventure. *New England Journal of Medicine.* **295**: 1479–80.

2 Moore A (1977) Medical humanities: an aid to ethical discussions. *Journal of Medical Ethics.* **3**: 26–32.

3 AcunaL E (2000) Don't cry for us Argentinians: two decades of teaching medical humanities. *Medical Humanities.* **26**: 66–70.

4 Cassell E (1984) *The Place of the Humanities in Medicine.* The Hastings Center Institute of Society, Ethics and Life Sciences, New York.

5 Pellegrino E (1984) The humanities in medical education; entering the post-evangelical era. *Theoretical Medicine and Bioethics.* **5**: 253–66.

6 Self D (1993) The educational philosophies behind the medical humanities programs in the United States: an empirical assessment of three different approaches to humanistic medical education. *Theoretical Medicine.* **14**: 221–9.

7 Grant VJ (2002) Making room for medical humanities. *Medical Humanities.* **28**: 45–8.

8 Brody H (2011) Defining the medical humanities: three conceptions and three narratives. *Journal of Medical Humanities.* **32**: 1–7.

9 Wear D and Aultman JM (2005) The limits of narrative: medical student resistance to confronting inequality and oppression in literature and beyond. *Medical Education.* **39**: 1056–65.

10 Scally J (1976) Transvaluing: the humanities in a technical–vocational curriculum. *Journal of Higher Education.* **47**: 217–26.

11 Weatherall D (2006) Science in the undergraduate curriculum during the 20th century. *Medical Education.* **40**: 195–201.

12 Leydon G, Boulton M, Moynihan C *et al.* (2000) Cancer patients' information needs and information seeking behaviour: in depth interview study. *British Medical Journal.* **320**: 909–13.

13 Maguire P and Pitceathly C (2002) Key communication skills and how to acquire them. *British Medical Journal.* **325**: 697–700.

14 Schuwirth L and van der Vleuten C (2003) *Written Assessment. In:* ABC of Teaching and Learning in Medicine. *British Medical Journal.* **326**: 643–5.

15 Corderre S, Harasym P, Mandin H and Fick G (2004) The impact of two multiple-choice question formats on the problem-solving strategies used by novices and experts. *BioMed Central Medical Education.* **4**: 23.

16 Kuhl D (2002) *What Dying People Want: Practice Wisdom for the End of Life.* Perseus Books, Cambridge, MA.

17 Dittrich L (2003) The humanities and medicine: reports of 41 US, Canadian and international programs: preface. *Academic Medicine.* **78**: 951–2.

18 Friedman LD (2002) The precarious position of the medical humanities in the medical school curriculum. *Academic Medicine.* **77**: 320–2.

19 Kamien M (1997) The reform of medical education. *Medical Journal of Australia.* **158**: 226–7.

20 General Medical Council (2009) *Tomorrow's Doctors.* GMC, London.

21 Ludmerer K (1999) *Time to Heal: American Medical Education from the Turn of the Century to the Era of Managed Care.* Oxford University Press, New York.

22 Cruess R and Cruess S (1997) Teaching medicine as a profession in the service of healing. *Academic Medicine.* **72**: 941–52.

23 American Board of Internal Medicine Foundation (2002) Medical professionalism in the new millennium: a physician charter. *Annals of Internal Medicine.* **136**: 243–6.

24 Royal College of Physicians (2005) Doctors in Society: medical professionalism in a changing world. Report of a Working Party of the Royal College of Physicians of London. RCP, London.

25 Hafferty F (2006) Professionalism – the next wave. *New England Journal of Medicine.* **355**: 2151–2.

26 Gordon J and Lyon P (1998) As others see us: students' role models in medicine. *Medical Journal of Australia.* **169**: 103–5.

27 Turner L (2002) Medical facilities as moral worlds. *Medical Humanities.* **28**: 19–22.

28 Apker J and Eggly S (2004) Communicating professional identity in medical socialization: considering the ideological discourse of morning report. *Qualitative Health Research.* **14**: 411–29.

29 Shem S (1978) The House of God. Richard MarekInc. New York.

30 Mercurio J (2002) *Bodies*. Jonathan Cape, London.

31 Whittebols J (1998) *Watching M*A*S*H, Watching America: A Social History of the 1972–1983 Television Series*. Mcfarland and Co, Jefferson NC.

32 Gull SE (2005) Embedding the humanities into medical education. *Medical Education*. **39**: 235–6.

33 Shapiro J and Lie D (2000) Using literature to help physician-learners understand and manage 'difficult' patients. *Academic Medicine*. **75**: 765–8.

34 Shapiro J and Rucker L (2003) Can poetry make better doctors? Teaching the humanities and arts to medical students and residents at the University of California, Irvine, College of Medicine. *Academic Medicine*. **78**: 953–7.

35 Pickering N (2000) The use of poetry in health care ethics education. *Medical Humanities*. **26**: 31–6.

36 Pellegrino E (1974) Medical practice and the humanities. *New England Journal of Medicine*. **290**: 1083–5.

37 Downie R, Hendry R, Macnaughton R and Smith B (1997) Humanizing medicine: a special study module. *Medical Education*. **31**: 276–80.

38 Meakin R and Kirklin D (2000) Humanities special studies modules: making better doctors or just happier ones? *Medical Humanities*. **26**(1): 49–50.

39 Kirklin D (2003) Responding to the implications of the genetics revolution for the education and training of doctors: a medical humanities approach. *Medical Education*. **37**: 168–73.

40 Lazarus PA and Rosslyn FM (2003) The arts in medicine: setting up and evaluating a new special study module at Leicester Warwick Medical School. *Medical Education*. **37**: 553–9.

41 Jacobson L, Grant A, Hood K *et al.* (2004) A literature and medicine special study module run by academics in general practice: two evaluations and the lessons learnt. *Medical Humanities*. **30**: 98–100.

42 Bolton G (2005) *Reflective Practice: Writing and Professional Development*. Sage Publications, London.

43 Marton F and Saljo R (1976) On qualitative differences in learning 1: outcome and process. *British Journal of Educational Psychology*. **46**: 4–11.

44 Biggs J (2003) *Teaching for Quality Learning at University*. Open University Press, Buckingham.

45 Shapiro J and Talbot Y (1991) Applying the concept of the reflective practitioner to understanding and teaching family medicine. *Family Medicine*. **23**: 450–6.

46 General Medical Council Education Committee (1993) *Tomorrow's Doctors: Recommendations on Undergraduate Medical Education*. GMC, London.

47 Evans D (2001) Imagination and medical education. *Medical Humanities*. **27**: 30–4.

48 Louis-Courvoisier M and Wenger A (2005) How to make the most of history and literature in the teaching of medical humanities: the experience of the University of Geneva. *Medical Humanities*. **31**: 51–4.

49 Fadiman A (1998) *The Spirit Catches You and You Fall Down*. Farrar, Strauss & Giroux, New York.

50 Horowitz H (1996) Poetry on rounds: a model for the integration of humanities into residency training. *Lancet*. **347**: 447–9.

51 Kleinman A and Benson P (2006) Anthropology in the clinic: the problem of cultural competency and how to fix it. *Public Library of Science – Medicine*. **3**(10): 1673–6.

52 Greenhalgh T (2006) *What Seems to Be the Trouble? Stories of illness and healthcare*. The Nuffield Trust, London.

53 Spencer J, Blackmore D, Heard S *et al.* (2000) Patient-oriented learning: a review of the role of the patient in the education of medical students. *Medical Education*. **34**: 851–7.

54 Almy T, Colby K, Zubkoff M *et al.* (1992) Health, society and the physician: problem-based learning and the social sciences and humanities. *Annals of Internal Medicine*. **116**: 569–74.

55 Gaita R (2000) *A Common Humanity: thinking about love and truth and justice*. Routledge, London.

56 Aull FB (ed.) (2003) *Editor's Choices from the Literature, Arts and Medicine Database: 10th Year Anniversary*. New York University, New York.

57 Dittrich L (2001) *Ten Years of Medicine and the Arts: 100 Selections from Academic Medicine*. Association of American Medical Colleges, Washington, DC.

58 Vannata J, Schleifer R and Crow S (2004) *Medicine and Humanistic Understanding: The Significance of Literature in Medical Practice [DVDROM]*. University of Pennsylvania Press, Philadelphia, PA.

59 Macnaughton J (2000) The humanities in medical education: context, outcome and structures. *Medical Humanities*. **26**: 23–30.

60 Evans H and Macnaughton R (2006) A 'core curriculum' for the medical humanities? *Medical Humanities*. **32**: 65–6.

61 Gordon J (2003) Fostering students' personal and professional development in medicine: a new framework for PPD. *Medical Education*. **37**: 341–9.

62 Evans M (2001) The medical body as philosophy's arena. *Theoretical Medicine and Bioethics*. **22**: 17–32.

63 Rudnick A (2004) An introductory course in philosophy of medicine. *Medical Humanities*. **30**: 54–6.

64 Louhiala P (2003) Philosophy for medical students – why, what, and how. *Medical Humanities*. **29**: 87–8.

65 Dufflin J (1999) *History of Medicine: A Scandalously Short Introduction*. University of Toronto Press, Toronto.

66 Dufflin J (1995) Infiltrating the curriculum: an integrative approach to history for medical students. *Journal of Medical Humanities*. **16**: 155–73.

67 Porter R (1998) *The Greatest Benefit to Mankind: A Medical History of Humanity*. WW Norton & Co, London.

68 Porter R (2002) *Blood and Guts: A Short History of Medicine*. Allen Lane, London.

69 Porter R (ed.) (2006) *The Cambridge History of Medicine*. Cambridge University Press, Cambridge.

70 Evans M (2003) Roles for literature in medical education. *Advances in Psychiatric Treatment*. **9**: 380–5.

71 Hawkins A (1993) *Reconstructing Illness: Studies in Pathography*. Purdue University Press, West Lafayette, IN.

72 Friedman L (1995) See me, hear me: using film in health care classes. *Journal of Medical Humanities*. **16**: 223–8.

73 Lepicard E and Fridman K (2003) Medicine, cinema and culture: a workshop in medical humanities for clinical years. *Medical Education*. **37**: 1039–40.

74 Charon R (2001) Narrative medicine: a model for empathy, reflection, profession, and trust. *Journal of the American Medical Association*. **286**: 1897–902.

75 Singer R and Singer P (2005) *The Moral of the Story*. Blackwell Publishing, Oxford.

76 Shapiro J, Duke A, Boker J and Ahearn CS (2005) Just a spoonful of humanities makes the medicine go down: introducing literature into a family medicine clerkship. *Medical Education*. **39**: 605–12.

77 Toombs S (1992) *The Meaning of Illness: A Phenomenological Account of the Different Perspectives of Physician and Patient*. Kluwer, Boston, MA.

78 Charon R (2004) Narrative and medicine. *New England of Journal of Medicine*. **350**: 862–4.

79 Greenhalgh T and Hurwitz B (1999) Narrative based medicine: why study narrative? *British Medical Journal*. **318**: 48–50.

80 Gysels M, Richardson A and Higginson I (2004) Communication training for health professionals who care for patients with cancer: a systematic review of training methods. *Supportive Care in Cancer*. **13**: 356–66.

81 Clark JA and Mishler EG (1992) Attending to patients' stories: reframing the clinical task. *Sociology of Health & Illness*. **14**: 344–72.

82 Lingard L and Haber R (1999) Teaching and learning communication in medicine. *Academic Medicine.* **74**: 507–10.

83 Bardes CL, Gillers D and Herman AE (2001) Learning to look: developing clinical observational skills at an art museum. *Medical Education.* **35**: 1157–61.

84 Tapajos R (2003) HIV/AIDS in the visual arts: applying discipline-based art education (DBAE) to medical humanities. *Medical Education.* **37**: 563–70.

85 Elder N, Tobias B, Lucero-Criswell A and Goldenhar L (2006) The art of observation: impact of a family medicine and art museum partnership on student education. *Family Medicine.* **38**: 393–8.

86 Rabow M (2003) Drawing on experience: physician artwork in a course on professional development. *Medical Education.* **37**: 1040–1.

87 Kirklin D, Meakin R, Singh S and Lloyd M (2000) Living with and dying from cancer: a humanities special study module. *Medical Humanities.* **26**: 51–4.

88 Easterbrook P, Berlin J, Gopalan R and Matthews D (1991) Publication bias in clinical research. *Lancet.* **337**: 867–72.

89 Shapiro J, Rucker L and Beck J (2006) Training the clinical eye and mind: using the arts to develop medical students' observational and pattern recognition skills. *Medical Education.* **40**: 263–8.

90 Dolev JC, Friedlaender LK and Braverman IM (2001) Use of fine art to enhance visual diagnostic skills. *Journal of the American Medical Association.* **286**: 1020–1.

91 Karkabi K and Cohen Castel O (2006) Deepening compassion through the mirror of painting. *Medical Education.* **40**: 462.

92 Dalhousie University (2006) *Humanities in Medicine: A Program of the Division of Medical Humanities.* Dalhousie University, Halifax, Nova Scotia.

93 Evans R (2003) Patient centred medicine: reason, emotion, and human spirit? Some philosophical reflections on being with patients. *Medical Humanities.* **29**: 8–14.

94 Anderson M, Cohen J, Hallock J *et al.* (1999) Learning objectives for medical student education – guidelines for medical schools. Report 1 of the Medical Schools Objectives Project. *Academic Medicine.* **74**: 13–8.

95 Fortin A and Barnett K (2004) Medical school curricula in spirituality and medicine. *Journal of the American Medical Association.* **291**: 2883.

96 Berlinger N (2004) Spirituality and medicine: idiot-proofing the discourse. *Journal of Medicine and Philosophy.* **29**: 681–95.

97 Ernst E, Cohen MH and Stone J (2004) Ethical problems arising in evidence based complementary and alternative medicine. *Journal of Medical Ethics.* **30**: 156–9.

98 Diamond J (2001) *Snake Oil and Other Preoccupations.* Vintage, London.

99 Weinstein A (2003) *A Scream Goes Through the House: what literature teaches us about life.* Random House, New York.

100 Magee B (1998) *Confessions of a Philosopher.* Phoenix, London.

Further reading

Books

Ahlzen R (2010) *Why Should Physicians Read? Understanding Clinical Judgement in Relation to Literary Experience.* Universitetstryckeriet, Karlstad.

Bamforth I (2003) *The Body in the Library: A Literary Anthology of Modern Medicine.* Verso, London.Barash DP and Barash NR (2005) *Madam Bovary's Ovaries: A Darwinian Look at Literature.* Random House, New York.

Coulehan J and Coles R (eds) (2003) *Chekhov's Doctors.* Kent State University, Kent, OH.

Downie R (2000) *The Healing Arts: An Oxford Illustrated Anthology.* Oxford University Press, Oxford.

Evans M and Finlay I (2000) *Medical Humanities.* BMJ Books, London.

Greenhalgh T (2005) *What Seems to Be the Trouble?* Radcliffe Publishing, Oxford.

Helman C (2002) *Doctors and Patients.* Radcliffe Publishing, Oxford.

Kirklin D and Richardson R (2001) *Medical Humanities: a practical introduction.* Royal College of Physicians, London.

Middleton J and Middleton E (2005) *Doctors and Paintings.* Radcliffe Publishing, Oxford.

Nadelhaft R and Bonebakker E (eds) (2008) *A Literature and Medicine Anthology.* University of Hawaii Press, Hawaii.

Salinsky J (2002) *Medicine and Literature.* Radcliffe Publishing, Oxford.

Singer P and Singer R (2005) *The Moral of the Story.* Blackwell Publishing, Malden, MA.

Journals

Journal of Medical Humanities. Springer. (http://springerlink.com/content/1041-3545, accessed 7 December 2012).

Medical Humanities. BMJ. (http://mh.bmj.com/, accessed 7 December 2012)

Literature and Medicine. The Johns Hopkins University Press. (http://www.press.jhu.edu/journals/literature_and_medicine, accessed 7 December 2012).

17 Patient involvement in medical education

John Spencer[1] and Judy McKimm[2]
[1]Newcastle University, UK
[2]College of Medicine, Swansea University, UK

 KEY MESSAGES

- Patient involvement in medical education is embedded within a broader health services policy agenda.
- There is a growing literature on patient involvement but much of it remains descriptive.
- A wide variety of initiatives and settings has been described.
- A wide range of benefits has been shown for all stakeholders.

- There is a need for appropriate support, training and remuneration for all involved.
- 'Patients' include patients themselves, patient groups, and patient representatives and advocates.
- There is a need for further research, including assessment of the strengths and weaknesses of different approaches, evaluation of long-term impact and factors influencing sustainability.

Introduction

My method (is to) lead my students by hand to the practice of medicine, taking them every day to see patients in the public hospital, that they may hear the patient's symptoms and see their physical findings. Then I question the students as to what they have noted in their patients and about their thoughts and perceptions regarding the causes of the illness and the principles of treatment. Sylvius (1614–1672)(1)

In the early 17th century Sylvius' teaching methods would have been unusual, indeed it would have been considered distinctly eccentric to involve patients in medical education to such a degree. Whilst the traditional physician apprenticeship – dating back (at least) to Hippocrates – relied on contact with sick people, by the time medical education was formally established in the universities of Europe in the 13th century, the patient had all but 'disappeared'. It was not until after the Renaissance that universities began to introduce bedside experience. And by the 18th century it was, in the words of one author, 'axiomatic' that students should supplement their book learning by spending time 'walking the wards',(2) although examination of patients as a component of assessment did not appear until the following century. Clinical experience through patient contact gradually assumed its place at the centre of medical education such that by the turn of the 20th century, Sir William Osler's assertion that 'it is a safe rule to have no teaching without a patient for a text, and the best teaching is that taught by the patient himself'(3) had become part of the rhetoric of a modern medical education.

Despite this evolving centrality, the role of the patient in clinical education has historically been a passive one. At worst a hapless hospital inmate unable to say 'No' to a gaggle of students at the foot of the bed; 'imposition' more than 'involvement' (think Sir Lancelot Spratt in the film *Doctor in the House* (4)). Even at best, the patient, though treated with courtesy, was often no more than a medium, 'an interesting case', through which clinical teaching took place.

This chapter considers the importance of the active involvement of patients in the education of doctors and other health professionals, explores aspects of the growing literature on the subject, including evidence of benefits and disadvantages, describes models of involvement, discusses problems and challenges, and identifies areas for further inquiry. Before doing that, however, it is important that we first consider terminology.

Patients, users and consumers

Labelling in this area is a source of controversy and confusion, and the issues are complex. The language used generates strong emotions, affecting communication and collaboration between interested groups, and may even impair scholarly activity, such as searching and reviewing the literature.(5,6) Views vary greatly about how people prefer to be described, and preferences and language change over time.(6) For simplicity's sake we will mainly use the term 'patient' (and, where relevant, 'carer') throughout this chapter, because, for all its limitations, it is probably the most widely recognised term in **medical** education – although terminology differs amongst user groups as well as different professionals and countries (*see* Box 17.1). We

Understanding Medical Education: Evidence, Theory and Practice, Second Edition. Edited by Tim Swanwick.
© 2014 The Association for the Study of Medical Education. Published 2014 by John Wiley & Sons, Ltd.

> **BOX 17.1 Terminology**
>
> 'User' or 'service user' is commonly used in the UK, but in North America may be more associated with illicit drug use. However, 'user' does imply a degree of active participation.
>
> 'Lay' is also used frequently; it implies the person is not necessarily either sick or under active care. However, 'lay' defines a person essentially not by any positive attributes, but by what they are not (i.e. 'professional') and what they do not have (i.e. medical expertise).
>
> 'Consumer', 'client' or 'customer' connote health as a commodity and health care as a market, thus a commercial relationship.
>
> 'Survivor' is a term mostly restricted to use in relation to cancer and mental health.
>
> 'Patient' is probably the most unambiguous term, although it implies that the person is sick and under active care; the term connotes passivity; and the care relationship is medicalised.

use it to mean both people with health problems, whether or not they are currently receiving care, and healthy people, although we recognise that this may be contentious and will not acknowledge everyone's preference. We also recognise that 'on the ground' it is important to recognise the power of language.(5)

Context of patient involvement

If we take the UK as an example, involving patients in the development, delivery and management of health care has been an important aspect of government policy since the 1980s, developing through the 1990s to the point where it became enshrined as an underlying principle of health care reform in a 'patient-led National Health Service (NHS)'. The intended aim was to make health services more responsive to the needs of individuals and communities, and it became a statutory requirement that 'patient and public involvement should be part of everyday practice in the NHS and must lead to action for improvement'.(7) The principle was carried forward into the most recent (highly controversial) UK health reforms, with all agencies required to 'promote involvement of patients, carers and representatives (where necessary) in decisions about care', reflected in the catch-phrase 'no decision about me, without me'.(8) This inevitably encompasses involvement in the education and training of health professionals.(9) Indeed the most recent iteration of the General Medical Council's (GMC) standards for undergraduate medical education, *Tomorrow's Doctors 2009*, contained specific, if somewhat cryptic, recommendations about public and patient involvement, later expanded in 'supplementary guidance'.(10) The GMC now requires medical schools to develop systems 'which give patients an opportunity to feed back on quality of teaching, as well as individual students' performance'. These trends are not confined to undergraduate medical education nor indeed to the UK.(11)

Angela Coulter has suggested eight distinct policy areas in which patients and citizens could make an important contribution to maximising health, as follows:(12)
- improving care processes
- building health literacy
- selecting treatments
- strengthening self-care
- ensuring safer care
- participating in research
- shaping services
- training professionals.

There is, however, a broader educational context, that of 'social accountability'. This has been defined by the World Health Organization as: 'The obligation [of medical schools] to direct their education, research and service activities towards addressing the priority health concerns of the community, region, and/or nation they have the mandate to serve'.(13) Social accountability has evolved as a major contemporary discourse embracing concepts such as 'the social contract' (between professions and society), 'social responsibility' (of doctors and other health professionals) and 'social responsiveness' (of institutions). Woollard and Boelen (14) highlight the challenge for medical schools 'to strive for and demonstrate greater impact on health through their bonds with society', which, they contend, is the very purpose of social accountability. They argue that medical schools must demonstrate a commitment to social accountability in both formal programmes and the 'hidden curriculum' At the same time, and influenced by similar social and political forces, the concept of 'professionalism' has been revisited and redefined, with obvious implications for education.(15–17)

These developments have occurred in parallel with changes in public expectations of health care and of doctors, changes often described as part of the move from paternalism to partnership. With the decline in an uncritical deference to the professions, the rise of consumerism and a greater understanding of what health care can achieve, many patients expect to have their concerns addressed and their requests heard, and to be fully informed about their condition, briefed about risks of treatment, involved in decisions about their care, and educated and supported to manage their own conditions.(18)

Aside from changes in expectations, there is now a greater appreciation of the psychological and social consequences of ill health and health care treatments, and the need for new models to guide practice, such as the 'bio-psychosocial model' and 'patient-centredness', which put the patient's perspective and priorities at the centre.(19,20) Increased knowledge about variation between patients in values, preferences and responses to illness and their effect on treatment outcomes has brought the health care professional's interaction with the patient to centre stage. And whilst the technical complexity of medicine increases apace, with greater choice of diagnostic tests and treatments, and more complex interventions, financial constraints often lead to doctors having to navigate their way through the tensions between expectations and feasible options.

Such circumstances make working with patients even more demanding – for example, supporting patients to exercise choice in situations of uncertainty, enabling them to understand the options available and the risks and dangers involved, and helping them appreciate restrictions on choice. Learning how to do all these things needs input from patients and challenges educators to seek the most appropriate ways of enabling students and trainees to learn, whilst respecting the rights and needs of patients.(21) We go on to explore some of the issues involved.

Scope of patient involvement

Most people would probably assume that 'patient involvement in the curriculum' means direct involvement in teaching, learning and assessment; indeed, these areas are the main focus of this chapter. Nonetheless, there is potential for people to make a contribution to *all* aspects of the educational process. These include the following:

- student selection and admission
- curriculum development
- course management
- faculty development
- practice placements
- programme evaluation.

However, several recent major literature reviews highlight that patient involvement in most of the above areas is still relatively unusual. A number of frameworks help us explore the potential scope of patient involvement, and

here we describe three: Tew *et al.*'s (22) 'ladder of patient involvement', the 'Cambridge framework'(23) and a taxonomy of active involvement described by Towle *et al.*(6)

Ladder of patient involvement
Tew *et al.*(22) describe a 'ladder of involvement', which they propose can be used to establish and monitor patients' involvement within individual programmes and institutions. The tool was developed in the context of mental health education and training, but could be applied across the educational spectrum, whether undergraduate or postgraduate (*see* Box 17.2).

The Cambridge framework
Spencer *et al.* (23) reviewed the patient's role in medical education and suggested a framework (the 'Cambridge framework') to facilitate discussion about patient involvement. The framework is based on four sets of attributes of contexts in which patients, students and teachers interact, under the headings 'Who?', 'How?', 'Where' and 'What?', providing a checklist against which patient involvement can be planned or evaluated (*see* Boxes 17.3, 17.4 and 17.5).

Who?
This reflects the individual background, culture, experience and expectations of each patient, their family and carers. Patients vary immensely in terms of the clinical problems with which they present, as well as their age, gender,

---

BOX 17.2 Ladder of patient involvement(22)

Level	Description of involvement
1 No involvement	The curriculum is planned, delivered and managed with no consultation or involvement of service users or carers
2 Limited involvement	Outreach with local service user or carer groups. Service users/carers invited to 'tell their story' in a designated slot and/or be consulted about course planning or management, student selection, student assessment or programme evaluation. Payment offered but no opportunity to participate in shaping the course as a whole
3 Growing involvement	Service users/carers contribute regularly to at least two of the following: planning, delivery, student selection, assessment, management or evaluation. Payment at normal visiting lecturer rates. However, key decisions on matters such as curriculum content, learning outcomes or student selection made in forums in which service users/carers are not represented. Some support before and after sessions, but no consistent programme of training and supervision. No discrimination against service users and carers accessing programmes as students
4 Collaboration	Service users/carers involved as full team members in at least three of the following: planning, delivery, student selection, assessment, management or evaluation. Underpinned by a statement of values. Service users/carers contribute to key decisions on matters such as curriculum content. Facility for contributors to the programme to meet and regular provision of training, supervision and support. Positive steps to encourage service users and carers to access programmes as students
5 Partnership	Service users, carers and staff work together systematically and strategically across all areas, underpinned by an explicit statement of partnership values. All key decisions made jointly. Service users and carers involved in the assessment of practice learning. Adequately funded infrastructure to provide induction, support and training. Service users and carers employed as lecturers on secure contracts and/or contracts established between programmes and independent groups. Positive steps made to encourage service users and carers to join learning sessions, even if not (yet) in a position to achieve qualifications

---

BOX 17.3 'How' patients may be involved in medical education(23)

Brief contact	Prolonged contact
Passive role	Active role
Time limited	Time committed
Trained	Untrained
Inexperienced ('novice')	Experienced ('expert')
Planned encounter	Unplanned encounter
Simulated situation	Real situation
'Questioning'	'Informing'
Known patient	Unknown patient
Focused learning	Holistic learning
Tutor involved	Tutor not involved

BOX 17.4 'Where' to involve patients(23)

'Our place'	'Your place'
Community	Hospital
'My culture'	'Your culture'
'My clothes'	'Your clothes'
Service setting	Educational setting
Real environment	Simulated environment
Multiprofessional setting	Uniprofessional setting

BOX 17.5 'What' to involve patients in(23)

Undifferentiated problem	Defined problem
Straightforward	Challenging
High impact	Low impact
General	Specific
Clinical science	Basic science
Minor	Major
Simple skills	Complex skills
'Revealed' attitudes	'Hidden' attitudes
Particular focus	Generic approach

---

ethnicity, sexual orientation, emotional and intellectual capacity, and socio-economic status.(24)

How?

Students and trainees work in a wide range of settings (such as hospital wards, hospital and community ambulatory clinics, emergency departments), which present different educational opportunities. These depend on factors such as whether encounters are planned or opportunistic, pressures of time, available supervision and so on. The issues under this heading (*see* Box 17.3) may help teachers to plan how patients may be involved, and to relate this to the intended learning outcomes and the setting. In fact, most of the issues apply to all patient encounters.

Where?

Recognising that health care takes place in a wide range of locations and settings, and that context will inevitably influence the nature and quality of learning, questions addressed under this heading explore issues to do with place, safety, identity and power relationships. The 'Where?' also includes whether it is a 'real or 'simulated environment', such as a training ward, and the contrast between 'uni-professional' or 'multi-professional' settings to distinguish between situations in which doctors alone are learning with patients and those in which a range of health and social care professionals are learning and working (*see* Box 17.4).(24)

What?

This set of attributes deals with 'content': the clinical problems presented, the specific skills and knowledge that may be learned, and underlying attitudes and values. Consideration of these should help teachers realise the maximum potential of particular situations and assess the likely impact on both patients and learners (*see* Box 17.5).

Taxonomy of active patient involvement

Although there are many different contexts in which students may encounter patients, historically this tended to be restricted to opportunistic contact with 'real' patients in the wards and clinics of a teaching hospital. In the past two-to-three decades, however, a number of other ways of providing patient contact have evolved in response to changes in health care delivery, the changing characteristics of patients in hospital, and increasing recognition of the need to protect patients from harm, including, most recently, the challenges of infection control. This has led to the use of new environments, notably 'the community', where patient encounters take place either in primary care clinics or in people's homes, inevitably changing the dynamics and power balance. The shift of clinical education into the community is a worldwide phenomenon, has been shown to be effective(25) and community-based learning is now a core component of undergraduate programmes.

Towle *et al.*(6) propose a taxonomy combining elements of both the 'Cambridge Framework' and 'ladder of involvement', which they argue helps both clarify the patient's role and makes communication of research findings easier to articulate, synthesise and compare. Their classification considers the wide variety of ways other than real patients in the workplace in which patients may be encountered, describing a continuum of involvement grounded in five attributes at six levels (*see* Box 17.6).

Levels of patient involvement

In this section, we describe some of the issues that may arise for medical educators under each of the levels described in Box 17.6.

BOX 17.6 A taxonomy of patient involvement(6)

Degree to which the patient is actively involved in the learning encounter *N.B.In all instances patients are 'real' and assumed to be representing themselves*	Duration of contact with learner	Patient autonomy during the encounter	Training for the patient	Patient involvement in planning the encounter and curriculum	Institutional commitment to patient involvement in education
1 Paper-based or electronic case or scenario Patient is focus of a paper-based, electronic or web-based case or scenario	None	Not applicable	Not applicable	None	Low
2 Standardised/volunteer patient in clinical setting Patient encounter with student is scripted and serves as an example to illustrate or reinforce learning (e.g. teacher asks patient to provide student with history or student practices a clinical exam)	Encounter-based	None	None	None	Low
3 Patients share their experience with students within faculty-directed curriculum Patient is invited to share experience; faculty plan the encounter but patient determines personal comfort and level of participation	Encounter-based	None–low	Brief, simple	None	Low
4 Patient teacher(s) involved in teaching and/or evaluating students Patient is given preparation for specific teaching role, may actively question students and may be involved in giving feedback and evaluating their performance	Variable	Moderate	Structured, extensive	Low–moderate	Low–moderate
5 Patient teacher(s) as equal partners in student education, evaluation and curriculum development Patients are involved in many aspects of educational delivery, development and evaluation, beyond specific courses to the curriculum as a whole – a true partnership in which patients make meaningful and valued contributions to decision-making	Moderate–extensive	High	Extensive	Moderate–extensive	Moderate
6 Patient(s) involved at the institutional level in addition to sustained involvement as patient teacher(s) in education, evaluation and curriculum development for students As(5) above but there are also institutional policies that ensure involvement in decision-making bodies within undergraduate, graduate and continuing health professional education	Extensive	High	Extensive	High	High

1   Electronic or paper-based case or scenario

Paper-based cases have long been used to supplement real patient contact, with video-based and electronic cases increasing in use as the technology has developed. The use of virtual patients was first described in the early 1970s. A virtual patient (VP) has been defined as a: 'specific type of computer program that simulates real-life clinical scenarios: learners emulate the roles of health care providers to obtain a history, conduct a physical examination, and make diagnostic and therapeutic decisions'.(26)

A critical literature review concluded that the evidence base to inform the use of virtual patients was very weak, at least in published form,(26) with wide variation, for example, in degree of interactivity, amount of feedback provided and use in assessment. In terms of effectiveness, evidence suggested that virtual patient interventions are more likely than *no* intervention to improve learning, are better at promoting more technical knowledge-based aspects than interpersonal skills, and possibly more effective and better accepted as triggers in problem-based learning than paper cases. However, a more recent discussion paper contended that much progress had been made in the thoughtful application of VPs, to the point where their use has become embedded in curricula, including areas such as problem-based learning cases, interactive lectures and seminars, and in both formative and summative assessments,(27) The main drivers for these developments include international collaboration, decreasing costs, better authoring systems and greater ease of dissemination. Although not intended to replace contact with real patients, the use of VPs appears to be able to usefully complement clinical experience – in particular, from both theoretical and empirical perspectives, in the development of clinical reasoning, which requires exposure to multiple cases and their variations.(27,28) However, there has still been relatively little high-quality research into, for example, the most effective design, sequencing or balance within the curriculum. Consideration of the evidence-based principles that underpin effective instructional design in the related field of simulation-based education may be helpful. These include range of difficulty, repetitive and distributed practice, cognitive interactivity, multiple learning strategies, individualised learning, mastery and feedback.(29,30) (*See* Chapter 13.)

Fast-evolving computer technology enables the building of VPs with far greater realism. This holds exciting potential. As Poulton and Balasubramaniam note, 'It is now possible to consider the extension of the current relatively lightweight VP into a truly interactive patient simulation, an 'e-human' or 'digital avatar . . .offering authentic patient management, clinical and communication skills training, and the potential capability to mimic the health or disease of any citizen'.(28) This development will need to draw on new collaborations between medical educators, content experts and learning technologists.

On a more holistic level, there have been increasing calls to adopt a narrative approach in all aspects of health care, clinical practice, research *and* education, with potential benefits claimed for all parties.(31,32) Guy Widdershoven, of Maastricht University, notes that 'we dream in narrative, daydream in narrative, remember, anticipate, hope, despair, believe, doubt, plan, revise, criticise, construct, gossip, learn, hate and love by narrative'.(31)

One kind of narrative account is what Aronson(33) called the 'autopathography', more simply referred to as a 'patient's tale', or perhaps more cynically, the 'medical confessional'. Over ten years ago he analysed and classified characteristics of nearly 300 such book-length tales. Reading and reflecting on such stories may help health professionals, both in training and in practice, better understand and empathise with their patients, and 'teach them things they won't learn from textbooks',(33) indeed 'that cannot be arrived at by any other means'.(31)

There are many ways in which such resources may be used educationally. Powley and Higson(34) suggest the following simple process for using written narratives in teaching:

- read
- discuss
- facilitate and analyse responses
- discuss applications.

Questions such as 'What is the story about?' and 'What effect did it have on me?' promote reflection and help learners focus on key messages and apply in new contexts. Grounding the exercise in reality reinforces relevance, which in turn helps motivate learners. Sufficient time must be allowed for reflection and discussion. In terms of choice of text, Aronson's own criteria for recommending a book are 'that it should provide a judicious balance between emotional expression and analytical discourse, and that it should have informed, and above all entertained me'.(33) He suggested a 'top ten' books in his article, but many more have been and continue to be published since he wrote.

Another common source of such stories is the internet. 'Google' any disease, common or rare, and a significant proportion of 'hits' will be personal blogs about the problem, as either patient or carer. Resources such as the 'Patient Voices' programme or Healthtalkonline (*see* 'Further Resources' section) are freely available. Others can be purchased or developed by teachers and learning technologists to suit specific purposes, although the cost, time and expertise required to do this should not be underestimated. Examples include interactive tutorials on various topics, such as epileptic seizure classification(35) or breaking bad news.(36)

Such resources can be included in face-to-face or e-learning tutorials, or lectures (e.g. embedded in Power-Point presentations), providing illustrative or trigger scenarios about different clinical conditions or situations. These are particularly helpful when it is inappropriate or difficult for learners to work with real patients – for example, patients with rare conditions, terminally ill patients or patients with mental health problems. Learning technologies can also enable a more standardised approach to assessment. For example, the Royal College of Paediatrics and Child Health has developed an assessment of clinical skills using videos of very ill children; the Royal College of Ophthalmologists also uses video assessments in examinations, and personal digital assistants (a handheld or palmtop computer) have been used as an assessment tool.(37) Another category of website has burgeoned recently in the UK, namely, sites soliciting patient feedback, one of the best known being Patient Opinion (https://www.patientopinion.org.uk/). One innovative way of using such a site in teaching is to treat the narratives as critical incidents to promote discussion about responding to complaints and preventing error (Jones A, *personal communication*).

2 Standardised or volunteer patient in a real clinical setting

Learning from real patients in a clinical setting has been the mainstay of clinical education, enabling students and trainees to consolidate and synthesise learning from a range of sources. Indeed, 'bedside teaching' is the only setting in which the full panoply of technical and non-technical skills, attitudes and applied knowledge that constitute 'doctoring' are modelled by clinical teachers and can be learnt as an integrated whole.(38)

Ramani reminds us that 'the bedside is the perfect venue for unrehearsed and unexpected triangular interactions between teacher, trainees and patient ... physician teachers should be vigilant about grabbing teachable moments'(39) during these encounters. McKimm's(40) clinical 'trialogue' – a 'discussion or conversation in which three persons or groups participate'(41) that attends to the developing relationships between all three 'players', rather than consciously trying to think about teaching and clinical practice – is a useful model that may help teachers plan and work actively with patients and learners.

Whenever clinical teaching occurs, patients are usually the most vulnerable of the parties involved. Notwithstanding, most find clinical teaching rewarding and are willing participants, often commenting that they recognise that students 'have to learn'. However, it should not be tacitly assumed that patients will engage in teaching; patients' feelings should always be respected, and they should know that, whatever their decision, their treatment and care will not be affected. Patients must always be informed that learners may be present and may be providing care, whatever the setting. This allows them to prepare for the initial encounter and to raise any anxieties (*see* 'Ethical Issues' section). There are also potential educational benefits from briefing patients explicitly about a session's aims, what teacher and learners hope to get out of it, and what may be expected of the patient, for example, whether they will be asked to give feedback.(38) Patients need to be aware of the number and level of the learners who may be present, each person's role should be clarified and verbal or written agreement obtained and recorded as appropriate.

3 Patients share their experience with students within faculty-directed curriculum; *and*

4 Patient teacher(s) involved in teaching and/or evaluating students

Selecting real patients for teaching is often opportunistic. A more structured approach employing trained patients is being increasingly used within undergraduate and postgraduate training. Expert patients or patient educators can

be drawn from many settings, including areas where concerns might be expressed about potential harm to patients, such as those who are terminally ill or have mental health problems.

The idea of the expert patient is also enshrined in the wider patient involvement agenda. The 'expert patient initiative was . . . part of the government's commitment to place patients at the heart of healthcare which is . . . part of the transformational focus of the clinical governance agenda'.(42) This initiative was primarily targeted at people with chronic conditions to help them 'become key decision makers in their own care'.(42) The expert patient initiative was supported by an educational programme for the patients themselves, and there is some evidence that it resulted in changes in confidence and self-efficacy in relation to self-management of symptoms (such as pain, tiredness and depression).(43) However, results of several randomised controlled trials looking at outcomes of such programmes in the UK failed to show any effect on use of health care.(44)

There are a number of advantages in involving patients in education who are not under current active care. Using such people can be particularly helpful when teaching inexperienced learners when more time needs to be taken than clinical demands allow. Patient educators have the benefits of being:

- motivated individuals with an interest in medical training
- 'real' (as opposed to simulated) with authentic clinical histories and possibly clinical signs
- able to give structured feedback from a patient's perspective, such as the pressure of the hands or the way in which a history was taken.

Patient instructors with rheumatological conditions comprise the most well-described group. A review article contended that most studies showed they can be as effective as clinicians in enhancing learners' knowledge and skills, especially, and unsurprisingly, in communicating the impact of living with the condition.(45) Another distinctive category of patient teacher is the gynaecology teaching associate, women trained to teach pelvic and breast examination, who are themselves examined. They are widely used in North America and Scandinavia, but are still a relative rarity in the UK, despite much contemporary debate around issues surrounding students performing intimate examinations.(46) Such teaching can help free up clinical tutors as, once trained, they need little assistance in running sessions or participating in clinical assessments. They have been found to be acceptable and effective – in one comparative study students taught by associates had better skills in an end-of-attachment assessment than students who were not.(47) A call was made by the authors for wider use of associates to complement existing teaching programmes.

Well-managed patient involvement in clinical teaching can benefit both patients and learners. The challenge is to be sensitive to both patients' and learners' needs and to identify suitable patients who feel equipped to participate. Sometimes, however, it is neither possible nor appropriate to involve real patients in learning, and this is where one needs to adopt alternative strategies.

5 Patient teacher(s) as equal partners in student education, evaluation and curriculum development

It is unusual in medical education to find this level of involvement, with some notable exceptions, but models have been developed in other disciplines, particularly (non-psychiatric) mental health and social care education. Guidelines and recommendations derived through a variety of processes have been published,(5,22,48–51) and UK guidance about involving patients in research highlights issues that may be relevant to professional education.(52) Both the GMC and British Medical Association have published advice about active patient involvement in medical education and training.(10,53)

6 Patient(s) involved at the institutional level in addition to sustained involvement as patient teacher(s) in education, evaluation and curriculum development for students

Involvement at this level is even rarer than Level 5. One of the best examples in the UK is the Universities/Users Teaching and Research Action Partnership (UNTRAP) based at Warwick University,(54) which is a partnership between Warwick and Coventry universities, users of health and social care services and their carers, and the NHS. Patients are involved at different levels, some in one-off events, others more heavily. The central philosophy of UNTRAP is that everyone will benefit if service users, carers, academics and professionals share their experience. Other institutional approaches have also been described.(22)

Benefits and disadvantages

The thought of training doctors *without* direct patient contact would nowadays be considered absurd (although in some undergraduate medical education systems in mainland Europe contact with patients is still minimal). Medical schools aspire to maximise it, teachers and administrators strive to deliver it, students demand as much as possible, and patients seem only too willing to help. At the postgraduate level, with increasing emphasis on in-service training grounded in clinical practice, patient contact is obviously crucial. A significant literature has accumulated (one of the most comprehensive bibliographies(6) identified nearly 300 relevant papers), providing corroboration for some of the theoretical benefits. Contact between patients and learners is generally very well received, with relatively few apparent adverse effects or disadvantages for the former, and even fewer for the latter. Patients intuitively recognise the contributions they can make – for example, by acting as 'experts' in and/or exemplars of their condition, showing and telling, aiding the development of professional skills and attitudes, and boosting learners' confidence.(55) The majority of studies report distinctive, largely positive outcomes for patients, which include altruistic feelings ('giving something back'), personal satisfaction, being better informed and improved relationships with health professionals (*see* Box 17.7) However, one study of the views of students and faculty demonstrated concerns about possible emotional and psychological impact on both patients (*and* students) of recounting painful and traumatic experiences, and 'professionalisation' of some patients through repeated telling of their stories.(56) Another study using a phenomenological approach, showed that involvement in clinical teaching for most patients was, in fact, often characterised by its ordinariness.(57) Generally speaking, however, benefits appear to far outweigh any disadvantages.

Much of the research informing this literature, however, is descriptive, with relatively 'soft' evaluations (for example, at the level of participant reaction – i.e. 'how was it for you?') often based on self-report, with all the limitations of such an approach. There is often insufficient information about the actual educational intervention and the research design used; there have been few attempts at evaluating long-term impacts. Little research so far appears to have been informed by theory (exceptions include Rees *et al.*'s(5) study that used socio-cultural theory). Finally, people have published in disparate outlets, which, along with problems posed by use of different terms, has bedevilled searching and synthesis of the literature.(6) Nevertheless, several comprehensive reviews have been published over the past few years showing, on the whole, consistent findings about benefits and disadvantages (*see* Boxes 17.7 and 17.8).(6,9,23,58–62)

BOX 17.7 Benefits of increased patient involvement

Based on theoretical considerations(23) and published evidence the main benefits to students are:

- motivation through relevance
- increased empathy
- development of professional skills and attitudes
- increased confidence
- social responsibility
- development of clinical reasoning
- new insights and understanding
- recognition of cultural diversity and lifestyle factors
- improved performance in examinations.

For patients, the benefits appear to be:

- satisfaction at contributing to student learning
- improved relationships with professionals
- altruistic feelings, for example, giving something back to 'the system'
- being valued and increased self-esteem
- development of own skills
- catharsis
- increased knowledge about their own condition
- getting a better service from their clinicians, for example, 'a good going over'
- companionship and relief from social isolation.

Principles and practice

In this section we explore general principles for active patient involvement, focus on three important ethical issues and consider the challenge of representativeness.

General principles

As described above, a number of reports supporting and guiding patient involvement have been published, and these invariably also highlight barriers and challenges. From this growing literature we have distilled a set of principles to inform practice (*see* Box 17.9). We have not explored barriers and challenges in any detail, but these are argued to include the following:

- different, sometimes conflicting, values and expectations
- power imbalances
- perceptions of intimidation (such as unfamiliar even hostile environments)
- lack of consent, choice and confidentiality
- time constraints
- institutional inertia
- inadequate resourcing
- lack of training, support and debriefing
- problems with language and communication.

Ethical issues

Ethical issues to be considered when involving patients can be summarised as the 'three Cs': consent, choice and confidentiality. The main message emerging from policy documents, good practice and the literature is that simply assuming that patients will be involved in teaching and learning without making this explicit through formal systems, professional conversations and ethical practice is no longer acceptable.

Consent

> A mindset shift needs to occur within the medical profession to enable informed partnership rather than informed consent (patient).(63)

This quote from the body that oversees postgraduate training in the UK highlights issues discussed earlier. Medical law and ethics enshrine the principle of informed consent, which should guide patient involvement routinely, not just those encounters involving intimate examinations or invasive procedures.(53) 'Arguments for not informing patients in advance seem to be based more on prejudice than on empirical evidence',(64) and providing information about learner involvement before the clinical encounter does not appear to adversely influence patients' decisions about participation. Perhaps unsurprisingly, there is evidence that patients are more positive about involvement when consent *is* obtained.(65) Obtaining consent should be 'a continuous process that begins with the first contact the service has with the patient',(53) and all patients should be informed that students may be present and, as appropriate, involved in care. It is important to recognise that the presence of a student will inevitably change the dynamics of a consultation, although there is little, if any, evidence of significant negative effects on quality of care.(66) An interesting argument has been made that there should be an expectation that all patients should be willing to contribute to medical education as a default stance, the *quid pro quo* being that all trainees should be required to demonstrate competence in the relevant task in simulation before being 'let loose'.(67)

Choice

Facilitating patient choice is challenging when students and trainees need to learn within the 'turbulent here and now of care delivery',(67) with little time to ensure that each encounter is set up as people would prefer. Promoting active choice about involvement shows basic respect but also acknowledges that the patient is an expert about the way his or her own condition affects them. It moves clinicians away from 'operating from within the safety of a powerful expert role and performing habitual and ritualized tasks that depersonalize the transaction of caring'.(68)

Informing patients and seeking consent about teaching should ideally be done without the learner in attendance, then confirmed in their presence.(50) Building in 'moment-to-moment' opportunities for patients to say 'No' is another way of empowering them and acknowledging their needs.(24) Patients should be informed about the level of experience and identity of any learner intending to carry out a procedure on them. Lack of personal power and space, and the more urgent need for treatment, mean that a different approach may need to be taken in hospital settings compared with primary care, where there is usually a more intimate relationship, more privacy and patients have greater autonomy.(69)

Confidentiality

Confidentiality in relation to patients involved in education has, in the past, been somewhat lax. This is clearly unacceptable, and institutions must develop strategies to ensure confidentiality is maintained. Some patients express concerns 'about students' access to their case notes and whether discussions about patients occurred after they had left the consulting room',(70) which raises questions about how aspects of choice, consent and confidentiality should be raised with patients.

Practical steps include the following:

- providing sufficient information so that patients can understand the boundaries of confidentiality
- reassuring patients that learners are bound by the same duty to respect confidentiality as are 'fully fledged' health professionals
- involving patients in discussions
- remembering that curtains around a bed or cubicle are not soundproof (!)
- finding private spaces to discuss intimate or distressing issues
- raising issues of confidentiality routinely with learners as part of preparation and debrief.

When patient information is being used in teaching, permission must be obtained for the use of images, sound recordings and extracts from case notes, particularly identifiable information. Increasing use of electronic records and mobile communications and technologies is creating new challenges. In the UK in future, students are likely to only have access to clinical records using a smartcard.(71)

Medical ethics and law is complex and ever-changing, and all clinicians have a responsibility to keep up to date and informed. Clinical teachers are key role models; keeping the 'three Cs' – consent, choice and confidentiality – in mind ensures that these are seen as fundamental pillars of good medical practice, not as options. Embedding these principles in institutional practices and policies is an important step.(53)

Patient representation

It is easy to forget that the vast, ubiquitous population of people who might fall under the general heading of 'patient' is by no means homogeneous; indeed, diversity is the norm. 'Patients' do not think alike any more than professionals do, yet much of the literature on 'involvement' sidesteps this issue and, if only by an act of omission, seems to treat all users, carers, survivors, clients, patients, etc. as the same. Charlotte Williamson(72) of Picker Institute, Europe, proposes the following three broad categories of 'patient' who might get involved.

- **Individual patients** who can (obviously) describe their own experience but cannot necessarily speak for others, which raises questions about the generalisability of their experience.
- **Patient group members** who usually *do* know about the experiences of others like themselves, but may still have a narrow perspective. Consulting all relevant groups in a locality is important.
- **Patient representatives or advocates** who generally have broader experience, perhaps of working with several groups, wider knowledge about issues at strategic and policy levels, and understand 'the bigger picture'.

Ideally consultation with 'patients' should involve all three categories using appropriate methods. In Williamson's words: 'The patient side of health care is complex but not mysterious. Consulting the "right" patients can be feasible and rewarding'.(72)

Simulated patients

We end our discussion with a brief word on simulated patients, as they both fall outside, and cut across the taxonomy used to structure the previous sections of this chapter. Simulation is increasingly used to complement both classroom and clinical learning. It cannot replace 'authentic experiential learning in the real world of clinical practice', but can 'prepare practitioners for the real world, providing a structure for deliberate practice . . . clinical reasoning and professional judgement'.(31) Simulated, or 'standardised', patients were first introduced by Barrows and Abrahamson(73) in the 1960s and are now well established in the mainstream of health professional education. They were originally real patients trained to present standardised representations of their own problems;(73) nowadays, in the words of Barrow himself, a simulated patient will generally be 'a well person, with or without a thespian background, trained to simulate a patient's illness'.(74) The significant difference is that they usually portray a range of scenarios *outside* their own experience (Silverman J and Britten N, *personal communication*).

The advantages of using simulated patients include the following:

- authenticity
- consistency

- predictability
- customisation
- convenience
- efficiency.

Using simulated patients allows exploration and rehearsal of challenging situations such as breaking bad news or communicating about sensitive issues, when the use of real patients would not be appropriate. Simulated patients can also teach, give feedback and contribute to assessment. Based on a survey of Belgian and Dutch medical schools, researchers described six of the more common ways in which simulated patients are used. These are: start-stop method; training on the job; dramatic role playing; carousel model with role rotation; individual simulated encounters; and assessment. The authors emphasised there is no 'one and only simulated patient-method'.(75) Research has shown that people generally cannot easily distinguish between real patients and well-trained simulators.(76,77) There is variability in the use of the terms 'standardised' and 'simulated'. They are often used interchangeably, which can cause confusion – for example, when trying to identify good practice or interpret research findings. A useful way of thinking about the difference is that situations involving a *simulated* patient focus predominantly on authenticity, whereas with a standardised patient the emphasis is on consistency. Of course, a standardised patient encounter is always a simulated encounter, whereas a simulated encounter is often unstandardised.(78)

The use of simulated patients has been shown to be acceptable to learners and faculty, and effective, reliable and valid in both instruction and assessment. There is now wide international experience of using simulated patients, although some mental health and paediatric problems, as well as those of the very elderly, may be difficult to simulate and thus may be under-represented, as may certain patient groups, for example, ethnic minorities.

There is a continuum between real patients and highly trained simulators, and the choice of which approach to use in a particular setting will be determined by a range of factors, including the nature of the phenomena to be simulated, intended aims and learning outcomes, local circumstances and available resources.(78) However, in the wider context of patient involvement and its aims, simulation's primary purpose is to enable skills development and rehearsal, *not* to ensure incorporation of the patient's voice (Silverman J and Britten N, *personal communication*).

The literature on the effects of simulation on simulated patients themselves is limited. There is potential for harm in some situations – for example, when portraying emotionally intense scenarios; indeed, it has been argued that only professional actors should undertake such demanding roles,(79) but the general consensus is that benefits outweigh any disadvantages so long as people are appropriately selected and supported in the role(s).(80) It is important to pay attention to recruitment, including exploring the person's reasons for wanting to get involved, training and support, and debriefing and de-roling.(64,78,80)

The use of simulation and simulated patients is discussed in more detail in Chapter 13.

Areas for further research

In light of the variable quality of much of the research in this area, a large research agenda has been identified looking at a wide range of aspects. Typical questions include the following.

- What are the drivers of patient involvement?
- What are the strengths and weaknesses of different approaches, and how do these vary between professions and disciplines, and between countries and across cultures?
- What factors influence what works, and why?
- How do structural and organisational factors such as location, access and safety influence development of programmes?
- What factors influence patients' experiences of involvement?
- What are the key outcomes, short *and* long term, for all parties?
- What factors influence sustainability of programmes?

Conclusions

From an early stage of training, students and trainees need to actively engage with patients, carers and families so they can learn to consolidate their learning and put learning from other contexts into practice in the real clinical environment. Appropriate involvement, carried out professionally and sensitively, provides immense benefits not only for the learners, but also for patients. Many patients want to 'give something back' to those who care for them, and engaging in medical education at all levels is one of way of so doing.

Teachers and learners need to be aware when learning on 'real' patients is inappropriate. However, there are many alternatives available ranging from paper case scenarios to high-fidelity simulations. The greater emphasis on professionalism, including attending to legal and ethical issues, and the changing agendas relating to patient empowerment and social accountability mean that, for a host of reasons, educators need to pay close attention to seeking active, informed involvement in educational activities from patients and carers. This approach will help put the rhetoric of 'patients as partners' centrally into practice in the teaching and learning environment.

References

1 Jolly B (1998) Historical and theoretical background. In: Jolly B and Rees L (eds) *Medical Education in the Millennium*, pp. 171–87. Oxford University Press, Oxford.

2 Rosner L (1997) The growth of medical education and the medical profession. In: Loudon I (ed.) *Western Medicine*, pp. 147–59. Oxford University Press, Oxford.

3 Osler W (1905) In: Osler W, *Aequanimitas*, p. 332. PK Blakiston's Son & Co, Philadelphia.

4 *Doctor in the House*. 1954. [Film] Directed by Ralph Thomas. Rank Organisation, UK.

5 Rees CE, Knight LV and Wilkinson CE (2007) User involvement is a sine qua non, almost, in medical education: learning with rather

than just about health and social care service users. *Advances in Health Sciences Education.* **12**(3): 359–90.

6 Towle A, Bainbridge L, William Godolphin W *et al.* (2010) Active patient involvement in the education of health professionals. *Medical Education.* **44**: 64.

7 Department of Health (2005) *Creating a patient-centred NHS.* (http://icn.csip.org.uk/_library/Creating_a_patient-led_NHS.pdf; accessed October 2012).

8 Secretary of State for Health (2010) *Equity and excellence: liberating the NHS* (http://webarchive.nationalarchives.gov.uk/+/www.dh.gov.uk/en/MediaCentre/Pressreleases/DH_117360

9 Morgan A and Jones D (2009) Perceptions of service user and carer involvement in healthcare education and impact on students' knowledge and practice: a literature review. *Medical Teacher.* **31**: 82–95.

10 General Medical Council (2010) *Patient and Public Involvement in Undergraduate Medical Education. Advice supplementary to Tomorrow's Doctors*, p. 2009. GMC, London. (http://www.gmc-uk.org/Patient_and_public_web.pdf_40939542.pdf; accessed September 2012).

11 Crawford MJ, Rutter D, Manley C *et al.* (2002) Systematic review of involving patients in the planning and development of health care. *British Medical Journal.* **325**: 1263.

12 Coulter A (2011) Patients – the greatest untapped resource? Ch 10. In: Coulter A (ed.) *Engaging Patients in Healthcare*, pp. 184–91. Open University Press, Maidenhead, Berkshire.

13 Woollard RF (2006) Caring for a common future: medical schools' social accountability. *Medical Education.* **40**: 301–13.

14 Woollard B and Boelen C (2012) Seeking impact of medical schools on health: meeting the challenges of social accountability. *Medical Education.* **46**: 21–7.

15 Royal College of Physicians (2005) *Doctors in Society – Medical Professionalism in a Changing World.* RCP, London.

16 Medical Professionalism Project (2002) Medical professionalism in the new millennium: a physicians' charter. *Lancet.* **359**: 520–1.

17 Hilton S and Southgate L (2007) Professionalism in medical education. *Teacher and Teacher Education.* **23**: 265–79.

18 Coulter A and Ellins J (2007) Effectiveness of strategies for informing, educating and involving patients. *British Medical Journal.* **335**: 24–7.

19 Engel GL (1989) The need for a new medical model: a challenge for biomedicine. *Journal of Interprofessional Care.* **4**: 37–53.

20 Stewart M, Brown JB, Weston WW *et al.* (2003) *Patient-Centred Medicine. Transforming the Clinical Method* (2e). Radcliffe Medical Press, Oxford.

21 Hasman A, Coulter A and Askham J (2006) *Education for Partnership.* Picker Institute, Oxford.

22 Tew J, Gell C and Foster S (2004) *Learning from Experience: Involving Service Users and Carers in Mental Health Education and Training.* Mental Health in Higher Education/NIMHE West Midlands/Trent WDC, York.

23 Spencer J, Blackmore D, Heard S *et al.* (2000) Patient-oriented learning: a review of the role of the patient in the education of medical students. *Medical Education.* **34**: 851–7.

24 McKimm J (2008) *Involving Patients in Clinical Teaching.* London Deanery, London. (http://www.faculty.londondeanery.ac.uk/e-learning/involving-patients-in-clinical-teaching; accessed August 2009).

25 Spencer J (2002) What can undergraduate education offer general practice? In: Harrison J and van Zwanenberg T (eds) *GP Tomorrow* (2e), pp. 49–66. Radcliffe Medical Press, Oxford.

26 Cook DA and Triola MM (2009) Virtual patients: a critical literature review and proposed next steps. *Medical Education.* **43**: 303–11.

27 Poulton T and Balasubramaniam C (2011) Virtual patients: a year of change. *Medical Teacher.* **33**: 933–7.

28 Eva K (2005) What every teacher needs to know about clinical reasoning. *Medical Education.* **39**: 98–106.

29 Issenberg SB, McGaghie WC, Petrusa ER *et al.* (2005) Features and uses of high-fidelity medical simulations that lead to effective learning: a BEME systematic review. *Medical Teacher.* **27**: 10–28.

30 Cook DA, Hamstra SJ, Brydges R *et al.* (2013) Comparative effectiveness of instructional design features in simulation-based education: systematic review and meta-analysis. *Medical Teacher.* **35**(1): e867–98.

31 Greenhalgh T and Hurwitz B (1999) Why study narrative? *British Medical Journal.* **318**: 48–50.

32 Engel JD, Zarconi J, Pethtel LL and Missimi SA (2008) *Narrative in Health Care. Healing Patients, Practitioners, Profession, and Community.* Radcliffe Publishing, Oxford.

33 Aronson JK (2000) Autopathography: the patient's tale. *British Medical Journal.* **321**: 1599–602.

34 Powley E and Higson R (2005) *The Arts in Medical Education. A Practical Guide.* Radcliffe Publishing, Oxford.

35 Farrar M, Connolly AM, Lawson J *et al.* (2008) Teaching doctors how to diagnose paroxysmal events: a comparison of two educational methods. *Medical Education.* **42**: 909–14.

36 Cleland J, Ford R, Hamilton NM *et al.* (2007) Breaking bad news: an interactive web-based e-learning package. *The Clinical Teacher.* **4**: 94–9.

37 van Schoor AN, Navsa N, Meiring JH *et al.* (2006) Perspectives on the use of PDAs as assessment tools. *The Clinical Teacher.* **3**: 170–4.

38 Spencer JA (2010) Teaching and learning in the clinical environment, Chapter 8. In: Cantillon P and Wood D. (eds) *ABC of Learning and Teaching in Medicine* (2e). John Wiley & Sons, Chichester.

39 Ramani S (2003) Twelve tips to improve bedside teaching. *Medical Teacher.* **25**: 112–5.

40 McKimm J (2008) The 'Trialogue': a new model and metaphor for understanding clinical teaching and learning and developing skills. Paper presented at the ASME Conference, Leicester, 10–12 September.

41 Dictionary.com, 2013 [online] Available at: http://dictionary.reference.com/browse/trialogue?s=t

42 Hardy P (2009) The Expert Patient Programme: a critical review. MSc Lifelong learning, policy and research. (http://www.pilgrimprojects.co.uk/papers/epp_msc.pdf; accessed August 2009).

43 Squire S and Hill P (2006) The expert patients programme. *Clinical Governance.* **11**: 17–21.

44 Griffiths C, Foster G, Ramsay J *et al.* (2007) How effective are expert patient (lay led) education programmes for chronic disease? *British Medical Journal.* **334**: 1254–6.

45 Hassell A (2102) Patient instructors in rheumatology. *Medical Teacher.* **34**: 539–42.

46 Rees CE and Monrouxe LV (2011) Medical students learning intimate examinations without vald consent: a multi-centre study. *Medical Education.* **45**: 261–72.

47 Pickard S, Baraitser P, Rymer J and Piper J (2006) Can gynaecology teaching associates provide high quality effective training for medical students in the UK? Comparative study. *British Medical Journal.* **327**: 1389–92.

48 Levin E (2004) *Involving Service Users and Carers in Social Work Education.* Social Care Institute for Excellence, London. (http://www.scie.org.uk/publications/guides/guide04/files/guide04.pdf; accessed October 2012).

49 Community Campus Partnerships for Health (2013) Community campus partnerships [online]. (http://depts.washington.edu/ccph/partnerships.html; accessed August 2009).

50 Howe A and Anderson J (2003) Involving patients in medical education. *British Medical Journal.* **327**: 326–8.

51 O'Keefe M and Jones A (2007) Promoting lay participation in medical school curriculum development: lay and faculty perceptions. *Medical Education.* **41**: 130–7.

52 Involve (National Institute for Health Research) (2013) Developing training and support [online]. (http://www.invo.org.uk/resource-centre/training-resource/; accessed October 2012).

53 British Medical Association (2008) Role of the Patient in Medical Education. (bma.org.uk/-/media/Files/PDFs/.../Role%20of%20 patient.pdf; accessed October 2012).

54 University of Warwick (2013) UNTRAP [online]. (http://www2 .warwick.ac.uk/fac/cross_fac/healthatwarwick/untrap/; accessed October 2012).

55 Stacy R and Spencer J (1999) Patients as teachers: a qualitative study of patients' views on their role in a community-based undergraduate project. *Medical Education.* **33**: 688–94.

56 Jha V, Quinton ND, Bekker HL and Roberts TE (2009) What educators and students really think about using patients as teachers in medical education: a qualitative study. *Medical Education.* **43**: 449–56.

57 McLachlan E, King N, Wenger E and Dornan T (2012) Phenomenological analysis of patient experiences of medical student teaching encounters. *Medical Education.* **46**: 963–73.

58 Wykurz G and Kelly D (2002) Developing the role of patients as teachers: literature review. *British Medical Journal.* **325**: 818–21.

59 Repper J and Breeze J (2004) A review of the literature on user and carer involvement in the training and education of health professionals. (http://www.shef.ac.uk/content/1/c6/01/34/62/ Finalreport.pdf; accessed August 2009).

60 Jha V, Quinton ND, Bekker HL and Roberts TE (2009) Strategies and interventions for the involvement of real patients in medical education: a systematic review. *Medical Education.* **43**: 10–20.

61 Moss B, Boath L, Buckley S and Colgan A (2009) The fount of all knowledge: training required to involve service users and carers in health and social care education and training. *Social Work Education.* **28**: 562–72.

62 Spencer J, Godolphin W, Towle A and Karpenko N (2011) Can patients be teachers? Involving patients and service users in health professionals' education. Health Foundation: London. (http://www .health.org.uk/public/cms/75/76/313/2809/Can%20patients%20 be%20teachers.pdf?realName=br0eQj.pdf; accessed October 2012).

63 Postgraduate Medical Education and Training Board (2008) *Training in Partnership: shaping the future of postgraduate medical education and training in the UK – the patient perspective, 2008.* PMETB, London. (available as pdf at: http://www.gmc-uk.org/PP_Background_ information_booklet.pdf_30377400.pdf; accessed October 2012).

64 Westberg K, Lynøe N, Löfgren M and Sandlund M (2001) Getting informed consent from patients to take part in the clinical training of students: randomized control trial of two strategies. *British Medical Journal.* **323**: 488.

65 Haffling A and Håkansson A (2008) Patients consulting with students in general practice: survey of patient's satisfaction and their role in teaching. *Medical Teacher.* **30**: 622–9.

66 Price R, Spencer J and Walker J (2008) Does the presence of medical students affect quality in general practice consultations? *Medical Education.* **42**: 374–81.

67 Draper H, Parle J and Ross N (2008) Medical education and patients' responsibility. Back to the future? *Journal of Medical Ethics.* **34**: 116–9.

68 Hardy P and Stanton P (2007) Cultivating compassion: seeing patient voices. *British Medical Journal.* **335**: 184–7.

69 Benson J, Quince T, Hibble A *et al.* (2005) Impact on patients of expanded, general practice based, student teaching: observational and qualitative study. *British Medical Journal.* **331**: 89.

70 O'Flynn N, Spencer J and Jones R (1997) Consent and confidentiality in teaching general practice: survey of patients' views on presence of students. *British Medical Journal.* **315**: 1142.

71 NHS Employers (2009) Medical student access to patient records [online] Available at: http://www.nhsemployers.org/PlanningY-ourWorkforce/MedicalWorkforce/Medical_Education_and_training/Pages/MedicalstudentsCRS.aspx.

72 Williamson C (2007) How do we find the right patients to consult? *Quality in Primary Care.* **15**: 195–9.

73 Barrows HS and Abrahamson S (1964) The programmed patient: a technique for appraising clinical performance in clinical neurology. *Journal of Medical Education.* **39**: 802–5.

74 Barrows HS (1993) An overview of the uses of standardized patients for teaching and evaluating clinical skills. *Academic Medicine.* **68**: 443–51.

75 Rethans J-J, Grosfeld FJM, Aper L *et al.* (2012) Six formats in simulated and standardized patients use, based on experiences of 13 undergraduate medical curricula in Belgium and the Netherlands. *Medical Teacher.* **34**: 710–6.

76 Kurtz S, Silverman J and Draper J (2005) *Teaching and Learning Communication Skills in Medicine* (2e). Radcliffe Medical Press, Oxford.

77 Thistlethwaite J and Ridgway G (2006) *Making it Real. A Practical Guide to Experiential Learning.* Radcliffe Publishing, Oxford.

78 Cleland JA, Abe K and Rethans J-J (2009) The use of simulated patients in medical education . AMEE guide no.42. *Medical Teacher.* **31**: 477–86.

79 Eagles JM, Calder SA, Wilson S, Murdoch JA and Sclare PD (2007) Simulated patients in undergraduate education in psychiatry. *The Psychiatrist.* **31**: 187–90.

80 Spencer J and Dales J (2006) Meeting the needs of simulated patients and caring for person behind them. *Medical Education.* **40**: 3–5.

Further resources

Coulter A (2011) *Engaging Patients in Healthcare.* Open University Press, Maidenhead. A definitive text by one of the most prolific champions and scholars of patient engagement in healthcare.

Association for Standardized Patient Educators (ASPE) (http://www.aspeducators.org). ASPE is the international organisation for professionals in the field of standardised patient methodology. It is based in the USA and the website provides good ideas around the use of simulated patients.

Healthtalkonline (http://www.healthtalkonline.org/). The information on Healthtalkonline is based on qualitative research into patient experiences, led by experts at the University of Oxford. These personal stories of health and illness will enable patients, families and health care professionals to benefit from the experiences of others.

Patient Voices (http://www.patientvoices.org.uk/). Patient Voices was founded in 2003, and 'aims to facilitate the telling and the hearing of some of the unwritten and unspoken stories of ordinary people so that those who devise and implement strategy in health and social care, as well as the professionals and clinicians directly involved in care, may carry out their duties in a more informed and compassionate manner.' It provides more than 100 digital stories from patients, carers and health workers on a range of topics.

Simulated Patients UK (http://www.simulatedpatients.co.uk). This site provides a one-stop resource for users of simulated patients throughout the UK.

UBC Division of Health Care Communication. Bibliography (http://www.chd.ubc.ca/dhcc/node/67). This is possibly the most comprehensive bibliography of relevant literature in the public domain.

Part 3
Assessment

18 How to design a useful test: The principles of assessment

Lambert WT Schuwirth[1] and Cees PM van der Vleuten[2]

[1] Flinders Innovation in Clinical Education, Flinders University, Australia
[2] School of Health Professions Education, University of Maastricht, The Netherlands

KEY MESSAGES

- Good assessment requires a variety of methods; no single method can test the whole of medical competence and performance.
- In a good assessment programme the whole is more than the sum of the parts. To achieve this:
  - each instrument must be chosen on the basis of its strengths and weaknesses
  - all decisions are based on rational arguments and/or scientific underpinning

  - rational decisions are made about to how to combine results
  - the whole programme is part of a total quality management system.
- Modern assessment in medical education is a matter of good educational design and not exclusively a psychometric measurement problem.

Introduction

Designing a system of assessment is not easy. Many different instruments have been described in the medical education literature, each with its own advantages and disadvantages. The volume of published research on assessment is huge, and research findings often contradict long-established practices based on tradition and intuition. Furthermore, the discipline has its own jargon and set of statistical concepts. In amongst all this, the responsibility regularly falls on medical teachers to set up fair assessment systems. The aim of this chapter is to explain the basic concepts behind assessment and thus help reduce this 'burden'. It is not a cookbook providing assessment 'recipes'; instead, we hope that after reading this publication the medical educator will be better equipped to make informed choices in matters of assessment.

What is assessment?

Although assessment is generally acknowledged to be fundamental to the educative process, there are many different constructions of the term, ranging from assessment as a certification procedure leading to a pass/fail decision, to assessment as an evaluative or feedback action in education. Here we will use 'any *purported* and *formal* action to obtain information about the competence and performance of a candidate' as our working definition of assessment.

Assessment is never undertaken without a specific purpose. This can be summative and/or formative. Summative means that the assessment has been conducted for decision-making or certification purposes, such as deciding who is admitted, progresses or qualifies. Formative relates to the feedback function of assessment or, more precisely, how the assessment informs the students about their performance.

Some people argue that formative and summative assessment purposes should not be mixed in one assessment, but in educational settings we tend to advise otherwise. Purely summative assessment ('pass' or 'fail' only) does not help students to plan their study. If a student fails, s/he does not know what s/he needs to work on in order to pass at the next attempt. On the other hand, purely formative assessment with no consequences at all is often not taken seriously.

How to choose the best approaches to assessment

A first step in setting up an assessment system is to choose the most appropriate methods. This is not an easy task. Over the past few decades, a wide variety of instruments have been developed and used in medical education, and often authors have claimed their instrument to be the best for all purposes. We may safely assume, however, that each method has its own strengths and weaknesses, and these

---

Understanding Medical Education: Evidence, Theory and Practice, Second Edition. Edited by Tim Swanwick.
© 2014 The Association for the Study of Medical Education. Published 2014 by John Wiley & Sons, Ltd.

must be weighed carefully against the desired purposes of the assessment. A testing authority whose purpose is licensing may demand different strengths from the methods from, say, a medical school. Several criteria that can be used in this evaluative process have been described in the literature.(1) The most popular ones are examined below.

Reliability

The reliability of a method pertains mostly to the *reproducibility* of its results, that is, how often the same result is obtained. Let us illustrate this with three examples.

1 John scores 83 per cent in a test. If John were given a different, but similar, test – a so-called parallel test – would he again score 83 per cent?

2 John is the best-scoring student in his class. Harry comes next, Peter's score is slightly lower and Jim's score is the lowest. If this class of students were given a parallel test, would the rank ordering of scores be the same as in the first test?

3 In another test, John passes. He scores 83 per cent and the cut-off score for the test was 50 per cent. If John were given a parallel test, would he pass again?

These examples illustrate three operational definitions of reliability. The first example is from a domain-referenced perspective. The test here aims to measure how much of a certain domain John knows. It may be intuitively clear that to be able to conclude that John's knowledge is *exactly* 83 per cent you need a very fine – highly reliable – measurement. The second example – from a norm-referenced perspective – is somewhat less demanding. Here we are not interested in whether John's score was exactly 83 per cent, but only whether his score was better than Harry's, Peter's and Jim's. The measurement can be slightly coarser. In the third case, demands on the measurement are even lower.

Now let us turn the concept around. If we have the test results of a class of students, depending on which of the three conclusions we want to draw, the test is more or less reliable. This is all very well in theory, but we do not have a parallel test, so how can we establish the parallel test score. A typical approach is to retrospectively divide the test into two halves randomly and treat them as parallel tests. Most of the well-known reliability tests in classical test theory, for example, Kuder–Richardson and Cronbach's alpha, build on this approach (*see* Box 18.1).

Why is it so hard to design a perfectly reliable test? The largest source of unreliability is sampling error. For pragmatic reasons, a test usually comprises a sample of questions from the whole domain of possible questions. But because items can differ in difficulty, and because different students find different items difficult – John does better on the myocardial infarction items and Harry does better on the arrhythmia items – sampling error arises. The same applies equally to other assessment modalities, such as the examiner's choice of questions in oral or short essay examinations. So if sampling error is such a major issue, it follows that brief assessments and assessments based on the judgement of only one examiner are very likely to be unreliable.

There is one final issue to discuss in relation to reliability, namely the relationship between reliability and objectivity. A common misconception is that subjective assessment is always unreliable and objective assessments are always reliable.(2) The following two illustrations demonstrate that this is not necessarily the case. The first example is a one-item multiple-choice examination. This is a so-called objective test, but as it has only one item, it is not reliable. On the other hand, suppose we were to write ten pieces of music ourselves and take, at random, ten pieces written by Mozart, and submit them all to a panel of experts who have to assess the musical artistry of the composer. The panel would reach the decision that Mozart is the better composer. It would not matter if we took another sample of our own compositions or another sample of Mozart's compositions or even another sample of experts, the decision would still be the same. Musical artistry, however, is not 'objective'; it is highly subjective. Yet the decision of the panel is highly reproducible and thus reliable.

In conclusion, reliability is a matter of careful sampling. It relies on a sufficiently large sample through all possible sources of error, for example, items, examiners and test occasions. But reliability is not the whole story.

Validity

Validity is defined as the extent to which the sort of competence the assessment claims to assess is actually being assessed. This is not always easy to demonstrate, and proving the validity of a particular test method is a matter of collecting evidence from different sources and perspectives.

The first step is to define exactly for what purpose the method is valid. In the way that a thermometer is a valid instrument to measure temperature and only temperature (not weight, for example), an assessment method is valid only for a certain aspect of competence. Any claim by a test developer that their instrument is a valid instrument for medical competence is therefore to be regarded with suspicion. Validity has been defined in numerous different ways. For the purposes of this publication, we will classify the different varieties of validity into two categories, as follows.(3,4)

Content validity (also referred to as *direct* validity)

Content validity refers to the judgemental type of evidence collected in the validation process. This can be expert judgement about the specific item construction, the necessary faculty development for judges, etc. One specific element in content validation is blue printing. This is done because an examination must be optimally representative of the whole testable domain. An examination on cardiology should not be composed only of items on myocardial infarction. To ensure adequate coverage, a test is typically constructed according to a blue print. The blue print is a matrix in which the test maker determines how many items per subject or category are to be asked. A subsidiary issue in content validity is the relevance of the items. Only relevant items contribute to the content validity of the examination.

Construct validity (also referred to as *indirect* validity)

Another category of validity arguments is based on the 'behaviour' of assessment scores; do they align with our

BOX 18.1 FOCUS ON: The measurement of reliability

Reliability is a central concept in test theory, as examiners and candidates want a test that gives a similar result on different occasions with different candidates. Test–retest analysis assesses the same candidate's performance in the same test on two separate occasions, whereas parallel testing assesses the same candidate using tests containing different questions that are thought to be equivalent. In each case, reliable tests should give very similar marks on both occasions. Mathematically, psychometricians *model* the responses of candidates in different ways, with three broad approaches.

Classical test theory (CTT)

This has been around for half a century or more. The main assumption is that a candidate has a true ability, or score, but because of measurement error, for whatever reason, the candidate does not obtain the exact same score, even if an identical test is used on two occasions. The similarity of marks on the two occasions is used to calculate the reliability, which becomes higher as measurement error becomes lower. A similar approach can be used for comparing parallel tests.

CTT works best with multiple-choice tests, where all candidates answer identical questions. Its major drawback is that reliability calculated from one group of candidates cannot be extrapolated easily to other groups. Apparent reliability of a test can be much inflated by including a few outstandingly bad candidates. CTT reliability is also very misleading as a description of the accuracy of a cut-off score (pass/fail boundary) in high-stakes examinations.

Generalisability theory (GT)

CTT does not work well with typical clinical examinations, where not all candidates can see all patients or be seen by all examiners. There is therefore variability due to examiners (e.g. hawks and doves) and clinical scenarios, as well as case-specificity, with some candidates doing better with some types of case than others. GT generalises CTT to include such

components. A measure equivalent to reliability ('generalisability') can be calculated; in effect, how similar would a candidate's mark be with different examiners and different scenarios?

GT allows sophisticated calculations of the effects of different types of exam – 'what if' questions – such as, 'Would the exam be more generalisable with more stations and fewer examiners per station'? The untested, perhaps unrealistic, assumption is that examiners and candidates will behave in precisely the same way in such new situations. As with CTT, GT estimates of generalisability cannot be easily extrapolated to new situations.

Rasch modelling (RM) and item–response theory (IRT)

IRT is a more complex variant of Rasch modelling. RM starts with the assumption that every test item has a particular difficulty, with the probability of a candidate answering an item correctly depending on the item's difficulty and the ability of the candidate. Mathematical modelling then allows the item difficulties to be calculated, as well as candidate abilities. A new test comprised of previously used items from an item bank used in different combinations can have its reliability calculated before the test is used. The reliability can also be calculated for candidates of differing ability (e.g. fourth-year students rather than third-year). IRT is an extension of RM that not only calculates the difficulty of items, but also calculates discriminative value and chance-guessing rates.

IRT requires large data sets and is best used for large-scale examinations with a thousand-plus candidates. RM, however, is robust with small numbers. RM cannot handle clinical situations with different scenarios and examiners, but these can be handled with Facet theory. The major problem for RM and IRT is not the conceptual basis, which is rigorous, powerful and realistic, but the mathematical and statistical skills of most biomedical examiners.

---

expectations about the type of competence we want to assess? A competency is in principle a construct or latent trait. This is a personal psychological characteristic that cannot be observed directly but which is assumed to exist. A typical example is 'intelligence'. We assume this construct to have certain characteristics: more intelligent people can learn faster, have superior memory skills and are better able to solve problems than less intelligent people. If we were to design a new test to measure intelligence, we would hope that people who learn faster outperform people who learn more slowly, and demonstrating this would contribute to the validity of our new test. So the scores on the intelligence test would 'behave' according to our – theoretical – assumptions. Applying this principle to tests for, e.g., medical problem-solving means that for a test

to have good construct validity, it would be necessary for people who solve problems more expertly to outperform those who are less good problem-solvers.

There are many other types of validity evidence: weak correlations between two tests that are supposed to measure different constructs; strong correlations between two tests that are assumed to measure the same construct; and so on. Although they are sometimes labelled as different forms of validity, in effect they all contribute to the evidence for the validity of a test for a specific construct.

The concept of validity has engendered a wide variety of viewpoints. Some claim that only construct validity is worthwhile and dismiss content and face validity as just a collection of opinions.(5) Some take the usability of the test and the relationship between the test and its user as an important element of validity.(6) Others take a more holistic view, and we think that Kane (quoting Messick) strikes an intelligent balance in taking a definition of validity as 'the degree to which empirical evidence and theoretical rationales support the adequacy and appropriateness of inferences and actions based on test scores or other modes of assessment'.(7) 'Inferences' and 'actions' bring us neatly to considering the educational consequences of the test.(8)

Educational impact

The saying 'Students don't do what you expect, students do what you inspect' epitomises the educational impact of assessment. Although there is still a need for more empirical underpinning of this notion, the emerging research does show that assessment has a major impact on students' study behaviour.(9–13) Often the standard response of teachers is to blame students for this strategic approach to learning, but a more rational response is for the assessment developer to capitalise on this behaviour. It is normal human behaviour and it is not going to go away; indeed, we are all susceptible to these kinds of external motivators. More importantly, the driving influence of assessment is a powerful tool to ensure that students learn what, and how, teachers want them to learn. To maximise the effectiveness of this alignment, it is important to realise that assessment influences student learning in several ways: through its content, its format, the scheduling of examinations and the regulatory structure of the assessment programme.

The influence of *content* is obvious. Topics that come up repeatedly in the examinations will be perceived by students as the most important. When it comes to *format*, the literature gives different views. Some studies seem to indicate that students prepare differently for different formats, especially multiple-choice versus open-ended examinations.(14) Others indicate that this is only the perception of students, whereas in fact they prepare similarly.(15) As a rule of thumb, we advocate using a variety of formats in an assessment programme. This way, students will not become used to one type of preparation.

A typical problem of *scheduling* concerns, for instance, annual examination periods. If several examinations are held during the same few weeks, students will not be able to prepare adequately for all of them. They will then have to select strategically the examinations for which they will prepare well and those for which they will not. From the faculty's point of view this is a waste of resources, as effort is put into constructing a high-quality examination that is not taken seriously. Better, therefore, to spread examinations rather than to cluster them. The assessment programme *as a whole* defines academic success. The credit points attributed to each part, the way scores are combined, the minimum number of points needed to progress and so on, all define how students will study or prepare for the examinations.(11–13) Programmes with continuous assessment will promote continuous learning; pinpoint assessments will promote cramming behaviour. Because educational impact is such a major effect of assessment, it is often also seen as a part of validity, specifically termed 'consequential validity'.(8)

Cost-effectiveness

This seems an easy and obvious issue, but the practice sometimes differs from the theory. For example, a prerequisite for a cost-effective assessment programme is an explicit description of its goals, both in terms of *what* is to be assessed and *how* it is to be assessed. Only then can an evaluation be conducted into whether the programme is optimally cost-effective. The most important factors hampering cost-efficiency are misconceptions based on tradition and intuition, poorly supportive infrastructure and lack of collaboration.

Typical examples of the first are interviews, oral examinations and open-ended questions. The literature on unstructured interviews for selection for medical schools converges on the conclusion that their predictive validity is unacceptably low.(16–18) Their use therefore constitutes a cost-ineffective assessment procedure. The recent development in this in the form of multiple mini-interviews (MMIs) seem to address these concerns successfully and thus are not only an improvement in terms of reliability and validity but possibly have a huge impact on cost-effectiveness.(19) The same applies to many unstructured oral examinations.(20) Such orals have poor reliability and are often used to test simple factual knowledge, which can better be tested using more cost-effective methods. This is not to say that there is no place for oral examinations in an assessment programme, but they should be used only where they have an added value over other formats.(21) Similarly, there is an almost inextinguishable belief that open-ended questions test higher-order cognitive skills and multiple-choice questions do not. Again, the literature converges on the notion that in this matter the question format is quite unimportant, but the content of the question is.(22–24) Of course, in an assessment programme there may be indications to use open-ended questions – for example, if creativity or spontaneous generation of the answer is essential. In other cases there are more cost-effective alternatives.

Typical examples of poor infrastructure support are the lack of good item banking and the absence of a centralised management and administrative support for the logistics and administration of examinations. The consequences are that 'expensive' scientific staff members carry out work that could be done just as well – or even better – by administrative personnel.

The benefits of collaboration may perhaps be obvious. Many medical schools have comparable curricula with comparable end goals, and sharing test material would be a way to reduce costs, because it would mean not everybody has to reinvent the wheel.(25) This is not to say that collaboration is easy. Careful planning, commitment of all partners and some sort of pre-investment are all needed to make collaboration successful.(26)

Acceptability

Setting up an assessment system cannot be done in a vacuum. Sometimes a careful balance between what may be scientifically and educationally superior and what is acceptable to the stakeholders has to be struck. Even the best assessment method is useless if teachers and students will not subscribe to it. Some even go so far as to incorporate this issue into the argument for a test's validity.(6) This is not that strange a point of view because an instrument is valid only if it is used properly.

Popular assessment instruments

No single assessment instrument is perfect, and no single instrument can test all aspects of medical competence and performance. Each instrument has its strengths and weaknesses. A good assessment programme should therefore include a combination of various methods, each selected for a specific purpose, and each with its indications and contraindications.(27–30) This section describes the major strengths and weaknesses of different groups of commonly used assessment methods, using the five criteria described above: reliability, validity, educational impact, cost-efficiency and acceptability.

Written assessment instruments

There are many different written assessment instruments currently in use. Some are case-based, some are context-free. Some use open-ended questions, some use multiple choice.

As a general rule, the amount of time it takes to answer a question has a negative impact on the reliability of the test. As you may recall, a test can only sample from the whole domain of possible items, and, as such, the sample must be large enough to be reliable. It follows then that the more items a test contains, the more reliable it is likely to be. This immediately places open-ended questions at a disadvantage because they require more answering time. So, essays are generally less reliable *per hour of testing time* than short-answer questions.

Where reliability is a fairly straightforward issue in written assessment, validity is much more complex. There are some popular beliefs about the validity of different types of question. For example, it is often thought that open-ended questions test higher-order cognitive skills and that multiple-choice questions can test only factual knowledge. This is a widespread misconception: the question *format* is quite unimportant with respect to validity, whereas the question *content* is very important.(22–24) So, *what* you ask is important, not how you record the answer. Of course, some contents do not fit certain formats. It is best not to ask items that require the spontaneous and creative generation of possibilities in multiple-choice format, whilst items requiring a selection from a finite list of realistic options are best not asked in an open-ended format.

Thus, careful consideration of content is essential. A further and important distinction relates to context. Context-rich items contain a case description and questions that ask for (essential) decisions or an evaluation of the problem. Typical examples of these are extended-matching items or key-feature approach items.(31–33) Context-free items do not have a case description and simply ask for general knowledge. Context-rich approaches test application of knowledge and problem solving, but context-free items do

not.(34) Both, however, can be equally important aspects to assess; one is not superior to the other.

The idea that open-ended questions test superior cognitive skills over multiple-choice questions is also widespread among students. Although this may not actually be true, it will still influence students' perception and their learning. Using a variety of methods sends a clear message to students that they have to master the subject matter, irrespective of the assessment format.

Another aspect of educational impact is the influence that assessment has on test makers. If, for example, all tests have to be in multiple-choice format, examiners may construct only items that fit this format, and questions requiring spontaneous generation of the answer could be under-represented. On the other hand, if all items are of the open-ended format, the examiners may be burdened with the high workload of correcting tests and may start asking simple questions that are easy to score, which also means that important aspects may be neglected.

The use of multiple-choice-based assessments is highly cost-effective. They may be slightly more difficult to produce, but the use of Optical Mark Reading scanners certainly makes them easier to score. This is a particularly relevant consideration in medical schools with a large number of students per year class. Every pound, euro or dollar can be spent only once; therefore, money spent on unnecessarily expensive assessment methods cannot be spent on improving education. So, from the viewpoint of cost-efficiency, it is best to use open-ended questions only if more efficient formats will not suffice.

There might be a wealth of scientific literature proving that test format is unimportant, but sometimes beliefs may be so strong that stakeholders cannot be convinced. In such cases arguments will be used claiming that multiple-choice assessments are too easy, make students lazy and are not worthy of an academic environment, and that real life and real practice are not simply a question of selecting options from a list. Such arguments may seem incorrect from a sheer psychometric/rationalist view point, but they may be very strongly embedded in the teachers' and the institution's core values. It is important then to consider whether it is useful to contradict them. Sometimes these values are very strong, and it may be better to aim for high levels of acceptability of an assessment system first, and to postpone the 'battle'. Energy may be better spent on good teaching and good-enough assessment, and, more important, any test can be valid only if it is used correctly. For this, it has to be acceptable to all stakeholders. You can read more about written assessment in Chapter 19.

Objective Structured Clinical Examinations and simulated patients

Objective Structured Clinical Examinations (OSCEs) and simulated patient (SP)-based examinations have become very popular for the assessment of (practical) skills.(35,36) Both are based on a series of structured cases that must be addressed by the candidate. In an OSCE, a candidate enters a series of different rooms or stations in sequence. In each room there is a specified assignment (e.g. perform a resuscitation or take the blood pressure), a simulated patient or dummy, and an examiner with a checklist or rating scale. The candidate has to complete the assignment and his or her performance is scored against the checklist or rating scale. After a fixed period of time, a signal is given and the candidate proceeds to the next station.

OSCEs and SP-based examinations were developed in response to unstructured observations in practice. They are cleverly developed in that they address the inherent unreliability of observed practice in three ways. First, by adding some structure to the observations, they become more reliable. Second, by keeping each of the observations short (the original OSCEs had five-minute stations), many different observations can be made per hour, thus enabling wider and more effective sampling. Third, by having the candidate move from station to station, such assessments also sample across different examiners. The 'hawks' will be compensated for by the 'doves', or better still all candidates will be examined by the same panel of examiners. The second of these issues – that of sampling across many cases – is the most important, because the biggest threat to reliability is having too small a sample. The many reliability studies on OSCEs have demonstrated this over and over again. One of the practical implications is that it is better to have more stations with one examiner per station than fewer stations with two examiners per station. Despite the clever reliability approach, as a rule of thumb, OSCEs still require a minimum average of at least two hours of testing per candidate to achieve an acceptable reliability for summative decisions.

With respect to validity, two issues are of overriding importance: the length of the stations and the use of checklists versus global rating scales. One might be inclined to think that longer stations, that is, longer than five minutes, may be more (content) valid but less reliable, but this is not necessarily the case. Longer cases contain more information than shorter ones, and there seems to be an optimum balance between the length and the number of cases in an OSCE. Therefore, it is generally best to adapt the length of the stations to the content of the case, so durations of stations may be designed to vary from 5 to 20 minutes.(37)

Checklists are detailed lists of behaviours, and they describe precisely the actions to be taken – for example, 'washes hands', 'puts left hand on the sternum of the patient'; whereas rating scales allow for more interpretation by the examiner, describing in broad terms only the skills to be performed – for example, 'explores patient's concerns', 'comes to the correct conclusions'. So should checklists or rating scales be used?

One would be inclined to think that as checklists are more structured they would be more reliable, but this is not always the case.(38) The choice of whether to use checklists or rating scales should be made mainly on the basis of the type of skill to be assessed. Technical skills, such as taking blood pressure or performing resuscitation, can easily be tested with checklists, whereas more complicated skills, such as short patient contacts, seem to be better tested with rating scales. Many medical schools use short stations with checklists for technical skills in the more junior year groups, and integrated longer stations with rating scales in the more senior years.

In general, OSCEs are taken very seriously by students and have a high impact on student learning behaviour. This provides both a risk and an opportunity. The risk comes with detailed checklists. Even if they are not handed out officially, a 'black market' in old checklists may develop, and memorising these may be a successful study strategy for students. Memorising rating scales is less useful. The use of rating scales in OSCEs induces a study behaviour that is aimed more at practising the skill, and an opportunity here is to allow some time – about two minutes – at the end of each station for specific feedback. When the OSCE is solely for certification purposes, this is not desirable. In such cases, optimising the reliability (and thus the sampling) is more essential. However, most OSCEs are held within the educational environment of medical schools and can provide a wonderful opportunity for learning.

Unfortunately, OSCEs are very expensive to run. They require extensive resources and good logistics. It is therefore important to use OSCEs effectively, and using an extensive part of the OSCE time to explore general knowledge is not efficient. This does not mean that no knowledge should be tested in an OSCE, but that the knowledge tested should be background knowledge and should have a direct relationship to the case.

OSCEs are widely accepted and popular throughout the world. The only threat to their acceptability is when OSCEs are used to test highly technical skills with very detailed checklists. They then tend to become monkey tricks, and examiners may feel that their expertise is not being used or valued. A more detailed exploration of OSCEs and other structured assessments of clinical competence can be found in Chapter 21.

Oral examinations

Oral examinations come in various forms, ranging from the completely unstructured to the highly structured, case-based examination. The oral examination has tended to be discarded, being considered too unreliable and too expensive. However, recently opinion on the oral has shifted in a more favourable direction,(21) and the prevailing view is that there is room for an oral examination in an assessment programme, as long as it is used in the correct way and for the correct purpose.

This does imply, though, that to be acceptable, the oral examination must be constructed in such a way that it achieves sufficient reliability. For this, some structure – but not too much – is needed; a situation analogous to the OSCEs, where detailed checklists do not lead to higher reliabilities than rating scales. Reliability can be further enhanced by asking about a good variety of topics rather than homing in on only one. If multiple examiners are used, it is also better to 'nest' cases within examiners instead of using panels.(20)

There is a largely unsubstantiated view that orals are somehow more valid than written examinations. You may recall that in considering the validity of an assessment, the content is more important than the format. Often, the answers to oral questions require a good deal of (factual) knowledge, which can be assessed just as well by less expensive methods. If orals are to be used correctly, they have to be aimed at examining aspects that cannot be examined otherwise, such as hypothesis generation, explanations and the transfer of principles through various contexts. Another misapprehension is the perceived advantage that orals offer in following through on a certain topic – 'to see if they really understand it'. In such cases, the law of diminishing returns rules: the first question on a topic may prove a rich source of information about the candidate's competence, but the tenth question will add virtually nothing new.

Of course, just as with any type of examination, students will prepare strategically for the oral. In doing this they often try to get the lenient examiners or find out what the examiners' hobby horses are. It is therefore best to use a rotational approach in which students rotate from examiner to examiner, each of whom addresses a different, but predetermined, case or topic.

Despite the high costs of oral examinations, they are widely accepted in assessment programmes, and it is the experience at many institutes that the expert judgement emanating from orals is less frequently the subject of appeals and litigation as are written assessments.

Workplace-based assessment

Recent developments have placed the assessment in the authentic medical context once again. Where OSCEs were developed to test students in a simulated environment, instruments such as mini-CEX (Clinical Evaluation Exercise) and 360° feedback assess the candidate in their professional environment.(39,40)

Mini-CEX uses a generic form with rating scales, which an examiner uses to score the student's performance during a patient encounter. Items include history-taking, physical examination, professionalism, clinical judgement, counselling, organisation and efficiency, and an overall impression. The competence of the candidate is assessed by a series of direct observations. Another workplace-based approach, 360° feedback, uses standard lists of rating scale items, which are sent to various parties. So, not only colleagues, but also nursing staff and patients, are sent a form and asked to give their rating on the items. Examples of items include the following:
- ability to diagnose patients
- ability to use evidence-based medicine approaches in practice
- verbal communication with colleagues.

At first sight, both of these methods may seem like a step back to the old in-training judgements, but this is not the case. The mini-CEX draws on the lessons learnt from the OSCEs about structure and sampling. Observations in practice, such as mini-CEX, can become reliable, as long as the examiners have some criteria; a sufficient number (roughly seven to ten) of different cases are observed; and there is more than one observer.(41,42) The added value is that what is being assessed is more authentic than in a simulated environment. In many simulated assessments, certain symptoms cannot be simulated, but in real contexts these symptoms are present.

The 360° feedback method is not based on direct observations, but on a judgement in retrospect. Normally, this is ill advised, since such judgements tend to be very unreliable; but two aspects remedy this problem. First, many different people are asked, so a broad sample of observations is obtained. Second, judges are not asked for a global impression but to give a judgement about specific aspects of someone's strengths and weaknesses. In both cases judges need to be trained to use the instrument correctly.

Apart from being 'measurements' of performance, these instruments are also intended to provide the candidate with extensive feedback. This is essential to influence learning behaviour. So rather than being measurement-only instruments, they are also educational tools aimed at improving the performance of candidates. Furthermore, the supervisor cannot complete them, if he or she has not observed the candidate directly. So, in those educational environments where direct observation is not part of the educational culture, the use of these instruments may help to change the educational routine.

Using workplace-based instruments well does not have to be time-consuming, especially in those situations where frequent observation and feedback are already part of the teaching culture. However, it is important not to make the forms too long, as this will make such an approach less acceptable to users. Workplace-based assessment is considered in more detail in Chapter 20.

Portfolios

The word 'portfolio' is a container term used to describe all kinds of educational tools. From the assessment point of view, there are two approaches that it may be useful to discuss here, as follow:
- portfolio as an instrument to measure the *reflective ability* of the candidate
- portfolio as an instrument to *collate assessment information* from various sources.

In both cases the portfolio contains a 'dossier and an 'analysis'. The analysis contains a self-assessment of strengths and weaknesses, learning goals and a learning plan.

The reflective portfolio focuses on self-assessment; it is used to assess the extent to which the candidate's self-assessment demonstrates a good reflective ability. The second portfolio approach collates all assessment information about the student. The analysis section is used to evaluate current performance and to plan future learning. This approach is best compared to a patient chart, in which information from various sources, such as laboratory data, imaging data, and results from history-taking and physical examination, is collected, but it also contains a regular evaluation about the well-being of the patient and a plan for further diagnostic and therapeutic actions. So, the portfolio becomes not only an assessment but also an educational instrument.

It is difficult to say anything definitive about the reliability and validity of portfolios. Studies calculating reliability in the traditional psychometric way, using either generalisability theory or inter-rater agreement measures such as Cohen's Kappa, report moderate reliabilities at best.(43) Other authors suggest an organisational approach to rendering the portfolios dependable, using concepts from qualitative research methodologies, such as benchmarking, peer evaluation, member checking and stepwise replication.(44) In such cases, reliability cannot be expressed as a number but must be derived from the carefulness of the processes.

The validity of the portfolio approach requires further study. It is apparent that conventional construct validity methods do not apply here, so other methodologies need to be developed. Moreover, since portfolios are used for so many purposes, content validity cannot easily be established.

It may also be obvious that portfolios are expensive. They are time-consuming not only to produce, but also to assess, especially if more than one judge has to assess each portfolio. It is tempting then to try to produce a simple scoring list or rubric to increase efficiency, but this only serves to trivialise the assessment. Training of assessors and using global criteria for judging the portfolio is a better approach, and it may be more efficient to set up a procedure in which multiple judges are used only if there is doubt about the result, with only a very limited number of judges used in all clear cases.(44)

You can read more about portfolios in Chapter 14.

Computers in assessment

There are many different ways in which computers can play a role in assessment. The most obvious is computerised administration. But there are other, and more important, roles for computers in assessment, and these are discussed briefly below.

Administrative support

Item banks can be very powerful in supporting quality control. Indeed, this aspect is often more important than their role in enabling the re-use of old items. Attempts to build a complete item bank from which items can be drawn at random often prove unsuccessful. There are two reasons for this. First, an examination is more than a randomly generated set of items, even if the individual items are of good quality. There is always an extra quality control step needed to ensure that the combination of items is good. A second reason is concerned with the nature of medicine and other health sciences. In these disciplines, things evolve quite rapidly, quickly rendering items outdated. Also, ideas about what constitutes a good item may evolve. Item banks are therefore, more useful in tracking an item in the quality control process. They also provide the opportunity to scan the domain coverage quickly, so that production of redundant items is prevented, and under-represented subjects can be completed with specific new items.

There are many good commercial products available for item banking. For simple purposes it is also possible to use standard database software with self-produced scripts, shells or queries. Developing complete high-brow software systems is always more time-consuming than one would expect. When an item-bank system is needed, the best approach is to determine carefully the needs of the organisation, or the functional and operational specifications, and then determine which of the available software can meet these needs sufficiently.

Test analysis

In the quality control of tests, computers can be used to evaluate test results. The most well-known application is a standard item analysis with p-values, a-values, item–total or item–rest correlations and the calculation of reliabilities. The p-value represents the proportion of students answering the question correctly. As such, it is an indication of how difficult this item was for this particular group of candidates. A p-value of 1.00 means that every candidate answered the item correctly, whereas a p-value of 0.00 means that nobody gave the correct answer. The a-values indicate the proportion of candidates choosing each option in a multiple-choice question and, as such, are an indicator for the attractiveness of each distracter. The item–total and item–rest correlations indicate the extent to which the item was answered correctly by the high achievers on the test and answered incorrectly by the low scorers on the test. Standard statistical software, such as SPSS, often allows for such analyses, and such structured item analyses can be very valuable and may have a major impact on the quality of tests.

Computerised testing

There are many obvious advantages of computerised testing. Hand-scoring is not needed; the results can be calculated immediately; and data files for further analysis are easily available. Also, there are no added costs for reproduction of test booklets and answer sheets. Audio- and video-clips are possible and can help to improve the content validity of the test.

But there are also downsides to computerised testing. First, open-ended questions are difficult to score automatically and may need hand-scoring or at least verification of the computer scoring procedures. Although hand-scoring of typed text may be easier than that of – sometimes illegible – handwriting, this still nullifies the advantages of immediate results and availability of data files. This may lead test developers to use multiple-choice-type questions exclusively. Second, if there are many more candidates than there are computers available, equivalent test forms have to be developed. Although corralling of students is an option to prevent unwanted information exchanges, this is possible only to a limited extent. Producing extra equivalent tests is more expensive than reproduction costs. Third, the necessity of a systems administrator for the computer network adds to the costs. Fourth, reading from a computer screen is more tiring than reading from paper, which may limit the maximum test length. Finally, without sufficient back-up systems computer or network problems may disturb the test administration. Although with current technology these problems are rare, and despite the fact that things can also go wrong with paper-and-pencil administration, problems are still more likely to occur with computerised testing. So, before deciding to use computers to administer a test that could also be a pen-and-paper exercise, it is important to consider all the pros and cons very carefully.

Assessment possibilities unique to computer testing

There are some interesting and potential possibilities presented by computer-based assessment that are unique to the format and not merely logistical advantages. We discuss three of them here – namely, real-time simulations, sequential testing and computer-adaptive testing.

Real-time simulations are useful to test the management of cases in which time is essential in real life, such as emergency medicine. As a formative tool it can also be helpful to demonstrate to the candidate how much time they took to solve the case and where a gain in efficiency could be made. For summative testing it tends to complicate things, as one cannot simply add up response time and proficiency. So, to come to a pass/fail decision, one has to find a valid way of combining these different qualities into one single score, and this is not easy.

Sequential testing is an approach that enables a more efficient use of time and resources in assessment. It basically comes down to administering a short screening test to all candidates. Based on the reliability of this test, a (95 per cent) confidence interval can be calculated around the pass/fail score. For every candidate whose score is outside this interval, there is sufficient certainty ($p \leq 0.05$) to say that his or her score is either a pass or a fail. The remainder of the students must answer an additional set of questions. The scores of these are added to their scores in the first part of the test. This way, a longer test is presented only to those candidates where there is doubt about their passing or failing. Such an approach is feasible only if the scores and the confidence interval can be calculated quickly and an additional test is available on request.(45)

A further development is *computer-adaptive testing* (CAT). This approach is based on a so-called calibrated item bank – an item bank in which the precise difficulty of all items is known beforehand. For such a calibration, classical test theory (CTT) is often not sufficient. A more complicated statistical approach – item–response theory (IRT) – is used (*see* Box 18.1). Unlike CTT, the use of IRT allows the difficulty and discriminative power of items to be estimated, regardless of the specific group of candidates. The computer selects an item of moderate difficulty for the candidate. When the candidate answers the item correctly, the computer selects a slightly more difficult item, and when the answer is incorrect, an easier item is selected. This process is repeated either until a specified number of items have been answered or until a certain level of preciseness of the test is reached.(46) In the former, the precision proficiency estimate varies across candidates (but in the majority of cases is better than a standard test); in the latter, the precision is fixed, but the number of items needed may vary from candidate to candidate (in the majority of cases this will be fewer than in a standard test). Although CAT is a wonderful concept, the statistical requirements for achieving a well-enough calibrated item bank are quite heavy, often requiring considerable pre-testing of all items.(46)

Combining assessment methods

It is currently generally accepted that in order to obtain a complete picture of someone's competence and performance, one assessment instrument is not enough; a variety of well-chosen instruments is needed.(28–30) How then should assessment methods be combined? Essentially, there are two approaches, one quantitative, the other qualitative.

Quantitative methods:
- compensatory
- partially compensatory
- conjunctive.

Qualitative methods:
- expert judgement
- explicit procedures.

In a quantitative combination, results are somehow translated into numerical values. These values are then combined in a compensatory, partially compensatory or conjunctive manner.

Compensatory means that the results of the tests are averaged or summed and that the average or sum needs to be above the pass/fail score, regardless of the scores on the individual tests. For example, averaging the two sets of marks 4/10 and 8/10, and 2/10 and 10/10, gives a result of 6 in both cases. A model in which every test result contributes to a total score with a certain percentage – for example, test 1 accounts for 30 per cent and test 2 for 20 per cent, etc. – is also a compensatory model. Compensatory models often result in high reliabilities for the final decision, because such decisions are made on the basis of many items within multiple tests held on different occasions, so on sampling across many sources of error. The major downside, however, is that compensatory models may induce a minimalist study strategy. Some students may have such high scores on previous tests that they tend not to take the later tests (and the related courses) seriously.

A *partially compensatory* model corrects for this. Here, the scores can be averaged, but for each test there is an absolute minimum score, and if this is not reached, the student has to repeat the test. This is a compromise in that the combined reliability is somewhat lower than in a completely compensatory model, but the negative educational impact is also diminished.

A (completely) *conjunctive* model requires that the student achieves a score above the pass/fail score in all the tests in order to gain an overall pass. Such an approach stimulates students to take all the individual tests (and courses) seriously and to study hard for all of them, but it is less reliable overall. In every test there is a probability of a false negative result, that is, a student who fails who should in fact have passed. Such failure is then largely due to measurement error, rather than incompetence. And, as each failure leads to a consequence (which is the case in conjunctive but not in compensatory models), in fact the false-negative results of all individual tests are combined resulting in a lower overall reliability.

The results of some assessments are simply not quantitative in nature. So, it is not possible to add them up to form a total score. Although it is common practice to convert the results of qualitative assessments into numerical scores, we want to warn against this as a methodologically incorrect practice.(47) This is perhaps best illustrated by an analogy to medical practice. You do not add your first impression of 'very sick patient' to a sodium level of 133 mmol/l – these two pieces of information need to be combined qualitatively. The same applies to different observations with results such as 'performed extremely well' and 'good bedside manner'. These cannot be combined in a quantitative way but need to be evaluated qualitatively. Such a combination requires – again similar to medical practice – expert judgement and careful procedures. Good examples of such approaches are the General Medical Council's practice performance procedures and some portfolio assessments.(44,48,49)

Standard-setting

Perhaps the most heavily debated issue in assessment is the issue of standard-setting. It is the cut-off score that determines the consequences of the assessment, that is, who passes and who fails. It is an important issue because often quite small changes in cut-off scores represent substantial changes in the numbers of students who pass and fail. The Holy Grail is therefore the *true* cut-off score. Unfortunately, like its mythical counterpart, there is no such thing. The literature describes a wide variation of methods,(50) each of which has its own specific purposes, and a distinction is usually made between relative and absolute standards. There is no one single-best standard-setting method for all tests, but there is probably a most appropriate method for each individual test in a specific context.

No matter which method of standard-setting is used, it will always be arbitrary, as there will always be assumptions made about the required level. Relative methods are based on assumptions about the stability of the mean competence of large groups of students. Especially large year classes of medical students appear to be comparable across cohorts and universities in many, but not all, countries. Absolute methods are based on assumptions about the required level of competence, the teaching the candidates have received and the end goals of the curriculum. In every case, therefore, there must at least be an explicit rationale for the decisions about the standard-setting method. This is sometimes expressed in the aphorism 'standard-setting may be arbitrary, it may never be capricious'. Any standard must therefore be:

- explicable, through the rationales behind the decisions made
- defensible, to the extent that it can assure the stakeholders about its validity (an issue in this may be 'due diligence', that is, demonstrating that good effort was put into setting the standard)
- stable, as it is not defensible that the standards vary from year to year.(51)

Chapter 22 examines the subject of standard-setting in more detail and looks at the different approaches currently used by test developers.

Future directions

A section on future directions is always a dangerous one to write since so-called 'future developments' may, with hindsight, appear to have been flukes. Still, we would like to make some predictions.

The change from defining educational outcomes in constructs – such as knowledge, skills, attitudes and problem-solving skills – to actions, as described in Miller's pyramid (knows, knows how, shows how and does), and the further change from there into more or less complex tasks that require the timely availability of relevant knowledge, skills, attitudes and problem-solving ability, the so-called competencies, must have an influence on our way of thinking about assessment.

Also, the emergence of new assessment methods such as mini-CEX, 360° feedback and portfolio, in which the main goal is *not* to add up the individual items to give a total score, must have an influence on our way of thinking about assessment. We see the following three main developments here.

1 Assessment will be less viewed as an external measurement of the results of the educational process but more as an integral part of the process. Currently, it is still fairly common to take students out of the authentic educational context to be tested on their competence. Assessments such as mini-CEX take the assessment back into the authentic educational context. Current approaches to assessing professional behaviour even acknowledge that it is impossible to evaluate this outside the authentic context. This leads, in our view, to a second development.

2 Assessment is no longer seen exclusively as a psychometric measurement problem, but more as an educational design problem. This implies that the purpose of assessment is not merely to determine whether a candidate is up to standard, but more how the information about the candidate's competence can best be used to tailor the teaching or the courses to individual needs. So, instead of striving for a standardised curriculum with standardised testing, it will entail a development to tailored assessment with flexible curricula. This, in turn, may lead to a third development.

3 Standard psychometric approaches to issues such as fairness and defensibility of examinations will have to be expanded with other measures. For example, basic assumptions underlying the standard psychometric approach, such as stable and generic constructs, homogeneity of the universe (e.g. the total universe of possible items) and assumption of local independency of the observations, cannot always be met. Moreover, some modern instruments aim precisely at being locally dependent observations (mini-CEX, longitudinal testing), acknowledge the heterogeneity of the universe (360° feedback) and acknowledge the non-existence of traits in competence (portfolio). This does not make the issues of defensibility, fairness and carefulness go away but will require different – statistical – models.(52)

Epilogue

Designing assessment programmes and selecting the best instruments for each purpose is not easy. To complicate matters further, medical education is a rapidly evolving discipline. This may lead some to be dismissive of assessment science and argue that the truths of yesterday are obsolete and will be replaced with new ones. We would argue against this. Any evolving discipline questions truths critically and scientifically, and this is strength rather than a weakness. Medical education does not differ from medicine in this respect – what was true when we were students often no longer holds true today. The purpose of this chapter is to guide the reader through the field of assessment of medical competence and performance by providing background information and a few guidelines. The most important messages we have tried to convey are that in designing high-quality assessments, foundations are rational decisions based on the best available evidence and careful quality control.

Acknowledgement

With thanks to Professor Chris McManus of University College London for providing a lucid summary of approaches to the assessment of reliability in Box 18.1

References

1 Van der Vleuten CPM (1996) The assessment of professional competence: developments, research and practical implications. *Advances in Health Science Education.* **1**(1): 41–67.

2 Van der Vleuten CPM, Norman GR and De Graaf E (1991) Pitfalls in the pursuit of objectivity: issues of reliability. *Medical Education.* **25**: 110–8.

3 Cronbach LJ (1983) What price simplicity? *Educational Measurement: Issues and Practice.* **2**(2): 11–2.

4 Ebel RL (1983) The practical validation of tests of ability. *Educational Measurement: Issues and Practice.* **2**(2): 7–10.

5 Downing SM and Haladyna TM (2004) Validity threats: overcoming interference with proposed interpretations of assessment data. *Medical Education.* **38**(3): 327–33.

6 Guba EG and Lincoln YS (2001) Guidelines and checklist for constructivist (aka fourth generation) evaluation. (http://www.wmich.edu/evalctr/checklists; accessed 17 August 2004).

7 Kane M (2006) Validation. In: Brennan RL (ed.) *Educational Measurement*, pp. 17–64. ACE/Praeger, Westport, CT.

8 Messick S (1994) The interplay of evidence and consequences in the validation of performance assessments. *Educational Researcher.* **23**(2): 13–23.

9 Frederiksen N (1984) The real test bias: influences of testing on teaching and learning. *American Psychologist.* **39**(3): 193–202.

10 Newble DI and Jaeger K (1983) The effect of assessments and examinations on the learning of medical students. *Medical Education.* **17**: 165–71.

11 Cilliers FJ, Schuwirth LWT, Herman N, Adendorff HJ and Van der Vleuten CPM (2012) A model of the pre-assessment learning effects of summative assessment in medical education. *Advances in Health Sciences Education.* **17**: 39–53.

12 Cilliers FJ, Schuwirth LWT and Van der Vleuten CPM (2012) A model of the pre-assessment learning effects of assessment is operational in an undergraduate clinical context. *BMC Medical Education.* **12**(9).

13 Cilliers FJ, Schuwirth LWT, Adendorff HJ, Herman N and Van der Vleuten CPM (2010) The mechanisms of impact of summative assessment on medical students' learning. *Advances in Health Sciences Education.* **15**: 695–715.

14 Stalenhoef-Halling BF, Van der Vleuten CPM, Jaspers TAM and Fiolet JBFM (1990) A new approach to assessing clinical problem-solving skills by written examination: conceptual basis and initial pilot test results. In: Bender W, Hiemstra RJ, Scherpbier A and Zwierstra RJ (eds) *Teaching and Assessing Clinical Competence. Proceedings of the Fourth Ottawa Conference*, pp. 552–7. Boekwerk Publications, Groningen, The Netherlands.

15 Hakstian RA (1971) The effects of type of examination anticipated on test preparation and performance. *Journal of Educational Research.* **64**(7): 319–24.

16 Eva K, Rosenfeld J, Reiter H and Norman G (2004) An admissions OSCE: the multiple mini-interview. *Medical Education.* **38**(3): 314–26.

17 McManus IC, Iqbal S, Chandrarajan A *et al.* (2005) Unhappiness and dissatisfaction in doctors cannot be predicted by selectors for medical school application forms: a prospective longitudinal study. *BMC Medical Education.* (**5**):38.

18 Salvatori P (2001) Reliability and validity of admissions tools used to select students for the health professions. *Advances in Health Science Education.* **6**(2): 159–75.

19 Eva K, Rosenfeld J, Reiter H and Norman G (2004) The ability of the multiple mini-interview to predict preclerkship performance in medical school. *Academic Medicine.* **79**(10): S40–2.

20 Swanson DB (1987) A measurement framework for performance based test. In: Hart IR, Harden RM (eds) *Further Developments in assessing Clinical Competence* pp. 13–45. Can-Heal Publications, Montreal..

21 Wass V, Wakeford R, Neighbour R and Van der Vleuten C (2003) Achieving acceptable reliability in oral examinations: an analysis of the Royal College of General Practitioners membership examination's oral component. *Medical Education.* **37**: 126–31.

22 Maatsch J and Huang R (1986) An evaluation of the construct validity of four alternative theories of clinical competence. Proceedings of the 25th Annual RIME Conference, 69–74. Association of American Medical Colleges, Chicago.

23 Norman GR, Smith EKM, Powles AC *et al.* (1987) Factors underlying performance on written tests of knowledge. *Medical Education.* **21**: 297–304.

24 Schuwirth LWT, Van der Vleuten CPM and Donkers HHLM (1996) A closer look at cueing effects in multiple-choice questions. *Medical Education.* **30**: 44–9.

25 Van der Vleuten CPM, Schuwirth LWT, Muijtjens AMM *et al.* (2004) Cross institutional collaboration in assessment: a case on progress testing. *Medical Teacher.* **26**(8): 719–25.

26 Schuwirth LWT, Bosman G, Henning RH, Rinkel R and Wenink AC (2010) Collaboration on progress testing in medical schools in the Netherlands. *Medical Teacher.* **32**(6): 476–9.

27 Schuwirth LWT, Southgate L, Page GG *et al.* (2002) When enough is enough: a conceptual basis for fair and defensible practice performance assessment. *Medical Education.* **36**: 925–30.

28 Van der Vleuten CPM and Schuwirth LWT (2005) Assessing professional competence: from methods to programmes. *Medical Education.* **39**(3): 309–17.

29 Dijkstra J, Galbraith R, Hodges B *et al.* (2012) Expert validation of fit-for-purpose guidelines for designing programmes of assessment. *BMC Medical Education.* **12**(20).

30 Dijkstra J, Van der Vleuten CPM and Schuwirth LWT (2010) A new framework for designing programmes of assessment. *Advances in Health Sciences Education.* **15**: 379–93.

31 Bordage G (1987) An alternative approach to PMPs: the 'key-features' concept. In: Hart IR and Harden R (eds) *Further Developments in Assessing Clinical Competence, Proceedings of the Second Ottawa Conference*, pp. 59–75. Can-Heal Publications, Montreal.

32 Page G, Bordage G and Allen T (1995) Developing key-feature problems and examinations to assess clinical decision-making skills. *Academic Medicine.* **70**(3): 194–201.

33 Case SM and Swanson DB (1993) Extended-matching items: a practical alternative to free response questions. *Teaching and Learning in Medicine.* **5**(2): 107–15.

34 Schuwirth LWT, Verheggen MM, Van der Vleuten CPM *et al.* (2001) Do short cases elicit different thinking processes than factual knowledge questions do? *Medical Education.* **35**(4): 348–56.

35 Stillman P, Ruggill J, Rutala P and Sabers D (1980) Patient instructors as teachers and evaluators. *Journal of Medical Education.* **55**: 186–93.

36 Harden RM and Gleeson FA (1979) Assessment of clinical competence using an objective structured clinical examination (OSCE). *Medical Education.* **13**(1): 41–54.

37 Petrusa E (2002) Clinical performance assessments. In: Norman G, Van der Vleuten CPM and Newble DI (eds) *International Handbook of Research in Medical Education*, pp. 673–709. Kluwer, Dordrecht, Boston, MA, London.

38 Regehr G, MacRae H, Reznick R and Szalay D (1998) Comparing the psychometric properties of checklists and global rating scales for assessing performance on an OSCE-format examination. *Academic Medicine.* **73**(9): 993–7.

39 Norcini J, Blank LL, Arnold GK and Kimball HR (1995) The mini-CEX (Clinical Evaluation Exercise); a preliminary investigation. *Annals of Internal Medicine.* **123**(10): 795–9.

40 Garman AN, Tyler JL and Darnall JS (2004) Development and validation of a 360-degree-feedback instrument for healthcare administrators. *Journal of Health Care Management.* **49**(5): 307–21.

41 Williams M, Klamen D and McGaghie W (2003) Cognitive, social and environmental sources of bias in clinical performance ratings. *Teaching and Learning in Medicine.* **15**(4): 270–92.

42 Norcini JJ, Blank LL, Duffy FD and Fortna GS (2003) The mini-CEX: a method for assessing clinical skills. *Annals of Internal Medicine.* **138**(6): 476–81.

43 Roberts C (2002) Portfolio-based assessments in medical education; are they valid and reliable for summative purposes? *Medical Education.* **36**: 899–900.

44 Driessen E, Van der Vleuten CPM, Schuwirth LWT *et al.* (2005) The use of qualitative research criteria for portfolio assessment as an alternative to reliability evaluation: a case study. *Medical Education.* **39**(2): 214–20.

45 Smee S, Blackmore DE, Rothman AI *et al.* (1998) Pioneering a sequenced OSCE for the Medical Council of Canada: an administrative overview. In: Melnick D (ed.) Evolving assessment: Protecting the human dimension. Proceedings of the 8th International Ottawa Conference on Medical Education and Assessment. Held July 12–15, 1998 Philadelphia (PA) USA. National Board of Medical Examiners, Philadelphia, USA.

46 Clauser BE and Schuwirth LWT (2002) The use of computers in assessment. In: Norman GR, Van der Vleuten CPM and Newble DI (eds) *International Handbook of Research in Medical Education*, pp. 757–92. Kluwer, Dordrecht, Boston, MA; London.

47 Delandshere G and Petrosky AR (1998) Assessment of complex performances: limitations of key measurement assumptions. *Educational Researcher.* **27**(2): 14–24.

48 Southgate L, Cox J, David T *et al.* (2001) The General Medical Council's Performance Procedures; peer review of performance in the workplace. *Medical Education.* **35**(1): 9–19.

49 Southgate L, Campbell M, Cox H *et al.* (2001) The General Medical Council's Performance Procedures; the development and implementation of tests of competence with examples from general practice. *Medical Education.* **35**(1): 20–8.

50 Cusimano MD (1996) Standard setting in medical education. *Academic Medicine.* **71**(s10): S112–20.

51 Norcini J (2003) Setting standards on educational tests. *Medical Education.* **37**: 464–9.

52 Schuwirth LWT and Van der Vleuten CPM (2006) A plea for new psychometrical models in educational assessment. *Medical Education.* **40**(4): 269–300.

19 Written assessment

Brian Jolly
University of Newcastle, Australia

🔑 KEY MESSAGES

- Start early; at least six months before the examination for intra-school assessments.

- Review or construct an assessment blueprint for the course or unit that is being assessed.

- Decide on the objectives or domains in the blueprint that need to be assessed with written formats. These would normally involve recall of information, recognition of patterns of presenting symptoms, clinical decision-making, choice of investigations, analysis of data and synthesis of ideas, strategies and management.

- Decide whether a constructed response is necessary to assess the objective or whether a selected response would do.

- Choose the appropriate format for each item of the blueprint.

- Collect all the items into their format groupings.

- Arrange a workshop to develop the required formats, along the lines identified above.

- Once the test is proofed and prepared, arrange a further workshop to set standards, methods for which may vary depending upon item type and the setting.

- Deliver the test.

- Prior to result determination, thoroughly review the items using item-analysis software. Make sure that key personnel know how to interpret the output.

- Determine the final scores of candidates and cut scores for the test with all the poorly performing items eliminated.

Introduction

Assessment has become accepted as a critical part of educational and accreditation strategies used in health professions education. The senior guardians of those professions have traditionally had high standards and developed refined means of ensuring them.(1) With increased international concern for patent safety,(2,3) the need for efficient, reliable and valid assessment has become vital. In turn, this has led to a search for increasing levels of sophistication in testing, mostly targeted at the development of hi-fidelity simulations and work-based assessments.(4,5) However, health professionals operate across a very broad spectrum of human activity, from listening and talking to patients, to intricate and physically demanding interventions. Knowledge and thinking play a crucial role in these undertakings, and there is considerable evidence to suggest that knowledge, and its storage in clinically useful frameworks, are the most important attributes that divide the novice from the expert.(6,7)

One of the most useful ways of finding out what people know is to ask them a question. When such enquiries are written down or the person is required to give a written response, we are in the territory of written assessment. This paper introduces the reader to the use of written assessment in medical and health professions' education and covers the following four key areas:

- the placement of assessment within the curriculum
- different formats of written assessments
  - ○ constructed response
  - ○ selected response
  - ○ combined constructed and selected responses
- how well written test items do their job
- how to set appropriate standards for these assessments.

Historical background

Assessment, particularly in medicine, historically involved oral activities: general discussion, case discussion, demonstration, answers at the bedside, etc. In this tradition the long case was adopted, in 1858, by the newly established General Medical Council (UK), as a means of assuring the competence of physician apprentices.(8) However, with the post-Flexnerian (circa 1910) emphasis on scientific endeavour in medicine, the measurement of knowledge through reliable and explicit means became increasingly emphasised.(9) In general psychometric perspectives on assessment have reflected the need for efficiency, reliability and validity, whilst the educational perspective has stressed the need for appropriate influences on learning of assessment processes.(10,11) In recent years these two heritages have converged considerably.

Understanding Medical Education: Evidence, Theory and Practice, Second Edition. Edited by Tim Swanwick.
© 2014 The Association for the Study of Medical Education. Published 2014 by John Wiley & Sons, Ltd.

Research on assessment in medicine has been most productive in the last 25 years,(12) and I do not intend to present all of this research here; there are books available that summarise the area and will help the interested reader.(13–15) I will, though, try to provide a balanced overview of the field and consider the theoretical determinants of assessment in as much detail as is necessary for a newcomer to the field.

Assessment in the curriculum

Before designing any assessment event, it is useful to think through the purpose of assessment. Although we use the term 'assessment' quite loosely, each assessment that a learner undertakes usually has a particular function, which reflects the complexity of professional training. These functions include the following:
- measuring competence
- measuring performance
- diagnosing trainees' problems
- measuring improvement
- self-evaluation
- selecting individuals
- identifying effective learning/teaching
- showing effectiveness of curriculum
- measuring curriculum change.

Each of these purposes will have constraining influences on the content of the assessment, the strategy used and the techniques employed. For example, assessments used to certify competence need to be closely aligned to the core curriculum objectives, that is, demonstrate content validity. They also need to be reliable and focused at pre-specified levels of competence. However, an assessment used to select trainees into a restricted-entry postgraduate training programme may be targeted at a level of excellence, and may need to contain specific elements that predict success in that programme.(16)

One process for assuring the content validity of assessment is called 'blueprinting'.(17–19) Essentially, this needs to be done for the assessment regime or strategy of the whole course, *before* individual components are designed, because it is one way of ensuring that the content is appropriately assigned to those components with the best fit to the mental processes being assessed. For example, there will be specific domains of activity that are better suited to some types of assessment, and this will become apparent when a thorough blueprinting exercise, that reflects the complete assessment strategy, is conducted for the whole curriculum. Detailed descriptions of the rationale and technique of blueprinting can be found elsewhere.(17–19) Trying to design the written segments of an assessment process without adequate blueprinting of the whole assessment on the curriculum is likely to result in an imbalanced assessment.

Knowledge, reasoning and written assessment

When the blueprinting is complete, it will identify a set of attributes of a qualified health professional that reflect the cognitive domain of human endeavour – understanding, recalling, recognising, reasoning, inferring, deducing and deciding. Such attributes can be assessed in a number of ways, and there is little doubt that an effective clinician needs to be able to do all these things with patients and colleagues in clinical situations. However, not only is it impracticable to assess these attributes comprehensively or effectively in clinical situations, there is some evidence that it leads to contamination of the measurement process by other factors – these factors are generally referred to as 'construct-irrelevant variance'.(20) For example, oral examinations purportedly aimed at examining clinical reasoning can be reduced to the investigation of factual recall, frequently focus on minutiae, or can reveal examiners' 'cultural incompetence'.(21)

One way of avoiding these influences, was to decontextualise the assessment. In most of the 20th century this trend, and the recognition that, psychometrically, a minimum number of questions on a topic was needed to give a reliable estimate of a person's knowledge, gave rise to a number of developments in assessment. These included the multiple-choice question (MCQ), in its various guises, and the short-answer question (SAQ). However, over the last 20 years, researchers have rediscovered that context is a crucial element of thinking. Generally, it has an important function in the formation of memory(22) and in clinical reasoning in particular.(23) It has also been determined that expertise is significantly dependent on knowledge.(24) Moreover, the way that this knowledge is obtained and organised is much more important than its sheer volume. For clinicians, the usability of knowledge is critical, and this depends both on the efficiency of learning and where and how that learning has taken place. In brief, clinical reasoning depends on integrated knowledge preferably learnt or repeatedly accessed by the learner in complex clinical contexts, where appropriate scientific principles are articulated to address patient problems.(25) These findings mean that we now have new varieties of written assessments. In MCQ format, the extended matching item and the script concordance test both typically establish a clinical context for the assessees' activities. And new approaches to short-answer items include the key features item. At the same time, previously endemic item types such as the multiple true-false MCQ (X type MCQ) have come under cogent criticism.(26)

There is another dimension to written assessment that needs to be considered: the nature of the response. This can either be a selected response or one constructed by the test taker. In general, although there has been some dispute over this, it is thought that constructed responses require candidates to operate at a higher level than selected responses; for example, recall and synthesis vs. recognition and choice.

In the next section we look at each of the format types. There are exhaustive treatments of many of these available in the literature.(15,26) Here, I will abbreviate much of the extensive debate in order to help the newcomer to make some practical decisions about assessment.

Formats of written assessment

Usefully, Epstein(27) has summarised assessment techniques and their general potential usage. I have expanded his summary table slightly for the written assessment components in Box 19.1. I have also removed Epstein's column referring to where each method might be best used to allow more flexibility based on: the domains of activity or objectives that need to be assessed, the need to reflect the blueprint outcomes, and the need to encompass local requirements for assessment of certain attributes. The test maker needs to think carefully about all these factors and make choices appropriately.

Constructed response formats

The essay

An essay is: 'A test item which requires a response composed by the examinee, usually in the form of one or more sentences, of a nature that no single response or pattern of responses can be listed as correct, and the accuracy and quality of which can be judged subjectively only by one skilled or informed in the subject'.(28, p. 495)

On the face of it, essays are one of the most effective ways of ascertaining how good a student is at constructing a complex response to a challenging question. The other approaches that might be used would be oral examinations, projects, observation of discussion and many more. However, many of these are subject to variability due to extraneous serendipitous factors. For example, in orals there is no 'product', so judgements about performance are made 'on the run', unless the examination is recorded and analysed later, and this would significantly increase the burden of administration.

Essays can be delivered in two contexts 'unseen' or 'seen'. In the former a question, or usually a suite of questions, is prepared and delivered 'de novo' to students under examination conditions. In the latter a topic is provided to students, and they are given a time limit in which to address it. They may use any resources they can find. Occasionally, questions may be given to students in advance, but the essay is written under examination conditions.

The attributes of the essay and issues in its construction, delivery and marking are far from straightforward. The key questions to consider when choosing any assessment are as follows.
- What type of response is required? (a content-validity issue)
- What cognitive processes are involved? (a content- and construct-validity issue)
- How well do the response and the cognitive processes invoked map to the expectations of the assessor about student performance, and to the objectives of the curriculum? (a content-validity issue)

Clearly, in the unseen examination, critical components of a successful essay will depend on memory (both short and long term). The essay's quality will also depend on the ability of the student to construct sentences of the appropriate length that are unambiguous and grammatically correct, and to organise his or her knowledge in a way that addresses the question. If these abilities are all critical elements of the curriculum or of the environment into which this examination might be the entry point (e.g. internship), then the essay may be a rational assessment. If they are only pre-requisites and were assessed earlier, or if only knowledge and memory are important, would another assessment method be superior?

Constructing an essay question

Decide on the constellation of attributes that you need to assess and decide whether an unseen or a seen essay would be the most appropriate. For example, if most of the knowledge you require the student to have is basic, core and extensive, and must enable them to solve, manage and monitor a real clinical problem at some time in the future, and possess an in-depth knowledge of related or differential conditions, then probably the unseen essay would be appropriate. Then:
- Choose a problem or issue that can be addressed satisfactorily in the time allocated, or limit it in such a way as to make it answerable.
- Define the problem/issue and describe the task clearly.
- Describe the structure that the answer should take and its scope.
- Do not use complex language in the question such as double negatives, ambiguities and abbreviations.
- Use terms that cover the cognitive processes that you are expecting to be used in marshalling the answer: for example, compare, predict, prioritise, rather than examine, elucidate. (*See* Box 19.2.)
- Avoid questions where radically different answers will be acceptable for a given question. This is fine for a group discussion or debate, but it makes marking an essay difficult especially where assessors might favour one or other of the answers.
- For every question, preferably construct a model answer, or list the essential features that should be contained in the answer.
- Trial-run the questions on a group who should know the answers.
- Make sure that *all* the defined essential features appear in the trial group's answers as a whole, not necessarily in every member's answers.
- Proofread the paper three times using a different reader each time.

When marking, ideally each answer should be scored by a pair of assessors working independently. If that is not possible, the same marker should score the same question for all candidates. This minimises extraneous variance stemming from the different ways each examiner marks different questions. To help with quality control of marking, all examiners of a question should preferably see all, or at least the complete range, of answers to that question. Scores for a question should be the mean of all the examiners marking that question.

Although assessor training is desirable for most written assessments, a model answer is often better than attempts at calibration. In fact a series of model answers specifically written to be at the boundaries between two grades is a very useful way of enabling accurate classification. For example, in an A-E grade system, model answers should be at A/B and B/C boundaries. This enables most essays to be rated using two anchor points, since most will fall between the boundaries. A model answer is also useful when there is a common core of content that needs to be

BOX 19.1 Types of written assessments and their primary usages. From Epstein(27)

Constructed Response Formats

Method	Domain Usage/Response Mode	Design Factors	Limitations	Strengths
1a Essay – Traditional. The typical university essay, either seen or unseen, where the writer is required to describe, discuss and propose new perspectives on one or more issues. The answer may or may not be predetermined.	Any situation where lengthy explanation or detail is required. Detailed synthesis of information; interpretation of literature, evaluation of management options. Context frequently provided by the candidate.	Traditionally questions can vary from the blindingly obvious to the very obscure. Large number of dimensions to the constructed response. Getting questions right takes time. Model answers or protocols help marking. High marking workload.	Can be usurped into provision of lists, e.g. for treatments; can become memory dumps. Can be misinterpreted. Long testing time per topic, so limited coverage possible. Reliability variable and susceptible to rater and candidate bias	Total flexibility in question setting. Can avoid cueing. Regarded as using higher-order cognitive processes.
1b Modified Essay – Specifically developed for medicine – mostly used in general practice. Highly structured case vignette followed by questions on any aspect. Focused on candidates' management of a case or cases. Answer(s) usually predetermined.	Clinical management issues. Some cue identification and reasoning required to link, e.g. signs and symptoms to investigations and management. Context provided by the question.	Can move from one stage of clinical management to another easily, by using slightly different cases to address issues, e.g. patient management in one case, and ethics in a similar one. More efficient sampling of a wide area of knowledge possible	Needs careful design to avoid cueing. As a result can be patchy in sampling knowledge across cases.	Can avoid cueing. Context is controllable by question setter. Can demand wide range of cognitive processes. May be machine scoreable in next 5–10 years.
2a Short Answer – Traditional. A short question that asks for a constructed specific answer, usually requiring one word, a short phrase, or a line or two of text. Answers mostly predetermined.	Recall of specific facts or statements about biomedical or clinical processes. Context provided by the question.	Deceptively simple to construct. Can sample widely different domains of knowledge easily.	Very wide variety of formats and little research on their use and psychometric properties. Can lead to cueing across items. Context provided by question.	Scoring by machine becoming a reality. Can replace MCQs where recall is thought to be vital (e.g. decisions based on core knowledge and experience)
2b Short Answer – Extended. A question that asks for an extended answer, usually requiring a paragraph or two, that may address different aspects, or an extension, of the issue. Answers may be predetermined.	Recall of related groups of concepts or relatively short explanations. Context provided by the question.	Deceptively simple to construct. Can sample widely different domains of knowledge but in more depth than short answer.	As above. Scoring more difficult as depends on multiple attributes of answers involved in essay construction. Machine scoring not possible. Context provided by question. Recent research on analysis of answers can give more insight into level of functioning of candidate.	Total flexibility in question setting.

Selected Response Modes

1a MCQ – True/False. Typically a short statement or brief paragraph followed by several (3–6) options. Candidates are asked to identify which options are true and which ones false in relation to the initial statement.	Recognition of consonance between two facts, attributes or concepts. Can test recognition of clear-cut knowledge in many domains. Complex items requiring calculations or problem-solving have been used.	Requires all options to be absolutely true or false. Can test knowledge of contraindications through the 'false' option.	Difficult to write. The number used in most assessments can lead to cross-cueing. Can involve silly or irrelevant options due to lack of absolute falsehoods. Getting statements into an absolute true/false mode sometimes requires convolutions such as double-negatives. Extreme controversy over 'correction for guessing' as random choice of options results in 50 per cent score. Rapidly waning in popularity.	Can test range of knowledge in limited testing time. Machine scoreable. True/False requirement restricts applicability and engenders artificiality.
1b MCQ – 1 from N. Typically a short statement or brief paragraph followed by several (3–6) options. Candidates are asked to identify the option that best fits with or is the best outcome for the initial statement.	Recognition of consonance between two facts, attributes or concepts. Can reflect basic clinical decisions, basic science or hypothesis generation.	Easier to write than MCQ T/F. Choosing one best answer is more salient to most areas of medicine.	The number used in most assessments can lead to cross cueing. Need not involve a correction for guessing.	Efficient sampling of knowledge. Allow more subtle distinctions than T/F types. Machine scoreable.
1c MCQ – Extended matching. Typically a topic area (e.g. Headache), followed by many (6–26) options homogenous to a clinical grouping (e.g. diagnosis). There is a linked question asking candidates to choose the most likely diagnosis. Then one or more paragraphs each comprising a clinical case vignette, including e.g. headache presentation at various stages of progression each of which may indicate different 'best' diagnoses.	Recognition of consonance between (typically) clinical presentations and their underlying pathology, investigation and outcome; diagnoses, prognoses, tests, pharmacology etc Items appear to involve basic clinical reasoning. Students report fidelity to 'real' medicine.	Relatively easy to generate first drafts. Salient to most areas of medicine that depend on a clinical context.	Not easy to write in some areas of medicine, especially non-clinical ones, e.g. epidemiology. Some argue that the 'extended' list of options is not as useful as first thought – many options are redundant.	Seem to be more reliable than one-best-answer MCQs and T/F MCQs, due to increased difficulty. No corrections for guessing needed. Good discriminators at higher levels of ability.

(Continued)

BOX 19.1 (*Continued*)

Method	Domain Usage/Response Mode	Design Factors	Limitations	Strengths
Selected Response Modes				
2d MCQ – Script Concordance Typically a case vignette followed, for example in items on diagnosis, by statements that give an additional sign or symptom and a question that asks whether a specific diagnosis would be more or less likely if such an attribute were present in the case (*see* example in text) . For example, given a description of a 67-year-old man with chest pain, if pain radiating down the left arm were present, would the likelihood of myocardial infarction be 'strongly increased, ... , strongly decreased'.	Recognition of relationship between, and agreement with an expert group on, attributes of case presentations that are predictive of diagnoses, prognoses, findings on investigation, etc. Appears to involve basic clinical reasoning and personal probabilities.	New type of item, limited experience available of construction. Scoring generated by expert group. May have more than one answer that scores marks. Appears to discriminate effectively between experts and non-experts in some specialties.	Probably limited to diagnostic and prognostic decisions	More research needed, but does show high construct validity for clinical experience. Writing protocols and rules still in development.
Constructed and Selected Response				
1. Short Answer – Key Features. Usually a short case vignette followed by between one and three questions that investigate the taker's knowledge of the main aspects of the case. Answers may be constructed or selected, usually requiring words or short phrases.	Answers that attempt to focus **only** on the critical aspects of clinical cases e.g. key decisions and the factors underpinning those. Developed (1990's) to counter arguments that short answers led to isolated recall of facts and trivialisation. Context provided by the question.	Strict rules for design, done usually by a small team. Items may involve some **selected** responses as well as **constructed** ones. Can explore wide variety of cases. Can match response mode to attributes of the context – e.g. selecting the most important features in clinical investigation results. Shares some properties of Modified Essay Questions.	Scoring and standard-setting can be complex. For example, single word answers are common, there may be several answers to one question each differentially weighted. There may be totally inappropriate or dangerous answers given by test takers. Can be challenging to avoid cueing between different parts of the item.	Partial scoring by machine is now becoming a reality. Can replace MCQ style questions where recall is thought to be important (e.g. decisions based on core knowledge and experience). Has embedded quickly into assessment technology in medicine.

BOX 19.2 Words that can be used to drive learners towards certain cognitive processes

analyse	diagnose	justify
apply	explain	match
classify	evaluate	plan
compare	generate	predict
compose	identify	propose
defend	infer	summarise
develop	interpret	synthesise

BOX 19.3 Example: Guidelines for Scoring of Resident/Medical Student Essays

A. Content (25%)
Reviews major and relevant articles for topic
Content is Current; Content is Accurate
Thorough; sufficient detail to understand issues being discussed
Articles cited are salient to the discussion

B. Critical review (15%)
Critique of methodology used in studies cited
Assesses quality of studies cited and compares to population of interest
Presents differing views; compares and contrasts

C. Conclusion/Synthesis (25%)
Synthesises data presented
Clear recommendations with clinical and/or research implications; includes implications for clinical practice
Conclusions are based on critique

D. Organisation (20%)
Title reflects content of paper
Presence of an abstract and summary
Abstract is reflective of the paper; not simply a repeat of the introduction
Introduction includes statement of what will be covered in the essay
Sections follow each other in a logical order with use of headings and sub-headings

E. Style (15%)
Formal scientific writing style
Easy to read and follow line of thought.
Uses plain English, good sentence length, and good use of paragraphs
Avoids unnecessary jargon.

Adapted from Canadian Association for Physical Medicine, with permission

---

covered in the essay. And a model answer can help minimise extraneous variance from different examiners' perceptions or biases. For example, marking can be influenced by better or worse answers coming adjacent to the answer you have scored. This is minimised by grade boundary model answers; you can check where the current essay stands in relation to them. Another trick, if there are no model answers available, is to scan all the answers you have briefly before you start and pick out what appears to be a good, middle and poor answer as the first three you mark. If marking in a pair, sharing these same three essays can be useful as calibration.

Where students each write an individual assignment on a pre-assigned or selected topic, it may not be possible to have a model answer (there would have to be as many models as there are questions/students). In this case a process-based framework can be used (*see* Box 19.3). Papers should be marked anonymously. A procedure needs to be in place to address wide marking variations within one question.

Assessors are frequently urged to use the complete scoring range and avoid centralising tendencies. However, health profession students tend to be very high achievers, so it is not uncommon to have skewed distributions on tests. If high scores seem warranted, they should be given.

There are constraints on the essay. Many clinical teachers do not regard them as relevant, but others suggest that they give training in marshalling arguments and practice in writing. However, the practice that essays give may be that of 'bad' writing – rushed, unedited, poorly planned (because of time constraints) and incompletely organised.(29) Many authors like to let the issues sit in their minds for some time before launching into print (like the author of this article), but that is not possible in an examination essay and may be difficult even in a seen paper.

An essay question does not necessarily assess higher-order cognitive skills. It often merely assesses recall, dressed up as something more profound. This happens in two ways, caused either by the students or the teacher. Students can memorise vast tracts. Asking students how they went about answering the questions in a debriefing session will assist you in deciding how your essays performed. However, beware the bright student who unwittingly uses memory and reports he/she is 'thinking'. If you design an essay question meant to assess higher-order processing but then arrange the scoring framework in a way that allots marks to recall, or biases towards recall processes, you are not assessing higher-order cognition.

Finally, the major disadvantage of the traditional essay is that it samples a small area in depth and this restricts inferences that you can make, about a person's competence, to those specific areas.

Where's the evidence for essays?

There is a great deal of evidence about the impact of construct-irrelevant variance on essay and other qualitative assessments; however, little of this comes from tertiary sector medical and health sciences. Experiments that change the quality of writing but not the content show moderate influences of style or construction factors on assessments of language and writing, but not for other content areas such as science and mathematics.(30) In addition:

Content scores do not seem to be appreciably affected by writing style when the scoring is done by teachers who have been trained by scoring professionals. Ratings in reading, social studies, science, and mathematics should be unaffected by writing style, and the results indicate that the scorers were reasonably successful at assessing the content of these responses without meaningful confounding with writing style.(30, p. 26)

In a study on law essays, agreement amongst law professors in how they graded a single typical essay was 0.58 (intraclass correlation).(31) However, although the basis for this agreement was not investigated, and it was not clear in the paper whether these essays were marked anonymously, assessors' marks were higher for longer answers and for those written by brighter (higher grade point average) students. Notably, the measures of length of essay and intellectual ability were unrelated. However, a combination of these two factors yielded a very high correlation with the assessors' grades. In other words, longer essays were marked higher even if written by the poorer students, and long essays by more able students attracted even higher marks. Markers who had no law training generally assigned the same grades to the papers as did the law professors. It appeared, therefore, that both professors and lay markers could and did identify and reward those papers that presented a persuasive 'common sense' answer to the question.

A more refined study showed that the amount that a student wrote on major issues, the use of jargon, the use of transitional phrases and quality handwriting all had significant positive correlations with grade, and grammatical and construction errors both had significant negative ones.(32) Two further predictors of success were 'strength of argument for conclusions reached' and 'tendency to argue both sides of an issue'. In further studies quality of handwriting has been confirmed to be a factor.(33) However, on the whole handwritten essays tend to score higher than computer-generated ones.(34)

An experimental study of structuring the essay question in medicine showed that the reliability of the structured questions was higher, due to the reduced variance between examiners in this format, and the better agreement between scores on individual questions in the structured format.(35)

Modified essay questions

A modified essay question (MEQ) consists of a brief scenario or clinical vignette, followed by one or more short but searching questions. Test takers are required to construct answers, usually of a paragraph or two. Each question is designed to test a wide range of issues and the ability to think rationally and laterally. By way of illustration (and with acknowledgement to the UK Royal College of General Practitioners) here are two examples.

- *Daisy Boyd, aged 68 years, arrives late for her routine appointment smelling of urine. How would you manage this situation?*

The question could contain issues as diverse as the management of incontinence through to the management of time and the doctor's own feelings.

- *Mike Hornby, aged 44 years, is in the terminal phase of motor neurone disease. He says, 'Will you help me when the time comes?' What factors influence your response?*

Such a question could raise clinical, ethical, legal, referral and personal issues. It may require further qualification to limit the range of answers to the areas you want, or the length of response to one that could be reliably scored.

The MEQ was first developed in Australia and the UK to overcome the major restrictions of sampling and scoring pertaining to the traditional essay and to the now largely disused 'patient-management-problem' (PMP). The PMP had some potentially useful attributes; the technique required the candidate to fully explore a case from initial diagnosis to management and follow-up, through a series of largely selected responses. However, it was dogged by psychometric inadequacies.(36) The MEQ allows exploration of different aspects of a case, but using mostly constructed responses. Initially, whole cases were followed through, but the impact of cueing in this format is high and, in general, the principle now is to explore candidates' knowledge of cases and management through a wider sampling of content. There is a broad literature on MEQs,(37,38) and they are ideally suited to computer administration and response collection, and soon may be marked by computers.

The major difficulty involves the same issues that apply to essay marking – there is variability between markers on most constructed response types of question,(39,40) and score weighting can be problematic. Also because cueing is so difficult to eradicate in an MEQ, many assessment developers limit the scope of each clinical problem to just one or two issues, so that dealing with a whole case across a time frame (one of the original arguments for using MEQs) becomes impossible. This can be circumvented by computer presentation of the segments of the MEQ.

Constructing an MEQ

Decide first on the type of objectives that you wish to assess – diagnosis, decision-making, patient or self-management. In the example MEQs, the designer was looking for affective and professional components of the encounters as well as cognitive ones. With some examinees this requirement may need signposting more clearly.

Decide how far it is possible to delve down into the specific case without risking cueing and avoid vaguely worded questions. To illustrate these points here is a deliberately flawed example.

- *Mrs Brown, a 38-year old primary school teacher, complains about fatigue and tachycardia. She has been admitted to the general medical unit on which you work, for further investigation.*

Question 1: What are the three most likely diagnoses?
Question 2: List five specific questions which would help you distinguish between these possibilities.

- *A routine blood test reveals microcytic hypochromic anaemia with a haemoglobin level of 9.8 g/dl.*

Question 3: List two typical signs you would look for when you examine the patient.
Question 4: Did this information affect your first diagnosis? If yes, how (explain briefly)?

In this example, computer delivery, or physical removal of the answers, first, to Question 1, and then 2, before giving the information about anaemia and asking candidates Questions 3 and 4, would be required to avoid both backward and forward cueing. Q1 and Q2 test broad knowledge of such clinical presentations and initial diagnostic strategy. They require understanding of the clinical significance of the scenario. Question 3 tests linkage between data from investigation (that may not have been initially considered by a test taker) and subsequent questioning. Question 4 is vague and open to misinterpretation – for example, Question 1 asks for three likely diagnoses – which one does question 4 refer to? Is the test taker supposed to assume certain positive or negative outcomes from their examination of signs in Question 3? What does 'information' mean in Q4? What does 'affect' mean? What is the designer's rationale for asking Q3 after the delivery of the information about the blood test? Would this information be better after Q3?

Where's the evidence for MEQs?

Psychometric studies done on the MEQ in the 1980s showed that reliabilities ranged between 0.43 and 0.90 (Cronbach's alpha) for a 60-item test, depending on the content area.(38) However, one study suggested that over 50 per cent of MEQ items in a general test for undergraduates in medicine and surgery tested nothing more than factual recall.(39) This contrasts with the rationale for MEQs that emphasises their ability to reflect analysis, interpretation and clinical decision-making. A more recent study in the same institution has resulted in the removal of the MEQ from the undergraduate assessment programme.(40)

Short-answer question

Many educators use short-answer questions (SAQs) in some form. Frequently, they are used as means of gauging students' factual knowledge or understanding – for example, in lectures and ward rounds. In the verbal form they tend to be quite short, asking for one word or a few alternative answers, within a specific context, as in the following example:

- What is the most common feature of diabetic retinopathy we are likely to see in this patient?

The other major use of short-answer questions is in assessments. Various forms exist requiring the test-taker to complete the sentence or supply a missing line (a 'cloze test'), give short descriptive or analytical answers, or annotate diagrams. Such questions can demand a wide range of responses, from one or several words, a paragraph, to more than a page. The different forms of SAQ provide for great versatility in usage, but make classification difficult. An individual question can be used to assess a specific objective and unlike multiple-choice questions, short-answer questions have the advantage of requiring students to construct an answer, rather than choosing (or guessing) from provided options, so avoiding cueing (at least when SAQs are used sparingly).

SAQs are easier to mark than essay questions and usually involve a structured marking sheet that indicates all possible answers, and ones that should or should not get credit. Marking sheets should also indicate whether spelling needs to be perfect or which common misspellings are acceptable. One-word answers are computer scoreable. Currently programs are being developed for scoring that involves longer answers.(41)

Items should be marked with assessors blind to the identity of candidates and different markers allocated to different questions or sets of questions. In this way, examiner bias is diluted for each candidate. Some assessors report that having the marking done at one time in a large room with all examiners able to talk to each other as unexpected responses are discovered is beneficial to efficient and equitable scoring. Test designers need to be prepared to accept answers not on the score sheet, some of which may or may not have been predicted. There will need to be a system for referring these to the test convenor or committee – do not allow discretion at the marker level, some markers may be unable to make this judgement.

Marking poses the major difficulties with this form of assessment, although there is variability between markers on most constructed response types of question. Increasing the number of markers and number of questions can ameliorate the problem, but is frequently impractical.(42,43) Many educators allege that SAQs reduce the likelihood that students will look for the relations between objectives or sections of the subject whilst studying, and that complex issues cannot always be satisfactorily addressed in short answers. However, there is little empirical evidence for these assertions.

Constructing an SAQ

- Identify the specific learning objectives the item will cover. These are generally in the area of factual recall, comprehension, application or analysis. Higher levels such as evaluation or synthesis will probably require a longer test format, such as a modified essay.
- Choose the most appropriate SAQ format for the objective – a cloze or completion item, an open one-word or phrase answer, a series of answers or a question that requires a short paragraph.
- State the item concisely in clear, unambiguous simple language. A good SAQ tests factual knowledge or capacity to analyse and clinically interpret a scenario. Introducing an element of the test taker's ability to make sense of the question introduces construct-irrelevant variance into the assessment.
- Look at the draft item from a number of different perspectives – mentally try out adequate and inadequate responses. Ideally, an item aimed at one fact should have just one answer, and one aimed at alternatives (e.g. differential diagnoses) should have as many as are appropriate. However, what you may think of as a clear, straightforward question may frequently be answered in multiple ways, depending on how the reader reads it.
- It is good practice to give the test taker an indication of the length of answer required.
- Indicate how many marks are available for the question.
- Some research suggests that items asking for positive perspectives (e.g. knowing the best method, describing

good practice or identifying the most relevant facts) have greater educational significance (e.g. in terms of capacity to measure objectives) than knowing the poorest method, unsatisfactory practice or the least relevant issues. However, clinical science sometimes depends on the capacity to rule out rare or unlikely occurrences, so research done in general educational settings may not always apply in the health context. If you have to word an item negatively, it is advisable to use some form of emphasis for the negative words (e.g. 'What is *not* an appropriate management option in this situation?'), using italics, bold type or underlining to stress this for the test taker.

- Try to avoid grammatical cues to the answer or providing answer spaces that are equal or proportional to the lengths of the required responses.
- Where a numerical answer has to be supplied, for example from a calculation based on clinical data, indicate that both;
  a) the degree of precision expected (e.g. give your answer to one decimal place and answers within 5% of the correct value will be given credit) and
  b) the appropriate units must be indicated.

Not doing this will result in uncertainty for markers about whether the answers supplied are acceptable or not.

Where's the evidence for SAQs?

There is very little research on short-answer questions, particularly in medicine. However, there is some evidence from secondary education that constructed response short-answer questions measure exactly the same thing as MCQ items, as long as the stems are the same.(44) In other words, the cognitive task set to the test taker is more important than the response format. However, once the task diverges, even in the same content domain, the correlation between the two forms falls off. Also, SAQs are more reliably scored than essays,(45,46) largely because the pitfalls of scoring lengthy answers are avoided, and because SAQs can sample more widely in a given time. In addition, using SAQs may reduce the reported differences between men and women, and black and white racial groups on propensity to omit items in MCQ tests.(47) In medicine SAQs have successfully been used as a reliable alternative to MCQ items in a progress test in the Netherlands.(48) One study showed that SAQ tests could produce better retention of information over time, as long as the delayed test was a short-answer test. There was no difference between groups if the test was an MCQ test.(49)

Selected response formats

Multiple-choice questions: Multiple true/false formats

Multiple-choice testing was once seen as an enduring solution to the reliable and valid measurement of knowledge in 'knowledge rich' or knowledge-dependent environments such as medicine, bioscience and engineering. Invented in 1914 by Frederick Kelly, head of a training school in Kansas, USA, by 1926 the multiple-choice test had become the rite of passage for entering post-secondary edu-

---

BOX 19.4 Example of a multiple true/false item

Stem	Options	
The following present as chronic (>3 months) airspace disease on a chest radiograph.	A. Streptococcal pneumonia	T/F
	B. Adult respiratory distress syndrome	T/F
	C. Pulmonary oedema	T/F
	D. Asbestosis	T/F

---

cation in the USA. The MCQ was developed into several forms. One of these is the multiple true/false item, called an 'X type' item in North America, which has become a significant feature of assessment of knowledge in medicine and many other professions over the last 50 years.

In essence, an MCQ is a question that proffers several answers from which the correct one or ones must be chosen. In multiple true/false types a set of options, usually four to six, is given of which each can be either true or false, and the candidate is required to indicate which is correct for each option. An example is shown in Box 19.4.

Over the last few years the multiple true/false item has received a good deal of critical attention. Many examining bodies (for example, the National Board of Medical Examiners (NBME) in the USA) have given up using it altogether. The main reasons have been elucidated with a good deal of empirical evidence.(26) In brief, Case and Swanson(26) state that:

- the distinction between 'true' and 'false' is not always clear, and it is not uncommon for subsequent reviewers to alter the answer key
- reviewers rewrite or discard true/false items far more frequently than items written in other formats
- some ambiguities can be clarified, but others cannot
- to avoid ambiguity, item writers are pushed toward assessing recall of an isolated fact, which is not desirable in most testing situations
- application of knowledge, integration, synthesis and judgement questions can better be assessed by one-best-answer questions.

It is also the case that using true/false restricts the choice of answers, as discussed in the NBME guidance,(26) to a sub-set that can best be classified as completely true all of the time or completely false all of the time. For this reason this author will strongly recommend not using this type of item.

Multiple choice questions: Single-best answer

In single-best-answer questions a stem question asks the test taker to choose the one best answer typically from a set of four-to-five options. An example, taken from the NBME guidance,(26) is given in Box 19.5.

MCQ items are usually scored optically or directly by computer. There are standard programs for marking and analysing test data straight from a scanner. The answer 'key' – a line of data containing the correct option for each

BOX 19.5 Example of a one best answer item.
(26, p. 38)

Stem	Options
A 65-year-old man has difficulty rising from a seated position and straightening his trunk, but he has no difficulty flexing his leg. Which of the following muscles is most likely to have been injured?	**A.** Gluteus maximus **B.** Gluteus minimus **C.** Hamstrings **D.** Iliopsoas **E.** Obturator internus

item – is used in this process and should be double', or even triple-, checked before use. The most common reason for problems at the marking or item analysis stage is a key that contains wrong answers. This may be because the answer has been wrongly transcribed from the item writer's design or (and this not as rare as it should be) because he/she has not provided the best answer.

Most MCQs are scored 1 or 0 for correct or incorrect answers, respectively. Weighting is not necessary for best-answer items; it has very little impact on rankings of students and can reduce reliability. A so-called 'correction for guessing' need not be used.(50)

How to construct a single-best-answer question

Writing multiple-choice items involves following a series of basic rules that, for the most part, apply to all types. A sensible approach to item construction is to have item-writing workshops that force item writers to work in small groups(2,3) and then have their items immediately reviewed by a larger group. During the workshops the rules are as follows and *should* be applied as a test to each of the items that you construct. Each item should pass *all* the rules.

- Focus on an important (non-trivial) concept, typically a common or potentially serious clinical problem. Avoid trivial, 'tricky', or overly complex questions.
- Focus on how knowledge is applied to a clinical situation, not on recognising an isolated fact or association between concept and exemplar.
- The stem must state a clear question, and it should be possible to arrive at an answer with the options covered (the cover test). To determine if the question is clearly focused, cover up the options and read the stem to make sure it is lucid and that other item designers can supply an answer dependent only on reading the stem.
- All distractors and the correct answer should be homogeneous, that is, they should fall into the same category. For example, in an anatomy question all answers should be the same type of structure – bones, vessels, nerves, etc. In a clinical item they should all be diagnoses, tests, treatments, prognoses, and so on.
- All distractors should be salient and plausible. Order the options in numeric, or in alphabetical order (*see* Box 19.5).

- Try to write questions of moderate difficulty – if any of the item constructors have a problem with the item it is probably too difficult. Make sure the correct answer has a sufficiently different degree of correctness, when compared to the distractors across all the conditions identified in the stem. For example, let's assume we are testing knowledge of a condition that affects men, usually in later life. If an incorrect option (distractor) is a diagnosis that does sometimes occur in the age group that the question stem has identified, and the correct answer is one of the rarer diagnoses, the two options may not be far enough apart to make a distinction clear.
- Avoid technical item flaws. For example, all items and options should be grammatically consistent, logically compatible, and of the same (relative) length as the correct answer.
- Writing questions of the form 'Which of the following is correct?' followed by a set of brief, possibly unrelated postulates, one of which is correct, is not advisable. It is basically a true/false item masquerading as a one best answer. Furthermore, it is a good way of ensuring that the questions do focus on trivia. These questions will not be directed at course objectives in a coherent fashion and will contain multiple heterogeneous options.

Where's the evidence for MCQs?

There is far too much research on MCQs to summarise in this chapter. The interested reader should look at recent evidence based guidelines by Wood,(15) Downing(51) and Haladyna *et al.*(52) for comprehensive treatments of many issues. One interesting fact to emerge is that the number of options to use in a one-best-answer item for maximal reliability is more likely to be 2 or 3 than 4 or 5. There is long-standing theoretical and empirical evidence to support this position.(53) This is because this effect is generated when the additional distractors, usually put in to make up or provide a standard number of options are not performing adequately. In items where the 4 or 5 distractors are operating effectively, the item tends to have increased reliability, but this situation is unusual. There is also contradictory evidence that extended matching question distractors, usually a naturally occurring fairly large set of 10–15 (*see* below), may operate more effectively than 3 or 4 pre-selected ones.(26,54) We would hope that the processes that students use to answer one-best-answer MCQ items are at least analytical and at best reasoning-rich. However, evidence suggests that 'the problem with multiple-choice items is not that they are mere exercises in recognition, but that we are unable to predict the processes that will be evoked'.(55, p. S9)

Extended matching questions

Extended matching questions (EMQs) were developed in the early 1990s.(26) However, the kernel of the idea was first conceived by Sue Case in her PhD thesis as early as 1983.(56) She and David Swanson are credited with most of the development work on this format, whilst at the National Board of Medical Examiners. An EMQ is a selected response item in which the item stem has been extended, usually, to a short clinical vignette or scenario and the

BOX 19.6 Example of an extended matching item

Area: Abdominal pain – Diagnosis

Options

A. Abdominal aneurysm	K. Kidney stone
B. Appendicitis	L. Mesenteric adenitis
C. Bowel obstruction	M. Mesenteric artery thrombosis
D. Cholecystitis	N. Ovarian cyst – ruptured
E. Colon cancer	O. Pancreatitis
F. Constipation	P. Pelvic inflammatory disease
G. Diverticulitis	Q. Peptic ulcer disease
H. Ectopic pregnancy – ruptured	R. Perforated peptic ulcer
I. Endometriosis	S. Pyelonephritis
J. Hernia	T. Torsion

Lead In: *For each patient with abdominal pain described below, select the most likely diagnosis.*

Scenario/Stem: A 25-year-old woman has sudden onset of persistent right lower abdominal pain that is increasing in severity. She has nausea without vomiting. She had a normal bowel movement just before onset of pain. Examination shows exquisite deep tenderness to palpation in right lower abdomen with guarding but no rebound; bowel sounds are present. Pelvic examination shows a 7-cm, exquisitely tender right-sided mass. Hematocrit is 32%. Leukocyte count is 18,000/mm3. Serum amylase activity is within normal limits. Test of the stool for occult blood is negative.

Answer: __

[Next scenario in the domain (diagnosis of abdominal pain) would appear here.]

Source: National Board of Medical Examiners(26)

choices have been extended to include all potentially acceptable ones for the clinical problem or issue that is being addressed by the item. This format was originally targeted towards the application of clinical knowledge to diagnostic and management problems, but has been extended to other areas such as basic science. In the example, in Box 19.6 there are 20 options pertaining to the theme of diagnosis of abdominal pain. This is followed by one or more clinical vignettes. The options are all causes of abdominal pain. It is usual in such items to attempt to make all the questions and options homogenous in this way, so other issues concerning abdominal pain, such as initial management or investigations, are not included. An item should focus on a specific area of clinical cognitive activity that pertains to a specific phase of the clinical process – in this case diagnosis.

EMQs are usually scored 1 for a correct response and 0 for an incorrect one. It is sometimes possible to have more than one best answer – for example, when two (or more) diagnoses are equally likely, given the information in the vignette. However, the scoring of these requires more attention during the scanning process, as for optical scoring two

(or more) passes of the score sheets are necessary with each correct answer keyed on each pass. Unless it is clinically important to be able to recognise both potential diagnoses from the same vignette, such multiple responses are probably best avoided (for example, by removing one of the options from the list).

Investigations of the reliability and construct validity of EMQs suggest that they have good measurement properties, and correlate well with other measures of recall, recognition and cognitive functioning.(57) Recently, studies of experts and novices who talk aloud whilst trying to complete EMQ items have strongly suggested that EMQs have good construct validity for, and can be reliably used to assess, clinical reasoning,(58) even though novice and experts approach the same item with different strategies (backwards vs. forwards reasoning, respectively).(59) Furthermore, when used in pathology EMQs are more reliable, better discriminate the competent from the borderline student, and can be written definitively to test core content.(60)

EMQs seem to be easier to write than true/false or other types of one-best-answer items, because in that style of item the convolutions that writers go through to reduce the item set to a smaller number where each is true or false, or there is clearly one best answer, are not needed.(61) Clinicians from some disciplines such as public health, epidemiology and statistics have suggested that EMQs are difficult to write for these content domains, but recent articles suggest they have been adopted or are being developed in some of these hitherto unexplored areas (e.g. psychiatry(62)).

How to construct an EMQ

It is best to write these items first by considering the area or domain of the assessment blueprint for which items need to be written (e.g. abdominal pain in Box 19.6). Then a general question is posed, followed by all the possible answers to that question (e.g. 'What are the causes of abdominal pain in adults?'). After these have been identified, scenarios that pertain to one or more of the answers are constructed. Ideally, create items (particularly the stems/scenarios) in pairs of writers, at workshops of about 8–12 people in total (4–6 pairs), with review every two hours or so in a larger group. This is an effective, and in most examiners' experience, an enjoyable way of generating items. The stages are as follows.

- *Identify the domain or subject for the set.* The domain is an area of cognitive activity (e.g. diagnosis, management planning). The subject can be a presenting complaint in a body system or systems (e.g. abdominal pain, so that diagnosis is the focus of the item), or a pre-diagnosed condition (e.g. community-acquired pneumonia, so that management is the focus of the item). Sometimes it might be appropriate to move directly from a non-diagnosed presenting complaint (e.g. abdominal pain) to an investigative option (e.g. ultrasound) or management plan (e.g. restricted diet). However, the more cognitive steps involved in moving between the presenting complaint and the focus of the item (e.g. asking about management), the less will be known about why an examinee might have answered the item incorrectly. For example, the examinee might have thought a patient with ulcerative colitis had appendicitis and ordered surgical intervention.

- *Write the lead-in for the set* (e.g. *for each patient described below, select the most likely diagnosis* (Box 19.6)). The lead-in indicates the relationship between the stems and options. It must be a clear question for examinees. It is an essential component of an extended-matching set. Sometimes two lead-ins can be written at the same time – for example, one based on diagnosis and one on indications for investigations or management. Subsequent scenarios can be used, usually with only minor modification, with either lead-in. In summary, the lead-in should consist of a single, clearly formulated task so that the examinee could, if necessary, create an answer without looking at the options.
- *Prepare the list of options.* The list of options should be single words or very short phrases. This list is best developed in a whole-group format. It will be generated in a fairly random order, but the options should be rearranged in alphabetical order for the final item presentation. For example, the initial list for Box 19.6 should contain all the likely causes of abdominal pain as options. Sometimes there are specific causes that occur only or predominantly in a particular subset of the population – for example, in women (e.g. ectopic pregnancy), in men (testicular torsion), in the elderly (dementia). Such options can sometimes become 'zebras',(26) which stand out as so obviously applying to one subgroup of patients that their inclusion is ill advised. In Box 19.6 there are some such options, but there are also sufficient important differential diagnoses in the list to warrant their inclusion for the given scenario.
- *Write the stems.* The stems (items) within a set should be similar in structure. Most often, patient vignettes are appropriate. The scenario should contain all the information that one would normally expect to be available from any conscious patient: the presenting problem, the history (including duration of signs and symptoms), the physical findings, and then the results of any immediate diagnostic tests carried out. Sometimes, for a complex case, further data pertaining to development of symptoms over several days might also be given – for example, initial management and subsequent clinical changes. Scenarios can include a smaller set of information, but it is unwise to exclude the information that would normally be collected by or available to the test taker in the real clinical context at the time they were seeing this patient. Specifying this information in a standardised order makes shorter reading time and hence allows more items to be delivered in a given time.
- *Review the items.* Make sure there is only one 'best' answer for each question. Having two right answers is possible, but entails more marking effort than it is usually worth. Also make sure that there are at least four reasonable distractors for each item to minimise guessing effects. Evaluate the extent to which the lead-in clearly formulated task. See if the other examiners can create an answer without looking at the options. Satisfying this

'cover-the-options' rule is an important feature of a good question because, if the examinee cannot do that, it means the question is too vague, is not appropriately targeted to the skills the examination is testing, or exhibits some other flaw of test writing. As a final check, review the items (without the correct answer indicated) across other pairs in the writing group. If the pair has difficulty determining the correct answer, modify the option list or the item to eliminate the ambiguity.

Where's the evidence for EMQs?

There is evidence that some MCQs, of which the EMQ type seems to be the most suited to clinical tasks, can involve substantially more than recognition of knowledge learnt by rote memorisation.(55) These authors nevertheless suggest that unfocused items or those with negatively worded stems, as sometimes, of necessity, occur in the typical true/false or best of five types, do not appear to provoke problem-solving skills and forward-reasoning. Whilst the evidence for the link between item type and cognitive response is being developed, they suggest concentrating on items that are low-fidelity simulations of clinical situations with examinee tasks that are relevant for them (e.g. diagnosis and management). EMQs are ideally suited to this role. EMQs also substantially reduce the likelihood of obtaining a correct answer by chance alone.

Although this area is fraught with controversy, and not all of the options provided for any one EMQ stem will be active for that item, modelling suggests that EMQs with between 7 and 12 active distractors will provide good insulation against the need to be concerned about the so called 'guessing' factor in multiple-choice tests.(63) Research on EMQ formats has shown that a reduction in the length of item option lists, from the 15–20 previously thought necessary, is possible without much, if any, deleterious effects on item quality.(64,65) Eight options seem to be a reasonable minimum number. In general, items with more options are more difficult, require more time to complete, and nevertheless have similar discriminating properties to items with eight options. Reducing the whole list to a 'shortlist' of eight or so can be done by carefully constructing physician panels to select the most appropriate set. Moreover, providing the panel with item response statistics from the long item does not seem to improve option selection. The use of a smaller number of options reduces time spent on each item by candidates and therefore increases the number of items that can be used in a set time.(64,65) Swanson *et al.* advised, 'We plan to begin advising [examiners] to reduce the number of options included on option lists in order to make more efficient use of testing time'.(64, p. S95) That advice may now be prudent to implement, as student numbers in medical schools have increased dramatically in a number of countries in the last few years.

Script concordance items

Over the last 15 years interest has developed in constructing a multiple-choice test that can reflect clinicians' capacity to weigh evidence in a clinical encounter. This work has its foundations in a clearer understanding of how clinicians approach the diagnostic task and how this information is remembered.(66,67) Recently, this work has expanded dramatically; in the last five years more papers on this issue have been published than in the previous 15. The reason for this is probably that the value of appropriately and efficiently stored knowledge in clinical decision-making, and the need to assess these cognitive processes, have been accentuated through literature on poor decision-making and its relationship to patient safety.

Memory for clinically important information is developed in stages. As a student, possibly because of the pre-clinical/clinical divide in most educational programmes, biomedical knowledge dominates. Additional insight into clinical problems develops, as students gain more experience with patients and elaborate their knowledge into explanatory frameworks and linkages between symptoms, causes, basic mechanisms and management. With more experience of patients, these frameworks depend less on biomedical detail and more on 'illness scripts' that involve applied (functional) knowledge and relate to both common (easy) and uncommon (more difficult) patient presentations. Eventually 'owners' of these illness scripts use them to promote rapid recognition of patterns of patient presentation, and reconcile any unfamiliar presentations with previous presentations. However, when a challenging presentation occurs, expert clinicians muster their existing knowledge and strive to activate biomedical principles and knowledge (albeit usually tied to specific patient or contextual exemplars), but these occasions occur less frequently as expertise develops.(68) Previously, attempts to create tests that reflect this process through patient management problems and modified essay questions have foundered, primarily because clinicians disagree about these issues and this, coupled with the variety of constructed responses that such items can generate from the test takers, results in great difficulty in scoring them. Moreover, in a typical MCQ item when the test makers cannot agree on the best answer, either before or after it has been used, the item is usually removed from the test.

However, a group in Canada(67) have devoted a considerable amount of effort to the task of developing an item format that overcomes these problems – this is the script concordance item (SCI).

The SCI is a selected response item that depends on respondents choosing how well pieces of information contribute to a diagnostic or management strategy for a particular clinical problem. As described above, the script is the internal rubric that experts use to classify data and generate or choose a hypothesis quickly. In the SCI, concordance is the congruence of the takers' script with elements of rubrics deemed by 'experts' to be most plausible. The items estimate the relative likelihood of diagnoses, given a certain piece of clinical or biomedical information. The test items ask for choices to be made based on the subjective clinical probabilities of the test takers. However, they are scored in such a way that takes into account the degree of similarity (concordance) between the illness scripts of the test takers and the test makers. An example is shown in Box 19.7.

The marking scheme is based on the performance of an expert group, and there are various ways to derive the

---

BOX 19.7 Example of a script concordance item

A 25-year-old male patient is admitted to the emergency room after a fall from a motorcycle with a direct impact to the pubis. Vital signs are normal. The X-ray reveals a fracture of the pelvis with a disjunction of the pubic symphysis.

If you were thinking of	And then you find	This hypothesis can be rated: (circle best response)
Urethral rupture	Urethral bleeding	−2 −1 0 +1 +2
Retroperitoneal bladder rupture	Bladder distension	−2 −1 0 +1 +2
Urethral rupture	Perineal haematoma	−2 −1 0 +1 +2

Where:

−2 = the hypothesis is almost eliminated;

−1 = the hypothesis becomes less probable;

0 = the information has no effect on the hypothesis;

+1 = the hypothesis has become more probable;

+2 = the hypothesis is very likely to be correct

Source: Charlin et al(67)

---

marks. In one method a consensus is reached between the experts on the best answer for each item. In others, each response attracts a mark that is proportional to the frequency of its choice by the expert group. Recommendations for exactly how this is done vary according to source. Some authors suggest awarding 1 mark for the experts' modal answer and then giving marks for alternatives based on the frequency ratios for the other answers. For example, if a group of 20 experts opted 12, 6 and 2 for the options +2, +1 and 0 respectively in any one item, these options would be awarded 1, 0.5 and 0.167 marks, and the others zero marks. Other sources suggest awarding marks on a percentage distribution basis, so this would work out at 0.6, 0.3 and 0.1 per option for the three 'correct' options.

Another interesting feature of the marking scheme is that it can have more than one reference panel, depending upon the context in which the item is to be used; for example, in a metro or rural environment, a general practice, the emergency department or medical ward. This is because the probabilities of some decisions or hypotheses may change depending on the context.

A test made up of SCIs is therefore a very flexible one, and one capable of rewarding partial or incomplete knowledge to some extent. Data so far suggest that a test composed of SCIs is very efficient; good reliability can be achieved with relatively small numbers of items.(69) The way that SCIs are constructed clearly has implications for how best to use them. They are a specialised item suitable for investigating test takers' ability to formulate and progress specific diagnostic and management decisions.

A systematic review of approaches to SCI development has identified several useful strategies in writing and scoring SCIs,(70) which have implications for reliability and validity. The number of experts needed on the concordance-generating panel has also been researched. Samples of at least ten panelists provided satisfactory internal consistency, and there was little gain when panel sizes exceeded 20. Larger panels give rise to higher cohort mean scores, presumably because the larger the panel, the higher the chance of an option being awarded weight by panelists, especially when the cases intrinsically demonstrate high uncertainty.

In an SCI expert panel, some panelists may act in an idiosyncratic manner with their answer, choosing options that are deviant or clearly incorrect, especially in tests with high degrees of uncertainty. This may concern test-designers or users of the test information, even though credit awarded for these answers is small. Removing some discordant responses or all the responses from deviant or low-scoring panelists (because a low score would suggest that those experts were not so expert after all) has been suggested. However, the psychometric impact of excluding such panelists' responses in score derivation is minimal, as long as the panel has 15+ members. However, if educators wish to remove these answers, the available methods(70) to do so appear equivalent in terms of psychometric consequences.

How to write a script concordance item

An SCI is created in a similar fashion to an EMQ, except that the specific diagnostic decision is the key to the choice of vignette, rather than a list of potential diagnoses, and hence there may be fewer data in an SCI than an EMQ. There are two stages, as follows.

- A vignette is created containing data that present a challenging clinical situation. This is usually text, but other information such as the X-ray from the item in Box 19.7, or other pertinent data such as blood analysis, can be given, depending upon the test takers' clinical decisions that are being investigated. Not all the data needed are provided because these can be revealed as part of the item hypotheses–information links. Each of these clinically relevant pieces of information might help the clinician refine, improve, confirm or eliminate the clinical decisions or hypotheses made about what is happening. The response required from the test taker is to appraise the effect of each piece of new information on their hypothesis.
- Responses are pre-prepared using a five-point scale running from −2 (the hypothesis or decision is much less likely) to +2 (the hypothesis or decision is much more likely). To get the best out of the item, and to sample knowledge broadly, there should be no links (cues) between the different provided responses. Once designed, a group of experienced clinicians complete the SCIs, and their answers are collated. These answers are then used to decide on the marking scheme for scoring items.

Although it would seem relatively easy to design such items, Charlin and Van der Vleuten(71) warn that the expert group writing the items must be familiar with the tool and be able to choose cases that are complex enough to fit with the level of training being assessed. Also the item is designed to assess decision-making that is grounded in evidence, as opposed to received wisdom, so there must be enough data available on the clinical solution to the case and the links provided in the case must be widely known by experts in the area.

Where's the evidence for script concordance items?

For reliability and validity purposes, attention should be paid to both the number of cases sampled in the test and the number of items used per case.(70) In general, sampling between 25 and 36 cases, with approximately three items per case should result in an SCI test with reliability of between 0.75 and 0.86. Adding items (e.g. more than one per case), rather than cases, is more effective in increasing test reliability and can reduce the workload of test designers, but there appears to be a ceiling effect after three or four items per case.

SCIs focus to a large extent on clinical judgement in areas of uncertainty. This is what makes them 'content'- and 'construct'-valid for the measurement of clinical judgement and reasoning. Good construct validity has been shown in a number of studies. SCIs discriminate between different levels of surgical expertise and have also been used in pharmacy education.(72,73)

Because SCIs are used on cases that are often far from clear-cut, this may mean that SCIs are unsuited to junior students with less experience of clinical conundrums than trainees with more clinical experience. Indeed a study comparing SCIs to traditional MCQs showed that interns rated them higher as a method of assessment and also these items' reliability was higher in an intern, as opposed to a medical student, cohort.(74) An SCT test has also been shown to be a useful adjunct to a suite of tests designed to examine the performance of poorly performing doctors.(75)

Formats using both selected and constructed responses

Key-features items

The key-features item (KFI) is a short-answer question that can use both selected and constructed responses. The defining characteristic of a KFI is that it is aimed at assessing whether the test-taker can recognise, deduce or infer the most important features of a clinical problem and, if required, subsequently choose the most salient, urgent and effective management strategies for that clinical problem.(76)

Readers may think that it could be reasonably assumed that all short-answer questions would possess these properties. Unfortunately, in the 1970s and 1980s this was not the case.(77) Curricula and assessments were frequently designed from discipline or specialty perspectives, with each concentrating on unusual or esoteric aspects of their craft in order to discriminate between the truly well-grounded student and the rest. This led to a culture in which trivia, rare morbidity, atypical presentations and specialty specific issues dominated short-answer tests. It was also believed that decision-making skill was generic, so many short-answer tests focused on one or two problems, with the 'short' answers practically exhausting the available knowledge about that problem.(78)

Two researchers, Georges Bordage and Gordon Page coined the term 'key feature' after a critique of and further research on the nature and assessment of clinical decision-making skills.(79) Their central concept was that 'in any clinical case, there are a few unique, essential elements in decision making which, alone or in combination, are the critical steps in the successful resolution of the clinical problem'.(76, p. 1189) With funding from the Medical Council of Canada their concept led to the creation of a new format for assessing decision-making skills. Furthermore, by testing only critical steps, candidates were tested both on important objectives and on a much larger number of clinical problems than was the case with previous formats. A typical key feature item with the scoring key is shown in Box 19.8.

The key features tested by such questions are: a) the ability to synthesise presenting complaints for recognition of an important and life-threatening condition; b) the ability to identify essential areas to investigate in the history to confirm or rule out this hypothesis.

Questions 1 and 2 directly address each of these key features. Each item challenges the candidate to apply his or her knowledge in making clinical decisions. In this item there is a constructed response for Question 1, with only one answer required, and a selection of six options only from a list of 28 for Question 2.

Usually both Q1 and Q2 answers would be written by the test taker on an optical scoring sheet. There would be space for free text to Q1 and buttons or ovals to fill in for Q2.

KFIs require a scoring rubric that reflects the importance of the various key elements of the case. It helps to test out the scoring rubric with colleagues and a few 'dummy' test takers. Higher weighted scores for more important answers should be encouraged. In Box 19.8, the diagnosis was awarded one mark and the elements of the history a total of six marks. The scoring key shows that only seven of the 28 options would be considered appropriate, so the candidate must select six of these to score maximum marks. The question also weights aspects of the history more highly than obtaining the correct diagnosis. This may be because in this situation knowing the best questions to ask would probably result in a change of diagnostic preference, if an inappropriate answer was initially given to Question 1. There are very few question formats that truly assess clinical decision-making, but KFIs can make this claim. Certainly, the foundation work done on the validity and reliability of the format(79) would suggest that KFIs robustly measure these facets of competence, and test takers seem to like their salience to clinical practice. However, KFIs are difficult to construct well, and although scoring seems simple, some questions can be very difficult to weight appropriately. Standard-setting with KFIs can also be complex, as although both the modified Angoff and Ebel methods have been used, some assessors report that they do not work very well for this format. This is because the items are generally multi-dimensional and can include many aspects of a case, some of which are interdependent.

BOX 19.8 Example of key features item

Paul Young, a 56-year-old male, consults you in your surgery because of pain in his left leg which began two days ago and has been getting progressively worse. He states his leg is tender below the knee and swollen around the ankle. He has never had similar problems. His other leg is fine.

Question 1

What is your principal working diagnosis? List, in note form only, your single (1) diagnosis.

Answer 1. . . . .

. . . .

Question 2

To establish your diagnosis, what elements of his history would you particularly want to elicit? Choose up to six (6) from the following list.

1. Activity at onset of symptoms	15. Palpitations
2. Alcohol intake	16. Paraesthesia
3. Allergies	17. Paroxysmal nocturnal dyspnoea
4. Angina pectoris	18. Polydipsia
5. Anti-inflammatory therapy	19. Previous back problems
6. Cigarette smoking	20. Previous knee problems
7. Colour of stools	21. Previous neoplasia
8. Cough	22. Previous urinary tract infection
9. Headache	23. Recent dental procedure
10. Haematemesis	24. Recent immobilisation
11. Impotence	25. Recent sore throat
12. Intermittent claudication	26. Recent surgery
13. Low back pain	27. Wounds on foot
14. Nocturia	28. Wounds on hand

Answer 2

1.   2.   3.   4.   5.   6.

Scoring Key

Question 1

Deep venous thrombosis must be the differential diagnosis (Score 1)

(Total requested = 1. Total accepted = 1 Total score = 1.) More than 1 answer scores zero.

Question 2

Any six (6) of the following items are required:

Activity at onset of symptoms

Cigarette smoking

Previous knee problems

Previous neoplasia

Recent immobilisation

Recent surgery

Wounds on foot

(Each scores 1. Total requested = 6. Total accepted = 6 Total possible score = 6). More than 6 answers scores zero

Source: Royal Australian College of General Practitioners Key Features Practice Paper 2007

Making decisions about how borderline test takers would respond to such items is challenging.

How to write a KFI

- Select a clinical problem from the assessment blueprint in which analysis of the context, identification of clinical conditions and synthesis of the diagnosis and/or management (clinical decisions) are required objectives.
- Think of several real instances of the case in everyday practice. With respect to these cases, consider what the essential (necessary and sufficient) steps are to resolve this problem. This will allow you to focus solely on the most critical decisions for each case. Make an effort to distinguish between decisions or steps that are appropriate, but not critical, and those that are really vital. It can help to elucidate the case's key features by identifying the attributes of or inconsistencies in the presentation that are most likely to result in clinical errors in dealing with the case by the particular test takers.
- Any of the typical cognitive processes used or actions planned can be tested in KFIs – the scope depends on the objectives being tested and the case presentation. For example, framing initial hypotheses, looking for particular clinical findings, choosing tests, management options, or specific drugs are all possible.
- Select one of the real cases for development into a problem scenario and related questions. The attributes of the case can be written according to the same rules as for EMQ items (*see* p. 265), that is age, sex, setting of the encounter. When you have written the scenario, use the key features to frame the questions for the case. Usually only two-to-three questions are possible without invoking prompting or cueing. The more questions are asked about a particular case, the more opportunities arise for cueing. For example, in order to ask about management, further information may need to be given about test results that will strongly imply the diagnosis, so asking about differential diagnosis, history and investigations, management and follow-up all in the same item becomes difficult. (This is the same issue that arises in MCQs, *see* p. 264.)
- Select the response format, or formats – write-in (constructed) or option choice (selected). This needs to be done carefully. The guiding principle is that if the key feature entails a cognitive process that is or should be generated by the professional (e.g. recognition of a myocardial infarction and decision on immediate action), then the response should be write-in. The number of required answers must be stated. This is to inhibit 'blunderbussing' — the tendency of test takers to write down everything they can think of in the hope that the correct answer(s) are included in their responses. Exceeding the number required should be penalised. Write-in items need to be marked, whereas options can be electronically scored.

Where's the evidence for KFIs?

KFIs have been used for both summative and formative assessment in a number of different contexts.(80,81) The reliability of the KFI paper (26 items) of the Royal Austral-ian College of General Practitioners increased from 0.64 in 1999 to around 0.83, in 2005.(83) KFIs were rated adequate on tests of clinical decision-making skills by approximately 90 per cent candidates in the 2004 Fellowship examination. Colo-rectal surgeons (N = 256) found them useful as a means of self-assessment and nine KFIs were almost as reliable as 50 multiple-choice questions (0.95 vs. 0.97, respectively).(81)

Although research on KFIs has not kept pace with that on EMQs and SCIs, it is notable that the generation of key features for a wide range of common priority topics in family medicine has been the focus of work by the College of Family Physicians of Canada over a seven-year period.(83) The purpose of this work was to generate key features for use on other approaches to learning and assessment beyond the specific KFI methodology

Computer-based written assessment

With the advent of accessible computers with high processing power to individual teachers and assessors, a number of the assessments discussed in this chapter can now be designed, delivered and marked on a computer. Even the short-answer questions and perhaps essays will soon be markable by computers. Another feature open to computer-delivered written items is the possibility of individually adaptive tests. Both the NBME and the Australian Medical Council are already using these. Computers deliver items to examinees that are targeted towards candidates' ability level. Further items are titrated by the computer against that individual's difficulty level based on their answers to the previous question(s). This continues until the computer is satisfied (using pre-designed algorithms) that it has reliably identified the candidate's ability level, and it then stops the assessment process. This has enormous potential for delivering tailored assessment, protecting large item data banks from piracy or examinee recall, and being time-efficient because very few examinees would get the same test.

The computer also has the capacity to deliver immediate feedback. This has given rise to a new item format – the F-format – which is currently under development. F-type items(84) have been trialled to fill the gap left by the demise of patient management problems.(77) F-types are essentially a hybrid of extended matching and PMP styles. F-type tests present authentic patient management scenarios that develop over time. Typically, two-to-three test items sit within one case. Each item addresses an objective relating to one or more clinical decisions that could be made during the case. The test items occur in a fixed sequence within the case; items start with patient presentation and end with management or resolution. Because the items within each case reflect the unfolding nature of the case over time, sometimes examinees learn about how successful their previous answers were from subsequent items. Because such cues might affect examinees' decisions, they are not permitted to revise their responses to earlier within-case items; the computer bars their access to going back to change responses. However, examinees can be given or not given feedback (depending on the item) after completing each item. Post-answer feedback on items allows all examinees to be kept on an equal footing, as the case develops. For example, when a clinical scenario is presented, examinees would be asked to identify the most appropriate next step in investigation. On the next test item, the scenario might be presented as if the correct next step had been taken, and the patient is being sent for a further definitive investigation. Presenting this updated information automatically 'gives away' the correct answer to the previous question but may enable someone who has previously answered incorrectly to get back on track with the new context. In this way examinees may improve their understanding of the case and/or be able to answer subsequent items without being disadvantaged by their previous inaccurate perceptions The items types are still in development but look quite promising for areas in which cases can be quite complex or for which it is difficult to write items without cross-item cueing, such as key-feature tests. These enormously exciting developments herald the possibility that there could be a whole new approach to item-writing that uses elements of different formats all in the same item.

Item analysis

After items have been used in a test, we wish to know how well each item has performed. There are two parts to this – first, did the item cover its own cognitive territory appropriately? And second, how did it do in relation to its contribution to the test as a whole? In essence we want to know the following.

(a) Did the item do its job in the understanding of an individual on that particular element of the content of the test? This would include identifying any problems with its construction that led to misinterpretation by test takers. For selected response items, distractors might have been included that did not work effectively, or were too close to the correct response to allow even good candidates to make an appropriate choice.

(b) Did it have demonstrable relationships with the content of other items on the test and with the content of the test as a whole? This would include looking at inter-item correlation, looking at item-test correlation, looking at relationships with other parts of an assessment regime – for example, other assessments of the same domain, and other assessments in different domains, such as procedural skills.

These questions can be answered in a number of ways. One way to approach problem (a) is to read every item on the test again. Of course, most items will have been read many, many times already, and after reading hundreds of items, test designers will have become immune to the potential inadequacies of the items.

Another way is to use basic item analysis. However, all item-analysis data must be interpreted with extreme caution and with reference to the overall purpose of the test. Rules of thumb about deleting or modifying items (for example, based on poor discrimination indexes for items) should probably be avoided.

Many programmes are available to process item data, and most operate in similar ways. The core of item analysis is to look at a set of parameters for each item that describe its performance as an item, its relationship to the test as a whole and its contribution to the performance of the current cohort on that test. In a selected response test such parameters include the following.

- The difficulty of the item – how many takers got the item correct?
- Which of the options were chosen most frequently?
- Which options were chosen by high, medium and low performers on the test as a whole?
- How did success on each item correlate with performance on the test as whole?
- What were the inter-item correlations? (this might be particularly important for short answer and key features questions)

This section demonstrates how to use a typical set of item analysis data to make inferences about these questions. The particular one shown here is from the IDEAL Consortium item analysis software, but many others provide analogous output.

Consider the item in Box 19.9 which is item 87 from a 100-item MCQ Test on Emergency Care for Year 3 Medical Students. A cohort of 148 students (*see* the N for TOTAL in Box 19.10) took this item as part of a 100-item test on emergency management. The item was chosen because it was thought that students needed to be aware of the repeated changes to guidelines over the years and that recognition of the correct guideline was a vital decision. Some previously recommended ratios were included as distractors. The output from the analysis software for this item is shown in Box 19.10

Box 19.10 shows a number of item parameters in the top row, then below this row it can be read as a table comparing the proportions of whole cohort (row TOTAL) and tertile groups' (rows HIGH, MID and LOW) who selected each of the options in the test. The final three rows describe param-

---

BOX 19.9 Example item for analysis (i)

Item 87

In Melbourne, Australia, a man collapses in the presence of a single health care worker who, after careful assessment of the patient, and whilst waiting for the paramedic team, decides to deliver cardio-pulmonary resuscitation (CPR).

Choose the most appropriate ratio for breaths:compressions with which the health worker should commence CPR.

A. 1:30

B. 2:30

C. 2:15

D. 3:15

E. 3:30

*The correct answer (Australian Resuscitation Council Guidelines) is **B**

BOX 19.10 Item analysis data for Item 87

DIF = 0.90, RPB = −0.039, CRPB = −0.075, (95%CON = −0.298, 0.157)
 RBIS = −0.068, CRBIS = −0.130, IRI = −0.012

GROUP	N	INV	NF	OMIT	A	B	C	D	E
TOTAL	148	0	0	0	0.03	0.90	0.01	0.03	0.03
HIGH	38	0			0.05	0.84	0.05	0.05	0.00
MID	64	0			0.00	0.97	0.00	0.00	0.03
LOW	46	0			0.04	0.87	0.00	0.04	0.04
TEST SCORE MEAN %					68	68	79	69	67
DISCRIMINATING POWER (D.P.)					0.01	−0.03	0.05	0.01	−0.04
STANDARD ERROR OF D.P.					0.07	0.11	0.05	0.07	0.05

---

eters of the various groups who selected the different distractors.

Returning to the areas we need to investigate the following.

- Did the item do its job in capturing the understanding of an individual on that particular element of the content of the test?

Well, the item was completed by all test takers. (The values for INV, the number of examinees not providing a valid response to this item, and for OMIT, the number of examinees omitting this item, was zero). Furthermore, the number of examinees not finishing the test from this item onwards (NF) was also zero. Takers did not get 'stuck' answering this item and not have time to finish as a result. As this item was number 87 of 100, we can probably conclude that all candidates finished the test, and we already know that all did this item. Most test takers got it right – 90 per cent in fact, expressed in this table as 'DIF' (the proportion of candidates who got the item right, 0.90. In some data analysis packages the difficulty index is often more appropriately called the 'facility' index). This number also appears in the box for the proportion of the TOTAL test takers who identified B as the correct answer – 0.90 in Column B. So if this item covers core knowledge the indications are that this was achieved in the vast majority of candidates.

How did the item work? Well, as we have seen, there were very few takers who got the item wrong (only 15 of 148; 0.10 as a proportion). The proportions choosing each of the distractors varied between 0.03 and 0.01 (*see* the other proportions in the TOTAL row of the table). Because of the low numbers choosing distracters, it is not possible to confidently say that any one of the distractors was more or less attractive than the others. The TEST SCORE MEAN % is the mean score on the total test of those candidates giving the indicated response to this item. Variation in this row would indicate that perhaps there was one, or more, distractors that was attractive to a high- or low-scoring group. If a particular distractor was chosen by a group that collectively did well on the test overall, there may have been some teaching that impacted on this issue for those students. This may have been the case for the 5 per cent of the cohort choosing C, the old guideline, who collectively

scored 79 per cent on this test. However, the very small numbers involved would make this interpretation risky.

Now we will consider the second issue:

- Did the item have demonstrable relationships with the content of other items on the test and with the content of the test as a whole?

This would include looking at inter-item correlation, and looking at item-test correlation.

RPB is the point bi-serial correlation between item 87 and the score on the whole test, including the present item. Point bi-serial correlations are used to determine the co-variation of a continuous variable (the total score on the test) with one that has a truly dichotomous distribution (in this case item 87). The point bi-serial is mathematically equivalent to a Pearson correlation coefficient in which one variable has only two values. The RPB for this item is almost zero. If the purpose of this test was to make discriminations between individual test takers, there would be a case for excluding this item, because it does not separate good from less good candidates. However, the focus of this item is to assess a core piece of knowledge that everyone should know – which is, in fact, what the item analysis shows the item does.

CRPB is the corrected point bi-serial. In this calculation the present item is removed from the test total, whilst the correlation is calculated. This is done because in some test situations the inclusion of the analysed item (Item 87) in the test total can inflate this value and introduce additional co-variation. This problem is more troublesome when short-answer questions are being analysed. Typically each short answer has a weight greater than 1 mark and so variation in the item can make a large difference to the total score and hence to differences between the corrected and uncorrected versions of the statistic, with the uncorrected score being somewhat inflated (more positive). Even in the data for item 87, we can see considerable variation between the RPB and the CRPB.

RBIS and CRBIS are the 'non-point' versions of the previously discussed correlations. Strictly speaking the bi-serial coefficient is used where the dichotomous variable in fact has an underlying continuity and has been separated or recoded into a dichotomous one. The RBIS and CRBIS are always larger than their respective 'point' values, and may give an inflated value for variables where the continuity does not in fact exist.

IRI is the item's overall reliability index, which is virtually zero. However whether it is retained in future tests depends upon the purpose of the test. As we discussed above, if the test is designed to be a test of competence in decisions around emergency medicine, then excluding all the items on which students scored highly might defeat the object of the test. If the test has some selective purpose – for example, identifying students who might be competing for an elective in emergency medicine in later years – then excluding Item 87 might be appropriate.

In summary, the item is correctly answered by almost all the cohort, has little discriminating power as a predictor of total test score, appears to reflect the possibility that the previous CPR guideline (Option C) was being used by a few individuals, whilst the majority were aware of the new recommendation to use 2:30 in single bystander CPR.

Item analysis is a relatively quick way to identify problems with items, especially when such problems reside with their distractors. It is surprising how often items are identified as having distractors that are chosen by a significant proportion of students and then issues are discovered with the validity of the 'correct' option or with ambiguous wording of the question.

It is crucial that one or more of the group of academics/clinicians who designed the items understand how to interpret item analysis software, and that they appreciate the need to tailor decisions about items to the purpose of the test. Indiscriminate use of the item parameters as a criterion for exclusion is highly undesirable, even though this may appear more 'objective' it will introduce more problems than it solves.

In Box 19.11, we have another item in the test; item 46, and in Box 19.12, the item analysis data for that item. See if you agree with my interpretation.

In brief this shows that there is competition in the cohort's mind as to which is the correct answer with sport and alcohol being the two main contenders, with a minor one, hereditary. The item is not worded particularly well, as the options do not all follow grammatically from the stem. This may introduce some bias in the option choices. It is also double negatively worded. It might have been better to ask, 'Which one of the following is *not* a predisposing factor for osteoarthritis?"

The difficulty is 0.50 – only half the cohort answered the item correctly. As it happens, items with difficulties within the 0.45–0.55 range are usually the most discriminating (this is a mathematical function), although of course they can be negatively discriminating (this is rare in well-chosen content, and is usually the result of an error in keying the correct answer). Here the discrimination is good: nearly half (0.48) of the third tertile chose 'A' as the correct answer, but roughly a tenth (0.11) of the top tertile did too. Perhaps this is because sport is featured so strongly in health promotional literature that some students believe it has few side-effects. Although the item is discriminating, and has good item-test correlations in both corrected and uncorrected versions, one might argue that in an emergency setting this knowledge might be less relevant; perhaps it would be much more appropriate in a musculoskeletal clinic or in general practice assessment. The overall item reliability is good – a test of 100 similar items would provide a highly discriminating test, though with a pass mark of around 50 per cent and may not defensible from a blueprinting perspective. If all such items were of 50 per cent difficulty, it would be difficult to argue that the knowledge they contained had been treated as core by test takers.

BOX 19.11 Example item for analysis (ii)

Item 46

Predisposing factors for osteoarthritis include all of the following, EXCEPT?

A. Sport

B. Alcohol abuse

C. Manual occupation

D. Obesity

E. Hereditary

*The correct answer is **B**

BOX 19.12 Item analysis data for item 46

DIF = 0.50,   RPB = −0.438, CRPB = 0.378, (95%CON = 0.164, 0.559)
   RBIS = 0.549, CRBIS = 0.474, IRI = 0.219

GROUP	N	INV	NF	OMIT	A	B*	C	D	E
TOTAL	148	0	0	0	0.23	0.50	0.07	0.08	0.12
HIGH	38	0			0.11	0.68	0.05	0.05	0.11
MID	64	0			0.12	0.63	0.06	0.09	0.09
LOW	46	0			0.48	0.17	0.09	0.09	0.17
TEST SCORE MEAN %					64	72	66	65	67
DISCRIMINATING POWER (D.P.)					−0.37	0.51	−0.03	−0.03	−0.07
STANDARD ERROR OF D.P.					0.14	0.15	0.08	0.08	0.11

Standard-setting for written assessment

In the previous section we noted that the purpose of the test is a fundamental consideration in how to interpret item-analysis data. We noted that our main example item was answered correctly by 90 per cent of the cohort. So what should be an appropriate passing score on the test which this item comes from? The mean score on the test was 69 per cent and the standard deviation was 5.7, the highest score was 91 per cent and the lowest 52 per cent, so even the one student scoring 3 SDs below the mean obtained more than 50 per cent.

There has been much recent interest in trying to define standards for written tests, because 'standards are always arbitrary but should not be capricious"', a quote often attributed to Ronald Berk, but which is borrowed from the USA legal system for appeals.(85) There seems nothing quite as arbitrary in a test of high-quality health professionals as a pass mark of 50 per cent – is this doctor half-full or half-empty of the knowledge needed to perform in practice?

Consequently effort has gone into describing what the appropriate level of performance on any test should be. Clearly, this might vary from test to test and year to year, as knowledge changes, items have different inherent difficulty and expectations change. Standard setting is discussed in detail in Chapter 22, and there are some good, practically focused treatments elsewhere.(86) However, there are some important principles as they relate to written assessment, as follows.

1. Production of all written high stakes tests should entail effort to set 'a priori' standards. This is perfectly possible in both 'objective' and other types of written items such as SAQs.
2. Usually, these standards should be based on careful consideration of test content and its appropriateness to meet course/professional requirements, by a group of judges familiar with the cohort, the curriculum, the content and the context. Research has shown that including a discussion phase on the standard-setting panel reduces the minimum number of judges required and can improve the reliability of test standards. The minimum number of judges to obtain a reasonable standard error of measurement on a test is ten or more judges without discussion, or six or more judges after discussion. This is a significant efficiency on some previous estimates (10–15 judges required.)(87)
3. Standard-setting methods that best fit the purpose of a test should be chosen. Setting a minimum standard of competence may be a different purpose to selecting students to enter an advanced course, or certifying to a specialty. Giving feedback to students is a different purpose to accrediting them to lead the advanced life support team.
4. Norm referencing is unacceptable for written items used in competency licensing tests. These tests are focused on candidates' safety to practise, amongst other things. A clear and defensible standard needs to be identified.
5. Usually, for written assessments, the minimum acceptable standard should be decided before the test. In this setting (high stakes examinations, and patient safety concerns) variation in test, and hence item, difficulty is a critical issue. Standards should be set for each test, item by item, using item-focused methods such as Angoff, modified Angoff or Ebel.(88,89) *See* Chapter 22.
6. The final choice of method will be governed by the available resources and the consequences of misclassifying examinees as having passed or failed.
7. In general setting standards for selected-response single-best-answer-questions is less complex than setting standards for script concordance and, particularly, for key features items. This is because, especially in the latter, decisions in one part of a key feature may have impact on responses to other parts, and each may also be weighted quite differently. This problem is still being discussed.(80)
8. The most robust methods are invariably also the most time-consuming, but frequently result in excellent insights into test construction flaws because each item or response is carefully examined.

Summary

Written assessment is the most commonly used form of testing in tertiary and professional education. Huge amounts of research have been carried out on multiple-choice item formats, and essay assessments. There are many variations of these methods used for assessment in the health professions. Newer formats, such as F-type and script concordance items, are still very much in development. Here I have presented the basic principles behind the most commonly used ones. Whilst there are many other topics that could be discussed in relation to written assessment, these are addressed by other chapters in this book.

Assessments of the types we have discussed here usually happen at the end of a term or year. However, they require a significant amount of time to prepare well, as each item needs to be written, reviewed, verified against the blueprint, and compiled into the whole test. Then the test needs to be reviewed to check for cross-cueing or repetition between items, and optical score sheets prepared to reflect the different categories of responses in the test (e.g. for key features items) and then printed for the assessment. This can require between two and six months for a complex and/or comprehensive assessment.

Faculty development is a key component of improvements in assessment strategies. Some written assessments are deceptively simple, when given a cursory glance, but their quality is dependent on expertise, in the discipline, as an educationalist, and in item-writing. Good items also require detailed preparation and extensive trialling and analysis of items.

Finally, it is clear that there are different uses for different items. It is unlikely that a good assessment of cognitive skills in health disciplines can be undertaken with an MCQ'. It will require a carefully chosen group of items, matched to the curriculum, using an array of different response modes to reflect the complexity of health care in the 21st century.

References

1 Dauphinee D (2002) Licensure and certification. In: Norman G, van der Vleuten C and Newble D (eds) *International Handbook of Research on Medical Education* (vol. 2), pp. 835–82. Kluwer, Dordrecht.

2 Smith J (2004) The Shipman Inquiry – 5th Report. Safeguarding patients: lessons from the past – proposals for the future. HMSO. (http://www.the-shipman-inquiry.org.uk/fifthreport.asp, accessed 01 January 2009).

3 Walton M, Shaw TJ, Barnet S and Ross J (2006) Developing a national patient safety education framework for Australia. *Quality and Safety in Healthcare*. **15**: 437–42.

4 Scalese RJ, Obeso VT and Issenberg SB (2008) Simulation technology for skills training and competency assessment in medical education. *Journal of General Internal Medicine*. **23**(Suppl 1): 46–9.

5 Norcini JJ (2003) ABC of learning and teaching in medicine: work based assessment. *BMJ (Clinical Research Ed.)*. **326**: 753–5.

6 Glaser R (1984) Education and thinking: the role of knowledge. *American Psychologist*. **39**: 93–104.

7 Boshuizen HPA and Schmidt HG (1992) On the role of biomedical knowledge in clinical reasoning by experts, intermediates and novices. *Cognitive Science*. **16**: 153–84.

8 Newble DJ (1991) The observed long case in clinical assessment. *Medical Education*. **25**: 369–73.

9 Hubbard JP and Clemens WV (1961) *Multiple-Choice Examinations in Medicine*. Lea and Febiger, Philadelphia, PA.

10 Newble DI and Swanson DB (1988) Psychometric characteristics of the objective structured clinical examination. *Medical Education*. **22**: 325–34.

11 Newble DI and Jaeger K (1983) The effect of assessments and examinations on the learning of medical students. *Medical Education*. **17**: 165–71.

12 Norman G (2002) Research in medical education: three decades of progress. *BMJ (Clinical Research Ed.)*. **324**: 1560–2.

13 Newble DI, Jolly BC and Wakeford RE (eds) (1994) *Certification and Recertification in Medicine: Issues in the Assessment of Clinical Competence*. Cambridge University Press, Cambridge.

14 Norman G, van der Vleuten C and Newble D (eds) (2002) *International Handbook of Research on Medical Education* (vol. 2). Kluwer, Dordrecht.

15 Wood R (1991) *Assessment and Testing*. Cambridge University Press, Cambridge.

16 Newble DI and Cannon R (2001) *A Handbook for Medical Teachers* (4e). Springer., New York, NY.

17 Dauphinee D (1994) The content of certifying examinations. In: Newble DI, Jolly BC and Wakeford RE (eds) *Certification and Recertification in Medicine: Issues in the Assessment of Clinical Competence*, pp. 92–104. Cambridge University Press, Cambridge.

18 Hamdy H (2006) Blueprinting for the assessment of health care professionals. *Clinical Teacher*. **3**: 175–9.

19 Kane MT (1992) The assessment of professional competence. *Evaluation and the Health Professions*. **15**: 163–82.

20 Downing SM (2002) Threats to the validity of locally developed multiple-choice tests in medical education: construct irrelevant variance and construct under-representation. *Advances in Health Sciences Education*. **7**: 235–41.

21 Roberts C, Sarangi S, Southgate L *et al.* (2000) Oral examinations – equal opportunities, ethnicity, and fairness in the MRCGP. *BMJ (Clinical Research Ed.)*. **320**: 370–5.

22 Hobus PP, Schmidt HG, Boshuizen HP and Patel VL (1987) Contextual factors in the activation of first diagnostic hypotheses: expert-novice differences. *Medical Education*. **21**: 471–6.

23 Bowen JL (2006) Educational strategies to promote clinical diagnostic reasoning. *New England Journal of Medicine*. **355**: 2217–25.

24 Mylopoulos M and Regehr G (2007) Cognitive metaphors of expertise and knowledge: prospects and limitations for medical education. *Medical Education*. **41**: 1159–65.

25 Croskerry P and Norman G (2008) Overconfidence in clinical decision making. *American Journal of Medicine*. **121**: 24–9.

26 Case S and Swanson D (1998) *Constructing Written Test Questions for the Basic and Clinical Sciences* (3e). National Board of Medical Examiners, Philadelphia, PA. (http://www.nbme.org/publications/index.html#iwman; accessed 1 December 2012).

27 Epstein R (2007) Assessment in medical education. *New England Journal of Medicine*. **356**: 387–96.

28 Stalnaker JM (1951) The essay type of examination. In: Lindquist EF (ed.) *Educational Measurement*, pp. 495–530. George Banta, Menasha, WI.

29 Ebel RL and Frisbie DA (1991) *Essentials of Educational Measurement* (5e). Prentice-Hall, Englewood Cliffs, NJ.

30 Schafer WD, Gagné P and Lissitz RW (2005) Resistance to confounding style and content in scoring constructed-response items. *Educational Measurement: Issues and Practice*. **24**: 22–8.

31 Klein SP and Hart FM (1968) Chance and systematic factors affecting essay grades. *Journal of Educational Measurement*. **5**: 197–206.

32 Linn RL, Klein SP and Hart FM (1972) The nature and correlates of law school essay grades. *Educational and Psychological Measurement*. **32**: 267–79.

33 Markham LR (1976) Influences of handwriting quality on teacher evaluation of written work. *American Educational Research Journal*. **13**: 277–83.

34 Powers D, Fowles M, Farnum M and Ramsey P (1994) Will they think less of my handwritten essay if others word process theirs? Effects on essay scores of intermingling handwritten and word-processed essays. *Journal of Educational Measurement*. **31**: 220–33.

35 Verma M, Chatwal J and Singh T (1997) Reliability of essay type questions – effect of structuring. *Assessment in Education*. **4**: 265–70.

36 Grosse ME and Wright BD (1988) Psychometric characteristics of scores on a patient-management problem test. *Educational and Psychological Measurement*. **48**: 297–305.

37 Lim E, Hian C, Seet H *et al.* (2007) Computer-based testing of the modified essay question: the Singapore experience. *Medical Teacher*. **9**: e261–8.

38 Feletti GI (1980) Reliability and validity studies on modified essay questions. *Journal of Medical Education*. **55**: 933–41.

39 Palmer E and Devitt PG (2007) Assessment of higher order cognitive skills in undergraduate education: modified essay or multiple choice questions? Research paper. *BMC Medical Education*. **7**: 49–53.

40 Palmer E, Duggan P, Devitt P and Russell R (2010) The modified essay question: its exit from the exit examination? *Medical Teacher*. **32**(7): 300–7.

41 Jordan S and Mitchell T (2009) E-assessment for learning? The potential of short free-text questions with tailored feedback. *British Journal of Educational Technology*. **40**(2): 371–85.

42 Smith B, Sinclair H, Simpson J, van Teijlingen E, Bond C and Taylor R (2002) What is the role of double marking? Evidence from an undergraduate medical course. *Education for Primary Care*. **13**: 497–503.

43 Cannings R, Hawthorne K, Hood K and Houston H (2005) Putting double marking to the test: a framework to assess if it is worth the trouble. *Medical Education*. **39**: 299–308.

44 Edwards BD and Arthur W Jr (2007) An examination of factors contributing to a reduction in subgroup differences on a constructed-response paper-and-pencil test of scholastic achievement. *Journal of Applied Psychology*. **92**: 794–801.

45 Rodriquez MC (2003) Construct equivalence of multiple-choice and constructed-response items: a random effects synthesis of correlations. *Journal of Educational Measurement*. **40**: 163–84.

46 Grant DL (1957) Studies in the reliability of the short-answer essay examination. *The Journal of Educational Research*. **51**: 109.

47 Matters G and Paul C (2003) Psychological predictors of the propensity to omit short-response items on a high-stakes achievement test. *Educational and Psychological Measurement*. **63**: 239–56.

48 Rademakers J, Ten Cate THJ and Bar PR (2005) Progress testing with short answer questions. *Medical Teacher.* **27**: 578–82.

49 Gay LR (1980) The comparative effects of multiple-choice versus short-answer tests on retention. *Journal of Educational Measurement.* **17**: 45–50.

50 Downing SM (2003) Guessing on selected-response examinations. *Medical Education.* **37**: 670–1.

51 Downing SM (2002) Assessment of knowledge in written test forms. In: Norman G, van der Vleuten C and Newble D (eds) *International Handbook of Research on Medical Education* (vol. 2), pp. 647–72. Kluwer, Dordrecht.

52 Haladyna TM, Downing SM and Rodriquez MC (2002) A review of multiple-choice item writing guidelines for classroom assessment. *Applied Measurement in Education.* **15**: 309–34.

53 Haladyna TM and Downing SM (1993) How many options is enough for a multiple-choice test item? *Educational and Psychological Measurement.* **53**: 999–1009.

54 Case SM, Swanson DB and Ripkey DR (1994) Comparison of items in five-option and extended-matching format for assessment of diagnostic skills. *Academic Medicine.* **69**(Suppl): S1–3.

55 Skakun E, Maguire T and Cook D (1994) Strategy choices in multiple choice items. *Academic Medicine.* **69**(Suppl): S7–9.

56 Case SM (1983) The development and evaluation of a new instrument to assess medical problem solving. *Dissertation Abstracts International.* **44**: 1764.

57 Bhakta B, Tennant A, Horton M, Lawton G and Andrich D (2005) Using item response theory to explore the psychometric properties of extended matching questions examination in undergraduate medical education. *BMC Medical Education.* **5**: 9.

58 Beullens J, Struyf E and Van Damme B (2006) Diagnostic ability in relation to clinical seminars and extended-matching questions examinations. *Medical Education.* **40**: 1173–9.

59 Beullens J, Struyf E and Van Damme B (2005) Do extended matching multiple-choice questions measure clinical reasoning? *Medical Education.* **39**: 410–7.

60 Fenderson BA, Damjanov I, Robeson MR, Veloski JJ and Rubin E (1997) The virtues of extended matching and uncued tests as alternatives to multiple choice questions. *Human Pathology.* **28**: 526–32.

61 McCoubrie P (2004) Improving the fairness of multiple-choice questions: a literature review. *Medical Teacher.* **8**: 709–12.

62 George S (2003) Extended matching items (EMIs): solving the conundrum. *Psychiatric Bulletin of the Royal College of Psychiatrists.* **27**: 230–2.

63 Zimmerman DW and Williams RHA (2003) New look at the influence of guessing on the reliability of multiple-choice tests. *App Psych Meas.* **27**: 357–71.

64 Swanson DW, Holtzman KZ, Clauser BE and Sawhill AJ (2005) Psychometric characteristics and response times for one-best-answer questions in relation to number and source of options. *Academic Medicine.* **80**(Suppl): S93–6.

65 Swanson DB, Holtzman KZ and Allbee K (2008) Measurement characteristics of content-parallel single-best-answer and extended-matching questions in relation to number and source of options. *Academic Medicine.* **83**(Suppl): S21–4.

66 Charlin B, Brailovsky C, Leduc C and Blouin D (1998) The diagnosis script questionnaire: a new tool to assess a specific dimension of clinical competence. *Advances in Health Sciences Education.* **3**: 51–8.

67 Charlin B, Brailovsky C, Roy L, Goulet F and van der Vleuten C (2000) The script concordance test: a tool to assess the reflective clinician. *Teaching and Learning in Medicine.* **12**(4): 189–95.

68 Schmidt H, Norman G and Boshuizen H (1990) A cognitive perspective on medical expertise: theory and implications. *Academic Medicine .* **65**: 611–21.

69 Gagnon R, Charlin B, Roy L *et al.* (2006) The cognitive validity of the script concordance test: a processing time study. *Teaching and Learning in Medicine.* **18**: 22–7.

70 Dory V, Gagnon R, Vanpee D and Charlin B (2012) How to construct and implement script concordance tests: insights from a systematic review. *Medical Education.* **46**: 552–63.

71 Charlin B and van der Vleuten C (2004) Standardised assessment of clinical reasoning in contexts of uncertainty: the script concordance approach. *Evaluation and the Health Professions.* **27**: 304–19.

72 Sibert L, Darmoni SJ, Dahamna B, Hellot MF, Weber J and Charlin B (2006) On line clinical reasoning assessment with script concordance test in urology: results of a French pilot study. *BMC Medical Education.* **6**: 45–7.

73 Meterissian S, Zabolotny B, Gagnon R and Charlin B (2007) Is the script concordance test a valid instrument for assessment of intraoperative decision-making skills? *American Journal of Surgery.* **193**: 248–51.

74 Kelly W, Durning S and Denton G (2012) Comparing a script concordance examination to a multiple-choice examination on a core internal medicine clerkship. *Teaching and Learning in Medicine.* **24**: 187–93.

75 Goulet F, Jacques A, Gagnon R, Charlin B and Shabah A (2010) Poorly performing physicians: does the script concordance test detect bad clinical reasoning? *Journal of Continuing Education in the Health Professions.* **30**: 161–6.

76 Farmer EA and Page G (2005) A practical guide to assessing clinical decision-making skills using the key features approach. *Medical Education.* **39**: 1188–94.

77 Norman G, Bordage G, Curry L *et al.* (1985) Review of recent innovations in assessment. In: Wakeford R (ed.) *Directions in clinical assessment. Report of the Cambridge Conference on the Assessment of Clinical Competence,* pp. 8–27. Office of the Regius Professor of Physic, Cambridge University School of Clinical Medicine, Addenbrookes Hospital, Cambridge.

78 McGuire CH, Solomon LM and Bashook PG (1976) *Construction and Use of Written Simulations.* Psychological Corporation of Harcourt, Brace, Jovanovich, New York, NY.

79 Page G and Bordage G (1995) The Medical Council of Canada's key features project: a more valid written examination of clinical decision-making skills. *Academic Medicine.* **70**: 104–10.

80 Fischer M, Kopp V, Holzer M, Ruderich F and Junger J (2005) A modified electronic key feature examination for undergraduate medical students: validation threats and opportunities. *Medical Teacher.* **27**: 450–5.

81 Trudel JL, Bordage G and Downing SM (2008) Reliability and validity of key feature cases for the self-assessment of colon and rectal surgeons. *Annals of Surgery.* **248**: 252–8.

82 Farmer EA and Hinchy J (2005) Assessing clinical decision making skills in general practice: the key features approach. *Australian Family Physician.* **34**: 1059–61.

83 Lawrence K, Allen T, Brailovsky C *et al.* (2011) Defining competency-based evaluation objectives in family medicine Key feature approach. *Canadian Family Physician.* **57**: E373–80.

84 Baldwin P, Baldwin SG and Haist SA (2011) F-type testlets and the effects of feedback and case-specificity. *Academic Medicine.* **86**: S56–9.

85 Cizek GJ (ed.) (2001) *Setting Performance Standards. Concepts, Methods and Perspectives.* Lawrence Erlbaum Associates, Mahwah, NJ.

86 Norcini JJ (2003) Setting standards on educational tests. *Medical Education.* **37**: 464–9.

87 Fowell SL, Fewtrell R and Mclaughlin PJ (2008) Estimating the minimum number of judges required for test-centred standard setting on written assessments. Do discussion and iteration have an influence? *Advances in Health Sciences Education.* **13**: 11–24.

88 Cizek GJ (1996) Standard setting guidelines. *Educational Measurement: Issues and Practice.* **15**: 13–21.

89 Ebel RL (1972) *Essentials of Educational Measurement* (2e). Prentice-Hall., Englewood Cliffs, NJ.

20 Workplace assessment

John J Norcini

Foundation for Advancement of International Medical Education and Research (FAIMER), USA

 KEY MESSAGES

- Assessment in the setting of clinical training is not well developed, but methods based on observation of routine encounters offer a rich and feasible alternative.
- A framework for assessment based on observation has two dimensions: the grounds on which judgements are made (single encounter or routine performance) and the nature of the judgements themselves (occurrence, quality or suitability).
- Tools such as the mini-CEX, DOPS, CbD and mini-PAT offer valid assessment.

- Faculty development is a key to the successful use of the methods.
- The opportunity for educational feedback as part of these methods is as important as their contribution to the assessment process.
- A series of challenges remains, including reliability, equivalence, stakes, relationships, the need for other forms of assessment and feasibility.

Introduction

Assessment in the context of medical education has changed dramatically over the past 50 years.(1) From near exclusive reliance on the essay question and the clinical viva, assessment methods have proliferated, particularly those appropriate to use in the setting of undergraduate medical education. These newer methods cover more of the competencies of a doctor, and there is a much better understanding of how to deploy them to produce scores that are valid and reliable.

Assessment in the setting of clinical training, particularly postgraduate training, is not as well developed as assessment in the undergraduate arena. The curriculum in most clinical training settings is less structured, and the trainees often have more responsibility. Consequently, assessment needs to pose a broader range of patient problems and include more complex and acute care, multi-system disease and procedural skill. Moreover, the focus is more often on the assessment of integrated skills rather than on specific aspects of competence. Compared with practising doctors, trainees in clinical settings are not yet completely responsible for patients, and they have not differentiated within specialty. As a result, assessment needs to focus on the potential to practise, not actual practice, so assessments of work products are likely to be less useful.(2) Moreover, the results of an assessment programme need to support the educational enterprise.

It is difficult to develop high-quality written or performance-based assessments locally, especially in the context of postgraduate training. There are small numbers of trainees and staff; resources are fragmented across the specialties; and assessment expertise is rare. There is also a need to address sophisticated content and skills, which are difficult to simulate at the level of advanced trainees.

Despite these challenges, there are two aspects of training in a clinical setting that offer significant advantages for assessment. First, there are routine interactions among members of the health-care team and between trainees and patients, so the clinical material that can serve as the basis for assessment is readily available. Second, there are skilled clinician-educators in the setting who, with some training, can act as judges. Consequently, assessment methods that are based on observation of routine encounters are most feasible in the setting of clinical training. In addition, the use of these methods supports the educational process because they offer the opportunity for formative feedback and the development of a plan for remediation when it is needed.

In 1990, Miller proposed a structure, in the form of a pyramid, for categorising methods of assessment.(3) Knowledge (knows) is at the lowest level of the pyramid followed by competence (knows how), performance (shows how) and action (does) (*see* Figure 20.1). Assessments based on observation in the setting of work are representative of the top two levels of the pyramid. Miller distinguished between these two levels depending on whether trainees were in an artificial testing situation (i.e. they were aware that they were being assessed). Underlying this distinction is the reasonable but unproven assumption that the assessment methods that come closest to capturing a doctor's unobserved, routine functioning will yield the most valid

Understanding Medical Education: Evidence, Theory and Practice, Second Edition. Edited by Tim Swanwick.
© 2014 The Association for the Study of Medical Education. Published 2014 by John Wiley & Sons, Ltd.

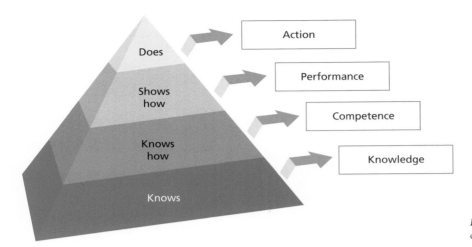

Figure 20.1 Miller's pyramid for assessing clinical competence.

results. Of course, capturing authentic performance has problems as well since the clinical context poses a number of threats to validity (e.g. differences between doctors in case mix and the severity of illness of their patients).(2)

A framework for assessment based on observation

In the work context, assessors are asked to make a number of different kinds of judgement based on their observations. For the purpose of this chapter, a two-dimensional framework will be used to describe these judgements.(4,5) The first dimension relates to the grounds on which the judgements are made – a single encounter or routine performance. The second dimension relates to the nature of the judgement – whether it is occurrence, quality or suitability.

Grounds for judgement

Single encounter
In this instance, the assessors base their judgements on observation of a single event. For example, a faculty member might observe the trainee in interaction with a particular patient, patient record or procedure, and then provide an evaluation of it. The traditional clinical viva illustrates this. A trainee examines and interviews a patient, draws conclusions and then presents all of this to one or more assessors. Judgements about the trainee are made on the basis of that one event.

The advantage of basing judgements on single events is the reassurance that the assessor has actually observed the performance and is focused on reaching a conclusion about it. Theoretically, this reduces the biasing effects of previous contact and clarifies what is to be evaluated. The disadvantage is that the performance of doctors is case or task specific.(6) This means that performance on one event does not predict with high accuracy performance on another. Therefore, several different events need to be sampled to obtain a generalisable estimate of performance (Box 20.1).

Routine performance
In this instance, the assessors base their judgements on observations they have made over a period of time. This is one of the most common types of assessment, and most training programmes in the US and UK ask faculty members to periodically complete rating forms that attest to the competence of their trainees.

The major advantage of this basis for judgement is that it should include observations of the trainee on a number of different occasions. In this way, it reduces, to some degree, the problems of case specificity of performance. However, assessors sometimes offer evaluations of aspects of performance they do not observe. For example, Pulito *et al.* found that faculty members primarily observe cognitive skills and professionalism and have little basis for assessing other aspects of competence.(7) Moreover, Silber *et al.* found that faculty members tend to assess competence along the two dimensions of medical knowledge and interpersonal skills, and do not make distinctions among other aspects of competence.(8)

Nature of the judgement
Based on their observations of single encounters or routine performance, the nature of judgements assessors are asked to make falls into three categories:
- occurrence – whether particular behaviours were demonstrated
- quality – the 'goodness' of the performance
- fitness or suitability – whether the performance was good enough for a particular purpose.

Occurrence
Assessors are sometimes asked to indicate whether they have observed a particular behaviour, and they are often given a checklist on which to note the occurrence. For instance, Martin *et al.* developed procedure-specific checklists containing 22–32 task steps.(11) They were applied by assessors to their observation of procedures done by trainees. Each time one of the steps on the checklist was completed, the assessor noted it, and after the procedure, the marks were tallied.

BOX 20.1 FOCUS ON: How many encounters are needed?

In most assessment programmes, the same number of encounters is required of all trainees.

For example, the Foundation Programme calls for each trainee to have four to six mini-clinical evaluation exercise (mini-CEX), direct observation of procedural skills (DOPS) and case-based discussion (CbD) encounters over the course of a year. These estimates balance traditional estimates of reliability against feasibility. Depending on the purpose of the assessment, however, this may be too few or too many encounters for certain trainees. Use of the standard error of measurement (SEM) permits the application of a more refined strategy for making this decision.

The SEM is an alternative to traditional measures of reliability, and it can be used to construct a 95% confidence interval around scores.(9) For example, data from a study of the mini-CEX indicate that the 95% confidence interval for the overall rating of clinical competence is ±1.2 after two encounters and ±0.8 after four encounters, and it continues to decrease more slowly with additional encounters.(10) These data are based on a nine-point scale where 1–3 is unsatisfactory, 4–6 is satisfactory and 7–9 is superior. Thus, we can be 95% confident that the true score of a trainee student with an average rating of 4 on two encounters lies between 2.8 and 5.2.

If the purpose of assessment is simply to identify which trainees are unsatisfactory, two encounters are probably sufficient for many trainees, certainly those with average ratings of 6 or better. On the other hand, for trainees with averages between 2.8 and 5.2, additional encounters are needed. As encounters are added, the width of the confidence interval shrinks and the number of good decisions increases. Thus, limited assessment resources can be focused where they do the most good.

The assessment advantages of this strategy go together with significant educational advantages. Borderline trainees will have more encounters, and since each is accompanied by feedback, those who need it most will receive more intense educational interventions.

Simply noting the occurrence of behaviours is often viewed as objective, leaving less to the judgement of the observer. It structures the task of the assessor and ensures that it is more focused and consistent over observations and assessors. If they are clinician-educators, however, simply asking the assessor to note the occurrence of particular behaviours does not make best use of their ability to discriminate among performances.

Quality

More often, assessors are asked to make a judgement about the quality of the performance they observe. They typically record these judgements on a rating scale. For example, in the study by Martin *et al.*, observers were also asked to complete a seven-item global rating form that captured the quality of the trainees' procedural skills on a five-point scale.(11) The same form was used for all procedures, and after the examination the ratings were tallied.

In the Martin *et al.* study, the global assessments of quality were strongly correlated with the checklists, which simply noted the occurrence of aspects of performance.(11) This is not an unusual finding, and it suggests that they are capturing the same aspects of competence.(12) However, the global ratings tend to be a bit more valid. For instance, in the Martin *et al.* study, they discriminated among levels of training, while the checklists did not.

Fitness

In some instances, assessors are asked to determine whether a performance is satisfactory or fit for purpose. For example, in the Martin *et al.* study, the assessors were also asked to make a pass/fail judgement.(11) In essence, this required them to make two judgements in sequence. They needed to first establish the quality of a performance, and then they had to decide whether it was good enough for a particular purpose. In the Martin *et al.* study, pass/fail results were not correlated with other measures (e.g. year of training) because so many of the participants passed.(11)

The simultaneous decision-making underlying a single judgement about fitness is very efficient in academic settings where it is important to identify individuals for advancement and remediation. However, it combines two somewhat unreliable judgements into one and renders the meaning of the results unclear to a degree. For example, a failing judgement can be rendered because the performance was poor or the assessor had high standards. Since it is not possible to disentangle these, it is best to ask for judgements about quality and fitness separately, as they did in the study by Martin *et al.*(11)

Common methods

A number of different methods of assessment based on observation have been used in the setting of clinical training. Four common assessment methods are the:
- mini-clinical evaluation exercise (mini-CEX)
- direct observation of procedural skills (DOPS)
- chart-stimulated recall (CSR)
- multi-source feedback (MSF).(13)

Often, these methods are gathered into a portfolio that trainees complete and this collection forms the basis for making judgements about educational progress. These four methods will be the focus of this section.

Mini-CEX

In the mini-CEX, a faculty member observes a trainee interact with a patient in a clinical setting.(13,14) The trainee engages in a clinical activity (e.g. taking a focused history and performing relevant aspects of the physical examination) and afterwards summarises the encounter (e.g. provides a diagnosis and/or treatment plan). The faculty member scores the performance and then provides educational feedback. The encounters are intended to take about

15 minutes, and trainees are expected to be evaluated several times and by different faculty members.

The method was originally devised for use in internal medicine postgraduate training programmes in the US. Individual faculty members were responsible for deciding when trainees were to be assessed and for identifying appropriate patients. Ratings were gathered on a nine-point scale, where 1–3 was unsatisfactory, 4–6 was satisfactory and 7–9 was superior. The dimensions of performance observed and evaluated were interviewing skill, physical examination, professionalism, clinical judgement, counselling, organisation and efficiency, and overall competence. Not every encounter permitted assessment of all of these dimensions. Depending on the purpose of the assessment, the ratings were aggregated across dimensions and encounters for each trainee.(13,14)

Given its structure, the ground for judgements underpinning the mini-CEX is always the single encounter. Depending on how it has been deployed, however, the nature of the judgements has varied depending on the purpose of the assessment. For instance, in the US, assessors were asked to judge both the quality (ranking from 1 to 9) of the performance and its fitness (unsatisfactory versus satisfactory–superior) for a first-year postgraduate trainee.

In the US, the mini-CEX has been used in a number of different inpatient, outpatient and emergency department settings. In these settings, the mini-CEX has been applied to a broad range of patient problems. For example, in a study by Norcini *et al.*, the presenting complaints included abdominal pain, chest pain, cough, dizziness, fever, headache, low back pain, shortness of breath and weight gain. Common internal medicine problems, such as arthritis, asthma, chronic obstructive pulmonary disorder, congestive heart failure (CHF), coronary artery disease, diabetes and hypertension, formed the basis for assessment, as well as other common problems, such as seizure, substance abuse, depression, dementia and rash. The mini-CEX was also applied to trainees assessing patients with multiple problems, such as CHF, hypertension and diabetes, and with acute problems such as sepsis and myocardial infarction.(10)

The mini-CEX is analogous to a classroom test for the clinical setting. It is intended to identify the few trainees whose performance is wholly unsatisfactory and to provide documentation of their shortcomings. This documentation serves as the evidence in support of a later educational decision about the trainee. More importantly however, for the vast majority of trainees it provides an opportunity for ongoing formative assessment and feedback. It is also designed to ensure that the clinical skills of trainees have been observed and evaluated by faculty members. Unfortunately, observation and feedback occur far too rarely in the context of many busy clinical placements.(15)

The mini-CEX is not intended for use in a high-stakes examination setting, nor should it be used to compare or rank trainees across different programmes.

Although more work remains, a recent systematic review finds a number of studies that provide evidence of the validity of the mini-CEX.(16) For example, in the undergraduate setting, Kogan *et al.* found that mini-CEX scores had modest correlations with examination scores, inpatient clerkship ratings, outpatient clerkship ratings, and final course grades.(17) In a postgraduate setting, Durning *et al.* found correlations between the individual components of the mini-CEX and the corresponding monthly evaluations by faculty members, as well as the results of an in-training examination.(18) In a study by Boulet *et al.*, videotapes of standardised patient (SP)–student encounters were evaluated by faculty using the mini-CEX form.(19) The SP checklists predicted faculty global ratings, and SP ratings of doctor–patient communication correlated with faculty ratings of communications. Finally, Holmboe *et al.* scripted videotapes of trainees whose performance was unsatisfactory, satisfactory or superior. Using the mini-CEX form, faculty successfully discriminated among the three levels of performance.(20)

Since its initial development, the mini-CEX has been modified for use in a number of different settings and the original forms have been translated into several different languages. The competencies assessed have been tailored to particular needs (e.g. the Professionalism Mini-Evaluation Exercise) and to a variety of undergraduate and postgraduate disciplines and clinical settings.(21–23) The rating scales have been modified as well, with changes in both the number of points on the scale, the definitions of those points, and in some instances the replacement of the ratings with written comments. All of these modifications are appropriate, and they ensure the relevance of the method to the setting in which it is being used.

The assessment portion of the UK Foundation Programme provides an example in which the mini-CEX has been appropriately modified to make it more relevant to a particular setting.(13) Trainees are assessed several times throughout the year with different faculty members for each encounter. Both the assessor and the patient are selected by the trainee, but the assessor must agree that the encounter is appropriate. Assessors include consultants, experienced specialist registrars, staff grade and associate specialists, and general practitioners. There is a list of core problems as part of the curriculum, and trainees are expected to sample from them. The immediate feedback given after the encounter includes strengths, weaknesses and an action plan for further effort. Initially, ratings of performance were gathered but more recently these have been replaced by the provision of text comments.

Figure 20.2 shows a typical assessment form. The descriptors require the assessors to judge both the quality of the trainee's performance and whether it meets expectations for completion of the year of training.

DOPS

Direct observation of procedural skills (DOPS) is a variation on the mini-CEX, which was originally designed by the Royal College of Physicians to assess and provide feedback on procedural skills.(24) Just as with the mini-CEX, trainees are observed with real patients, but in DOPS they are conducting procedures. After the encounter, the faculty member rates the trainee's performance and provides educational feedback. The encounters are necessarily brief (usually less than 15 minutes, with 5 minutes for feedback),

Please refer to www.hcat.nhs.uk for guidance on this form and details of expected competencies for F1

Mini-Clinical Evaluation Exercise (CEX) – F1 Version

Please complete the question using a cross: ☒   Please use black ink and CAPITAL LETTERS

Doctor's Surname

Forename

GMC Number: **GMC NUMBER MUST BE COMPLETED**

Clinical setting:	A&E ☐		OPD ☐		In-patient ☐		Acute Admission ☐		GP Surgery ☐

Clinical problem category:	Airway/ Breathing ☐	CVS/ Circulation ☐	Gastro ☐	Neuro ☐	Pain ☐	Psych/ Behav ☐	Other

New or FU:	New ☐	FU ☐	Focus of clinical encounter:	History ☐	Diagnosis ☐	Management ☐	Explanation ☐

Number of times patient seen before by trainee:	0 ☐	1–4 ☐	5–9 ☐	>10 ☐	Complexity of case:	Low ☐	Average ☐	High ☐

Assessor's position:	Consultant ☐	GP ☐	SpR ☐	SASG ☐	SHO ☐	Other

Number of previous mini-CEXs observed by assessor with any trainee:	0 ☐	1 ☐	2 ☐	3 ☐	4 ☐	5–9 ☐	>9 ☐

Please grade the following areas using the scale below:	Below expectations for F1 completion		Borderline for F1 completion	Meets expectations for F1 completion	Above expectations for F1 completion		U/C*
1. History Taking	☐	☐	☐	☐	☐	☐	☐
2. Physical Examination Skills	☐	☐	☐	☐	☐	☐	☐
3. Communication Skills	☐	☐	☐	☐	☐	☐	☐
4. Clinical Judgement	☐	☐	☐	☐	☐	☐	☐
5. Professionalism	☐	☐	☐	☐	☐	☐	☐
6. Organisation/Efficiency	☐	☐	☐	☐	☐	☐	☐
7. Overall clinical care	☐	☐	☐	☐	☐	☐	☐

*U/C Please mark this if you have not observed the behaviour and therefore feel unable to comment.

Anything especially good?   **Suggestions for development**

Agreed action:

Have you had training in the use of this assessment tool?: ☐ Face-to-Face ☐ Have Read Guidelines ☐ Web/CDrom

Assessor's Signature:

. . . .

Date (mm/yy): M M Y Y

Time taken for observation: (in minutes)

Time taken for feedback: (in minutes)

Assessor's Surname

Assessor's registration number:

Please note: Failure of return of all completed forms to your administrator is a probity issue
Acknowledgements: Adapted with permission from American Board of Internal Medicine

Figure 20.2 Typical mini-CEX assessment form.

and trainees are expected to be evaluated several times and by different faculty members.

An example of DOPS is its use in the UK Foundation Programme. Trainees must select from an approved list that contains many of the procedures used routinely in practice.(13) For example, it includes various injections, intubation, electrocardiogram, nasogastric tube insertion, venepuncture, cannulation and arterial blood sampling. Trainees are assessed on their understanding of indications, anatomy, technique, aseptic technique, proper analgesia, communication and other important aspects of procedural skill. They are also asked how often they have performed the procedure. More recently, the ratings have been removed and the trainee is offered free text assessment and feedback.

Trainees are to be assessed several times throughout the year with different procedures and faculty members for each encounter.(13) As with all the tools used as part of this programme, the timing, procedure and assessor are selected by the trainees, but the assessor must agree that the procedure is appropriate. Like the mini-CEX, assessors include consultants, experienced specialist registrars, staff grade and associate specialists, and general practitioners. However, nurses and other appropriate allied health professionals can also act as assessors. The immediate feedback given after the encounter includes areas of strengths and suggestions for development.

Since it is a variation, studies indicating the validity of the mini-CEX apply to DOPS as well. In addition, there is considerable research showing that global ratings of procedural skills can produce valid results.(25) For example, Goff *et al.* demonstrated that in an objective structured assessment of technical skills, judgements of occurrence, quality and fitness by two assessors were able to distinguish among levels of training.(26) Similarly, a study of actual performance by Winckel *et al.* found that both checklists and global ratings distinguished among levels of training for 41 operations (*see* Box 20.2).(27) More recently,

BOX 20.2 WHERE'S THE EVIDENCE: Checklists versus global ratings

There is a sizeable body of research on the use of checklists, which capture the occurrence of particular behaviours, and global rating scales, which capture the quality of a performance.(29–34)

Scores based on checklists are strongly correlated with scores based on global rating scales. Checklists are (i) perceived to be more objective and (ii) can produce slightly more reliable scores, but (iii) they may not be as good at capturing advanced levels of expertise. Global ratings are (i) perceived to be more subjective, but (ii) tend to be slightly more valid.

Doctors or trained patients can use checklists since they require only that behaviour to be noted. Only experts can use global ratings. Overall differences between checklists and global ratings are relatively small.

Marriott *et al.* found good validity, reliability and acceptability when using DOPS to assess trainees' skills in the operating theatre.(28)

CSR

Chart-stimulated recall (CSR) was developed by Maatsch for use by the American Board of Emergency Medicine.(35) A variation of it, called the Case-based Discussion, has been used in the Foundation Programme. In this setting, the trainee must select two case records from patients they have seen recently and in which they have made entries.(13) The assessor selects one of the two cases and explores one aspect of it with the trainee. For example, they might choose to focus on which investigations the trainee ordered or on the ethical issues raised by a particular patient. In all instances, the assessor is interested in understanding the reasoning behind the trainee's choices.

CSR is designed to offer an assessment of medical record keeping and to stimulate trainees to discuss why they acted as they did. In this way it offers the opportunity for assessment of the application of knowledge, decision-making and ethical issues. CSR uses single encounters as the grounds for measurement, and assessors are asked to make judgements about both the quality of the clinical assessment, investigation and referrals, treatment, professionalism, medical record keeping and overall clinical care, and about whether they meet or exceed expectations (i.e. fitness). An assessment form for the Case-based Discussion version of CSR is shown in Figure 20.3.

When used in the Foundation Programme, each encounter is intended to take 15 minutes, followed by 5 minutes of feedback, and there should be four to six encounters during the year.(13) Assessors include consultants, experienced specialist registrars, staff grade and associate specialists, and general practitioners. There is a list of core problems as part of the curriculum, and trainees are expected to sample from them. The feedback given after the encounter should include strengths, suggestions for development and an action plan that outlines a response to these suggestions.

The original work on the validity of the CSR was done in conjunction with the certification and recertification programmes of the American Board of Emergency Medicine.(35) When given to a sample of practising doctors, CSR score distributions and pass–fail results were consistent with those for initial certification. They were also correlated with scores from a variety of other methods, including an oral examination and an audit of practice records. Of all the methods used, CSR was considered most valid by practising doctors.

In a later study, Norman *et al.* applied several different assessment methods to a group of doctors, who were referred because of practice problems, and a group of volunteers.(36) CSR was correlated with an SP examination (0.74) and an oral examination (0.51) given to these same groups. In addition, CSR was able to distinguish the 'referred' from the volunteer group.

Finally, Solomon *et al.* gave CSR to a group of doctors eligible for recertification.(37) It was correlated with an oral exam (0.49), and when it was combined with the oral exam,

Please refer to curriculum at www.mmc.nhs.uk for details of expected competencies for F1 and F2

Case-based Discussion (CbD) – F2 Version

Please complete the question using a cross: ☒   Please use black ink and CAPITAL LETTERS

Doctor's	Surname																	

	Forename																	

GMC Number: ☐☐☐☐☐☐☐   **GMC NUMBER MUST BE COMPLETED**

Clinical setting: A&E ☐   OPD ☐   In-patient ☐   Acute Admission ☐   GP Surgery ☐

Clinical problem category: Pain ☐   Airway/ Breathing ☐   CVS/ Circulation ☐   Psych/ Behav ☐   Neuro ☐   Gastro ☐   Other ☐ _____

Focus of clinical encounter: Medical Record Keeping ☐   Clinical Assessment ☐   Management ☐   Professionalism ☐

Complexity of case: Low ☐   Average ☐   High ☐   Assessor's position: Consultant ☐   SpR ☐   GP ☐

Please grade the following areas using the scale below:	Below expectations for F2 completion		Borderline for F2 completion	Meets expectations for F2 completion	Above expectations for F2 completion		U/C*
	1	2	3	4	5	6	
1 Medical record keeping	☐	☐	☐	☐	☐	☐	☐
2 Clinical assessment	☐	☐	☐	☐	☐	☐	☐
3 Investigation and referrals	☐	☐	☐	☐	☐	☐	☐
4 Treatment	☐	☐	☐	☐	☐	☐	☐
5 Follow-up and future planning	☐	☐	☐	☐	☐	☐	☐
6 Professionalism	☐	☐	☐	☐	☐	☐	☐
7 Overall clinical judgement	☐	☐	☐	☐	☐	☐	☐

*U/C Please mark this if you have not observed the behaviour and therefore feel unable to comment.

Anything especially good?   **Suggestions for development**

Agreed action:

	Not at all									Highly
Trainee satisfaction with CbD	1☐	2☐	3☐	4☐	5☐	6☐	7☐	8☐	9☐	10☐
Assessor satisfaction with CbD	1☐	2☐	3☐	4☐	5☐	6☐	7☐	8☐	9☐	10☐

What training have you had in the use of this assessment tool?:   ☐ Have Read Guidelines ☐ Face-to-Face ☐ Web/CD rom

Time taken for discussion: (in minutes) ☐☐

Assessor's Signature: ....   Date: ☐☐ / ☐☐ / ☐☐

Time taken for feedback: (in minutes) ☐☐

Assessor's Surname: ☐☐☐☐☐☐☐☐☐☐☐☐☐☐☐☐

Assessor's GMC Number: ☐☐☐☐☐☐☐

Please note:
Failure of return of all completed forms to your administrator is a probity issue

2466400642

Figure 20.3 Typical CbD assessment form.

CSR had correlations with written and oral exams administered 10 years earlier (0.45, 0.37).

MSF

Making judgements about the performance of colleagues has formed the basis of the referral process in medicine and other professions for centuries.(38) In recent years, these judgements have been collected in a systematic fashion and aggregated to provide an assessment of performance. There are several variations of the process, the assessors (e.g. peers, seniors, patients), and the forms that are used, but as an example, this chapter focuses on the mini-PAT.

Trainees nominate assessors who are consultants, experienced specialist registrars, staff grade and associate specialists, general practitioners, nurses or allied health personnel. Each is sent a questionnaire, which, after completion, is returned to a central location for processing. This ensures that the trainee does not know the views of their assessors. The trainee self-assesses and submits the questionnaire for processing as well. Figure 20.4 shows the mini-PAT questionnaire. It contains 16 questions addressing the categories of:
- good clinical care
- maintaining good medical practice
- teaching and training – appraising and assessing
- relationships with patients
- working with colleagues
- an overall assessment.

Unlike the other methods that are described in this chapter, the judgements underpinning the mini-PAT are grounded in routine performance rather that performance on a specific encounter. As with the other methods, however, assessors are asked to make judgements about both quality and fitness.

It is most efficient if the questionnaires are collated electronically in a central location, and feedback is prepared for the trainee. The reports to trainees typically provide self-ratings, the mean ratings of the assessors and the national mean ratings. All comments are included verbatim, but they are anonymous. The trainee and their educational supervisor review the results together and agree on strengths, areas for development and an action plan. This process can be repeated as often as makes sense in the context of training.

Multisource feedback (MSF) programmes of this type have been used at a number of different institutions. For 30 years, medical students in the obstetrics/gynaecology and internal medicine clerkships at the University of Missouri-Kansas have been asked to evaluate the professionalism of their peers.(39) The programme has evolved over the years, but recently most of the negative reports about professional behaviours received by the promotions committee emanated from peers.(40)

Similarly, the University of Florida uses an MSF assessment system to identify those medical students whose professionalism is outstanding.(41) The information is included in the Dean's letter of recommendation for postgraduate training, and there are reports that it has enabled some students to acquire a more desirable post.(40)

There is a growing body of evidence supporting the validity of these assessments. A study of certification in the US by Ramsey *et al.* compared certified internists and non-certified internists who were 5–10 years past certification or training.(42) Several assessments were collected, and the certified doctors had higher peer ratings, even though their peers did not know their certification status. The results were also correlated with written examination performance.

In a follow-up study, Ramsey *et al.* focused only on practising internists who were 5–15 years past certification.(43) Two lists of peers were solicited, one from the participants and one from their medical supervisors. In addition, the questions on the assessment form were divided into two scales, one for cognitive/technical skills and one for professionalism. The source of the peers (participant versus medical supervisor) did not affect the ratings. Further, a written examination had a statistically significant correlation with the cognitive/technical scale but not the professionalism scale.

The mini-PAT is a shortened form of the Sheffield Peer Review Assessment Tool, which was studied with paediatricians.(44) Results of that work indicate that it was feasible, produced scores with reasonable reliability and was not significantly influenced by extraneous factors, such as occupation of assessor, length of working relationship and the clinical setting in which the relationship took place. Moreover, it was able to distinguish between doctors of different grades. It was used in the Foundation Programme at its inception but has since been replaced with the Team Assessment of Behaviour (TAB), which is shorter and so more practical.(45)

Portfolios

A portfolio is simply a collection of information (methods for the purposes of this chapter) that is intended to demonstrate achievement. However, there are many variations on this simple theme. Portfolios can include a number of different types of information, both single-encounter and routine performance. In some instances, the content of the portfolio is left wholly to the trainee, while in others they must all include exactly the same information. Typically, the portfolio is reviewed by assessors, who are asked to make judgements about it.

A portfolio for use in postgraduate training might include several components or sections. For instance, it may contain a section devoted to the educational experiences of the trainee, such as procedure and patient logs, participation in didactic sessions, clinical rotations, research papers and critical incidents. A second section might contain the results of workplace-based assessments such as the mini-CEX, DOPS, CSR and MSF, plus scores on written knowledge examinations. A third section could be devoted to the trainee's reflections on these educational experiences and ongoing self-appraisal. A final section might contain all of the signoffs necessary to support a decision about the trainee's promotion.

Please refer to curriculum at www.mmc.nhs.uk for details of expected competencies for F1 and F2

mini-PAT (Peer Assessment Tool) – F1 Version

Please complete the question using a cross: ☒   Please use black ink and CAPITAL LETTERS

Doctor's   Surname

Forename

GMC Number:

How do you rate this Doctor in their:	Below expectations for F1 completion		Borderline for F1 completion	Meets expectations for F1 completion	Above expectations for F1 completion		U/C*
	1	2	3	4	5	6	
Good Clinical Care							
1 Ability to diagnose patient problems	☐	☐	☐	☐	☐	☐	☐
2 Ability to formulate appropriate management plans	☐	☐	☐	☐	☐	☐	☐
3 Awareness of their own limitations	☐	☐	☐	☐	☐	☐	☐
4 Ability to respond to psychosocial aspects of illness	☐	☐	☐	☐	☐	☐	☐
5 Appropriate utilisation of resources e.g. ordering investigations	☐	☐	☐	☐	☐	☐	☐
Maintaining good medical practice							
6 Ability to manage time effectively / prioritise	☐	☐	☐	☐	☐	☐	☐
7 Technical skills (appropriate to current practice)	☐	☐	☐	☐	☐	☐	☐
Teaching and Training, Appraising and Assessing							
8 Willingness and effectiveness when teaching/training colleagues	☐	☐	☐	☐	☐	☐	☐
Relationship with Patients							
9 Communication with patients	☐	☐	☐	☐	☐	☐	☐
10 Communication with carers and/or family	☐	☐	☐	☐	☐	☐	☐
11 Respect for patients and their right to confidentiality	☐	☐	☐	☐	☐	☐	☐
Working with colleagues							
12 Verbal communication with colleagues	☐	☐	☐	☐	☐	☐	☐
13 Written communication with colleagues	☐	☐	☐	☐	☐	☐	☐
14 Ability to recognise and value the contribution of others	☐	☐	☐	☐	☐	☐	☐
15 Accessibility/Reliability	☐	☐	☐	☐	☐	☐	☐
16 Overall, how do you rate this doctor compared to a doctor ready to complete F1 training?	☐	☐	☐	☐	☐	☐	☐

Do you have any concerns about this doctor's probity or health?   ☐ Yes   ☐ No
If yes please state your concerns:

*U/C Please mark this if you have not observed the behaviour and therefore feel unable to comment.   **6927534062**

Figure 20.4 The mini-PAT questionnaire.

Because portfolios used for different purposes might contain different forms of assessment, it is not reasonable to extrapolate the validity of one portfolio from another. However, it is sensible to extrapolate the validity of the portfolio from the validity of the contents (i.e. mini-CEX, DOPS, CSR, MSF) and the quality of the process used to make decisions based on those contents.

Regardless of the particular application, the use of portfolios in assessment requires that one or more experts make judgements about their contents. Applying the framework presented above, these judgements can be made about occurrence (e.g. whether a trainee has had the required number of mini-CEX encounters), quality (e.g. whether the mini-CEX results indicated good performance) and fitness (e.g. whether the mini-CEX results indicated satisfactory completion of a year of training). There are several factors that will contribute to the quality of these judgements, and they are similar to those for all assessments based on observation.

First, the purpose of the portfolio must be clear (e.g. it is intended for summative use). Second, it is important to be specific about what each portfolio must contain and to have as much commonality across them as possible; this enhances the ability to make comparisons both among trainees and against standards. Third, the portfolios should be based on as many independent assessments of performance as is feasible. This is equivalent to having a number of different encounters in the mini-CEX or DOPS. Fourth, several examiners should be involved in making judgements about each portfolio; this reduces the effects of examiners who differ significantly in stringency. Portfolio-based learning and assessment is covered in more detail in Chapter 14.

Influence on learning

The workplace offers a rich environment for assessment, and the observational methods described above can be of considerable use in this regard. It is perhaps more important, however, that several of them offer the opportunity for formative assessment and feedback at the same time. Unfortunately, there are data suggesting that a sizeable majority of postgraduate trainees are never observed in a patient encounter.(15) Not only do the methods described above require that observation, but in addition to summative assessment, the observations are intended to serve as a basis for formative assessment and educational feedback (*see* Chapter 23).

Holmboe *et al.* have developed an excellent programme for providing feedback.(34) At the completion of the assessment process, the observers need to provide an evaluation of the trainees' strengths and weaknesses while enabling them to react to these. Faculty members then need to encourage self-assessment and develop action plans that will enable the trainees to address any deficiencies. These components are sometimes documented on the mini-CEX, DOPS and CSD forms that are used as part of workplace assessment. Feedback between the educational supervisor and trainee is also an important part of MSF.

Faculty development

Faculty development is one key to the success of workplace assessment based on observation. Holmboe *et al.* have developed an excellent workshop, which has applicability to a variety of observational methods.(46) It consists of three major pieces. First, there is training in behavioural observation, including knowing what to look for, preparing the trainee and patient, and minimising intrusiveness and interference. Second, there is performance dimension training, in which faculty members decide on the dimensions of performance that are important. Finally, there is frame of reference training, where faculty members practise to improve their accuracy and discrimination and reduce differences in stringency.

The workshop consists of didactic mini-lectures, small group and videotape evaluation exercises and practice with standardised trainees and patients. A randomised control trial of this model showed that faculty members who underwent training thought it was excellent, felt more comfortable performing direct observation and were more stringent than the control group faculty members.

In addition to the focus on assessment, faculty development efforts should also be provided for the provision of educational feedback. This goes well beyond the methods presented here, but given the few times trainees are actually observed in their work, workplace-based assessment offers an opportunity that should not be missed.

Challenges for workplace-based assessment

For the methods described above, as well as others that are based on observation, there is a series of challenges to the assessment process. Among them are reliability, equivalence, stakes, relationships, the need for other forms of assessment, feasibility and future research.(38)

Reliability

If the same trainee were examined on different occasions with different patients by different assessors, we would want their results to be the same. This is called reliability or reproducibility. In the observation of clinical performance, three major factors affect reliability: the number of encounters observed (both single encounters and routine performance), the number of assessors and the aspects of performance being evaluated.(47)

Seminal work by Elstein *et al.* in the mid-1970s indicated that doctors' performances were case specific; performance on one case only weakly predicted performance on others.(6) This finding has been replicated several times. Consequently, it is important to observe trainees with a number of different patients before having confidence in the results of their assessment. All of the methods used in the Foundation Programme require multiple encounters with patients.

Likewise, there is research showing that experienced assessors, even when observing exactly the same encounter, differ in their opinions about its difficulty and quality.(48)

More importantly, they interact with each encounter along the lines of their own strengths, weaknesses and experiences. Consequently, it is important to include assessments from different faculty members to achieve reliable results. Again, all of the methods used in the Foundation Programme require multiple observers and a different assessor for each different encounter.

Finally, there is research indicating that more reliable results are obtained when assessors are asked to judge a number of aspects of a performance rather than making a single overall judgement about it.(43) At the same time, asking for too many judgements does little to improve reliability and adversely affects feasibility. The exact number will, of course, vary with the characteristics of the performance and the nature of the judgements being made (more for quality and fitness, less for occurrence), but generally 5–10 questions should be sufficient.

Some factors, such as the exact wording of the questions and the number of points on the scale, have only a very modest influence on reliability. But because these things are obvious and easy to change, some users spend considerable effort on them. Assuming that reasonable care has been taken, this effort would better be spent recruiting and training assessors or observing additional encounters.

Equivalence

An important issue in the use of observational methods is whether the assessments of trainees are equivalent to one another. In most of the methods described above, different patients or their records serve as the basis for assessment, and these may differ in complexity. Likewise, different faculty members and different peers act as assessors for the trainees, and they are not equally stringent. In portfolios that do not have strict requirements for what is included, there is considerable variability in the basis for assessment. As a consequence, it is not clear whether trainee differences are due to their ability or to the difficulty of the encounters and assessors that trainees face.

This is less of a problem within each training programme, where presumably the assessors and clinical settings are similar. It is also less troublesome when the stakes are lower and there is an emphasis on feedback and formative assessment. However, the observational assessments of the type described above do not yield comparable scores at the regional or national level because faculties can differ appreciably, as do the clinical settings for training. Using a common problem list, involving a number of assessors for each trainee and providing good faculty development will lessen the impact of these problems, but they remain significant.

Stakes

Although it has not been studied extensively, there is some evidence to indicate that assessments based on observation are influenced by what is at stake. Certainly, authors have found that when used for an important purpose (e.g. promotion, continued certification), grades tend to be very high and very few trainees are considered unsatisfactory.(49–51) Although it is possible that doctors in these studies are well above average, it is more likely that peers and faculty members are reluctant to provide negative assessments when the stakes are moderate or high.

There is no way to avoid this problem completely, but there are some things that will lessen its effect. The use of external examiners reduces the amount of prior information available and lessens the assessors' personal stake in the trainee. For both external assessors and internal assessors, faculty development is important and has been shown to increase the stringency of the grades they provide.(52) For any sort of MSF, anonymity is crucial. Where appropriate, it is also helpful to restrict the nature of the judgements to occurrence or quality rather than fitness. The latter requires a high-stakes decision, and these are often better made using other faculty members and other methods.(53)

Relationships

The relationship between trainees and their observers can adversely affect the validity of the assessments. In the Foundation Programme, these effects might be exacerbated by the fact that trainees choose their assessors.(13) In addition, when assessors are faculty members, their role as educator is in conflict with their role as evaluator. Likewise, the relationships between the trainee and those peers who complete the MSF questionnaires are varied and might influence the results.

Although there is no way to avoid the effects of relationships, there are some steps that might decrease their influence. Where feasible, using external assessors reduces some of the concerns. Similarly, ensuring anonymity in the context of MSF is important. It may also be useful if the assessor selects the trainee, the patients and the peers rather than having them chosen by the trainee. However, the effect of self-selection of assessors versus selection by others did not make a difference when studied by Ramsey *et al.*(43)

Need for other forms of assessment

Observation in the workplace constitutes a powerful tool for assessment and feedback. However, it does not serve all purposes, and other forms of assessment are better suited to some functions. For example, differences in assessors and clinical material make it unwise to compare trainees regionally or nationally. Consequently, assessment based on observation in the workplace should not be the sole basis on which to rank trainees and select them for additional educational experiences. Likewise, this form of assessment alone is not suitable for making high-stakes end-of-training decisions such as those for certification in the US. In both instances, assessment based on observation in the workplace needs to be supplemented with a national programme that includes tests of knowledge and clinical skill.

In addition to national ranking and achievement testing, observation in the workplace is best suited to an assessment of integrated skills in the context of patient care. Where problem trainees are identified, this form of assessment is neither ideal nor efficient in determining relative areas of strength and weakness. For diagnostic purposes, it is best to follow with assessments of medical knowledge and clinical skill.

Feasibility

There are significant resource constraints in the workplace setting, and the methods described here were designed to be as efficient as possible given this context. Nonetheless, there remain serious challenges to carrying out this form of assessment. Clearly, the centralisation of functions, such as collecting and reporting data for MSF, significantly enhances the feasibility of the method. Likewise, a national programme of faculty development is useful.

Despite these efficiencies, local administration strategies are still needed. In the case of the Foundation Programme, trainees are given responsibility for ensuring that the assessments are completed.(13) This is effective but creates challenges based on the assessor–trainee relationship. In the US, the assessors have chosen the trainee and patient, but enlisting the cooperation of busy clinician-educators is difficult. This is an area that requires more attention to ensure the validity and feasibility of the methods.

Future research

Although observation and feedback has been central to education for millennia, research on systematic observation and feedback in the medical workplace is in its infancy. A recent systematic review of direct observation concluded that although there are numerous methods, studies of their validity and outcomes are limited.(16) Similarly, a systematic review of the impact of workplace-based assessment on doctors' education and performance found subjective reports of educational impact, but no research in the area.(54) Going forward, addressing these deficits in the literature will be essential even though studies of this type are difficult to do well. In the meantime, there is considerable support in the general education literature for the central role of feedback in achievement.(55) Also, feedback is not possible without observation and assessment.

Summary

Assessment in the setting of clinical training, particularly postgraduate training, is not as well developed as assessment in the undergraduate arena. Over the past decade, several methods based on the observation of routine trainee–patient encounters and interactions with colleagues have been proposed. These methods have been used in the UK, the US and other countries around the world.

The mini-CEX, DOPS and CSR are based on the observation of a single performance with a patient or a medical record, while MSF captures routine performance. In all instances, judgements about the quality and fitness of the performance(s) are made by the assessor(s), and there is considerable research supporting the validity of these methods.

The opportunity for educational feedback as part of these methods is as important as their contribution to the assessment process. At the completion of each assessment, the observers need to provide an evaluation of the trainees' strengths and weaknesses while enabling them to react to these. Faculty members then need to encourage self-

assessment and develop action plans, which will enable the trainees to address any deficiencies. In a sense, the methods bring together summative and formative assessment and create a teaching moment that skilled faculty members can grasp.

A portfolio is a collection of a variety of different assessments and experiences. Because of the variability in their contents, it is not reasonable to generalise from studies of the validity of one portfolio to another. However, it is possible to extrapolate the validity of the portfolio from the validity of the contents (i.e. mini-CEX, DOPS, CSR, MSF) and the quality of the process used to make judgements about it.

Faculty development is a key to the successful use of these methods. A model workshop would consist of training in behavioural observation, performance dimension training and frame of reference training, along with considerable practice. Periodic but shorter versions of the workshop are needed to maintain faculty involvement and proficiency. In addition, the provision of educational feedback should be an important part of the overall faculty development effort.

Finally, a series of challenges remains, including reliability, equivalence, stakes, relationships, the need for other forms of assessment and feasibility. Given the nature of the methods, some (e.g. equivalence) will be very difficult to surmount. Consequently, it will be important to deploy these methods appropriately and to ensure that they are only one piece of a larger assessment programme.

Acknowledgements

The Foundation Programme assessment examples are reproduced here with grateful acknowledgement to the American Board of Internal Medicine (mini-CEX), the Federation of Royal Colleges of Physicians (DOPS), the American Board of Emergency Medicine (CSR) and the University of Sheffield (mini-PAT). Further information can be found at http://www.mmc.nhs.uk

References

1 Norman GR (2002) Research in medical education: three decades of progress. *British Medical Journal.* **324**: 1560–2.
2 Norcini JJ (2005) Current perspectives in assessment: the assessment of performance at work. *Medical Education.* **39**: 880–9.
3 Miller GE (1990) The assessment of clinical skills/competence/performance. *Academic Medicine.* **65**(9): s63–7.
4 Norcini JJ (2003) Peer assessment of competence. *Medical Education.* **37**: 539–43.
5 Norcini JJ (2006) Faculty observations of student professional behaviour. In: Stern D (ed.) *Measuring Professionalism*, pp. 147–58. Oxford University Press, Oxford.
6 Elstein AS, Shulman LS and Sprafka SA (1978) *Medical Problem-Solving: An Analysis of Clinical Reasoning.* Harvard University Press, Cambridge, MA.
7 Pulito AR, Donnelly MB, Plymale M and Mentzer RM Jr (2006) What do faculty observe of medical students' clinical performance? *Teaching and Learning in Medicine.* **18**(2): 99–104.

8 Silber CG, Nasca TJ, Paskin DL *et al.* (2004) Do global rating forms enable program directors to assess the ACGME competencies? *Academic Medicine.* **79**(6): 549–56.

9 Brennan RL (2001) *Generalizability Theory.* Springer-Verlag, New York.

10 Norcini JJ, Blank LL, Duffy FD and Fortna G (2003) The mini-CEX: a method for assessing clinical skills. *Annals of Internal Medicine.* **138**: 476–81.

11 Martin JA, Regehr G, Reznick R *et al.* (1997) Objective structured assessment of technical skill (OSATS) for surgical residents. *British Journal of Surgery.* **84**(2): 273–8.

12 Norcini JJ and Boulet JR (2003) Methodological issues in the use of standardized patients for assessment. *Teaching and Learning in Medicine.* **15**(4): 293–7.

13 Davies H, Archer J, Southgate L, Norcini J (2009) Initial evaluation of the first year of the Foundation Assessment Programme. *Medical Education.* **43**: 74–81.

14 Norcini JJ, Blank LL, Arnold GK and Kimball HR (1995) The mini-CEX (clinical evaluation exercise): a preliminary investigation. *Annals of Internal Medicine.* **123**: 795–9.

15 Day SC, Grosso LG, Norcini JJ *et al.* (1990) Residents' perceptions of evaluation procedures used by their training program. *Journal of General Internal Medicine.* **5**: 421–6.

16 Kogan JR, Holmboe ES and Hauer KE (2009) Tools for direct observation and assessment of clinical skills of medical trainees. *Journal of the American Medical Association.* **302**(12): 1316–26.

17 Kogan JR, Bellini LM and Shea JA (2003) Feasibility, reliability, and validity of the mini-clinical evaluation exercise (mCEX) in a medicine core clerkship. *Academic Medicine.* **78**(s10): S33–5.

18 Durning SJ, Cation LJ, Markert RJ and Pangaor LN (2002) Assessing the reliability and validity of the mini-clinical evaluation exercise for internal medicine residency training. *Academic Medicine.* **77**(9): 900–4.

19 Boulet JR, McKinley DW, Norcini JJ and Whelan GP (2002) Assessing the comparability of standardized patient and physician evaluations of clinical skills. *Advances in Health Sciences Education.* **7**: 85–97.

20 Holmboe ES, Huot S, Chung J, Norcini J and Hawkins RE (2003) Construct validity of the miniClinical Evaluation Exercise (miniCEX). *Academic Medicine.* **78**: 826–30.

21 Cruess R, McIlroy JH, Cruess S *et al.* (2006) The professionalism mini-evaluation exercise: a preliminary investigation. *Academic Medicine.* **81**(s10): S74–8.

22 Hatala R, Ainslie M, Kassen BO *et al.* (2006) Assessing the mini-clinical evaluation exercise in comparison to a national specialty examination. *Medical Education.* **40**(10): 950–6.

23 Kogan JR and Hauer KE (2006) Brief report: use of the mini-clinical evaluation exercise in internal medicine core clerkships. *Journal of General Internal Medicine.* **21**(5): 501–2.

24 Wragg A, Wade W, Fuller G *et al.* (2003) Assessing the performance of specialist registrars. *Clinical Medicine.* **3**(2): 131–4.

25 Larson JL, Williams RG, Ketchum J *et al.* (2005) Feasibility, reliability and validity of an operative performance rating system for evaluating surgery residents. *Surgery.* **138**(4): 640–7.

26 Goff BA, Nielsen PE, Lentz GM *et al.* (2002) Surgical skills assessment: a blinded examination of obstetrics and gynecology residents. *American Journal of Obstetrics and Gynecology.* **186**(4): 613–7.

27 Winckel CP, Reznick RK, Cohen R and Taylor B (1994) Reliability and construct validity of a structured technical skills assessment form. *American Journal of Surgery.* **167**(4): 423–7.

28 Marriott J, Purdie H, Crossley J and Beard JD (2010) Evaluation of procedure-based assessment for assessing trainees' skills in the operating theatre. *British Journal of Surgery.* **98**(3): 450–7.

29 Martin JA, Reznick RK, Rothman A *et al.* (1996) Who should rate candidates in an objective structured clinical examination? *Academic Medicine.* **71**(2): 170–5.

30 Hodges B, McNaughton N, Regehr G *et al.* (2002) The challenge of creating new OSCE measures to capture the characteristics of expertise. *Medical Education.* **36**(8): 742–8.

31 Hodges B, Regehr G, McNaughton N *et al.* (1999) OSCE checklists do not capture increasing levels of expertise. *Academic Medicine.* **74**(10): 1129–34.

32 Rothman AI, Blackmore D, Dauphinee WD and Reznick R (1997) The use of global ratings in OSCE station scores. *Advances in Health Sciences Education.* **1**: 215–9.

33 Regehr G, MacRae H, Reznick RK and Szalay D (1998) Comparing the psychometric properties of checklists and global rating scales for assessing performance on an OSCE-format examination. *Academic Medicine.* **73**(9): 993–7.

34 Regehr G, Freeman R, Robb A *et al.* (1999) OSCE performance evaluations made by standardized patients: comparing checklist and global rating scores. *Academic Medicine.* **74**(s10): S135–7.

35 Maatsch JL, Huang R, Downing S and Barker B (1983) *Predictive validity of medical specialty examinations.* Final report for Grant HS 02038-04, National Center of Health Services Research. Office of Medical Education and Research and development, Michigan State University, East Lansing, MI.

36 Norman GR, Davis D, Painvin A *et al.* (1989) Comprehensive assessment of clinical competence of family/general physicians using multiple measures, In: *Proceedings of the Annual Conference on Research in Medical Education*, p. 75. Association of American Medical Colleges, Washington, DC.

37 Solomon DJ, Reinhart MA, Bridgham RG *et al.* (1990) An assessment of an oral examination format for evaluating clinical competence in emergency medicine. *Academic Medicine.* **65**(s9): S43–4.

38 Norcini JJ (2003) Peer assessment of competence. *Medical Education.* **37**: 539–43.

39 Arnold L, Willoughby L, Calkins V and Eberhart G (1981) Use of peer evaluation in the assessment of medical students. *Medical Education.* **56**: 35–42.

40 Arnold L and Stern D (2006) Content and context of peer assessment. In: Stern D (ed.) *Measuring Professionalism*, pp. 175–94. Oxford University Press, Oxford.

41 Small PA, Stevens B and Duerson MC (1993) Issues in medical education: basic problems and potential solutions. *Academic Medicine.* **68**: S89–98.

42 Ramsey PG, Carline JD, Inui TS *et al.* (1989) Predictive validity of certification by the American Board of Internal Medicine. *Annals of Internal Medicine.* **110**(9): 719–26.

43 Ramsey PG, Wenrich MD, Carline JD *et al.* (1993) Use of peer ratings to evaluate physician performance. *Journal of the American Medical Association.* **269**: 1655–60.

44 Archer JC, Norcini JJ and Davies HA (2005) Peer review of paediatricians in training using SPRAT. *British Medical Journal.* **330**: 1251–3.

45 Whitehouse A, Hassell A, Bullock A *et al.* (2007) 360 degree assessment (multisource feedback) of UK trainee doctors: field testing of team assessment of behaviours (TAB). *Medical Teacher.* **29**: 171–6.

46 Holmboe ES, Hawkins RE and Huot SJ (2004) Effects of training in direct observation of medical residents' clinical competence: a randomized trial. *Annals of Internal Medicine.* **140**(11): 874–81.

47 Norcini JJ (2001) The validity of long cases. *Medical Education.* **35**: 735–6.

48 Noel GL, Herbers JE, Caplow MP *et al.* (1992) How well do internal medicine faculty members evaluate the clinical skills of residents? *Annals of Internal Medicine.* **117**: 757–65.

49 Hay JA (1995) *Tutorial reports and ratings. Evaluation Methods: A Resource Handbook.* McMaster University, Hamilton, Ontario.

50 Ramsey PG, Carline JD, Blank LL and Wenrich MD (1996) Feasibility of hospital-based use of peer ratings to evaluate the performance of practicing physicians. *Academic Medicine.* **71**: 364–70.

51 Hall W, Violato C, Lewkonia R *et al.* (1999) Assessment of physician performance in Alberta: the physician achievement review. *Canadian Medical Association Journal.* **161**: 52–7.

52 Holmboe ES, Yepes M, Williams F and Huot SJ (2004) Feedback and the mini clinical evaluation exercise. *Journal of General Internal Medicine.* **19**(5 Pt 2): 558–61.

53 Norcini JJ (2005) Standard setting. In: Dent JA and Harden RM (eds) *A Practical Guide for Medical Teachers*, pp. 293–301. Elsevier Churchill Livingston, Edinburgh.

54 Miller A and Archer J (2010) Impact of workplace based assessment on doctors' education and performance: a systematic review. *British Medical Journal.* **341**: c5064.

55 Norcini JJ (2010) The power of feedback. *Medical Education.* **44**: 16–7.

21 Structured assessments of clinical competence

Katharine AM Boursicot[1], Trudie E Roberts[2] and William P Burdick[3]

[1] St George's, University of London, UK
[2] University of Leeds, UK
[3] Foundation for Advancement of International Medical Education and Research (FAIMER), USA; Drexel University College of Medicine, USA

KEY MESSAGES

- Objective Structure Clinical Examinations (OCSEs) have become widespread in the assessment of clinical competence.
- Authenticity is important in enhancing the validity of the test.
- Developing high-quality OSCE stations takes time and effort.
- OSCEs are often complex and costly to run, but they are a fair and reliable method of assessing clinical skills.

- OSCEs should be blueprinted to the learning outcomes of the curriculum.
- Training of simulated patients is essential for high levels of consistency.
- Future developments of OSCEs are likely to be in the area of acute medical simulations, which are difficult to test by other means.

Introduction

The reliable and valid assessment of clinical competence has become an increasingly important area of concern in medical education. Various stakeholders, with legitimate interests in the clinical competence of graduates from medical schools and of postgraduate trainees, require evidence that assessments are discriminating between the sufficiently and insufficiently competent at all levels of medical training and education.

While clinical competence is based on a thorough base of specialist medical knowledge,(1) the term *clinical competence* also encompasses other professional practice elements such as history taking and clinical examination skills, skills in practical procedures, doctor–patient communication, problem-solving ability and management skills, relationships with colleagues and ethical behaviour.(2–4)

Unsuited to testing by written examination, the assessment of clinical competence has historically involved the direct observation of candidates by professional colleagues. With the development of work-based learning methods to assess clinical performance in a more authentic and naturalistic way, there is the potential for confusion over terminology. For the purposes of this chapter we will consider assessments of clinical competence to be measures of what doctors can do in *controlled representations of professional practice*, i.e. under examination conditions. We will restrict the use of performance assessment to measurements of what doctors do in their professional practice.(5) In other words, we shall consider competency-based assessments to be those assessments undertaken outside the 'real' clinical environment and performance-based assessment to be those administered within the natural clinical setting.

A variety of formats for assessing clinical competence have been developed over the years and in this extended chapter we review the more 'classical' long- and short-case formats, and also describe newer formats such as the Objective Structure Clinical Examination (OSCE) and Objective Structured Long Case Examination Record (OSLER). We discuss the stages of planning and implementing OSCEs and offer practical advice on blueprinting, station development, examiner training, simulated/standardised patient training, organisational issues and standard setting. We do not discuss workplace-based assessment instruments as these are covered comprehensively in Chapter 20.

The long case

In the traditional long case, candidates spend up to 1 hour with a patient, during which they are expected to take a full formal history and perform a complete examination. The candidate is not observed. On completion of this task the candidate is questioned for 20–30 minutes about the case, usually by a pair of examiners, and may be taken back to the patient to demonstrate clinical signs.

Holistic appraisal of the examinee's ability to assess and manage a real patient is a laudable goal of the long case. However, there are some shortcomings in using one or two long cases as a measure of clinical competence, related to issues of reliability pertaining to examiner and patient factors.(6) The lack of measurement consistency caused by

Understanding Medical Education: Evidence, Theory and Practice, Second Edition. Edited by Tim Swanwick.
© 2014 The Association for the Study of Medical Education. Published 2014 by John Wiley & Sons, Ltd.

examiner bias and variations in examiner stringency is a major argument against the long case. Reliability is further compromised when there is little prior agreement between pairs of examiners as to what constitutes acceptable competence. Unstructured questioning and global marking without anchor statements compounds the problem. Reliability in the long case encounter is diminished by variability in degree and details of information disclosure by the patient, as well as variability in patients' demeanour, comfort and health. Furthermore, some patients' illnesses may be straightforward, whereas others may be extremely complex. Examinees' clinical skills also vary significantly across tasks (i.e. task or case specificity),(7) so that assessing examinees on one patient will not provide generalisable estimates of their overall ability.(6,8,9)

While the authenticity of a long-case examination is one of the strengths of the genre, inferring examinees' true clinical skills in the time-constrained environment of actual clinical practice from a 1-hour long-case encounter is debatable. Additionally, given the evidence of the importance of history taking in achieving a diagnosis(10) and the need for students to demonstrate good patient communication skills, the omission of direct observation in this process is a significant weakness.

Objective Structured Long Case Examination Record

In an effort to address these shortcomings, while at the same time attempting to retain the concept of seeing a 'new' patient in a holistic way, the Objective Structured Long Case Examination Record (OSLER) was developed by Gleeson in the 1990s.(11)

The OSLER has 10 key features:
- it is a 10-item structured record
- it has a structured approach – there is prior agreement on what is to be examined
- all candidates are assessed on identical items
- construct validity is recognised and assessed
- history process and product are assessed
- communication skill assessment is emphasised
- case difficulty is identified by the examiner
- it can be used for both criterion- and norm-referenced assessments
- a descriptive mark profile is available where marks are used
- it is a practical assessment with no need for extra time over the ordinary long case.

The OSLER consists of 10 items, which include four on history, three on physical examination, and three on management and clinical acumen. For any individual item, examiners decide on their overall grade and mark for the candidate and then discuss this with their co-examiner and agree on a joint grade. This is done for each item and also for the overall grade and final agreed mark. The recommended time allocation for the OSLER examination is 30 minutes.(12)

There is evidence that the OSLER is more reliable than the standard 'long case'.(13) Most recently, Wass *et al.* dem-

onstrated that assessments using structured long cases could be highly reliable (predicted Cronbach's alpha of 0.84),(14) but this required 10 separate cases and 20 examiners raising major issues of practicality.

Short cases

In traditional tests of clinical competence, candidates undertook a series of (usually three to six) short cases. In this type of test, they were taken to a number of patients with widely differing conditions, and asked to examine individual systems or areas and give differential diagnoses of their findings, or to demonstrate abnormal clinical signs or produce spot diagnoses. Although in some ways similar to an OSCE in that they provided a wider range of cases on which the examiner was able to base his or her opinion of the student's ability, there are important differences. Different candidates rarely saw the same set of patients, cases often differed greatly in their complexity and the same two assessors examined the candidate at each case. These cases were not designed to test communication skills, but instead concentrated on clinical examination skills, with communication with the patients merely incidental. The examination was not structured and the examiners were free to ask any questions they wanted. Like the long case there was no attempt to standardise the expected level of performance. For all these reasons OSCEs have superseded this type of assessment.

Objective Structured Clinical Examinations

The remainder of this chapter relates to the OSCE, an assessment format in which the candidates rotate sequentially around a series of structured cases located in 'stations', at each of which specific tasks have to be performed. The tasks usually involve a clinical skill, such as history taking, examination of a patient or a practical skill. The marking scheme for each station is structured and determined in advance. There is a time limit for each station, after which the candidates have to move on to the next task.

The basic structure of an OSCE may be varied in the timing for each station, the use of a checklist or rating scale for scoring, the use of a clinician or standardised patient as examiner and the use of real patients or manikins, but the fundamental principle is that every candidate has to complete the same assignments in the same amount of time and is marked according to a structured marking schedule.

The terminology associated with the OSCE format can vary – in the undergraduate arena they are more consistently referred to as OSCEs, but in the postgraduate setting a variety of terminology exists. For example, in the UK, the Royal College of Physicians' membership clinical examination is called the Practical Assessment of Clinical Examination Skills (PACES), while the Royal College of General Practitioners' membership examination is called the Clinical Skills Assessment (CSA).

Rationale

The use of OSCEs in the quantitative assessment of competence has become widespread in the field of undergraduate and postgraduate medical education(15–19) since they were originally described,(20) mainly due to the improved reliability of this assessment format. This has resulted in a fairer test of candidates' clinical abilities, since the score has become less dependent on who is examining the candidate and which patient is selected for the encounter. The criteria used to evaluate any assessment method are well described(21) and summarised in Chapter 13. We will examine these criteria – reliability, validity, educational impact, cost-efficiency and acceptability – in some detail, as they relate to OSCE design.

Reliability

Essentially, the OSCE was developed to address the inherent unreliability of classical long and short cases. OSCEs are more reliable than unstructured observations in four main ways:

- Structured marking schedules allow for more consistent scoring by examiners according to predetermined criteria; hence reliability is improved.
- Candidates have to perform a number of different tasks across clinical, practical and communication skill domains – this wider sampling across different cases and skills results in a more reliable picture of a candidate's overall competence. The more stations or cases each candidate has to complete, the more generalisable the test is.
- The reliability of the total test score increases with increasing number and increasing homogeneity of stations or cases. Reliability of sub-scores must be carefully reviewed before reporting.
- As the candidates move through all the stations, each is examined by a number of different examiners, so multiple independent observations are collated. Individual examiner bias is thus attenuated.

It is worth bearing in mind that sampling across different cases makes the most important contribution to reliability; the more stations in an OSCE, the more reliable it will be. However, increasing the number of stations has to be balanced with the practicability of an OSCE exercise. Practically, to enhance reliability it is better to have more stations with one examiner per station than fewer stations with two examiners per station.(22,23)

Validity

Validity assessment asks the question 'What is the degree to which evidence supports the inference(s) made from the test results?' Each separate inference or conclusion from a test may require different supporting evidence. Note that it is the inferences that are validated, not the test itself.(24,25)

Inferences about ability to apply clinical knowledge to bedside data gathering and reasoning, and to effectively use interpersonal skills, are most relevant to the OSCE model. Inferences about knowledge, rather than clinically relevant application of knowledge, or clinical and practical skills, are less well supported by this method.(26)

Types of validity evidence include *content validity* and *construct validity*. Content validity (sometimes referred to as *direct validity*) of an OSCE is determined by how well the sampling of skills matches the learning objectives of the course or degree for which that OSCE is designed.(26,27) The sampling should be representative of the whole testable domain for that examination purpose. The best way to ensure an adequate spread of sampling is to use a *blueprint* method, which we will describe later in the chapter.

Construct validity (sometimes referred to as *indirect validity*) of an OSCE would be the implication that those who performed better at this test had better clinical skills than those who did not perform as well. In an OSCE testing situation, we can only make inferences about a candidate's clinical skills in actual practice, as the OSCE is an artificial situation.

To enhance the validity of inferences from an OSCE, the length of any station should be best fitted to the task to achieve the best authenticity possible. Thus, for example, a station in which blood pressure measurement is tested would authentically be achieved in 5 minutes, whereas taking a history of chest pain or examining the neurological status of a patient's legs would be more authentically achievable in 10 minutes.(28)

Educational impact

The impact on students' learning resulting from a testing process is sometimes referred to as *consequential validity*. The design of an assessment system can reinforce or augment learning, or undermine learning:(29,30) it is a well-recognised phenomenon that students focus on their assessments rather than the learning objectives of the course. Explicit, clear learning objectives allied with clinical skills assessment content and format can be a very effective way of encouraging students to learn the desired clinical competencies. Objectives that include action verbs like 'demonstrate' or 'perform', which are then linked to OSCEs that measure ability to demonstrate or perform certain skills, will encourage students to practise these skills. By contrast, an assessment system that measures students' ability to answer multiple-choice questions about clinical skills will encourage students to focus on knowledge acquisition. Neither approach is wrong – they simply demonstrate that assessment drives education and that assessment methods need to be thoughtfully applied. There is a danger in using detailed checklists as this may encourage students to memorise the steps in a checklist rather than learn and practise the skill. Rating scale marking schedules encourage students to learn and practise skills more holistically.

OSCEs may be used for formative or summative assessment. When teaching and improvement are a major goal of an OSCE, time should be built into the schedule at the end of each station to allow the examiner to give feedback to the student on their performance, providing a very powerful opportunity for student learning. For summative certification examinations, expected competencies should be clearly communicated to the candidates so they have the opportunity to learn the skills prior to taking such examinations.

Cost-efficiency

OSCEs can be very complex to organise. They require meticulous and detailed forward planning, and engagement of considerable numbers of examiners, real patients, simulated patients, and administrative and technical staff to prepare the circuits and station materials and manage the examination. It is therefore most cost-effective to use OSCEs to test clinical competencies and not knowledge, which can be tested more efficiently in a different examination format. Effective implementation of OSCEs requires thoughtful deployment of resources, with attention to production of examination material, timing of sittings, suitability of facilities, catering, and collating and processing of results. Other critical logistics include examiner and standardised patient recruitment and training. This is possible even in resource-limited environments.(31)

Acceptability

The increased reliability of the OSCE format over other formats of clinical testing and its perceived fairness by candidates has helped to engender the widespread acceptability of OSCEs among test takers and testing bodies.

Since Harden's original description in 1979,(20) the use of OSCEs has become widespread in the undergraduate level of testing of clinical competence,(17,18,32,33) as well as increasingly in postgraduate assessment.(16–19,34–39) More recently, OSCEs have been used to replace traditional interviews in recruitment processes in both undergraduate and postgraduate settings.(40,41) For example, for recruitment to general practice training schemes in the UK, candidates go through an OSCE format of scenarios in assessment centres where different exercises are assessed by trained assessors, who observe various job-related competencies, including communication skills, team involvement and problem-solving ability.

In North America, clinical skills assessment has been accepted on a massive scale. In 1992, the Medical Council of Canada (MCC) added a standardised patient component to its national licensing examination because of the perception that important competencies expected of licensed physicians were not being assessed.(40) Since inception, approximately 2500 candidates per year have been tested at multiple sites at fixed periods of time during the year throughout Canada. The MCC clinical skills examination uses physicians at each station to score the encounter.

In the US, the Educational Commission for Foreign Medical Graduates (ECFMG) instituted a performance-based examination in 1998 to assess bedside data gathering, clinical reasoning, interpersonal skills and spoken English communication skills of foreign medical graduates seeking to enter residency training programmes. From 1998 to 2004, when it was incorporated into the United States Medical Licensing Examination (USMLE), there were 43 642 administrations, including 37 930 first-time takers, making it at the time, the largest high-stakes clinical skills examination in the world.(42) The 11 scored encounters had a standardised format, with each requiring the candidate to elicit a medical history, perform a physical examination, communicate in spoken English with a patient in a clinical setting and generate a written record of the encounter. In each station, the candidate encountered a unique standardised patient – a lay person recruited and trained to give a realistic portrayal of a patient with a standardised medical and psychosocial history, and standardised findings on physical examination. Each case had a case-specific checklist containing the elements of medical history and physical examination considered pertinent to that particular case. Simulated patients were trained to recognise appropriate queries and/or physical examination manoeuvres, including acceptable equivalents or variants, and to document each checklist item achieved by the candidate. Simulated patients also evaluated each candidate's interpersonal skills and spoken English proficiency. After each encounter, the candidate generated a patient note on which the pertinent positive and negative elements of history and physical examination were recorded, a differential diagnosis constructed and a diagnostic work-up plan proposed. Performance was evaluated by averaging scores across all encounters and determining the mean for the integrated clinical encounter (data gathering combined with the patient note score) and communication (interpersonal skills and spoken English). Generalisability coefficients for the two conjunctively scored components of CSA were approximately 0.70–0.90.(43)

In 2004, the USMLE adopted the ECFMG clinical skills assessment model and began testing all US medical graduates in addition to foreign medical graduates seeking ECFMG certification.(44) Additional computer and standardised patient training infrastructure was included to ensure comparability across all centres.

The USMLE Step 2 (Clinical Skills) uses 12 standardised patient encounters, each 15 minutes in length followed by 10 minutes to write a patient note. As in the ECFMG CSA examination, standardised patients document the items asked in the history and performed in the physical examination to specified criteria, and evaluate interpersonal skills and spoken English skills, while physician raters score the patient note. Approximately 35 000 administrations take place each year.

OSCE design

We turn now to the elements of good OSCE design, which are summarised in Box 21.1.

Blueprinting

For any particular OSCE, the content – clinical tasks chosen for the stations – should map onto the learning objectives of the course and the candidates' level of learning. It is only reasonable to test candidates on what they have been taught.(27)

To map the assessment to the learning objectives, the categories of skill to be tested should be mapped on one axis and the elements of the course being tested should be mapped on the other. Usually in OSCEs, the skills domains are categorised into clinical examination skills, practical skills and communication skills, which can be further subgrouped into history-taking skills and other doctor–patient/colleague interactions. The subject content of the

OSCE will be determined to a certain extent by how the elements of the course are categorised, that is, by subject discipline or systems.

Blueprinting is a powerful tool that helps to focus the OSCE designers on the exact nature of what they wish to test and relate this to the teaching. Once this blueprint or framework for an OSCE is agreed, the individual stations can be planned and classified according to this blueprint. This ensures adequate sampling across subject area and skill, in terms of numbers of stations covering each skill and the spread over the subjects/systems of the course being tested.

The feasibility of testing a particular task also needs to be considered. Real patients with clinical signs can be used to test clinical examination skills, while simulated patients are best for testing communication skills. Simulated patients can also simulate a number of clinical signs (e.g. loss of visual field, localised abdominal pain). Healthy volunteers can be used when testing the technical process of a clinical examination. There are many manikins on the market for testing invasive practical skills, e.g. intravenous cannulation, urethral catheterisation and arterial blood gas sampling.

BOX 21.1 Elements of Objective Structure Clinical Examination design

Blueprinting

Ensuring the test content maps across the learning objectives of the course

Station development and piloting

Writing stations that function well

Examiner training

Engaging examiners, ensuring consistency of marking contributes to reliability

Simulated patient training

Consistent performance ensures each candidate is presented with the same challenge

Organisation

Making detailed plans well in advance. Be prepared!

It is essential to use a blueprint to plan the content of an OSCE as this helps to ensure that different domains of skill are tested equitably and that the balance of subject areas tested is fairly decided. An example is provided in Box 21.2.

Station development

It is important to write out station specifications well in advance of the examination date so the stations can be reviewed and trialled prior to the actual assessment. Sometimes stations that seem like a good idea at the time of writing may turn out to be unfeasible in practice. When writing a station specification, the following aspects should be considered:

- *Construct:* a statement of what that station is supposedly testing, e.g. this station tests the candidate's ability to examine the peripheral vascular system.
- *Clear instructions for the candidate:* to inform the candidate exactly what task they should perform at that station.
- *Clear instructions for the examiners:* including a copy of the candidate instructions, to assist the examiner at that station to understand his or her role and conduct the station properly.
- *List of equipment required.*
- *Personnel requirements:* whether the station requires a real patient or a simulated patient and the details of such individuals (e.g. age, gender, ethnicity).
- *Simulated patient scenario:* if the station requires a particular role to be played.
- *Marking schedule:* this should include the important aspects of the skill being tested, a marking scheme for each item and how long the station should last. The marking schedule may be either a checklist or a rating scale as there is good evidence that, despite the apparent objectivity of structured checklists, global rating scales have been shown to be equally as reliable (*see* Box 20.2). Items can be grouped into the broad categories of process skills, content skills and clinical management skills.

Process skills

For clinical examination stations with a real or simulated patient, these could include introduction and orientation, rapport, professional manner and communicating with the patient appropriately during examination.

BOX 21.2 Example of a system-based blueprint

	History	Explanation	Examination	Procedures
Cardiovascular	Chest pain	Discharge drugs	Cardiac	BP
Respiratory	Haemoptysis		Respiratory	Peak flow
Gastrointestinal	Abdominal pain	Gastroscopy	Abdominal	PR
Reproductive	Amenorrhoea	Abnormal smear	Cervical smear	
Nervous	Headache		Eyes	Ophthalmoscopy
Musculoskeletal	Backache		Hip	
Generic	Pre-op assessment	Consent for post-mortem		IV cannulation

THIS IS A 10-MINUTE STATION	Good	Adequate	Not done/ Inadequate
1 Introduction and orientation (name and role, explains purpose of examination, confirms patient's agreement)	[ ]	[ ]	[ ]
2 Rapport (shows interest, respect and concern, appropriate body language)	[ ]	[ ]	[ ]
3 Appropriately exposes the patient and positions them at 45 degrees		[ ]	[ ]
4 Looks at hands, commenting on peripheral stigmata (i.e. cyanosis, clubbing, splinter haemorrhages, etc.)		[ ]	[ ]
5 Checks the radial pulse, commenting on the rate and rhythm		[ ]	[ ]
6 Asks for patient's blood pressure **Examiner please give correct BP**		[ ]	[ ]
7 Looks for central stigmata of cardiovascular disease (i.e. anaemia, central cyanosis, hyperlipidaemia)		[ ]	[ ]
8 Examines the JVP correctly (positions the patient's chin and neck; assesses the waveform in the correct area) and comments on findings		[ ]	[ ]
9 Palpates the carotid or brachial pulses, commenting on the character		[ ]	[ ]
Inspects and palpates the praecordium: 10 Localises the apex beat, commenting on the position		[ ]	[ ]
11 Examines for RVH		[ ]	[ ]
12 Auscultates in all four cardiac areas		[ ]	[ ]
13 Moves patient to left side and sits patient forward in expiration	[ ]	[ ]	[ ]
14 Comments on heart sounds and times heart sounds against central pulse	[ ]	[ ]	[ ]
15 Comments on any murmurs		[ ]	[ ]
16 Listens to the lung bases		[ ]	[ ]
17 Candidate attempts to assess peripheral pulses **Examiner please stop candidate**		[ ]	[ ]
18 Checks for ankle/sacral oedema		[ ]	[ ]
19 Presents a brief summary and conclusions	[ ]	[ ]	[ ]
20 Communicates with patient appropriately during examination (explain what they are doing, gains patient's co-operation)	[ ]	[ ]	[ ]
21 Examines patient in a professional manner (gentle, watches for pain, maintains dignity and privacy)	[ ]	[ ]	[ ]
22 Closure (thanks patient, leaves patient comfortable)	[ ]	[ ]	[ ]
23 Candidate cleans hands after examination		[ ]	[ ]

Figure 21.1 Example checklist mark sheet for cardiovascular examination.

For history-taking stations, these could include introduction and orientation, listening skills, questioning skills, demonstration of empathy and appropriate closure.

For explanation stations, these could include introduction and orientation, rapport, establishing what the patient knows/understands, demonstration of empathy, appropriate organisation of explanation, checking the patient's understanding and using clear language, avoiding jargon.

Content skills

These include appropriate technical steps or aspects of the task or skill being tested.

Clinical management skills

It may be appropriate to ask the candidate some set questions in relation to the specific case.

Figures 21.1 and 21.2 provide examples illustrating the checklist and rating scale marking schedules, respectively.

Piloting

Ideally, stations should be piloted before they are used in examinations to ensure that all stations are functional in terms of the following:

- *Timing:* can the candidates realistically perform the task in the time allotted?

	Clear fail	Borderline fail	Borderline pass	Clear pass	Excellent
1 Physical examination: inspection, pulses, JVP, carotids, palpation of precordium, auscultation of valve areas	☐	☐	☐	☐	☐
2 Identification and interpretation of physical signs: identifies and interprets signs correctly; makes reasonable diagnosis	☐	☐	☐	☐	☐
3 Management: suggests appropriate investigations, treatment and follow-up	☐	☐	☐	☐	☐

Figure 21.2 Example rating scale mark sheet for cardiovascular examination.

- *Difficulty:* how difficult is the station?
- *Equipment:* is all the equipment required available and on the list?
- *Is an additional helper required* to assist the examiner, e.g. for catherisation, suturing stations?
- *Candidate instructions:* do the instructions tell the candidate exactly what the task is?
- *Examiner instructions:* do the instructions tell the examiner how to conduct the station? Does the examiner know what the candidate has been told to do?
- *Real patient specifications:* are the medical conditions specified?
- *Simulated patient scenario:* is the age/gender/ethnicity specified? Is there enough information for the simulated patient to learn and play the part effectively?
- *Construct validity:* is the station testing what it is meant to test? Does the marking schedule reflect the elements of the task appropriately?

Simulated patient training

For consistent performances, particularly at communication skills stations, it is best to use well-trained simulated patients. Depending on location, it may be possible to organise a database of actors who assist in the teaching as well as assessment of communication skills. It is desirable to have people across a range of ages and ethnicities, as well as a balanced gender mix. Training and monitoring simulated patients is essential to ensure consistent performance – a significant factor in the reliability of the examination. The simulated patients should be sent their scenarios in advance and then asked to go through their roles with other simulated patients playing the same role, while being supervised by a communication skills teacher and/or a clinician, to develop the role to a suitable standard.

Examiner training

OSCEs require large numbers of examiners. This can be a strength, as candidates are observed and scored by clinicians, but it is also one of the potential weaknesses of OCSEs, as inconsistency between examiners will reduce fairness and reliability.

Considerable resources are devoted to examiner training. Structured face-to-face training sessions are good for introducing new examiners to OSCEs and scoring processes. The programme for these events is interactive and very much acknowledges the inherent expertise that experienced clinicians bring to the assessment process. These training sessions cover:

- principles of OSCEs
- role of examiners (i.e. to assess not to teach; to conduct vivas, adhere to marking schedules and respect the role of the simulated patient)
- marking video-recorded OSCE stations, followed by assessment with the clinicians of their marking and getting them to think through their mark allocation
- marking 'live stations' with group members playing the candidate, the assessor and the simulated patient. This demonstrates how stressful this assessment is for the candidate and how difficult it can be to play the part of a good simulated patient

- standard-setting procedure used. This can be crucial when using a student-centred approach, and all the examiners are integral to the standard-setting process. The more the assessors understand their vital role in this process the more likely they are to do it in a satisfactory way. The use of non-clinicians in assessment is discussed in Box 21.3.

Once examiners have had initial training, it may be helpful to refresh examiners' scoring and standards via interactive on-line courses, with videos of candidate performance and feedback on examiner scoring.

Working with real patients

Patients do not always give the same history each time they are asked to repeat it; they can become tired or unwell and they may develop new signs and symptoms to the ones they originally reported; they may even lose previous clinical findings. However, they can be a most valuable resource and need to be treated as such. Using 'real' patients in OSCEs adds greatly to the validity of the assessment. Ideally, patients should be used to assess the detection of common chronic clinical signs. For each clinical sign assessed several patients will be needed and even the most stoical patient should not be expected to be examined by more than 10 students in the course of a day. Ideally, patients should be swapped in and out of the station to allow them to have sufficient rest time.

Practical considerations

The smooth running of OSCEs is highly dependent on the detail of the practical arrangements made in advance and it is worth putting some effort into this to ensure a tolerable day of examinations. There are many aspects to consider.

Prior to the OSCE

Suitable venue

Depending on the number of stations and candidates, more than one circuit may need to be conducted simultaneously. There are advantages (less noise, more privacy for patients) to conducting each station in a separate room (e.g. in an outpatient department), but larger halls divided up with soundproofed partitions can also be suitable. Venues may need to be booked well in advance of examination dates. Appropriate adjacent rooms to the OSCE circuits are required for the gathering of the students, where they can be registered and briefed prior to the examination. Rooms may be required for patients to rest in between each examination. A floor plan of the stations and rest rooms is an invaluable aid to planning.

Video cameras to record encounters may be useful for quality assurance, training of simulated patients and examiners, and standard setting. This is particularly important when attempting to standardise encounters and examiners across different sites.

Recruitment of examiners

Busy clinicians and other teachers will need advance notice to enable them to attend and play the vital role of assessors at each station. It is helpful to send out a grid of dates and

 BOX 21.3 FOCUS ON: Simulated patients as assessors

Scoring standardised patient examinations can be done by third-party observers (usually physicians) or by the standardised patients themselves. Physician examiners enhance the validity of the assessment because they can apply holistic judgements and integrate subdomains of sequence, logic and other factors that may be difficult for a non-professional completing a binary checklist to capture. Boulet *et al.*(45) however, demonstrated that holistic judgements from physician examiners are similar to aggregate scores from trained standardised patients, at least in assessing a general, entry-level physician. Physician evaluator models using holistic scoring models may have greater utility in capturing higher levels of expertise – something that checklist models may not be able to do. Any examiner, whether simulated patient or physician, must be thoroughly trained and then monitored to ensure consistent use of the score scale, since variability diminishes reliability.(46)

Ratings of interpersonal and communication skills provide a unique challenge in determining who is best able to provide the ratings. Although the assessment of doctor–patient communication skills can be accomplished by a physician or other observers, and can be done 'live' or via video-taped reviews, it is unclear whether someone watching the interplay between a doctor and a patient can adequately measure the complex, multi-dimensional nature of the communication. Many aspects of this communication, especially those that are non-verbal, are best assessed by the patient or the person trained to be the patient.(44)

Spoken English is another domain that might be better scored by non-physicians. The generalisability coefficient of this component of the Educational Commission for Foreign Medical Graduates Clinical Skills Assessment (CSA), scored by standardised patients, was 0.94.(47)

From a logistical and cost perspective, the examinee volume for the CSA and now the United States Medical Licensing Examination Step 2 (CS) (approximately 35 000 per year) makes it effectively impossible to entertain using physician examiners. Cost analysis also needs to account for training time and quality assurance for standardised patients or physician raters as well as the different nature of the training needed by each group. It may also be harder to standardise a large number of highly educated, typically independently thinking physicians across five test centres in a year-round testing model.

Currently in the UK, at both the undergraduate and postgraduate levels, examiners are clinicians or other health-care professionals. It would probably need a considerable shift in cultural acceptance to move to standardised patients as the sole assessors of clinical competence.

times so people can tick the sessions they wish to attend. This is best done by central coordination.

Recruitment of simulated patients

Once the OSCE has been blueprinted, the simulated patients required should be listed and actors contacted to engage them for the dates of the exam.

Running order of the stations

Stations should be numbered to avoid confusion over mark sheets, equipment and people involved. Rest stations should be provided: usually one rest per 40 minutes in a circuit is suitable. If many candidates are sitting the OSCE, running multiple circuits of the same stations enables more candidates to be examined at any one time.

Using stations of different lengths

It is best to group stations of the same length together and to run these circuits separately. If there are 5-, 10- and 15-minute stations, then the candidates should be asked to attend on three separate occasions to undertake each circuit. Mixing stations of different timings in one circuit is possible, but can lead to confusion.

List of all the equipment required

Detailed by station, this is vital for the preparations to be successful. Arrange to go round the circuit the day before the OSCE and to check that all the equipment is correctly set up.

Production and processing of mark sheets

Calculate the numbers required for each station and allow extra for spoilage. Allow time for proofreading. If there are a large number of candidates, it may be worth looking into using sheets that can be processed by electronic scanning after the OSCE. Alternatively, marking by hand will require the organisation of people to mark and ensure that results are entered correctly. Computer systems for automated collection and analysis of station data may be purchased or developed. If a computer system is used, a paper backup should always be available in case the network goes down.

Liaison with clinical skills centre staff

Close cooperation with clinical skills centre technical and teaching staff is vital in the planning. It is useful to draw up a circuit plan to indicate the layout required and for the numbering of the stations to be agreed (*see* Figure 21.3).

On the day of the OSCE

Signs

It is very helpful to put up signs indicating the rooms for the candidates, patients and the examination, so that people unfamiliar with the venue can find their way easily. Large signs should be used to number all the stations to help candidates follow the circuit successfully.

Timing

An electronic timing programme is the ideal, but a reliable stopwatch and loud manual bell is an acceptable alterna-

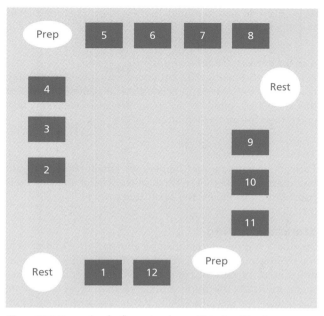

Figure 21.3 Example of a floor plan for an Objective Structure Clinical Examination in a large room.

tive. It is important to ensure that all candidates and examiners can hear the bell so the candidates move onto the next station promptly.

Helpers/marshals

A vital part of the smooth running of OSCEs depends on having a small army of helpers to direct the candidates, examiners, simulated patients and patients to ensure everyone is in the right place at the right time. This should include looking after the welfare of all the people involved on the day.

Catering

Examining, acting, being examined and helping at OSCEs can be tiring and sometimes stressful work. The very least one can do is provide refreshments for all participants – water for the candidates at rest stations, drinks for all other staff and lunch for those who spend the whole day assisting or being examined.

Briefing

It is helpful to gather all candidates in a room where they can be registered and briefed about the practical arrangements for the day. Examiners, even if they have attended a training session, should be reminded about how to score the mark sheets and conduct the stations appropriately, and also to switch off their mobile phones.

After the OSCE

Collection of mark sheets

Collection should be organised meticulously, as missing sheets can be very prejudicial to a candidate's overall score. It is also helpful to check the sheets for completeness of scoring and to ask examiners to check they have completed the sheets before leaving.

Care of patients/simulated patients

A system to ensure that patients have transport to take them home is always appreciated. Arrangements to ensure the simulated patients are paid are also welcome and encourage future participation.

Thank-you letters

Patients, examiners and helpers are much more likely to take part again if they receive acknowledgement of their contribution to the examination process.

Standard setting

Standard setting or establishing the pass mark is critical for determining who passes and who fails any particular assessment of clinical competence. The standard or pass mark indicates the minimum score that every candidate has to reach to pass the OSCE. While it is difficult to quantify a concept as complex as clinical competence, the reality is that examinations such as OSCEs are used to discriminate between those who have sufficient clinical skills and those who do not, for a particular level or purpose.

The fundamental principle underlying all standard-setting methods is to reach a consensus on professional values and standards.(48) There are many standard-setting methods described in the literature,(49–52) but many of the traditional ones were developed for multiple-choice questions. It is debatable whether it is appropriate for these methods to be used for complex performance-based examinations such as OSCEs.

Norcini, in his comprehensive review of standard setting,(48) suggests that the Fixed Percentage and Hofstee methods can be applied to OSCEs directly, while the Angoff method can be used in a modified version.(53) The issue for examination setters is whether they are prepared to use relative methods such as Fixed Percentage or compromise methods such as Hofstee rather than absolute or criterion-referenced techniques such as Angoff and the Borderline Group methods. As experience has grown, it is the latter that has become the favoured method of standard setting for OSCEs.(54–57) It does require some expertise in processing the data, and is more reliable if the examiners are trained(56), but overall has become regarded as the 'gold standard' for OSCEs.(57) For a full discussion of standard setting methods see Chapter 22.

Conclusions

Assessment of clinical competence is a crucial part of the basis on which decisions are made about the ability of clinicians and doctors in training. But any method of assessing clinical skills should be considered in the context of a wider programme of assessment, which should include the assessment of knowledge, clinical examination skills, practical procedure skills, doctor–patient communication, problem-solving ability, management skills and relationships with colleagues, as well as professional attitudes and behaviour.

One of the most important aspects of assessing clinical skills is the range of sampling across a candidate's skill base; this has to be taken into account when designing any assessment. OSCEs can assess clinical, communication and practical skills but are still situated in the context of an examination setting. To assess doctors in the context of their professional practice requires the use of different formats in the workplace.

As workplace-based assessment becomes more widespread, the focus of testing in OSCEs may be directed towards earlier stages of clinical skill acquisition and technical proficiency. Sequential OSCE design may become more common in an effort to control costs and improve efficiency (*see* Box 21.4). Another development might be that OSCEs become more specialised, possibly focusing on acute clinical scenarios, which would be difficult to assess reliably *in vivo*. Complex high-fidelity team-working scenarios are being developed in some areas and may become more appropriate as interprofessional training in the postgraduate arena becomes more common.

Acknowledgement

Some of the material used in this section has previously been published in an article by one of the authors in *The Clinical Teacher*(60) and is reproduced here with permission.

BOX 21.4 FOCUS ON: Sequential testing in OSCE administration

The majority of health-care institutions use models of test–short-term remediation–retest for underperforming students. Whilst these models are typically associated with short-term improvement in candidate performance at retest, such models are costly to deliver (particularly for performance retest with OSCEs). There is increasing evidence that these traditional models are associated with longitudinal underperformance of candidates. Recent work has shown that whilst students often pass the OSCE retest, in the longer term those who have failed continue to perform weakly compared to their peers within a programme of assessment, and often deteriorate.(58) Rather than a traditional OSCE model, sequential testing involves a smaller 'screening' test format, with a further 'sequential' test for candidates who fail to meet the standards of the screening test. Overall pass/fail decisions are then made on the full sequence of tests. This can be used effectively to improve the efficiency of performance assessments like OSCEs that can be very expensive to run.(59)

References

1 Miller G (1990) The assessment of clinical skills/competence/performance. *Academic Medicine.* **65**(s9): S63–7.

2 General Medical Council (2003) *Tomorrow's Doctors.* GMC, London.

3 General Medical Council (2013) *Good Medical Practice.* GMC, London.

4 Frank JR, Jabbour M and Tugwell P (1996) Skills for the new millennium: report of the Societal Needs Working Group, CanMEDS 2000 Project. *Annals of the Royal College of Physicians and Surgeons of Canada.* **29**: 206–16.

5 Rethans JJ, Norcini JJ, Baron-Maldonado M *et al.* (2002) The relationship between competence and performance: implications for assessing practice performance. *Medical Education.* **36**: 901–9.

6 Norcini JJ (2001) The validity of long cases. *Medical Education.* **35**: 720–1.

7 Swanson DB, Norman GR and Linn RL (1995) Performance based assessment: lessons learned from health professions. *Education Research.* **24**(5): 5–11.

8 Norcini JJ (2002) The death of the long case? *British Medical Journal.* **324**: 408–9.

9 Norcini JJ (2001) Does observation add to the validity of the long case? [letter]. *Medical Education.* **35**: 1131–3.

10 Hampton JR, Harrison MJG, Mitchell JRA *et al.* (1975) Relative contributions of history taking, physical examination and laboratory investigations to diagnosis and management of medical outpatients. *British Medical Journal.* **2**: 486–9.

11 Gleeson FA (1997) Assessment of clinical competence using the objective structured long examination record (OSLER). *Medical Teacher.* **19**: 7–14.

12 Gleeson FA (1994) The effects of immediate feedback on clinical skills using the OSLER. Proceedings of the Sixth Ottawa Conference in Medical Education, 412–5.

13 van Thiel J, Kraan HF and van der Vleuten CPM (1991) Reliability and feasibility of measuring medical interviewing skills. The revised Maastricht history and advice checklist. *Medical Education.* **25**: 224–9.

14 Wass V, Jones R and van der Vleuten CPM (2001) Standardized or real patients to test clinical competence? The long case revisited. *Medical Education.* **35**: 321–5.

15 Reznick RK, Blackmore D, Cohen R *et al.* (1993) An objective structured clinical examination for the licentiate of the Medical Council of Canada: from research to reality. *Academic Medicine.* **68**(s10): S4–6.

16 Sloan DA, Donnelly MB, Schwartz RW and Strodel WE (1995) The Objective Structured Clinical Examination. The new gold standard for evaluating postgraduate clinical performance. *Annals of Surgery.* **222**: 735–42.

17 Cohen R, Reznick RK, Taylor BR *et al.* (1990) Reliability and validity of the objective structured clinical examination in assessing surgical residents. *American Journal of Surgery.* **160**: 302–5.

18 Davis MH (2003) OSCE: the Dundee experience. *Medical Teacher.* **25**: 255–61.

19 Newble D (2004) Techniques for measuring clinical competence: objective structured clinical examinations. *Medical Education.* **38**: 199–203.

20 Harden RM and Gleeson FA (1979) Assessment of clinical competence using an Objective Structured Clinical Examination (OSCE). *Medical Education.* **13**: 41–54.

21 van der Vleuten CPM (1996) The assessment of professional competence: developments, research and practical implications. *Advances in Health Science Education.* **1**: 41–67.

22 Swanson DB (1987) A measurement framework for performance-based tests. In: Harvey I and Harden RM (eds) *Further Developments in Assessing Clinical Competence*, pp. 13–45. Can-Heal, Montreal.

23 van der Vleuten CPM and Swanson DB (1990) Assessment of clinical skills with standardized patients: state of the art. *Teaching and Learning in Medicine.* **2**: 58–76.

24 Messick S (1994) The interplay of evidence and consequences in the validation of performance assessments. *Educational Researcher.* **23**(2): 13–23.

25 Downing SM and Haladyna TM (2004) Validity threats: overcoming interference with proposed interpretations of assessment data. *Medical Education.* **38**: 327–33.

26 Downing SM (2003) Validity: on the meaningful interpretation of assessment data. *Medical Education.* **37**: 830–7.

27 Biggs J (1999) *Teaching for Quality Learning at University.* Open University Press and Society for Research into Higher Education, Buckingham.

28 Petrusa E (2002) Clinical performance assessments. In: Norman GR, van der Vleuten CPM and Newble DI (eds) *International Handbook of Research in Medical Education*, pp. 673–709. Kluwer, Dordrecht, Boston and London.

29 Kaufman DM (2003) ABC of learning and teaching in medicine: applying educational theory in practice. *British Medical Journal.* **326**: 213–6.

30 Newble DI and Jaeger K (1983) The effect of assessments and examinations on the learning of medical students. *Medical Education.* **17**: 165–71.

31 Vargas AL, Boulet JR, Errichetti AM, van Zanten M and Lopez MJ (2007) Developing performance-based medical school assessment programs in resource-limited environments. *Medical Teacher.* **29**(2–3): 192–8.

32 Adamo G (2003) Simulated and standardized patients in OSCEs: achievements and challenges 1992–2003. *Medical Teacher.* **25**: 262–70.

33 Newble DI (2004) Techniques for measuring clinical competence: objective structured clinical examinations. *Medical Education.* **38**: 199–203.

34 Townsend AH, McIlvenny S, Miller CJ and Dunn EV (2001) The use of an Objective Structured Clinical Examination (OSCE) for formative and summative assessment in a general practice clinical attachment and its relationship to final medical school examination performance. *Medical Education.* **35**: 841–6.

35 Hodges B (2003) Validity and the OSCE. *Medical Teacher.* **25**: 250–4.

36 Hodges B, Turnbull J, Cohen R *et al.* (1996) Evaluating communication skills in the OSCE format: reliability and generalizability. *Medical Education.* **30**: 38–43.

37 Mavis BE and Henry RC (2002) Between a rock and a hard place: finding a place for the OSCE in medical education. *Medical Education.* **36**: 408–9.

38 Reznick RK, Blackmore D, Dauphinee WD *et al.* (1996) Large-scale high-stakes testing with an OSCE: report from the Medical Council of Canada. *Academic Medicine.* **71**(s1): S19–21.

39 Rymer AT (2001) The new MRCOG Objective Structured Clinical Examination – the examiners' evaluation. *Journal of Obstetrics and Gynaecology.* **21**: 103–6.

40 Eva KW, Rosenfeld J, Reiter HI and Norman GR (2004) An admissions OSCE: the multiple mini-interview. *Medical Education.* **38**: 314–26.

41 Lane P (2005) Recruitment into training for general practice – the winds of change or a breath of fresh air? *British Medical Journal Career Focus.* **331**: 153.

42 Whelan GP, Boulet JR, McKinley DW *et al.* (2005) Scoring standardized patient examinations: lessons learned from the development and administration of the ECFMG Clinical Skills Assessment (CSA). *Medical Teacher.* **27**: 200–6.

43 Boulet JR, Ben David MF, Ziv A *et al.* (1998) High-stakes examinations: what do we know about measurement?: using standardized patients to assess the interpersonal skills of physicians. *Academic Medicine.* **73**(10): S94–6.

44 Whelan GP, McKinley DW, Boulet JR *et al.* (2001) Validation of the doctor–patient communication component of the Educational Commission for Foreign Medical Graduates Clinical Skills Assessment. *Medical Education.* **35**: 757–61.

45 Boulet JR, McKinley DW, Norcini JJ and Whelan GP (2002) Assessing the comparability of standardized patient and physician evaluations of clinical skills. *Advances in Health Sciences Education: Theory and Practice.* **7**: 85–97.

46 Noel GL, Herbers JE Jr, Caplow MP *et al.* (1992) How well do internal medicine faculty members evaluate the clinical skills of residents? *Annals of Internal Medicine.* **117**: 757–65.

47 Boulet JR, van Zanten M, McKinley DW and Gary NE (2001) Evaluating the spoken English proficiency of graduates of foreign medical schools. *Medical Education.* **35**: 767–73.

48 Norcini JJ (2003) Setting standards on educational tests. *Medical Education.* **37**: 464–9.

49 Norcini JJ and Shea JA (1997) The credibility and comparability of standards. *Applied Measurement in Education.* **10**: 39–59.

50 Livingstone SA and Zeiky MJ (1982) *Passing Scores: A Manual for Setting Standards of Performance on Educational and Occupational Tests.* Educational Testing Service, Princeton, NJ.

51 Zeiky MJ (2001) So much has changed. How the setting of cutscores has evolved since the 1980s. In: Cizek GJ (ed.) *Setting Performance Standards: Concepts, Methods, and Perspectives*, pp. 19–52. Lawrence Erlbaum Associates, Mahwah, NJ.

52 Cizek GJ (2001) *Setting Performance Standards: Concepts, Methods, and Perspectives.* Lawrence Erlbaum Associates, Mahwah, NJ.

53 Angoff WH (1971) Scales, norms and equivalent scores. In: Thorndike RL (ed.) *Educational Measurement*, pp. 508–600. American Council on Education, Washington, DC.

54 Cohen R, Rothman AI, Poldre P and Ross J (1991) Validity and generalizability of global ratings in an objective structured clinical examination. *Academic Medicine.* **66**: 545–8.

55 Dauphinee WD, Blackmore DE, Smee SM *et al.* (1997) Using the judgements of physician examiners in setting standards for a national multicentre high stakes OSCE. *Advances in Health Science Education.* **2**: 201–11.

56 Hodges B (2003) Analytic global OSCE ratings are sensitive to level of training. *Medical Education.* **37**: 1012–6.

57 Smee SM and Blackmore DE (2001) Setting standards for an objective structured clinical examination: the borderline group method gains ground on Angoff. *Medical Education.* **35**: 1009–10.

58 Pell G, Fuller R, Homer M and Roberts T (2012) Is short-term remediation after OSCE failure sustained? A retrospective analysis of the longitudinal attainment of underperforming students in OSCE assessments. *Medical Teacher.* **34**: 146–50.

59 Pell G, Fuller R, Homer M and Roberts T (2013) Advancing the Objective Structured Clinical Examination: sequential testing theory and practice in action. *Medical Education.* **47**: 569–77.

60 Boursicot K and Roberts T (2005) How to set up an OSCE. *The Clinical Teacher.* **2**: 16–20.

Further reading

Boursicot KL, Etheridge SZ, Sturrock A *et al.* (2011) Performance in assessment: consensus statement and recommendations from the Ottawa conference. *Medical Teacher.* **33**(5): 370–83.

22 Standard setting methods in medical education

André F De Champlain
Research and Development, Medical Council of Canada, Canada

KEY MESSAGES

- Standard setting is a crucial activity for any assessment programme that must render a judgement as to the competency of candidates, whether at the school level or for licensure and certification purposes.

- There is no such thing as a 'gold standard' in determining a cut-score value for a test. Selecting and implementing a rigorous process by which a cut-score value can be arrived at, with appropriate supporting documentation and empirical evidence, is what needs to be defended.

- For the vast majority of medical education assessments, criterion-referenced methods are more appropriate than their norm-referenced counterparts, as the former are based on expert judgement of what constitutes minimal competency. Norm-referenced standards are defensible for selection decisions only.

- For multiple-choice examinations, test-centred standard setting methods, such as the Angoff and Bookmark

procedures, are most appropriate given the nature of the task. For performance assessments, examinee-centred methods are preferable given the complex, multi-dimensional nature of OSCEs and workplace-based assessments.

- Regardless of the standard setting method selected, it is imperative to properly document all phases of the exercise, including the objective of the examination, the selection and composition of the panel, as well as the definition of the borderline or minimally proficient candidate.

- Providing evidence to support the stability of the cut-score is integral to supporting *internal* validity. Documenting the impact of applying a cut-score on pass/fail rates, as well the relationship to decisions on other similar assessments, is at the core of the *external* validity argument for the standard.

The need to make decisions

The need to make decisions that assign people, objects or things into 'classifications' permeates all aspects of daily life, from the mundane to the most significant. For instance, passing an examination to obtain a driver's licence requires meeting a certain level of proficiency with regard to knowledge of traffic laws and performance (passing, parallel parking, etc.). The aim of such a classification is to keep unsafe drivers from getting behind the wheel of a vehicle. Similarly, a jury that renders a verdict in a criminal trial is charged with 'classifying' a defendant as 'guilty' or 'not guilty', after carefully weighing the evidence of a case, i.e. analysing relevant data. The jury analogy seems particularly relevant to standard setting in assessment on a number of counts:

- Both activities require a sufficiently large and representative participant group from the population (whether a citizenry or a profession).

- Both activities necessitate a decision that will be used for classification purposes (rendering a verdict or setting a pass/fail standard).

- The intended use of the information is very similar in each instance (incapacitation and/or rehabilitation in a criminal trial and the corresponding protection of the public and remediation considerations in standard setting).

The need to make a decision is also part-and-parcel of all phases of a physician's professional life, from undergraduate medical education to revalidation. Key decisions occur when awarding or denying an unrestricted licence to practice medicine,(1,2) granting or withholding a credential,(3–5) granting or denying entry into a professional body,(6,7) as well as at the medical school level.(8–12) These decisions are arrived at through a process that is referred to as *standard setting*. Cizek(13) describes standard setting as 'the proper following of a prescribed, rational system of rules or procedures resulting in the assignment of a number to differentiate between two or more states or degrees of performance' (e.g. pass/fail). This activity is especially critical within the health professions, given the need to ensure the public that graduates as well as holders of certificates and licences possess the knowledge and skill sets that permit safe clinical practice.(14,15) In spite of this,

Understanding Medical Education: Evidence, Theory and Practice, Second Edition. Edited by Tim Swanwick.
© 2014 The Association for the Study of Medical Education. Published 2014 by John Wiley & Sons, Ltd.

BOX 22.1 Definitions

- A *standard* is a qualitative description of a level of performance and can be viewed as a conceptual definition of competence.
- A *cut-score* or passing score corresponds to a number that reflects this standard and can be viewed as an operational definition of competence.

BOX 22.2 Key considerations

- There is no 'gold standard' in standard setting.
- A standard and accompanying cut-score should reflect expert judgement as to what constitutes competence, supported by several sources of evidence.
- A standard setting panel should be composed of experts who broadly represent all key examination stakeholders with respect to gender, age, specialty, geographical area, etc.
- Thoroughly training panellists on all aspects of the exercise is a task critical to the success of any standard setting exercise, regardless of the method adopted.

---

a basic misconception still persists regarding the terms *cut-score* and *passing standard* (*see* Box 22.1).

Standard versus cut-score

The primary use of any test score in a criterion-referenced setting is to determine whether a candidate has mastered a set of competencies presumed to underlie performance on the examination. Whether at the school level or for licensure and/or certification decisions, standard setting exercises are routinely carried out to identify a passing standard, which is treated as an indicator of mastery or competency in the skill areas deemed important and measured by an examination.

Kane[16] defines a passing standard as a qualitative description of an acceptable level of performance and knowledge required in practice. As such, the passing standard can be viewed as a conceptual or qualitative definition of competence. For example, in a final year undergraduate OSCE, a standard might stipulate that the borderline candidate demonstrate the data gathering, physical examination and communication skills necessary for entry into supervised practice. The cut-score, on the other hand, is a number along the score scale that reflects the standard. It is an *operational definition of competence*. In our previous example, expert panellists might decide that a candidate who scores at or above 65% has met the performance standard for the final-year undergraduate OSCE.

Key considerations in standard setting

Standard setting is a process that allows human judgements to be synthesised in a rational and defensible way to facilitate the partitioning of a score scale into two or more categories. Given the emphasis on expert judgement, it is important to underscore that all standards are intrinsically subjective in nature. Consequently, there is no 'gold standard' when it comes to setting a cut-score on an examination. Cut-scores can and will vary as a function of several factors, including, but not limited to, the method selected to set the standard and the panel of participating judges.[17–21] Jaeger[18] best summarised this point by stating that 'a right answer [in standard setting] does not exist, except, perhaps, in the minds of those providing judgement'. Following a systematic process that is supported with appropriate empirical evidence can help standard setting panels translate (policy-based) judgement onto a score scale in a defensible manner, but no method can be used to estimate

some 'true' cut-score that perfectly separates masters from non-masters or passers from failers.

In view of the inherent subjectivity of any standard setting process, best practice dictates selection of a panel of judges that broadly represents the target examination population, with respect to background and educational characteristics.[22,23] The composition of the standard setting panel becomes even more relevant given the complexity of assessments in medical education. Despite their seniority and level of expertise, extensive training of panellists is essential to ensure that the resulting cut-score is reasonable given the objectives of the assessment.[24] If nothing else, training is necessary to ensure that all panellists are in harmony with one another in regard to the goal of the assessment, the purpose of the standard setting exercise, the task that they are asked to complete and a general definition of what constitutes minimal proficiency or a borderline performance.[25] A typical standard setting training session requires a number of steps including: (i) the provision of sample examination materials to panellists; (ii) a clear presentation of the task that participants are being asked to complete; (iii) a period of discussion allocated to the definition of the borderline candidate; (iv) judgements on a set of exemplars; (v) a discussion period to clarify any misconceptions amongst participants; and (vi) a post-exercise survey on all aspects of training.[22]

Despite these caveats, the methods outlined in this chapter will provide systematic steps that can be followed to ensure that the resulting cut-score is defensible and based on informed, rather than capricious, judgements on the part of the expert panel. The difference between a norm-referenced and criterion-referenced standard will first be reviewed prior to an overview of common methods for determining a cut-score on an examination. (*see* Box 22.2.)

Norm- versus criterion-referenced standards

At a very high level, standards can be classified as either norm-referenced or criterion-referenced in nature.[26] A norm-referenced standard is a *relative* standard in that the cut-score is derived from the performances of a comparative group of candidates. There are many examples of norm-referenced standards, such as setting the cut-score at one standard deviation above the mean of the class or fixing the cut-score at the 90th percentile rank of a distribution. The fundamental notion is that the cut-score is set solely as a function of the relative performances of a comparative group. We pass or fail a candidate on an examination purely based on how well (or badly) other test takers performed.

On the other hand, within a criterion-referenced framework, the standard is typically set as a function of the amount of knowledge of the domain that the candidate needs to demonstrate, irrespective of group performance. As such, it is an *absolute* standard. For example, a panel of medical experts might determine that a candidate needs to master 70% of the domain to be deemed minimally competent, based on their professional judgement and the objectives of an examination.

For professional examinations, criterion-referenced standards are generally preferred for a number of reasons. First, a norm-referenced standard tells little to nothing about what a given candidate knows or does not know, since it is entirely based on the relative performance of the group. Second, and more importantly, the cut-score selected in a norm-referenced standard setting exercise will vary as a function of the ability level of the group. Lower cut-scores will result from the performances of less proficient candidates, whereas higher cut-scores will be set with more able cohorts. This, in turn, produces cohorts of candidates who vary in regard to their level of competence. For example, setting a cut-score at one standard deviation below the mean will result in failing about 16% of any cohort, irrespective of what candidates may or may not know. However, it is conceivable that these groups could differ drastically in their knowledge of the domains. Scoring 'near the average' of a distribution can have quite a different meaning if the class is composed of high ability candidates versus less able students. That is, the meaning of a passing performance (and consequently 'minimal compe-

tence') can vary as a function of when and with whom the candidate passed.

Consequently, a norm-referenced approach to setting a passing standard is untenable from both political and professional perspectives. The only instance in which it may be acceptable to use a norm-referenced standard is when the selection of a small number of candidates is necessary (e.g. for a restricted number of postgraduate training slots).

Criterion-referenced methods for setting a standard are appealing because they overcome many of these limitations. A cut-score that is set using a criterion-referenced method reflects a level of proficiency that experts representing wide sectors of a given profession agree is indicative of a candidate who possesses the skills and knowledge required for safe practice. For this reason, criterion-referenced methods for setting cut-scores have been successfully employed and defended for several years in the medical licensing arena as well as with other health profession examination programmes.(1,2,27–29) The following two sections briefly describe the criterion-referenced standard setting methods in most common use. (*see* Box 22.3.)

Test-centred methods

Criterion-referenced test-centred methods are appealing for setting a pass mark on knowledge assessments, such as multiple-choice examinations (MCQs). In this form of standard setting, experts are asked to judge the level of performance required on each item of the test or task to meet the standard (e.g. minimal proficiency). Common and frequently used test-centred methods include the Angoff, Ebel, Nedelsky and Bookmark procedures.(30) (*see* Box 22.4.)

BOX 22.5 Angoff standard setting example

In this five-item test, three judges are involved in standard setting and are asked to estimate, on an item-by-item level, the proportion of 'minimally proficient' candidates who would answer each item correctly.

Judge	1	2	3
Item 1	0.65	0.60	0.75
Item 2	0.60	0.40	0.60
Item 3	0.25	0.10	0.35
Item 4	0.10	0.05	0.55
Item 5	0.30	0.20	0.40
Overall cut-score	1.9 (or 2/5)	1.35 (or 1/5)	2.65 (or 3/5)

Overall cut-score = 1.9 + 1.35 + 2.65 = 5.9/3 = 1.97/5 or 2/5

BOX 22.6 Ebel standard setting example

In this 50-item test, the standard setting panel is invited to consider both the relevance and degree of difficulty of items before estimating the proportion of questions that the minimally proficient candidate would correctly answer in each cell.

Content relevance	Level of difficulty		
	Easy	Average	Difficult
Essential	0.85 (five items)	0.65 (10 items)	0.25 (five items)
Important	0.75 (five items)	0.55 (five items)	0.15 (five items)
Acceptable	0.65 (three items)	0.45 (four items)	0.10 (three items)
Questionable	0.65 (two items)	0.40 (two items)	0.05 (one item)

Cut-score = 0.85(5) + 0.65(10) + 0.25(5) + 0.75(5) + 0.55(5) + 0.15(5) + 0.65(3) + 0.45(4) + 0.10(3) + 0.65(2) + 0.40(2) + 0.05(1)

=25.45/50 (50%)

Angoff method

In the Angoff procedure, panellists are asked to estimate, on an item-by-item level, the proportion of minimally proficient candidates that *would* answer each item correctly.(31) Effectively this constitutes an assessment of the degree of difficulty of each component part of the test based on expert judgement. These proportions are then summed for each expert judge. Typically, the mean or median sum of item proportions across judges is treated as the cut-score on the examination. Box 22.5 provides a simple illustration of the Angoff procedure based on a five-item examination with three panellists. In this example, panellist cut-scores ranged from 1.35 (or 1/5) to 2.65 (or 3/5). An overall cut-score equal to 1.97/5 (or 2/5) could therefore be selected as the final cut-score.

Modified Angoff methods have also been proposed for determining a standard.(9,32–35) One adaptation of the Angoff method allows panellists to modify their judgements following a general discussion.(36) Other revisions entail providing normative data (e.g. item difficulty and discrimination indices) following the initial round of ratings in order to provide panellists with a 'reality performance check' against which to gauge their initial judgements and modify them, if so desired, in a final round.(37)

Advantages and limitations

One main advantage of the Angoff family of methods is that they have been used extensively with a host of examinations, including both MCQ and performance-based assessments.(34) As such, a wealth of evidence and information is available to any researcher interested in carrying out such an exercise. Also, the Angoff method holds a certain amount of intuitive appeal in that panellists are required to review test items and offer judgements based on their expert knowledge of the material and candidates. Finally, the Angoff method is amenable to streamlining such as through the 'Yes/No' method,(38) which can simplify the task even more.

On the downside, the Angoff methods have come under heavy criticism due to the inherent nature of the two main tasks that panellists are required to complete, namely to articulate what constitutes minimal proficiency and then consistently estimate proportions of minimally proficient candidates who would correctly answer each test item.(35) Shepard(39) argued that the task presented to panellists was too cognitively challenging and probably beyond the capability of most participants. Others, however, have refuted this claim and ascribed these difficulties to insufficient training of panellists or the absence of performance data to guide judgements.(40) Research conducted by Plake *et al*.(41) also showed that item performance estimates were consistent within and across panels, as well as within and across years for a high-stakes certification examination. These findings once more underscore the importance of selecting appropriate panels of judges for standard setting exercises and, more importantly, offering extensive training to all experts to eliminate any misconceptions regarding the nature of the task at hand. Despite these limitations, the Angoff family of methods continues to be one of the most prevalent, longstanding and well researched set of procedures for setting a cut-score on an examination.(30)

Ebel method

The procedure outlined by Ebel extends Angoff's method by asking panellists not only to provide difficulty estimates for each item but also content relevance, given the domains that are presumed to underlie the examination.(42) The cut-score is computed by adding the cross-products of the difficulty and relevance judgements. Box 22.6 provides a simple example of a two-dimensional Ebel grid. In this example, judges felt that five of 50 items were essential to the content and 'easy' level of difficulty. In a similar vein, panellists were asked to estimate the proportion of items, in each content relevance/difficulty cell, that the minimally proficient candidate would correctly answer. The resulting cut-score is the sum of the relevance/difficulty cell cross-products. In this example, candidates would need to correctly answer 25/50 items (50%) to pass the examination.

Advantages and limitations

Ironically, one advantage of the Ebel method for setting a standard, namely that item relevance, in addition to difficulty, can be factored into panellists' judgements, is also its chief weakness. Berk,(43) for example, questions the ease with which panellists can separate content (difficulty) and relevance judgements during an exercise, largely based on the argument that these two dimensions are often correlated quite highly. From a test development standpoint, one could also question the merits of including test items that are not relevant in an examination. In most contexts, the total score is interpreted as an overall reflection of candidates' competencies on a composite of (interrelated) domains. Consequently, items that are deemed irrelevant contribute little to nothing in informing inferences about overall competency (e.g. pass/fail) or standing.

Nedelsky method

Nedelsky(44) outlined a standard setting method based on the premise that when answering MCQs, minimally proficient candidates first eliminate options that they identify as incorrect based on their knowledge of the material, and then randomly guess amongst remaining choices. The actual cut-score corresponds to the sum across items of the reciprocal of the remaining number of alternatives. To illustrate; assume that a group of panellists estimates that the following number of options would be eliminated, respectively, by the minimally proficient candidate on a five-item, five-option MCQ examination: 2, 1, 3, 3, 4, across each of the items. The Nedelsky cut-score would therefore correspond to:

$$(1/3 + 1/4 + 1/2 + 1/2 + 1/1) = 2.58/5 \text{ or } 3/5 \ (60\%)$$

Advantages and limitations

The main advantage of the Nedelsky method is that allows panellists to factor in the quality of the distractors when making their judgements, that is, any partial knowledge that the minimally proficient candidate may possess when answering an MCQ. However, the procedure also suffers from a number of well-documented shortcomings. First, the task imposed on panellists is much more onerous that what is expected in either an Angoff or Ebel exercise. Panellists must not only estimate the probability of a correct response on the part of the minimally proficient candidate, but they must do so in light of options they believe the latter test taker can eliminate either due to poor distractors or partial knowledge. Additionally, probability values that are provided by panellists are *de facto* restricted due to the nature of the procedure. For example, with a five-option MCQ, the only plausible estimates that judges can provide are: 0.20, 0.25, 0.33, 0.50 and 1.00.(43) That is, the minimally proficient candidate can eliminate either 0, 1, 2, 3 or 4 options as non-plausible. Finally, and most importantly, the

Nedelsky method assumes that the test-taking behaviour of minimally proficient candidates is identical, i.e. they guess in the same fashion from those alternatives not eliminated as implausible. This assumption has been seriously called into question given risk behaviours, differential partial knowledge and other factors.(45,46) Though modifications of the procedure have been proposed to address these limitations,(47) the Nedelsky method has waned in popularity over the past few decades due to its inherent complexity and few practical benefits over more popular methods.

Bookmark method

The Bookmark method is also used quite regularly to set a cut-score due to its intrinsic simplicity.(48) With this approach, test items are presented to panellists by order of difficulty from least to most difficult (one item per page in a booklet). Though the original intent of the method was to sequence the items as a function of item response theory (IRT)-based difficulty estimates, it is also possible to adapt the method and order the MCQs by simple *p*-values (proportion of correct responses). Each panellist is required to place a bookmark (a stopping rule) beyond which a minimally proficient candidate would not be expected to correctly answer remaining items. Note that the Bookmark method is also frequently employed for multiple judgements (e.g. determining levels of *basic*, *proficient* and *advanced*). The final cut-score, in its simplest application, would correspond to the median number of items at the bookmark across panellists. It is important to point out that the original Bookmark procedure also translated this cut-score to the underlying IRT ability metric.(48) Extensions of the method that entail adding the use of performance benchmarks have also been proposed.(49,50) Readers wishing to obtain more details on these revisions are encouraged to consult these references.

Advantages and limitations

The main advantage of the Bookmark method is its simplicity and the relatively light cognitive load that is imposed on panellists, at least in comparison to other test-centred methods. Test items are ordered according to difficulty (again, unbeknownst to participants) and panellists are required to place one or several bookmarks to delineate two or more proficiency categories. Another attractive feature of the Bookmark method is that it can be readily applied to multiple-choice and performance examinations as well as mixed-format assessments. Finally, its traditional link to an IRT proficiency metric also holds great appeal given that the majority of large-scale testing programmes implement IRT-based methods for a host of activities, including test construction, scoring, scaling and equating. As such, the Bookmark standard setting method can easily be integrated into a unified IRT framework.

Despite these advantages, the Bookmark standard setting method does possess a number of limitations that the practitioner should be aware of. First and foremost, the cut-score in a Bookmark standard setting exercise is inextricably linked to the difficulty of the test form. To illustrate, consider a test that is very 'easy' in relation to the proficiency level of candidates. This is often the case with medical licensing and certification examinations where over 90% of first-time test takers typically pass.(27) This 'mis-targeting' can make it impossible for panellists to set an appropriate bookmark. In certain instances, it is plausible that even the last item in a booklet is too easy to distinguish between masters and non-masters when the candidate sample is highly able. As others have mentioned,(30) this problem could also crop up with other test-centred methods. The Bookmark approach, by virtue of item difficulty ordering, makes any such problems glaringly obvious. Another practical limitation of this standard setting method is that booklets (i.e. test items if there is one item per page) need to be re-ordered if some items are deleted due to poor performance. A final limitation is that items may not, and in fact are probably not, evenly spaced in terms of differences in difficulty from low to high throughout a test form. Thus, it might be difficult for panellists to identify an actual point along the scale that best discriminates between masters and non-masters, i.e. the bookmark might not be identifiable given gaps in item difficulty. While these limitations do not invalidate the Bookmark method, practitioners should be aware of these potential issues and plan accordingly prior to the actual standard setting exercise.

Examinee-centred methods

Criterion-referenced examinee-centred methods, on the other hand, involve setting a standard based on global judgements of performance by a group of qualified expert panellists. Given the integrated, multi-dimensional nature of performance assessments in medical education, the latter methods are particularly well suited for setting a cut-score on OSCEs, for example.(51) Two popular examinee-centred standard setting methods are the contrasting groups method and the borderline group method.(52,53) (*see* Box 22.7.)

Contrasting groups method

In the contrasting groups method, panellists are asked, for each candidate, to review a performance profile (e.g. checklists and rating scales on an OSCE station) and determine whether the test taker is qualified or unqualified to pass the examination. OSCE station scores for both groups of candidates (unqualified and qualified) are then plotted on a graph. The score that best discriminates between both groups of test takers is typically selected as the cut-score.(52–54) A sample contrasting-groups plot is shown in Figure 22.1. In this example, the mid-point of the intersection zone could be selected as the cut-score value if false-positive and false-negative decisions were of equal importance. However, if the intent of the exam is to protect patients from malfeasance, a value in the upper part of the intersection zone would be chosen (minimising false-positive decisions, i.e. passing candidates who do not possess the clinical skills necessary to pass).

Borderline group method

In the borderline group method, panellists are also asked to review a performance profile for each candidate and identify unacceptable as well as acceptable performances. Additionally, panellists must designate those candidates that are deemed to lie just at a borderline acceptable performance level. The scores of these borderline acceptable examinees are then plotted on a graph. Typically, the median score value is chosen as the cut-score on the examination.(1,53) One limitation that has been raised with this approach is that the size of the borderline acceptable group might be quite small, thus contributing to a very unstable cut-score (e.g. median) value.

> **BOX 22.7 FOCUS ON: Standard setting for performance assessments**
>
> - For performance examinations, such as OSCEs and workplace-based assessments, examinee-centred methods are generally used to set a standard. Common examinee-centred standard setting methods include the contrasting groups and borderline group methods.
>
> - These methods are appealing and well-suited to performance assessment as they allow panellists to provide overall holistic judgements of performance. They require panellists to assign candidates to two or more proficiency categories (e.g. master/non-master, unacceptable, borderline acceptable, clearly acceptable, etc.).
>
> - While appealing, these methods inherently treat the panel as the 'gold standard'. Ample training is therefore necessary to ensure that the task is well understood as well as the definition of borderline performance.
>
> - A number of technical issues need to be considered when implementing any examinee-centred standard setting method, including: (i) determining the costs associated with false-positive and -negative classifications; (ii) ensuring that the borderline acceptable group is composed of a sufficiently large number of candidates; and (iii) for the contrasting groups method, assuring that panellists are able to assign candidates to one of two categories.

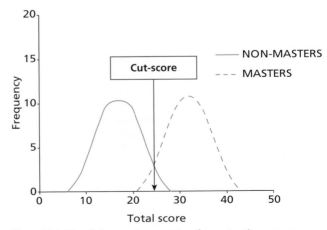

Figure 22.1 Identifying a cut-score using the contrasting-groups method.

As a means of addressing this shortcoming, the *borderline regression method* was proposed as an alternative, related standard setting method. As it implies, this procedure uses linear regression modelling to predict the cut-score on the score scale as a function of the rating categories (e.g. unacceptable, borderline acceptable, acceptable). That is, the pass mark for a given OSCE station is obtained by regressing candidate scores (e.g. checklist scores) onto the global ratings. Unlike the more traditional borderline group method, all data points are used in determining the cut-score, not only those associated with borderline acceptable candidates.(55)

Advantages and limitations

The contrasting groups and borderline group methods are very similar in that they require panellists to make holistic judgements on the overall performance of candidates by classifying them into two (or more) categories. In fact, one could conceive of the borderline group method as a generalisation of the contrasting groups approach where experts not only need to determine whether a performance is acceptable or unacceptable, but also 'on the cusp', i.e. borderline acceptable. Given the high degree of similarity between the methods, it should come as little surprise that they carry the same advantages and limitations.

On the plus side, both methods are often preferred for performance assessment such as OSCEs and workplace-based assessments as they require panellists to complete a task that is more 'intuitive', i.e. classify candidates as either unacceptable, acceptable or borderline acceptable. They are also well suited to these complex assessments given that dimensions on which to make classification judgements are often highly related. As such, these methods provide panellists with the latitude to incorporate all of their considerations when arriving at a classification decision with a candidate. The greater level of flexibility that is afforded by both approaches also potentially constitutes their chief limitation. Both methods treat panellist judgements as intrinsically reliable and valid, i.e. as *the* gold standard. Any factor that can detract from the panellists' ability to provide such judgements will bias the ultimate cut-score value in a way that is difficult to predict and will lead to a standard that is most certainly unfair to subgroups of candidates. Consequently, the moderator plays a critical role in ensuring that the training offered to panellists can at least minimise this effect to ultimately assure a defensible process for all stakeholders. It is easy to envisage a scenario where panellists, who might very well be familiar with the candidates who they are evaluating, are affected by construct irrelevant factors when providing their judgements. Such construct irrelevant factors might include gender, ethnicity, dress, personality, work habits and a myriad of other extraneous features that are unrelated to 'competency', as broadly defined by the examination.

Both the contrasting groups and borderline group methods also rest on the central premise that a sufficiently large group of representative professionals in the field can be identified for an exercise and also trained to complete the task at hand as instructed. Inadequate training can lead to a number of undesirable outcomes, including the pro-

pensity to assign disproportionally large number of candidates to the borderline acceptable group.(56,57) While this may sound appealing, given that the cut-score is derived from the performances of the latter group, classifying nearly all candidates as borderline acceptable seriously raises questions about the quality of the examination, instruction, and other factors, while yielding a cut-score that is again biased in ways that are difficult to ascertain. Related to this point, the borderline group method does require that the latter group be composed of a sufficiently large number or the resulting cut-score, whether the median score in the simplest case or a predicted value based on more complex statistical modelling (e.g. logistic regression, latent class analysis, etc.), will be unstable and inappropriately reflect 'minimal competency'. Given the dichotomous nature of the task that is required in a traditional contrasting groups standard exercise, it might also be difficult for panellists to classify candidates as either unacceptable or unacceptable, with no option for a borderline acceptable performance. Plake and Hambleton,(56) among others, proposed an extension of the method that does allow for a finer gradation of the decision scale. Finally, it is critical, for both methods, that the medical educator clearly set a policy that outlines the consequences of misclassifying a candidate. Treating both false-positive (passing a candidate who should have failed) and false-negative (failing a candidate who should have passed) decisions equally might be quite undesirable in instances where protection of the public is of prime consideration. Under the latter scenario, minimising false-positive classifications is of greater concern. Conversely, in lower-stakes settings, minimising false-negative errors could be perfectly acceptable as a policy. All of the potential limitations associated with the contrasting groups and borderline regression methods, given the immense responsibility that is conveyed upon panellists, again underscore the critical role that the moderator needs to play in such standard setting exercises. Indeed, it is not an exaggeration to state that the moderator can 'make or break' a borderline group or contrasting groups standard setting exercise.

Hofstee method

The use of criterion-referenced approaches for setting a standard can lead to unacceptable outcomes in the absence of political considerations associated with the decision. That is, the cut-score arrived at following a standard setting exercise should not result in failing or passing an unacceptably large or small proportion of candidates. To illustrate, assume that a given medical specialty examination has consistently failed around 15% of candidates. Further assume that this population is very comparable, ability wise, from year to year. If the cut-score set after an Angoff exercise results in failing 50% of candidates, the standard is unrealistic and might very well be unacceptable from a policy standpoint.

As a means of providing a 'reality check', Hofstee(58) proposed a 'compromise' method that involves asking panellists the following questions, the answers to which are subsequently graphed in a (Hofstee) plot:

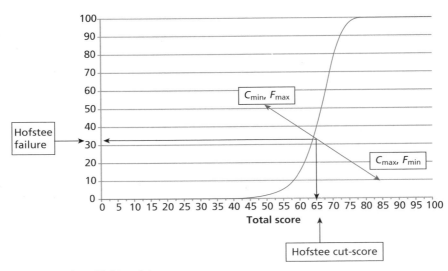

Figure 22.2 Identifying a cut-score using a Hofstee plot.

- Considering the content as a whole, what are the maximum and minimum tolerable cut-scores? These are typically labelled C_{min} and C_{max} on the Hofstee plot.
- What are maximum and minimum tolerable failure rates? These are usually listed as F_{max} and F_{min} on the Hofstee plot.

An example of a Hofstee plot is provided in Figure 22.2. In order to create this plot, a cumulative percentage-correct score distribution needs to first be computed. This distribution outlines the cumulative percentage of candidates who would fail at each point along the score scale. Then, the coordinates (C_{min}, F_{max}) and (C_{max}, F_{min}) are plotted and joined by a straight line, as illustrated in Figure 22.2. The point of intersection between this line and the frequency distribution corresponds to the Hofstee cut-score. The cut-score is illustrated by the 'cut' value shown on the x-axis. In the example outlined in Figure 22.2, panellists felt that the cut-score should be no lower than 55 (C_{min}) and no higher than 85 (C_{max}). Similarly, they indicated that the failure rate should be at least 10% (F_{min}) but not higher than 50% (F_{max}). Linking both sets of coordinates and drawing a line down to the x-axis yields a Hofstee cut-score value of 65, which would result in failing about 35% of the candidate cohort. The aim of the Hofstee method is generally to determine whether criterion-referenced standards fall within the vicinity of the Hofstee based value, i.e. whether they are consistent with political considerations and global impressions of cut-score values and failure rates.(59)

Advantages and limitations

The primary advantage of the Hofstee method is that it allows panellists to offer holistic judgements on cut-score values and failure rates with few to no constraints. Based on their experience, knowledge of the test content and objective of the examination, panellists must define performance parameter limits. The flexibility and ease with which one can implement the Hofstee method also constitutes its chief limitation. That is, it is not generally viewed

BOX 22.8 HOW TO: Choose a standard setting method

- No standard setting method can yield an 'optimal' cut-score value as this is based on experts' internal construction of what constitutes competence.
- The extent to which a process is systematically implemented and supported with appropriate sources of evidence is much more important than the selection of any standard setting method.
- However, several factors can be considered in the choice of a standard setting method, including the format of the examination (MCQ versus performance assessment).
- Combining several methods will not yield a 'better' standard as the choice of any cut-score is ultimately a policy decision based on a number of considerations.

as a primary standard setting method but rather as a 'reality check' or fall-back method meant to complement other approaches, whether test- or examinee-centred. Within this supporting context, the Hofstee method can provide valuable information that can help the practitioner gauge whether a cut-score set with a more traditional method gibes with the general expectations of panellists. However, it should generally not be used as a standalone measure given its *ad hoc* nature.

The next section provides some practical guidelines to aid in the selection of a standard setting method.

Selecting a criterion-referenced standard setting method

The American Educational Research Association 'Standards for Educational and Psychological Testing'(60, p.53) clearly state that 'there can be no single method for determining cut-scores for all tests or for all purposes, nor can there be any single set of procedures for establishing their defensibility'. Along these lines, Angoff(61) also noted that 'regarding the problem of setting cut-scores, we have observed that the several judgemental methods not only fail to yield results that agree with one another, they even fail to yield the same results on repeated application'.

Despite the fact that no single method can lead to the identification of an 'optimal' cut-score value, as the latter is always embedded in professional judgement, there are nonetheless a number of factors that the medical educator might wish to consider when selecting a standard setting approach. An overview of these factors is presented next.

The extent to which a clear standard setting process is adhered to has the greatest impact on the cut-score. This process, regardless of the method adopted, should include a clear definition of the objective of the examination as well as the standard setting exercise; extensive training of panellists to minimise any misconceptions, as well as a clear outline of what constitutes minimal proficiency or a borderline acceptable performance. However, a number of factors can be considered to select a standard setting method that might be most suitable given the intended aims of the examination and the associated decision that the test score user wishes to make.

First, what is the complexity level of the examination? For knowledge-based examinations (e.g. MCQs), test-centred methods are most appropriate given the task that panellists are asked to complete, i.e. estimate a cut-score based on a review of the actual test items. Conversely, for performance assessments, such as OSCEs and workplace-based tasks, examinee-centred methods are more suitable for setting a standard given the complex, multi-dimensional nature of performance. The latter typically entail holistic judgements of performance. Second, the user may also wish to consider the format of the examination. For example, some standard setting methods (e.g. the Nedelsky method) were developed exclusively for use with MCQs. While some methods can be used with different formats (e.g. Angoff methods), certain assumptions are made that may or may not meet expectations. For example, the Angoff method and its offshoots assume that performance is compensatory in nature, i.e. candidates can compensate for doing poorly in certain parts of the examination by doing well in other sections. These methods would therefore be inappropriate in a conjunctive setting, where different components need to be successfully and independently completed. Other methods (Hofstee, contrasting groups) were developed as test format invariant.

One erroneous belief that is often promulgated is the one that suggests that combining a multitude of methods when setting a standard will provide a 'better cut-score'. It is important to reiterate that standard setting and the selection of a cut-score are ultimately policy decisions, albeit derived from informed judgement. There is little evidence to suggest that combining multiple methods will lead to a 'better' standard.(57) Since there is no 'correct' cut-score, how can policy makers synthesise results from multiple approaches? This strategy also requires significantly more resources. It is always better to systematically implement one standard setting method rather than provide results from several (poorly) carry out approaches. Again, the process that is followed when arriving at a cut-score is ultimately what needs to be defended. The latter includes properly documenting all phases of a standard setting exercise, clearly describing the selection and training of panellists, as well as providing empirical evidence to support the use of a cut-score. These data typically include the impact of sources of variability (judges, panels, etc.) on the cut-score value as well as the consequences of implementing a cut-score (e.g. the appropriateness of pass/fail rates in light of historical trends). The importance of validating any cut-score is underscored in the next section. (*see* Box 22.8.)

Gathering validity evidence to support a cut-score

Regardless of the standard setting method adopted, gathering evidence to validate the resulting standard is a critical step.(61,62) As stated throughout this chapter, what is ultimately of importance with any standard setting exercise is the extent to which a process is systematically adhered to and can be defended using a number of evidential sources.

First and foremost, evidence to support *procedural validity* needs to be clearly documented in the standard setting report. The latter usually comprises the first part of any standard setting report and entails a thorough account of each step of the exercise including:

- An overview of the targeted examination and its purpose.
- A clear articulation of the selected standard setting method implemented with a supporting rationale.
- The process used to select the panel of expert judges, as well as a description of their qualifications and the extent to which they represent the profession as a whole.
- An outline of all phases of the exercise, including the training process, definition of the performance standard and how data were collected.

Surveying panellists on various aspects of the standard setting exercise constitutes a final important piece of supporting procedural validity evidence. How confident are the panellists in the process and more importantly, in the resulting cut-score? Evaluating judges' impressions of the training phase as well as the cut-score can provide strong confirmation for any standard setting exercise.

Evidence to support the *internal validity* of the cut-score is also of great importance given the high-stakes nature of most criterion-referenced examinations. That is, how precise is the estimate of the cut-score and how reproducible is it across any facet of interest? With regard to precision, if the cut-score is relatable to an item response theory ability metric, the (conditional) standard error of the proficiency estimate associated with a cut-score can provide a straightforward indication of the stability of the latter value. With an observed score scale (e.g. number-right, percentage-correct, etc.), the practitioner can also estimate the amount of error associated with a cut-score using a compound binomial model.(63)

Additionally, the extent to which the cut-score is impacted as a function of the judges participating in an exercise, the panel of judges (if multiple groups are involved), the items/stations selected, etc. can be readily assessed using generalisability theory.(8,64) This framework allows the medical educator to estimate the amount of variability in scores (including the cut-score) that can be ascribed to any facet or potential source of measurement error as listed above. Similarly, IRT-based rating scale models(65) can also provide useful information with respect to the ability distribution of candidates, difficulty of items/stations, as well as stringency of raters. Regardless of the complexity of the models utilised to gather evidence of internal validity, the aim of this critical source of information is to provide an indication of the stability or precision with which a cut-score is estimated, primarily to provide some boundaries to the practitioner in order to minimise its misuse.

Evidence to support the *external validity* of a cut-score should also be part of any standard setting effort as this relates directly to the impact of implementing a standard. Assessing the reasonableness of the cut-score in light of its impact on failure rates is generally at the core of external validation efforts. For example, assume that a graduation OSCE has typically failed between 10% and 12% of a class. A failure rate of 55%, following a standard setting exercise, would warrant considerable scrutiny of the cut-score and its appropriateness, assuming that the cohort is of comparable ability to past groups and the OSCE of a similar difficulty level.

A comparison of results to other assessments constitutes another important source of external validity for any proposed cut-score. For example, how comparable are pass/fail rates to grades or the status of students on other examinations measuring similar constructs (e.g. a prior OSCE)? Though we would not expect two examinations to measure exactly the same combination of domains, they should nonetheless yield a comparable standing for most candidates.

Conclusions

Standard setting is an intrinsic part of all assessment activities in medical education, from undergraduate training to physician revalidation efforts. Determining whether a candidate has mastered any number of competencies underlying an examination is a key outcome used not only to render individual judgements but also to evaluate programme effectiveness, teaching efficacy, etc.(66,67)

First and foremost, it is important to reiterate that there is no gold standard and that all cut-scores ultimately reflect informed judgement from a group of content experts on what level of performance constitutes 'competency'. Systematically following a standard setting process and supporting its use with appropriate empirical evidence is therefore central to any such exercise.

This chapter has described a number of standard setting methods that the medical educator might wish to consider based on the nature of their examination as well as practical and financial concerns. Irrespective of the method selected to arrive at a cut-score on an examination, several issues need to be addressed prior to undertaking a standard setting exercise. First, the panel of judges should be viewed as a microcosm of all exam stakeholders and as such should mirror any characteristic deemed important by the profession, be that geographical area, medical school location, specialty, gender or ethnicity. Convening such a broad panel will ensure that views from most members of the profession are incorporated in the exercise, and ultimately, the standard.

Determining a suitable number of panellists for any standard setting panel is also critical. Inviting too few panellists is ill-advised, as the judgements of a single dissenting judge could have an undue impact on the value of the final cut-score. On the other hand, assembling a large panel may not be cost-effective. Consequently, clearly identifying the desired characteristics of the group, as outlined above, can provide valuable information for determining the panel's optimal size. Once set, it is also important that the cut-score for any examination be periodically revisited to ensure its continued appropriateness in light of any changes that may have occurred in the profession, whether political or content-based in nature. Finally, it is important to restate that different standard setting methods will produce different cut-score values. The central aim in any standard setting exercise should be to: (i) defend the choice of a particular method, (ii) meticulously document all steps followed throughout the exercise and (iii) base the selection of the standard on as much empirical evidence as possible, factoring in global impressions as well as the consequences of adopting a given cut-score. Hopefully, this chapter provides a convenient guiding framework for any medical educator who needs to identify a cut-score for an examination and highlights some of the issues to consider when conducting a standard setting exercise, irrespective of the method adopted.

References

1 Dauphinee WD, Blackmore DE, Smee S, Rothman AL and Reznick R (1997) Using the judgments of physician examiners in setting the standards for a national multi-center high stakes OSCE. *Advances in Health Sciences Education: Theory and Practice.* **2**: 201–11.

2 Melnick DE, Dillon GF and Swanson DB (2002) Medical licensing examinations in the United States. *Journal of Dental Education.* **66**: 595–9.

3 Norcini JJ (1994) Research on standards for professional licensure and certification examinations. *Evaluation and the Health Professions.* **17**: 160–77.

4 Hess BJ, Weng W, Lynn LA, Holmboe ES and Lipner RS (2011) Setting a fair performance standard for physicians' quality of patient care. *Journal of General Internal Medicine.* **26**: 467–73.

5 Sturmberg JP and Hinchy J (2010) Borderline competence – from a complexity perspective: conceptualization and implementation for certifying examinations. *Journal of Evaluation in Clinical Practice.* **16**: 867–72.

6 Mucklow J (2011) Development and implementation of the specialty certificate examinations. *Clinical Medicine.* **11**: 235–8.

7 Lee RP, Venkatesh B and Morley P (2009) Evidence-based evolution of the high stakes postgraduate intensive care examination in Australia and New Zealand. *Anaesthesia and Intensive Care.* **37**: 525–31.

8 Lagha Richter RA, Boscardin CK, May W and Fung CC (2012) A comparison of two standard-setting approaches in high-stakes clinical performance assessment using generalizability theory. *Academic Medicine*. **87**: 1077–82.

9 Jalili M and Norcini JJ (2011) Comparison of two methods of standard setting: the performance of the three-level Angoff method. *Medical Education*. **45**: 1199–208.

10 Cohen-Schotanus J and van der Vleuten CP (2010) A standard setting method with the best performing students as point of reference: practical and affordable. *Medical Teacher*. **32**: 154–60.

11 Ricketts C, Freeman AC and Coombes LR (2009) Standard setting for progress tests: combining external and internal standards. *Medical Education*. **43**: 589–93.

12 Boursicot KA, Roberts TE and Pell G (2006) Standard setting for clinical competence at graduation from medical school: Comparison of passing scores across five medical schools. *Advances in Health Sciences Education: Theory and Practice*. **11**: 173–83.

13 Cizek GJ (1993) Reconsidering standards and criteria. *Journal of Educational Measurement*. **30**: 93–106.

14 Kane MT, Crooks TJ and Cohen AS (1999) Designing and evaluating standard-setting procedures for licensure and certification tests. *Advances in Health Sciences Education*. **4**: 195–207.

15 Norcini JJ and Shea JA (1997) The credibility and comparability of standards. *Applied Measurement in Education*. **10**: 39–59.

16 Kane MT (2001) So much remains the same: conception and status of validation in setting standards. In: Cizek GJ (ed.) *Setting Performance Standards: Concepts, Methods, and Perspectives*, pp. 53–88. Lawrence Erlbaum Associates, Mahwah, NJ.

17 Impara JC and Plake BS (2000) *A comparison of cut scores using multiple standard setting methods*. Paper presented at the meeting of the American Educational Research Association, New Orleans, LA, April 24–28, 2000.

18 Jaeger RM (1989) Certification of student competence. In: Linn RL (ed.) *Educational Measurement* (3e), pp. 485–514. Macmillan, New York.

19 Livingston SA and Zieky MJ (1989) A comparative study of standard setting methods. *Applied Measurement in Education*. **2**: 121–41.

20 Longford NT (1996) Reconciling experts' differences in setting cut-scores for pass–fail decisions. *Journal of Educational and Behavioral Statistics*. **21**: 203–13.

21 Norcini JJ and Shea J (1992) The reproducibility of standards over groups and occasions. *Applied Measurement in Education*. **5**: 63–72.

22 Hambleton RK and Pitoniak MJ (2006) Setting performance standards. In: Brennan RL (ed.) *Educational Measurement* (4e), pp. 433–70. Macmillan, New York.

23 Jaeger RM (1991) Selection of judges for standard setting. *Educational Measurement, Issues and Practice*. **10**: 3–6, 10, 14.

24 Raymond MR and Reid JB (2001) Who made thee a judge? Selecting and training participants for standard setting. In: Cizek GJ (ed.) *Setting Performance Standards: Concepts, Methods and Perspectives*, pp. 119–57. Lawrence Erlbaum, Mahwah, NJ.

25 Skorupski WP and Hambleton RK (2005) What are panelists thinking when they participate in standard setting studies? *Applied Measurement in Education*. **18**: 233–56.

26 Norcini JJ (1994) Research on standards for professional licensure and certification examinations. *Evaluation and the Health Professions*. **17**: 236–41.

27 Swanson DB, Case SM, Waechter D *et al.* (1993) A preliminary study of the validity of scores and pass/fail standards for USMLE steps 1 and 2. *Academic Medicine*. **68**: s19–21.

28 Wendt A and Kenny L (2007) Setting the passing standard for the National Council Licensure Examination for Registered Nurses. *Nurse Educator*. **32**: 104–8.

29 De Champlain AF (2004) Ensuring that the competent are truly competent: an overview of common methods and procedures used to set standards on high-stakes examinations. *Journal of Veterinary Medical Education*. **31**: 61–5.

30 Cizek GJ (2012) *Setting Performance Standards: Foundations, Methods and Innovations*. Routledge, New York.

31 Angoff WH (1971) Scales, norms, and equivalent scores. In: Thorndike RL (ed.) *Educational Measurement* (2e), pp. 508–600. American Council on Education, Washington, DC.

32 Plake BS and Impara JC (1997) Standard setting: an alternative approach. *Journal of Educational Measurement*. **34**: 353–66.

33 Downing SM, Lieska NG and Raible MD (2003) Establishing passing standards for classroom achievement tests in medical education: a comparative study of four methods. *Academic Medicine*. **78**: s85–7.

34 Hambleton RK and Plake BS (1995) Using an extended Angoff procedure to set standards on complex performance assessments. *Applied Measurement in Education*. **8**: 41–55.

35 Ricker KL (2006) Setting cut-scores: a critical review of the Angoff and modified Angoff methods. *The Alberta Journal of Educational Research*. **52**: 53–64.

36 Jaeger RM (1978) *A proposal for setting a standard on the North Carolina high school competency test*. Paper presented at the meeting of the North Carolina Association for Research in Education, Chapel Hill, NC.

37 Norcini JJ (1988) The effect of various factors on standard setting. *Journal of Educational Measurement*. **25**: 57–65.

38 Plake BS and Cizek GJ (2012) Variations on a theme: the modified Angoff, extended Angoff, and yes/no standard setting methods. In: Cizek GJ (ed.) *Setting Performance Standards: Foundations, Methods and Innovations*, pp. 181–99. Routledge, New York.

39 Shepard L (1995) Implications for standard setting of the National Academy of Education evaluation of National Assessment of Educational Progress achievement levels, In: *Proceedings of the Joint Conference on Standard Setting for Large-Scale Assessments* (vol. II), pp. 143–60. US Government Printing Office, Washington, DC.

40 Hambleton RK, Brennan RL, Brown W *et al.* (2000) A response to 'setting reasonable and useful performance standards' in the National Academy of Sciences' Grading the Nation's Report Card. *Educational Measurement, Issues and Practice*. **19**: 5–14.

41 Plake BS, Impara JC and Irwin PM (2000) Consistency of Angoff-based predictions of item performance: evidence of the technical quality of results from the Angoff standard setting method. *Journal of Educational Measurement*. **37**: 347–56.

42 Ebel RL (1972) *Essentials of Educational Measurement*. Prentice-Hall, Englewood Cliffs, NJ.

43 Berk RA (1986) A consumer's guide to setting performance standards on criterion-referenced tests. *Review of Educational Research*. **56**: 137–72.

44 Nedelsky L (1954) Absolute grading standards for objective tests. *Educational and Psychological Measurement*. **14**: 3–19.

45 Gross LJ (1985) Setting cutoff scores on credentialing examinations: a refinement in the Nedelsky procedure. *Evaluation and the Health Professions*. **8**: 469–93.

46 Melican GJ and Plake BS (1985) Are correction for guessing and Nedelsky's standard setting method compatible? *Journal of Psychoeducational Assessment*. **3**: 31–6.

47 Smith RM and Gross LJ (1997) Validating standard setting with a modified Nedelsky procedure through common item test equating. *Journal of Outcome Measurement*. **1**: 164–72.

48 Lewis DM, Mitzel HC, Green DR and Patz RJ (1999) *The Bookmark Standard Setting Procedure*. McGraw-Hill, Monterey, CA.

49 Barton PE (2009) *Contents for a new NAEP report: The five largest states*. Paper presented for the National Assessment Governing Board. (http://www.nagb.org/publications/reports-papers.htm; accessed 15 March 2013).

50 Pashley PJ and Phillips GW (1993) *Toward world-class standards: A research study linking international and national assessments*. Educational Testing Service, Princeton, NJ.

51 Boulet J, De Champlain A and McKinley D (2003) Setting defensible performance standards on OSCEs and standardized patient examinations. *Medical Teacher*. **25**: 245–9.

52 Berk RA (1976) Determination of optimal cutting scores in criterion-referenced measurement. *Journal of Experimental Education*. **14**: 9475–69.

53 Livingstone SA and Zieky MJ (1982) *Passing scores: A manual for setting standards of performance on educational and occupational tests.* Educational Testing Service, Princeton, NJ.

54 Clauser BE and Nungester RJ (1997) Setting standards on performance assessments of physicians' clinical skills using contrasting groups and receiver operator characteristic curves. *Evaluation in the Health Professions*. **20**: 215–38.

55 Wood TJ, Humphrey-Murto S and Norman GR (2006) Standard Setting in a small scale OSCE: a comparison of the Modified Borderline-Group Method and the Borderline Regression Method. *Advances in Health Sciences Education*. **11**: 115–22.

56 Plake B and Hambleton R (2001) The analytic judgment method for setting standards on complex performance assessments. In: Cizek GJ (ed.) *Setting Performance Standards: Concepts, Methods, and Perspectives,* pp. 283–312. Erlbaum, Mahwah, NJ.

57 Cizek GJ and Bunch MB (2007) *Standard Setting: A Guide to Establishing and Evaluating Performance Standards on Test*. Sage Publications, Thousand Oaks, CA.

58 Hofstee WKB (1983) The case for compromise in educational selection and grading. In: Anderson SB and Helminck JS (eds) *On Educational Testing,* pp. 107–27. Jossey-Bass, San Francisco, CA.

59 De Gruiiter D (1985) Compromise models for establishing examination standards. *Journal of Educational Measurement*. **22**: 263–9.

60 American Educational Research Association (1999) Standards for educational and psychological testing (1999). American Educational Research Association, American Psychological Association, National Council on Measurement in education, Washington, DC.

61 Angoff WH (1988) Validity: an evolving concept. In: Wainer H and Braun H (eds) *Test Validity*, pp. 19–32. Erlbaum, Hillsdale, NJ.

62 Kane MT (1994) Validating the performance standards associated with passing scores. *Review of Educational Research*. **64**: 425–61.

63 Lord FM (1984) *Standard errors of measurement at different score levels* (Research Report RR-84-8). Educational Testing Service, Princeton, NJ.

64 Verhoeven BH, van der Steeg AF, Scherpbier AJ, Muijtjens AM, Verwijnen GM and van der Vleuten CP (1999) Reliability and credibility of an Angoff standard setting procedure in progress testing using recent graduates as judges. *Medical Education*. **32**: 832–7.

65 Andrich D (1978) A rating scale formulation for ordered response categories. *Psychometrika*. **43**: 561–73.

66 Brandon PR (2005) Using test standard-setting methods in educational program evaluation: addressing the issue of how good is good enough. *Journal of MultiDisciplinary Evaluation*. **2**: 1–29.

67 Bennett J, Tognolini J and Pickering S (2012) Establishing and applying performance standards for curriculum-based examinations. *Assessment in Education: Principles, Policy & Practice*. **19**: 321–39.

Further reading

American Educational Research Association (1999) Standards for educational and psychological testing (1999). American Educational Research Association, American Psychological Association, National Council on Measurement in education, Washington, DC.

Cizek GJ and Bunch MB (2007) *Standard Setting: A Guide to Establishing and Evaluating Performance Standards on Test*. Sage Publications, Thousand Oaks, CA.

23 Formative assessment

Diana F Wood

University of Cambridge School of Clinical Medicine, UK

KEY MESSAGES

- Formative assessment promotes a number of desirable educational outcomes, including learner self-regulation and the development of lifelong learning skills.
- Students with a high level of self-regulation are more effective learners, showing increased resourcefulness, resilience, persistence and success.
- A well-designed programme of formative assessment linked to overall curriculum aims and the teaching and learning goals of individual modules enhances the learning experience for students.

- Effective feedback is central to the process of formative assessment.
- Teachers in medical education identify the development of constructive feedback skills as the most important aspect of their professional development.
- Formative assessment linked to curriculum design should be an essential component of medical education at all levels.

Introduction

Assessment forms a major element of any teaching and learning programme and should be recognised as integral to the whole educational enterprise, not just delivered as an 'add-on' at the end of a course. Traditionally, in medical education, assessment was used to demonstrate that information had been transmitted in some way from the teacher to the learners, the latter memorising notes diligently and reproducing them as necessary in formal examinations requiring factual recall.

One of the most obvious developments in medical education over the past 20 years or so has been a greater understanding of assessment and the way it can be used to enhance both students' learning and the overall quality of the educational experience. At its most pragmatic level, this reflects our recognition that 'assessment drives the curriculum'.(1) Students learn what is needed to pass examinations and use weighting of assessments as a means to rank the importance of various parts of the syllabus. If assessments are developed independently and added on to the teaching programme to test 'what students have learned' (usually by factual recall), then well-meaning attempts to foster deep learning and understanding of a subject will founder.

Furthermore, students expect to be assessed and tend to use grading systems that compare them with their peers as a means of evaluating the amount of work required of them to perform well in the course.(2) This in itself has provided a challenge to many medical educators faced with intro-

ducing minimum-competency 'pass/fail' assessments in which students are not ranked against their peers but against pre-set, minimal-competency guidelines.

The key is to align assessment with the educational desires of the faculty and the aims of curriculum planners. In a well-designed curriculum, faculty are aware of their educational goals from the outset and build in the design and timing of assessments to ensure that these goals are addressed by the teaching programme.

This chapter predominantly relates to the use of formative assessment in undergraduate medical education. However, the principles described are derived from a variety of sources, including the general educational literature, and can be extrapolated to all levels of medical education. In many cases, the formative assessment methods described here can be directly transferred to the postgraduate arena with correction only for the level of the learners in relation to the educational goals.

The following areas will be considered:
- definitions of formative and summative assessment
- teacher and learner perspectives on formative assessment and some of the research evidence underpinning them
- the role of feedback in formative assessment, including examples from experiential learning settings in communication skills teaching
- how formative assessment may be used within a curriculum
- examples of formative assessment in different teaching and learning environments.

Understanding Medical Education: Evidence, Theory and Practice, Second Edition. Edited by Tim Swanwick.
© 2014 The Association for the Study of Medical Education. Published 2014 by John Wiley & Sons, Ltd.

BOX 23.1 Some functions of assessment

Assessment may be used to:

Measure student learning	Against a pre-set criteria
Grade students	Against a standard
	Against a comparative group
Summarise achievement	For the student
	For the faculty
	For other interested bodies, e.g. university, potential employer, etc.
Indicate readiness to progress	
Provide feedback	On learning
	On why a mark was given to teaching staff
Diagnose specific misunderstandings	
Motivate students to learn	
Focus and direct student learning	
Help students learn more effectively	
Inform the teaching programme	Review what students do not know or understand
	Review teaching and learning methods
Promote staff development	Ensure that faculty are aware of the curriculum goals and understand how assessment forms part of the programme
Contribute to education quality assurance	

Assessment is a complex construct, and recognition of its various purposes will help ensure that an individual educational programme achieves its multiple goals (*see* Box 23.1). Classically, assessment has been divided into two categories: *formative* and *summative*. In essence, formative assessment provides feedback to learners about their progress, whereas summative assessment measures the achievement of learning goals at the end of a course or programme of study. In undergraduate medical education, summative assessments are used at various points in the course to determine progression, to signify the need for remediation in one or more areas and ultimately for graduation, allowing registration with national medical certification bodies and progression into postgraduate and continuing medical education. In general, little feedback is provided to students from summative assessments except in the case of failure. In recent years, particularly in postgraduate medical education, the distinction between formative and summative assessment has become blurred, with essentially formative workplace-based assessments being collated and used for summative purposes. This trend has presumably been driven by a desire to reconnect assessment with learning.

Much of the literature related to formative assessment derives from studies in secondary schools and in general higher education. However, a focus on the development of learner self-regulation and lifelong learning means that the general principles described below can be related to medical education at all levels.

Assessment can be thought of as serving three main functions; *assessment of learning*, *assessment for learning* and *assessment for quality assurance*. Whilst summative assessment fits most neatly into the first category and formative assessment into the second, in a well-designed educational programme, there is considerable overlap such that the results of ongoing, formative assessment can be used both to measure student learning and to inform institutional quality assurance procedures.

Characteristics of formative assessment

Formative assessment refers to any assessment that is designed specifically to provide feedback. It has been defined as follows:

'. . . encompassing all those activities undertaken by teachers, and/or by their students, which provide information to be used as feedback to modify the teaching and learning activities in which they are engaged.'((3), p.8)

More recently, the same authors refined this definition to include five features of formative assessment that should be more directly applicable in medical education:(4)

- clarifying and sharing learning intentions and criteria for success
- engineering effective classroom discussions and other learning tasks that elicit evidence of student understanding
- providing feedback that moves learners forward
- activating students as instructional resources for one another
- activating students as the owners of their own learning.

Some characteristics of formative assessment that reflect these features are shown in Box 23.2. Feedback is central to effective formative assessment. In general, formative assessment should be ongoing, frequent, non-judgemental and carried out in informal settings. For students, the availability of a regular, dynamic interaction with their tutors

BOX 23.2 Characteristics of formative assessment

General	Informal
	Ongoing and frequent
	Dynamic
	Non-judgemental
	Part of the overall teaching and learning process
Effects on students	Allows detailed feedback
	Promotes self-directed learning
	Raises self-esteem
	Engages students in the learning process
	Encourages deep learning and understanding
	Motivates learning
	Identifies insecurities
	Offers help with specific remediation
Effects on staff	Allows detailed feedback
	Promotes self-directed learning by the students
	Fosters interactive teaching and learning methods
	Encourages varied and challenging teaching methods
	Identifies students in difficulty early in the curriculum
	Develops teaching skills
	Evaluation feeds into curriculum development

helps them engage with the learning process, acting as a motivator and encouraging deep learning and understanding. Furthermore, it offers them the opportunity to identify their learning difficulties in a safe environment and to take up remedial assistance if appropriate.

For teachers, formative assessment encourages the development of skills associated with the promotion of self-directed learning in the student. Teachers are motivated by better understanding of their students' needs and by helping them become more self-regulated in their learning. Review of the teaching and assessment programme feeds into curriculum development and forms part of ongoing curriculum evaluation.

Overall, consideration of the effects of formative assessment on students and teachers suggests that it should be a positive experience for both groups. Students are encouraged to engage in active learning and teachers to develop skills with which to provide a challenging educational experience in a supportive environment.

Formative assessment can play a major role in the acquisition of lifelong learning skills by helping students self-regulate their learning activities. A well-designed series of formative assessments can make a major contribution to the educational impact of an overall assessment programme, a characteristic that is as important as the reliability and validity of the individual assessments themselves.(5) Thus, in the ideal situation, formative assessment is a two-way process between learner and teacher, placing the student at the centre of the activity.

In reality, assessment is usually seen as the province of teachers, many of whom regard feedback primarily as a means of transmitting information to students. Often, little thought is given to how feedback information received during formative assessment is processed by students. In this respect, assessment has not kept pace with other developments in teaching and learning in higher education, where the emphasis has shifted towards a dialogue between teacher and student, fostering self-direction and motivation to learn. An assessment process that focuses solely on the teacher's role overlooks the need to help students gain the skills of self-regulation necessary for lifelong learning and ignores the way in which feedback interacts with students' motivation and beliefs. To understand how formative assessment can be most effective, it is therefore necessary to consider the process from the point of view of both teacher and students.

Teacher perspectives

From the teacher's perspective, the formative assessment process could be described in the following three steps:
1 Review the student's work.
2 Evaluate the work against a reference framework that reflects the pre-set learning objectives and the level expected of students at a particular stage in the course.
3 Make a judgement on the work and provide verbal or written feedback to the student on that judgement.

The apparent simplicity of these steps is misleading, mainly because it disguises the expertise of individual teachers and their differing levels of skill and experience, particularly in giving feedback. Such 'teacher factors' were reviewed by Sadler;(6) he identified six important characteristics that highly competent teachers bring to the assessment process. These characteristics are summarised in Box 23.3.

Highly competent teachers are not only knowledgeable but also bring a positive attitude to teaching, with their ability to empathise with their students and desire to see them improve. Such teachers are reflective about their own skills and show concern for the integrity of the judgements they make. They demonstrate skill in constructing assessments using a variety of methodologies and are aware of assessment criteria and the standards expected of students at different levels within the curriculum. They learn from their experience in assessment and develop expertise in giving constructive feedback.

Clearly, in any given faculty, the level of expertise will vary between teachers. The importance of the skills of individual teachers in formative assessment reinforces the requirement for assessment to be designed as part of an institutional educational programme, particularly in relation to staff development and appraisal.

Student perspectives

From the student perspective, formative assessment should be a means to improve performance and aid development

BOX 23.3 Characteristics of highly competent teachers that affect the quality of formative assessment

Characteristic	Effect on formative assessment
Knowledge	Greater knowledge base and understanding of the subject matter than the students
Attitude to teaching	Empathy with students, ability to communicate educational goals, desire to help students improve, concern for the integrity of their own judgements
Skill in constructing assessments	Use of varied assessment tools to develop different skills in students
Knowledge of assessment criteria and appropriate standards	Awareness of standards and appropriate expectations of students' performance at a certain level within the curriculum based on learning outcomes and previous experience of student achievement
Evaluative skills	Ability to make qualitative judgements informed by experience as assessors
Expertise in giving feedback	Identification of strengths and weaknesses, evaluative comments in relation to criteria, suggestions for alternative learning methods, examples of different ways to achieve the goals

Adapted from Sadler.(6)

as self-directed and motivated learners. The term 'self-regulation' is used to describe the way in which students monitor their learning behaviour by setting and achieving goals, managing resources and adapting to external feedback. In doing so, students generate their own internal feedback, helping them evaluate their progress towards goals and to adapt their learning processes in the face of obstacles or changes in motivation. Self-regulated learners are aware of their own knowledge, beliefs and cognitive skills, and they use these to interpret external feedback effectively.(7) Self-regulated learning is discussed in detail in Chapter 15.

Nicol and Macfarlane-Dick reviewed the literature relating to formative assessment and self-regulated learning, elaborating the student's role in developing internal feedback mechanisms and modelling the relationship between internal and external feedback (Figure 23.1).(8) This model is useful as it illustrates the way in which a task set by the teacher acts as a trigger for internal regulatory processes within the student, drawing on prior knowledge and motivation to learn. The process generates a set of internal outcomes, such as increased understanding or changes in motivational state, in addition to the external outcomes reflected in a piece of work submitted for assessment. External and internal outcomes are linked by external feedback requiring the student to engage actively with such input. Evidence from the literature suggests that students with a higher level of self-regulation are more effective learners, showing increased resourcefulness, persistence and success.

This student-centred approach to formative assessment described in the general educational literature is consistent with the constructivist approach to learning widely adopted in medical education through formal problem-based learning and other forms of problem-orientated learning and assessment.(9) Translation of social constructivist theories into practice places the relationship between teacher and student and the effective use of feedback at the centre of the educational endeavour.(10,11)

Feedback

Feedback provides the route by which assessment becomes a tool for teaching and learning, and it is central to the concept of formative assessment. Feedback following assessment encourages the student and teacher to work together to improve the student's understanding of a subject. The teacher shows that they are interested in the student's opinions, seeks clarification where appropriate and, where necessary, encourages the student to approach a topic in a different way. Feedback provided in a non-judgemental and open fashion allows the student to feel more confident to discuss their difficulties and plan better approaches to learning where necessary.

It has been recognised for many years and across all educational sectors that effective feedback is positively correlated with student achievement,(12) although it is also clear from early studies that the quality of feedback is vital. Poor-quality feedback may have no effect or may even be detrimental.(3)

Effective feedback

Feedback can be defined as a way in which learners become aware of the gap between their current level of knowledge or skill and the desired goal. It provides guidance towards reaching the goal, but effective feedback is achieved only when the student takes action to narrow the gap.(13,14) This implies not only that the educational goals are clearly described, but also that students are able and empowered to take the necessary action to achieve them. This in turn means that effective feedback is a collaboration between teachers and learners rather than just a function of teaching *per se*.

Nicol and Macfarlane-Dick propose seven principles of good feedback that can facilitate the development of self-regulation (*see* Box 23.4).(8) These emphasise the need for learner and teacher to work together towards learner self-regulation. They clarify the teacher's role in providing information to the student about their performance and

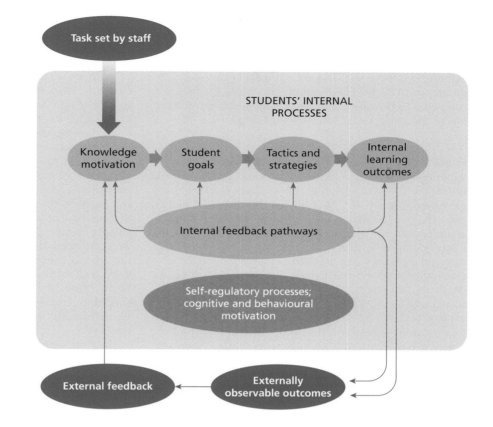

Figure 23.1 A model of self-regulated learning illustrating the relationship between external factors and internal self-regulation in the student. Adapted from Nicol and Macfarlane-Dick.(8)

BOX 23.4 Good feedback practice

- Helps clarify what good performance is
- Facilitates the development of self-assessment (reflection) in learning
- Delivers high-quality information to students about their learning
- Encourages teacher and peer dialogue around learning
- Encourages positive motivational beliefs and self-esteem
- Provides opportunities to close the gap between current and desired performance
- Provides information to teachers that can be used to help shape teaching

Adapted from Nicol and Macfarlane-Dick.(8)

---

also, crucially, about what is expected of them and how to recognise the gap between current and expected attainment. These principles raise a number of issues pertinent to undergraduate medical education that can be considered under the heading 'Education for feedback'.

Education for feedback

On entry into medical school, students are generally very well motivated and academically capable, having achieved high standards in national school exit examinations, prior higher degrees and/or medical school selection examina-

tions. Despite this, some students experience early failure, contributing to internal demotivation and a cycle of further failure. Paradoxically, for the small number of students who underachieve in medical school, the learning habits developed to produce high-level performance in premedical school examinations may be the reason for their failure at the undergraduate level.(15) In particular, students who have learnt previously in a didactic teaching environment and become successful at memorising facts may be challenged by small group learning, problem-solving, dealing with 'grey areas' of knowledge and scoping vast amounts of information to contain their learning goals within reasonable limits.

A programme of formative assessment and feedback introduced early in a course can go a long way towards preventing the onset of the cycle of failure and demotivation in these students. A well-designed formative assessment programme will ensure that students are aware of their goals and the ways in which these might be achieved. However, it is incumbent on the faculty to explain this process to the students at the beginning of the course. Individual and group feedback can be difficult for students and, if handled badly, can be detrimental to their progress. Educating students about formative assessment and feedback is essential to ensure maximum gain from the process. This in itself requires planning and thought – it is unlikely that a single lecture at the start of a course will be effective. Integrating the educational process with early feedback sessions and modelling good feedback within a learning group is more likely to be educationally valuable.(16)

Much of the research into feedback in medical education comes from the field of teaching communication skills, and these principles have been carried forward into other experiential and reflective learning environments. In the following section, two well-known approaches to feedback developed in the field of communication skills teaching are compared to provide examples of how effective feedback can be used in practical teaching situations.

Feedback in experiential learning settings

Experiential learning in one-to-one or small group settings forms the basis of communication skills teaching programmes, usually in the form of observed simulated consultations. Students learn through frequent practice accompanied by feedback and reflection. This type of teaching can be particularly challenging for students who may feel exposed when required to perform difficult communication tasks in front of their tutors and peers. It places demands on teachers, who need to be aware of the dynamics within a learning group and who need to be trained and capable of handling students' responses and reactions. In these situations, feedback should not only be constructive, but is best delivered within a framework that is known and accepted by both teachers and students.

One widely used set of guidelines for providing feedback during teaching about consultation skills was described by Pendleton *et al.* in 1984(17) and has become known as 'Pendleton's Rules'. The stimulus for developing these guidelines was primarily the observation that feedback in medical education is traditionally negative, pointing out students' errors while failing to draw attention to their strengths and successes. Application of this type of feedback to the experiential learning settings being introduced in communication skills teaching was more destructive than constructive, leading students to develop negativity about the whole teaching process and resent the use of role play and other observational teaching methods. In experiential learning it is clearly important that students should feel that they are in a safe environment. Actions must be confidential to the teacher and the learning group, and students should be supported in identifying their own strengths and weaknesses and helped in addressing areas of concern.

Pendleton's Rules stress the need for safety in the learning environment by emphasising the need to discuss the learners' strengths before commenting on their weaknesses, and to make recommendations rather than criticise. Furthermore, in each part of the process, the learner makes the first comments – this self-evaluation not only encourages them to develop skills of reflection but also enables the teacher to assess these skills and address any difficulties students may have in self-reflection.

Pendleton's Rules applied to a small group learning session following a simulated consultation model can be summarised as follows from the teacher's point of view:
- clarify any issues of fact
- ask the learner to comment on what went well and why
- ask the group to discuss what went well and why, and add comments

- ask the learner to comment on what went less well and how it could be done differently
- discuss what could be done differently and how with the whole group.

There are a number of advantages to this approach to feedback. From the student's point of view, it provides a consistent framework in a safe environment – the student knows what to expect at the end of an observed consultation. The emphasis on self-assessment helps the student become more reflective about learning. The 'rules' force the student to think about positive aspects of their performance and to become aware of their individual strengths in communication. The requirement for positive comments by the student, the teacher and the group means that no student receives only negative feedback, and any adverse comments must be presented in a constructive way as recommendations for change. The overall effect is that the feedback experience should enhance motivation to learn and encourage the development of self-regulation. Finally, from the teacher's point of view, it provides a simple structure within which much can be achieved – this is particularly important for relatively inexperienced teachers.

There are, however, a number of disadvantages to Pendleton's Rules, mainly related to their enforcement of a strict order for the way in which feedback is given. By ensuring that each student receives positive feedback at the beginning of the process, the individual student's own agenda may be overlooked – students themselves feel that within the time available during a teaching session, there is little opportunity for the constructive criticism they desire. Interestingly, this may reflect much-needed change in the culture of teaching and learning in medical schools over recent years, and the improved methods used by teachers for experiential learning activities. Increasingly, students expect their opinions to be sought by the faculty, and the culture of persistently negative feedback prevalent at the time of the development of Pendleton's Rules is disappearing. Students appreciate the opportunity to reflect on their successes, but are anxious to receive advice on how they might improve their performance.

The agenda-led outcome-based analysis (ALOBA) of the consultation, described by Silverman *et al.* in 1996,(18) provides an alternative mechanism for giving feedback in small group and one-to-one experiential learning situations. The ALOBA approach is built around the students' own agenda, allowing them to identify their individual problems in the context of their own and the patient's desired outcomes for a consultation. It provides opportunities for a group to give feedback, thus encouraging the development of feedback skills in all the learners in a small group setting. Finally, it allows the teacher to introduce a wider discussion of theoretical concepts and research evidence. The principles of the ALOBA method are shown in Box 23.5.

For a teacher using the ALOBA method, the task can be divided into three sections:
- organising the feedback
- group feedback
- ensuring that feedback leads to greater understanding.

BOX 23.5 Agenda-led, outcomes-based analysis of the consultation (ALOBA)

Task for the teacher	Reason
Organise the feedback	
Identify the learner's agenda	Helps the learner to express their views on the consultation and describe what help they would like from the group
Discuss the outcomes that both learner and patient were trying to achieve	The learner starts to recognise the importance of their own desired outcomes and those of the patient
Allow the learner to comment first	Encourages self-assessment and reflection
Involve the whole group in problem-solving	All students become more analytical of the consultation and reflect on how they might perform in the same situation
Group feedback	
Invite feedback from all members of the group	Helps all students develop feedback skills, including making specific non-judgemental comments
Ensure balanced feedback	Allows all students to support the learner by considering both what went well and what was less successful
Suggest alternatives rather than make prescriptive comments	The learner can consider alternative approaches and how they might work
Be supportive, act as a role model	All students can observe the use of constructive feedback
Ensure that feedback leads to greater understanding	
Rehearse suggestions	Allows the learner time to try out alternatives and for group comment on the effects
Use the consultation as learning material	All group members can contribute to the session and can learn as much as the learner under observation
Develop a wider discussion	Allows the introduction of concepts and research evidence to the group
Structure, summarise and record	Provides structure for the teaching allowing maximum learning benefits for the students; record the learning to inform future sessions

Adapted from Silverman *et al.*(18)

Following a real or simulated consultation, the feedback process is organised in terms of the learner's agenda, requiring them to identify the problems they have encountered and the help they would like from the group. The student should first identify what outcomes they wished to achieve from the consultation and, with the rest of the group, should consider the patient's agenda in terms of outcomes (this part of the process may include the opinions of simulated or trained patients where present). The learner can then be asked to comment on the process, and the whole group is asked to join in the problem-solving process, identifying the issues, feeding them back to the learner and generating solutions.

In the second part of the process, specific feedback is invited from all members of the group. It is the teacher's responsibility to ensure that feedback is balanced, non-judgemental and descriptive in nature, and that the group offers suggestions and alternatives rather than prescriptive comments. This is a particular opportunity for the teacher to be seen as a role model, providing constructive criticism in a supportive environment.

In the final part of the process, the teacher has more freedom to optimise the learning opportunities of the session. Thus, the learner may be given time to rehearse suggestions made by the group, allowing other group members to see the effects of their suggestions. The teacher may take the opportunity to widen the discussion, introducing aspects of their own experience or drawing on the research evidence for a particular aspect of the consultation. Finally, the teacher should summarise the session, providing structure and offering suggestions for further learning within an appropriate conceptual framework. Recording the learning that has occurred in a session is another useful activity that can form the foundation of future sessions.

The advantages of the ALOBA method for providing feedback are, paradoxically, that having placed the individual student and their own agenda at the centre of each learning experience, the session becomes of more value to all the students involved. By offering the opportunity for students to consider the problems inherent in a consultation and engage in problem-solving, all participants are more involved in the learning process. Whereas Pendleton's Rules may result in the learner becoming the passive recipient of feedback from all the other participants, the ALOBA technique ensures that everyone is equally engaged in the process. From the teacher's point of view, the ALOBA method also provides an opportunity to introduce some of the concepts underlying good communication skills, providing a theoretical structure for the students to understand their learning. However, the ALOBA method does require more experienced teachers and may be daunting for the less skilful.

Other methods for giving feedback in experiential learning have been described,(19–21) all of which contain aspects of the models described above.

Helpful and unhelpful feedback

Feedback is central to the process of formative assessment. Constructive feedback can enhance the learning experience

BOX 23.6 How to: Give helpful feedback in experiential learning

Unhelpful feedback	Reason	Helpful feedback	Reason
'Your body language wasn't very good at the start'	Judgemental	'At the beginning you were looking at the computer screen records and not at the patient as she started to tell her story'	Descriptive, detailed, behavioural
'You weren't very empathetic'	Non-specific	'You didn't acknowledge the problems she has dealing with her husband's illness'	Identifies specific problem
'You're very abrupt'	Personality issue	'You interrupted a lot, for example. . .' (give specific points in consultation)	Behavioural, specific
'I think it would be better if you did it this way'	Advice	'Have you thought about trying it like this?'	Generating alternatives
'I don't think you heard everything with your hearing problem'	Hearing problem not resolvable in this situation	'You have always discussed your hearing problems with us. Was there any point at which you thought it was affecting the consultation?'	Supportive, possibly can be changed by altering the environment
'You didn't notice how upset she was'	Judgemental	'At one point she was looking down and appeared quite upset. You quickly continued by asking her direct questions about her medication and she never returned to the problem of what was upsetting her. Did you notice that?'	Descriptive, non-judgemental, specific
'It was really good'	Non-specific	'At the start you asked an open question and then allowed her to tell her story. You left silences so that she continued in her own words'	Positive, specific, descriptive

and develop learner self-regulation; destructive feedback can have profoundly negative effects on learning. For many teachers in medical education, the development of constructive feedback skills is seen as the most important aspect of their professional development.(22) The principles of constructive feedback for experiential learning situations have been described elsewhere(23–25) and are summarised in Box 23.6. In essence, helpful feedback is specific, non-judgemental, behavioural and descriptive, and is provided within a supportive educational environment close to the time of the learning experience.

Similar criteria can be applied to feedback given in other formative assessments. For example, when marking written pieces of work, simply giving a grade or making a comment such as 'Good work' is less helpful to the learner than a description of why the work is good and suggesting other issues that might have been included or arguments that might have been presented. A number of systems for classifying students' responses have been described, of which the most well known is the structure of the observed learning outcome (SOLO) taxonomy(26) (*see* Box 23.7). The levels described in this scheme are not content specific and can be applied to students' work at any stage in a curriculum, assuming the teacher is aware of the aims of the module and the level of attainment expected. Student work that scores in levels 4 and 5 shows evidence of categorising

BOX 23.7 The SOLO taxonomy to classify the structural complexity of students' written work

Level	Descriptor
1 Prestructural	Use of irrelevant information or no meaningful response
2 Unistructural	Answer focuses on one relevant aspect only
3 Multistructural	Answer focuses on several relevant features, but they are not coordinated
4 Relational	The several parts are integrated into a coherent whole: details are linked to conclusions; meaning is understood
5 Extended abstract	Answer generalises the structure beyond the information given: higher-order principles are used to bring in a new and broader set of issues

From Biggs and Collis.(26)

and structuring knowledge, characteristics associated with deep learning. Feedback offered to the students within this (or a similar) framework is more helpful to their learning than simple judgemental statements.

Finally, it is useful to check with the students that they have understood the feedback they have been given and that their interpretation of the feedback is correct. The students' perception of the feedback they have received may vary greatly from that of the teacher who gave the feedback(27) and only by checking can these discrepancies be addressed.

Formative assessment in the curriculum

A programme of formative assessment with effective feedback can be used to develop self-regulation in learners, leading to better outcomes in terms of their learning and overall success. Formative assessment should be considered as part of a teaching institution's assessment strategy alongside summative assessments. The following section reviews the way in which a programme of formative assessment can be designed within a curriculum and considers some examples of different types of formative assessment used in medical education.

Formative assessment and module design

A programme of formative assessment should be built into the design of a teaching module that has explicit learning outcomes (which can be assessed). The module design should show clearly how evaluation of teaching, learning and assessment will be performed, allowing development of the teaching programme in the future. A number of schemata for module design incorporating assessment,

feedback and evaluation have been described, such as the one shown in Figure 23.2.

This basic pattern of module design is appropriate for all types of learning in medical education, including classroom-based activities and experiential learning.(28) The example given in Figure 23.2 is based around threshold criteria (pass/fail assessments) but can be adapted to include grading, where appropriate. The model takes into account not only the aims of the teaching module but also the level of attainment expected at the particular point in the curriculum. Module designers can therefore translate the level descriptors into learning outcomes and hence threshold assessment criteria. At that point the assessment methods are designed alongside the teaching and learning strategy for the module. Having delivered the module and performed the assessment as designed, evaluation of the module includes the teaching methods and the appropriateness of the learning outcomes and assessments used.

Using this format for curriculum design, assessment forms an integral part of the teaching programme and can easily be blueprinted against curriculum content and teaching methodologies. This 'constructive alignment' of the curriculum ensures that assessments facilitate learning by being linked explicitly to the learning outcomes such that internally coherent assessments (both formative and summative) are embedded in curriculum design and review.(29,30) Linking the assessment programme explicitly to the design and evaluation of a single module should ensure that evaluation of the assessment process itself is not overlooked.(31)

Examples of formative assessment in undergraduate medical education

Recognition of the value of formative assessment as a means of enhancing teaching and learning in medical edu-

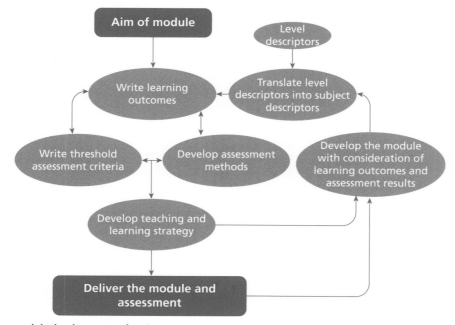

Figure 23.2 Curriculum module development and review. Adapted from Moon.(28)

cation has led to an increase in its use in undergraduate programmes. The ability of formative assessment to identify students with difficulties and then to offer them remedial teaching is an important feature of the widening use of formal formative assessment. The principles of good formative assessment can be applied to all areas of assessment in medical education, including:

- knowledge testing
- testing competence – practical, communication and clinical skills
- experiential learning settings – hospital clinical placements, general practice, community placements
- portfolios.

Often the most appropriate formative assessments includes elements of different learning activities [e.g. an Objective Structure Clinical Examination (OSCE) plus written work], allowing the faculty to give a rounded assessment of student performance and provide help in specific areas. This section focuses on examples of formative assessment in three areas of undergraduate medical education:

- hospital clinical placements
- teaching consultation skills in general practice
- assessment of portfolios and reflective writing.

Hospital clinical placements

Much of the teaching and learning in medical schools occurs in the context of hospital clinical placements (clerkships). One of the most well-recognised and disheartening aspects of traditional medical education programmes was the ability of students to pass through a clinical teaching programme and only be identified as having problems when they failed a summative assessment or even their final examinations (often not to the surprise of teaching staff). Formative assessment can identify struggling students earlier in the course and, coupled with appropriate identification of the learning difficulties and additional teaching, can result in improved student performance.(15)

Most medical schools expect students on clinical placements to receive feedback on their performance, usually in the form of a grade, which is regarded as highly subjective by the students. Furthermore, learners report a lack of regular feedback or describe feedback that they perceive to be poorly given or unfair, and they may become defensive, especially to feedback given by non-medical clinicians such as nurses or paramedical staff.(32) It is less common to have a formative assessment process in which the 'firm grades' form part of the overall assessment. In my own medical school, we have established a major assessment at the end of the first stage in the clinical programme that combines formative and summative elements and which is supplemented by additional teaching tailored to students' needs (Box 23.8). Other schools have made similar changes to their assessment programmes with improved student performance.(15,33)

However, the format of the assessment programme is crucial – the introduction of an in-training assessment (ITA) consisting of a range of assessment formats to an internal medicine clerkship was not found to increase the number of supervisions or the quality of feedback received by the

Box 23.8 HOW TO: Combine formative and summative assessment

The University of Cambridge standard undergraduate medical course is a 6-year programme. In the first 3 years the emphasis is on core medical sciences and all students undertake a first degree, usually (but not exclusively) in one of the biomedical sciences. The final 3 years of the course focus on clinical medicine. This programme is divided into three stages: Clinical Method, The Life Course and Preparing for Practice. At the end of Stage 1 a combined formative/summative assessment identifies those students with difficulties and enables them to receive additional teaching in the area of concern.

The assessment consists of:

- Eighteen station OSCE: including practical, communication and clinical examination skills – clinical and communication skills stations are summative, contributing towards ranking of graduates.
- Written paper: comprising multiple choice and extended matching questions.
- Four case histories: one written in each of the four clinical placements and including reflective pieces related to one of the main curriculum themes.
- Review of feedback from clinicians who have taught the student.
- One-to-one interview with senior member of the teaching faculty and their clinical supervisor (a junior doctor who teaches clinical method to small groups of students on a weekly basis).

Students are given the results of the OSCE and the written paper in advance of the interview. Detailed feedback is given to them in the light of their own reflection on their performance and the views of the clinical supervisor who knows each student well. Students who identify specific difficulties, such as in practical or communication skills, are then referred for additional tuition during the succeeding part of the course. A record is made of the interview and students followed up by the faculty.

The advantages are that:

- Each student is provided with a detailed review of their progress.
- A range of assessment modalities is used to inform the discussion.
- Detailed knowledge of each student's performance held by the clinical supervisor is acknowledged and relayed to senior faculty members.
- Students are able to 'benchmark' themselves and evaluate the amount and type of work they need to do in order to succeed in clinical medicine.
- Students with difficulties are clearly identified and can be offered additional targeted support.

students.(34) The ITA was complex, requiring the student to undertake a number of supervised encounters or presentations related to 13 core competencies, and was accompanied by feedback. The commitment of the senior clinicians to such a programme needs to be very high as it is ongoing and time-consuming. Asking too much of busy clinicians by way of formative assessment and feedback may be counterproductive. It may prove to be more valuable to organise centralised assessment formats assessing competence, which can be used in either formative or summative ways, and to ask for workplace-based assessment only where it is absolutely vital in the assessment of performance. Workplace-based assessment is discussed in Chapter 20.

Consultation skills in general practice

General practice placements often provide particularly good environments for formative assessment with appropriate feedback. In general, students are attached to a practice in small numbers and may be given the opportunity to see patients on their own or in observed consultations. A wide range of assessment methods for postgraduate trainees in general practice have been described, including observed consultations, review of video-taped consultations, multi-rater assessment and evaluation by peers and patients. General practitioner teachers are therefore skilled in assessment and feedback, and many of these methods can be extended to the undergraduate curriculum. Work reported from the Department of General Practice in Leicester suggests that postgraduate assessment methods can be transferred successfully with high levels of reliability, validity and educational impact.(35)

Portfolios

Much has been written about the use of portfolios in medical education, and there remains a debate about what the term actually means and what should be contained in a medical student's learning portfolio. To some, it is a repository for assessment grades, written pieces of work and lecture notes. Others have tried to harness the potential of portfolio learning to encourage students to develop reflective practice and adult learning skills.(36,37) Online learning portfolios have the potential to enhance the progression towards adult learning.

Portfolios lend themselves to use in formative assessment as they can be the centre of discussion at student progress meetings. Inclusion of a variety of assessments within a portfolio is helpful if they have been marked according to appropriate criteria and with effective feedback given as part of the overall formative assessment programme. The attraction of the portfolio as a means of assessment is strong – the collection of a series of pieces of work or assessments of competencies together with self-reflective pieces and evidence of professional development is a unique addition to the assessment opportunities open to medical educators. Portfolios are now increasingly used in formative assessment, and it may be possible to combine this with a summative element in the portfolio assessment.(38,39) For a full discussion of portfolios in medical education *see* Chapter 14.

Conclusions

A programmatic approach to assessment within a curriculum that is constructively aligned and with staff and students who understand the learning outcomes and the goals of each assessment is desirable and can address all three of the overarching aims of assessment.(40,41) In medical education, formative assessment is a valuable part of the assessment programme. A well-designed programme of formative assessment linked to overall curriculum aims and the teaching and learning goals of individual modules enhances the learning experience for students and promotes desirable educational outcomes, including learner self-regulation and the development of lifelong learning skills.

References

1 Newble DI and Jaeger K (1983) The effect of assessments and examinations on the learning of medical students. *Medical Education.* **17**: 165–71.

2 Rust C (2002) The impact of assessment on student learning: how can research literature practically help to inform the development of departmental assessment strategies? *Active Learning in Higher Education.* **3**: 128–44.

3 Black P and William D (1998) Assessment and classroom learning. *Assessment in Education.* **5**: 7–74.

4 Black P and William D (2009) Developing the theory of formative assessment. *Educational Assessment, Evaluation and Accountability.* **21**: 5–31.

5 van der Vleuten C (1996) The assessment of professional competence: developments, research and practical implications. *Advances in Health Science Education.* **1**: 41–67.

6 Sadler DR (1998) Formative assessment: revisiting the territory. *Assessment in Education.* **5**: 77–84.

7 Butler DL and Winne PH (1995) Feedback and self-regulated learning: a theoretical synthesis. *Review of Educational Research.* **65**: 245–81.

8 Nicol DJ and Macfarlane-Dick D (2006) Formative assessment and self-regulated learning: a model and seven principles of good feedback practice. *Studies in Higher Education.* **31**: 199–218.

9 Schuwirth LWT and van der Vleuten CPM (2004) Changing education, changing assessment, changing research? *Medical Education.* **38**: 805–12.

10 Rushton A (2005) Formative assessment: a key to deep learning? *Medical Teacher.* **27**: 509–13.

11 Wood DF (2012) Formative assessment. In: Walsh K (ed.) *Oxford Textbook of Medical Education.* Oxford University Press, Oxford.

12 Hattie JA (1987) Identifying the salient factors of a model of student learning: a synthesis of meta-analyses. *International Journal of Educational Research.* **11**: 187–212.

13 Ramaprasad A (1983) On the definition of feedback. *Behavioural Science.* **28**: 4–13.

14 Sadler DR (1989) Formative assessment and the design of instructional systems. *Instructional Science.* **18**: 119–44.

15 Sayer M, Chaput de Saintonge M, Evans D and Wood D (2002) Support for students with academic difficulties. *Medical Education.* **36**: 643–50.

16 Henderson P, Ferguson-Smith AC and Johnson MH (2005) Developing essential professional skills: a framework for teaching and learning about feedback. *BMC Medical Education.* **5**: 11. (http://www.biomedcentral.com/1472-6920/5/11; accessed 27 July 2013).

17 Pendleton D, Schofield T, Tate P and Havelock P (1984) *The Consultation: An Approach to Learning and Teaching*. Oxford University Press, Oxford.

18 Silverman JD, Draper J and Kurtz SM (1996) The Calgary–Cambridge approach to communication skills teaching. 1. Agenda-led outcome-based analysis of the consultation. *Education for General Practice*. **7**: 288–99.

19 Neher JO, Gordon K, Meyer B and Stevens N (1992) A five-step 'microskills' model of clinical teaching. *Journal of the American Board of Family Practice*. **5**: 419–24.

20 Brukner HA, Altkorn DL, Cook S *et al.* (1999) Giving effective feedback to medical students: a workshop for faculty and house staff. *Medical Teacher*. **21**: 161–5.

21 Wall D (2004) Giving feedback effectively. In: Mohanna K, Wall D and Chambers R (eds) *Teaching Made Easy: A Manual for Health Professionals*. Radcliffe Medical Press, Oxford.

22 Hewson MG and Little ML (1998) Giving feedback in medical education: verification of recommended techniques. *Journal of General Internal Medicine*. **13**: 111–6.

23 Ende J (1983) Feedback in clinical medical education. *Journal of the American Medical Association*. **250**: 777–81.

24 Kurtz S, Silverman J and Draper J (2005) *Teaching and Learning Communication Skills in Medicine*, pp. 123–9. Radcliffe Publishing, Oxford.

25 Roy Chowdhury R and Kalu G (2004) Learning to give feedback in medical education. *The Obstetrician and Gynaecologist*. **6**: 243–7.

26 Biggs JB and Collis KF (1982) *Evaluating the Quality of Learning: The SOLO Taxonomy*. Academic Press, New York.

27 Sender Liberman A, Liberman M, Steinart Y, McLeod P, Meterissien S. (2005) Surgery residents and attending surgeons have different perceptions of feedback. *Medical Teacher*. **27**: 470–2.

28 Moon JA (2004) *A Handbook of Reflective and Experiential Learning*, pp. 149–57. Routledge Falmer, London.

29 Biggs JB (2003) *Teaching for Quality Learning at University* (2e). Open University Press/SRHE, Buckingham.

30 Gitomer DH and Duschl RA (2007) Establishing multilevel coherence in assessment. *Yearbook of the National Society for the Study of Education*. **106**: 288–320.

31 Fowell SL, Southgate LJ and Bligh JG (1999) Evaluating assessment: the missing link? *Medical Education*. **33**: 276–81.

32 Higgins RSD, Bridges J, Burke JM *et al.* (2004) Implementing the ACGME general competencies in a cardiothoracic surgery residency program using 360-degree feedback. *Annals of Thoracic Surgery*. **77**: 12–7.

33 Denison AR, Currie AE, Laing MR and Heys SD (2006) Good for them or good for us? The role of academic guidance interviews. *Medical Education*. **40**: 1188–91.

34 Daelmans HEM, Hoogenboom RJI, Scherpbier AJJA *et al.* (2005) Effects of an in-training assessment programme on supervision of and feedback on competencies in an undergraduate internal medicine clerkship. *Medical Teacher*. **27**: 158–63.

35 McKinley RK, Fraser RC, van der Vleuten C and Hastings A (2000) Formative assessment of the consultation performance of medical students in the setting of general practice using a modified version of the Leicester Assessment Package. *Medical Education*. **34**: 573–9.

36 Snadden D (1999) Portfolios – attempting to measure the unmeasurable? *Medical Education*. **33**: 478–9.

37 Hays RB (2004) Reflecting on learning portfolios. *Medical Education*. **38**: 800–4.

38 Friedman Ben David M, Davis MH *et al.* (2001) AMEE Medical Education Guide 24. Portfolios as a method of student assessment. *Medical Teacher*. **23**: 535–51.

39 Driessen E, van der Vleuten C, Schuwirth L *et al.* (2005) The use of qualitative research criteria for portfolio assessment as an alternative to reliability evaluation: a case study. *Medical Education*. **39**: 214–20.

40 Schuwirth LW and van der Vleuten CP (2011) Programmatic assessment: from assessment of learning to assessment for learning. *Medical Teacher*. **33**: 478–85.

41 van der Vleuten CPM, Schuwirth LWT, Driessen EW *et al.* (2012) A model for programmatic assessment fit for purpose. *Medical Teacher*. **34**: 205–14.

Part 4
Research and Evaluation

24 Thinking about research: Theoretical perspectives, ethics and scholarship

Jan Illing
Centre for Medical Education Research, Durham University, UK

 KEY MESSAGES

- Research is a practice of critical or scientific inquiry.
- Research differs from audit and evaluation; research is about discovering the right thing to do, audit, ensuring that it is done right and evaluation, the assessment of worth or value.
- Theoretical perspectives provide the assumptions and frameworks that guide research.
- A theoretical perspective encompasses ontology, epistemology and methodology.
- Research projects sometimes combine qualitative and quantitative research methods, a study design for which

differing theoretical perspectives provide both support and challenge.

- Researchers are expected to minimise the risk of harm or discomfort to people, which in educational or social research is more likely to take the form of psychological distress than physical injury.
- Research that aims to be published requires an ethical review.

Introduction

Quantitative, qualitative, positivism, post-positivism, post-modern, naturalistic, interpretivism, constructionism, participatory, grounded theory, ethnography, phenomenology, hermeneutics, conversation analysis and narrative. A plethora of research approaches and methods; words that may leave the novice researcher feeling rather overwhelmed; that it's all 'too heavy'.

To make matters worse, authors will often confuse the use of terms,[1,2] sometimes relabelling research approaches[3] themselves. Without a map to organise and sort the labels into meaningful groups it can be quite a challenge to make any sense of these theoretical concepts at all. This chapter aims to provide such a map and will focus on the fundamental theoretical concepts associated with research and practical issues for the researcher to consider before starting out on their project.

What is research?

Research has been defined as 'a search or investigation directed to the discovery of some fact by careful consideration or study of a subject; a course of critical or scientific inquiry'.[4] This definition may sound straightforward, in that most researchers would agree that they are involved in a critical inquiry of something, but some would argue that their aim is not to establish facts but to increase or change understanding about something.

How does research differ from audit?

Research is concerned with discovering the right thing to do, and audit, with ensuring that it is done right.[5] Following this definition, audit focuses on what is given and asks questions about the given, while research has the freedom to ask questions about the given, including 'Is this the best or only way to do something?'

How does research differ from evaluation?

According to Clarke,[6] what differentiates evaluation from research is the question of purpose. 'An evaluation is action orientated. It is conducted to determine the value or impact of a policy, programme, practice, intervention or service, with a view to making recommendations for change'. Robson[7] states that 'to evaluate is to assess the worth or value of something'. Following this definition, evaluation is about setting out to make a judgement. Going back to our definition of research, there is no mention of research leading to judgement, but to the discovery of findings by critical inquiry. Evaluation research is part of research, but in evaluation the aim involves assessing the worth of something. *See* Chapter 27.

Theoretical frameworks in education and the social sciences

Kneebone[8] published a personal view about his attempt to engage with the education and social science literature. He wrote, 'At first and to my great surprise I found this

Understanding Medical Education: Evidence, Theory and Practice, Second Edition. Edited by Tim Swanwick.
© 2014 The Association for the Study of Medical Education. Published 2014 by John Wiley & Sons, Ltd.

literature almost impenetrable, of course it was peppered with unfamiliar words . . . I had the disquieting sensation of moving into alien territory, where familiar landmarks had disappeared'. Kneebone came to the realisation that all his medical training had been based within one view of science, the positivist paradigm, and that this was a very narrow and limited view. He ended with a plea to include an exploration of what the humanities have to offer the medical curriculum, and also with explicit guidance on how to gain access to this world. The aim of this chapter is to make this other 'world' penetrable.

The focus of this particular section is to present some of the frameworks within which quantitative and qualitative research in education and the social sciences is conducted. Quantitative research in education and social science is typically represented by the social survey and experimental methods, whereas qualitative research uses techniques such as observation and interview. Deciding on which method to choose is integral to the research question being posed, but each type of approach signals to the reader the framework within which the research is expected to be read and judged. Research methods are addressed in detail in Chapters 25 and 26.

In the past, the scientific method applied to the study of the natural sciences was considered appropriate and desirable for the study of education and the social sciences. Early textbooks focused on the scientific method, and other methods such as participant observation were deemed less scientific and weak by comparison, and consequently of lower status. From the 1970s, the debate over the appropriateness of the natural science model for social sciences inquiry gained momentum. Arguments centred on the differences in focus; people in education and the social sciences, and objects in the natural sciences. There was an increase in philosophical ideas and debate on the key issue of whether scientific method was appropriate for the study of people. The terms 'qualitative' and 'quantitative' signified more than different methods of collecting data; they indicated different assumptions about research in the social world.

The debate may have gathered momentum following Kuhn's(9) work on the history of science. Of particular importance is Kuhn's idea of a *paradigm*, a set of beliefs and dictats that influence what should be studied, how the research should be conducted and how the results should be interpreted. Here, a paradigm is a set of basic beliefs or assumptions about the social world. It can be compared to viewing the social world through a particular lens and encompasses ontology, epistemology, theory and methods. Paradigms cannot be proven but rely on argument, persuasion and usefulness. A paradigm is defined as 'a conceptual or methodological model underlying the theories and practices of a science or discipline at a particular time; [hence] a generally accepted world view'.(4)

Apart from positivism, all the other paradigms discussed below are still in their formative stages of development; hence some of the changes in nomenclature referred to above. So from this point on I shall refer to theoretical perspectives rather than paradigms. Each perspective has important consequences for the research that follows in terms of procedure and interpretation of findings, and suggests to the reader how the research should be read and in which framework it sits.

Theoretical perspectives in research

Theoretical perspectives are taken here to mean the philosophical stances that lie behind the research methodology. The theoretical perspectives are the starting point from which assumptions about the research are based; they influence how the study is conducted, the researcher's role and the type of knowledge that is produced. Each perspective will also have a particular set of criteria to be used in evaluating a piece of research. There has been a great deal written about the different perspectives, and much of it has focused narrowly on only one perspective without guiding the reader on where each perspective sits in relation to others. What is offered here is an overview in which I will cover the conventional positivist and post-positivist perspectives, and then other, more emergent, perspectives. For more detailed exposition, see Guba and Lincoln,(1,10) Heron and Reason,(11) and Crotty.(12)

Each theoretical perspective takes a particular *ontological* and *epistemological* position that informs the resulting research methods. *Ontology* is the study of being, and is concerned with the nature of existence and the structure of reality. It raises questions about the nature and form of reality and what can be known about it. In the social world is there a 'real' and single reality? Are there multiple realities dependent on whose view is taken? *Epistemology* focuses on the nature of the relationship between the researcher and what is to be known. The epistemological question is dependent on the answer to the ontological question. For example, when reality is assumed to be 'real', then what can be known about it can be independent of any relationship between the researcher and the subject of inquiry, and knowledge can be said to be objective. Therefore, the concept of objectivity in research assumes the existence of a 'real' world. However, if the answer to the ontological question is that reality is socially constructed and there is no 'real' version, then the answer to the epistemological question becomes subjective, as each researcher has his or her own version of reality and there is no true version, only a socially constructed reality. The methodological approach taken comes secondary to the answers to the ontological and epistemological questions (and focuses on the methods by which knowledge can be acquired on the subject of inquiry). If a 'real' reality is assumed, then this implies that the researcher can collect objective data and the ability to control variables becomes feasible (*see* Box 24.1).

Positivism

Positivism has been the dominant perspective in the physical and social sciences, going back to the Enlightenment in the 17th century, and is identified with quantitative methods. Positivism is linked to empirical science, offering assurances that knowledge is unambiguous, accurate and certain. 'Positive' comes from '*something that is posited*', a science that is firmly grounded, not something that is

BOX 24.1 'Heavy' words*

- *Epistemology:* the theory of knowledge, its origins and nature, and the limits of knowledge.
- *Ontology:* the study of being. It is concerned with the nature of existence and the structure of reality. With regard to social inquiry, this is often taken to mean the assumptions that a particular theoretical perspective makes about the nature of social reality.
- *Methodology:* the research design or plan that shapes the methods to be used in the study. The methodology provides a rationale for the choice of methods used in a study.
- *Methods:* the techniques used for data collection.
- *Theoretical perspective:* the philosophical framework and assumptions that lie behind the methodology.

*'Heavy words' is the title of a poem by Julia Darling that, although about a different medical subject entirely, begins; 'Dear Doctor, I am writing to complain about these words you have given me. . .'

arrived at from speculation. Auguste Comte (1798–1857) is attributed as the founder of positivism, although the ideas on establishing scientific laws from observation and experiment are reported much earlier in the work of Francis Bacon (1561–1626). What is posited in positivist science is what is scientifically observed following use of the scientific method. Comte's positivism bids us to look for regular characteristics, constant relationships to facts and to laws that can be scientifically established using the scientific method of observation, experimentation and comparison. The 'verification principle', which became a central tenet of positivism, is attributed to Ludwig Wittgenstein (1889–1951). The verification principle focuses on the importance of verifying statements via the experience of the scientific method. Today, positivism is still linked to empirical science. The confidence in science is reflected in the belief that science is both accurate and certain, in contrast to values, opinions and feelings, which are empirically unverifiable and of no interest to positivism.

Ontology, epistemology and methodology

The ontology of positivism is realism. Reality is assumed to exist in an 'absolute' sense, and the aim is to explain the social world in terms of laws, often including cause and effect. The epistemology of positivism is objectivism. Positivism maintains that objects in the world have meaning both prior to and independently of any consciousness of them. Positivism maintains that there are 'facts' that can be accurately collected about the social world, which are independent of individual interpretation and are 'true'. Researchers can be objective in the collection and interpretation of data. It is assumed that the researcher is capable of investigating the object of study without influencing it or being influenced by it. This differs from our subjective understanding, which constitutes a different form of knowledge from knowledge made up of scientific facts.

Positivist methodology is usually deductive and the aim is often concerned with the prediction and control of phenomena, and involves testing hypotheses to support or disprove a theory. Research procedures need to be followed rigorously to prevent values and biases from affecting the data. Methods are reported in detail to enable others to repeat the study and show that the results are reproducible by others. The methods used are mainly quantitative, involving experimental or manipulative research designs. Results are generally reported using statistics to show that any differences are beyond mere chance. The aim is to generalise findings to a larger population than the study sample.

For positivists (and post-positivists), the important aspects of research are:

- the aim
- testing hypotheses
- cause and effect
- generalisability
- adding to existing knowledge
- research rigour, in particular validity and reliability.

These are the main areas where research rooted in other perspectives is attacked. Quality is assessed by internal (findings are congruent with reality) and external (findings are generalisable) validity, and reliability (findings are stable) and objectivity (researcher has not influenced findings).

Knowledge, values and ethics

Knowledge from positivist research is built up like building blocks, by adding new knowledge to old. Knowledge is viewed to identify patterns and determine where new knowledge fits with existing old knowledge, and frequently aims to form rules and laws such as cause and effect. While the reporting of scientific knowledge is acceptable, criticisms focus on claiming that scientific knowledge is the only valid form of knowledge and that it is completely objective and accurate. Ethics and values are important for all types of research, although treated differently by them.(1) Values are excluded in positivism. Positivism claims to be value-free as a result of its epistemological position that research can be objective if rigour is applied. Positivists view values as confounding variables that need to be controlled and excluded from the study. The methodology is designed to isolate and remove subjectivity and bias. Research ethics, although of importance in positivism, is largely viewed as something external to the research itself. Ethics is seen as something that would be applied to the research, possibly by an external research ethics body or a professional body that may advise on the professional conduct of researchers.

The positivist researcher

The researcher is often in the role of 'expert'. The researcher takes on the role of independent observer, who is impartial to the study findings and reports them objectively, using them to inform decisions and recommendations. Positivists maintain that research is a specialist activity that needs to be carried out by trained and qualified 'scientists'. The novice researcher is trained in quantitative methods, research design and measurement. The aim is to be objective and any personal bias has no part in the research.

Is there conflict with other perspectives?

Proponents of positivism take a *reductionist* stance, in that it is assumed that at some point in the future a structure will be identified on which questions of difference can be considered and explained. This position assumes that the other perspectives are measurable or can be measurable by the same standards and therefore comparison can be made. There is much disagreement about this from proponents of critical theory and constructivism. Positivists would see action research as a contamination of both the research process and research findings.

Post-positivism

Post-positivism emerged following a realisation that the scientific method could not be applied to all scientific theory and much of what was accepted as 'fact' was theory and had not been observed at all or the act of observation had changed the subject. The work of the physicist Heisenberg (1901–1976) highlights this. He claimed that it was impossible to determine the position and momentum of a subatomic particle with any real accuracy, as the very act of observing it changed it. Popper (1902–1994) introduced the principle of *falsification*, where the emphasis moves from proving a theory is correct to being unable through repeat testing to prove it is wrong. Popper maintained that no theory could ever be proven, only disproved, and if a theory or hypothesis was not open to refutation from experimentation or observation, then the claims or theories made were not truly scientific.

Kuhn (1922–1996) identified a disparity between Aristotelian and Newtonian physics and noted that the differences were so extreme that a revolution in scientific thinking must have occurred. Kuhn questioned the objectivity and value neutrality of the scientific method and findings that could not be explained within the positivist paradigm, which led him to question the adequacy of the paradigm and call for a 'paradigm shift' and a shift in the way scientists view reality. The post-positivist perspective is less absolute; probability has replaced certainty; a level of objectivity has replaced absolute objectivity; and approximate truth has replaced absolute truth.

Ontology, epistemology and methodology

The ontology of post-positivism is critical realism. Like positivism, reality is assumed to exist, but unlike positivism, reality cannot be truly 'known'. Access to reality is imperfect due to weaknesses in the human as researcher and the complexity of the inquiry. Post-positivist epistemology is objectivist; objectivity is the ideal, but the data are subject to critical review. The post-positivist perspective acknowledges that no matter how much rigour is applied to the scientific method, research outcomes are never totally objective or certain, and claims are tempered. Emphasis is placed on collecting more than one type of data (triangulation) and on the falsification of hypotheses rather than con-

firmation. Post-positivism aims to address some of the problems of positivist research by collecting data in natural settings and collecting the insider views. Aims are achieved by using both quantitative and qualitative methods. Like positivism, quality is assessed by internal validity (the findings are congruent with reality), external validity (the findings are generalisable), reliability (the findings are stable) and objectivity (the researcher or the study procedure has not influenced the findings).

Knowledge, values and ethics

Knowledge consists of hypotheses that thus far have not been falsified and is made up of facts and laws that are probably 'true'. But as with positivism, knowledge is built by adding new knowledge to old to fit into existing patterns and form generalisations or rules such as cause and effect. As in positivism, post-positivist values are excluded and claim to be value neutral. Values are perceived as confounding variables that need to be excluded from the study. Research ethics is again an area of importance but is viewed as something largely external to the research itself.

The post-positivist researcher

The post-positivist researcher is more often in the role of 'expert', and the aim of the study is to provide an explanation and, when possible, prediction and control of phenomena. Again the researcher takes on the role of independent enquirer, who is impartial to the study findings and reports them objectively, using them to inform decisions and recommendations. Positivists maintain that research is a specialist activity that needs to be carried out by trained and qualified 'scientists'. The novice researcher is trained in the same way as the positivist researcher, but with the addition of qualitative methods, so that more detail is added to the meaning of the data, and data are no longer 'context stripped' but put in context. The minority and the individual voices are presented as well as the majority voice.

Is there conflict with other perspectives?

Proponents of this perspective take the same reductionist stance as positivism. It is assumed that at some point in the future a structure will be identified upon which questions of difference can be considered and explained. This position assumes that the other perspectives are measurable by the same standards and therefore comparison can be made. There is much disagreement about this from proponents of critical theory and constructivism.

Critical theory and related ideological positions

In contrast to positivist or post-positivist perspectives oriented to understanding or explaining the world, critical theory is oriented towards critiquing and changing society as a whole. Critical theory is used here as a blanket term, which includes, among others, the feminist and Marxist perspectives, used here as illustrative examples.

Feminist research starts with criticism of science, stating that it is incomplete and reflects a male distortion of the social world. Although it is more accurate to talk of feminisms, as there is not one unified body of thought, Tong(13) categorises seven forms of feminism. However, there is agreement that society has marginalised women and that this is reflected in research practice. Science perpetuates the myth of the superiority of men to women. Gender, as a significant issue in dealing with explanations of social phenomena, has largely been absent. The feminist perspective maintains that perpetuating a male view of science narrows ideas and limits understanding of the social world, and that if the male viewpoint were not dominant, a different research model would be dominant. Positivist research has stressed the importance of emotional separateness of researchers from their research participants to maintain objectivity. The feminist perspective maintains that research is a two-way process and detachment and objectivity are impossible. It does not acknowledge how the researcher is affected by the research and how the researcher's own biography becomes a fundamental part of the research process.(14)

The Marxist perspective, like the feminist, is not merely seeking to understand and accept the status quo, but to challenge, to recognise conflict and oppression, and to bring about change. Marx perceived a basic conflict between capital and labour between the bourgeoisie and the proletariat, and believed similar class struggles were part of earlier society. Marx maintained that economic forces determine how we think. Thoughts and consciousness come from our social being, itself the result of economic forces. Marx maintained that those who held economic power also held the intellectual power. The ruling classes ruled as thinkers, producers of ideas, and regulated the production and distribution of ideas.(15) He described an oppression that penetrated deep into human life, resulting in the alienation from work and finally from others. The proposed solution was for the proletariat to emancipate itself in a revolt, destroying their inhuman existence and all other inhuman conditions in society.

Ontology, epistemology and methodology

The ontology of critical theory is historical realism. Reality is assumed to be captureable, but has been shaped over time by social, cultural, gender, ethnic, political and economic factors, and changed into a reality that 'has set' over time. The epistemology is transactional and subjectivist: the researcher and the object of the research are assumed to be linked by the values of the researcher and relevant others who influence the study. Findings or knowledge are value dependent; they are mediated by the values of the researcher and the relevant others. It is the epistemological position that sets it apart from positivism and post-positivism. Methods require a dialogue between investigator and the subjects of inquiry. The aim of the research is to critique and change factors that constrain and exploit individuals. Quality is assessed by the historical context of the study, that is whether it takes account of social factors of the studied situation, and the extent to which the study acts to remove a lack of knowledge, and acts as a stimulus for action in the sense of bringing about a change in the existing structure.

Knowledge, values and ethics

Knowledge is made up of historical or structural insights that will transform with time. Transformations occur following informed insight. Knowledge grows and changes with historical revision as ignorance is eroded. Generalisations occur when the mix of social demographics, circumstances and values are similar. Values play a central role in critical theory and are important in shaping research outcomes. Excluding values would go against the interests of any minority or powerless group who were part of the study. The aim is to give the weak and powerless groups a platform and let their voice be heard along with any others who may be more dominant. Unlike the positivist and post-positivist perspectives, ethics is more internal than external to the research study. The critical theorist takes more of a moral standpoint in revealing full details about the study to ensure the study participant can be fully informed prior to consent and with no deception.

The critical theorist researcher

In critical theory, the researcher takes on the role of facilitator, raising not only their own level of consciousness about the object of study but also that of others. The researcher may facilitate change in the study group by providing greater insight into their situation and provide a stimulus for members of the community to take control of their future and initiate action and change. The novice critical theory researcher must first be 're-socialised' from previous exposure to the positivism. This involves conscious re-educating about positivism and post-positivism and its limitations. New researchers need to understand the perspective differences and understand both quantitative and qualitative methods so that they can understand how the perspectives differ and how the research is conducted. New researchers also need to understand the role that social issues have in the research context and structure and uphold the values of empowerment and altruism in their work.

Is there conflict with other perspectives?

Critical theory and constructivism (see below) agree that they are in conflict with positivist and post-positivist perspectives. The epistemological position of critical theory sets it apart from the positivist and post-positivist perspective; research can be value-free or it cannot; and a single model cannot support both tenets.

Constructivism

Guba and Lincoln's(1) constructivism is a broad eclectic framework that embraces interpretive, phenomenological and hermeneutic perspectives (*see* Box 24.2). Space does not permit me to cover each of these, and for more detail I recommend Guba and Lincoln,(10) Crotty(12) and Schwandt.(17) Constructivism is the view that knowledge, and therefore all meaning, is not discovered but socially constructed. Meaning is not created but constructed out of the world that is already there, and objects in that world. The world and its objects may have no intrinsic meaning,

BOX 24.2 FOCUS ON: Hermeneutics

The word 'hermeneutics' derives from the name of the Greek god Hermes, the messenger and interpreter of the gods. Hermeneutics is a branch of philosophy concerned with the understanding and the interpretation of texts, although the concept of 'text' has, in recent years, been extended beyond the written word to speech, performances, works of art and even events.

A hermeneutic defines a method for interpretation, or a specific theory of interpretation. In contemporary usage it has been widely used to denote the study of the general principles of biblical interpretation. Hermeneutics assumes that the text remains as written, painted or recorded, but that its interpretation changes with time and across contexts.

In critical hermeneutics the interpreter constructs the context as another form of text, which can then, of itself, be critically analysed so that the meaning construction can be understood as an interpretive act. In this way, the hermeneutic interpreter is simply creating another text on a text, and this recursive creation is potentially infinite. Every meaning is constructed, even through the very constructive act of seeking to deconstruct, and the process whereby that textual interpretation occurs must be self-critically reflected upon.(16)

but they are partners in the generation of meaning. Crotty(12) states that constructivism mirrors intentionality (meaning reaching out into directedness) in that consciousness is directed towards an object such that the object becomes shaped by consciousness and what comes to the fore is the interaction between subject and object. From this, meaning is born. The acceptance of intentionality therefore means the rejection of both objectivism and subjectivism.

It is accepted, even by the positivists, that social realities are socially constructed. The difference between constructivists and positivists is that the former maintain that all meaningful reality is socially constructed. A table may have a real existence irrespective of whether anyone is consciously aware of it. However, it exists as a table only if it is recognised as a table by our consciousness. The table is also constructed through social life, and our culture informs how we see these objects and in some cases whether to see them at all. Throughout our lives we learn about the social and natural worlds and interpret them, not as separate worlds but as one human world. Schwandt(17) draws the distinction between constructivism, meaning that the individual mind constructs the meaning, and constructionism, meaning the society or culture the individual belongs to has constructed the meaning. This highlights the depth of human social constructions.

Ontology, epistemology and methodology

The ontology of constructivism is relativism; this assumes multiple and sometimes conflicting realities that are socially and experientially based and dependent on individuals for their form and content. There is no 'real' world that pre-exists and is independent of human consciousness. People could therefore inhabit very different worlds based on different sets of meaning. Constructions change as their associated realities change and become more informed rather than 'true'. The ontological position of constructivism is crucial in terms of separating it from other perspectives. The answer to the epistemological question of 'How do I know what I know?' is that reality is subjective. The researcher and the research object are assumed to be related, such that the research findings or knowledge are created from the relationship between the researcher and the subject of study. It is the epistemological position of constructivism that sets it apart from positivism and post-positivism. Guba and Lincoln(18) maintain that the inquiry methodology is a two-way process of listening to the constructions of both the researcher and the research participant. The optimum process of developing joint constructions is via 'hermeneutic-dialectic', meaning that the researcher compares and contrasts different constructions to achieve a consensus. For Guba and Lincoln, the researcher cannot and should not be separated from the research participant, and hence the research outcomes are a joint construction of the research process. The aim of the research is understanding or reconstruction of the constructions that are held by the subjects and the researcher about the study topic. Two sets of criteria are used to assess quality: *trustworthiness* (parallels internal validity), *transferability* (parallels external validity), *dependability* (parallels reliability) and *conformability* (parallels objectivity) make up the first set. These criteria are analogous to those used to judge quality in positivist research. The second set consists of authenticity criteria of fairness: *ontological authenticity* (develops and enhances personal constructions), *educative authenticity* (leads to improved understanding of others), *catalytic authenticity* (provides the stimulus to action) and *tactical authenticity* (the research empowers action) [*see* Guba and Lincoln(18)]. The second set of criteria share some common ground with critical theory.

Knowledge, values and ethics

Knowledge consists of constructions about which there is relative consensus. Multiple constructions can coexist and be of equal weight, depending on interpretation and factors that influence interpretation such as social, political and gender issues. For constructivism, values play a central role in creating and shaping the research outcomes. Constructivism views the role of researcher as the producer and facilitator of the research and acknowledges their central role in the research process. The role of ethics, like values, is central to constructivism. The researchers' role is to recognise their own constructs and values and, as in critical theory, inform the study participants fully about the research prior to taking consent, work towards uncovering the constructs of the study participants and work towards improving constructs. The methodology involves close personal interactions and as a result may raise some difficulties with confidentiality and anonymity.(19)

The constructivist researcher

The researcher takes on the role of participant or facilitator. Increasingly, constructivists aim to involve research participants to take an active part in the study, that is, by suggesting questions and outlets for research findings. The researcher is both facilitator and participant, who uncovers the constructs of self and others and reconstructs the 'multi-voice' into more informed constructs. Change is facilitated when the reconstructions are formed and participants are stimulated to act on them. As in critical theory, the new researcher must first be re-socialised from previous exposure to the dominant perspective of positivism. Again, this involves re-educating about positivism and post-positivism and the limitations of these perspectives. New researchers need to understand how this perspective differs from others, and be trained in quantitative and qualitative research methods to be able to understand how the research is conducted within this perspective.

Is there conflict with other perspectives?

The ontological stances of constructivism and critical theory are in conflict with the positivist and post-positivist perspectives. Either there is a 'real' reality or there is not; it is either value-free or it is not. The concept of reconciling both of these positions in one system seems impossible.

Participatory action research

Participatory action research is a form of action research that involves practitioners as both subjects and co-researchers. It is based on the proposition put forward by Kurt Lewin (1890–1947) that causal inferences about human behaviour are more likely to be valid if the relevant humans participate in building and testing them. Participatory action research arose partly out of recognition that a gap often exists between the completion and publication of high-quality research and the implementation of findings. Researchers do their job and wait for the findings to be acted on by someone else. The view espoused by participatory action research is that it is important for the advancement of science to devise strategies in which research and action are closely linked. Participatory action research involves research participants in the research process working alongside the researchers from the first steps of designing the study through to research outcomes.(19) The participatory perspective was added by Heron and Reason(11) to Guba and Lincoln's(1) lists of the major paradigms that frame research, and was later included by Guba and Lincoln themselves.(18) The participatory perspective underpins forms of action research.

Ontology, epistemology and methodology

The ontology of participatory action research is subjective–objective. Heron and Reason explain this:

> 'When I hold your hand, my tactual imaging both subjectively shapes you and objectively meets you. To encounter being or a being is both to imagine it in my way and to know that it is there'.(11, p.274)

From the participatory perspective, the mind is actively participating in a primordial reality, such that what emerges as reality is the result of an interaction and how the mind has engaged with it. The epistemological position of participatory action research is that the knower participates in the knowing in at least four different ways:

- experiential knowing – by direct encounter with feedback from the real world in real time
- presentational knowing – the artistic rehearsal process through which we craft new practices
- propositional knowing – knowing in conceptual terms that something is the case
- practical knowing – knowing how to do something.

The methodology is a collaborative form of action inquiry and is explained in terms of knowing: people collaborate to define the questions they wish to explore and the methodology for that exploration (propositional knowing); together or separately they apply this methodology in the world of their practice (practical knowing); which leads to new forms of encounter with their world (experiential knowing); and they find ways to represent this experience in significant patterns (presentational knowing) which feeds into a revised propositional understanding of the originating questions.(11)

Heron and Reason argue that cooperative inquiry has two participatory principles: first, that the research outcome is grounded in the researcher's own experiential knowledge, and second, that research participants have a right to participate in research that is about them. They argue that researchers are also research participants and vice versa, and the co-researchers are also the co-subjects. These two principles do not apply within constructivism (where there is no identified epistemological role for experiential knowing); researchers are not also subjects and the findings are grounded in the experiential knowing of others. Heron and Reason argue that participatory research differs from other forms of qualitative research in that research participants inform the research design and inform how knowledge is generated about them. They also argue that the purpose of research within the participatory perspective is closer to the purposes of critical theory – 'the critic and transformation of social, political, economic, ethnic and gender structures that constrain and exploit humankind' – than constructivist, where the aim is about 'understanding and reconstruction'. The aim therefore is to create a situation in which participants give and receive valid information and are committed to the outputs of the study.

Social scientists are frequently faced with the dilemma of rigour or relevance. From the participatory action research perspective the aim is to define the standards of appropriate rigour and then meet them without loss to the relevance of the study. Validity is enhanced by the research process of participation and cycling several times through the four forms of knowledge in order to enrich congruence in articulating a subject–object reality.

Generalisations do occur, but they remain within local contexts, such as describing the thematic patterns in one context and suggesting how they might apply in a similar context, but would require a further study to confirm their relevance.

Knowledge, values and ethics

Knowledge is the result of collaboration and is built up from this collaborative relationship. Participatory action research emphasises the importance of a 'living knowledge' that is linked to the practical knowing (how to do something) that comes from being grounded in the situation within which an action occurs. Participatory action research maintains that research subjects have a basic human right to be engaged in research that intends to gather knowledge about them. The roles of values and ethics are embedded into the study; the subjects are also the researchers and the researchers also the subjects.

The participatory action researcher

The research voice is the result of 'aware self-reflective action'.(11, p. 294) The participatory action research researcher takes on the role of collaborator engaged with the practitioners and may need training to understand the relevant issues involved in the research. The researcher can act as research trainer to the practitioners to facilitate the research process. The novice researcher needs to acquire facilitator skills to work alongside their co-researchers. The researcher needs to acknowledge the skills and knowledge of the practitioners in the working partnership and, where appropriate, use this knowledge to understand the ongoing research. Participatory action research researchers need to be trained in both qualitative and quantitative research methods.

Is there conflict with other perspectives?

Participatory action research relates closely to both critical theory and constructivism, but uses the same type of measurement and standards as positivism and post-positivism. Arguably, the movement towards action research has come about as a result of non-utilisation of research findings and a desire to conduct research that will result in recommendations being implemented.

Reconciling and combining research frameworks

The type of framework in which a piece of research is conducted has implications for how the research is conducted, who has control of the study, how quality is assessed, how values and ethics are viewed, and, ultimately, the type of knowledge that is produced and what is done with that knowledge. The researcher's role differs depending on the perspective influencing the study.

Guba and Lincoln(10) point out that: 'Within the last decade the borders and boundary lines between these paradigms and perspectives have begun to blur'. Rather than theoretical perspectives working in competition, they are more often combined into one study to inform the arguments of another perspective. It is more useful to identify how the inquiry perspectives are similar and how they differ. Perspectives can be blended together into two main groups: first, the positivist and post-positivist, who share important elements; and second, the critical theory, constructivist and participatory perspectives, which also share important elements. However, these two main groups are not easily combined into one model as their assumptions about reality and objectivity are contradictory.

Positivism has been the dominant research perspective for many centuries. However, in more recent years the superior status of quantitative research approaches within education and the social sciences has been challenged. Criticisms of quantitative approaches have included arguments about 'context stripping' (taking data out of context and thereby removing much of the associated meaning), that the focus is on the majority or dominant view and important messages from the minority are ignored, and that even in well-controlled experiments researchers and subjects can influence each other and bias the results. In 1994, Guba and Lincoln reported that the dominant perspective was the post-positivist perspective. Post-positivists tend to have power and influence in numerous professional decision-making processes, namely research funding, journal publications and committees for promotion. Proponents of critical theory and constructivism have gained ground and recognition over the past 30 or so years, with more journal publications, journals and qualitative research. Participatory action research is also emerging as a perspective. In 2005, Guba and Lincoln acknowledged that 'the number of qualitative texts, research papers, workshops, and training materials has exploded', and pointed out the distinct turn towards the emerging perspectives.

Writers such as Guba and Lincoln suggest that the use of a particular method implies commitment to a particular perspective and its associated ontology and epistemology. This position assumes that a methodology is necessarily indicative of particular assumptions about knowledge. This position is challenged by Bryman,(20, p. 433) who suggests:

'if we accept that there is no perfect correspondence between research strategy and matters of epistemology and ontology the notion that a method is inherently or necessarily indicative of certain wider assumptions about knowledge and the nature of social reality begins to founder.'

Bryman argues that research methods are more 'free-floating' in terms of ontology and epistemology than is often proposed. Bryman quotes the work of Platt, who conducted historical research on American sociology and reported no clear association between positivism and the social survey. Platt stated:

'Research methods may on the level of theory, when theory is consciously involved at all, reflect intellectual *bricolage* or *post hoc* justifications rather than the consistent working through of carefully chosen fundamental assumptions . . . in many cases general theoretical/methodological stances are just stances: slogans, hopes, aspirations, not guidelines with clear implications that are followed in practice.' [Platt 1996, quoted in Bryman(20, p.619)].

Bryman continues that the link from methodology to certain assumptions is not absolute and suggests that research that combines both qualitative and quantitative approaches in one study illustrates that these research methods can be autonomous. Patton(21) concurs with the views of Bryman, commenting first on the parallel status of qualitative to quantitative research and on the increased use of multiple methods.

'Signs of détente and pragmatism now abound. Methodological tolerance, flexibility, eclecticism, and concern for appropriateness rather than orthodoxy now characterise the practice, literature and discussions of evaluation. Several developments seem to me to explain the withering of the methodological paradigms debate.'(21, p.302)

Patton goes on to list several developments that explain the change towards combined methods. For example, the importance of methodological appropriateness rather than paradigm orthodoxy, that the strengths and weaknesses of both qualitative and quantitative approaches are better understood, advances in methodological sophistication, support for methodological eclecticism and increased advocacy for combining approaches (*see* Box 24.3). Maxwell(22) discusses the use of quantifying qualitative themes, moving away from the use of vague terms such as 'some' and even conducting statistical analysis on the number of themes reported.(23)

The work on realistic evaluation by Pawson and Tilley(24, p.24) is of interest as they report that realistic evaluation sits between positivism and constructivism, that social reality cannot be measured directly (due to the weakness of the human researcher and because it is processed by individuals) but can be known indirectly. This approach is close to the post-positive ontology but with a pluralist epistemology: 'one can imagine the attractions of a perspective which combines the rigour of experimentation with the practical nous on policy making of the pragmatists, with the empathy for the views of the stakeholders of the constructivist'. The perspective of the constructivists is valued by acknowledging that access to the phenomenon being studied is imperfect and plural due to the human researcher and the research subject, but is criticised for limiting the findings of a study only to the sample studied. Participants such as doctors share structural similarities such as working in the NHS, the grade of doctor and the specialty, all of which will share common contextual features: 'Constructivism suffers from. . .the inability to grasp those structural and institutional features of society which are in some respects independent of the individuals' reasoning and desires. The social world (and thus policies and programs) consists of more than the sum of people's beliefs, hopes and expectations'(24, p.23). A realist synthesis is effectively a qualitative approach to a literature review in that it seeks to identify patterns and themes in the data that provide a deeper understanding about why interventions work, but also in what context and what triggers the outcome. The process of identifying the relevant literature starts very systematically, but ends iteratively searching for evidence that will help to confirm or refute a theory to explain the findings, and shares many similarities with grounded theory (discussed below).

The competing theoretical perspectives associated with *grounded theory* make for an interesting example. Grounded theory methods were based on the work of Glaser and Strauss.(25) Glaser applied his positivistic methodological training from Columbia University to the development of qualitative data analysis, while Strauss brought symbolic interactionism following Blumer, from his training at the University of Chicago. Hence, Glaser brought epistemological assumptions and methodological terms, and Strauss brought the study of process and meaning.(26) Charmaz *et al.*(1,26,27) place grounded theory in the post-positivist✓ perspective. They argue that Glaser's position comes close to a traditional positivist stance with assumptions of an objective, external reality and a researcher who remains neutral and discovers data. The position of Strauss and Corbin is considered post-positive as they propose giving a voice to the respondents. Yet, Strauss and Corbin(28) quote the study by Orona, which is constructivist in stance, and comment that it is 'a textbook' example, suggesting Strauss has a constructivist stance, which Bryman reports is evident in Strauss's earlier work.(20) Charmaz suggests that researchers can develop a constructivist ground theory by seeking the meaning of both respondents and researchers and by looking more for beliefs and values as well as acts and facts. Bryant and Charmaz(29) viewed the positivist stance as a weakness and repositioned grounded theory within social constructivism.

This example highlights that the linkage of perspective to methodology is not always clear, and if certain changes are made to the methodology, then it can become compatible with another theoretical perspective.

Box 24.4 illustrates how two contrasting research perspectives can illuminate the same research area, and

---

BOX 24.3 HOW TO: Combine qualitative and quantitative research

- *Triangulation:* use qualitative research to cross check findings from quantitative research or vice versa.

- *Provide hypotheses:* use qualitative research to identify hypotheses that can be tested using quantitative research.

- *Aid measurement:* use qualitative research to inform survey questions.

- *Screening:* use quantitative research to screen for people with specific characteristics for in-depth qualitative study.

- *Fill gaps:* one methodology will not provide all of the needed information.

- *Snapshot versus process:* quantitative research will provide a single snapshot of the social, whereas qualitative research provides information on process.

- *Where two types of data are required:* sometimes both data about meaning and data about a set of issues are required.

- *Quantification:* use qualitative research to identify problems and quantitative research to quantify the problem.

- *Explaining the relationship between variables:* quantitative research frequently needs to explain the relationship between variables; this can be explored further by a follow-up qualitative study.

- *Exploring the micro and macro:* use of both methodologies allows a study to explore the different levels of a problem.

- *Solving a problem:* a different research strategy to the one already employed to explore unexpected or puzzling outcomes.

See Bryman(20) for further discussion on the subject.

BOX 24.4 Comparison of two linked studies

Quantitative study

O'Cathain A, Walters SJ, Nicholl JP, Thomas KJ and Kirkham M (2002) Use of evidence based leaflets to promote informed choice in maternity care: randomised controlled trial in everyday practice. *British Medical Journal.* 324: 643–6.

This study was a randomised controlled trial with the aim of assessing the effect of leaflets on promoting informed choice in women using maternity services. The sample was clearly defined as women reaching 28 weeks' gestation before the intervention took place. Outcomes were assessed using a postal questionnaire. Various means were used to test the validity of the questionnaire, and a power calculation was used to identify the sample size needed to detect a 10% difference between the intervention and the control groups. Results included response rates (reported in numbers and percentages) and further analysis to identify any differences that could be related to age, social class, parity, pain relief and type of delivery. There was an attempt to examine confounding factors that would bias results, such as having been given the leaflets on another occasion prior to the start of the study.

The conclusion was that the evidence-based leaflets were not effective in promoting informed choice in the women. The authors reported on the limitation of the study and expressed concerns over their measurement of informed choice and the power of the study to detect a difference. Authors referred to the qualitative findings below for further explanation.

Qualitative study

Stapleton H, Kirkham M and Thomas G (2002) Qualitative study of evidence based leaflets in maternity care. *British Medical Journal.* 324: 639.

The stated aim was to examine the use of evidence-based leaflets on informed choice in maternity services. The design involved both non-participant observation of antenatal consultations, and in-depth interviews with both the expectant mothers and the health professionals. The sample was initially opportunistic (depending on which staff were doing the clinic and which women agreed to be involved), but progressed to be more selective to ensure that women from all childbearing ages, social class, minority groups and current and past obstetric histories were represented. Observations were used to help identify how the leaflets were used, and field notes made on the setting, actions, words and non-verbal cues. Semi-structured interviews were conducted using an interview guide. A grounded theory approach was used(25,31) so, as the interview progressed, interviewees were selected to help confirm or refute emerging theory, until no new information was gathered (theoretical saturation). Validity and reliability were said to be ensured by using several researchers and experts, to 'guard against any researcher dominating the analytical process'. Results were reported in terms of emerging themes, and quotes were used to illustrate them. The qualitative study revealed that time pressures and competing demands within the clinical setting undermined the intervention.

The observations revealed that health professionals rarely differentiated the leaflets from other information that they offered or discussed with them. The interviews identified that the women confused the leaflets with other information they had been given or denied having received them. The midwives reported that hierarchical power structures resulted in obstetricians defining the choices possible, resulting in informed compliance rather than informed choice.

---

provides a summary of two papers by O'Cathain *et al.*(30) and Stapleton *et al.*(31) These abstracts show quantitative and qualitative methods both being used within the same study and highlight some of the differences behind the qualitative and quantitative traditions.

It is possible to identify the post-positivist stance of the quantitative study, which attempted to control variables while manipulating others. There was concern with numbers and measurement and reporting findings in terms of statistical differences. There was also concern about using the 'correct' measurement, and fears were expressed about contamination of the intervention by earlier exposure to the leaflets.

The qualitative study referred to grounded theory, which originates from symbolic interactionism,(32) and leans towards critical realism, with the researcher seeking the meaning in the data. However, grounded theory acknowledges that reality cannot be known but is interpreted, shifting towards relativism [Strausserian approach(33)], and shares a constructivist epistemology. The qualitative study was less concerned with numbers and measurement and

more concerned with gaining a wider range of views and identifying all of the issues related to the intervention from many viewpoints. Observed behaviour was used to identify how the intervention was implemented, and findings were generated from observer notes. Analysis was conducted by looking for common themes in the data. The quantitative study reported that the intervention was not effective, and the qualitative study explained why.

Having an understanding of what each perspective is aiming to achieve can increase our understanding and provide an appreciation of the different types of knowledge produced rather than viewing one approach as superior to others. The theoretical perspectives of research are helpful as they form a backdrop to a study (grand theories). However, grand theories remain theoretical and cannot be used to explain the data that are produced – such theories are termed mid-range theories. Our use and understanding of theoretical perspectives in research is still developing. Methodologies that were once based in one perspective have been transposed to another and perspectives that have been in conflict have been combined.

Practical considerations when starting research

The research question

Most researchers have little problem identifying the general field in which they wish to conduct their research, but have more difficulty finding a focus and pinning down a research question. Punch(34) makes a distinction between general research questions and specific research questions. The hierarchy offered by Punch can be illustrated using the study by O'Cathain *et al.*(30) which can be summarised as follows (*see also* Box 20.4).

Research area	Maternity care
Research topic	Informed choice
General research question(s)	Does informed choice change behaviour?
Specific research question(s)	To assess the effects of leaflets on promoting informed choice in women using maternity services
Data collection question(s)	– Do women who receive the intervention answer 'yes' more often to the question 'Have you had enough information to make choice on . . .?' – Do the women who receive the intervention report greater satisfaction with antenatal information – Do the women report being given at least one leaflet?

Novice researchers sometimes confuse data collection questions and research questions.(35) A research question is the question that the research is attempting to answer, whereas the data collection question is asked to collect data that will be used to answer the research question.

Coming up with a research topic is about following your interests (it is difficult to sustain interest if it is not there from the start). Looking around, listening or experiencing something or being aware of current issues are all sources of inspiration. Think about what is known and what is not known about something. O'Leary,(2) in her book for novice researchers, suggests the use of concept maps to help identify an area of interest. Once identified, the general area of interest needs to be narrowed down. A good research question needs to be feasible; this relates to the research expertise and resources available and, indeed, whether the question is capable of being answered at all. This last point involves checking with those who have more expertise in research and knowledge of the field of study.

Bell,(36) in her guide, advises that a good first step is to simply talk over your research ideas with a colleague. Gaining another perspective early on can be very valuable. A good research question not only gives the research focus and direction, but also sets boundaries. Boundaries are particularly important for novice researchers, who have more difficulty estimating how much research time is required to undertake a study and may need to limit both the size and the focus more than anticipated. Defining the terms used within the research question identifies the criteria of concern and by exclusion sets some boundaries on the study. Specifying a research question involves identifying the concepts or variables of interest and, where possible, identifying suitable indicators for the variables of interest. It is important to check that any assumptions made by the question are correct. Getting to the stage of identifying a good research question involves exploration of the topic in the literature to gain knowledge on what is already known (although for some study designs familiarity with the literature may come later, so that the researcher does not limit his or her view of the research area) and where the gaps are, or asking questions in a new context. Deciding on whether you need to frame your question as a hypothesis depends on the theoretical perspective the research will be framed in, and on the type of question being asked. Research within the positivist and post-positivist perspectives is more likely to contain a hypothesis, but the key question is whether the research question forms a testable statement about the relationship of one or more variables to others. Research that is exploratory or framed within the new perspectives is unlikely to start with a hypothesis. The research question should be a pointer to the methods to be used and indicate what type of data will be needed to answer the question.

The research proposal

All research should start with a proposal, also referred to as a *protocol*. Again, like the application for ethical review, it can be helpful for novice researchers to see another research protocol first to identify what is required.(34) A proposal is a plan of action, a communication on which approval to commence the study is given, and is a contract between the researcher and supervisor, university, any funding source and ethics committee.(35) The proposal describes the research background, including relevant literature, the research question, methods and details about recruitment of the intended sample and how the data will be analysed. All applications for ethics review will also need a proposal. The protocol starts with the relevant literature by 'setting a scene' or 'telling a story' of what is known, how the knowledge has built up to form our current understanding. The research question follows; this should extend that understanding.

Ideally, the background literature should present the context of the study, what is known already and what is needed – ideally this will match your study aim, but it could provide part of a much larger question. Literature searches are mainly conducted online using databases such as Medline, Education databases and Ovid, and key articles selected following searches on keywords or authors. Punch(34) reports that two common criticisms of literature reviews in dissertations are that they are not thematic, tending to be chronological or presented serially, and they are not properly integrated with the study. These criticisms can be addressed by creating a conceptual framework into which the literature can be organised.

The research question should suggest the types of method needed to collect the data required to answer the question. The two studies presented in the O'Cathain paper had the research question: 'To assess the effects of leaflets on promoting choice in women using maternity services'. The

---

BOX 24.5 HOW TO: Write a research protocol

Title

- Provide a clear title that articulates the aim or research question

Relevant background literature

- Summarise the work that has already been done in this area
- Search the relevant databases as well as journals, books and policy documents, if relevant
- Write up thematically if meaningful, or chronologically if the topic changed and developed over time
- Identify what is missing, what new research should be conducted. Add any relevant educational or clinical theory that is relevant to this area of study
- Include all references at the end of the document

Research question

- Provide a clearly worded research question (aim)
- Keep it feasible; set boundaries for study and think realistically about the available resources you have, e.g. time, staff and level of expertise
- Define what you mean by the terms used
- Consider including a secondary research question (something of a lower order which you would also like to explore)
- Consider including some stated objectives – questions that are driven by data collection that help you to answer the research question

Methods

- Study design (e.g. randomised trial, grounded theory)
- Sampling
  - sampling strategy (e.g. opportunistic, purposive)

- define target sample, i.e. demographic details, how selected and recruited to study
  - sample size (reason for size, is it informed by power calculation?)
- Data collection
  - details of any instruments to be used and references to existing tools
  - details about validity, reliability, e.g. randomisation, piloting of questionnaires
  - outline stepwise procedures including pre-testing and piloting of tools
  - data collection methods (e.g. via postal questionnaire, field notes, interviews)
- Data analysis
  - details of how data will be analysed (e.g. statistical tests, type of qualitative analysis)
  - details of computer programs to be used in analysis

Ethical considerations

- state if approval from ethics committee has been received or is in progress

Plans for dissemination of findings

References

- from literature review, methods, instruments, etc.

Appendices

- costings
- research instruments (e.g. questionnaire, interview schedule, consent forms)
- flow chart summarising study plan with a timeline

---

question suggests measurement in the use of the term 'assess', the leaflets were defined as '10 pairs of Informed Choice leaflets', the women were defined as 'women reaching 28 weeks' gestation' and so on. 'Effects' were measured using a questionnaire. Assessment came in the design of comparing a control group with the women who received the leaflets. For the qualitative part of the study the research question was: 'To examine the use of evidence-based leaflets on informed choice in maternity services'. The term 'examine' suggests 'look at' rather than 'measure', and again the leaflets and maternity service were defined. Outcome measures were views and responses from the expectant mothers and the staff. Exactly how the methods are arrived at will be influenced not only by the research question, but also by the interest and expertise of the researcher, supervisor and team.

The protocol should include details about who will be recruited into the study and from where, how recruitment will take place and the numbers involved (this may require

a power calculation for research designs). This should be followed by a detailed description of the research procedure. A plan or flow diagram will be useful if the procedure is complex. Details of how the data will be collected and analysed, and any planned statistical tests, should be included, and a timeline or Gantt chart is useful to work out when each activity is planned to start and finish. A breakdown of the costs involved in the study for staff and research activities, among others, is also needed, as well as plans for the dissemination of findings(2,34,37,38) (*see* Box 24.5).

Ethics in research

What is ethics?

Ethics is concerned with rules of conduct and principles relating to moral behaviour. Researchers are responsible for ethical decisions from formulation through to the dissemination of research. As discussed above, the type of research framework influences how ethics is regarded in the study, as well as appreciating other 'realities' and empowering voices otherwise not heard. All types of study involve making ethical decisions about what is right for the research participant, as well as considering the interests of the researcher, the funding body and the study itself. Ethical decisions are based on the values of the researchers and the research community, and those who hold access to the data the researchers hope to gather. Although there are codes of ethics covering all types of professional research, it is not possible to provide a list of rules that should be applied to every study as each piece of research will be individual and will require different solutions.

The emergence of research ethics came about after the end of the Second World War, when details of horrific medical experiments came to light during the Nuremberg trials. The Nuremberg Code (1947) was published 2 years later, followed by the Declaration of Helsinki (1964) and the World Medical Association(39) (which amended the declaration of Helsinki), which established ethical principles for research involving humans.

Social research has proceeded in two ways:
- deontological approaches to morality (Immanuel Kant 1724–1804)
- consequentialism (Jeremy Bentham 1748–1832).

Deontological approaches to ethics follow a set of principles that guide research. One such principle is that of 'informed consent', which was enshrined in the Nuremberg Code. Informed consent includes providing all relevant information about the study and what taking part will involve, including risks. The research subject must be able to comprehend the information and be competent to make a decision about involvement, and agreement to take part should be voluntary, free of coercion or influence. This also involves taking steps to ensure the participant is protected from any consequences of being in the study by ensuring that the research protects the identity of the participant. Deontological approaches reject the notion that what is morally right can be considered by assessing consequences.

Consequentialism is not concerned with whether an act is morally right, but with the consequences of the act. For research this translates to potential ethical dilemmas that the researcher may have to respond to and the consequences of their actions. Classic utilitarianism is a form of consequentialism. Classic utilitarianism is consequentialist rather than deontologist because it denies that moral 'rightness' depends on anything except the consequences of an act. The consequences, not the intention, of an action determine its merit. Critics of consequentialism have commented on the difficulty of anticipating all the potential outcomes that might result from an act. Important areas to be considered are:
- informed consent
- confidentiality
- anonymity.

Informed consent has two components: the research participants need to understand what taking part will involve; and agreement to take part needs to be voluntary. Gener-

ally, consent will be obtained by asking the research participant to confirm their consent by signing a consent form, by giving recorded verbal consent or by returning a questionnaire. Gaining consent may involve gaining approval from many more people than those directly involved in the study, that is, the host care organisation, in order to access patients. Consent needs to be voluntary, free from coercion, manipulation and any threat. There is also some evidence that response rates improve as interviewees are given more details about what the study involves.(40) Gaining consent can provide an important part in negotiating the researcher's relationship with participants. This should involve participants being told about any risks of taking part and having the opportunity to ask questions about the study.

Consent to take part in research may be given on the basis that the information obtained about the participants will only be used by the researcher and only in particular ways. The information is offered to the researcher in confidence. Beauchamp and Childless(38) argue that the right to privacy rests on the principle of respect for autonomy. On this basis people have the right to decide who knows what about them. Research should uphold this principle. Confidentiality means protecting the identity of those who agree to take part in research, maintaining the data in a form such that the identity of the participant is protected. This implies keeping names and data separated by using a code that is only accessible to the researchers, and reporting data in a format that does not lead to individuals being readily identifiable. For example, it may involve removing or changing details to protect individuals who would otherwise be identifiable because of their unique characteristics or experiences.

Anonymity goes further than confidentiality, as the researchers do not collect named data at all. This means the researcher cannot identify which respondent gave the data (e.g. postal survey). This type of data allows participants to make any negative comments more freely without fears or concerns that anything they do report might be attributed to them with unknown consequences. For researchers, this might be difficult or impossible to achieve if the methods involve interviewing, and problematic if they wish to send reminders only to those who have not already agreed to participate. For a full discussion on ethics in research, see Israel and Hay(40) and Punch,(41) and for ethical dilemmas in qualitative research, see Welland and Pugsley.(42)

Returning to our example, ethics questions that may have been addressed before the Stapleton *et al.* study was carried out include:
- Will the midwives and expectant mothers be given all the information they require to give their informed consent?
- Is there any pressure or coercion to take part?
- How will consent be taken?
- How will confidentiality of the interaction of midwife and mother be assured?
- How will collected data be anonymised, particularly with reference to the use of quotes?
- Who will have access to the data?
- Have the researchers anticipated all that could go wrong? How would they respond if they did?

In conclusion, researchers are expected to minimise the risk of harm or discomfort to people, to conduct research in a manner that upholds certain principles such as informed consent and to consider any consequences or harm that may result from the research. Harm from educational or social research is more likely to take the form of psychological distress than physical injury. Conversely, many researchers aim to provide benefit by conducting research that empowers participants, such as in feminist research.

Statutory ethical review

Israel and Hay(40) commented that novice researchers rarely seriously consider the ethical implications of their research and that it is only when compelled to respond to the research ethics committee requirements that any detailed consideration is given to ethical issues. It is at this point that the novice researcher may confront considerable ethical difficulties. The formal mechanism can offer the opportunity to consider ethical issues, and this process can be helped by adapting tools that are available as guidance. Novice researchers may falsely anticipate that gaining approval for a study necessitates conforming to certain procedures, that is, written consent and providing a written participant information sheet, even when their study may not require such documentation, effectively making the study more difficult to conduct.

Processes for ethical 'approval' vary in their rigour and administration from country to country, but in the UK, it is necessary to make an application to the Integrated Research Application System (IRAS) for ethical review before starting research, if the research involves NHS patients or clients or prisoners.(43) The IRAS was set up as a single system for applying for the permissions and approvals for health and social care/community care research in the UK. The system enables information about the project to be put into one application instead of duplicating information in separate application forms. The system uses filters to ensure that the correct permissions and approvals are requested depending on the type of data collected.

The IRAS captures the information needing approval from the following bodies:

- Administration of Radioactive Substances Advisory Committee (ARSAC)
- Gene Therapy Advisory Committee (GTAC)
- Medicines and Healthcare products Regulatory Agency (MHRA)
- Ministry of Justice
- NHS/HSC R&D offices
- NRES/NHS/HSC Research Ethics Committees
- National Information Governance Board (NIGB)
- National Offender Management Service (NOMS)
- Social Care Research Ethics Committee.

Ethical review is one of a series of safeguards intended to protect individuals, and these are described in the 'Governance arrangements for research ethics committees'.(44) The primary function of the Research Ethics Committee, when considering a proposed study, is to protect the rights, safety, dignity and well-being of all actual or potential participants. Completing the IRAS form for the first time may seem rather daunting and having sight of a couple of successful applications first can be helpful. The number of additional supporting documents (i.e. the protocol, contact letters, consent forms, any questionnaires, etc.) may seem burdensome because they are required upfront rather than developed at each stage of progress. However, this is all documentation required to proceed with the study. There are some advantages in preparing supporting documents early and getting feedback on them. The IRAS regulations state that the time from receiving a valid application to notification of final opinion from the committee must not exceed 60 days. The biggest hold-up is the time taken for applicants to respond to the questions raised by the committee. All applicants are invited to attend the committee meeting. This can be very useful, as it provides the opportunity for the committee to ask questions and clarify points that have not been fully understood. This can speed up the process by reducing the need to ask further questions later.

In 2007(45,46) papers were published expressing concern about the need for medical education research to require full ethical review, particularly with regard to students' projects. Concern focused on the new process of requiring ethical review being so onerous as to compromise postgraduate clinical research;(46) however, concern also focused on medical education projects, maintaining that students' projects were delayed, over burdened by a lack of clarity and suffered from contradictory opinions as to what constituted 'research' and therefore required ethical review. In 2011 there was a change in the IRAS regulations and there is no longer a requirement to seek ethical review for a study that is focused only on NHS staff; however, R&D approval (discussed below) is still required.

In addition to ethical review, an application must also be made for research management and governance approval (this is usually referred to as R&D approval) to each NHS organisation in which the research will be carried out. This has now been integrated within IRAS and for each site the applicant needs to generate a Site Specific Information (SSI) form. SSI forms provide local information specific to a particular NHS site. The SSI form asks two main questions: is the site suitable and is the principal investigator qualified to do the research? The system is in the process of being introduced as an electronic application system. Parts of the system are already fully electronic and the rest is moving towards this. The NIHR Coordinated System for gaining NHS permission (CSP) in England and the multi-centre review system in Scotland (NHS Research Scotland) only receive applications made through IRAS. Some R&D offices set a time limit for responding to applications, but not all, and there is no standard time limit set, unlike for IRAS, and therefore R&D approval could take longer than IRAS.

Ethical approval of research in medical education

In 2001, Morrison and Prideaux(47) asked whether research in medical education should be exempt from the ethical considerations that govern other research involving humans. The authors argued that it may be ethically wrong not to evaluate educational interventions, but then questioned at what point evaluation becomes research. They suggested that the crucial point is if the study is aimed at producing generalisable results with the intention of publishing in refereed literature. It is at this point that ethical approval must be gained and the following statement now makes this very clear. The journal *Medical Education* conforms to contemporary standards on ethical publication. It requires evidence of approval by an appropriate human research ethics committee for all papers that report research involving human subjects.(48) However, journals such as this, that accept research from an international community, require a certain acceptance of local standards of ethical review, which will mean accepting a variable ethical standard.(42) There has been a debate about the appropriate place to review educational research. This stemmed from a recognition that educational research does not incur the same level of potential risks as biomedical research, and from a concern that ethics committees that were originally established to review biomedical research may not fully comprehend educational research.(48,49) This concern has already been realised from educational research submitted to statutory ethics committees who reclassed the study as audit and therefore not requiring ethical review.(48) There are problems when submitting research classed as audit rather than research to journals, as there is no ethical review of the study. Possible solutions to the problem include gaining retrospective ethical consent and having studies reclassified as research;(50) embedding consent into the delivery of the curriculum; and providing independent evidence that participants gave informed consent to data collection and that risk of harm to the participants was unlikely.(48,50) Another way of avoiding this problem would be by ensuring that researchers from the field of educational research are members of statutory ethics committees or by setting up alternative ethics committees within faculties to monitor educational research.(47,49,50)

Scholarship

Boyer(51) discussed the trend towards a singular view of scholarship as research and publication, and proposed reconsidering the priorities of the professoriate by broadening the definition of scholarly work. He argued that the definition of scholarship should be wider and proposed three additional areas of endeavour that should be viewed as scholarship, in addition to the discovery of new knowledge. These are:
- the integration of knowledge by placing isolated research into a larger context and making connections within or between disciplines
- the teaching of knowledge, stimulating others to become active learners and encouraging students to be critical, creative thinkers, with the capacity to go on learning after their college days are over
- the application of knowledge – how theory and practice vitally interact to inform each other.

Discovery of new knowledge
This chapter has focused on scholarship as discovery of new knowledge. The first section explained how the frame-work in which the research is set influences the type of knowledge that is created and how it should be evaluated. Power is still held by the post-positive perspective, although over the past 10 years or so there have been more studies from the new perspectives and more that are informed from more than one perspective. The critical theorists inform us that other knowledge has been dominated by evidence from positivism and post-positivism perspectives, which has been influenced by men in positions of power, but that other forms of knowledge are valid. The two studies used to illustrate a quantitative and qualitative approach highlight the importance of using different approaches to the discovery of new knowledge.

Integration of knowledge
Integration of knowledge can be achieved by collaboration across disciplines in primary research, but equally important is the appraisal of existing knowledge to evaluate progress in a particular field or inform another. Unless literature reviews are conducted in a standardised way, they run the risk of being subjective and biased. To address these weaknesses, there has been increased interest in conducting literature reviews in a systematic way.

A systematic literature review is conducted using a transparent process such that the reader could replicate the study and arrive at the same findings. Far greater precision is required in a systematic review, which requires definitions of terms used, clearly written research questions, publication of the search strategy used, including search terms and databases used, and the incorporation of a complete list of inclusion and exclusion criteria. Papers initially selected by the search but excluded from the review are also listed with reasons for exclusion.(52,53)

Teaching of knowledge
Scholarship in teaching is the legacy of handing on knowledge to the next generation. Scholarship is said to occur when it is public, open to evaluation and presented in a format that others can build on.(54) However, while a clinical teacher may be informed about contemporary research in their area of clinical expertise, this is less common with regard to education, where change is more opinion than evidence led.(37)

Best Evidence in Medical Education (BEME)(55) is a collaboration of individuals and institutions that support the need to develop a systematic approach to the review of evidence about clinical teaching. The website shares information about completed and ongoing systematic reviews. Mennin and McGrew(56) stress that research in teaching and learning as applied to the clinical setting is in the early stages of development. BEME, and initiatives like it, represents an opportunity for medical education to become more evidence based.

Application of knowledge
The application of knowledge is a crucial part of scholarship; otherwise research becomes an end in itself. There has been recognition that there is a delay from research findings to implementation, which evidence-based medicine in particular has tried to address.(57) The participatory action

research perspective recognises the delay in implementing research findings and has resolved this problem by making the research part of the change programme.(19)

Implementation is the end point of research, but as Boyer(51) reminds us, this is only until new issues arise and are fed back into research and the cycle begins again.

Conclusions

Theoretical perspectives determine the assumptions that are made about reality and what can be known. Positivism became the dominant perspective after the Enlightenment, but following the realisation that all research did not fit into this paradigm, a shift in thinking occurred. This brought about a new way of thinking about social science, and new and competing theoretical perspectives emerged.

The arguments against combining qualitative and quantitative research centre on the acceptance that research strategies are committed to particular theoretical perspectives(2) or the view that they are autonomous.(20) A growth in the preparedness to view research methods as techniques for data collection and a movement away from concerns about ontology and epistemology has resulted in more research using a combination of both qualitative and quantitative research methods.(21)

Getting started in research involves identifying a good research question. After this, consideration needs to be given to the type of data that needs to be collected to answer the question. A plan or proposal needs to set out how the research will be conducted, with milestones. Consideration needs to be given to ethical questions that affect the research and how these can be dealt with. Educational scholarship brings it all together. New knowledge is created, integrated and applied, and through dissemination, discussion and critical appraisal, new questions are generated. This in turn leads to the formulation of new research questions and the circle of scholarly inquiry is complete.

References

1 Guba EG and Lincoln YS (1994) Competing paradigms in qualitative research. In: Denzin DK and Lincoln YS (eds) *Handbook of Qualitative Research*, pp. 105–17. Sage, Thousand Oaks, CA.

2 O'Leary Z (2004) *The Essential Guide to Doing Research*. Sage, London.

3 Alvesson M (2002) *Postmodernism and Social Research*. Open University Press, Buckingham.

4 Oxford English dictionary. (2013) (http://www.oed.com; accessed 16 July 2013).

5 Smith R (1992) Audit and research. *British Medical Journal*. **305**: 905–6.

6 Clarke A (1999) *Evaluation Research*. Sage, London.

7 Robson C (2000) *Small-Scale Evaluation: Principles and Practice*. Sage, Thousand Oaks, CA.

8 Kneebone R (2002) Total internal reflection: an essay on paradigms. *Medical Education*. **36**: 514–8.

9 Kuhn TS (1970) *The Structure of Scientific Revolutions*. University of Chicago Press, Chicago.

10 Guba EG and Lincoln YS (2005) Paradigmatic controversies, contradictions and emerging confluences. In: Denzin DK and Lincoln YS

(eds) *Handbook of Qualitative Research* (3e), pp. 191–215. Sage, Thousand Oaks, CA.

11 Heron J and Reason R (1997) A participatory inquiry paradigm. *Qualitative Inquiry*. **3**: 274–94.

12 Crotty M (2003) *The Foundations of Social Research: Meaning and Perspective in the Research Process*. Sage, London.

13 Tong R (1995) *Feminist Thought: A Comprehensive Introduction*. Routledge, London.

14 Steier F (1991) Introduction: research as self-reflectivity, self-reflexivity as social process. In: Steier F (ed.) *Research and Reflexivity*. Sage, London.

15 Marx K (1961) *Selected Writings in Sociology and Social Philosophy*. Edited with an Introduction and notes by Bottomore TB and Rubel M. Watts, London.

16 Ricoeur P (1974) *The Conflict of Interpretations: Essays in Hermeneutics*. Northwestern University Press, Evanston, IL.

17 Schwandt TA (1994) Constructivist, interpretivist approaches to human inquiry. In: Denzin DK and Lincoln YS (eds) *Handbook of Qualitative Research*, pp. 118–37. Sage, Thousand Oaks, CA.

18 Guba EG and Lincoln YS (1989) *Fourth Generation Evaluation*. Sage, Newbury Park, CA.

19 Whyte WF (1991) *Participatory Action Research*. Sage, London.

20 Bryman A (2001) *Social Research Methods*. Oxford University Press, Oxford.

21 Patton MQ (2002) *Qualitative Research and Evaluation Methods* (3e). Sage, London.

22 Maxwell J (2010) Using numbers in qualitative research. *Qualitative Inquiry*. **16**: 475–82.

23 Rees C and Monrouxe L (2011) Medical students learning intimate examinations without valid consent: a multicentre study. *Medical Education*. **45**: 261–72.

24 Pawson R and Tilley N (1997) *Realistic Evaluation*. Sage, London.

25 Glaser B and Strauss A (1967) *The Discovery of Grounded Theory*. Aldine, New York.

26 Charmaz K (2003) Grounded theory: objectivist and constructivist methods. In: Denzin DK and Lincoln YS (eds) *Strategies of Qualitative Inquiry*, pp. 249–91. Sage, Thousand Oaks, CA.

27 Harris I (2002) Qualitative methods. In: Norman GR, van der Vleuten C and Newble D (eds) *International Handbook of Research in Medical Education*, pp. 45–96. Kluwer Academic, London.

28 Strauss A and Corbin JM (1997) *Grounded Theory in Practice*. Sage, Thousand Oaks, CA.

29 Bryant A and Charmaz K (2007) *The Sage Handbook of Grounded Theory*. Sage, London.

30 O'Cathain A, Walters SJ, Nicholl JP et al. (2002) Use of evidence based leaflets to promote informed choice in maternity care: randomised controlled trial in everyday practice. *British Medical Journal*. **324**: 643–6.

31 Stapleton H, Kirkham M and Thomas G (2002) Qualitative study of evidence based leaflets in maternity care. *British Medical Journal*. **324**: 639–42.

32 Blumer H (1969) *Symbolic Interactionism*. Prentice Hall, Englewood Cliffs, NJ.

33 Strauss AL and Corbin J (1990) *Basics of Qualitative Research: Grounded Theory Procedures and Techniques*. Sage, London.

34 Punch K (2000) *Developing Effective Research Proposals*. Sage, London.

35 Loche LF, Spirduso WW and Silverman SJ (1993) *Proposals that Work* (3e). Sage, Newbury Park, CA.

36 Bell J (1999) *Doing Your Research Project: A Guide for First-Time Researchers in Education and Social Science* (3e). Open University Press, Buckingham.

37 Tarling R (2006) *Managing Social Research: A Practical Guide*. Routledge, London.

38 Beauchamp TL and Childless JF (2001) *Principles of Biomedical Ethics* (4e). Oxford University Press, New York.

39 World Medical Association (2002) World Medical Association Declaration of Helsinki: ethical principles for medical research involving human subjects. (http://www.wma.net/en/30publications/10policies/b3/; accessed 16 July 2013).

40 Israel M and Hay I (2006) *Research Ethics for Social Scientists*. Sage, London.

41 Punch M (1994) Politics and ethics in qualitative research. In: Denzin DK and Lincoln YS (eds) *Handbook of Qualitative Research*, pp. 83–98. Sage, Thousand Oaks, CA.

42 Welland T and Pugsley L (2002) *Ethical Dilemmas in Qualitative Research*. Ashgate, Hampshire.

43 NHS National Research Ethics Service (NRES). (http://www.nres.nhs.uk/; accessed 16 July 2013).

44 UK Health Departments (2011) Governance arrangements for research ethics committees: a harmonised edition, DH.

45 Pugsley L and Dornan T (2007) Using a sledgehammer to crack a nut: clinical ethics review and medical education research projects. *Medical Education*. **41**: 726–8.

46 Robinson L, Drewery S, Ellershaw J et al. (2007) Research governance: impeding both research and teaching? A survey of impact on undergraduate research opportunities. *Medical Education*. **41**: 729–36.

47 Morrison J and Prideaux D (2001) Ethics approval for research in medical education. *Medical Education*. **35**: 1008.

48 Prideaux D and Rogers W (2006) Audit or research: the ethics of publication. *Medical Education*. **40**: 497–9.

49 Evans A (2002) Ethics approval for research in medical education. *Medical Education*. **36**: 394.

50 McLachlan JC and McHarg J (2005) Ethical permission for the publication of routinely collected data. *Medical Education*. **39**: 944–8.

51 Boyer EL (1990) *Scholarship, Reconsidered: Priorities of the Professoriate*. Princeton University of New Mexico, Princeton, NJ.

52 Albanese M and Norcini J (2002) Systematic reviews: what are they and why should we care? *Advances in Health Sciences Education: Theory and Practice*. **7**: 147–51.

53 Reeves S, Koopel I, Barr H et al. (2002) Twelve tips for undertaking a systematic review. *Medical Teacher*. **24**: 358–63.

54 Hutchings P and Shulman LS (1999) The scholarship of teaching: new elaborations, new developments. *Change*. **Sept/Oct**: 11–5.

55 Best Evidence Medical Education. (http://www.bemecollaboration.org; accessed 24 August 2013).

56 Mennin SP and McGrew MC (2001) Scholarship in teaching and best evidence medical education: synergy for teaching and learning. *Medical Education*. **2**(5): 468–72.

57 Sackett DL, Rosenberg WMC, Gray JAM et al. (1996) Evidence-based medicine: what it is and what it isn't. *British Medical Journal*. **312**: 71–2.

Further reading

Research practice

Cohen L, Manion L and Morrison K (2007) *Research Methods in Education*. Routledge, London.

Green J and Browne J (2005) *Principles of Social Research*. Open University Press, Buckingham.

Locke LF, Spirduso WW and Silverman SJ (2007) *Proposals that Work: A Guide for Planning Dissertations and Grant Proposals*. Sage, London.

Punch K (2000) *Developing Effective Research Proposals*. Sage, Thousand Oaks, CA.

Theoretical perspectives

Bryman A (2008) *Social Research Methods*. Oxford University Press, Oxford.

Bunnis S and Kelly DR (2010) Research paradigms in medical education. *Medical Education*. **44**: 358–66.

Burr V (1995) *An Introduction to Social Constructionism*. Routledge, London, New York.

Cuff EC and Payne GCF (1979) *Perspectives in Sociology*. Unwin Hyman, London.

Gergen K (1999) *An Invitation to Social Construction*. Sage, London.

Kemmis S and McTaggart R (2003) Participatory action research. In: Denzin DK and Lincoln YS (eds) *Strategies of Qualitative Inquiry* (2e), pp. 271–330. Sage, Thousand Oaks, CA.

Kincheloe JL and McLaren PL (1994) Rethinking critical theory and qualitative research. In: Denzin DK and Lincoln YS (eds). *Handbook of Qualitative Research*, pp. 138–57. Sage, Thousand Oaks, CA.

May T (2001) *Social Research: Issues, Methods and Process*. Open University Press, London.

25 Quantitative research methods in medical education

Geoff Norman¹ and Kevin W Eva²
¹Clinical Epidemiology and Biostatistics, McMaster University, Canada
²Centre for Health Education Scholarship, University of British Columbia, Canada

---

 KEY MESSAGES

- There is much more to good research than rigorous design.
- The appropriateness of a particular research design is dependent on the question to be addressed.
- The hierarchy of research methods commonly applied to clinical studies is inappropriate when judging the strength of research strategies in educational domains.

- The value of critical, synthesising, theoretically oriented and empirically-based reviews of the literature cannot be overstated.

The quantitative paradigm

Quantitative research methods have been central to physical science for centuries, dating back as far as the astonishing developments in astronomy in the 1500s. Indeed, it is difficult to envision natural science without quantification, and it is even more difficult to delve into some of these accomplishments without feeling an overwhelming sense of wonderment at the ability of the scientist, whether we ponder on our understanding of the very big (e.g. cosmology) or the very small (e.g. particle physics), or closer to home, as we reflect on the rapid evolution of digital electronics in our lifetime. For those old enough to remember a computer card, a 1 GB flash drive contains as much memory as 10 000 000 computer cards – about the volume of a one-car garage. But quantitative methods are not a panacea. Many would claim that social scientists have been too quick to adopt the methods of natural science unquestioningly and have not given adequate recognition to the complexity of social situations, which are not evidently reducible to a few numbers. In Chapter 24, Illing reviewed the history of the adoption of quantitative methods into social science, and the subsequent uneasy integration (or partitioning) with qualitative methods. It is not surprising that the quantitative 'dust bowl empiricism' led to a counter reaction. It is embarrassingly easy to find examples in medical education that, on a moment's reflection, exemplify the silliness of attempts to reduce the complexity of human interaction in an educational setting to a 'treatment' that half receive and half do not, and an 'outcome' such as pass or fail on an examination.(1) Although we are personally wedded to quantitative approaches to social science research, such studies, which, as Illing points out, reduce the people in the study to 'objects' that are supposed to absorb exactly the same dose of the educational drug, amount to little more than unintended '*reductio ad absurdum*'.

Little is served by identifying specific examples. The larger question is the extent to which quantitative methods have been aligned with recognised progress in the field. There is simply no dispute that the methods of the natural sciences, from the electron microscope to the wet lab and the clinical trial, have led to enormous advances in medicine with direct consequences for human longevity and welfare. Clearly, it would be specious to try to make similar claims in the small and impecunious field of medical education. Nevertheless, the past three decades of research have seen substantial advances in medical education, much of it directly related to the application of sophisticated quantitative methods,(2) particularly in the area of student assessment.

In writing a paper on quantitative methods our goal is not to promote these methods over qualitative research strategies or even to contrast the two, but rather, to provide some guidance for those trying to better understand the variety of quantitative methods available. As Bordage notes,(3) the community should move on from the qualitative–quantitative debate because 'this oft-repeated debate is not productive. . .each approach is useful in its own right and is often most productive when complementary'. In fact, lost in the qualitative–quantitative debate is the complexity of both qualitative and quantitative methods.

Much is written about the various schools of qualitative research; Illing, as one example, cites post-positivism, critical theory, constructivism and participatory action as various *genres* in qualitative research. To our knowledge, no similar taxonomy exists for quantitative research.

BOX 25.1 Quantitative research traditions

- Experimental
- Epidemiological
- Psychometric
- Correlational
- Reviews and meta-analyses

Indeed, many critics of quantitative methodology appear to presume that quantitative methods in educational research amount to testing hypotheses using randomised experiments that are proven or disproven by application of statistical methods. This is a woefully inadequate description of, for example, the psychometric methods that have led to such significant advances in assessment methods.

In this chapter, we will distinguish four research traditions – experimental, epidemiological, psychometric and correlational – exploring some basic principles of measurement and statistical inference along the way. Finally, we will describe the methods of meta-analysis and systematic reviews, and contrast these strategies with those of reviews that are better defined as critical and theory-oriented. We begin, though, with a commentary on the importance of precisely focusing one's research question, emphasising that while good studies require good methods, the quality of a study is not completely defined by its methodological rigour (Box 25.1).

The research question

In the previous section, we noted that many authors equate quantitative research with hypothesis testing. In our view, not only is this association simplistic, but it gives insufficient attention to the nature and adequacy of the research question. Far too frequently, when students do discuss the research question, much effort is expended in learning how to convert a practical, commonsense question into a formal research hypothesis or, even better, a 'null hypothesis' that frames it as no difference, no effect or zero correlation. Such efforts, by promoting precision of planning, can enable one to ensure that the research question is ultimately answerable. Much of that precision, however, becomes evident in any case as the research design and methods are devised, thereby leading us to believe that much of this effort is stylistic and does little to fundamentally improve the research. It really is of little consequence if a question is framed as a question, a research hypothesis or a null hypothesis.

In any case, the idea of a research hypothesis only applies well to some kinds of quantitative research. The development of a new evaluation instrument will proceed by a very different route, with studies of reliability and validity. To frame a reliability study as a null hypothesis would look something like: *The reliability of the new written test of reflective practice will be less than 0.5.*

This framing simply does not adequately capture the goal of the research. While our views may not represent a majority position, we believe that we should focus effort on an adequate research *question*, and forget about the niceties of null hypothesis creation. In the end, the goals of the research question are to reduce the possibility of *post-hoc* explanations, to specify or constrain the methods used to answer the question, and to enable careful analysis of whether or not the focus of the research is achievable. As human beings we are remarkably good at generating explanations for any pattern that is presented to us, so scientists try to avoid drawing conclusions without some *a priori* reason to have predicted the result. That is not to say that *post-hoc* speculation is not useful when unanticipated findings arise, but it is to say that further study should be engaged to confirm the result before running to the printers. Style is unimportant, but precision is invaluable to avoid wasting time and resources in pursuit of ultimately unanswerable questions.

So how do we ensure that the research question is good? Compared to the many approaches that exist to determine if the research methods are good, there is relatively little written about what constitutes a good research question. What does exist tends to focus on the technicalities of what information should be present in the question.(4) There is good reason for this. The worth of a research question cannot be judged in isolation, but can only be viewed in the context of the specific research domain in which it arises. Research is about discovery, and there is little point in discovering what is already known (Box 25.2).

'Discovery' is a useful way to think about the potential contribution of a research study, but the word implies such large leaps from current understanding that we prefer to think of the act of discovery in terms of knowledge building. Arguably, the value of a study is directly related to the extent to which it reveals some new understanding of the world – it 'discovers' some new insight or builds on existing knowledge in a meaningful way. Quantitative research is judged, in large part, by the extent to which the lessons learned can be generalised to other contexts. But what advice can we give the beginning researcher to help him or her identify research questions that are most likely to yield knowledge-building discoveries? Very simply, this is the role of the literature review.

The latter point is worth reinforcing – this emphasis on using the literature is not meant to imply that there are no practical (potentially atheoretical) questions that need to be addressed; rather our view is that grounding one's study in the existing literature is a valuable strategy for ensuring that even purely practical research projects have a decent chance of being successful and contributing to the generalisable knowledge base of the community. Too frequently, the literature review reads like a child recounting a playground fight: 'Johnny did this. Then Sally did that. Then Bob came along and said this other thing.' The literature review is not, and should not be, a chronological recounting of who did what to whom, but rather, should establish a conceptual framework within which the present study will reside.(5)

BOX 25.2 HOW TO: Select an issue worthy of research

When contemplating which research ideas are worth developing into more fully fledged projects, there are a variety of criteria that should be used. Here are just a few guiding principles:

- *Novelty:* Has the study been done before? It is insufficient to say 'to our knowledge this has never been done' without a concentrated effort to determine whether or not it has been done. Talk with experts, be they local or international, and scour the literature for other studies aimed at similar issues. At this point in history it is inconceivable that no one has ever written anything of relevance to whatever topic you care to study. Only after a careful search of a variety of literatures can you make a compelling argument for how your particular study could advance understanding in some meaningful way beyond what has already been done.

- *Importance:* Medical education is an applied field. As a result, while any given study might not yield immediate practical implications, it should be possible to conceive of ways in which the research efforts might beneficially impact on the field in the future. Use your 'on-the-ground' experiences to inform your research questions just as much as you use the literature.

- *Programmatic:* Too often we in applied fields think of research in terms of projects as opposed to programmes. The latter term, put forward by the Hungarian philosopher of science Imre Lakatos, should draw attention to the fact that real advances are typically made through systematic and long-term study of a particular issue.(5)

- *Guided:* What is the conceptual framework within which your study fits?(5) Which theories speak to the issue with which you are trying to grapple? Do they contradict one another in a way that you could inform through your research efforts? Is your theory/hypothesis falsifiable (i.e could your study design yield an answer that would counter the theory you are using as a guide)?

- *Grounded:* Related to some of the previous points, we use the term 'grounded' to indicate that the study should be grounded in the context of what is already known such that the context is used to determine which of the various possible research directions is most appropriate (i.e. most likely to provide meaningful results to the community) at this point in history. One may not be able to predict this with perfect accuracy, but the issue should be considered through broad consultation and reflection.

The literature review should clearly identify knowledge gaps, and the gaps should be substantive enough to warrant filling; statements such as 'this study has never been done in our country/city/university/discipline' are weak justification. The emerging conceptual framework should be such that it helps the researcher – and eventually his or her readers – focus on the bigger picture (the 'state of the art'), and should clearly delineate how the present study adds to this knowledge. This implies that the researcher should begin every study with a formal literature review, from which all unanswered questions will become as evident as a full moon on a clear night. Of course, research does not proceed in such a linear fashion, but one characteristic of mature research programmes (i.e. long-term and systematic exploration of a domain;(6) is that situations where a study is created *de novo* from a literature review are the exception. When a programme of research is ongoing, new study questions arise from existing study findings.

So what can be done to ensure the quality of the research question? One way to answer this question is to draw on the notion of 'theory'. In contrast to a research hypothesis, which ultimately leads to only two conclusions: (a) it worked, or (b) it did not, a research theory involves an understanding of the interaction of multiple variables. Such theory-based research is conspicuously in the minority within our field.(7) Only about half the articles in a recent review were identified as having a conceptual framework(8) let alone a testable theory. Yet another 'study' showing that students gave your new course in anatomy an average rating of 4.5/5 is unlikely to provide any new insights into teaching and learning. But application of a novel theoretical perspective may alter the way the community thinks about the issue and reveal insights that are relevant to various curricular strategies. Although educational theories typically do not make quantitative predictions, they nevertheless often involve the interplay of several variables and may get people thinking about the problem in a more refined manner. That is the importance of theory; by the time the theory has been subjected to a critical test, inevitably involving a few to a few dozen studies, we can gain good insight into the limits and generality of the findings (thanks to an accumulation of evidence) rather than being stuck with a series of only superficially related results.

It is worth noting here that a defining property of scientific theory is, to use Popper's words,(9) that it is falsifiable, i.e. it can be proven wrong. As such, studies that use theory as a basis for knowledge building have a more dynamic quality than typical invocations of theory as context. Scientific theories are not permanent and immutable; we expect them to change and evolve (and increase in explanatory power) as new evidence arises. This stands in stark contrast to the use of theory as justification implied by statements such as: 'The curriculum was designed to be consistent with theory Y.' Such statements are not terribly useful, as many theories can be implemented in countless ways and other theoretical positions might also promote the same types of learning activities.(10) More critically, many theories are framed in such sweeping generalisations as to be virtually unfalsifiable. Just because a set of data 'is consistent with' one theory does not in any way amount to an accumulation of knowledge unless the data can be shown to be inconsistent with some alternative theory or unless they lead to revision and refinement of the theory being utilised.

It might also be noted that, while some notions of theory-building remain firmly rooted in a positivist tradition,

		Considerations of Use	
		Low	High
Quest for Understanding	Yes	Pure basic research e.g. Bohr	Use-inspired research e.g. Pasteur
	No	-	Pure applied research e.g. Edison

Figure 25.1 Pasteur's quadrant [from Stokes(12)].

theory is probably best used when it moves some towards the recognition that the world is not adequately described by a single 'it worked/it did not' reductionistic package.(11) Further, as we alluded to earlier, the fact that research is theory-based does not mean it is irrelevant to practice. On the contrary, as Stokes(12) has convincingly described, theory-based basic science and practically-oriented research efforts should not be construed as lying at separate ends of a continuum. Rather, he argues, the two agendas should be considered orthogonal continua in their own rights, with the best research lying in what he called 'Pasteur's quadrant', to reflect the great strides Louis Pasteur made in advancing fundamental knowledge about bacteriology, while simultaneously having practical, real-world, impact in the wine and silk industries, and of course, medicine (Figure 25.1).

Research designs

When the phrase 'research design' is mentioned, many individuals who grew up in an educational research environment automatically think about experimental designs, quasi-experimental designs, and Cook and Campbell.(13) Those who are closer to clinical research are more likely to think of the epidemiological classifications of case–control study, cohort study and randomised trial. Both are inadequate taxonomies. Within medical education, much of our quantitative research, in particular psychometric and correlational research methods, does not fit neatly into any of these pigeonholes. Furthermore, which tradition one adopts should be tailored to the specific research questions one is trying to address.

In addition, different research design traditions arise from different kinds of question. In the remainder of this chapter we will examine various issues related to selecting a particular research design. The next section deals with the experimental tradition by exploring a set of methodologies primarily aimed at testing questions of causality (e.g. 'Does increasing test frequency cause better retention of studied material?'). A related tradition that we will then examine briefly is the epidemiological approach. Because many methodological reviews address research design on the continuum of case–control study, cohort study and ran-

domised trial, we will define these terms and show some (limited) applications in medical education.

The subsequent section will focus on the psychometric tradition, a method of study primarily directed (at least within educational circles) at the development of better measures of various aspects of competence or other outcomes of the educational process. These studies do not speak of interventions, control groups, outcomes and the like. Instead, the preoccupation is with issues of reliability and validity, which are indices of the ability of the instrument to differentiate between individuals in a defensible manner.

Finally, we will look at correlational research designs that tend to be used when the desire is to seek understanding by examining relationships among measured variables. As these measurements are frequently gathered from surveys and rating forms, we will also examine some basic principles of questionnaire design.

As can be seen from this introduction alone, each tradition has different aims, and the design conditions necessary for one may be exclusionary of another. As one example, which we will elaborate on later, correlational research requires individual variation in order to see relationships, while experimental research does its best to eliminate individual differences in order to detect treatment effects. There are other differences: experimental research is almost by definition prospective, whereas correlational research is often conducted on existing databases. Use of existing data, while often necessary, can encourage an attitude where the questions are driven by the available data, rather than the reverse, adding little in the way of advancing understanding. That danger noted, it is certainly true that prosaic questions are not proprietary to any one research approach, and conversely, some of the most interesting research has arisen from retrospective analysis of large institutional databases.(14,15)

The experimental tradition

The act of discovery, which is central to science as we discussed earlier, is often, although not entirely, directed at identifying causal relationships among things (variables). The experimental tradition exemplifies this agenda. The basic notion of an experiment is that there is a relationship between the independent variable, which is usually under the control of the experimenter, and the dependent variable, which is observed to change as a consequence of the intervention. Many methodological discussions focus on devising studies that can allow one to unambiguously infer causal relationships between experimenter-controlled independent variables and observed dependent variables. Statements like:

- the absorption of a neutron by the P^{32} nucleus decreases its stability, making it radioactive and leading to decay to S^{32} by emission of a β particle
- excess sodium chloride in the diet leads to hypertension that results in increased risk of stroke
- a half-day nutrition workshop given to patients with transient ischaemic attacks increased compliance with a restricted salt diet

exemplify the causal goal of the experimenter. Yet while all these statements imply causation – an independent variable that 'causes' a change in a dependent variable – none mentioned the word 'cause'. Further, the meaning of causation is very different as we proceed from top to bottom, and the steps one must take to ensure a valid test of the inference are correspondingly more and more complex. For the neutron, there is no ambiguity. Everyone in atomic physics knows what a neutron is, how to 'make' one and how to get a phosphorus nucleus to absorb it. It is relatively easy to create a neutron target that is 100% phosphorus. The methods to detect β particles are clear and well understood. Further, the relationship is absolutely causal – if the P nucleus absorbs a neutron, it will eventually emit a β particle (with a known half-life of 14.28 days); if it does not, it will not. No control group of other phosphorus atoms that do not receive neutrons is necessary. While philosophers of science may challenge the reality of a neutron or a β particle, physics practitioners are unlikely to share their concern. However, there is much more uncertainty in the second statement. 'Excess' is not defined, nor is stroke, although there are probably fairly unambiguous criteria for the latter. 'Hypertension' has a definition, but this has drifted lower over the years and is somewhat cohort-dependent.(16) Nonetheless, it is not simply a definitional problem. The causal relationship in this example is far more probabilistic; reduction of salt intake has a fairly small effect on blood pressure, and hypertension is only one contributor to stroke, so excess salt may only 'cause' a small proportion of strokes.

The final causal statement is even more vague. It is difficult to unambiguously define compliance with a diet, and it is more difficult to attempt to define a cut-off point that unambiguously separates 'compliant' from 'non-compliant' patients. Further, it is well-nigh impossible to identify what aspect of the workshop was the causal variable in inducing change, nor, for that matter, is it even likely that any single variable was causal for everyone in the workshop. If the 'causal' relationship is confirmed, this may simply be a stimulus for more research to establish the 'active ingredient' (or combination of ingredients) that led to the change.

Of course, much of educational research resembles the final rather than the first example. This has two critical implications for our understanding of the role of experimental research in education. First, in contrast to physical sciences, the relationships we seek are inevitably probabilistic, and the signal of a causal relation is almost always swimming in a sea of noise. It is for this reason that we must impose such strategies as control groups, randomisation and inclusion criteria. Second, the complexity of the relationships may well stifle any serious attempt at understanding processes and mechanisms. To the extent that experiments are directed at, and useful for, discovering lawful causal relationships, it may well be the case that experimental methods like randomised controlled trials (RCTs), which tend to focus on curriculum-level interventions, are over- rather than under-used in education.(17) That is, although many recent reviews have decried the paucity of good randomised trials in education,(8,18) it makes little sense to conduct elegant studies of interventions that are so complex in their idiosyncrasies as to be unreplicable.(19) Still, much can be learnt from good experimentation in appropriate settings.

Study designs

The essence of the experimental approach is a comparison – between one group of individuals who received an intervention and another who did not. In an ideal situation, the participants in the two groups are as alike as possible before the intervention (which is why randomisation is used in an effort to achieve equivalence), so that any differences observed later can be unambiguously attributed to the intervention and nothing else.

However, although the two-group, intervention–control study design is ubiquitous, it is far from unique. Books on research design dating back over several decades have described many increasingly complex designs,(20) and we will discuss some of the more common variants.

One group: Pre-test–post-test and post-test only

A recent review in medical education showed that a single-group pre-test–post-test design was the most commonly reported experimental methodology (32% of 105 studies) followed by a one-group post-test-only design (26%).(8) It is easy to see why this is the case. These designs can easily be incorporated into an ongoing curriculum or course change. All one needs to do is teach something to students taking the course and measure them at the beginning and the end. By contrast, comparisons with a control group require identification of a comparable control group of participants who will volunteer to be tested but will only receive a sham intervention or none at all. Regrettably, one-group designs, labelled 'pre-experimental' by Campbell and Stanley,(20) have very limited scientific value. The problems are myriad. Logically, there is no way that whatever changes are observed from beginning to end can be ascribed to the intervention as opposed to competing hypotheses such as maturation, co-intervention or any number of other plausible explanations.

Further, while the logical flaws may appear parochial, there is a more fundamental educational problem. If one shows a change in performance before and after an intervention, the comparison is against zero change, which implies a comparison against no education at all. While it may well be useful to determine whether, for example, a homeopathic remedy has any effect whatsoever,(21) we can pretty well assume that an hour or two of education is going to result in more learning than none – although not always.(22) In the end, a demonstration that students learnt something after a course reveals nothing about the contribution of any specific aspect of the course.

Two groups: Randomised controlled trials and cohort studies

This difficulty with identifying a causal agent in one-group designs naturally leads to RCTs. The standard RCT involves randomising participants to two groups, so that at the end of the study the only difference between the two groups (except for chance variation) should be that one group received one intervention and the other did not (or received a second intervention). Randomisation is intended to ensure equivalence at inception; standardisation of interventions facilitates interpretation; blinding avoids bias as does complete follow-up, and so on. In this manner, if a difference is observed, it can unequivocally be attributed to the intervention alone short of the omnipresent influence of chance.

The criteria in Box 25.3 are easy to understand but much more difficult to put into practice. Some aspects, such as random assignment, are not too difficult. Blinding of participants however, so they do not know what educational intervention they received, is effectively impossible. Indeed, if a student does not know whether he or she received problem-based learning (PBL) or lectures, one would worry about the student, the intervention, or both. Standardisation is much easier with drugs than curricula – what does 300 mg of PBL t.i.d look like? We might recall that teacher differences typically account for twice as much variance in learning as curriculum differences, and it is not clear how one standardises teachers.(23)

Let us critically examine these aspects in more detail, and in doing so, identify the art of the possible.

BOX 25.3 FOCUS ON: The randomised controlled trial

The randomised controlled trial has only a few critical elements:

- it has two (usually) or more (occasionally) groups
- participants are randomly assigned to each group
- the study is conducted prospectively
- all study participants are blinded to what group they are in
- the intervention(s) are standardised and under experimenter control
- outcome assessment is performed blind on all participants (i.e the person collecting the data does not know to which group the participants were assigned)
- complete follow-up of participants is achieved.

Randomisation, quasi-randomisation and intact groups

One methodological *sine qua non* of the experimental approach is randomisation, assignment to groups using a random process. But randomisation is difficult to achieve at times – a student may sign up for the Tuesday tutorial because he or she plays piano on Monday, and may not take kindly to a Monday tutorial assigned by a random number. We forget that randomisation is a means to an end; if students select a tutorial or a hospital rotation in some manner that is highly unlikely to have an impact on their ultimate performance, what we might call 'quasi-randomisation', that may well be good enough. Further, safeguard against bias must scale against the likely size of the treatment effect; if the treatment effect is large, concern about bias can be reduced. Lipsey and Wilson(24) analysed 319 systematic reviews of educational and psychological interventions and showed: (a) an average effect size of 0.45 (effect sizes of clinical interventions are much smaller; one study of aspirin in preventing myocardial infarction had a computed effect size of 0.02)(25) and (b) no influence of randomisation on effect size; the effects were of equal magnitude (on average) whether randomisation took place or not. Under such circumstances, the potential bias from 'quasi-randomisation' is negligible.

Sometimes randomisation of individuals is just not possible. Students are in one section or another of the course; they are assigned to one hospital or another. A variant of randomisation to deal with this situation is called 'cluster randomisation' – where clusters (e.g. classes) are assigned to one treatment or another. Note that the analysis must account for clusters, and this may have an impact on sample size.

On the other hand, many studies use *intact* groups – turning them into what epidemiologists would call *cohort* studies (which we will discuss later). As one example, many studies have looked at PBL versus lecture-based curricula. Most of these studies involved between-school comparisons. A few, usually from the 1970s, involved within-school comparisons, where the school ran a parallel track. Fewer still randomised students to the two tracks. In considering any differences that emerge, between-school comparisons must be viewed with caution, because different schools differ on myriad variables, from the admissions criteria to the cost of tuition. Within-school comparisons may be better, although often students were selected using different criteria in the two tracks or may have self-selected one track or another. Thus, the finding that PBL students have better interpersonal skills(26,27) must be tempered by the likelihood that the PBL school may well select students for interpersonal skills, or that students with good interpersonal skills may prefer the small group focus of the PBL track.(28) More recently, Schmidt *et al.* have provided empirical data suggesting that the PBL intervention might alter drop-out rate, leaving groups at the end of the programme that are no longer comparable even were randomization at the start perfectly effective.(29)

The conclusion about allocation is a conditional one. In some circumstances there is a good likelihood that non-random assignment can be viewed as equivalent. In others, this may lead to serious confounding. To make an informed decision about which is most likely to be the case, researchers should gather as much information as possible on dimensions relevant to the question of interest from both groups and judge whether or not differences exist that are strong enough to account for differences observed in the outcome.

Placebo or usual care

The choice of control group in educational research is rarely given sufficient attention. This is hardly surprising. Programme evaluation is often initiated by someone who has put time and energy into a new curriculum, course or learning module. It hardly seems worth the effort to now put equal time into a second intervention that is only there for comparison. Consequently, it is often the case that students receiving the innovation are compared with students at another hospital, say, who receive the regular instruction – what epidemiologists may refer to as 'usual care'. A variant is where the intervention is made available to some students but not others.

Such comparisons may be of limited value, regardless of how well other methodological criteria are accomplished. If usual care consists of, for example, lectures that are examined to ensure that the same content is covered, this is fair. If, however, the intervention amounts to a greater amount of time spent studying the to-be-learnt material relative to the control group (a situation that often arises when one simply adds the innovation, such as a high-fidelity simulation, to the curriculum in the treatment arm), then we again find ourselves in the awkward situation of concluding simply that the more they study, the more they learn. From a scientific perspective, a 'usual care' group is about as valuable as none at all, unless the specific aspects of the control intervention can be described as accurately as the experimental arm. Similarly, comparing two groups where one had access to additional resources and the other did not amounts to comparing (A + B) to A; again it amounts to a 'no treatment' comparison.

It is far more informative to compare two experimental interventions where it is possible to standardise for total time of instruction, quality of instruction or other confounders. As one excellent example of how this strategy would work, Cook(30) has discussed the many studies of e-learning and argued for studies that make comparisons within medium (e.g. both arms of the study use the computer) so that pedagogical variables can be systematically manipulated (i.e. controlled) and the specific medium is not confounded. In deciding on a comparison, one must be careful also to avoid over-controlling the study by equating the two groups with respect to the very variables that are likely to make a difference. The literature on class size, in trying simply to test the impact of size, is a case in point; many studies control the very features of small class discussions (e.g. the opportunity to interact with the professor) that may yield benefits.(31)

Blinding

As we said before, one criterion of a good RCT is that all participants – teachers, students and researchers – are 'blind' as to who is in which group. It may be possible to have outcome measurement performed with blinded assessors or with objective tests, it seems highly unlikely that students and teachers will be blinded. But the issue is broader than that. Implicit in the experimental method is that the participant is an 'object', whose motivation and ability is under experimental control. Orwell's vision of 1984 was never achieved, fortunately, and we are left with students who are unlikely (in the extreme) to knuckle under to a researcher's whims. Does this negate the experimental agenda? Not necessarily. But it does ring a cautionary note. To ensure the validity of the study we must make some calculated guesses about the effect of the inevitable unblinding. Failure to do so may lead to false interpretation. As one example, all medical students in North America are highly motivated to pass the licensing examination, for obvious reasons. Consequently, it makes little sense, in our view, to use a licensing examination as a criterion to evaluate a PBL curriculum because student performance on the licensing examination is likely to reflect many hours of study activity unrelated to the curriculum. The outcome may be of interest if it shows a difference, but the numerous studies showing no difference add little to our understanding, and are certainly no basis for any claim of equivalent curricula.

The perils of pre-tests

One variant on the RCT is a two-group, pre-test–post-test design. The usual reason for considering a pre-test, to correct for baseline differences, turns out not to be logically defensible, and the potential side effects of a pre-test often go unrecognised. The issues surrounding use of change scores are quite complex, and we can only highlight some.(32)

The problem with baseline differences is this. If the two groups were created by random assignment, then any difference between groups arose by chance, and to some extent can be adequately dealt with by statistical procedures, which explicitly examine the role of chance in any observed difference. Pre-tests *may* serve a useful role in identifying whether or not there are baseline differences that should factor into one's interpretation; however, if this is a consequence of non-random allocation, no amount of pre-test correction can control for such differences, simply because any correction involves strong assumptions about the relation between pre-test and post-test. In education, pre-tests have one further serious liability. There is no better way to inform students about what the final test will look like than to give them a parallel pre-test. The pre-test becomes part of the curriculum and has the potential to completely eliminate curriculum differences. In fact, the pedagogical value of testing has become a topic of considerable research in medical education in recent years. Using exactly the same test, both pre- and post-intervention simply magnifies the concern, as highlighted by Larsen *et al.*'s findings,(33) which suggest that the material one is tested on becomes particularly memorable (a phenomenon known as test-enhanced learning or testing effects). One solution that explicitly recognises this issue is called the Solomon Four Group Design. In this design there are four groups:

- pre-test, intervention, post-test
- pre-test–post-test
- intervention–post-test
- post-test.

It is then theoretically possible to disentangle the effect of pre-test from the intervention itself.

Outcomes: Self-assessed versus performance-based, and short term versus long term

The choice of the appropriate outcome is perhaps the most difficult part of study design. It almost inevitably represents a compromise between what would be assessed in an ideal world and what can reasonably be assessed with the inevitable constraints of time, money, and acceptability. Moreover, the simple fact is that many outcomes of interest in education (like the CanMEDS roles that have been broadly adopted) are theoretical constructs rather than absolute objective entities.(34) Of course, we would like to show that ultimately the educational innovations we are studying have an impact on patient outcomes, and editors of four journals in the field have argued that this is a goal to be seriously entertained.(35–38) But realistically, with rare exceptions,(14) few studies will last long enough to examine patient outcomes. In any case, we agree with Gruppen(39) that such a quest is ill-advised for the more fundamental reason that there are so many intervening variables between educational treatment and patient outcome that it is unlikely any educational intervention will lead to detectable differences.

There is, however, another reason to seek more immediate measures, which aligns with the philosophical commitment to theory-based, programmatic research. While demonstrating that an intervention leads to a (small) increment in performance in, say, a final exam or a licensing examination may be of some practical value, these outcomes are subject to so many confounders that they are unlikely to reveal a cause–effect relationship with the intervention. It is helpful to think of a causal chain where an intervention at each level will have maximal effect on proximal outcomes, and less impact as the chain lengthens. (It is possible that the effects are additive or even multiplicative – the rich get richer – but this appears unlikely in the situations we have examined.) For example, if an intervention can be shown to improve knowledge levels in the first year of medical school and first-year performance is shown to be predictive of clerkship performance, clerkship performance is found to relate to scores received on a national licensing exam, and so on, then we can develop a richer picture of what variables have an impact at each stage, and make more informed decisions regarding the educational activities that should be undertaken. Our recent work on testing the validity of various admissions procedures provides an example of this approach.(40) As an aside, while it is difficult to show enduring effects of curricula, some recent studies have shown that individual differences in students, either in performance or ethical behaviour,(14,41) may have long-term effects that are consequential.

A second issue to consider when deciding on outcome measures is the source. Satisfaction scales, completed by learners, are ubiquitously used as measures of programme effectiveness, probably because of their ease of administration. However, it is difficult to imagine how someone who has spent the time and money to take a course would perceive that they had learnt nothing and it was all a waste – even though some highly touted courses are exactly that.(42) Satisfaction with teaching is moderately related to performance gains;(43) however, this may be a chicken–egg phenomenon as the strongest relations result when students know their scores. Worse still, self-reported judgements of competence have been shown repeatedly to have minimal relationship with observed competence,(44–46) thereby making it important that self-assessments are not used as surrogate markers of an individual's performance. That said, recent data do suggest that consideration of self-assessments in the aggregate (i.e. averaged across many individuals) can offer reliable information regarding which aspects of an educational intervention (i.e. a curriculum) have been particularly effective in yielding performance improvement.(47)

The optimal choice must be a measure that, on the one hand, is sufficiently close in time and context to be sensitive to intervention effects and to permit causal inferences, but is sufficiently relevant, in some absolute sense, to be viewed as a valid and important outcome. This latter point requires careful consideration, consultation and pilot testing to ensure that one is looking at outcomes that are likely to represent the changes that could conceivably be occurring. Again, one should use both theory and experience to interpret whether the intervention is likely to impact upon measures of affect, behavioural outcomes or cognitive indicators of ability (the ABCs of outcomes). Finally, note for now that the measures must be psychometrically sound, with proven evidence of reliability and validity. We will have more to say on this topic in the next section.

Three or more groups, and factorial designs

Apart from feasibility, there is rarely any reason to restrict a study to only two groups. Certainly, when one abandons the simplistic approach of a placebo or usual care control and seeks better explanation through systematic manipulation of a number of independent variables, there is good reason to consider multiple groups. Analytical methods are straightforward: analysis of variance (ANOVA) followed by some *post-hoc* procedure. The primary disadvantage is that each additional group requires an additional sample of participants. However, an alternative design strategy, using 'factorial designs', has the remarkable property that one can address multiple hypotheses with very small penalty in sample size. An example is a study of e-learning in brain anatomy by Levinson *et al.*(48) There were two variables: key views (front, back, top, section) versus multiple views (where the visualised brain could assume multiple positions) and active versus passive control over the presentation (one group had control over the time the computerised image was presented in each of the various orientations, the other did not). This made four groups:

- active–key
- active–multiple
- passive–key
- passive–multiple.

	Key views	multiple views
Active control	(a)	(b)
Passive control	(c)	(d)

Figure 25.2 Example of a two-group comparison: e-learning in brain anatomy.(44)

These four groups can be thought of as lying within a 2 × 2 table (Figure 25.2).

Now, suppose that 25 students are in each group. The data would be analysed with a two-way ANOVA, giving a significance test for active versus passive based on two groups of 50, key versus multiple based on two groups of 50, and the interaction between them (i.e. whether or not the effect of active versus passive control is the same for both levels of the views variable), based on four groups of 25. In terms of the two main hypotheses, the comparison is virtually as powerful as the test using only two groups with 50 subjects per group.

Further, one cannot assess an interaction without including both variables in a single research study, and the interaction is often where the most interesting findings lie. Such was the case in the Levinson study in that the best group was the passive–key view participants, the worst was the passive–multiple view participants, and the two active groups were intermediate with respect to their performance at test.

This is the simplest of factorial designs. In our view, these designs, with their capability to examine multiple hypotheses simultaneously and to explore interactions among variables at almost no cost in sample size, are underutilised in education research.

Sample and effect sizes

Given that the previous section argued for the value of multifactorial designs, in part on the basis that one can get more information with very small penalty in terms of sample size, it would be remiss of us not to include an answer to the ubiquitous question of 'How many people do I need?' Of course, questions are usually ubiquitous when the answer is 'it depends', but we will provide an indication of what it depends on by highlighting issues that should be considered when engaging with experimental research paradigms.

There are two central issues to take into account in determining the required sample size. The first is statistical and is related to the concept of 'power' alluded to in the last section. In educational research, there is always variability related to differences among learners. Some students will learn more than others. Regardless of whether one is learning via large-group lecture or small-group tutorial (to name one example of a comparison that has been made *ad nauseum*) there will be variability in the amount learnt, and

the distribution of one group is likely to overlap (often substantially) with the distribution of the other group. As such, statistics are required to determine the probability that the differences observed in the mean scores achieved by both groups are unlikely to have arisen simply by chance. The standard of '$p = 0.05$' means that the likelihood that an observed difference (or association as we will discuss later) arose due to chance is less than 5%, so the odds are good that the intervention, and not random variation, resulted in the differences between the groups. Because it is based on probabilities, the conclusion is fallible – one can falsely conclude that there is a difference when there is none.

'Power' reflects the opposite concern; concluding that no difference exists when in fact there is an underlying effect of the intervention. It is the probability that a study has a large enough sample to detect an educationally important effect. Specific calculations for sample size are beyond the scope of this chapter as the formulae differ depending on the statistical test one needs to perform, but it should be noted that in all cases sample size calculations are dependent on predictions of how large a difference and how much variability in the sample one would expect. The predictions should be based on the best information available, but inevitably the calculations will be guesstimates to some degree. If one is able to find a statistically significant difference, however, then by definition the study was sufficiently powered (i.e. had a large enough sample size). One could debate the representativeness of the sample and whether or not the effect might disappear with greater sampling, making replication an invaluable strategy for confirming the accuracy of the results, but whether or not the study had sufficient power (i.e. was statistically 'big enough') is not debatable. Power calculations are only relevant before a study has ended or if significance was not obtained, but like sample size calculations these require an assumption of the magnitude of difference one wanted to detect. Big differences require smaller samples than small differences.

The second issue to consider is implicit in the preceding discussion. Very large samples can yield the opposite problem to small samples. An intervention can have a statistically significant effect even if it is of no practical importance, simply because the study had a very large sample size. For this reason, it is wise to consider not only the statistical significance, but also the size of the effect, typically defined as the difference between group means divided by the standard deviation (see any statistical text for more detail). The larger the effect size, the easier it is to argue that the findings are 'clinically important'. By convention, effect sizes of 0.2, 0.5 and 0.8 (i.e. differences that amount to 20%, 50% and 80% of the standard deviation) are considered small, medium and large.(49)

Summary

For many, experimental research is held up as the gold standard for which we should strive when addressing all research questions. Clearly this is simplistic, but it is true that experimental designs, when applied appropriately, can have great impact on our ability to understand the extent to which causal relationships exist between variables (i.e.

if one variable changes, does it cause another to change?). But such inferences rarely arise from curriculum-level interventions, which contain many variables and covariates. It is often more informative to design a series of small-scale experiments that tease apart the active ingredients, thus building knowledge of which elements are critical for learning. However, when one is interested in testing the relationship between naturally occurring variables that cannot easily be manipulated, then methodologies drawn from the epidemiological or correlational traditions may be more appropriate, as discussed in the following sections.

The epidemiological tradition

The term RCT has been used repeatedly in this chapter, referring to what is commonly viewed as the optimal experiment, in which subjects are randomly assigned to different groups that receive different treatments, and are then compared on some outcome measure. The RCT has a position of honour at the top of a hierarchy of research designs derived from epidemiology. While other designs in this hierarchy are rarely explicitly used in educational research, they may occasionally have a very useful role, as we shall point out.

Because many epidemiological investigations are based on a dichotomous outcome (dead or alive, improved or worsened, diseased or disease-free) as well as a dichotomous classification at inception (drug/placebo, risk factor present/absent, e.g. smoker/non-smoker), the easiest way to think about these designs is as a 2 × 2 table.

We have already discussed the RCT, the design of which is shown in Box 25.4. Respondents are randomised to rows (i.e. to the drug or placebo group) and the outcome (the columns) is tabulated. A *cohort* study looks the same, except that participants are not randomised to the two groups; rather, they are members of each cohort as a result of processes beyond the experimenter's control and, as such, the word 'intervention' should be replaced by 'exposure' or some other descriptor appropriate to the particular focus of the study.

Many studies of PBL versus lecture-based curricula can be classified as cohort studies, because students are in one cohort or the other through non-experimental factors such as self-selection or differential admissions policies. They may then be followed forward to determine, for example, success rates on licensing examinations or acceptance into primary care residency programmes. One example is the study by Woodward *et al.*(26) of billing patterns of McMaster graduates matched to graduates from the rest of Ontario.

A *case–control* study can be illustrated in the same way, but the method of allocation runs in the opposite direction. Cases are selected by the outcome – they had the disease, or they failed the examination – and controls are selected by who did not have that outcome. The study then looks back to determine whether the cases were more likely to be exposed to some risk (e.g. smoking or PBL). A case–control study, therefore, looks the same as the RCT with the exceptions that:

- the rows are better labelled as risk factors (present/ absent)
- subjects are assigned to the columns rather than by the rows as the researcher looks for different rates of risk factor across the columns.

The important study by Papadakis *et al.*(14) of predictors of disciplinary action by a medical board is a good example of a case–control study. They identified a group of cases: 235 graduates from three medical schools who had some kind of disciplinary action as physicians and matched them to 469 controls, who were comparable demographically (i.e. were matched), but who had no record of disciplinary action. They then looked back at both groups' undergraduate records to determine whether they had episodes of unprofessional behaviour in medical school, and found that 92/235 cases (39%) revealed problems as a student, whereas only 90/469 controls (19.2%) revealed similar issues. One must consider base rates to determine the consequences of acting on such differences,(50) but these compelling findings draw appropriate attention to the types of behaviour that should be considered in the context of professionalism.

Summary

Perhaps ironically, the most applicable study design from this hierarchy is the last. There are many examples of studies that resemble cohort studies or RCTs, and it is not particularly helpful to single these out with a new label. However, the case–control study is uniquely useful in situations analogous to its application in clinical medicine, where the outcome is categorical (disciplinary action yes/ no), the prevalence of the outcome is low and the time delay until it occurs is long. Because it is usually retrospective, the case–control study may well be the only, or at least the most efficient, response to the concern to link educational interventions to patient outcomes; any alternative is likely to be too large, too costly and too inefficient to show any yield (Box 25.5).(41)

The psychometric tradition

As alluded to in the last section, the RCT is frequently held up as the 'best' research design with accompanying con-

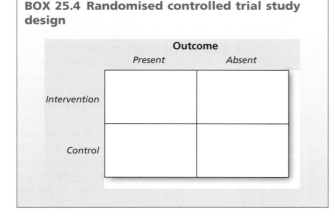

BOX 25.4 Randomised controlled trial study design

	Outcome	
	Present	*Absent*
Intervention		
Control		

BOX 25.5 FOCUS ON: Quasi-experimental designs

Quasi-experimental designs including cohort and case–control studies have the following characteristics:

- they include two (usually) or more (occasionally) groups
- they enrol participants who are assigned to each group based on some predetermined characteristic on which it is not possible to randomise (e.g. presence of disease or risk factor)
- they are conducted retrospectively (usually)
- participants are not blinded to the group they are in
- complete follow-up of participants is rarely achieved.

sternation regarding how few studies in medical education use an RCT. Such an attitude is, in our view, amazingly myopic.(17) One need not leave the quantitative domain to recognise that many of the most important questions and issues in the field cannot, *and should not*, be addressed with an RCT or, for that matter, any other experimental or quasi-experimental design.

Arguably, the most significant advances in our field have been in assessment, where medical education has, quite literally, led the world(51) in developing authentic, yet psychometrically defensible, measures like the Objective Structure Clinical Examination (OSCE).(52) Assessment methods are analogous to diagnostic tests, designed to identify those who have a lot or a little of the characteristic of interest, and perhaps to eventually create a cut-off to label a disease, in this case, 'incompetence'. Just as the starting point in developing a diagnostic test (e.g. a new radiographic procedure) is to assemble a group of patients, administer the test and look at (a) inter-rater agreement and (b) relation to some other measure of the same characteristic, we would set about testing a new assessment method by assembling a group of students, administering the test and examining reliability and then validity. Any radiologist who introduced a new diagnostic procedure by conducting a multicentre trial to see whether patients who had the test lived longer before they first proved that radiologists had adequate inter-rater agreement and that the test results converged on other measures of disease would be at risk of psychiatric referral. Similarly, while we might like to eventually use an experimental method to show that students who get a new assessment method eventually perform better than those who are assessed using some conventional method, this is hardly the first step.

Because so much research in medical education is directed towards the development and testing of assessment methods, this section is devoted to a discussion of basic issues in psychometric methods. The discussion is necessarily brief; for a substantial elaboration, we refer you to Streiner and Norman.(53)

Basic concepts

Psychometric methods are designed to ensure that data are sufficiently trustworthy to enable appropriate interpretations and accurate decision-making. Medical educators and the lay public are bombarded with 'data-based' claims every day, but it goes without saying that not all such claims should be treated equally. Most threats to validity require us to formalise this intuitive scepticism and devise ways to test whether or not our measurement instruments are indeed measuring what we intend them to be measuring.

These strategies can be applied to any number of domains, including but not limited to assessments of the quality of admissions decisions,(54) research into the relation between personality and professionalism(55) or use of a questionnaire to measure the extent to which learners demonstrate self-directed learning.(56) In each case it is easy to collect information and make decisions, but much more is involved in determining whether or not those conclusions stand up to proper scrutiny. To understand this statement it is of course necessary to define 'proper scrutiny'. For any measurement instrument to provide useful information, be it an objective indication of some physical state (as would be measured with thermometers) or a subjective claim about a more ethereal construct (like one's perceptions of one's own abilities), it is necessary to ensure that the tool satisfies the four '-*ities*' of good measurement:

- feasibility
- acceptability
- reliability
- validity.

The first two need no explanation in that it seems fairly straightforward to suggest that a tool should only be used to the extent that it can be used (feasibility) and to the extent that people will use it (acceptability). How to assess these -ities requires some thought as part of acceptability, for example, entails demonstrating that the measure does not show undue bias against particular subgroups of the population. However, it is the latter two -ities that likely require elaboration. Before we begin, a disclaimer: while we will discuss *the* psychometric properties of measurement instruments, we do so simply for the sake of useful shorthand, as it is inaccurate to make acontextual claims about such properties in relation to any instrument. That is, the utility (*see* Chapter 18) of an instrument is based entirely on the population and context within which the instrument is to be used. While a grading system based on sad and smiling faces might be appropriate for school-age children, it is unlikely to be accepted in the context of national licensing exams in medicine; a survey that asks people to answer questions about their sexual activity levels may elicit accurate responses in some respondent cohorts, but may not be answered (and may cause offence) in others; a clinical skills examination that requires blood pressure to be taken may discriminate among beginner medical students but may be useless with medical residents. As we will see, these contextual variables can have significant impact on the assessment of reliability and validity.

Reliability

Reliability may be the most misused word in all of medical education. It does not mean agreement (although agreement is relevant), it does not mean variability (although variability is relevant) and it is not indicated by consistency of mean scores calculated for a group of individuals (although one would expect such consistency if the tool is reliable). Reliability is a statistical term indicating the extent to which a measurement instrument *consistently differentiates* between *individual* subjects of interest. The subjects may be learners, teachers, courses, schools, survey respondents or any other group of individual entities. As attempts to differentiate between students are most common within our community, we will use that domain as an example. Were one interested in developing a tool to assess knowledge of professional responsibilities, it would not be hard to generate items that result in variability of responses. That, in fact, would be a predominant goal as, presumably, if everyone were to provide the same responses there would be little reason to administer the test. That variability, however, could be attributable to any number of factors. Our hope is that scores on the test reflect true or consistent differences between students, with respect to their knowledge of professional responsibilities. Some portion of the variability, however, will be attributable to error of measurement because systematic biases and random forces can be expected to impact on the scores assigned to students.

While there are an infinite number of sources of error, the primary question is how much of the variability in scores can be attributed to error in relation to actual differences between the students? In other words, if we were to re-administer the test (or have different examiners rate the responses or use a parallel test), how consistent would individuals' scores be from one administration to the next? Mathematically, the simplest way to represent this concept is with the following equation:

$$Reliability = \frac{\sigma^2_{subjects}}{\sigma^2_{subjects} + \sigma^2_{error/n}}$$

σ^2 is the conventional symbol used to express variance, so the numerator indicates the amount of variance attributable to differences between the students themselves and the denominator represents the total variability observed in the scores. This equation is not presented to scare away the innumerate, and we will not elaborate here on how one would calculate reliability. Rather, the formula is presented because it enables us to illustrate some fundamental points about reliability and, in turn, research in the psychometric tradition (*see* Box 25.6).

Within the psychometric tradition readers of educational journals will also encounter the notion of *generalisability*, a close cousin of the concept of reliability. Generalisability theory is a way of expressing the extent to which the scores assigned to individual subjects generalise to the scores assigned in another context (with another rater, at another time, etc.).(52) If that sounds familiar, it is because generalisability theory is simply an extension of classic test reliability theory that provides the mathematical infrastructure to enable multiple sources of error variance to be considered simultaneously. The fundamental advantages are that one need not complete multiple studies to assess the relative error contributions of multiple variables and that, as a

result, one can determine the relative benefits of increasing the number of observations collected across one variable relative to the benefits that can be gained by increasing the number of observations collected across another.

Validity

Historically, most descriptions of validity have used one taxonomy or another to differentiate various ways in which one can consider the trustworthiness of a set of ratings.(58) *Content validity* is considered to be the extent to which the items in a tool adequately sample the domain of interest without extending beyond it (i.e. are the questions sufficient and relevant?); *criterion validity* refers to the extent to which the measure correlates well with another measure of the same underlying construct; and *construct validity* indicates the extent to which the scores derived from the instrument align with expectations based on understanding of the underlying construct that the tool was intended to measure (e.g. a new measure of height should result in higher scores for basketball players relative to jockeys). Other taxonomies have been used, but in our minds it is all just validity (i.e. an indication of whether or not the scores derived from the use of the instrument vary in conjunction with the extent to which the amount of construct in the individual being measured varies). In fact, some have argued that reliability is simply one aspect of validity rather than a separate concept, the argument being that if the amount of underlying construct is not expected to have changed across administrations of the instrument, then the scores should not change either.(59) The various taxonomies that have been published may be useful to generate ideas as to how the validity of an instrument can be tested, but one should not allow the taxonomy to distract from awareness that proper validity testing requires systematic study, preferably with a variety of methodologies.

That said, one aspect of what Messick calls '*consequential validity*' is worth highlighting.(58) Any time we put in place an instrument to assess students, we must worry about the extent to which the measurement instrument has an impact on behaviour. Assessment has long been known to have a steering effect on the learning activities of students.(60) As a result, to ensure the utility of an assessment instrument it is necessary to engender a match between the learning activities one hopes to promote and the learning activities stimulated by the tool.(60) As these five principles of good measurement (the four '-*ities*' and educational impact) that form a tool's utility do not always align (and, in fact, often run counter to one another), it is almost inevitably necessary to decide on an appropriate compromise, the balance of which should be determined by the specifics of the situation.

Most will start their study of the validity of an instrument by testing its reliability as described above, for the simple reason that if a tool is not reliable, it cannot be valid. For example, in studying the consistency of ratings provided to medical school applicants during panel-based interviews, Harasym *et al.*(61) noted that over 50% of the variance in scores could be attributed to the person doing the interview, thereby fundamentally calling into question both the reliability and the validity of the panel-based interview process, as that process is intended to provide infor-

BOX 25.6 FOCUS ON: Reliability

- *Reliability is not a fixed property of the measurement instrument.* If a test of professionalism knowledge, as described above, is designed to provide an assessment of second-year residents, then its reliability (i.e. its ability to consistently differentiate between subjects) must be tested on a sample of second-year residents. To recruit a more heterogeneous sample (e.g. by enrolling first-year undergraduates and practising ethicists) will result in artificial inflation of the numerator, and as a result, artificially inflated estimates of the reliability of the tool. Researchers must make a concerted effort to specify the context within which they want to use their instruments and test by recruiting a sample of respondents representative of those working in that context.

- *Repeated measurement across the variables of interest is required to estimate the reliability of a tool.* If raters are liable to disagree about the strength of a student's performance, then multiple raters should be asked to rate the student's performance. If performance varies across the cases (content specificity), then students should be assessed on multiple cases. Simply administering a test and revealing that the scores are normally distributed tells us absolutely nothing about the extent to which the tool consistently differentiates between subjects because the variation can result from true differences between students or measurement error.

- *The more observations per individual one is able to average across, the more reliable the instrument will tend to be.* The n under the error term represents the number of observations collected (be they from multiple test questions, multiple raters, multiple administrations of the exercise or some other source of error variance). An average over multiple observations provides a better estimate of the amount of the construct held by the individual than any one score because random positive sources can cancel out random negative forces. Of course if a particular source of variance does not contribute error to a particular measurement, averaging across multiple observations collected across that source will have no impact

(dividing zero by anything still leaves one with zero). An important aspect of psychometric analysis, therefore, is to determine how many observations one must collect for the total to achieve reasonable levels of reliability – if the answer is too many to be feasible, it suggests that the tool should be modified or abandoned.

- *A tool that does not discriminate is useless for assessment.* There may be other aspects of utility (specifically, motivating individuals to engage in desired study behaviour – educational impact) that warrants use of a particular measurement instrument, but generally, claims of utility rely on evidence of reliability and, if everyone receives the same score, from an assessment perspective one may as well assume the result and do something better with one's time than administer the test.

- *Claims that the mean score of a group did not change over time (or across raters) provide no evidence of reliability.* One would find a stable mean even if the rank ordering of individuals within the sample perfectly reversed from one test administration to the next (i.e. if there was absolutely no consistency in the scores assigned and, as a result, all variance could be attributed to error). A random number generator can be expected to result in equivalent means on different occasions, but random number generators can hardly claim to provide reliable measures of performance.

- *Occasionally, the claim is made that reliability of a measure is irrelevant because validity is more important.* Such a statement is simply illogical. One can view reliability as the correlation between a measure and itself (on repeated occasions). One aspect of validity expresses the correlation between a measure and some external (preferably 'gold') standard. It is axiomatic that a measure cannot correlate with something better than it correlates with itself. Hence, reliability is not dissociated from validity; instead, it sets an upper limit on possible claims to validity. And, in fact, modern models of psychometrics consider reliability to simply be one aspect of validity.(57)

---

mation on the quality of applicants, not the stringency of the interviewers.

However, reliability is insufficient. Just because something can be measured consistently does not mean that the measurements are valid. It is easy to measure the circumference of an individual's head in a consistent and reliable manner. Those data, however, are completely useless if one is trying to assess the empathy levels of the subjects given that phrenology was discredited a century ago.(62) A more direct example comes from the literature on OSCE testing formats. As most readers of this chapter will be familiar with the OSCE, we will note simply that it is a 'bell ringer' type of examination in which examinees interact with multiple patients in sequence while striving to demonstrate their clinical skills. The 'O' in OSCE stands for objective, to indicate the initial idea that one could evaluate performance by generating a checklist of appropriate behaviours

and noting which were undertaken by the examinee. Indeed, such checklists have been shown to robustly provide very reliable measurements of individuals' performance.(63) In various studies, however, they have been seen to bear no relation to experience, an important variable if one wants to make claims about measuring ability. In contrast, global ratings of performance do tend to correlate with experience levels, suggesting that while checklists may provide a valid measure of comprehensiveness, subjective judgement provides a more valid measurement of clinical expertise in many domains.(64,65)

One could go on *ad nauseum* about the variety of methodologies that can be used to study validity. Comparing average scores received by different groups that can be anticipated to differ in amount of the construct, correlating individual scores with other continuous variables that are expected to be related to the underlying construct, and examining the change in scores that takes place after an intervention expected to change levels of the underlying construct provide three broad classes of approach that might be adopted. Interesting examples include the work of Tamblyn *et al.*, which revealed a relationship between performance on the Canadian licensing examination and professional behaviours during practice as a physician;(41) the work of Ramsey *et al.*,(66) which revealed that specialist certification based on multiple-choice testing is predictive of peer ratings 10 years into practice; and the work of Davis *et al.*,(46) which has continued a line of inquiry that casts doubt on the validity of self-assessments as indicators of performance. In fact, many of the methodologies included in other sections of this chapter (as well as those not included) could be deemed strategies for testing validity.

Instead of trying to generate a comprehensive list of strategies we will close this section by simply noting that one can rarely expect to prove validity in any absolute sense. It is important to test validity because claims that a measure provides information that should be allowed to guide decision-making rest on the balance of evidence. In essence, validity testing is theory testing; each new test that reveals a positive result supports both the theory and the validity of the instrument, but each new test that reveals a negative result should lead one to question (and study) whether the theory is incorrect or the tool provides an inadequate measure of the construct.

Summary

The overarching theme of research undertaken within the psychometric tradition is that researchers, educators, clinicians, and the lay public for that matter, need to strive to be sure that the data that guide our thinking and decision making are sufficiently trustworthy to warrant using them to draw conclusions. This is not simply an academic issue, as too often people's lives are altered (by admittance to/rejection from/advancement within their chosen profession, by decision-making within the legal system, or by personal life/marriage counsellors) on the basis of 'data' of dubious validity. Ensuring the validity of one's research instruments and assessment strategies is an ethical imperative.(67) It is not easy and there are certainly factors that need to be considered beyond psychometric properties, but the methods and concepts outlined here hopefully provide a good start and, if nothing else, should provide a basis for reasoning about these types of problem.

The correlational tradition

A significant proportion of research in medical education is derived from survey questionnaires. These may cover a potentially vast array of topics, from intrapersonal issues such as learning styles or emotional intelligence, to observer ratings of achievement or other aspects of observable behaviour, to satisfaction measures. It would be unrealistic to attempt to cover this vast, heterogeneous and complex field; instead this section will be devoted to a number of common issues related to scoring, research design and

analysis. Questionnaire 'design' is addressed by Lovato and Wall in Chapter 27, but we would remind the reader that proper questionnaire-based research is not easy, and reliability and validity must still be ensured. In general, questionnaires are useful for systematically determining a large group of individuals' perceptions and attitudes towards a particular issue they have experienced. Beyond that, however, one must always be aware of the limitation that people are notoriously bad at accurately judging the cause of their behaviour,(68) or the adequacy of their own performance.(45,46)

Scoring

Quite commonly, responses from individual items are to be summed into a score. Much effort is sometimes expended to decide what weight should be given to each item comprising the score. As it turns out, an extensive literature dating back to at least 1976 is absolutely consistent – an equal weighting model, where all items are simply summed together, is as reliable and valid as *any* alternative.(69) There is one cautionary note: a simple sum assumes that the items are similar in means and standard deviations. It would be no more appropriate to add together items, some of which are binary (0 or 1) and some of which are on seven-point scales, than it would be to add an interview score based on seven-point scales to grades out of 100, or for that matter, to add weight in kilograms to height in metres as a measure of overall size. When the individual items are on different scales, the correct approach is to convert to Z scores [(score – mean)/standard deviation] before combining scales, but the combination should still retain equal weights.

One other point about scoring is that there is extensive debate about whether the scores assigned to the sorts of scale described here should be summed to calculate a mean given that, technically, the data are ordinal in nature (i.e. they indicate rank order without any guarantee of there being equal intervals between all pairs of sequential points).(70) In practice, the parametric statistical tests that require interval-level data tend to be quite robust to deviations from normality(71–73) and their ease of application provides great advantage in most situations.

Validation

The validation methods described in the section on psychometric methods are appropriate for survey instruments and should be considered carefully to avoid making decisions based on survey data that might not be trustworthy for the purpose for which they were intended.

Analysis

The correlational approach is based on a search for relationships among variables, and analysis typically begins (and all too often ends) with every variable being correlated with every other, and then *post-hoc* stories being constructed around the few 'significant' correlations. The problem with the strategy is researchers appear to forget the meaning of '$p = 0.05$' – the likelihood that an observed relationship of this magnitude could have arisen by chance *if there was in fact no relationship.* In other words, for every 20 correlations that are calculated, one will be significant by chance at the 0.05 level (actually, there is a 64.2% chance that at least one will be significant). It is worth noting here that this applies to any statistical analyses, including ANOVAs, *t*-tests and other strategies that rely on *p*-values to determine whether or not the data can be accounted for by chance alone. An obvious solution to this 'data dredging' is to begin with a substantive theory about what relationships are expected. At a minimum, this can direct attention to specific correlations rather than using a 'shotgun' approach. Further, as it is likely that the researcher will still be interested in more than one correlation, the critical *p*-value should be set at $0.05/n$ where 'n' is the total number of statistical tests – a 'Bonferroni correction'.(74)

A more sophisticated approach than correlations involves multivariate methods such as multiple regression, factor analysis and structural equation modelling. Strictly speaking, the term 'multi-variate' should only apply to a situation with multiple *dependent* variables. So multiple regression is a univariate procedure, factor analysis and structural equation modelling are multi-variate. Multiple regression involves predicting a single dependent variable with multiple independent variables, e.g. predicting licensing exam performance with a combination of variables like undergraduate grades, gender and Medical College Admission Test (MCAT) score. Factor analysis seeks underlying associations among clusters of variables, which are called 'factors'. More sophisticated is the family of multi-variate methods, including confirmatory factor analysis, hierarchical linear models and structural equation models. In all these methods, the researcher begins with a theory about the relationship among variables (e.g. *good tutors* succeed by increasing *motivation* of students, and this, in combination with their *prior achievement*, predicts their *final exam performance*). Different causal models are fitted to the data set and the degree of fit computed. Challenges for these approaches include: (a) all of these methods are sample intensive, and the rule of thumb is that the sample size should be at least 5–10 times the number of variables; (b) as the complexity of the model increases, it becomes less and less clear what it actually means to say that this model fits the data but that model does not; and (c) because it is unlikely that any two studies will use the same combination of variables, the concern remains that the causal theory, whatever it may be, is unique to the data set on which it is based.

Nevertheless, these approaches do represent a considerable advance over the mindless cranking out of dozens of correlation coefficients that is all too frequently the norm in correlational research. As in the discussion on effect size presented in the experimental studies section, we urge a focus on the correlation coefficient, not the associated *p*-value. With large samples, even small correlations (e.g. $r = 0.1$) can be statistically significant. The coefficient of variation (r^2), however, reveals that $r = 0.1$ describes a relationship that accounts for only 1% of the variance in the data. As a result, r^2 should always be used to judge the 'clinical' importance of a correlation. We will return to this issue in the final section (Box 25.7).

BOX 25.7 FOCUS ON: Common statistical tests

Statistical tests are based on two broad classes.

Parametric tests

Applied to data on which it makes sense to calculate means and standard deviations.

Used for comparing means:

- *t-test:* one independent variable with two groups, or two related observations (such as before–after).
- *Analysis of variance (ANOVA):* one or more independent variables, each containing two or more groups ('levels').
- *Repeated measures ANOVA:* a special case of ANOVA in which repeated observations are taken within an independent variable on the same subjects. Also used for reliability and generalisability studies.

Used for examining relationships:

- *Pearson's correlation:* provides relation between two measured continuous variables.
- *Multiple regression:* provides relation between multiple predictor variables and a single *continuous* dependent variable.
- *Factor analysis:* provides relations (underlying factors) for a large number of related variables.

Non-parametric tests

Used for frequency counts:

- *Chi-squared:* compares proportions in two or more related categories (e.g. 2 × 2 tables).
- *Logistic regression:* provides relation between multiple predictor variables and a single *dichotomous* independent variable.

Cronbach's 'two disciplines'

At the outset of this chapter, we pointed out that many research questions cannot *and should not* be answered with experimental designs. The methodology that is most appropriate, whether choosing between quantitative and qualitative designs or between experimental and correlational methods, is dependent on the question the researchers want to address. In promoting theory-based and programmatic research efforts, we advocate using a variety of methods to enable triangulation on a problem, thereby developing a richer understanding of the underlying relationships than any one methodology would allow. However, the choice is not quite as value-free as might be imagined. Lee Cronbach first recognised a fundamental duality in a classic paper published in 1957(75) called the 'The two disciplines of scientific psychology'.

The essence of the dichotomy is this: Correlational methods, including psychometrics, are critically dependent on individual differences. It begins with the reliability coefficient, which is zero if everyone is alike (i.e. if there is no subject variance). If we want to examine the relation between some individual attribute such as intelligence quotient or premedical grades and some outcome such as licensing examination performance, unless some students are high or low on each measure there can be no correlation. By contrast, if we were to do an experiment to see whether a supplementary course can help students achieve higher scores on a standardised admissions test, ideally we would like to begin with a cohort of students whose abilities, as measured by undergraduate grades, are exactly the same. To the extent that some students are already very good at biology, physics, etc., and others in the course have little knowledge or aptitude, this will lead to large variability in the scores of students in the experimental and control groups. This variability will, in turn, end up in the denominator of any statistical test designed to show that the treatment was statistically significant (i.e. will add 'noise' to the data).

To the experimentalist, any variation between people will dilute the chances of finding a treatment effect. To the correlationalist, the goal is explicitly to understand the differences between people. Thus it is literally the case that one person's signal is the other's noise.

Given this dichotomy, it makes no more sense to argue which is 'better' methodologically than to try to find evidence that red is better than blue, irrespective of the use to which the colours are to be put. They are not better or worse, except in relation to what one is trying to achieve; they are just different. The situation was nicely summarised recently by a wag who declared that, 'Randomised controlled trials are the best design of all to find out if a treatment works, and the worst design to find out who it works for.'

Reviews

As mentioned earlier, any primary research study will have flaws; even if the perfect study could be designed, there is no way to completely control for the powerful forces of random variation. As a result, it is important to consider the balance of evidence available when deciding how to use the information that has accumulated in the literature. This is the key reason that scholarly reviews of a field are so valuable – when done well, they synthesise the available evidence in a way that can refine the readers' understanding of the focal problem and help them better understand the implications of the literature for their own practices or their own knowledge-building research efforts. We have already noted that every research effort should be informed by a review of existing literature. Here we provide some insights into the creation and interpretation of more formal efforts, starting with systematic reviews, as they represent a form of review on which emphasis has been growing in recent years.

Systematic reviews and meta-analysis

In part as a consequence of the Best Evidence Medical Education (BEME) movement, initiated by Harden *et al.*,(76) systematic reviews have become increasingly popular in the medical education literature. To some degree they epitomise the reductionistic approach to quantitative research

– the goal is to determine the one number that best specifies how well 'it' works. Although many might assume that medical education has adopted the technology of systematic reviews from clinical research, where systematic reviews of, for example, the risk reduction for stroke from beta-blocker therapy are commonplace, in fact the path is more tortuous than that. The first proponent of systematic reviews and the accompanying meta-analyses were educational statisticians, Smith and Glass, whose 1977 article in *American Psychologist*(77) is usually cited as the first publication of the type.

What is a systematic review? The goal is, more or less, to identify *all* of the empirical literature on a particular question, and to then use statistical methods to best estimate the effect (or non-effect) of a particular intervention in a way that is relatively free of bias compared with less comprehensive strategies. There are, therefore, three aspects of 'systematic':
- a systematic search for all the literature relevant to a topic
- a systematic review to select the subset of articles achieving at least minimal quality and relevance
- a systematic summary using specific statistical methods to arrive at the best estimate of the effect in question.

It is clear that these aspects, while equally important, are separable. First, careful computer algorithms to search electronic databases must be devised and then supplemented with manual searches. Once the key articles have been located they must be reviewed in detail to ensure methodological rigour, often using a detailed reporting form that enables a quality score for each study. Finally, each study is typically analysed to estimate an 'effect size' indicating the strength of the intervention in each instance in which it was used.

In meta-analyses these effect sizes are then combined, using a weighting by sample size, to arrive at an overall (i.e. average) effect size and a statistical test of significance. It is at this point that the second 'systematic' emerges – a systematic statistical averaging of all the individual effects into an overall unbiased estimate. This is the whole point of the exercise: to determine whether a particular intervention affected a particular outcome. One example might be the effect of PBL on national licensing examinations.(78) Another is the recent BEME review of the predictive validity of undergraduate assessment instruments predicting licensing examination performance.(79)

Problems with systematic reviews

While wonderful in theory, there are at least three problems with trying to put these methods into practice.

Quality of the evidence

It seems that an inevitable consequence of the systematic review is a note of despair about the poor quality of the studies, based on the number of criteria that were not fulfilled. It has almost reached the point of there being a standard disclaimer in systematic reviews: 'The authors take no responsibility for any personal damage resulting from the quality of the studies that went into this review.'

This disparaging of the quality of published papers seems a bit strange because, for the most part, the articles had all satisfied peer reviewers. Either the peer reviewers are not very good at their jobs, or they are basing their judgements on different criteria altogether than the systematic reviewers. We sense the latter; as editors, we rarely judge the worth of a paper by the number of methodological criteria it fulfilled(80,81) and, indeed, Bordage(82) has shown the same to be the case on the part of peer reviewers. Just as the OSCE literature has found that global judgements are superior to checklists, Bordage's examination of the peer-review process suggests that the methodological components of a paper provide a poor indication of its overall value. Further, a preoccupation with quality might be tempered by the finding of Lipsey and Wilson,(24) mentioned earlier, that there was no relation between judged study quality and treatment effect, nor did randomised trials yield systematically different treatment effects than non-randomised studies.

Heterogeneity of the outcome
While the use of effect sizes enables putting various measures *of the same construct* on a common metric, it appears that systematic reviews are rarely able to reduce the outcome to one measure such as examination performance. In fact, in the recent review of learning portfolios(83) there was commonality among studies only at the broad level of classification (e.g. learning versus assessment) and no attempt was made to try to average outcomes across studies. Instead, the review reported findings along the lines of 'two studies reported that portfolios contributed to reflective learning'.

Undoubtedly, the most careful and comprehensive approach to systematic reviews in medical education has been mounted by the BEME group. Very careful quality control is exercised at every step of the process, and the group of collaborators goes to enormous lengths to ensure consistent quality. The first review, of high-fidelity simulation, by Issenberg *et al.*(84) began with over 600 abstracts that were then reduced to 109 studies for detailed analysis. The review concluded: 'Heterogeneity of research designs, educational interventions, outcome measures, and time frame precluded data synthesis using meta-analysis.' The authors then went on to describe the conditions that led to effective use of simulation. This approach, where a systematic search on many abstracts yields a small number of suitable studies, which in turn are combined with too many potential outcomes to permit any quantitative synthesis or meta-analysis, emerges as the norm for these reviews.

Low yield of studies
Systematic reviews can be enormously labour-intensive, primarily because the yield of useful articles is so low. Examples drawn from the BEME monographs can be given. The study of early community experience(85) catalogued 23 outcomes from 73 studies (out of 6832 abstracts) and no quantitative synthesis was possible. Perhaps the worst example of 'needle in a haystack' was the synthesis of interprofessional education(86) that began with 10 495 abstracts and ended with 12 worthy of detailed review. Interestingly,

a hand search added a further nine, despite beginning with only 46. Again, the results consisted of counts of what kind of intervention led to what kind of result. To avoid some of these problems, while admittedly creating others, many scholars choose to engage in generating critical rather than systematic reviews. In the following section we will strive to compare the two strategies, highlighting strengths and weaknesses of both approaches.

Critical reviews

In our initial discussion of the research question, we described the characteristics of a good literature review, namely that it represents a critical synthesis of a literature, identifying what is well established, what is only poorly understood and what remains to be understood. It may, when done well, bring together several disparate literatures and, as a result, offer a new perspective. It should *not* end up as a chronological 'blow-by-blow' account, with one paragraph per study and no real synthesis. There is no pretence in a critical review that the cited literature represents all the relevant literature in the field, so there may be less of a tendency to provide a one-paragraph summary of every related study; the author is bound by an unwritten moral code to represent the various perspectives fairly, but that is all.

To our knowledge little is written about how to go about such reviews, which is somewhat strange, as there is little doubt that some of these papers become, over time, the 'citation classics' of the field. Far and away the most cited papers in the area of PBL are three old chestnuts: Albanese and Mitchell,(87) Vernon and Blake(78) and Norman and Schmidt;(88) two of the three are critical reviews. What distinguishes a good critical review from a poor one? One expects that it has little to do with comprehensiveness or systematicity. Instead, the cited reviews appear to be those that present unique perspectives and marshal evidence convincingly to support the claims. Rather than scouring the nooks and crannies of the literature for every paper that is relevant to a narrow question, successful critical reviewers explore a variety of literature, mining for gold nuggets that often alter the way the community fundamentally defines the question.

In practice, critical and systematic reviews in education have often led to similar conclusions, in part because, while no one would debate that the goal of systematicity – to eliminate bias in the data one draws on – is laudable, to some extent the mantle of systematicity is just a guise of credibility. If one cannot combine the findings in some systematic way as a result of heterogeneity of outcomes to the point of having to describe each study independently, then the only thing separating systematic reviews from critical narrative reviews is the amount of time and resources spent searching for information. Given the typical low yield of studies, it is questionable whether or not that effort proves a worthy use of resources or serves as a key arbiter of quality. Again, this is not meant to imply that systematicity is bad or that all systematic reviews have been thoughtless – the examples used in this chapter make it clear that is not the case. It is to say though, that too often the claim of systematicity is applied thoughtlessly as a criterion by which quality is judged, when in fact true advances in the field are as often gained from critical syntheses of diverse ideas rather than systematicity itself.(89) That said, we in no way mean to imply that systematic reviews are not useful when done well as there are many exemplary examples in the literature.(90,91)

Problems with critical reviews

Despite the arguments expounded above, critical reviews too are not without their own problems.

Author bias

The strengths of critical reviews are also their weaknesses. When literature is marshalled to support a unique perspective, there is the vague disquiet that the selected literature may be, consciously or unconsciously, biased in favour of the claim. The author is under no explicit mandate to present all the evidence for and against, only to be unbiased in his or her conclusions. But such a stricture may not be realistic; if we were aware of our biases, we may well not be biased, so it is not uncommon for two critical reviews to come to diametrically opposite conclusions. Such is the fodder for academic debate.

Biased sampling of literature

A second problem is that if the purpose of the review is really to obtain a best estimate of the value of something like the predictive value of standardised aptitude tests or the effect of PBL on outcomes such as standardised examinations, or the effectiveness of faculty development programmes in changing faculty teaching competence, the synthesis methods used in critical reviews, if used at all, are primitive at best. They often reduce to a summary like '22/30 studies showed a positive effect'. That is precisely what systematic reviews do best – sometimes.

Finally, critical reviews can also assume a mantle of academic dithering. Such reviews rarely conclude with a final 'it works/it does not work', instead providing far more nuanced discussion than purely systematic reviews, with an inevitable self-fulfilling call for more research. Again, however, we would emphasise that where one might call this a weakness we consider it a strength, as this sort of academic dithering can enable much more refined appreciation for issues than was available in the field before the review was generated.

Summary

In the examples cited, the distinction between systematic review and critical review becomes vanishingly small. While each type of review may be stimulated by differing goals (Does it work? versus How does it work?), inevitably, as the systematic review identifies subgroups and subgoals, the additional knowledge is more of the form of revealing how different circumstances may influence the results. And while the critical review may be directed at advancing a theory, the reality is that there are very few theories in this field, so it is more likely that it will be focusing on the various things that may influence the effect under review. So it would seem that the ecology of the

domain may be forcing a convergence between the two approaches.

Discussion

For about three decades, educational research has been embroiled in the 'qualitative–quantitative' debate, to the detriment of both. A careful read of this chapter and Chapter 25 on qualitative methods, reveals that there is probably as much divergence in goals, design and methods within each tradition as there are differences between the two camps.

Is there any way to resolve the differences? The insight was, we believe, again provided by Lee Cronbach. In his 'Two disciplines' paper that we described earlier,(75) he advocated a search for aptitude–treatment interactions – using more complex quantitative methods such as analysis of covariance to relate aspects of the individual learner (aptitudes) to curriculum design factors (treatments). As one recent example, a series of studies of learning anatomy from a computer showed that students with high spatial ability had a small benefit from being presented views of an animated specimen at multiple angles, but that students with poor spatial ability were seriously handicapped by multiple views.(92) The current use of methods such as confirmatory factor analysis and structural equation models is a logical extension of this aptitude–treatment interaction approach. However, after two decades, failures have far exceeded successes, and in our view, the more powerful methods now in vogue follow in this tradition, yielding little in the way of substantive theoretical explanation.

Cronbach's resolution in a later paper(93) was to abandon attempts at greater experimental control in favour of more careful observation:

> '[This paper will] explore the consequences of attempting to establish in psychological experimentation, empirical generalisations in a world in which most effects are interactive. While the two scientific disciplines of experimental control and systematic correlation are designed to answer pre-stated formal questions, the time has come for more open-ended, inquisitive investigation that will more fully explore the richness of scientific reality.'

Another way to think about the intent of an individual study is a categorisation developed by Schmidt,(94) who described three goals for studies.

- *Description*, which focuses on the first step of the scientific method – observation. An approach is described, but no comparison is performed.
- *Justification* represents the opposite extreme, where the goal is to justify a particular approach by a careful experimental study showing it is superior to some alternative. The problem, as identified by Cook *et al.*,(95) is that without sufficient theory specification the results may have limited application.
- *Clarification* studies are modelled on the scientific method, beginning with observation, proceeding to careful theory building, testing and elaboration.

In an initial study, Schmidt found that 64% of 850 medical education studies reviewed were description studies, a further 29% were justification studies and only 7% were directed at clarification.(94) Cook *et al.* looked at a different database of experimental studies only and found that 16% were description, 72% justification and 12% clarification.(95) However desirable theory-based research is, it is a small minority of educational research studies. We hope that by drawing attention to these issues, this chapter may, in some small way, help to redress the balance.

References

1 Dolmans D (2003) The effectiveness of PBL: the debate continues. Some concerns about the BEME movement. *Medical Education.* **37**: 1129–30.

2 Norman G (2002) Research in medical education: three decades of progress. *British Medical Journal.* **324**: 1560–2.

3 Bordage G (2007) Moving the field forward: going beyond quantitative-qualitative. *Academic Medicine.* **82**: S126–8.

4 Meltzoff J (1998) Research questions and hypotheses. In: *Critical Thinking about Research*, pp. 13–30. American Psychological Association, Washington, DC.

5 Bordage G (2009) Conceptual frameworks to illuminate and magnify. *Medical Education.* **43**: 312–9.

6 Eva KW and Lingard L (2008) What's next? A guiding question for educators engaged in educational research. *Medical Education.* **42**(8): 752–4.

7 Albert M, Hodges B and Regehr G (2007) Research in medical education: balancing service and science. *Advances in Health Sciences Education: Theory and Practice.* **12**: 103–15.

8 Cook D, Beckman TJ and Bordage GE (2007) Quality of reporting of experimental studies in medical education: a systematic review. *Medical Education.* **41**: 737–45.

9 Popper K (1959) *The Logic of Scientific Discovery.* Hutchinson and Co., London.

10 Norman GR (1999) The adult learner: a mythical species. *Academic Medicine.* **74**: 886–9.

11 Regehr G (2010) It's NOT rocket science: rethinking our metaphors for research in health professions education. *Medical Education.* **44**(1): 31–9.

12 Stokes DE (1997) *Pasteur's Quadrant: Basic Science and Technological Innovation.* Brookings Institution Press, Washington, DC.

13 Cook TD and Campbell DT (1979) *Quasi-Experimentation: Design and Analysis for Field Settings.* Rand McNally, Chicago, IL.

14 Papadakis MA, Teherani A, Banach MA *et al.* (2005) Disciplinary action by medical boards and prior behavior in medical school. *New England Journal of Medicine.* **353**: 2673–82.

15 Hojat M, Paskin DL, Callahan CA *et al.* (2007) Components of postgraduate competence: analyses of thirty years of longitudinal data. *Medical Education.* **41**: 982–9.

16 Rose G (2001) Sick individuals and sick populations. *International Journal of Epidemiology.* **30**: 427–32.

17 Norman GR (2003) RCT = results confounded and trivial. *Medical Education.* **37**: 582–4.

18 Schuwirth LW and van der Vleuten CP (2006) Challenges for educationalists. *British Medical Journal.* **333**: 544–6.

19 Norman GR, Eva KW and Schmidt HG (2005) Implications of psychology-type theories for full curriculum interventions. *Medical Education.* **39**: 247–9.

20 Campbell DT and Stanley JC (1963) *Experimental and Quasi-Experimental Designs for Research on Teaching.* Rand McNally, Chicago, IL.

21 Goldacre B (2007) A kind of magic? (http://www.guardian.co.uk/science/2007/nov/16/sciencenews.g2; accessed 16 July 2013).

22 Norman GR and Shannon SI (1998) Effectiveness of instruction in critical appraisal (evidence-based medicine) skills: a critical appraisal. *Canadian Medical Association Journal.* **158**: 177–81.

23 Schmidt HG and Moust JHC (1995) What makes a tutor effective? A structural equations modeling approach to learning in problem-based curricula. *Academic Medicine.* **70**: 708–14.

24 Lipsey MW and Wilson DB (1993) The efficacy of psychological, educational, and behavioral treatment. Confirmation from meta-analysis. *American Psychologist.* **48**: 1181–209.

25 Meyer GJ, Finn SE, Eyde LD *et al.* (2001) Psychological testing and psychological assessment: a review of evidence and issues. *American Psychologist.* **56**: 128–65.

26 Woodward CA, Cohen M, Ferrier BM *et al.* (1989) Correlates of certification in family medicine in the billing patterns of Ontario general practitioners. *Canadian Medical Association Journal.* **141**: 897–904.

27 Koh GC-H, Khoo HE, Wong ML and Koh D (2008) The effects of problem-based learning during medical school on physician competency: a systematic review. *Canadian Medical Association Journal.* **178**: 34–41.

28 Colliver JA and Markwell SJ (2007) Research on problem-based learning: the need for critical analysis of methods and findings. *Medical Education.* **41**: 533–5.

29 Schmidt HG, Rotgans JI and Yew EH (2011) The process of problem-based learning: what works and why. *Medical Education.* **45**: 792–806.

30 Cook DA (2005) The research we still are not doing: an agenda for the study of computer-based learning. *Academic Medicine.* **80**: 541–8.

31 Ehrenberg RG, Brewer DJ, Gamoran A and Willms JD (2001) Does class size matter? *Scientific American.* **285**: 79–84.

32 Norman GR and Streiner DL (2007) *Biostatistics: The Bare Essentials* (3e). BC Decker, Hamilton, ON.

33 Larsen DP, Butler AC and Roediger HL (2008) Test-enhanced learning in medical education. *Medical Education.* **42**: 959–66.

34 Lurie SJ, Mooney CJ and Lyness JM (2009) Measurement of the general competencies of the accreditation council for graduate medical education: a systematic review. *Academic Medicine.* **84**: 301–9.

35 Whitcomb ME (2002) Research in medical education: what do we know about the link between what doctors are taught and what they do? *Academic Medicine.* **77**: 1067–8.

36 Bligh J (2003) Editorial. *Medical Education.* **37**: 184–5.

37 Colliver JA (2003) The research enterprise in medical education. *Teaching and Learning in Medicine.* **15**: 154–5.

38 Norman GR (2006) Outcomes, objectives and the seductive appeal of simple solutions. *Advances in Health Sciences Education.* **11**: 217–20.

39 Gruppen L (2007) Improving medical education research. *Teaching and Learning in Medicine.* **19**: 331–5.

40 Eva KW, Reiter HI, Trinh K, Wasi P, Rosenfeld J and Norman GR (2009) Predictive validity of the multiple mini-interview for selecting medical trainees. *Medical Education.* **43**(8): 767–75.

41 Tamblyn R, Abrahamowicz M, Dauphinee D *et al.* (2007) Physician scores on a national clinical skills examination as predictors of complaints to medical regulatory authorities. *Journal of the American Medical Association.* **298**: 993–1001.

42 Werner LS and Bull BS (2003) The effect of three commercial coaching courses on Step One USMLE performance. *Medical Education.* **37**: 527–31.

43 Cohen PA (1981) Student rating of instruction and student achievement: a meta-analysis of multisection validity studies. *Review of Educational Research.* **51**: 281–309.

44 Eva KW and Regehr G (2005) Self-assessment in the health professions: a reformulation and research agenda. *Academic Medicine.* **80**: S46–54.

45 Gordon MJ (1991) A review of the validity and accuracy of self-assessments in health professions training. *Academic Medicine.* **66**: 762–9.

46 Davis DA, Mazmanian PE, Fordis M *et al.* (2006) Accuracy of physician self-assessment compared with observed measures of competence: a systematic review. *Journal of the American Medical Association.* **296**: 1094–102.

47 Peterson LN, Eva KW, Rusticus SA and Lovato CY (2012) The readiness for clerkship survey: can self-assessment data be used to evaluate program effectiveness? *Academic Medicine.* **87**: 1355–60.

48 Levinson AJ, Weaver B, Garside S *et al.* (2007) Virtual reality and brain anatomy: a randomised trial of e-learning instructional designs. *Medical Education.* **41**: 495–501.

49 Cohen JJ (1988) *Statistical Power Analysis for the Behavioral Sciences.* Erlbaum, Hillsdale, NJ.

50 Colliver JA, Markwell SJ, Verhulst SJ and Robbs RS (2007) The prognostic value of documented unprofessional behavior in medical school records for predicting and preventing subsequent medical board disciplinary action: the Papadakis studies revisited. *Teaching and Learning in Medicine.* **19**: 213–5.

51 Swanson DB, Norman GR and Linn RL (1995) Performance based assessment: lessons from the professions. *Educational Research.* **24**: 5–11.

52 Harden RM and Gleeson FA (1979) Assessment of clinical competence using an objective structured clinical examination (OSCE). *Medical Education.* **13**: 41–54.

53 Streiner DL and Norman GR (2003) *Health Measurement Scales: A Practical Guide to Their Development and Use* (3e). Oxford University Press, Oxford.

54 Eva KW, Rosenfeld J, Reiter HI and Norman GR (2004) An admissions OSCE: the multiple mini-interview. *Medical Education.* **38**: 314–26.

55 Hodgson CS, Teherani A, Gough HG *et al.* (2007) The relationship between measures of unprofessional behavior during medical school and indices on the California Psychological Inventory. *Academic Medicine.* **82**: S4–7.

56 Mamede S and Schmidt HG (2004) The structure of reflective practice in medicine. *Medical Education.* **38**: 1302–8.

57 Kane MT (2006) Validation. In: Brennan RL (ed.) *Educational Measurement.* Praeger Publishers, Westport, CT.

58 Messick S (1989) Validity. In: Linn RL (ed.) *Educational Measurement,* pp. 103–4. Macmillan, New York.

59 Downing SM (2003) Validity on the meaningful interpretation of assessment data. *Medical Education.* **37**: 830–7.

60 Newble DI and Jaeger K (1983) The effect of assessments and examinations on the learning of medical students. *Medical Education.* **17**: 165–71.

61 Harasym PH, Woloschuk W, Mandin H and Brundin-Mather R (1996) Reliability and validity of interviewers' judgements of medical school candidates. *Academic Medicine.* **71**: S40–2.

62 Paul A (2004) *The Cult of Personality: How Personality Tests are Leading Us to Miseducate Our Children, Mismanage Our Companies, and Misunderstand Ourselves.* Free Press, New York.

63 Hodges B, Turnbull J, Cohen R *et al.* (1996) Evaluating communication skills in the OSCE format: reliability and generalizability. *Medical Education.* **30**: 38–43.

64 Hodges B, Regehr G, McNaughton N *et al.* (1999) OSCE checklists do not capture increasing levels of expertise. *Academic Medicine.* **74**: 1129–34.

65 Eva KW and Hodges BD (2012) Scylla or Charybdis? Can we navigate between objectification and judgement in assessment? *Medical Education.* **46**: 914–9.

66 Ramsey PG, Carline JD, Inui TS *et al.* (1989) Predictive validity of certification by the American Board of Internal Medicine. *Annals of Internal Medicine.* **110**: 719–26.

67 Norman GR (2004) The morality of medical school admissions. *Advances in Health Sciences Education.* **9**: 79–82.

68 Bargh JA and Chartrand TL (1999) The unbearable automaticity of being. *American Psychologist.* **54**: 462–79.

69 Wainer H (1976) Estimating coefficients in linear models: it don't make no nevermind. *Psychological Bulletin.* **83**: 213–7.

70 Jamieson S (2004) Likert scales: how to (ab)use them. *Medical Education.* **38**: 1217–8.

71 Glass GV and Stanley JC (1970) *Statistical Methods in Education and Psychology.* Prentice Hall, Englewood Cliffs, NJ.

72 Carifio J and Perla R (2008) Resolving the 50-year debate around using and misusing Likert scales. *Medical Education.* **42**: 1150–2.

73 Norman G (2010) Likert scales, levels of measurement, and the "laws" of statistics. *Advances in Health Sciences Education.* **15**: 625–32.

74 Wikipedia (2010) Bonferroni correction. (http://en.wikipedia.org/wiki/Bonferroni_correction; accessed 16 July 2013).

75 Cronbach LJ (1957) The two disciplines of scientific psychology. *American Psychologist.* **12**: 671–84.

76 Harden R, Grant J, Buckley G and Hart I (2000) Best evidence medical education. *Advances in Health Sciences Education.* **5**: 71–90.

77 Smith ML and Glass GV (1977) Meta-analysis of psychotherapy outcome studies. *American Psychologist.* **32**: 752–60.

78 Vernon DT and Blake RL (1993) Does problem-based learning work? A meta-analysis of evaluative research. *Academic Medicine.* **68**: 550–63.

79 Hamdy H, Prasad K, Anderson MB *et al.* (2006) BEME guide no. 5: predictive values of assessment measurements obtained in medical schools and future performance in practice. *Medical Teacher.* **28**: 103–16.

80 Eva KW (2009) Broadening the debate about quality in medical education research. *Medical Education.* **43**: 294–6.

81 Eva KW (2012) The state of science 2012: building blocks for the future. *Medical Education.* **46**: 1–2.

82 Bordage G (2001) Reasons reviewers reject and accept manuscripts: the strengths and weaknesses in medical education reports. *Academic Medicine.* **76**: 889–96.

83 Driessen E, van Tartwijk J, van der Vleuten C and Wass V (2007) Portfolios in medical education: why do they meet with mixed success? A systematic review. *Medical Education.* **41**: 1224–33.

84 Issenberg SB, McGaghie WC, Petrusa ER *et al.* (2005) Features and uses of high-fidelity simulation that lead to effective learning: a BEME systematic review. *Medical Teacher.* **27**: 10–28.

85 Dornan T, Littlewood S, Margolis S *et al.* (2006) How can experience in clinical and community settings contribute to early medical education? A BEME systematic review. *Medical Teacher.* **28**: 3–18.

86 Hammick M, Freeth D, Koppel I *et al.* (2007) BEME guide no. 9: a best evidence systematic review of interprofessional education. *Medical Teacher.* **29**: 735–51.

87 Albanese MA and Mitchell S (1993) Problem-based learning: a review of literature on its outcomes and implementation issues. *Academic Medicine.* **68**: 52–81.

88 Norman GR and Schmidt HG (1992) The psychological basis of problem-based learning. *Academic Medicine.* **67**: 557–65.

89 Eva KW (2008) On the limits of systematicity. *Medical Education.* **42**: 852–3.

90 Cook DA, Hatala R, Brydges R *et al.* (2011) Technology–enhanced simulation for health professions education: a systematic review and meta-analysis. *JAMA: The Journal of the American Medical Association.* **306**: 978–88.

91 Cook DA and West CP (2012) Conducting systematic reviews in medical education: a stepwise approach. *Medical Education.* **46**: 943–52.

92 Garg A, Norman GR, Spero L and Maheshwari P (1999) Do virtual computer models hinder anatomy learning? *Academic Medicine.* **74**: S87–9.

93 Cronbach LJ (1975) Beyond the two disciplines of scientific psychology. *American Psychologist.* **30**: 116–27.

94 Schmidt HG (2005) *Influence of research on practices in medical education: the case of problem-based learning*. Paper presented at the Association for Medical Education in Europe, Amsterdam, The Netherlands, September.

95 Cook DA, Bordage G and Schmidt HG (2008) Description, justification and clarification: a framework for classifying the purposes of research in medical education. *Medical Education*. **42**: 128–33.

Further reading

Bowling A (1997) *Research Methods in Health: Investigating Health and Health Services*. Open University Press, Philadelphia.

Chalmers A (1999) *What is this Thing Called Science?* (3e). Open University Press, Buckingham.

Norman GR, van der Vleuten CPM and Newble DI (eds) (2002) *International Handbook of Research in Medical Education* (vol. 7). Springer International Handbooks of Education, New York.

Norman GR and Streiner DL (2007) *Biostatistics: The Bare Essentials* (3e). BC Decker, Hamilton, ON.

Streiner D and Norman GR (2003) *Health Measurement Scales: A Practical Guide to Their Development and Use* (3e). Oxford University Press, Oxford.

26 Qualitative research in medical education: Methodologies and methods

Stella Ng¹, Lorelei Lingard², and Tara J Kennedy³

¹Centre for Faculty Development, St Michael's Hospital, Canada; Faculty of Medicine, University of Toronto, Canada
²Schulich School of Medicine & Dentistry, Western University, Canada
³Stan Cassidy Centre for Rehabilitation, Canada

KEY MESSAGES

- Qualitative research explores social, relational and experiential phenomena in their natural settings.
- Qualitative research methods can contribute to theory building and to the study of complex social issues in medical education.
- Qualitative research encompasses multiple research methodologies, including case study, grounded theory, phenomenology, hermeneutics, narrative inquiry and action research.

- Qualitative data collection methods and qualitative analysis strategies must be selected for their suitability to a particular research question and methodology.
- Principles of rigour, specific to qualitative research, have been developed and can be used as a framework on which to build a qualitative research study or in the appraisal of its quality.

Paradigms and purposes of qualitative research

What is qualitative research in medical education?

Qualitative researchers study social, relational and experiential phenomena in their natural settings. For questions about group interactions, social processes or human experience, a qualitative approach is appropriate. *How* and *what* questions are particularly suited for exploration through qualitative research (*see* Box 26.1).

The term 'qualitative research' encompasses a broad range of philosophical and theoretical traditions, methodologies and methods, which the following sections will take up in detail. Common to all qualitative approaches are some basic principles. Qualitative research explores the object of study within its natural environment, by observing and interacting with the people and places experiencing the phenomenon. Qualitative research seeks to understand and represent complexity, to offer a richly textured account of social or human phenomena. Also, qualitative research attends carefully to the role of context, to produce situated accounts that are anchored in space and time. As a consequence of these principles, the goal of qualitative research is the careful understanding of instances. It does not make claims to generalisability; rather, it values contextualised understanding and theory building. Qualitative research is frequently used to understand subjective experiences and perspectives; it can also be used to understand empirical networks or sequences of

activity, with potential to explicate tacit or hidden elements of such activity.

Origins of qualitative research in medical education

Qualitative research comes to medical education from the social sciences and humanities, from disciplines such as anthropology, sociology, education and history. At various points, each of these disciplines used medical education as a site for research shaped by their own disciplinary questions and theories. Now, medical education researchers use tools from these disciplines to explore questions arising in the domain of medical education.

According to Harris,(1) the importation of methods from these disciplines into medical education began in the 1980s amid calls for more prescriptive theory building to complement the dominant paradigm of controlled experiments. Interestingly, these calls persist as reviews of the medical education research field continue to identify a need for increased theory building and qualitative strategies of inquiry to grapple with complex social questions.(2,3)

Qualitative research paradigms

Discussions of qualitative research often begin with discussions of research paradigms. As Denzin and Lincoln(4) explain, paradigms are basic sets of beliefs that guide action; Harris describes them as 'cognitive road maps, taken-for-granted assumptions within communities of scholars'(1) that orient researchers towards meaning and the research endeavour. Paradigms encompass ontology

---

Understanding Medical Education: Evidence, Theory and Practice, Second Edition. Edited by Tim Swanwick.
© 2014 The Association for the Study of Medical Education. Published 2014 by John Wiley & Sons, Ltd.

BOX 26.1 Examples of qualitative research questions

- What is the nature and impact of social group interaction?
- How are decisions made in problem-based learning groups?
- How do team members learn from each other when they confront new situations?
- What do people think about an experience?
- How do medical students respond to professional dilemmas?
- How do paediatric residents approach 'difficult' patients?
- How does a social process work?
- How do international medical students acquire a sense of professional identity as residents in a Canadian programme?
- How do clinical teachers balance the duties of education and clinical care?

and epistemology. Ontology refers to the study of being and nature of existence and is linked to epistemology, which refers to the theory of knowledge. Ontology can be thought of as questions of 'what is' and epistemology as questions of 'what it means to know'.(5) For example, the ontology most commonly associated with medical research is realism, which assumes one true reality exists. Realism implies an epistemology of objectivism, which asserts that we can accurately and directly attain knowledge of the one true reality through perception. The most congruent paradigm for a realist–objectivist position, then, would be positivism, which attempts to empirically measure reality and asserts that it can, or more commonly today, post-positivism.(5)

Post-positivism, a common paradigm in medical education research, shares with positivism the belief that there is an objective reality that can be discovered if the correct research procedures are in place. What distinguishes post-positivism from positivism is the acknowledgement that complex human behaviour is shaped by individual motivations and cultural environments, and research must represent these complexities rather than elide them in search of a contextual 'essence' or truth. Irby's account of how clinical teachers make decisions about what to prioritise in their round exchanges with students represents the post-positivist paradigm in his search for the essence of teachers' decision-making while paying attention to the contextual and individual features that shape this process.(6)

Constructivism, another common paradigm in medical education research, departs from post-positivism in its acceptance of reality and meaning as relative, produced through the interaction between researcher and researched. Research in the constructivism paradigm acknowledges the subjectivity of the researcher, producing accounts of a social phenomenon that reflect the researcher's interaction with the phenomenon. Lingard's accounts of tension, collaboration and socialisation within operating room teams

provide an example of this approach, as she views team communication through her training as a rhetorician and blends this perspective with those of study participants and 'insider informants' engaged in the collaborative analysis process.(7–10)

Also becoming apparent in medical education research is work within the critical inquiry paradigm, which is identifiable by its goal of revealing power dynamics in studied phenomena and fostering empowerment through the careful description and analysis of these dynamics. Albert's account of tensions within the medical education research community uses critical theorist Bourdieu's theoretical notion of field to explore the configuration of power relations in this research community.(11)

Two less frequently discussed elements of paradigm worth mentioning are axiology and rhetorical structure.(12,13) Axiology refers to the place or role of values, and rhetorical structure to the use of language in 'writing up' the research. For example, a study drawing on feminist theory might be written in the first person and include explication of the researcher's own experience and position relative to the research, including explication of biases. In contrast, a study informed by a post-positivist paradigm may adopt language that is more in line with the objectivist scientific tradition, such as third person narration and passive voice.

Although contrasting examples are useful to highlight the nuances of each paradigm, the researcher's paradigm does not inflexibly dictate one's methodological choice. A thoughtful consideration of research question and paradigmatic position will guide the qualitative researcher in selecting the most appropriate methodology for inquiry. The best methodological approach for a particular study depends on the research question, the nature of the research setting and the objective of the research. These factors also determine what the best methods are. The selection of a well-aligned and well-justified paradigmatic position, methodological approach and methods relative to the research question is a primary marker of methodological rigour in qualitative research. This notion of 'best fit' is a more philosophically appropriate marker of quality and rigour in qualitative medical education research than a ranking based on a biomedical hierarchy of evidence.(14)

For a more detailed discussion of research frameworks and paradigms, see Chapter 24.

Relationship between qualitative and quantitative research

Historically, in medical education, the relationship between qualitative and quantitative research has tended to be represented as a dichotomy. A situation that probably arises from strong paradigmatic differences between researchers working within these two approaches. Experimentalists have tended to espouse a positivist belief system, thus the intent to control variables in order to see the essence of a phenomenon, and the use of statistical analyses to reveal and represent knowledge. By contrast, qualitative researchers in medical education have been more likely to adopt post-positivist, constructivist and critical world views.

There has been a gradual recognition that such polarisation is distorting and unhelpful and scholars have consistently urged the medical education community to reconsider this position; from Irby's invited address in 1990 [cited by Harris(1)] to Norman's editorial in 1998,(15) to Lingard's in 2006(16) and to O'Sullivan and Irby's plea to reframe faculty development research in 2011.(17) These calls emphasise the generative potential of considering qualitative and quantitative research depending on 'best fit' with purpose. Certain kinds of research questions are suited to certain paradigms, certain methodologies and methods,(18) and a dichotomous or hierarchical view may be severely limiting.

Together, the components of a research paradigm should be congruent with the methodology. So, one's ontology informs one's epistemology, which together shape one's paradigm, which guides their selection of methodology, which guides their use of particular methods. Methodology and methods are described next.

As in quantitative research, in qualitative research there is a distinction and synergistic relationship between methodology and method. Methodology refers to the theory of how inquiry should proceed, including assumptions, principles and procedures governing the use of particular methods.(19) Methods are the specific investigative tools or procedures used to gather and analyse data.(19)

Qualitative research methodologies

Qualitative research encompasses an eclectic group of research methodologies, which are linked by their common aim to explore social processes through interpretation or representation of qualitative data. These methodologies, or 'systems of inquiry', are, according to Denzin and Lincoln,(4) 'a bundle of skills, assumptions, and practices' that the researcher employs to generate and address their research questions. The various qualitative methodologies stem from different philosophical and/or theoretical perspectives, with resultant implications for the research process. Although there can be a significant overlap between them, and some qualitative methodologists may creatively and effectively employ combinations of methodologies, the following section provides a brief overview of seven major qualitative research approaches (summarised in Box 26.2), with examples of their contribution to medical education research.

Ethnography

The tradition of ethnography originates in the field of anthropology, in which a researcher would travel to study an 'exotic' tribe.(20,21) Current-day ethnography often rejects the traditional notion of a privileged researcher, and ethnographic studies are now more likely to occur in local subcultures (such as a medical school or an operating room) than in far-flung locations. However, ethnographic studies carry on the practice of long-term engagement in a study setting, and the collection, through observation and conversational interviews, of data that are analysed to understand the meaning inherent in the everyday activities of a particu-

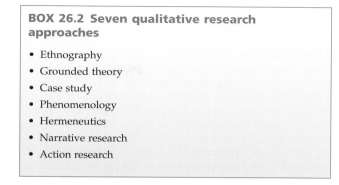

BOX 26.2 Seven qualitative research approaches

- Ethnography
- Grounded theory
- Case study
- Phenomenology
- Hermeneutics
- Narrative research
- Action research

lar social group.(22) There are a number of classic ethnographies in the domain of medical education, including Becker's *The Boys in White*,(23) a study of the nature of student culture in medical school, and Bosk's *Forgive and Remember*,(24) a study of the treatment of medical error in postgraduate surgical education. An example of a variant, critical approach to ethnography within medical education research is Mykhalovskiy's investigation of the social organisation of evidence-based medicine using institutional ethnograpy.(25)

Grounded theory

Grounded theory research explores social phenomena through the development of theoretical explanations that are 'grounded' in (i.e. derived from) the practical experience of study participants.(26) Grounded theory was developed by two sociologists, Glaser and Strauss, in the 1960s, to provide a systematic approach to the analysis of qualitative data that would live up to the standards of 'rigour' imposed by the quantitative paradigm and that would focus on theory generation rather than theory testing.(26) Since its inception, three main methodological schools of grounded theory have gained popularity:(27,28) a post-positivist or classicist approach,(26) pragmatist(29) and constructivist.(30) Key elements that are common across all 'schools' of grounded theory include:

- *iterative* study design (cycles of simultaneous data collection and analysis, in which the results of the ongoing data analysis inform the subsequent data collection)
- *purposeful or theoretical* sampling (purposeful selection of data sources for their ability to provide data that would confirm, challenge or expand an emerging theory)
- *constant comparison* approach to data analysis (through which incidents or issues of interest in the data are compared against other examples for similarities and differences)(31–33)
- *theoretical saturation or sufficiency* – the end point of data collection for a particular study, which occurs when no new codes or concepts are found in newly collected data; sufficiency has been proposed as the more appropriate term by some grounded theorists, particularly constructivists, who assert that saturation must be declared cautiously.(30,34)

In the domain of medical education research, Ginsburg has used grounded theory to develop a behavioural theory of professionalism.(35–40) Watling has used grounded theory to theorise feedback in medical education.(41)

Case study

Case study research involves an in-depth analysis of a 'bounded system' (a programme, an event, an activity, a process, a group, etc.).(42) The case study can have intrinsic value or can be used as a means of gaining understanding of a larger process.(43) Case study research has roots in sociological tradition as well as in the medical case report.(42) One hallmark of case study methods is triangulation, which is the use of multiple data collection tools or data sources to gain rich insight into the study phenomenon from multiple perspectives (*see* Principles of rigour, below). An example of a qualitative case study in medical education is Perley's study of a group of primary care physicians to explore their use of the 'curbside consultation' with colleagues as a continuing education tool.(44)

Phenomenology

Phenomenology arose early in the 20th century from philosophical reflections on consciousness and perception. Phenomenological research aims to understand the essence of a social phenomenon from the perspective of those who have experienced it.(45) Phenomenology with a descriptive intent involves the 'bracketing' (or putting aside) of the researcher's own preconceptions and perspectives in order to understand the 'lived experience' of the research participants.(45) Phenomenological studies often involve an in-depth exploration of the experiences of a relatively small number of individuals. Bearman has used phenomenology to explore the experiences of medical students during interactions with virtual patients.(46)

Hermeneutics

The term hermeneutics historically refers to the interpretation of biblical texts. In the domain of qualitative research, hermeneutics uses the lived experience of participants as a means of understanding their political, historical and sociocultural contexts.(47) Hermeneutic analysis involves a cyclical process called the 'hermeneutic circle': movement back and forth between the consideration of the meaning of individual parts of a data set and the meaning of the whole text.(48) Addison has explored how medical residents cope with their training through a hermeneutic approach.(49)

Narrative research

Narrative research stems from the ancient practice of storytelling as a method of communicating, arranging and interpreting human experience. Narrative inquiry is a qualitative approach that 'solicits and analyzes personal accounts as stories',(50) using these stories as a means of understanding or making sense of a particular experience or situation. Narrative analysis seeks meaning in the content, structure, context and relational aspects of a story.(51) Narrative methods have been promoted as an educational tool for teaching empathy and communication skills to medical students,(52) but are also being used to address research questions in medical education. Ventres has used narrative case reports of patient interviews conducted by residents to compare differences between patients' and physicians' perspectives.(53)

Action research

Action research has its roots in the social activism movements of the mid-20th century. Key principles of action research are the explicit aim of producing social change through the research process and the direct engagement of research participants in the research process.(54) Action research classically occurs through sequential cycles of planning a change, implementing the change while observing the process and reflecting on the consequences of the change.(55) Participants collaborate with researchers to construct the results of the research and implement social change. An action research approach was employed successfully in the design and implementation of a new general practice curriculum in Dundee, Scotland.(56)

Qualitative research methods

Qualitative research studies are carried out through a set of tools for data collection and analysis. In the following section, methods for data collection and approaches to data analysis will be reviewed separately. This separation of data collection from analysis is somewhat artificial in qualitative research for two reasons. First, many qualitative studies employ an iterative study design,(1) in which cycles of data collection and analysis occur simultaneously. In an iterative research process, preliminary analysis of data collected early in the study process affects decisions about how to go about the next phase of data collection by revealing questions that require clarification or new ideas that require further exploration in subsequent data collection and analysis cycles.(26) The second way in which data collection and analysis are linked in qualitative research practice is the way in which the choice of data collection methods necessarily informs the choice of the analytical approach and vice versa. For example, an exploration of the educational impact of the choice of language used during case presentations (*see* Discourse analysis section) requires access to audio-recorded data that can be transcribed for analysis. For the sake of clarity, in this chapter, data collection methods (including interviews, focus groups, observations and assembly of textual documents) and data analysis methods (including thematic analysis and discourse analysis) are considered separately.

General questions relating to ethics have been dealt with in Chapter 24, but particular ethical issues arise in the collection and analysis of qualitative data. These include both procedural ethics (how the research is conducted to protect research participants from harm) and situational ethics [how the researcher conducts himself or herself in what Guillemin and Gillam call 'ethically important moments'(57)]. Reflexivity is encouraged in qualitative research; it is a way to identify, articulate and consider the influences shaping research.(58) It is asserted as a sensitising concept researchers can use as they negotiate ethical

BOX 26.3 FOCUS ON: Ethical issues in qualitative research

Subjectivity of the researcher:

- Who are you in relation to your participants?
- What power dynamics are inherent in your relationship to your research subject and participants?
- How can these be managed appropriately to safeguard confidentiality and anonymity, and to avoid harm?

Emotionality of research participation:

- Will your research provoke powerful emotions in participants sharing their stories and experiences?
- How can you provide appropriate support and negotiate the evolving balance between harms and benefits in individual research interactions?

Minimal disclosure:

- Have you used minimal disclosure in your informed consent process (offering generic rather than specific study information to help minimise observer effect in field observations)? Such studies must include a mechanism for full disclosure when appropriate, and the ability to exclude data if participants decline participation following full disclosure.

BOX 26.4 HOW TO: Choose a data collection tool

Consider a hypothetical research programme about professionalism in medical students. The following potential research questions are matched with an appropriate data collection tool.

1 How do medical students' characterise professional behaviour in themselves and other members of the interdisciplinary health-care teams?
   In-depth interviews could provide a rich understanding of the students' conceptualisations of professional behaviour in multiple contexts, derived from detailed descriptions of relevant personal experience.

2 What are medical students' impressions of the professional behaviour of their clinical supervisors?
   Focus groups could provide an affirming environment where the accounts of other students' similar experiences might promote disclosure of relevant anecdotes. Discussion between students could make evident the range of relevant experience.

3 Do patient-care discussions on medical teaching teams promote professionalism in novice physicians?
   Observations of case presentations or teaching rounds could provide 'real-life' data that would permit analysis of the language used by medical students and their supervisors.

4 What messages about professionalism are being conveyed through the clinical evaluations of medical students?
   Textual analysis of the narrative comments on clinical evaluation forms could provide insight into the types of behaviour that are being promoted through the evaluation process.

tensions that may arise in their interactions with participants in the field (*see* Box 26.3).

Data collection methods

The various qualitative research methodologies have in common a set of data collection tools. Although certain qualitative approaches are classically associated with particular data collection or analysis methods (e.g. ethnography with participant observation or hermeneutics with document analysis), contemporary qualitative researchers commonly choose from the available methods the one(s) that is (are) best suited to address the research question at hand (*see* Box 26.4).(3)

Interviews

Individual interviews are probably the most familiar and the most often used form of data collection in qualitative medical education research.(1,59) Interviews provide access to participants' personal perspectives and relevant experiences on an unlimited number of topics.(60) The qualitative interview standard is the 'in-depth interview',(60) which provides a rich and detailed exploration of a research question and generally lasts between 45 minutes and a few hours.(61) Qualitative research interviews often follow a 'semi-structured' format.(59) The semi-structured interview is guided by a predetermined set of open-ended questions, but the researcher and participant are free to pursue additional relevant topics as they arise (*see* Box 26.5 for a sample interview script). Qualitative interviews are usually audiotaped and later transcribed to facilitate analysis, but

BOX 26.5 Sample semi-structured interview script

Research question: How do medical students characterise professional behaviour in themselves and other members of interdisciplinary health-care teams?

1 Could you give me an example of a time when you acted professionally? *(prompt for rich contextual details)* What is it about this behaviour that was professional? *(elicit further examples as appropriate, for this and all subsequent questions)*

2 Could you give me an example of a time when you acted unprofessionally? What is it about that behaviour that was unprofessional?

3 Could you give me examples of times when your medical student colleagues acted professionally or unprofessionally?

4 Could you give me examples of time when a nurse working with your team acted professionally? Unprofessionally? *(repeat question for other members of the health-care team: therapists, social workers, staff physicians, etc.)*

5 What, in your understanding, are the important elements of professional behaviour for a medical student? For a nurse? For a physiotherapist? *(repeat for other relevant members of the health-care team)*

recent advances in analysis software allow analysis directly from a digital audio or video recording.

The main disadvantage of the interview method of data collection is the fact that the information provided is filtered through the memory of the participant and is influenced by the social context of the interview.(62) Interview researchers must be careful to avoid leading questions (consider, for example, the potential difference in responses to the questions 'What barriers to the mentorship process have you encountered?' and 'What have your experiences with the mentorship process been like?'). Researchers must also attend to the power dynamics of the interview. For example, candid opinions from medical students about their experiences during clerkship are unlikely in an interview conducted by the clerkship director.

Focus groups

Focus groups have recently become well known as a marketing research tool, but they have a long history in the domain of social sciences research. Focus groups are sessions involving 4–12 participants and a moderator or facilitator who guides the group discussion of a topic relevant to the research question.(63) Focus groups provide access to multiple stories and diverse experiences in an efficient manner. More importantly, focus groups provide a dynamic and interactive exchange that can stimulate exploration of contrary opinions, reflection on group norms and common practices and exposure of taken-for-granted values.(64) Like individual interviews, focus group discussions often follow a semi-structured format and are audio-recorded and transcribed for analysis. The focus group moderator also records notes on group dynamics and interactions.

Researchers using focus groups must consider whether their topic would benefit from exploration in the synergistic and dynamic focus group format (e.g. some deeply personal topics might be more safely or productively explored in an individual interview). Attending to power dynamics is also critical in focus group methodology: one influential, opinionated group member can monopolise the discussion.(63)

Focus groups have been useful in exploring medical education questions such as the ethical implications of providing medical education in public and private hospital settings.(65)

Observation

Observation of study participants as they go about their regular activities can provide powerful insights into social processes. Researchers conducting observations have access to data on what participants do and not just on what they recall or say they do.(66) Qualitative researchers conducting observations make records called 'field notes' (*see* Box 26.6 for an illustrative example), which can be structured to capture details such as the content of conversations, the context of discussions, the participants and intended audience for relevant comments and the nonverbal nuances that accompany these interchanges.(67) Observations are sometimes accompanied by audio recording of 'naturalistic' conversations, which are later transcribed for analysis.

BOX 26.6 Sample field note

Research question: Do patient-care discussions on medical teaching teams promote professionalism in novice physicians?

Reflective notes*	Observation notes* Morning rounds, 31 Jan, ward 5C nursing station Present: AP, MS1, JR, SR, CN
MS2 is flustered, out of breath AP – good natured sarcasm MS2 doesn't appear upset by the comment Note respect for patient through use of name rather than diagnosis	MS2 arrives 5 minutes after rounds have started AP: Nice of you to join us! (laughter) MS2: Sorry, I ran into the asthmatic's mom in the hall – she wanted to know about the chest x-ray AP: You mean J's mum . . . MS2: Right AP: Did you tell her? MS2: Yeah, that it was clear. AP: Thanks . . .

*Two-column format is often used to facilitate recording of observation notes (containing details of the observed events) and reflective notes (containing the researcher's comments about the context and process of the observation, as well as emerging analytical ideas).

Abbreviations used to distinguish participants without identifying personal information: AP = attending physician, MS = medical student, JR = junior resident, SR = senior resident, CN = charge nurse

---

Observational researchers must deal with 'observer effect', which is the fact that the presence of the observer has an impact on the behaviours of study participants. There are a number of ways to deal with observer effect.(66) Some researchers will spend long periods of time in the field to allow participants to become accustomed to their presence. Others will not reveal the specific focus of their observations to prevent participants from altering specific behaviours (e.g. a researcher might obtain consent to observe all clinical teaching in an intensive care unit without revealing to participants that the research question related specifically to the teaching of technical skills).(68) Still, others will take care to document evidence of the impact of their presence and then reflect on and write about the significance of this impact on their results.

Another consideration in observational research is the likelihood that relevant data will be obtained. Observations are a useful tool for gathering data about common events and activities, but they are inefficient when the event in question is uncommon or difficult to predict. For example, observations of teaching clinics would be an inefficient way to collect data about failing students if only one or two students fail their clinical rotations each year.

Observational research has a long tradition in medical education. Observational researchers in medical education, as in other fields, must decide to what degree they will participate in the activities around them. The term 'non-participant observation' has been used to signify an observer who remains uninvolved in the activities of their study participants, taking the role of a passive observer. Stern used non-participant observation of internal medicine teaching teams to investigate the hidden ethics curriculum being taught on the wards.(69) Observational research in the ethnographic tradition takes the form of 'participant observation', in which the researcher becomes fully engaged in the daily activities of the study participants: Sinclair, a sociologist from London, enrolled in medical school and completed a medical degree as he conducted his ethnographic research.(70)

Assembly of textual documents

In the domain of medical education, a myriad of documents is used and created on a daily basis, many of which can yield important insights into educational processes. Sources of text for analysis include course curricula, assignments and examinations, student and faculty evaluations, clinical notes and policy documents. More recently, texts from websites, email correspondence and even digital images and video have been included in qualitative analyses.(71) Analysis of pre-existing documents can be a quick and inexpensive data collection method, and because they were created for purposes other than research, the content of these data is not influenced by the research process.(72) Assembly of textual documents, however, does not allow the researcher to take full advantage of the powerful qualitative process of iterative inquiry (see above), in which ongoing analysis informs the data collection process because the data collection occurs one step prior to the analysis. However, analysis of one type of collected document may point to another as potentially useful for the research.

Perhaps the most common use of textual documents for qualitative analysis in medical education is the analysis of documents produced as course assignments by students. For example, Olney analysed written 'experience summaries' created by medical student participants in a community service project to explore learning outcomes.(73)

Data analysis methods

Qualitative data analysis is the process of making sense of a qualitative data set. As previously emphasised, qualitative data analysis does not often mean sifting through hundreds of pages of text in one sitting, but is rather an ongoing process of reading, reflecting on and questioning the meaning of the data as they are collected. Qualitative data analysis can be conducted individually or as part of a research team that analyses as a group or meets to compare and discuss results of individual analytical work.

Although the different qualitative approaches involve somewhat different analytical procedures, there are some basic processes that are common to most qualitative analyses. The most common of these is coding. Coding is a process of sorting or organising the data into categories representing similar trends.(26)

The first step in the coding process is the selection of the unit of analysis. For example, analysis of medical student interviews about professionalism might involve coding for the settings in which professional lapses occurred, or for types of professional behaviour or for specific words or phrases used by participants to describe unprofessional acts. Coding for more than one of these different units of analysis might occur over time. As the data are being sorted into categories or codes, names or labels are created for the codes that describe the essence of the category, and memos or reflective notes are written to document the process of the analysis and record reflections and analytical ideas as they arise. Qualitative software can be used as a data management tool to keep track of the coding process as it proceeds, but the cognitive work of categorising data, identifying trends and interpreting meaning is still done by the researcher(s).

The specific approaches to data analysis in qualitative research are wide ranging. They are illustrated below in broad clusters of approaches to thematic analysis and approaches to discourse analysis.

Thematic analysis

The most commonly used qualitative analysis approach in the domain of medical education is the organisation of data according to topics, ideas or concepts, often called themes. Variations of thematic analysis are used in many of the qualitative approaches, and a number of different systems of thematic analysis have been developed [e.g. content analysis(74) and constant comparative analysis].(26,32) The basic process of thematic analysis is to identify instances in the data set that are similar in concept. As further related examples are identified, a progressively rich understanding of the concept is developed, and as other important concepts are identified in the data, the relationships between concepts or themes are explored. The set of themes can then be used for description, theory development or interpretation (*see* Interpretation, below). Thematic analysis has been used to explore many complex issues in medical education, e.g. Burack's study of the process of medical students' decision-making on specialty choice.(75)

It is important to note that the manner and extent to which thematic analysis is closely tied to the data or abstracted beyond depends on the methodological approach. For example, in constructivist grounded theory, initial codes are at the level of very concrete and representative of the data. As coding progresses, codes should become progressively more conceptual and abstract, with multiple initial codes being clustered or categorised together to form a broader conceptual code or theme, which will eventually be incorporated into the developed theoretical model.(30) Contrastingly, in a post-positivist action research project, the development of theory is not imperative, but rather the grass-roots adoption of practices that will result in positive change in a local context. Themes may thus be useful at the level of description and identification of practical challenges and creative solutions.(76)

Discourse analysis

Discourse analysis is an approach to qualitative research that analyses data at the level of language. Discourse is a term meaning 'socially situated language'.(77) The aim of discourse analysis is to make explicit what is normally taken for granted about language use or to show what talking accomplishes in a particular social context. Discourse analysis is an umbrella term that references a number of different approaches to the analysis of socially situated language use. Some discourse analysts, often in the domains of linguistics or conversation analysis, work to understand the complex mechanisms and structures of social language. Others, in fields like sociolinguistics or critical discourse analysis, use talk as a source of evidence about social processes. In critical discourse analysis, a central concern is the explication of power relations, with analysis focusing on identification of that which is constructed as 'truth' within a particular discourse and how those truths, from a socio-historical perspective, came to be.(78) Discourse analysis has an extensive history in the study of physician–patient communication,(79) but has been more recently applied to the domain of medical education. Hekelman *et al.* conducted a discourse analysis to investigate the changes in language use in the teaching encounters of a physician–teacher who was enrolled in a peer-coaching programme intended to improve clinical teaching skills.(80,81)

Interpretation and writing

The final stage of qualitative analysis is the process of interpretation, or finding the pivotal meaning in a data set. Without interpretive work, qualitative research produces merely a catalogue of ideas or themes. Important as those ideas may be, qualitative studies that do not take the next step of exploring the meaning at an interpretive level have not fully exploited the power of qualitative research.

There are different approaches to interpretation in qualitative research. In some qualitative approaches, the production of a thick, rich description of a social phenomenon is the goal of the research process (e.g. phenomenology). In other approaches, the development of a novel theoretical explanation of a social process is the aim (e.g. grounded theory). In still other qualitative approaches, the meaning of a data set is considered through the lens of pre-existing theory, such as feminist, rhetorical or Marxist theory.

The process of 'writing up' has been posited as an important tool in the toolkit of methods that qualitative researchers employ.(82) In a constructivist paradigm, writing can be considered a part of the interpretive inquiry process at the stage of coding, when memos are written by researchers to document the analytical process and associated reflective thinking as it unfolds. These memos, iteratively refined, may ultimately lead to the published written form of the qualitative work, and the act of memo writing is thus an intrinsic part of the interpretive inquiry process.(83)

Principles of rigour

Qualitative researchers both within and outside the domain of medical education have sought to articulate criteria for judging the quality of a qualitative report. Journals have published papers with checklists,(84–87) and qualitative leaders have offered overarching concepts such as 'trust-worthiness',(88) 'utility'(89,90) and authenticity.(91) Position papers on the state of medical educational research assert a need for education and attention to rigour in qualitative research.(92,93)

Specific methodologies will often develop and suggest their own methodology-specific quality criteria. For example, in constructivist grounded theory, Charmaz(83) asserts four main criteria for rigour for her constructivist approach to grounded theory: credibility, originality, resonance, and usefulness. In phenomenology, a hallmark quality criterion is termed the 'phenomenological nod', which refers to the resonance of the research findings with the reader's own experience, such that the reader might nod his/her head in recognition.(94)

While there is growing debate about the politics of such criteria and their feasibility given the vast spectrum of activity housed within the term qualitative research,(95) this debate will not be taken up here. Rather, this section outlines and illustrates, using positive examples, some basic principles of rigour to assist the newcomer in their appreciation of 'quality' in qualitative research. These principles are drawn from an extensive literature outlining guidelines for excellence in qualitative research. They can serve either as a framework for critical appraisal of qualitative research studies in the literature or as a starting point for considering how to design a qualitative project (*see* Box 26.7).

Sampling: Adequacy and appropriateness

Sampling in qualitative research is not just about 'how many' subjects to include in the study. Because qualitative research explores social and experiential phenomena, deciding whom to include and exclude is a critical step in the sampling logic. A social phenomenon often engages a wide variety of participants, and the researcher must justify

---

BOX 26.7 HOW TO: Achieve rigour in qualitative research

Adequacy and appropriateness of the sample:

- Are the right people/activities being sampled?
- Is the sample size likely to yield sufficient insight?
- Does disconfirming data need to be sought?
- Does theoretical or purposive sampling need to be conducted to further explore a developing or emerging concept or theme?

Quality of the data collected:

- Is the researcher's relationship to the participants/setting considered and explicated?
- Are interview and observation techniques likely to capture naturalistic data?

Clarity of the analysis process:

- Can the analysis be audited?
- Were member checking techniques or considerations of representation of participants appropriately considered?

their decisions about who best to observe/interview and who to leave out of their study boundaries. In some qualitative research methodologies, sampling refers not only to individuals but also to groups, concepts or documents.(83) In other qualitative research methodologies, e.g. in institutional ethnography, the term 'sampling' is a slight misnomer, because the goal of selecting participants or informants for the research is not to report on a particular population's perceptions and experiences, but rather to learn from the informants about the actualities, work processes, and social coordination of a particular phenomenon.(96) However, overall, qualitative research seeks to sample with the aim of achieving a robust exploration of the study questions.

The following questions can help in assessing the nature and extent of a study sample and evaluating its adequacy:

- Who?

  Can this sample provide data that answer the research question?

  Does the sample tap into all relevant participants in the research setting?
- Why?

  The choice of subjects must be justified, particularly if it does not represent all potentially relevant groups.
- How much?

  Sample size is not a matter of mere numbers: it is a matter of a thorough exploration of a culture or phenomenon. Often, such thoroughness is referred to as 'saturation', which means that data collection was considered complete when dominant themes/trends were recurrent and no new issues were arising from subsequent data collection. For instance, if after 10 interviews the researcher is not hearing anything new on the topic and recurrent themes are similar across interviews, saturation is said to have been reached, and data collection may be stopped using this rationale.

Sample estimations may be justified by reference to method-based estimates (e.g. in-depth interviews),(61) sampling strategy (e.g. theoretical, confirming/disconfirming, snowball)(97) or past research findings. Methods need to reflect sampling strategy (e.g. confirming/disconfirming sampling requires data analysis to proceed alongside data collection).

Box 26.8 illustrates a number of issues relating to sampling through an extended example. The nature of the sample is specified, and justification is provided for the types of participant sampled, which include various kinds of problem-based learning (PBL) tutors and students who may perceive conflict resolution from different perspectives. Sampling strategies are well articulated. There is no explicit reference to saturation, although reference to the dominant themes implies this. A range of perspectives in faculty and students appears to be explored, suggesting that triangulation is adequate.

Data collection: Authenticity and reflexivity

Because the qualitative researcher engages with their research participants in the collection of data, their role in the construction of meaning must be considered. As part of this, their relation to the participants, and the ways in

---

BOX 26.8 Example: Sampling

To explore how conflict resolution is achieved in problem-based learning (PBL) groups in medical school, we conducted both individual interviews and focus groups in the final month of the 1999–2000 academic year. Faculty interviews were conducted with 15 PBL tutors with at least 3 years' experience in the tutor role, to ensure an information-rich population. Purposeful sampling of faculty was employed, in order to include both non-clinical tutors ($n = 5$) and tutors from a variety of clinical disciplines, including medicine ($n = 4$), paediatrics ($n = 2$), psychiatry ($n = 1$) and surgery ($n = 3$). Students were sampled using two strategies: convenience sampling for the first six students interviewed, and then a confirming/disconfirming strategy in which interviewed students were asked to recommend potential participants who might: (a) have a similar experience/viewpoint to their own; and (b) have a divergent experience/viewpoint from their own. Using this sampling method, 11 additional students were recruited for voluntary participation. Following preliminary analysis of the interview transcripts, dominant themes were returned for discussion to three student focus groups comprised of both interview participants and new subjects.

---

which that relationship may shape the data that are being collected, requires careful thought both when deciding how to collect the data and when considering constraints on their interpretation. In educational settings, hierarchical relationships between researchers, who may be medical faculty members, and participants, who may be trainees, can have a distorting effect on the authenticity of the data collection. Participants in vulnerable positions may alter their observed behaviour or tailor their interview responses to safeguard themselves, to please the researcher or to advertise their membership in a group. Data collection processes must take such participant motives and actions into account, and researchers must both strategise to maximise the authenticity of their data and reflect on the ways in which the data are a construction of a research relationship in a hierarchical situation.

A common strategy used by qualitative researchers to maximise the quality of their data set is 'triangulation'. Triangulation is a term from cartography, which refers to the process of finding one's position on a map with reference to multiple other mapped positions. In a qualitative research study, the process of triangulation involves collecting data from multiple 'positions', so that the researcher can gain insight into the studied phenomenon from multiple perspectives, thus realising a more refined and comprehensive understanding by the end of the research. Triangulation requires the selection of the most relevant data sources and their integrated analysis, exploring how they confirm or disconfirm one another.

The following questions can help when considering the factors related to the quality of the data collected:

- Has the researcher considered his or her relation to the study setting and subjects?

- Are the interview script and processes non-leading?
  How was the script developed?
  Was it piloted?
  Were questions appropriate to capture relevant insights?
- Has the Hawthorne effect been considered?
  The Hawthorne, or observer, effect is seen when observed participants act differently from how they would act if the observer were not present.(98)
  Were mechanisms to minimise the Hawthorne effect used, e.g. prolonged engagement in the field, time taken to establish trust and rapport, and observer comportment (e.g. dressing like an insider)?
  Was there a process for recording/reflecting on the Hawthorne effect; e.g. field notes should record any references to observer presence, such as jokes made about being observed.
- Are data triangulated for maximal richness?
- Are complementary data sets collected?
- Are different forms of data/subject populations accessed?

Continuing our worked example, Box 26.9 illustrates how rigour is achieved in data collection. The relationship of the observers to participants has been considered, and steps have been taken to minimise the impact of the observer on the observed activities. Triangulation among methods (observations, interviews and case note analysis) and groups (students and faculty) will assist in creating a more in-depth portrait of this activity.

BOX 26.9 Example: Data collection

Eleven students and 10 faculty participated in the observational phase. Students included five women and six men, while faculty included five women and five men. Faculty experience ranged from those within their first 5 years of appointment ($n = 4$) and those with 20+ years of teaching experience ($n = 4$). Nineteen oral case presentations and the teaching exchanges related to them were observed and audio-recorded by trained research assistants during morning rounds. Observers had no prior relationship with the study participants. All participants were observed at least once, with repeat observations purposefully distributed across the sample to maximise its range and richness. A pocket-sized digital recording system and clip-on microphone worn by the observer were used to record data, and written field notes were compiled. Attempts to minimise the Hawthorne effect included the unobtrusiveness of the recording equipment, the duration of the observation phase (4 months) and the observers' abilities (through similar dress, age and comportment) to blend into the team on rounds. The notes that students created as they prepared for their case presentations were also collected, anonymised and transcribed. Individual interviews were conducted with all students and faculty, using open-ended questions and asking participants to comment on two case presentation scenarios derived from the observational data.

Data analysis: Clarity and audit trails

Although a challenging task, given its iterative nature, the analysis process in qualitative research should be described such that there is little or no 'mystique' surrounding how the researchers went from a pile of transcripts to a list of conceptual or thematic categories. This is not to suggest that there is no 'art' to qualitative analysis; there is, of course, and it includes serendipitous, imaginative links, just as it may in the analysis of experimental data. However, on the whole, the steps involved in the analysis process can be made explicit, and they should be both in a published manuscript and in the researchers' own journals, which can form the basis of an 'audit trail' to review their analytical journey. Reflexivity may be a helpful tool in the elaboration of what may otherwise seem like 'conceptual leaps'.(99) Questions to consider include the following:

- Is the analysis process well described?
  Can you tell what was done, by whom and how?
  Were insider experts used to verify coding samples?
- Were the following key aspects of analysis evident?
  Is 'constant comparison' evident?
  How were discrepancies resolved?
- Was an attempt made to engage participants or other stakeholders in reflecting on the results of the analysis?
  Was 'member checking' or 'return of findings', processes that provide participants or other informants an opportunity to weigh in on findings and interpretations, conducted? How?
- Was a software program used?
  Was its use appropriately described?

Box 26.10 and our worked example illustrate attempts to address these questions. The analytical process makes clear who conducted the analysis, the steps involved, the iterative process of data collection and analysis, the strategy in place for keeping an audit trail and the effort to engage participants in refining the analytical concepts.

As suggested earlier, some qualitative researchers would argue that the broad application of any of these proceduralist principles is a sub-optimal way of measuring quality. As Eakin argues, this approach can oversimplify and distort the complex and non-formulaic nature of qualitative inquiry. Instead, the notion of a paper's 'so what' factor – its ability to contribute to the understanding of a social phenomenon – is offered as the most important criterion.(100) Similarly, Sandelowski(90) has proposed a study's 'utility', its power to 'be of use' in the world, as another holistic principle for consideration when evaluating qualitative research. The utility of a study is related to how it is 'written up'. Charmaz(30) and Richardson(82) encourage researchers to attend closely to the aesthetics of the written product of qualitative research in order to maximise understanding and potential impact. These more holistic approaches build upon other principles, such as sampling and authenticity, while trying to avoid the pitfalls of a naïve, checklist approach to quality in qualitative research.

Role of theory

A final note regarding data analysis relates to theory. A beginner qualitative researcher should be aware that theory

BOX 26.10 Example: Data analysis

All interviews were audio-taped and fully transcribed. Initial themes were identified and developed by both authors in an iterative process of reading and re-reading transcripts. These initial themes were further explored, clarified and iteratively refined alongside ongoing data collection. Although *a priori* ideas existed in the form of literature review, research questions and the researchers' general familiarity with the topic, systematic attempts were made to be open to unexpected findings through searches for disconfirming examples, reflexive dialogue and reflexive memos. The development of themes and the framework for analysis were based on and driven by the original accounts and observations of the study's participants. Interviews and analyses, concurrently conducted, continued until no new themes emerged and data saturation was felt to be complete. The trustworthiness of the data was enhanced by the transparent process of analysis, the involvement of two independent researchers who read and compared ideas on the transcripts, and by searching for disconfirming evidence of the developing themes. An analytical journal was kept to record memos of ongoing analytical decisions, definitions of themes and researcher reflexivity. All interviewees were sent a copy of the primary analysis in order to elicit their comments on the representation of the data.

may play a differing role in the various stages of a qualitative study depending on the methodological approach. That is, depending on the underlying assumptions of a given paradigm and methodology, theory may be more or less involved from the initial phases of developing a research question and designing a study, to the final stages of analysing data and writing up findings. So, how does one know if theory has been appropriately employed? Generally, when assessing the rigour of a qualitative study with regard to the use (too much, or not enough?) of extant theory, the principle of 'best fit' applies again. Have the authors justified their approach in a cogent manner? If breaking from a methodological tradition or trend with regard to the use of theory, has the break been convincingly explained? If drawing from extant theory, have the authors reproduced more of the same, missing the opportunity to develop new knowledge? A sound understanding of the paradigmatic theories that underlie a chosen methodological approach is beneficial, and most qualitative researchers would argue, obligatory.(12,30) Debates about the role of theory relate to two main considerations: (i) the interpretation of data through a theoretical lens or frame and (ii) the production of theory through qualitative research.

On the one hand, qualitative research can effectively use theory to inform analysis and interpretation; when this is done well, the research ultimately moves beyond extant theories to produce new ways of thinking.(83) For example, in constructivist approaches to grounded theory, which of

course aim to produce theory, 'sensitising concepts' have been proposed to provide a theoretical lens for data analysis.(101) Grounded theory is often cited as an ideal methodology for process-based questions for which there is little extant theory. Forcing data into pre-conceived categories is strongly opposed by classicist grounded theorists, who suggest that constructivist approaches legitimate such forcing.(102) Yet, despite such resistance, a methodology is evolving to engage existing theory in the analysis process.(103) The use of 'sensitising concepts' in grounded theory may make way, if controversially, for grounded theorists to expand existing theory or make use of extant theory to understand similar processes in different contexts.

On the other hand, some methodologies aim neither to use theory to guide analysis nor to produce theory as an outcome of the research. For example, descriptive phenemonology aims to remain true to a rich description of the 'essence' of the lived experience of a particular phenomenon,(94) and institutional ethnography aims to explicate the 'actualities' of every day work without imposing theory to explain this work, and without producing theory (but rather, enabling social change) from the explication.(96,104)

As an interdisciplinary field, medical education draws from myriad disciplines, which offer countless social theories that need not be completely re-invented. So, at times, drawing from extant theory can be the 'best fit' for a research purpose. Calls for more theory in medical education(3) implore the medical education research community to use rigorous theory-building approaches. At the same time, a value for theory does not hierarchise theory over description; such a hierarchy may create implicit pressure to claim theory when one has produced description, which in turn may undermine the rigour of some qualitative research.(105) Researchers need to be both thoughtful and transparent about their purposes and procedures with regard to theory building and theory use, in order to advance understanding of medical education through rigorous qualitative research.

Conclusions

Qualitative research has made important contributions to medical education research in the past few decades. This form of inquiry is situated within a particular set of paradigms and draws on recognisable approaches and methodological tools to build knowledge regarding the experiences and activities of teachers, trainees, patients and team members in medical education settings. Particular ethical issues must be considered in a qualitative project, as well as appropriate criteria for determining the most rigorous path for each individual study. Used properly, qualitative research promises to offer profound insights into the complex social and human aspects of how health professionals develop their identity, expertise and practice.

References

1 Harris I (2002) Qualitative methods. In: Norman G, van der Vleuten C and Newble D (eds) *International Handbook of Research in Medical Education*, pp. 45–95. Kluwer Academic Publishers, Dordrecht, The Netherlands.

2 Shea JA, Arnold L, Mann KV, Shea JA, Arnold L and Mann KV (2004) A RIME perspective on the quality and relevance of current and future medical education research. *Academic Medicine.* **79**: 931–8.

3 Regehr G (2010) It's NOT rocket science: rethinking our metaphors for research in health professions education. *Medical Education.* **44**: 31–9.

4 Denzin N and Lincoln Y (2000) Introduction: the discipline and practice of qualitative research. In: Denzin N and Lincoln Y (eds) *Handbook of Qualitative Research*, pp. 1–28. Sage Publications, Thousand Oaks, CA.

5 Crotty M (1998) *Foundations of Social Research: Meaning and Perspective in the Research Process.* Sage Publications, Thousand Oaks, CA.

6 Irby DM (1992) How attending physicians make instructional decisions when conducting teaching rounds. *Academic Medicine.* **67**: 630–8.

7 Lingard L, Espin S, Whyte S *et al.* (2004) Communication failures in the operating room: an observational classification of recurrent types and effects. *Quality & Safety in Health Care.* **13**: 330–4.

8 Lingard L, Garwood S and Poenaru D (2004) Tensions influencing operating room team function: does institutional context make a difference? *Medical Education.* **38**: 691–9.

9 Lingard L, Espin S, Rubin B *et al.* (2005) Getting teams to talk: development and pilot implementation of a checklist to promote safer operating room communication. *Quality & Safety in Health Care.* **14**: 340–6.

10 Lingard L, Reznick R, DeVito I and Espin S (2002) Forming professional identities on the health care team: discursive constructions of the 'other' in the operating room. *Medical Education.* **36**: 728–34.

11 Albert M (2004) Understanding the debate on medical education research: a sociological perspective. *Academic Medicine.* **79**: 948–54.

12 Ponterotto JG (2005) Qualitative research in counsling psychology: a primer on research para-digms and philosophy of science. *Journal of Counseling Psychology.* **52**: 126–36.

13 Creswell JW and Plano Clark VL (2007) *Mixed Methods Research.* SAGE, Thousand Oaks, CA.

14 Morse J, Swanson JM and Kuzel AJ (2001) *The Nature of Qualitative Evidence.* Sage Publications, Inc, Thousand Oaks, CA.

15 Norman G (1998) Editorial. *Advances in Health Science Education.* **3**: 77–80.

16 Lingard L (2007) Qualitative research in the RIME community: critical reflections and future di-rections. *Academic Medicine.* **82**: S129–30.

17 O'Sullivan PS and Irby DM (2011) Reframing research on faculty development. [Research Support, Non-U.S. Gov't]. *Academic Medicine.* **86**: 421–8.

18 Sandelowski M (2001) Real qualitative researchers do not count: the use of numbers in qualitative research. *Research in Nursing & Health.* **24**: 230–40.

19 Schwandt TA (2007) *The Sage Dictionary of Qualitative Inquiry* (3e). Sage Publications, Thousand Oaks, CA.

20 LeCompte M and Schensul J (1999) *Designing and Conducting Ethnographic Research. An Ethnographers Toolkit.* Alta Mira Press, Lanham, MD.

21 Hammersley M and Atkinson P (1995) *What is Ethnography? Ethnography: Principles in Practice.* Routledge, London.

22 Atkinson P and Pugsley L (2005) Making sense of ethnography and medical education. *Medical Education.* **39**: 228–34.

23 Becker H, Geer B, Hughs E and Strauss A (1961) *The Boys in White: Student Culture in Medical School.* University of Chicago Press, Chicago, IL.

24 Bosk CL (2003) *Forgive and Remember: Managing Medical Failure.* University of Chicago Press, Chicago, IL.

25 Mykhalovskiy E (2003) Evidence-based medicine: ambivalent reading and the clinical recontextualization of science. *Health.* **7**: 331–52.

26 Glaser B and Strauss A (1967) *The Discovery of Grounded Theory: Strategies for Qualitative Research.* Aldine Pub Co., Chicago, IL.

27 Meston CN and Ng SL (2012) A grounded theory primer for audiology. *Seminars in Hearing.* **33**: 135–46.

28 Watling C and Lingard L (2012) Grounded theory in medical education research: AMEE Guide No. 70. *Medical Teacher.* **34**: 850–61.

29 Corbin J and Strauss A (2008) *Basics of Qualitative Research: Techniques and Procedures for Developing Grounded Theory* (3e). Sage Publications, Inc, Los Angeles, CA.

30 Charmaz K (2006) *Constructing Grounded Theory: A Practical Guide through Qualitative Analysis.* Sage Publications, Inc, London.

31 Corbin J and Strauss A (1990) Grounded theory research: procedures, canons, and evaluative criteria. *Qualitative Sociology.* **13**: 3–21.

32 Strauss A and Corbin J (1998) *Basics of Qualitative Research.* Sage Publications, Thousand Oaks, CA.

33 Kennedy TJ and Lingard LA (2006) Making sense of grounded theory in medical education. *Medical Education.* **40**: 101–8.

34 Dey I (1999) *Grounding Grounded Theory: Guidelines for Qualitative Inquiry.* Academic Press, San Diego, CA.

35 Ginsburg S, Kachan N and Lingard L (2005) Before the white coat: perceptions of professional lapses in the pre-clerkship. *Medical Education.* **39**: 12–9.

36 Ginsburg S, Regehr G and Lingard L (2004) Basing the evaluation of professionalism on observable behaviors: a cautionary tale. *Academic Medicine.* **79**: S1–4.

37 Ginsburg S, Regehr G and Lingard L (2003) The disavowed curriculum: understanding students' reasoning in professionally challenging situations. *Journal of General Internal Medicine.* **18**: 1015–22.

38 Ginsburg S, Regehr G and Lingard L (2003) To be and not to be: the paradox of the emerging professional stance. *Medical Education.* **37**: 350–7.

39 Ginsburg S, Regehr G, Stern D and Lingard L (2002) The anatomy of the professional lapse: bridging the gap between traditional frameworks and students' perceptions. *Academic Medicine.* **77**: 516–22.

40 Ginsburg S, Regehr G, Hatala R *et al.* (2002) Context, conflict, and resolution: a new conceptual framework for evaluating professionalism. *Academic Medicine.* **75**: S6–11.

41 Watling C, Driessen E, van der Vleuten CP and Lingard L (2012) Learning from clinical work: the roles of learning cues and credibility judgements. *Medical Education.* **46**: 192–200.

42 Stake R (2005) Qualitative case studies. In: Denzin N and Lincoln Y (eds) *The Sage Handbook of Qualitative Research*, pp. 443–66. Sage Publications, Thousand Oaks, CA.

43 Aita V and McIlvain H (1999) An armchair adventure in case study research. In: Crabtree B and Miller W (eds) *Doing Qualitative Research*, pp. 253–68. Sage Publications, Thousand Oaks, CA.

44 Perley CM (2006) Physician use of the curbside consultation to address information needs: report on a collective case study. *Journal of the Medical Library Association.* **94**: 137–44.

45 Creswell J (1998) Chapter 4: Five qualitative traditions of inquiry. In: Creswell J (ed.) *Qualitative Inquiry and Research Design: Choosing among Five Traditions*, pp. 47–72. Sage Publications, Thousand Oaks, CA.

46 Bearman M (2003) Is virtual the same as real? Medical students' experiences of a virtual patient. *Academic Medicine.* **78**: 538–45.

47 Miller W and Crabtree B (1999) Clinical research: a multi-method typology and qualitative roadmap. In: Crabtree B and Miller W (eds) *Doing Qualitative Research*, pp. 3–32. Sage Publications, Thousand Oaks, CA.

48 Addison R (1999) A grounded hermeneutic editing approach. In: Crabtree B and Miller W (eds) *Doing Qualitative Research*, pp. 145–62. Sage Publications, Thousand Oaks, CA.

49 Addison RB (2006) Grounded interpretive research: an investigation of physician socialization. In: *Entering the Circle: Hermeneutic Investigation in Psychology*, pp. 39–56. State University of New York Press, New York.

50 Muller J (1999) Narrative approaches to qualitative research in primary care. In: Crabtree B and Miller W (eds) *Doing Qualitative Research*, pp. 221–38. Sage Publications, Thousand Oaks, CA.

51 Bleakley A (2005) Stories as data, data as stories: making sense of narrative inquiry in clinical education. *Medical Education*. **39**: 534–40.

52 Pullman D, Bethune C and Duke P (2005) Narrative means to humanistic ends. s*Teaching and Learning in Medicine*. **17**: 279–84.

53 Ventres W (1994) Hearing the patient's story: exploring physician–patient communication using narrative case reports. *Family Practice Research Journal*. **14**: 139–47.

54 Thesen J and Kuzel A (1999) Participatory inquiry. In: Crabtree B and Miller W (eds) *Doing Qualitative Research*, pp. 269–90. Sage Publications, Thousand Oaks, CA.

55 Kemmis S and McTaggart R (2005) Participatory action research: communicative action and the public sphere. In: Denzin N and Lincoln Y (eds) *The Sage Handbook of Qualitative Research*, pp. 559–604. Sage Publications, Thousand Oaks, CA.

56 Mowat H and Mowat D (2001) The value of marginality in a medical school: general practice and curriculum change. *Medical Education*. **35**: 175–7.

57 Guillemin M and Gillam L (2004) Ethics, reflexivity and 'ethically important moments' in research. *Qualitative Inquiry*. **10**: 261–80.

58 Mauthner NS and Doucet A (2003) Reflexive accounts and accounts of reflexivity in qualitative data analysis. *Sociology*. **37**: 413–31.

59 Dicicco-Bloom B and Crabtree BF (2006) The qualitative research interview. *Medical Education*. **40**: 314–21.

60 Miller W and Crabtree B (1999) Depth interviewing. In: Crabtree B and Miller W (eds) *Doing Qualitative Research*, pp. 89–107. Sage Publications, Thousand Oaks, CA.

61 McCracken G (1988) *The Long Interview*. Sage, Newbury Park, CA.

62 Reeves S, Lewin S and Zwarenstein M (2006) Using qualitative interviews within medical education research: why we must raise the 'quality bar'. *Medical Education*. **40**: 291–2.

63 Barbour RS and Barbour RS (2005) Making sense of focus groups. *Medical Education*. **39**: 742–50.

64 Brown J (1999) Focus group interviews. In: Crabtree B and Miller W (eds) *Doing Qualitative Research*, pp. 109–24. Sage Publications, Thousand Oaks, CA.

65 Maa A and McCullough LB (2006) Medical education in the public versus the private setting: a qualitative study of medical students' attitudes. *Medical Teacher*. **28**: 351–5.

66 Hammersley M and Atkinson P (1995) *Ethnography: Principles in Practice*. Routledge, London.

67 Bogdewic S (1999) Participant observation. In: Crabtree B and Miller W (eds) *Doing Qualitative Research*, pp. 47–69. Sage Publications, Thousand Oaks, CA.

68 Bannister SL, Hilliard RI, Regehr G and Lingard L (2003) Technical skills in paediatrics: a qualitative study of acquisition, attitudes and assumptions in the neonatal intensive care unit. *Medical Education*. **37**: 1082–90.

69 Stern DT (1998) In search of the informal curriculum: when and where professional values are taught. *Academic Medicine*. **73**: S28–30.

70 Sinclair S (1997) *Making Doctors: An Institutional Apprenticeship*. Berg, New York.

71 Heath C, Luff P and Sanchez SM (2007) Video and qualitative research: analysing medical practice and interaction. *Medical Education*. **41**: 109–16.

72 Creswell J (2003) Chapter 9: Qualitative procedures. In: Creswell J (ed.) *Research Design: Qualitative, Quantitative, and Mixed Methods Approaches*, pp. 179–209. Sage Publications, Thousand Oaks, CA.

73 Olney CA, Livingston JE, Fisch S and Talamantes MA (2006) Becoming better health care providers: outcomes of a primary care service-learning project in medical school. *Journal of Prevention & Intervention in the Community*. **32**: 133–47.

74 Krippendorf K (2004) *Content Analysis: An Introduction to Its Methodology*. Sage Publications, Thousand Oaks, CA.

75 Burack JH, Irby DM, Carline JD, Ambrozy DM, Ellsbury KE and Stritter FT (1997) A study of medical students' specialty-choice pathways: trying on possible selves. *Academic Medicine*. **72**: 534–41.

76 Finlay L (2006) Mapping Methodology. In: Finlay L and Ballinger C (eds) *Qualitative Research for Allied Health Professionals: Challenging Choices*, pp. 9–29. John Wiley & Sons Ltd., West Sussex, England.

77 Cameron D (2001) Chapter 1: What is discourse and why analyse it? In: Cameron D (ed.) *Working with Spoken Discourse*, pp. 7–18. Sage Publications, London.

78 Mills S (2004) *Discourse* (2e). Routledge, New York.

79 Maynard DW and Heritage J (2005) Conversation analysis, doctor–patient interaction and medical communication. *Medical Education*. **39**: 428–35.

80 Hekelman FP and Blase JR (1996) Excellence in clinical teaching: the core of the mission. *Academic Medicine*. **71**: 738–42.

81 Hekelman FP, Blase JR and Bedinghaus J (1996) Discourse analysis of peer coaching in medical education: a case study. *Teaching and Learning in Medicine*. **8**: 41–7.

82 Richardson L (2004) Writing: a method of inquiry. In: Nagy Hesse-Biber S and Leavy P (eds) *Approaches to Qualitative Research: A Reader on Theory and Practice*, pp. 473–95. Oxford University Press, New York.

83 Charmaz K (2004) Premises, principles, and practices in qualitative research: revisiting the foundations. *Qualitative Health Research*. **14**: 976–93.

84 Mays N and Pope C (2000) Qualitative research in health care. Assessing quality in qualitative research. *British Medical Journal*. **320**: 50–2.

85 Mays N and Pope C (1995) Rigour and qualitative research. *British Medical Journal*. **311**: 109–12.

86 Inui TS and Frankel RM (1991) Evaluating the quality of qualitative research: a proposal pro tem. *Journal of General Internal Medicine*. **6**: 485–6.

87 Rowan M and Huston P (1997) Qualitative research articles: information for authors and peer reviewers. *Canadian Medical Association Journal*. **157**: 1442–6.

88 Lincoln Y and Guba EG (1985) *Naturalistic Inquiry*. Sage Publications, Thousand Oaks, CA.

89 Sandelowski M (2004) Using qualitative research. *Qualitative Health Research*. **14**: 1366–86.

90 Sandelowski M (1997) 'To be of use': enhancing the utility of qualitative research. *Nursing Outlook*. **45**: 125–32.

91 Lincoln Y and Guba EG (2000) Paradigmatic controversies, contradictions and emerging confluences. In: Denzin N and Lincoln Y (eds) *Handbook of Qualitative Research*, pp. 163–88. Sage Publications, Thousand Oaks, CA.

92 Wolf FM (2004) Methodological quality, evidence, and Research in Medical Education (RIME). *Academic Medicine*. **79**: S68–9.

93 Britten N (2005) Making sense of qualitative research: a new series. *Medical Education*. **39**: 5–6.

94 van Manen M (1997) *Researching Lived Experience: Human Science for an Action Sensitive Peda-Gogy*. Althouse Press, London, ON.

95 Rolfe G (2006) Validity, trustworthiness and rigour: quality and the idea of qualitative research. *Journal of Advanced Nursing.* **53**: 304–10.

96 Campbell ML and Gregor FM (2002) *Mapping Social Relations: A Primer in Doing Institutional Ethnography.* Rowman Altamira, Aurora, Canada.

97 Kuzel AJ (1999) Sampling in qualitative inquiry. In: Crabtree BF and Miller WL (eds) *Doing Qualitative Research.* Sage, Newbury Park, CA.

98 Holden JD (2001) Hawthorne effects and research into professional practice. *Journal of Evaluation in Clinical Practice.* **7**: 65–70.

99 Klag M and Langley A (2012) Approaching the conceptual leap in qualitative research. *International Journal of Management Reviews.* **15**(2): 149–66. Available early online: doi: 10.1111/j.1468-2370.2012 .00349.x.

100 Eakin JM and Mykhalovskiy E (2003) Reframing the evaluation of qualitative health research: reflections on a review of appraisal guidelines in the health sciences. *Journal of Evaluation in Clinical Practice.* **9**: 187–94.

101 Bowen GA (2006) Grounded theory and sensitizing concepts. *International Journal of Qualitative Methods.* **5**: Article 2. (http://www .ualberta.ca/~iiqm/backissues/5_3/pdf/bowen.pdf; accessed 15 January 2012).

102 Glaser BG (2002) Constructivist grounded theory? *Forum, Qualitative Sozialforschung / Forum, Qualitative Social Research.* **3**: Art. 12. (http://www.qualitative-research.net/index.php/fqs/article/ view/825/1792; accessed 15 January 2012).

103 Morse J, Stern P and Corbin J (2008) *Developing Grounded Theory: The Second Generation.* Left Coast Press, Walnut Creek, CA.

104 Smith D (ed.) (2006) *Institutional Ethnography as Practice.* Rowman & Littlefield Publishers, Inc, Lanham, MD.

105 Sandelowski M (2000) Whatever happened to qualitative description? *Research in Nursing & Health.* **23**: 334–40.

Further reading

Britten N (2005) Making sense of qualitative research: a new series. *Medical Education.* **39**: 5–6.

Crabtree B and Miller W (eds) (1999) *Doing Qualitative Research.* Sage Publications, Thousand Oaks, CA.

Creswell J (1998) *Qualitative Inquiry and Research Design: Choosing among Five Traditions.* Sage Publications, Thousand Oaks, CA.

Crotty M (1998) *Foundations of Social Research: Meaning and Perspective in the Research Process.* Sage Publications, Thousand Oaks, CA.

Denzin N and Lincoln Y (eds) (2005) *The Sage Handbook of Qualitative Research.* Sage Publications, Thousand Oaks, CA.

Miles MB and Huberman AM (1994) *Qualitative Data Analysis: A Sourcebook of New Methods.* Sage Publications, Thousand Oaks, CA.

Schwandt TA (2007) *The Sage Dictionary of Qualitative Inquiry* (3e). Sage Publications, Thousand Oaks, CA.

Strauss A and Corbin J (1998) *Basics of Qualitative Research.* Sage Publications, Thousand Oaks, CA.

27 Programme evaluation: Improving practice, influencing policy and decision-making

Chris Lovato[1] and David Wall[2]

[1] Faculty of Medicine, University of British Columbia, Canada
[2] West Midlands Deanery, Birmingham, UK

 KEY MESSAGES

- Programme evaluation focuses on questions related to whether a programme is working as intended and if there are any unintended consequences.

- Evidence from programme evaluation is essential to enhance professional practice and to achieve the best medical education for students, trainees and doctors engaged in continuing professional development.

- There are important similarities and differences between research and evaluation.

- Evaluators have the same obligations as researchers in considering the ethical issues involved in implementing studies.

- The value of an evaluation rests on whether the information is useful. There are methods and techniques that can enhance impact.

- High-quality evaluation in medical education will ultimately contribute to quality patient care.

Introduction

This chapter covers the wide role of programme evaluation in medical education from micro to macro, from the evaluation of individual teaching episodes to entire curricula, for the purposes of improving pedagogy to influencing national policy.

The chapter is divided into four sections. We begin with some definitions and a discussion of the purposes of evaluation and the symbiotic relationship between programme planning and evaluation. Some key concepts are described and selected models and theories of evaluation are presented. This first section concludes by exploring the differences between evaluation and research. The second section focuses on evaluation practice. It describes ethics in evaluation, evaluation methods, sources of evidence and promoting the use of evaluation findings. The third section addresses ways in which an evaluation can be implemented to promote its use and the role of evaluation in change management. The chapter concludes with three examples of evaluation in medical education and selected further information resources.

What is programme evaluation?

Programme evaluation focuses on questions related to whether a programme is working as intended and if there are any unintended consequences. There are many differ-

ent definitions of evaluation in the literature. In this chapter we use an adapted version of the definition provided by Fink in her text on evaluation 'fundamentals':(1, p.4)

> 'Program evaluation is the diligent investigation of a program's characteristics and merits. In the context of health care, the purpose of program evaluation is to provide information about the effectiveness of programs, so as to optimize the outcomes, efficiency and quality of health care. An evaluation may analyse a program's structure, activities and organization as well as its political and social environment. It may also appraise the achievement of the program's goals and objectives and the extent of the program's impact and costs.'

The term 'program' (or programme) can refer to any organised action such as a curriculum, a course, session, student service, event, guidelines or a policy in medical education. The reasons for conducting an evaluation are varied and can include the desire to improve the implementation and effectiveness of a programme, manage limited resources, justify funding, support the need for increased funding, document social accountability and meet requirements for academic standards or accreditation.

Evaluation is much broader than merely handing out satisfaction surveys to students and trainees at the end of teaching sessions. Evaluation is vital for curriculum development and in determining if the curriculum is operating as intended and achieving the intended outcomes. Did the learners achieve the targeted knowledge and skills from the teaching programme? Evaluation may also be used to ensure that supporting programmes and services are meeting

Understanding Medical Education: Evidence, Theory and Practice, Second Edition. Edited by Tim Swanwick.
© 2014 The Association for the Study of Medical Education. Published 2014 by John Wiley & Sons, Ltd.

users' needs. It is often used to identify areas where the curriculum needs to improve. It is used to determine if an educational programme is of an acceptable standard and may be approved for training and accreditation purposes. It may be used to give feedback to instructors, administrators, managers and faculty on a broad range of programmatic services (e.g. library services, technology, admissions, and assessment) that support medical education. It may be used as part of the information presented at the annual appraisal process for medical teachers, and for promotion and career development. In terms of assessments, it may be used to gather outcome measures on pass rates for qualifying and professional examinations. And it can be used to determine long-term outcomes such as speciality choice and location of practice in rural, remote and underserved regions.

In addition, evaluation may be used to determine future educational policy in a curriculum, teaching and learning, or assessment. It may also be used as a tool to implement centrally determined policy through a number of covert and controlling processes. Examples of questions evaluators might therefore legitimately ask would include the following:

- Is there comparability between regional training sites?
- What is the educational climate like for medical students in the operating theatre?
- What are the facilitators and barriers to implementing the new integrated clerkship?
- What aspects of the faculty development course had a positive impact on teaching?
- How reliable was the shortlisting and interviewing for paediatric trainees?
- What do students and junior doctors think about career advice provided by support services?
- What is the practice location and speciality of trainees?

Programme evaluation generally consists of eight primary activities(1) (*see* Box 27.1). The practice of programme evaluation involves applying theory, research findings and the most rigorous methods possible to a real-world setting in order to address practical questions relevant to decision-makers and stakeholders. The tricky part is that evaluators working in medical education programme settings often do not have the same kind of control over study conditions as researchers might.

BOX 27.1 Eight primary activities in programme evaluation

1. Posing questions about the programme
2. Setting standards of effectiveness
3. Designing the evaluation
4. Selecting participants
5. Collecting data
6. Managing data
7. Analysing data
8. Reporting and disseminating results

Definitions: Evaluation, assessment and appraisal

In everyday life the terms *evaluation*, *assessment* and *appraisal* are often used interchangeably. This confusion is compounded by international differences in definitions. In North America, for instance, the word 'evaluation' is sometimes equated with the UK term 'assessment', to mean measurement of learners' skills.(2) An example of this is in the mini-clinical evaluation exercise – actually an 'assessment' tool for testing junior doctors' history-taking and examination skills.(3)

In this chapter, *assessment* is defined as 'the processes and instruments applied to measure the learner's achievements, normally after they have worked through a learning programme of one sort or another.(4) Assessment then is about testing the learners. *Appraisal* is 'a two-way dialogue focussing on the personal, professional and educational needs of the parties, which produce agreed outcomes'.(5,6) As noted earlier in this section, *evaluation* focuses on the design, implementation, improvement or outcomes of a programme rather than an individual or individuals.

Programme planning and evaluation

Programme planning and evaluation are highly interrelated. If there is not a good programme plan with clear goals and objectives, it is difficult and often impossible to carry out a credible evaluation. In developing a new programme it is important to identify goals and objectives that are measureable or 'evaluable'. and, over the life of the programme, planning and evaluation are both part of an ongoing cycle of ongoing improvement. The methods and approaches used in programme planning and evaluation occur throughout the lifecycle of a programme, including assessing needs, modifying approaches, identifying indicators and measures, determining effectiveness, identifying facilitators and barriers to implementation, and making recommendations for improvement. In practice, the process and methods used for curriculum development are the same for evaluation: for example, developing a programme description, specifying a target process and outcomes, identifying or developing measures, designing and collecting data, and disseminating results. Whether you are engaging in planning or evaluating, these processes involve the use of theory, research findings and the most rigorous methods possible in a medical education setting.

Theory in evaluation

In the literature on programme evaluation, theory is often used in two different ways. 'Theory-driven evaluation' refers to an evaluation study that is based on the programme's 'theory of change', which is most often represented as a logic model. In the second instance, theory refers to an evaluative approach, model or theory of practice.

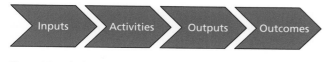

Figure 27.1 The basic components of a logic model. Redrawn from Cross TL, Barzon BJ, Dennis KW and Isaacs MR (1989) *Towards a Culturally Competent System of Care: A Monograph on Effective Services for Minority Children who are Severely Emotionally Disturbed.* CASSP Technical Assistance Center, Georgetown University Child Development Center, Washington, DC.

Logic models

An important tool for conducting theory-driven evaluation is logic modelling. A logic model provides a concise graphic representation that communicates the purpose of a programme, its components, the sequence of activities and outcomes anticipated. In effect it is a causal model that links inputs, activities, outputs and outcomes. The basic components of a logic model are shown in Figure 27.1. Inputs are defined as those resources dedicated to or consumed by the programme (e.g. money, staff, faculty, facilities, equipment), activities are the tactical actions (e.g. curriculum, support services) that occur to achieve the objectives of the programme, and outputs are what the programme does with the inputs to fulfil its mission (e.g. admit students to a programme, deliver courses, provide clinical training, provide student support services). Outcomes refer to the benefits for students during and after their training (e.g. knowledge, skills, licensing and practice) and they are often specified as short-term, intermediate and long term.(7)

Conceptual models and approaches

There are a variety of theories, models and approaches described in the evaluation literature. Typically, they differ based upon who is involved in the evaluation, what is evaluated, and why and how it is conducted. In the majority of evaluation studies these approaches are blended. As many as 13 different models and approaches to evaluation have been identified.(8) Examples of those most relevant to medical education include an objectives approach, expertise-accreditation approaches, utilisation-focused approaches, participatory collaborative approaches and organisation learning. Although there are many different models of evaluation described in the literature, we describe three widely used models that are well suited to medical education: utilisation-focused evaluation; Kirkpatrick's hierarchy; and participatory, collaborative and empowerment evaluation.

Utilisation-focused evaluation

Utilisation-focused evaluation is an approach associated with Michael Quinn Patton. This approach is decision-oriented and is based on the premise that 'an evaluation should be judged according to its utility and actual use'.(9) The evaluator focuses on developing and implementing an evaluation that places 'use' as the primary consideration in how the evaluation is planned and implemented, and findings reported. 'The focus in utilization-focused evaluation is on intended use by intended users'.(9)

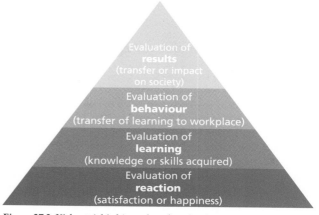

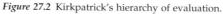

Figure 27.2 Kirkpatrick's hierarchy of evaluation.

In utilisation-focused evaluation, the evaluator works with decision-makers to design the evaluation. There is no particular evaluation method, approach or model associated with utilisation-focused evaluation. The assumption is that the most appropriate method, approach or model will be based on the needs of the primary intended users. A utilisation-based approach can be used in all types of evaluations (e.g. formative, summative, outcome, etc.) with both qualitative and quantitative data, and any type of design (e.g. experimental, quasi-experimental, and any qualitative design).

An important strength of this approach is that it increases the use of evaluation results. A potential downside to using this approach is that by focusing the evaluation primarily on the interests of the intended users of the results, the viewpoint of the target population can be overlooked.(10) Vassar *et al.*(11) encourage the application of utilisation-focused evaluation in medical education settings because it is a flexible and pragmatic approach to answering a wide variety of programmatic questions. It also actively includes key decision-makers, thus making it more likely that the results will be used.

Kirkpatrick's hierarchy

One of the most widely applied evaluation approaches in medical education has been Kirkpatrick's hierarchy, which was first described by Donald Kirkpatrick in 1967 as a series of levels of evaluation on which to focus questions. At the base (the lowest level) of the model is some indication of satisfaction with the teaching and learning. Next up the pyramid is a concern for what learning has taken place, followed by indication of behavioural change. The apex of the pyramid focuses on the impact of an intervention on society or a community (*see* Figure 27.2). Each is a legitimate level of evaluation, though it is generally agreed that movement up the pyramid provides increasingly credible findings about the impact of a programme or intervention on health-care outcomes.

Kirkpatrick's hierarchy(12) has been adapted for use in medical education.(13) Unfortunately, most educational evaluations are at the lower levels and few are at the apex of this adapted model. Belfield *et al.*,(13) for instance, found that in a study of 305 papers, only 1.6% had looked at health-care outcomes.

Participatory, collaborative and empowerment evaluation

Participatory, collaborative and empowerment all refer to the involvement of those who have a stake in the programme, including funders, policy-makers, students, faculty, staff, students and members of the community. Participatory evaluation methods are based on the foundations of community-based participatory research and participatory action research. While the level of participation can vary across studies using this approach, the focus is upon valuing and using the knowledge and expertise of those involved with or benefitting from the programme. Participation can include involving stakeholders in identifying evaluation questions, developing indicators and measures, collecting data, analysing and interpreting data, and disseminating results of the evaluation. In general, there has been an increased use of collaborative methods in evaluating education and social programmes with the movement toward wider accountability to government, citizens and students themselves.

There are many advantages to using collaborative approaches, including the empowerment of those involved, building evaluation capacity and re-inforcing organisational learning.(14) However, participatory evaluation is not always appropriate for every evaluation. There are a number of constraints to be considered such as the cost and time of involving individuals with a broad level of experience and understanding of evaluation. In addition, the process can sometimes be unpredictable, requiring an experienced evaluator who can negotiate the process. An important advantage of involving stakeholders in the evaluation is the significant increase in the chances that the findings will be used.

Fetterman *et al.*(15) describes the use of empowerment approaches when evaluating and transforming a medical school curriculum. Five tools are outlined as being central to implementing the approach: (i) developing a culture of evidence; (ii) using a critical friend; (iii) encouraging a cycle of reflection and action; (iv) cultivating a community of learners; and (v) developing reflective practitioners. Fetterman *et al.*(15) report that the application of these methods during a curriculum reform process fostered greater institutional self-reflection, an evidence-based model of decision-making and expanded opportunities for collaboration among faculty, students and staff.

Evaluation or research?

Evaluation and research in education are similar activities, and share many of the same methods. Programme evaluation is a systematic method for collecting, analysing and using information to answer questions about projects, policies and programmes, particularly about their effectiveness and efficiency. It is about providing practice-based evidence from the real world to address questions that are important to stakeholders, including funders, programme planners, implementers, decision-makers and consumers. The focus is upon stakeholder-generated questions versus questions that arise from theory, the literature or researcher curiosity.

The difference in perspective that evaluation brings to the study of problems has to do with intent. The intent of evaluation is to identify questions that are meaningful for making evidence-based decisions and establishing accountability. Those questions may or may not address a gap in the literature. The driving questions are always specific to the local context of the programme. This differs from research where the intent of the researcher is to undertake work that will contribute to a larger body of knowledge (i.e. the scientific literature). The questions are curiosity driven and typically arise from previous research or theory.

Evaluation is methods neutral within the broad domain of social science methods. Evidence can be gathered based on experimental, quasi-experimental and observational designs. Similar to research, evaluation uses qualitative, quantitative and mixed-methods; and evaluation and research use the same principles of design, data collection and analysis. However, when it comes to report writing and dissemination, an evaluative perspective is different from a research perspective in that evaluators use multiple forms of reporting and results that will not necessarily be published. Providing specific actionable recommendations is a focus in evaluation, and facilitating use of evaluation results is part of the role of an evaluator.

Evaluators address study questions that facilitate evidence-based decision-making and accountability. The work is often ongoing and cyclical, focusing on continuous improvement of programmes. Evaluation is about providing practice-based evidence from the real world to address questions that are important to programme planners, implementers, decision-makers and consumers.

With the growing interest in knowledge translation research, there has been a greater focus on the knowledge generated from evaluation studies. For the most part, this has been driven by the commitment to evidence-based practice and the strong call for better links between research and practice. More research funding agencies are encouraging researchers to address evaluation questions in their studies and to focus on questions related to programme implementation, adaptation of approaches, impact evaluation and knowledge use. By publishing their work on applying theories, methods and evidence, evaluators are in an excellent position to contribute to the knowledge base in medical education.

Ethics in programme evaluation

Evaluators have the same obligations as researchers in considering the ethical issues involved in implementing studies. However, the overlap between evaluation and research often causes confusion as to whether formal approval by an Institutional Review Board (IRB) is required. Bedward *et al.*,(16) in their editorial in *Medical Teacher* in 2004, discussed the lack of clarity on what requires ethical approval, the reliance on one procedure for all applications, confusion over the scope of responsibilities within trusts and the scale of the work involved.

In general, if there is intent to publish or otherwise disseminate findings, then IRB review is required. This is an important consideration for many evaluators working in medical education since the redefinition of scholarship by Boyer(17) emphasises the educational environment as a setting for academic inquiry.(18) It is recommended that medical education evaluators seek advice from their institution's IRB, as there is evidence that considerable variability exists in requirements for medical education research studies.(19)

Among the tips Egan-Lee *et al.*(20) provide for obtaining ethical approval for research in health professions' education are examining your intent, planning for early communication with your IRB, and determining if your study is exempt from review. As they note, many institutions exempt programme evaluation studies from requiring IRB approval. However, it is important to remember that it is the IRB that determines whether or not an evaluation study is exempt from review.

Morrison(21) describes ethical issues in evaluation practice as arising at any stage in the evaluation process, but most commonly during the entry and design phase, communication of results and utilisation of findings. Examples of issues include:

- stakeholders who have already decided what the findings 'should be'
- different expectations or purposes for the evaluation as viewed by different stakeholders
- leaving out certain stakeholder voices from the evaluation
- pressure by stakeholders to alter presentation of findings
- stakeholders who suppress or ignore findings
- stakeholders who misinterpret the findings.

Goldie(2) cites seven ethics standards for evaluators, drawn from a number of national bodies by Worthen *et al.*(22) (*see* Box 27.2). Ultimately though, it is the individual evaluator's responsibility to work ethically to bring to their work a principles-based or virtue-based approach rather than to merely follow external policies and procedures.

As in other professions, evaluators have developed standards and guidelines for practice that are informative in both anticipating and dealing with ethical issues that may arise in evaluation practice. Box 27.3 provides a synopsis and internet links for the UK Evaluation Society and American Evaluation Association guidelines for practice.

Evaluation methods

This section includes brief descriptions of several methods that may be used in programme evaluation, including questionnaires, interviews, focus groups, site visits, administrative records and group methods.

Several methods may be used serially, e.g. when a focus group is used to generate items for a questionnaire. Alternatively, methods may be used in parallel where multiple methods are adopted to tap into different data sources in order to build the richest possible picture of the educational initiative under study.

Questionnaires

There are several advantages of using a questionnaire for evaluation purposes. The questionnaire is feasible and economical in terms of time and effort to collect a range of

---

BOX 27.2 Ethical standards in evaluation(2)

- Service orientation
- Formal agreements
- Rights of human subjects
- Complete and fair assessment
- Disclosure of findings
- Conflicts of interest
- Fiscal responsibility

BOX 27.3 FOCUS ON: Good practice in evaluation

A number of organisations have defined standards for good evaluation practice. The European Evaluation Society lists the standards laid out by a number of European countries. The UK version spells out what constitutes good practice for:

- evaluators
- participants
- commissioners
- institutions conducting self-evaluation.

The UK Evaluation Society Guidelines for Good Practice in Evaluation can be downloaded from http://www .evaluation.org.uk

The American Evaluation Association has also produced guiding principles. These are built around five areas:

Systematic inquiry: Evaluators conduct systematic, data-based inquiries.

Competence: Evaluators provide competent performance to stakeholders.

Integrity/honesty: Evaluators display honesty and integrity in their own behaviour, and attempt to ensure the honesty and integrity of the entire evaluation process.

Respect for people: Evaluators respect the security, dignity and self-worth of the respondents, programme participants, clients and other evaluation stakeholders.

Responsibilities for general and public welfare: Evaluators articulate and take into account the diversity of general and public interests and values that may be related to the evaluation.

The full guidance can be viewed at: http://www.eval.org/ Publications/GuidingPrinciples.asp

views from the whole population to be studied, rather than sampling some parts of the population. Questionnaire data (especially for closed rating scale questions) may be analysed using statistical testing for significance and associations between different data, including data reduction techniques such as factor analysis.(23,24) In addition, it may be necessary to use statistical testing to assess reliability of the data, e.g.Kappa, Wilcoxon signed-rank test and repeated measures analysis of variance to assess test–re-test reliability, and Cronbach's alpha to assess internal consistency.(25) The questionnaire may also allow a search for new patterns by two methods. One is the use of open-ended questions and free comments, analysed by qualitative methods, where one may catch the 'gem' of information that may be missed by the closed question.(26) The other is the method of principal component factor analysis, a data reduction method to reduce the quantitative data from the Likert questions to a small number of factors with common characteristics.

There are, however, some disadvantages to the questionnaire method. There is a well-recognised problem with pre-coded responses, which may not be sufficiently comprehensive to accommodate all answers, forcing the candidate to choose a view that does not represent their views correctly.(27) We make assumptions that all respondents will understand the questions in the same way, and there is no way of clarifying the question as in a one-to-one interview. Non-response affects the quality of the data and thus the generalisability of the results. Responders may differ from non-responders, in that non-responders may be of lower social class,(28) or older and more ill than responders.(27) To overcome these problems, an evaluation questionnaire may be designed to include both open questions (to get at the gems), closed questions (yes/no), tick box questions with specified categories, scale items such as the Likert rating scale (agree to disagree points on a scale) and the opportunity for free comments to attempt to catch any other gems there may be.

Individual interviews

Cohen *et al.*(26) defined a research interview as a 'two-person conversation initiated by the interviewer, for the purpose of gathering research relevant information'. The interview has multiple uses within educational evaluation and research. It can be used:

- to gather information about the what evaluation questions to ask
- to develop ideas for new hypotheses or research questions
- as a primary source of data or in conjunction with other evaluation methods
- to validate results from a study
- to go deeper and explore new themes generated from other evaluation methods
- to test hypotheses that have already been generated.(26)

Also, the interview method is a powerful way to gain internal validity in case study work, to go deeper and explore new themes generated from other educational evaluation methods in this work.

Focus groups

The focus group is a form of group interview in which discussion and interaction within the group is part of the methodology.(29) People are encouraged to talk, exchange ideas, tell stories, comment on each other's ideas and ask one another questions. The method is useful in evaluation in exploring learners' knowledge and experiences, and also in determining what they think about the course and why. The idea of a focus group is that it may help to clarify ideas and views that might be less accessible in a one-to-one interview.

Krueger and Casey(29) give advice on group composition, running the group (four to eight people as an ideal number), analysis and writing up. It is highly recommended that the focus groups be recorded and transcribed for detailed analysis. Digital recording using a digital recorder and boundary microphone (for 360-degree capture of what people say) will give good sound quality. In addition, audio files may be stored on computer and burned onto compact disc and sent to participants and colleagues for further comments.

Group consensus techniques

A number of consensus techniques have been developed for the evaluation of educational events involving medium-to-large groups. Two commonly used approaches are described here.

Snowball review

This is a group-based evaluation(4) that uses a series of steps where comment and opinion are suggested, discussed, shared and agreed, before going on to the next step, until a final list of good and not so good points about a course has been agreed. The steps are as follows:

- Each individual alone lists, say, three good and three not so good points about the programme being evaluated.
- Participants form pairs and discuss their suggestions, and then come to an agreement as a pair.
- Each pair then forms a group of four, and this again debates the views and comes to an agreement.
- Two groups of four join up to form a group of eight. Again they debate and agree their conclusions.
- A reporter presents the group's views to the whole course.

This is a good method in that it involves everyone and ideally reaches a consensus and a conclusion, but it does take time.

Nominal group technique

This is another group-based consensus method. It differs from the snowball review (above) in that each person gives their views and then all the views are collected up and voted on. The steps are as follows:

- Each individual is asked in turn for feedback on the best and least good aspects of the course.
- Comments are collected and listed (once) on a flip chart, that is, if two members of the group thought that the catering was not very good, this is only listed once.
- The facilitator continues to go round the group until all (unique) comments have been exhausted.

BOX 27.4 Sources of evaluation evidence(22)

What	How	Who	Why
Student (learner) ratings	Rating scale	Students	Formative and summative
Peer ratings	Rating scale	Peers	Formative and summative
External expert ratings	Rating scale	Experts	Formative and summative
Self-ratings	Rating scale	Self	Formative and summative
Video recording of teaching	Rating scale	Self and peers	Formative and summative
Student interviews	Rating scale	Students	Formative and summative
Exit and alumni ratings	Rating scale	Graduates	Formative and summative
Employer ratings	Rating scale	Graduates' employer	Programme
Administrator ratings	Rating scale	Administrator	Summative
Teacher scholarship	Review	Administrator	Summative
Teaching awards	Review	Administrator	Summative
Learning outcomes measures	Exams	Administrator	Formative
Teaching portfolios	All above	Students' peers, administrator	Summative

---

- Group members are then allowed a set number of votes to distribute among the items listed.
- The result is a scored and ranked list of feedback comments to which all members of the group have contributed.
- An optional stage is to put people into groups to discuss some or all of the items derived from the voting.

Group consensus techniques carry a health warning. Both methods may achieve answers of good face validity but are of low order as far as Kirkpatrick's hierarchy is concerned and the results do not lend themselves to further analysis in terms of generalisability.

Sources of evaluation evidence

There are many potential sources of evidence for evaluating medical education programmes, including students, faculty, staff and clinical supervisors. We recommend that all those involved in the delivery of a programme be considered in gathering evidence to address evaluation questions. What follows focuses on the evaluation of teaching as an illustration of the use of different sources of evidence when conducting an evaluation. We chose teaching as our example because it is central to evaluating most medical education programmes.

Berk(30) commented that student ratings have dominated as the primary measure of the evaluation of teaching effectiveness for the past 30 years. Berk(30) made a plea for 'a variety of sources to define the construct and to make decisions about performance . . .'. Similarly, we wish to plea for the broadening and deepening of evaluation questions and sources of evidence. Berk suggested drawing on at least three sources of evidence, so that the strengths of one may compensate for the weaknesses of others (e.g. the different biases of peer ratings and student ratings) and suggested 13 sources of evidence, using a wide range of evaluation methods. These are listed in Box 27.4 and each is discussed in more detail below.

Student/learner ratings
Here, students or learners evaluate the teaching programme, often by means of evaluation questionnaires. These have been used for many years and are a necessary and essential part of evaluating teaching effectiveness. Research confirms that student ratings are an excellent source of evaluation evidence.(31) However, they should not be relied on by themselves when making important decisions.

Peer ratings
With peer ratings, colleagues look at a teaching programme, either by sitting in and observing, or reading and reviewing the teaching materials. Peer review of teaching and of teaching materials is useful, and covers aspects that the students as learners will not be in a position to evaluate. Since teaching is a scholarly activity, it should be subject to peer review (as with research). There is evidence that the results of peer review compare well with student ratings,(32) so peer ratings complement student ratings. Peer ratings are best used for formative rather than summative evaluation.(31)

External expert ratings
Here, an external expert will look at the teaching programme, as with peer evaluation. Such individuals will be very experienced and highly skilled with the ability to give really good and helpful feedback. This may be of great benefit to younger teachers, although in our experience this is not always the case.

Self-ratings
Self-evaluation is an important part of the evaluation of a teaching programme. However, much like assessment,

where there are differences between teacher and student assessment,(33) superior teachers provide a more accurate self-evaluation than do less highly rated teachers.(34) A highly effective, but rarely executed, evaluation strategy is to triangulate the three sources of evidence from students, peers and self.

Video recording of teaching

Berk(30) suggests that a video is one of the best sources of evidence for formative evaluation decisions. But who should evaluate it, and what methods and criteria should be used? A video recording of a teaching tutorial has been a requirement in UK general practice trainer approval for many years now. However, in hospital practice clinical teachers still seem to be wary of the video method, both in clinical work and in evaluation.

Student interviews

Interviews with groups of students are useful for evaluation purposes and may be considered more accurate and reliable than individual student ratings. Braskamp and Ory(35) suggested three types of group student interview:
- Quality control circle (e.g. a junior doctors' forum) that meets regularly to review the teaching and feedback comments and suggestions
- Classroom group interviews (with someone other than the usual teacher)
- Exit interviews with those who have completed the programme.

Exit and alumni ratings

A great strength of the alumni rating is that it can give valuable feedback but from a different perspective from that of current students. An example of the sort of question exit or alumni data can inform might be 'Was your medical school course fit for purpose?' We did precisely this study and found, perhaps not surprisingly, that it was good in some parts but not in others.(36) The young doctors and their consultant educational supervisors thought they were good at communication skills but less good at diagnosis, decision-making and prescribing. Elsewhere, graduates' opinions have been shown to correlate very highly with current students' views, even up to 4 years later.(37)

Employer ratings

Is the young graduate fit to do the job? What is their performance like once qualified? Studies in this area can evaluate the strengths and weaknesses of the programme, and again can give valuable feedback from another, different perspective. In the study above,(36) we also included the consultants. One common theme was that young doctors knew no anatomy, and though good at communicating, lacked the basic knowledge with which to communicate with patients.

Administrator ratings

Deans and those in senior positions may evaluate faculty in terms of criteria for promotion, merit awards, discretionary points and so on, as well as for teaching excellence awards. Often they will rely on secondary evidence, rather than direct observation themselves.

Teaching scholarship

By this we mean the academic contribution that people make to the growing body of knowledge in medical education, in terms of development of teaching programmes, research, published papers, books and presentations at conferences. This can discriminate the key educators or star performers from others.(38)

Teaching awards

An example of reward for teaching excellence is the system of awards at Toronto General Hospital devised by Posluns *et al.*(39) The authors developed a programme to recognise teaching excellence, using evaluations from trainees and departmental administrators. Awards were presented to teachers at a ceremonial event.

Learning outcomes measures

Claims are often made that success in professional examinations are a measure of how good the teaching was in a particular hospital. Superficially this might seem attractive, in view of the present emphasis on outcomes-based curricula.(40) But can we really infer teaching excellence from student performance? In fact, the correlation is low to moderate, only 0.4 in meta-analyses.(41) The big problem is how we isolate teacher input as the sole influence on students' performance at the end of their programme of study. There are many variables in addition to the teaching (such as student ability, motivation, examination standards) that also have an impact on the achievement of outcomes. So, in evaluating teaching effectiveness, learning outcome measures should be used with great caution.

Teaching portfolios

Currently portfolios seem to be everywhere in medical education, and increasingly these are 'electronic' and 'online'. Established practitioners use portfolios as collations of evidence towards an annual appraisal: doctors in the foundation and specialty training programmes use them as repositories for personal reflections and workplace-based assessments, and some medical schools have adopted portfolios as an integral part of the course. A teaching portfolio would ideally contain one's best work as a teacher, with evaluations from a variety of sources, and a reflective analysis on the different parts, together with appendices detailing some of the evidence. But how should such a portfolio of evidence be assessed? There are many approaches, with the assessment strategy chosen linked clearly to the portfolio structure (*see* Chapter 14 for a further discussion).

Promoting the use of evaluation findings

An essential question in judging the quality of an evaluation is 'are the results used'? No matter how beautifully designed the evaluation strategy, the key question for evaluators is: Can the results be fed back into the system and acted upon? 'Use' can mean different things to different people. There are five different types of 'use' described in the evaluation literature:(42)

1. *Instrumental use:* when an evaluation directly affects decision-making and influences change. Evidence for this type of use involves decisions and actions that come from the evaluation, including the implementation of recommendations.
2. *Conceptual use:* when the evaluation findings help individuals understand the programme in a new way or influence thinking in a general way without any immediate new decisions being made about the programme.
3. *Enlightenment:* related to conceptual use, but more focused on whether the evaluation findings add knowledge to the field and thus may be used by anyone, not just those involved with the programme or evaluation of the programme.
4. *Process use:* how individuals and organisations are impacted as a result of participating in an evaluation. It acknowledges that being involved in an evaluation can lead to changes in how people think, what they do and how they make decisions, which then result in cultural and organisational change.
5. *Symbolic use:* when evaluations are done as a requirement or political move, rather than serving an identifiable need. This is not an ideal or recommended use of evaluation.

There is a substantial amount of theoretical and empirical research on the use of results from evaluation studies. In a systematic review of the literature in this area, Johnson *et al.*(42) identified three broad categories of factors that increase the use of evaluation findings: (i) stakeholder involvement, (ii) characteristics-related implementation and (iii) characteristics of the decision or policy setting; the context in which the evaluation was implemented. Their findings are elaborated and discussed below.

The strongest evidence regarding use of evaluation falls under stakeholder involvement, including early involvement, inclusion of different stakeholder groups, and an evaluator who communicated well and sustained engagement throughout the evaluation.

Characteristics related to implementation included the quality and credibility of the evaluation approach, evaluator competence and timely/relevant reporting. However, the most critical factor in this category relates to evaluator/user communication. Frequency and quality of communication are important factors, as well as dissemination. The other interesting element in this category is the type of recommendations evaluators make; more specifically, if the recommendations are detailed and actionable items, they are more likely to result in changes, as compared to broad platitudes that have no practical significance.

The most important characteristics of context for increasing use are the personal characteristics of the individual(s) who will use the evaluation. To get the most value out of resources spent in conducting evaluations, the right decision-makers must engage with results. This means the organisational role of the decision-maker, the kind of authority they have, where they are in the organisational structure and their level of experience are critical to increasing the probability that results will be used. An important consideration for the evaluator is the 'information processing style' of the user – dissemination of some 'reports' verbally, in briefing style or by simply providing key findings and recommendations may be better than written reports.

Managing change

How do we manage change in a medical education system? There is a vast amount of literature in the area of change management that has been well summarised elsewhere.(43,44) Much of the early literature suggested a way of proceeding through the change process in a controlled and logical way. For example, by using a problem-solving approach we might identify a problem, agree the problem, suggest solutions, agree solutions, implement solutions and evaluate the changes, but rationale approaches do not always work (*see* Chapter 33).

To try to explain such events, it is helpful to rethink the linear model of change. Mintzberg(45) suggested that change can either be thought of as a pre-planned and logical series of steps or, perhaps more realistically, as an open-ended, ongoing and unpredictable process that aims to align and realign in response to change within society. Government departments, ministers, the Royal Colleges, the Postgraduate Medical Education and Training Board, the General Medical Council and the British Medical Association were all active players in the UK's *Modernising Medical Careers* process, a massive piece of educational change underpinned [with one or two small exceptions(46)] by almost no evaluation evidence.

So, what then is the relationship between evaluation and public policy? Weiss(47) and Swanwick(48) both discuss this interface and highlight that although researchers would wish for a direct and logical link, this is rarely the case. Policy-makers rarely base their new policies directly on evaluation decisions. Organisations do not often use knowledge directly to help organisational change. In fact, policy-makers tend only to cite evaluation studies that suit their particular line of policy. Direct influence of evaluation on policy is unusual. Instead, a more gradual process of change, the slow incorporation of ideas and methods into policy, is more common, a process that Weiss calls 'enlightenment'. New ideas seep in and percolate through the system, gain ground and may eventually become mainstream. Through this kind of process evaluation can have real and powerful consequences, challenging old ideas, offering new perspectives and helping to influence the policy.

Challenges in educational evaluation

There are several common pitfalls to try to avoid in any evaluation, some of which were mentioned earlier. The following are some common problems we have encountered in our careers as evaluators in medical education.

Timeliness

The timing of results is an important consideration. Too often planning and decision-making occur before data have been analysed or are even available. Providing a polished final report is not as important as providing results when planners and decision-makers need them. It is often necessary to provide rapid turnaround. Using alternate venues for reporting, such as presentations, memos or open discussion, are all good (and welcomed) alternatives to the long formal report.

Generalizability

Programme evaluation is often very local and the results may not be generalisable to other contexts. While the results may be useful at the local level, they may be challenging to publish. Because most evaluators working in medical education evaluation are academics, this represents an important challenge. It is impingent upon the evaluator to make a case for how the study contributes to the literature and to provide a thorough description of the context in which the work was conducted so that readers can determine its applicability to their context.

Standard of acceptability

E-*valu*-ation is about 'valuing' or 'judging' the success of a programme. Therefore, some standard of comparison is necessary. It can often be challenging to get stakeholders to define what will be considered 'successful'. Is it 100% of trainees achieving licensure? If 80% of trainees are satisfied, will that be considered successful?

Measuring only what is easy to measure

This may be related to following a certain methodology. It might be quite easy to send out a questionnaire and more difficult to do case studies where problems of bullying, negative feedback and so on are the main problem. It may also relate to gathering only one source of evidence, rather than trying to triangulate the evidence from three different areas.

Survey fatigue and low response rates

Trainees and students in medical education receive many surveys. Low response rates can pose a serious validity problem since a good response rate of at least 70% is standard for purposes of controlling bias. Do as much as you can to keep the number and length of surveys trainees reasonable. Providing incentives for special one-off surveys are worth considering as they can increase response rate, particularly amongst students.

Reliability of surveys

Some evaluation instruments have not been properly tested for reliability, or if they have, have been found wanting. The latter situation is very rare, and a lack of proper testing, or even lack of knowledge as to what should have been done, is far more common. It may then be impossible to derive any conclusions, or the conclusions obtained may be unreliable, which is worse when important conclusions are drawn from them.

Balancing the positive and negative

It is easy to fall into the trap of ignoring the positive accomplishments of a programme and to emphasise the negative. We have seen examples of this in evaluation studies and even on national quality assurance visits. Everyone is happy with the teaching except for one or two disaffected and sometimes dysfunctional individuals. The visiting team takes into consideration all of the concerns of those who are disaffected, to the exclusion of all other evidence. All of this appears in the report, but the emphasis on the negative, small though it may be, distorts the conclusions. Even if further investigations show much of this to be factually incorrect, the damage is done.

Conclusions

Evaluation is an essential part of medical education and needs to be carried out rigorously and systematically, all the while focusing on its utility. A good knowledge of many different areas is needed if we are to be able to carry out meaningful evaluations that can be fed back to improve medical education programmes. In the end, the ultimate goal is to design, implement and use evaluations that will produce improvements in patient care – an outcome that is at the pinnacle of Kirkpatrick's hierarchy – the very *raison d'etre* of medical education.

Examples of evaluations in medical education

Example 1: Evaluation of a course or curriculum

A widely known method for looking at course or curriculum content in medical education is what many call Harden's Ten Questions.(49) These questions can be used both in planning a course or curriculum, and to evaluate the course in a systematic way. The 10 questions are:

1. *What are the needs in relation to the product of the training programme?*
   Is the programme or curriculum fit for purpose? To evaluate this, one may consult experts, and look at errors in practice, critical incident reports, task analysis, morbidity and mortality figures, opinions and beliefs of star performers, existing curricula and views of recent students.
2. *What are the aims and objectives?*
   What will the student be able to do at the end of the course of study? Is this borne out by evaluation data?
3. *What content should be included?*
   Content should be put into a course if it directly contributes to the course objectives, forms a building block of skill or knowledge needed to tackle a later part of the course, allows development of intellectual abilities such as critical thinking and aids the understanding of other subjects on the course.
4. *How should the content be organised?*
   This relates to the order in which subjects are taught, and a theoretical plan of *why* the order is as it is.

5. *What educational strategies should be adopted?*
'Strategies' relate to the curriculum model being used, such as a spiral curriculum, an objectives model, a process model or an outcome-based model. Sometimes there is no obvious model at all.

6. *What teaching methods should be adopted?*
Student grouping may be one way, with, for example, whole class teaching by the lecture method, small groups, one-to-one bedside teaching and distance learning. Another way may be by teaching and learning tools, such as computer packages, web-based learning, simulators, skills laboratories and role play. The choice of methods needs to reflect the course aims and objectives. One would not choose to teach communication skills and breaking bad news to patients in a lecture-based course.

7. *How should assessment be carried out?*
This includes the choice of assessments used [such as essays, projects, portfolios, multiple-choice questions, Objective Structure Clinical Examinations (OSCEs), oral examinations, and long and short cases]. Question to ask include: Who will assess the work? Are there external examiners? Is there self-assessment? Will assessment be continuous throughout the course or at the end? What are the standards to be achieved? Are the assessment standards criteria referenced or norm referenced? How is the course evaluated? Is it by the students? Is there internal and external evaluation?

8. *How should details of the curriculum be communicated?*
Details have to be communicated to those teaching the course, the students attending the course, potential students and other bodies. How is this done? How do the subjects relate to each other and the final product?

9. *What educational environment or climate should be fostered?*
Does the environment encourage cooperation between students, students and teachers, scholarship, probity and support, or is it hostile, with teaching by humiliation, sexism and bullying?

10. How should the process be managed?
Who is responsible for planning, organising and managing the process? Can changes be made? How does this course relate to others? Is there student representation? Do the teaching staff know what is going on? Is there a course committee?

Example 2: Evaluation of the role of faculty development programmes

Does faculty development – teaching the teachers – really work? What is the evidence for this? This summary illustrates many different methods of evaluation that have been carried out seeking to answer this question. There is now good evidence that these courses do improve teachers' ability to teach, and do improve learning by trainees. Researchers in medical and dental education have shown that teaching the teachers initiatives really do work.

One of the few studies that tried to do this was undertaken by Whitehouse,(50) who followed up participants who had attended a 6-day educational teaching the teachers course. Participants did use the lessons learnt on the course and put many of these ideas into their own educa-

tion practice. Indeed, the group formed on this course continues to meet more than 10 years on from the original course.

In Turkey, Yolsal *et al.*(51) reported the impact of their Training of Trainers courses since 1997. They used a questionnaire at the end of their 6- to 9-day courses, and at 6 months post-course. Seventy-two per cent of their medical teachers said they had implemented the knowledge and skills acquired on the courses, and that students had given better feedback on their teaching. Many stated they now enjoyed their teaching more, and that they had set up a network of keen teachers after being on courses together. This study and these results are very similar to Whitehouse's study and results.(50)

Steinert *et al.*(52) at McGill University in Canada described a year-long faculty development programme to develop leaders in medical education. The course included educational knowledge and skills, in protected time, while maintaining the participants' other clinical, teaching and research responsibilities. A year after completing the programme, the authors found in a follow-up survey of 22 faculty members that many had joined new educational committees, taken up new leadership roles in medical education and developed new courses for students and doctors in training, and two had pursued further studies to Masters level. However, all three studies relied on self-reporting by the candidates rather than other evidence.

There are more recent studies that used different methodologies and end-point assessments to make similar points. Godfrey *et al.*(53) from Sheffield asked whether a teaching the teachers course did in fact develop teaching skills. They used a quasi-experimental design and compared a group of consultant teachers who attended a 3-day teaching the teachers course with a control group taken from the course waiting list. However, the candidates were not assigned to the taught group or the control group randomly. A questionnaire of teaching skills was applied to participants and controls before the course and at 8–10 months afterwards. Up to 63% of participants and 51% of controls replied to all aspects of this study. Candidates who had attended the course did significantly better and reported significantly greater improvements in self-reported teaching skills. These authors did discuss self-reporting as a source of bias, but argued that the control group in this research design did help overcome these issues.

In a Californian study, Morrison *et al.*(54) used an experimental design with an intervention group and a control group of medical residents to explore whether they could improve residents' teaching skills. Their research question was: 'Do trained teachers perform better then untrained control residents?' They ran a 13-hour teaching the teachers course over 6 months. This was a rigorously designed and carried out study. The two groups were similar in terms of gender, specialty and academic performance, and people were assigned randomly to each group, either to attend the course or be a control. The outcome measures included an eight-station, 3½-hour OSCE – previously validated – in which the participants were assessed by trained medical students. A subset of participants were interviewed 1 year later by two educational researchers, who did not know in advance who had attended the course and who was a control. Those residents in the teaching the teachers course group did significantly better in all eight stations of the OSCE, and people who were required to attend did as well as those who volunteered. Also, the interviews showed that the taught group showed greater enthusiasm for teaching, used learner-centred approaches, had more elaborate understanding of pedagogic principles and planned to teach after finishing their training.

In Alberta, Panderchuck *et al.*,(55) in another quasi-experimental study, looked at the effects of a 2-day teaching the teachers workshop. They compared a group of medical teachers who had attended the workshops with controls (who had not) by means of ratings by medical students on their teaching abilities before and after the workshops, using the standard University of Alberta student evaluation questionnaire. Their study used data from 1993 to 2002. Students' ratings of teachers' teaching abilities increased significantly for the teachers after the workshops, but remained unchanged for the control group, who had not attended the workshops.

In November 2006, evidence from the Best Evidence for Medical Education (BEME) review of faculty development initiatives by Steinert *et al.*(56), who reviewed 2777 papers and selected 53 of these papers for detailed analyses, showed:

- overall satisfaction with programmes was high
- participants reported positive changes in attitude to teaching
- increased knowledge of educational principles and of gains in teaching skills
- changes in teaching behaviours
- greater educational involvement and establishment of collegiate networks.

Key strategies for effective interventions to improve teaching effectiveness in medical education included:

- experiential learning
- feedback
- effective peer and colleague relationships
- interventions that followed the principles of teaching and learning
- use of a wide variety of educational methods.

In summary, much of the earlier literature is based on opinion from distinguished and senior individuals within the profession, both individually and in terms of organisations such as expert government committees, professional bodies and the regulators.(57,58) More recently, there have been examples of good evaluation studies that try to examine the effects of teaching the teachers courses by means of follow-up and self-reporting of changes, and of the effects of such initiatives on the learners, the medical students themselves. Here there is evidence that teaching the teachers courses do improve teaching ability, widen teachers' pedagogic approaches to teaching and increase enjoyment of teaching.

Example 3: Evaluation of the educational climate

The educational environment variously referred to as climate, atmosphere or tone is a set of factors that describe what it is like to be a learner within that organisation. Chambers and Wall(59) considered the educational climate in three parts:

- physical environment (safety, food, shelter, comfort and other facilities)
- emotional climate (security, constructive feedback, being supported and absence of bullying and harassment) *and*
- intellectual climate (learning with patients, relevance to practice, evidence-based, active par¬ticipation by learners, motivating and planned education).

The good clinical teaching environment(60) should ensure the teaching and learning is relevant to patients, has active participation by learners and shows professional thinking and behaviours. There should be good preparation and planning of both the structure and content, reflection on learning and evaluation of what has happened in the teaching and learning. Spencer(60) also goes on to describe some of the common problems with teaching and learning in the clinical environment, including lack of clear objectives, focus on knowledge rather than problem-solving skills, teaching at the wrong level, passive observation, little time for reflection and discussion, and teaching by humiliation.

Undermining, bullying and harassment is a big problem in the UK and other countries. Much of this relates to teachers' lack of awareness of educational skills and knowledge(61,62) and inability to promote a good, supportive educational climate for trainee learning.(57,58) Lowry(61) described disenchantment with medicine in the words of a young doctor as 'It could have been such a wonderful thing to be a doctor – but it's not. It's just a disaster.'

Sadly, there are many examples in the literature of bullying and harassment of junior doctors and medical students. Such studies show the practice is widespread, and at the individual level illustrate how destructive to confidence and well-being bullying and harassment can be. Wolf *et al.*(63) carried out a questionnaire study of medical students in the Louisiana State University School of Medicine. Of these, 98.9% reported mistreatment, with shouting and humiliation being most frequent. Over half reported sexual harassment, mainly by women students. There was a high level of remarks degrading doctors and medicine as a profession. Increased mistreatment was positively associated with a perceived increase in cynicism.

In Manchester, Guthrie *et al.*(64) used a postal questionnaire to measure the psychological morbidity and the nature and sources of stress in first-year medical students. Half the students reported a stressful incident, most of which related to medical training and the styles of medical teaching. They described being upset by the attitudes of tutors, including humiliation, shouting, ridicule, exposure of ignorance and a confrontational nature.

Metcalfe and Matharu(65) used a postal questionnaire study of medical students in Manchester to investigate student perceptions of good and bad teaching. Good examples were when there was active learning and teachers let students 'run the session'. Bad examples were mainly examples of bad behaviour of staff towards students, such as humiliation, sexism and ridicule.

Is this all in the past? In the 21st century, are all these problems behind us? The answer is probably no. Bullying and humiliation are still common within the medical profession. An anonymous author(66) described repeated bullying of a junior surgeon by a consultant. A questionnaire study by Quine(67) of bullying of junior doctors shows how common such behaviours still are. Of 594 doctors, 37% identified themselves as having been bullied in the past year, and 84% had experienced one or more bullying behaviours. Black and Asian doctors fared worse than white doctors, and women fared worse than men. The most common bullying strategies were attempts to belittle and undermine work, unjustified criticism, humiliation in front of colleagues, and intimidating use of discipline and competence procedures.

Despite this, the evaluations from the trainees at senior house officer level report good-to-excellent scores for induction, supervision and clinical experience in these posts. This is using the post-evaluation tool, developed and used every 6 months on all senior house officer posts within the West Midlands since 1997.(68) Also, evidence from our quality management visits to intensive care units has repeatedly shown that senior house officers value their time there very much, feel well supported and rate the jobs highly.

So can the education environment be measured using a practical, valid and reliable tool? The Dundee Ready Education Environment Measure was developed in Dundee by Roff *et al.*(69) It is a valid and reliable measure of the perceived education environment. It has been widely used in many countries throughout the world, including the Gulf States, Nepal, Nigeria, the West Indies, Thailand, China, Canada and the UK. It has been used for medical students, nurses, dentists, chiropractors and other professions allied to medicine.

From this original environmental measure, further postgraduate measurement scales have been developed. For the postgraduate medical education environment, the Dundee group has also developed a 40-item inventory for the various aspects of junior doctor training in the UK and Ireland, the Postgraduate Hospital Education Environment Measure.(70) The Anaesthetic Theatre Educational Environment Mea¬sure(71) has been developed and validated for teaching in anaesthesia in the operating theatre, and for junior surgeons in the operating theatre the Surgical Theatre Environmental Educational Measure(72) has been developed and validated.

In anaesthetic trainees, Holt and Roff(71) showed that there was a better educational climate perceived by first-year senior house officers than by specialist registrars, and these results were statistically significant. In the operating theatre, Nagraj *et al.*(73) showed that the educational climate was reasonably good for medical students and slightly less so for senior house officers. Only at specialist registrar level did the climate improve significantly. So, educational climate can be measured using a variety of well-researched, valid and reliable tools that are available free of charge in the public domain. One of the great assets of using these tools is that comparisons may be made of your own evaluations with others throughout the UK and indeed other parts of the international medical education community.

References

1 Fink A (2005) *Evaluation Fundamentals: Insights into the Outcomes, Effectiveness, and Quality of Health Programs* (2e). Sage, Thousand Oaks, CA.

2 Goldie J (2006) AMEE guide no. 29: evaluating educational programmes. *Medical Teacher.* **28**: 210–24.

3 Norcini JJ, Blank LL, Duffy FD and Fortna GS (2003) The miniCEX: a method of assessing clinical skills. *Annuals of Internal Medicine.* **138**: 476–83.

4 Mohanna K, Wall D and Chambers R (2004) *Teaching Made Easy – A Manual for Health Professionals* (2e). Radcliffe Medical Press, Oxford.

5 SCOPME (1996) Appraising Doctors and Dentists in Training. Standing Committee on Postgraduate Medical and Dental Education, London.

6 General Medical Council (2012) Good medical practice framework for appraisal and revalidation. (http://www.gmc-uk.org/static/documents/content/GMC_Revalidation_A4_Guidance_GMP_Framework_04.pdf; accessed 15 March 2013).

7 Knowlton LW and Phillips CC (2009) *The Logic Model Guidebook: Better Strategies for Great Results.* Sage, Thousand Oaks, CA.

8 Preskill H and Russ-Eft D (2005) *Building Evaluation Capacity.* Sage, Thousand Oaks, CA.

9 Patton MQ (2008) *Utilization-Focused Evaluation.* Sage, Thousand Oaks, CA.

10 Donaldson SI, Patton MQ, Fetterman DM and Scriven M (2010) The 2009 Claremont Debates: the promise and pitfalls of utilization-focused and empowerment evaluation. *Journal of Multidisciplinary Evaluation.* **6**: 15–57.

11 Vassar M, Wheeler DI, Davison M and Franklin J (2010) Program evaluation in medical education: an overview of the utilization-focused approach. *Journal of Educational Evaluation for Health Professions.* **7**: 1.

12 Kirkpatrick DI (1967) Evaluation of training. In: Craig R and Mittel I (eds) *Training and Development Handbook*, pp. 87–112. McGraw Hill, New York.

13 Belfield CR, Thomas HR, Bullock AD *et al.* (2001) Measuring effectiveness for Best Evidence Medical Education – a discussion. *Medical Teacher.* **23**: 164–70.

14 Fettermen DM, Wandersman A and Millett RA (2005) *Empowerment Evaluation Principles in Practice.* Sage, Thousand Oaks, CA.

15 Fetterman DM, Deitz J and Gesundheit N (2010) Empowerment evaluation: a collaborative approach to evaluating and transforming a medical school curriculum. *Academic Medicine.* **85**: 813–20.

16 Bedward J, Davison I, Field S and Thomas H (2005) Audit, educational development and research: what counts for ethics and research governance? *Medical Teacher.* **27**: 99–101.

17 Boyer EL (1990) *Scholarship Reconsidered: Priorities of the Professoriate.* Carnegie Foundation for the Advancement of Teaching, Menlo Park, CA.

18 Henry RC and Wright DE (2001) When do medical students become human subjects of research? The case of program evaluation. *Academic Medicine.* **76**: 871–5.

19 Dyrbye LN, Thomas MR, Mechaber AJ *et al.* (2007) Medical education research and IRB review: an analysis and comparison of the IRB review process at six institutions. *Academic Medicine.* **82**: 654–60.

20 Egan-Lee E, Freitag S, Leblanc V *et al.* (2011) Twelve tips for ethical approval for research in health professions education. *Medical Teacher.* **33**: 268–72.

21 Morrison M (2005) Ethics. In: Mathison S (ed.) *Encyclopedia of Evaluation.* Sage, Thousand Oaks, CA.

22 Worthen BL, Sanders JR and Fitzpatrick JL (1997) *Program Evaluation: Alternative Approaches and Practical Guidelines* (2e). Longman, New York.

23 Oppenheim AN (1992) *Questionnaire Design, Interviewing and Attitude Measurement*. Continuum, London.

24 Field A (2000) *Discovering Statistics Using SPSS for Windows*. Sage Publications, London.

25 Howitt D and Cramer D (2003) *A Guide to Computing Statistics with SPSS 11 for Windows*. Pearson Education, Harlow.

26 Cohen L, Manion L and Morrison K (2000) *Research Methods in Education* (5e). RoutledgeFalmer, London.

27 Bowling A (1997) *Research Methods in Health*. Open University Press, Buckingham.

28 Cartwright A (1988) Interviews or postal questionnaires? Comparisons of data about women's experiences with maternity services. *Milbank Quarterly*. **66**: 172–89.

29 Krueger RA and Casey MA (2009) *Focus Groups: A Practical Guide for Applied Research*. Sage, Thousand Oaks, CA.

30 Berk RA (2006) *Thirteen Strategies to Measure College Teaching*. Stylus Publishing LLC, Sterling, VA.

31 Arreola RA (2000) *Developing a Comprehensive Faculty Evaluation System: A Handbook for College Faculty and Administrators on Designing and Operating a Comprehensive Faculty Evaluation System* (2e). Anker, Bolton, MA.

32 Murray HG (1983) Low inference classroom teaching behaviours and student ratings of college teaching teac ing effectiveness. *Journal of Educational Psychology*. **71**: 856–65.

33 Falchikov N and Boud D (1989) Student self-assessment in higher education: a meta-analysis. *Review of Educational Research*. **59**: 395–430.

34 Barber LW (1990) Self-assessment. In: Millman J and Darling-Hammond L (eds) *The New Handbook of Teacher Evaluation*, pp. 216–28. Sage, Newbury Park, CA.

35 Braskamp LA and Ory JC (1994) *Assessing Faculty Work*. Jossey-Bass, San Francisco, CA.

36 Wall D, Bolshaw A and Carolan J (2006) Is undergraduate medical education fitting for purpose to be a pre-registration house officer? *Medical Teacher*. **28**: 435–9.

37 Overall JU and Marsh HW (1980) Students' evaluation of instruction: a longitudinal study of their stability. *Journal of Educational Psychology*. **72**: 321–5.

38 Harden RM (1986) Approaches to curriculum planning. *Medical Education*. **20**: 458–66.

39 Posluns E, Sharon Safir M, Keystone JS *et al.* (1990) Rewarding medical teaching excellence in a major Canadian teaching hospital. *Medical Teacher*. **12**: 13–22.

40 Harden RM, Crosby JR and Davis MH (1999) An introduction to outcomes based learning. *Medical Teacher*. **21**: 7–14.

41 Feldman KA (1989) The association between student ratings of specific instructional dimensions and student achievement: refining and extending the synthesis of data from multisection validity studies. *Research in Higher Education*. **30**: 583–645.

42 Johnson K, Greenseid LO, Tiak SA *et al.* (2009) Research on evaluation use: a review of the empirical literature from 1986 to 2005. *American Journal of Evaluation*. **30**: 377–410.

43 Handy C (1989) *The Age of Unreason*. Business Books, London.

44 Iles V and Sutherland K (1997) *The Literature on Change Management. Review for Healthcare Managers, Researchers and Professionals*. National Co-ordinating Centre for NHS Service Delivery and Organisation, London.

45 Mintzberg H (1987) Crafting strategy. *Harvard Business Review*. **65**: 66–75.

46 Walzman M, Allen M and Wall D (2009) General practice and the Foundation Programme: the views of FY2 doctors from the Coventry and Warwickshire Foundation School. *Education for Primary Care*. **19**: 151–9.

47 Weiss C (1999) The interface between evaluation and public policy. *Evaluation*. **5**: 468–86.

48 Swanwick T (2007) Introducing large-scale educational reform in a complex environment: the role of piloting and evaluation in modernizing medical careers. *Evaluation*. **13**: 363–73.

49 Harden RM (1986) Ten questions to ask when planning a course or curriculum. *Medical Education*. **20**: 356–65.

50 Whitehouse A (1997) Warwickshire consultants' 'training the trainers' course. *Postgraduate Medical Journal*. **73**: 35–8.

51 Yolsal N, Bulut A, Karabey S *et al.* (2003) Development of training of trainers' programmes and evaluation of their effectiveness in Istanbul, Turkey. *Medical Teacher*. **25**: 319–24.

52 Steinert Y, Nasmith L, McLeod PJ and Conochie L (2003) A teaching scholars program to develop leaders in medical education. *Academic Medicine*. **78**: 142–9.

53 Godfrey J, Dennick G and Welsh C (2004) Training the trainers: do teaching courses develop teaching skills? *Medical Education*. **38**: 844–7.

54 Morrison EH, Rucker L, Boker JR *et al.* (2004) The effect of a 13 hour curriculum to improve residents' teaching skills – a randomised trial. *Annals of Internal Medicine*. **141**: 257–63.

55 Panderchuck K, Harley D and Cook D (2004) Effectiveness of a brief workshop designed to im-prove teaching performance at the University of Alberta. *Academic Medicine*. **79**: 798–804.

56 Steinert Y, Mann K, Centeno A *et al.* (2006) A systematic review of faculty development initiatives designed to improve teaching effectiveness in medical education: BEME guide no. 8. *Medical Teacher*. **28**: 497–526.

57 SCOPME (1992) Teaching Hospital Doctors and Dentists to Teach: its role in creating a better learning environment. Proposals for Consultation - full report. Standing Committee for Postgraduate Medical Education, London.

58 SCOPME (1994) Creating a Better Learning Environment in Hospitals 1. Teaching Hospital Doctors and Dentists to Teach. Standing Committee on Postgraduate Medical Education, London.

59 Chambers R and Wall D (2000) *Teaching Made Easy: A Manual for Health Professionals*. Radcliffe Medical Press, Oxford.

60 Spencer N (2003) The clinical teaching context: a cause for concern. *Medical Education*. **37**: 182–3.

61 Lowry S (1993) Teaching the teachers. *British Medical Journal*. **306**: 127–30.

62 Lowry S (1992) What's wrong with medical education in Britain? *British Medical Journal*. **305**: 1277–80.

63 Wolf TM, Randall HM, Von Almen K and Tynes LL (1991) Perceived mistreatment and attitude change by graduating medical students: a retrospective study. *Medical Education*. **25**: 182–90.

64 Guthrie EA, Black D, Shaw CM *et al.* (1995) Embarking on a medical career: psychological morbidity in first year medical students. *Medical Education*. **29**: 337–41.

65 Metcalfe DH and Matharu M (1995) Students' perceptions of good and bad teaching: report of a critical incident study. *Medical Education*. **29**: 193–7.

66 Anon (2001) Personal view. Bullying in medicine. *British Medical Journal*. **323**: 1314.

67 Quine L (2002) Workplace bullying in junior doctors: questionnaire survey. *British Medical Journal*. **324**: 878–9.

68 Wall DW, Woodward D, Whitehouse A *et al.* (2001) The development and uses of a computerised evaluation tool for SHO posts in the West Midlands Region. *Medical Teacher*. **23**: 24–8.

69 Roff S, McAleer S, Harden RM *et al.* (1997) Development and validation of the Dundee Ready Educational environment Measure (DREEM). *Medical Teacher*. **19**: 295–9.

70 Roff S, McAleer S and Skinner A (2005) Development and validation of an instrument to measure the postgraduate clinical learning environment for hospital based junior doctors in the UK. *Medical Teacher*. **27**: 326–31.

71 Holt M and Roff S (2004) Development and validation of the Anaesthetic Theatre Educational Environment Measure (ATEEM). *Medical Teacher.* **26**: 553–8.

72 Cassar K (2004) Development of an instrument to measure the surgical operating theatre learning environment as perceived by basic surgical trainees. *Medical Teacher.* **26**: 260–4.

73 Nagraj S, Wall D and Jones E (2006) Can STEEM be used to measure the educational environment within the operating theatre for undergraduate medical students? *Medical Teacher.* **28**: 642–7.

Further reading

Andres L (2012). *Designing and Doing Survey Research.* Sage, London.

British Educational Research Association (2011) Ethical guidelines for educational research (2011). British Educational Research Association, Southwell. (http://content.yudu.com/Library/A1t9gr/BERA EthicalGuideline/resources/index.htm?referrerUrl=http%25253A%25252F%25252Fwww.yudu.com%25252Fitem%25252Fdetails%25252F375952%25252FBERA-Ethical-Guidelines-2011; accessed 16 March 2013).

Cohen L, Manion L and Morrison K (2000) *Research Methods in Education* (5e). RoutledgeFalmer, London.

Donaldson SI, Christie CA and Mark MM (2009) *What Counts as Credible Evidence in Applied Research and Evaluation Practice?* Sage, Thousand Oaks, CA.

Owen JM (2007) *Program Evaluation: Forms and Approaches* (3e). Guildford Press, New York.

Western Michigan University. Evaluation checklists site. (http://www.wmich.edu/evalctr/checklists/; accessed 12 March 2013).

Yarbrough DB, Shulha LM, Hopson RK and Caruthers FA (2011) *The Program Evaluation Standards: A Guide for Evaluators and Evaluation Users* (3e). Sage, Thousand Oaks, CA.

Part 5
Staff and Students

28 Selection into medical education and training

Fiona Patterson[1], Eamonn Ferguson[2] and Alec L Knight[3]

[1]University of Cambridge, UK
[2]University of Nottingham, UK
[3]Work Psychology Group, UK

KEY MESSAGES

- Historically, medical school admissions have relied primarily on indicators of academic achievement to select students.

- There is relatively little research investigating selection issues in medical education and training other than the prediction of exam performance.

- Assessment for selection is significantly different from summative assessments of education or training, such as written examinations.

- Best practice selection involves a thorough job analysis and the use of evidence from validation studies to drive continual improvement of accuracy and fairness.

- Establishing the predictive validity of a selection method presents many conceptual and practical problems. The validation process may take several years and piloting is essential.

- At postgraduate level, selection ratios for specialties differ widely. This has implications for the design of specific selection systems.

Introduction

After an individual submits his or her medical school application, selection is the first assessment he or she will undergo in the medical education and training pathway. The intention at this point is to predict who will become a competent doctor – and to identify those individuals who will successfully complete training – before training commences. Historically, when faced with limited student places and large numbers of applicants, most medical schools have tended to reply upon academic criteria in admission procedures. High academic achievement is a minimum entry requirement in medical school admissions almost universally. This assumes that with a high level of academic ability, the other skills and attributes required to be a competent doctor are trainable. However, research suggests that we should not assume that individuals with high academic ability can necessarily be trained to be good doctors.(1–3) In addition to high academic ability, it is vital that medical students also possess a range of other important skills and qualities.(4) This follows a deeper analysis of the so-called (and somewhat artificial) divide in criteria between the *cognitive* (e.g. clinical knowledge) and the *non-cognitive* (e.g. empathy, communication, integrity). Conceptually, a key issue is whether medical schools should aim to select individuals who will make successful students or those who will make competent clinicians.(5,6) Clearly, success as a student and competence as a doctor are not mutually exclusive, but the former is not necessarily a precursor of the latter.

Research evidence suggests that medical school selection criteria vary between schools both intra- and internationally. This diversity of entry criteria is at odds with recent job analysis research suggesting that there is good evidence for a large commonalty in the knowledge, skills and attributes required to be a competent doctor, irrespective of the specialty practised.(7)

In this chapter we explore why the variability in medical school selection criteria has arisen, and we provide recommendations about how to resolve this variability. An important consideration in designing selection systems is accounting for the reactions of key stakeholders to the criteria and methods used (e.g. reactions towards the use of interviews versus IQ tests). Patterson and colleagues(8,9) suggested that the *political* validity of selection system design is an important consideration. This notion refers to levels of acceptance of selection criteria and methods by a broad range of stakeholders. The reactions of applicants and recruiters are important, as are reactions from wider stakeholders, including government, regulatory bodies and the general public, which play an important role in decision-making at policy level.

Later in the chapter we outline the key concepts associated with selection processes and the relative accuracy of selection methods for medical education and training. We discuss why medicine provides a unique occupational

Understanding Medical Education: Evidence, Theory and Practice, Second Edition. Edited by Tim Swanwick.
© 2014 The Association for the Study of Medical Education. Published 2014 by John Wiley & Sons, Ltd.

context and summarise international perspectives on selection practices, referencing both undergraduate and postgraduate training. Key concepts underpinning selection research are described and we summarise the research evidence on the reliability and validity of current selection methods. Finally, some considerations for a future research agenda are presented.

The state of the art

Compared to many other professions, the length of training required to practise as a clinician in any given specialty is long and costly, normally taking in excess of 15 years from medical school through to senior appointment. When reviewing selection issues within the training pathway, a distinction must be drawn between selection into medical school (*pre-employment*) and postgraduate training (*employment*). Importantly, the latter is governed by specific employment law, for which there are also significant international differences.(10,11)

The assessment paradigm used to describe a selection context is different from that of professional examinations. In examinations, the aim is to assess end-of-training capability, where judgements are made by trained examiners about an individual's capacity to perform a job with competence. In theory, all candidates can pass the assessment. By contrast, in selection settings, if the number of candidates outweighs the number of available posts, then the assessment is geared towards ranking individuals effectively. Potentially, if the competition is very high, competent candidates may not be awarded a post.

Assessment in selection uses a 'predictivist paradigm', where the intention is to *predict* who will be a competent doctor (i.e. to identify those individuals who will successfully complete training, *before* training commences). Although there are several similarities, the parameters for designing and validating a robust selection system and selection tools are different from other assessment settings. Importantly, the criteria used to judge the effectiveness of a selection system are potentially more complex.

Selecting the wrong person for a job can have serious consequences for an organisation, the employee involved and, perhaps of most importance in medicine, the patient. For many occupational groups there exists a large body of international research investigating best practice selection. In medicine, there is a significant volume of research exploring predictors of performance at medical school. However, there is limited research exploring international selection practices. In particular, there is very little research exploring selection for entry into postgraduate training or into senior medical appointments.

Recently, leading figures in the field of health-care selection research from across the world came together to describe the current state of the art.(12) We would direct readers to this international consensus statement for a discussion of selection best practice based on contemporary international research findings. The statement is summarised in Box 28.1. In the following section, we provide a brief summary of the international context so as to high-

light international differences in training that are important to consider when interpreting research findings.

Context of medical selection

Undergraduate selection

Recently there has been considerable scrutiny of medical schools' admission processes, where policies vary internationally. As already mentioned, faced with limited student places and large numbers of applicants, most medical schools have traditionally relied upon academic criteria in admission procedures. Almost universally, high academic achievement is a minimum entry requirement. This assumes that with good academic ability, other skills required to be a good doctor are then trainable. However, researchers recognise that future clinicians should be selected on criteria other than academic performance alone.(1–3,6) There is increasing emphasis on assessing a candidate's personal characteristics and other abilities, such as communication skills, for admission to medical school.(13) For example, in the UK many applicants are offered a place based on a combination of academic competence, and performance in an interview and aptitude test [the UK Clinical Aptitude Test (UKCAT)]. In the USA, Canada and Australia, aptitude tests are also used, such as the Medical College Admission Test (MCAT),(14) the Graduate Australian Medical School Admission Test (GMSAT)(15) and the Undergraduate Medical and Health Science Admission Test (UMAT). However, with the possible exception of MCAT, there is relatively little published evidence on the reliability and validity of these tests.(16)

BOX 28.1 FOCUS ON: The 2010 Ottawa Consensus Statement(12)

There is an international consensus about assessment for selection for the health professions and specialty programmes but the areas of consensus are small. There is evidence for the predictive validity of the Medical College Admission Test (MCAT) and Grade Point Average (GPA). There is not strong evidence as yet for the credibility of newer tests introduced in countries outside of North America, such as Graduate Medical School Admisisons Test (GAMSAT), Undergraduate Medicine and Health Sciences Admission Test (UMAT) or UK Clinical Aptitude Test (UKCAT). Nor is there much evidence outside North America about GPA of prior study whether it be in the form of high school leaving grades or prior university study. There is an obvious need for more studies in these areas.

For other measures, there is evidence of the test–retest reliability and predictive validity of the Mini Multiple Interview (MMI) but not much else. Furthermore, there is evidence on this issue from outside North America. There is not much evidence of the credibility of interviews, personal statements and letters of reference.

Postgraduate medical selection

At postgraduate level selection criteria not only vary within and between countries, but also within and between specialties.

In the USA, medical students apply for residency positions in postgraduate specialty training through the National Resident Matching Program (NRMP).(17) Selection criteria usually comprise performance on the United States Medical Licensing Examination (USMLE), clinical rotation grades, class rank and interviews with faculty members.(18) Selection tools used by US admission panels have changed in the last 20 years.(19) In the 1970s, a survey of residency programme directors showed the interview to be the most important selection method.(20) Additional information used included the Dean's letter, other letters of recommendation and honours grades in clinical clerkships. Scores on the national board examination and membership of the Alpha Omega Alpha Honor Medical Society (AOA) were given less consideration in selection. A survey conducted in the 1980s(21) suggested that programme directors considered performance in selection interviews to be the most important selection criterion. Although less than half (46%) of the directors indicated that evidence for academic achievement was essential for the candidate to be admitted to interview, most directors (86%) declared they would not consider a candidate who had failed part 1 of the national board examination and had not passed it prior to interview.

More recent studies show measures of academic performance such as honours in the rotation of the chosen specialty or scores on USMLE Step I are viewed as being particularly important by programme directors in both primary care and non-primary care residencies.(22–26) Emphasis on indicators of academic success is more pronounced in more competitive specialties such as surgery.(24–26) Awareness that Deans' letters and other letters of recommendation do not always contain 'valid' information has led many programme directors to place less emphasis on data gathered from references.(26,27) In the USA, Crane and Ferraro(23) investigated selection criteria used by emergency medical residency committees. Results showed that, in order of reported importance, the interview was seen as the most important followed by clinical grades and then recommendations. Moderately important determinants of candidates' eligibility for training included: (i) elective completed at the programme director institution, (ii) USMLE Step II, (iii) interest expressed in programme director institution, (iv) USMLE Step I and (iv) awards/achievements.

In Canada, selection for admission to the various training programmes is made primarily on the basis of scholastic, personal and professional attributes as determined by academic records, personal interviews, letters of reference, choice of electives and in-training evaluation reports. The selection process is determined by each particular training programme, and admission to the postgraduate training year one for most programmes is conducted through a matching system.(11)

In the UK, a wide range of innovative practice has been piloted and adopted across the foundation programme and the 67 approved UK specialties (and 35 sub-specialties) since a wholesale reform of postgraduate medical education in 2005 known as *Modernising Medical Careers*. The use of selection centres is discussed later and Box 28.7 highlights one computerised selection method that is growing in use, the situational judgement test.

Key concepts

Selection process

Figure 28.1 provides a diagrammatic summary of the main elements involved in designing and implementing a selection process. The process starts by conducting a thorough analysis of the relevant knowledge, skills, abilities and attitudes associated with performance in the target role. This information is used to construct a person specification (and job description where appropriate). This is used to decide which selection instruments are best used to elicit applicant behaviour related to the selection criteria. In deciding to apply for a post (or a place at medical school), applicants will engage in *self-selection* where they can make an informed judgement about whether the particular role suits their skills and abilities.

This in-depth analysis is the cornerstone to producing an effective selection process as the aim is to identify appropriate selection criteria. In job analysis studies, researchers use various methods such as direct observation, and interviews with job holders.(28) Having defined these criteria at a level appropriate for the career stage (e.g. entry to specialty training), this information is used to guide choice of selection methods. Outputs from this analysis should detail the responsibilities in the target job and also provide information about the particular competencies and characteristics required of the job holder. Box 28.2 illustrates example outputs from a job analysis study to define selection criteria for those entering training in UK General Practice (Family Practice).

Once selection decisions are made and the accepted applicants enter training, information on the performance of trainees related to the original selection criteria should be used to examine the predictive validity of the selection instruments (i.e. to what extent are scores at selection associated with assessment of in-training and work performance)?

Figure 28.1 also shows that best practice selection is a 'two-way' selection process. In other words, in order to attract the best trainees, both medical schools and hospitals have become increasingly aware that evaluating candidates' reactions to the selection process is essential, particularly in relation to perceptions of fairness. Since large resources are often spent on selection procedures, the utility of the selection procedures should be evaluated. In addition, information collected at selection (i.e. entry point to training) can be used to design tailored development plans for trainees.

The rudiments of best practice selection are clear, yet research shows that there are two elements in the process that are often not conducted effectively. First, many organisations fail to conduct a thorough job analysis to identify

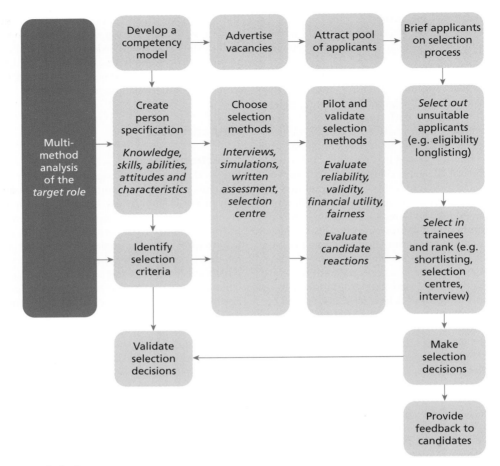

Figure 28.1 The process of selection.

the key knowledge, skills and behaviours associated with competent performance in the target job role. This is particularly important when exploring potential differences between medical specialties. Second, validation studies are rarely conducted in organisations as they are time consuming and difficult to administer. It often means tracking the performance of trainees over several years, from selection to medical school through to senior posts. In medical education and training, far more validation research has occurred in undergraduate selection. Here research has explored the predictive validity of various cognitive factors (prior academic performance or knowledge tests) with respect to exam performance.(30) The criteria used to judge performance at medical school are potentially more readily observed as there are standardised assessments involved, such as examinations. By contrast, the research literature is sparse when considering selection for either postgraduate training or non-cognitive factors.(30)

In summary, research clearly demonstrates that best practice selection is an iterative process. Results from evaluation and validation studies should be used to review the original selection criteria and the choice of selection methods. Thereby, feedback can be used to make continual improvements to selection systems to enhance their accu-

racy and fairness. Ideally, a selection system should have mutual feed-forward and feed-back connections.

Evaluative criteria

Before judging how well selection methods work, it is necessary to understand the framework used for determining best practice. Box 28.3 lists a number of criteria for judging the 'quality' of selection procedures. This should be reviewed when designing and implementing any selection system.

When choosing the selection method(s) it is important that the output (score) is consistent/stable (*reliable*) and relevant/precise/accurate (*valid*), and that the method is *objective, standardised*, administered by trained professional(s) and monitored. Evaluation of the system is essential to ensure that selection tools are also *fair, defensible, cost-effective* and *feasible*. Feedback is used to make continual improvements to the selection system to enhance accuracy and fairness. For postgraduate training there are legal reasons for ensuring accurate selection procedures are used, as is essential for compliance with employment law.

Validity

No single validation study will provide a definitive answer regarding the validity of any selection method. This is

BOX 28.2 Competency domains from a job analysis for UK general practitioners

Competency	Definition	Example positive behavioural indicators
Empathy and sensitivity	Patient is treated with sensitivity and personal understanding, asks patient about feelings. GP is empathetic, in control but not dominating, and creates atmosphere of trust and confidence. Focuses on the positive rather than negative, works to involve the patient, shows interest in the individual, gives reassurance and checks patient needs are satisfied	• Generates an atmosphere where the patient feels safe • Patient is taken seriously, treated confidentially • Picks up on patient's emotions and feelings • Encourages patient, gives reassurances • Use of 'I understand what you're saying' • Focuses on the positive • Is sensitive to feelings • Treats individuals as people • Checks patient needs are satisfied • Demonstrates a caring attitude
Communication skills	Active listening to patients, understands and interprets body language. Able to use different questioning styles and probe for information to lead to root cause. Matches patient language, uses analogy to explain, engages in social conversation, confident style. Clarity in both verbal and written communication.	• Demonstrates active listening skills • Is not patronising • Confident in approach • Able to form relationships with people and build rapport easily • Uses analogy to explain problems/complex issues • Restates information for understanding • Open body language and direct eye contact • Matches patient's language • Allows patients time to talk • Engages in social conversation • Refers to the patient by name
Clinical expertise	Able to apply and trust one's judgement (and other's) in diagnosing problems. Fully investigates problem before prescribing, able to anticipate rather than just react and to maintain knowledge of current practice. Doesn't allow patient to develop a dependency	• Trust in your clinical judgement • Clinical competence • Provides anticipatory care • Guards against dependency • Has courage to make decisions • Seeks to update clinical skills • Gives clear decision and diagnosis • Prescribes and checks medication • Provides clear explanation of facts and systems • Gets to the root of the problem • Encourages patient compliance

From Patterson et al.(29)

BOX 28.3 Evaluative criteria for selection procedures

1. Reliability and validity of selection tools
2. Employee/candidate reactions
3. Ease of interpretation
4. Generality of use
5. Minimising costs and maximising value
6. Practicality/administrative convenience
7. Legality
8. Availability of analytical expertise
9. Fairness
10. Educational impact
11. Mechanisms for generating feedback
12. Arrangements for ongoing validation, evaluation and development

---

BOX 28.4 FOCUS ON: Validity in selection

Faith validity	This is a 'blind' faith that a selection method works because someone plausible said so
Face validity	The selection tool content appears relevant to the target role
Content validity	The content of the selection tool is judged to be directly relevant to the target role by subject matter experts
Criterion validity: *Concurrent*	A form of criterion-related validity in which data on the predictor and criterion are obtained at the same time. High correlations between predictor and criterion scores indicate concurrent validity
Criterion validity: *Predictive*	This is the extent to which a predictor measure (e.g. a selection test score) is correlated to a criterion measure (e.g. work performance). High predictive validity indicates that a selection measure gives an accurate indication of candidates' future performance on the criterion
Incremental validity	This is an empirical issue to determine how much additional value using another assessment provides
Construct validity	An indication of the extent to which the test or procedure measures the construct that it is intended to measure (such as empathy, clinical expertise)
Political validity	An indication of the extent to which various stakeholders and stakeholder groups (such as employers, parents, government departments, society, the regulator) consider the tool(s) to be appropriate and acceptable for use in selection

---

because any particular study can be conducted on only a sample of relevant people and, of course, has to be conducted at a particular time, using particular measures. There are likely to be specific factors, such as the sampling, the measures, the timing of the study and so on, which influence the results in some way. To estimate the validity of a particular selection procedure, more than one study design is needed, so that error is minimised. Most selection systems combine several predictors (selection tools), such as an applicant's score on an interview and academic achievements.

In validation studies, a key question is how much does adding another predictor increase the predictive power of the selection process? This is known as *incremental validity*. Specifically, recruiters want to know how accuracy is improved, for example as a result of using a personality assessment (rather than relying solely on interview scores). Information on the incremental validity of a specific selection tool is extremely valuable as it allows organisations to conduct a cost–benefit analysis of using additional tools. Box 28.4 provides a list of the different forms of validity for reference.

Conducting validation studies is very complex in practical terms since researchers would rarely use one single predictor to make selection decisions, and applicants will usually be judged on multiple selection criteria. Given the multifaceted nature of the role of a doctor, recruiters are likely to design multiple selection tools to assess applicants. Therefore, recruiters must decide whether a job applicant must score highly on all selection criteria (non-compensatory) or whether high scores on some criteria can make up for low scores on another (compensatory). In practice, recruiters might assign different weightings to various selection criteria, depending on the nature of the job role. For example, if clinical knowledge is the most important criterion and an applicant does not achieve a certain score, their application may not be considered further.

Predictive validity and the 'criterion problem'

In theory, the way to collect criterion-related validity data (i.e. how well do scores on the selection measure predict some future outcome or criterion) is to use a predictive (or follow-up) design. This design involves collecting predictor information (e.g. interview ratings, test scores) for candidates and then following up to gather data on their performance (e.g. during their first year of employment or exams at medical school). Predictive validity is assessed by examining the correlation between scores at selection (Time 1) and criterion data collected at Time 2 (perhaps through relevant work-based assessments, examinations, etc.). Research shows it is unusual in field studies to obtain validity coefficients in excess of r = 0.5.(31) Nevertheless, validity coefficients that are considerably less than +1.0 can provide a basis for improved selection practices.(32)

Conducting validation studies in practice presents a variety of problems. One major problem is with regard to accessing the appropriate criterion (outcome) data to validate the selection process. Often the criteria used to measure

BOX 28.5 FOCUS ON: Sources of error in validation studies

1 *Sampling error*
   If relatively small samples are used in many validation studies, the results obtained may be unduly influenced by the effects of small numbers of people within the sample whose results may be unusual. As sample size increases, more reliable results are obtained.

2 *Poor measurement precision*
   The measurement of attributes at both the predictor (i.e. selection method) and criterion (i.e. job performance) stage of the validation process is subject to unsystematic error. This error (unreliability) in the scores obtained will reduce the ceiling for the observed correlation between predictor and criterion: the error is unsystematic and random, thus this element of the predictor or criterion score will not correlate systematically with anything. This means that as reliability decreases, the maximum possible correlation between predictor and criterion will decrease.

3 *Restricted range of scores*
   The sample of people used in a validation study may not provide the full theoretically possible range of scores on the predictor and/or criterion measures. A restricted range of scores has a straightforward statistical effect on limiting the size of the linear correlation between two variables. So, like unreliability, range restriction in a sample serves to reduce the magnitude of the observed correlation coefficient.

performance in the job role do not match the criteria used for selection. Conversely, sometimes the criterion and predictor are very similar (e.g. using the MCAT or other knowledge-based tests to predict exam performance in medical school), which may lead to problems of common method variance and content overlap. Ideally, predictor scores should not be used to take selection decisions until after a predictive validation study has been conducted. Practically, this is difficult to achieve and so piloting is essential to conduct an appropriate validation. Box 28.5 presents three sources of error that are important to consider when conducting validation studies in selection, including sampling, measurement precision and restriction of range issues. Note that this is not intended to be an exhaustive list of sources of error, which also includes issues such as selection bias, reverse causation and missing variable problems.

Candidate reactions

Candidate reactions to different recruitment methods are critically important.(33) Considerable research has attempted to determine applicants' views on selection methods. Research has tended to explain the different factors that affect applicant reactions using organisational theories of justice.

Distributive justice focuses on perceived fairness regarding equity (where the selection outcome is consistent with the applicant's expectation) and equality (the extent to which applicants have the same opportunities in the selection process). *Procedural justice* refers to the formal characteristics of the selection process, such as information and feedback offered, job-relatedness of the procedures and methods, and recruiter effectiveness.(34) Four main factors seem to account for positive applicant reactions. These are where selection methods: (i) are based on a thorough job analysis and appear job relevant, (ii) are not personally intrusive, (iii) do not contravene procedural or distributive justice expectations, and (iv) allow applicants to meet in person with the recruiters. Other research shows that applicants prefer multiple opportunities to demonstrate their skills (as in selection centres) and prefer selection systems that are administered consistently for all applicants. In particular, when competition ratios are high, applicant reactions and candidate expectations of 'fair play' are crucial.

Fairness

Fair selection and recruitment is based on (i) having objective and valid criteria (developed through an appropriate job analysis), (ii) accurate and standardised assessment by trained personnel and (iii) monitored outcomes. Research has explored the extent to which selection procedures are fair to different subgroups of the population (such as ethnic minorities or women). However, a test is not unfair or biased simply because members of different subgroups obtain different scores on the tests. Men and women have different mean scores for height: this does not mean that rulers are unfair measuring instruments. However, it would be unfair to use height as a selection criterion for a job, if the job could be done by people of any height, since it is important for selection criteria to be job related. Normally, of course, the extent to which a selection method is related to job performance can be estimated by validation research, and it is clear, therefore, that fairness and validity are closely related.

Selection methods

Researchers have reviewed the use of numerous selection methods across several different occupational groups.(35–37) Although some of these methods have been piloted for selection into medicine, the interview tends to be the most common method used in both undergradute and postgraduate selection. In the following section we provide an overview of the research evidence in relation to the most common selection methods.

Interviews

Interviews are ubiquitous in the selection processes of a variety of professions.(35) They can be used at different stages of the selection process, either as the sole method of selection, or in conjunction with other methods. Interviews vary in terms of (i) purpose, (ii) duration, (iii) mode of administration (telephone, face-to-face or video conference), (iv) number of interviewers (one-to-one or panel), (v) degree of structure (unstructured, semi-structured or

> ### BOX 28.6 HOW TO: Run a structured interview
>
> - Relate questions directly to the person specification (which should be based on a thorough job analysis)
> - Ask the same questions of each candidate, limit prompting, use follow-up and probing questions to elicit evidence
> - Use relevant questions and design as either situational, competency-based, biographical or knowledge questions
> - Use longer interviews, or a larger number of questions, to control the input of ancillary information
> - Do not allow questions from the candidate until after the interview (when the information to make selection decisions has been collected)
> - Rate each answer and use standardised rating scales (increase specificity)
> - Use detailed anchored rating scales and take detailed notes
> - Use multiple interviewers where possible (but ensure efficiency)

structured) and (vi) number of sessions (single or multiple). Research consistently shows that structured interviews tend to have much higher criterion-related validity than unstructured interviews, when they are based on thorough role analysis and have validated scoring criteria.(38–41) Box 28.6 provides a summary of best practice in designing structured interviews.

Meta-analytical studies (which statistically combine results from a number of studies to identify generalisable findings) have found structured interviews to be valid predictors of job performance.(40,42) Research evidence also suggests that structured interviews have incremental validity over cognitive ability tests(43,44) and that they generally yield small ethnic group differences.(45,46) Adding structure to an interview may also increase the chances of an organisation successfully defending a lawsuit.(47) A limitation of structured interviews involving multiple assessors is that inter-rater reliability may be modest, especially if assessors are not properly trained.(48) However, research suggests this method has an acceptable level of inter-rater reliability when assessors are properly trained, and when they make use of standardised questions and validated scoring criteria.(40,49–52)

Unstructured interviews are still widely used in many countries for selection into a variety of industries, despite their low reliability and predictive validity and, thus, their poor legal defensibility.(10,53,54) Unstructured interviews are prone to bias and error, including (i) stereotyping, (ii) making a judgement solely on first impressions rather than allowing all candidates the chance to demonstrate their skills (e.g. *'I know if he or she is the right person immediately'*), (iii) halo and horns effects (i.e. selectors being unduly influenced by one positive or negative characteristic of the applicant) and (iv) similar-to-me bias, where interviewers rate most favourably interviewees who are similar to them-

selves.(55) Moreover, unstructured interviews may assess different characteristics for different candidates, meaning the content validity of the method can be variable.(56) All of these factors are likely to distort interviewers' ratings of candidates.(51)

In recent years, Multiple Mini-Interviews (MMIs) have become increasingly popular in medical selection. The MMI is an interview format comprising multiple stations, which is based on the format of the Objective Structured Clinical Examination (OSCE). MMIs typically involve a one-to-one interview, as well as role-play and interactive tasks, focused on a range of domains and lasting for 5–10 minutes each.(57) Some evidence exists to suggest that graduate and female applicants may outperform school-leavers and male applicants on MMIs, respectively.(58) However, the weight of research on this method suggests MMIs often have a good level of reliability.(58–61) Accordingly, MMIs have now been incorporated into medical school and postgraduate medical selection systems in many countries.(60,62–65) Moreover, research suggests that candidate reactions to MMIs are also favourable.(58,59,61, 63,64,66–68)

The ultimate criterion of a selection instrument is the relationship between performance at selection and subsequent job performance (i.e. predictive validity). Some evidence suggests that interview methods may not always be strong predictors of performance at medical school.(69,70) Other research suggests that performance on MMIs offers good predictive validity in relation to licensure examinations.(12,58,71–75) Currently, the extant research literature provides support for the validity, reliability and acceptability of MMIs and some structured interviews in medical selection, but comparatively less evidence supports the use of less structured interview methods. Nevertheless, reliability, validity and acceptability are not the only criteria that are important in determining whether a particular selection method should be used as part of a selection process. Further research on MMIs may be necessary to assess group differences in performance, and the relative financial feasibility of the selection method.(57)

References and referees' reports

Large-scale empirical studies consistently show that references tend to be unreliable and ineffective at predicting job performance.(76–79) Despite these rather pessimistic findings, references are widely used in selection in a variety of occupations, including medicine, and it is likely that they will continue to be used as an additional guide to the selection process.(80,81) In practice, employers tend to value references, but often ratings tend to be poor at differentiating between candidates fairly. Anecdotal evidence suggests that low scores on reference reports can be informative; further research is warranted in this area. Research on the content of references suggests that the writers of reports tend to apply positive and negative attributions homogenously across applicants, making it impossible for admissions committees to differentiate between applicants on the basis of these data.(76)

In the UK, references for undergraduate applicants are used. A 2006 study found that the vast majority of medical schools in England used referees' reports as part of their selection process.(71) However, their reliability is often questionable given recent changes in data legislation, which removed the confidentiality that existed previously.(2) In studying predictive validity, Ferguson *et al.*(77) showed that references obtained though UCAS (the central organisation that processes applications for full-time undergraduate courses at UK colleges and universities) did not predict pre-clinical or clinical performance. However, medical schools differ in terms of the weight they place on references obtained through the UCAS application. Some medical schools may actually ignore information contained in referees' reports for fear of unduly biasing selection decisions.(71) Despite the inherent limitations of using referees' reports, they remain widespread in medical student selection.(71,82) Moreover, despite evidence of poor reliability and validity, referees' reports may still be viewed positively by some medical selection professionals.(82) This finding contradicts the prevailing opinion among researchers in the field that referees' reports are not an appropriate method to use in medical student selection.(71,79,82,83)

Personal statements and autobiographical submissions

Personal statements, essays and other autobiographical submissions are often included in application forms, as an alternative to curriculum vitae, in order to facilitate shortlisting of candidates. The information obtained through application forms is collected in a systematic way, making it easier for employers to assess the candidates' suitability for a given post objectively, and make fair comparisons across applicants.(84) Application forms may include questions on biographical information, educational background, previous work experience and competencies identified through a job analysis. Application forms are a crucial part of the selection process and the quality of information obtained varies according to the design of the form. Some research evidence suggests that medical school application forms may be predictive of subsequent performance.(83,85) However, other evidence suggests that application forms have low reliability compared to other selection methods.(74) Other researchers suggest that application forms are not predictive of performance in the clinical aspects of medical training or performance at medical school overall.(77,86) The reliability and validity of application forms that are not completed under invigilated examination conditions may be contaminated by factors such as the length of time spent completing the form, and the potential influence and assistance of third parties. Therefore, it has been concluded that application forms are not likely to reflect the genuine nature of medical school candidates as well as selection methods like interviews or observations.(74) This conclusion is supported by research findings that medical school applicants present themselves in application forms in ways that they perceive to be desirable and that are not necessarily accurate.(87,88) These findings contrast with the intended function of application forms, which is to provide objective data that can be used to make selection decisions.

Academic records

Academic criteria are a major component of selection to medical school in most countries. Traditionally, in the UK for example, selection for admission to medical school is based on predicted or actual A-level results (a school-end examination designed to assess knowledge in various chosen subjects). One problem associated with using A-level grades for selection is in discriminating amongst students who obtain similarly high A-level results.(89) Another concern is that entry into medical school is socially exclusive, partly because A-level results might reflect type of schooling and 'social class'.(90) In addition, research suggests that predicted A-level grades may be inaccurate in more than 50% of cases.(91) In the USA and Canada, students apply to medical school at postgraduate level (graduate entry). However, academic grades such as Grade Point Average (GPA) remain the main criterion for selection, although they are usually considered in combination with other predictors, such as the MCAT.

Some authors have shown that academic criteria such as A-level grades correlate with drop-out rates, career progression, postgraduate membership and fellowship exams.(30,92–96) These findings are in contrast with earlier studies that questioned the long-term predictive validity of academic records.(3) Whilst pre-admission academic grades such as A-level or GPA are undoubtedly related to academic performance at medical school, their relationship with long-term outcome measures of a doctors' performance is less obvious, partly because of the 'criterion problem', discussed earlier.(84,94) In addition, there is some evidence that candidates from the highest academic performance group are more likely to be rated negatively by interviewers as unsuitable for medicine.(97) Other researchers have presented evidence that candidates selected purely on high academic performance are much more likely to drop out than candidates selected using a series of selection methods aimed at exploring commitment to studying medicine.(98) Therefore, use of academic records as a method of selecting candidates into medicine is complicated by a number of factors, including grade inflation, bias towards higher socio-economic classes and an uncertain relationship between academic attainment and subsequent performance as a doctor.

General mental ability and aptitude tests

Tests of *general mental ability* (GMA) and tests of specific cognitive abilities (e.g. numerical, verbal and spatial reasoning) are increasingly popular in selection processes both in the USA and in the UK.(31,81) Internationally, GMA and cognitive ability tests are robust predictors of job performance and training success across a wide range of occupations.(99,100) However, there are concerns regarding fairness since GMA tests can produce adverse impact, with marked racial differences in test performance.(101–103) Specific ability tests tend to show smaller group differences.(102)

Aptitude tests are typically defined as standardised tests designed to measure the ability of a person to develop skills or acquire knowledge. They are used to predict future performance in a given activity.(104) Like tests of GMA, aptitude tests measure an individual's overall performance across a broad range of mental abilities. In addition, aptitude tests also often include items that measure more specialised abilities (such as verbal and numerical skills) that predict academic, training or job performance.

Aptitude tests that include specific ability tests and a knowledge component are increasingly popular in medicine. In the UK, concerns over the discriminatory power of A-levels has led to the introduction of additional selection methods such as specific medical knowledge tests(89) and intellectual aptitude tests (e.g. the Oxford Medicine Admission test). The UKCAT, which comprises reasoning tests and tests of decision-making and situational judgement, is now used in selection by many medical and dental schools in the UK. The use of aptitude tests for medical school selection is also increasing in several other countries.(65) The outlook is somewhat different at postgraduate level where aptitude tests are rarely (if at all) used. This is not surprising given that most applicants, in the USA particularly, have already passed an aptitude test for entry into medical school. Therefore, there is a danger of obtaining redundant information. At this stage, arguably, cognitive ability is a necessary but not a sufficient condition to predict who will be a competent physician.

In a selection context – especially with respect to widening access – it is important to distinguish between GMA in terms of *crystallised* intelligence (i.e. knowledge-based acquired via schooling) and *fluid* intelligence (i.e. biologically-based cognitive skills such as processing speed, inductive reasoning, etc.)(105,106) It has been argued that tests of fluid intelligence should be used in medical school selection to widen access (i.e. to identify 'raw talent' independent of education). There are, however, various problems with approach. Research shows most commonly used tests of 'intelligence' assess crystallised intelligence(106) and such knowledge-based measures are good predictors of exam performance.(89) In addition, assuming it is possible to assess 'raw talent', unless this is combined with an assessment of the desire to study medicine and the other necessary non-cognitive skills (as determined by a job analysis), a student may fail, drop-out or under-perform at medical school.

Recent research evidence suggests, for example, that the UKCAT has predictive validity in relation to performance in the first 2 years of medical school.(107) Similarly, there is evidence that the MCAT, which is widely employed in North America, has significant predictive validity.(108–110) Finally, there is some evidence that the BioMedical Admissions Test, which is used by some UK universities to select medical students, may have a degree of predictive validity in relation to subsequent performance.(111) Despite this evidence of significant predictive validity, the strength of the predictive relationship between aptitude tests and subsequent performance is often relatively weak.(108,109,112) High quality, longitudinal studies are required to examine the precise relationship between scores on selection aptitude tests, and subsequent performance in medical school and as a doctor.

Personality inventories

The last 20 years have seen a substantial increase in the use of personality and related tests in personnel selection for a broad spectrum of jobs.(113) Personality assessments generally make use of self-report inventories that require candidates to respond to questions or statements by rating the extent to which they agree, or by indicating how accurate an item is as a description of their personality. Over many decades of research, personality researchers have agreed a general taxonomy of personality traits, the 'Big Five' model, which is based on five factors or traits: *extraversion* (i.e. outgoing, sociable, impulsive), *emotional stability* (i.e. calm, relaxed), *agreeableness* (i.e. trusting, cooperative, helpful), *conscientiousness* (i.e. hardworking, dutiful, organised) and *openness to experience* (i.e. artistic, cultured, creative).

Some research has shown that important relationships exist between measures of personality and job or academic performance.(113) For example, personality traits defined as "dysfunctional" have been found to be significantly associated with negative outcomes for medical students, such as lower academic performance.(114,115) Other researchers have found that another personality inventory, the Personal Qualities Assessment, may also be a useful addition to medical school selection procedures and is predictive of performance at medical school.(116) Significant associations have also been reported between some Big Five personality traits and performance across various aspects of medical school performance.(117) Conscientiousness, for example, has been shown to be a positive predictor of pre-clinical knowledge and exam results(77,86,118) and to offer incremental validity over knowledge-based assessments.(77,86) However, while positively associated with pre-clinical knowledge, conscientiousness has also been found to be a significant negative predictor of clinical skill.(77) Therefore, the relationship between personality traits and performance in medical education and training may be complex and possibly non-linear.

Other researchers have presented evidence suggesting that personality measures were not useful predictors of medical school performance. For example, no significant association was reported between the Myers–Briggs Type Indicator and performance on the MCAT.(119) Similarly, the PQA has been reported not to be correlated with success as a medical student.(120) These mixed findings are perhaps best interpreted in light of recent findings that certain personality characteristics may have differential costs and benefits over time. For example, recent evidence suggests that the validity of personality measures in predicting medical school grades increases over the course of medical education and training.(121) For example, while there may not be any advantages to being open and extraverted for early academic performance, these traits may gain importance for later academic performance. Similarly, conscientiousness may be an increasing asset over time for medical students. Therefore, in assessing the usefulness of personality assessment in medical student selection, earlier studies may have misestimated the predictive value of some personality traits. Other researchers agree that certain personality traits, such as conscientiousness, change in importance over the course of medical education and training, but disagree as to whether the trait increasingly becomes a benefit. Currently there is no consensus among researchers about whether conscientiousness is increasingly advantageous or disadvantageous over the course of medical education and training, with recent research presenting contradictory findings.

The use of personality tests to assess characteristics of job applicants remains controversial. Critics argue that the predictive validity of personality traits for job performance is often low and badly understood.(122) Further, personality tests used by organisations are often poorly chosen,(123) and 'faking' can compromise the validity of personality tests.(124–126) However, there is also evidence to suggest that faking or responding in a socially desirable way does not compromise the predictive validity of personality tests.(127,128) In medicine, concerns over the strong reliance on academic predictors have led to the search for alternative selection methods. Specifically, there is a growing interest in the role of personality tests in selection at undergraduate level. Best practice currently suggests that personality assessment should be used to drive more focused questioning at interviews, and that personality inventories should not be used in isolation to make selection decisions.

Selection centres

Selection centres (SCs), also known as assessment centres, are a selection method used widely in non-medical selection contexts. They involve a combination of selection techniques, such as written exercises, interviews and work simulations, to assess candidates across a number of key skills, attitudes and behaviours (e.g. empathy) required by the job as identified in the job analysis. Candidates are usually assessed in groups or individually by multiple assessors. The SC is different from an OSCE. In an OSCE, each station assesses a candidate on *one* key skill, and is usually observed by one assessor. By contrast, the SC allows the candidate *multiple* situations (interview, work simulation, written exercise, etc.) in which to demonstrate a key skill, and to be observed by a number of trained assessors. Thus, a fairer (multiple opportunities to perform) and more reliable (multiple observations of key behaviours by multiple observers) assessment can be made. With careful design, the increased reliability should result in greater validity and more positive candidate reactions.

SCs were first used during World War II to select military personnel. However, it was not until the American company AT&T applied SCs to identify industrial managerial potential in the 1950s that the idea developed as a selection method. Since this time, SCs have become widely used as a tool for recruitment.(129) SCs are especially popular for graduate recruitment, with the Inland Revenue Service (IRS) estimating that over half of recruiters and over 95% of large organisations employing more than 10 000 individuals use selection centres for graduate recruitment.(130) However, it is only recently that this approach has been used in medicine.(131) In the UK, Patterson *et al.* have pioneered the use of SCs, initially in the selection of general practitioners. The results have shown good predictive validity.(28,132) This work has been extended to select doctors for postgraduate training in other specialties such as obstetrics and gynaecology, and paediatrics.(133–135) The design process followed a thorough multi-method job

analysis study of the target specialty. Patterson *et al.* have also piloted the use of SCs in the UK for graduate entry to medical school, in addition to other academic assessments.(136) SCs have also been piloted for medical student selection internationally, with positive reports on the reliability and internal validity of the method.(65,137,138) Provisional evidence is emerging as to the predictive validity of the SC when used in medical specialty training,(135) but further research is required to determine the predictive validity of SCs in medical student selection. Such research may be constrained by the financial cost and logistical complexity of implementing SCs.(137)

Research shows that a carefully designed and administered SC can be highly effective at predicting job performance across a wide range of occupations.(44,139–141) As described above, gains are made in reliability and validity because SCs make use of a combination of different exercises (using a multi-trait, multi-method approach) and use standardised scoring systems to measure the selection criteria. Scoring should be directly linked to the selection criteria (not the exercise scores) and the information gathered should be interpreted in context by appropriately trained assessors. Unfortunately, many fail to understand this fundamental difference between OSCE-style examinations and SCs in the selection context. Well-executed SCs have incremental validity over cognitive ability tests,(142–144) and tend to be viewed positively by candidates.(145, 146) Careful design and implementation of a SC is crucial for the assessment to live up to its reputation and to be cost-effective.(147)

Situational judgement tests

Situational judgement tests (SJTs) are assessments designed to measure candidates' judgement in role-relevant settings (*see* Box 28.7). Tests present candidates with a scenario and a list of possible responses. The candidate is asked to consider the situation and make judgements about the possible responses. The candidates' responses are scored against expert responses. An example of a SJT item used for health-care selection purposes is displayed in Box 28.8. For a review of the research evidence relating to the use of SJTs and their relevance for selection into the health-care professions we direct readers to Patterson *et al.*'s recent article.(148)

Recently in the UK, the use of SJTs in medical selection and assessment has become widespread. Numerous high quality meta-analyses, review articles and cross-sectional studies have been published that assess the effectiveness of SJTs.(7,36,149–152) These studies suggest SJTs have criterion validity and incremental validity over academic ability and personality assessment. Moreover, evidence suggests SJTs have low adverse impact against minority groups, and are perceived favourably by candidates.

Other researchers have reported procedural issues in the use of SJTs in medical student selection. For example, the mode of administration may impact on the validity of an SJT.(151) Similarly, the response instructions included in an SJT and the construction of different SJT forms may impact on their validity.(153,154) Other researchers have presented contradictory evidence on the susceptibility of SJTs to coaching, faking and practice effects.(149,155) However, it

BOX 28.7 FOCUS ON: Situational Judgement Tests in UK medical selection

In 2009, a review of the methods by which UK medical students are selected into foundation training was recommended. Although the existing system worked well, several concerns needed to be dealt with regarding the use of personal statements on the application from. Concerns about the use of personal statements included low reliability, a lack of adequate standardisation, plus the risk of plagiarism and costs in terms of the time it takes to score them.

The recommendations were to design a Situational Judgement Test (SJT) to assess several non-academic professional attributes and employability for a training post (to replace the application form questions and personal statement). The SJT was recommended to be used in conjunction with a measure of educational performance to assess academic competence, clinical knowledge and skills.

Pilots of the SJT involving more than 1000 UK students showed it to be a valid and reliable method of selection in this context. The SJT was based on a multi-method job analysis of the role and was developed in consultation with clinicians who work with junior doctors and with junior doctors themselves. This was to ensure that the scenarios are relevant, realistic and fair. The SJT targets five professional attributes: commitment to professionalism, coping with pressure, effective communication, patient focus and working effectively as part of team. The test was launched successfully for live recruitment in 2013 and further information can be found at http://www.isfp.org.uk/

In the SJT there are two item formats:

1. Rank five possible responses in the most appropriate order
2. Select the three most appropriate responses for the situation.

The choice of response options reflects the scenario content and is the appropriate format to both provide and elicit the information needed. For example, the nature of some scenarios and the possible responses to them lend themselves to ranking items (requiring the ability to differentiate between singular actions that vary in appropriateness in response to a scenario), whereas some scenarios lend themselves to multiple-choice items (where it is necessary to do more than one thing/tackle more than one aspect in response to a scenario).

Applicants must answer what they 'should' do in the scenario described, not what they 'would' do. This is because research into SJTs shows that questions asking an applicant what they 'would' do are more susceptible to coaching.

Box 28.8 provides an example of an SJT multiple-choice item. Applicants should select the three most appropriate responses to tackle the dilemma in the scenario. Remember that these responses should not be viewed in isolation, but in combination.

BOX 28.8 Situation Judgement Test: Question example

You review a patient on the surgical ward who has had an appendicectomy done earlier on the day. You write a prescription for strong painkillers. The staff nurse challenges your decision and refuses to give the medication to the patient.

Choose the THREE most appropriate actions to take in this situation A Instruct the nurse to give the medication to the patient B Discuss with the nurse why she disagrees with the prescription C Ask a senior colleague for advice D Complete a clinical incident form E Cancel the prescription on the nurse's advice F Arrange to speak to the nurse later to discuss your working relationship G Write in the medical notes that the nurse has declined to give the medication H Review the case again Answer: B C H

Rationale: Ensuring patient safety is key to this scenario. It is important that the nurse's decision is discussed with her as there may be something that was missed when first reviewing the patient (B). Therefore, it would also be important to review the patient again (H). Also relating to this is the importance of respecting the views of colleagues and maintaining working relationships, even if there is disagreement. As there has been a disagreement regarding patient care, it is important to seek advice from a senior colleague (C).

is important to note that SJTs are a measurement method and that they can be designed to minimise coaching effects in high-stakes selection settings such as in medicine.

In terms of the pragmatics of selection systems, research suggests that SJTs can often usefully and feasibly be incorporated into existing selection systems.(7,149,156–158) SJTs tend to have high face validity, and are rated favourably by candidates.(149,159–161) Tentative (indirect) evidence has also been provided that SJTs are a cost-effective option in medical selection.(149) In summary, adoption of SJTs in medical student selection is supported by the weight of published research evidence on this selection method. Although the research base is relatively small in comparison to more established selection methods, there is a good degree of consensus at to the reliability, validity and utility of SJTs as selection tools in the medical arena. Direct evidence on the predictive validity of SJTs in medical student performance and in postgraduate selection is now available. Further research on this selection method should be directed at the finding that the predictive validity of SJTs increases throughout medical education and training(36) and the predictive validity of medical school entrance SJTs on subsequent performance as a doctor.

Opportunities for further research

Box 28.9 summarises the research evidence on the predictive validity of different selection tools. The evidence on

Selection method	Evidence for criterion-related validity	Applicant reactions	Extent of use
Structured interviews	High	Moderate to positive	High
Cognitive ability	High	Negative to moderate	Moderate
Personality tests	Moderate	Negative to moderate	Moderate
Work sample tests	High	Positive	Low
Selection centres	High	Positive	Moderate
Handwriting	Low	Negative to moderate	Low
References	Low	Positive	High
Situational judgement tests	High	Positive	Moderate

each of the techniques listed also includes an estimate of extent of usage across all occupational groups, and likely applicant reactions to each. Note that there are international differences in the extent of usage for various techniques, which in turn is governed by international differences in employment law.

Research into medical selection though is relatively new and there remain many unchartered territories for exploration. Medicine continues to change rapidly and the skills relevant to many specialties are changing. For example, in surgery, the use of laproscopes and other technologies has transformed many surgical procedures. With international developments in technology and new treatment regimens, it is likely that the pace of change will increase in future. Since the career path for a physician is long and complex, it is difficult to define appropriate selection criteria for the physicians of the future. Going forward, research must involve more job analysis studies to define the knowledge, skills, abilities and attitudes relevant for physicians in general, and to explore any differences between specialties. In many countries, the enhanced focus on patient satisfaction has highlighted the requirement for empathy and communication skills for example, where physicians work in partnership with patients.

The selection gateways to progressing in medical training should be accompanied by accurate careers information for individuals. The process of self-selection is crucially important and further research is clearly warranted in this area. When exploring the selection literature, it is notable that very little research exists at more senior level appoint-

ments. Future research must address this area, particularly at the consultant level, where competencies required may also include leadership of multi-professional teams, resource management and political awareness, amongst others.(162) Chapter 29 addresses this issue in more detail.

More research is needed in the area of candidate reactions with respect to medical education and training. What combination of selection tests is seen as fair and valid by candidates? What are the implications for widening access to the profession of medicine? What is the effect of candidate reactions (emotional, anxiety, perceived justice and fairness) on test performance and test validity? Whilst there is a growing research literature on these topics in other professions,(33,163) they have not been explored within medicine.

Future research should also explore how a selection system is best designed across the whole training pathway. There may be generic skills required across all specialities (i.e. the basic skills for being a doctor, including cognitive, non-academic and behavioural skills). These should guide the design of selection criteria used to recruit to undergraduate medical courses at the outset of training. It should not be assumed that one part of medical career path (e.g. undergraduate to initial specialty training) should fully equip an applicant with all the skills to progress from one stage to the next (e.g. from specialty training to senior appointments), especially if candidates are not selected to have the core aptitude at the outset. Indeed, a selection centre approach could be adopted for undergraduate selection, in addition to academic assessments, to address this issue.

Designing an accurate selection system is a complex process. It should be acknowledged that medical education and training is a continual process, and that the predictive validity of selection tests may not be consistent at different points in the career pathway. In other words, a factor may be identified as an important predictor for undergraduate training but may not be predictive for aspects of specialty training. For example, the personality factor *conscientiousness* may be a positive predictor for undergraduate preclinical training but a negative predictor for undergraduate clinical performance.(77) Similarly, evidence shows *openeness to experience* is important to general practitioner training performance, but is not important for undergraduate training performance. The real challenge is to integrate this knowledge and develop selection systems that are internally reliable from undergraduate selection through to selection for specialty training.

Future research must account for established theoretical models of adult intellectual development and skill acquisition, which attempt to integrate cognitive and non-cognitive factors. One such model is PPIK theory,(164) which asserts that adult intellectual ability is a function of *process* (basic mental capacities such a processing speed), *personality* (e.g. extraversion, conscientiousness), *interests* (e.g. preferences for science or art) and *knowledge* (e.g. factual knowledge as contained in A-levels). PPIK theory specifically proposes a developmental trajectory to understand adult intellectual functioning, where personality, intellect and interests operate in tandem. For example, the interests a person may express influences the types of knowledge they seek out. This approach may help us to understand what motivates people to study medicine and also their choice and aptitude for a specialty later in training. The idea of trait complexes (overlapping cognitive and non-cognitive traits) should be considered in medical selection.(105,164) Clusters of traits may be identified that overlap to define areas of competence and preference. In future, it may be possible to identify trait complexes that are unique to success in undergraduate medical education and in later specialty training.(86)

There are many opportunites for research in the area of medical selection. To summarise these, we propose that key topics for a future research agenda in selection to undergraduate and postgraduate medical education are job analysis, longitudinal validity studies, organisational justice, exploring trait overlaps, and the temporal dynamics of training.

References

1 Greengross S (1997) What patients want from their doctors. In: Allen I, Brown P and Hughes P (eds) *Choosing Tomorrow's Doctors*, pp. 12–9. Policy Studies Institute, London.

2 Hughes P (2002) Can we improve on how we select medical students? *Journal of the Royal Society of Medicine*. **95**: 18–22.

3 Reede JY (1999) Predictors of success in medicine. *Clinical Orthopaedics and Related Research*. **362**: 72–7.

4 Patterson F and Ferguson E (2010) Selection for medical education and training. In: Swanwick T (ed.) *Understanding Medical Education*, pp. 352–65. Wiley-Blackwell, Oxford.

5 Patterson F and Ferguson E (2012) Testing non-cognitive attributes in selection centres: how to avoid being reliably wrong. *Medical Education*. **46**(3): 240–2.

6 McManus IC (2003) Commentary: how to derive causes from correlations in educational studies. *British Medical Journal*. **326**: 432.

7 Patterson F, Baron H, Carr V, Plint S and Lane P (2009) Evaluation of three short-listing methodologies for selection into postgraduate training in general practice. *Medical Education*. **43**(1): 50–7.

8 Patterson F, Lievens F, Kerrin M, Zibarras L and Carette B (2012) Designing Selection Systems for Medicine: the importance of balancing predictive and political validity in high-stakes selection contexts. *International Journal of Selection and Assessment*. **20**(4): 486–96.

9 Patterson F and Zibarras LD (2011) Exploring the construct of perceived job discrimination in selection. *International Journal of Selection and Assessment*. **19**(3): 251–7.

10 Klehe UC (2004) Choosing how to choose: institutional pressures affecting the adoption of personnel selection procedures. *International Journal of Selection and Assessment*. **12**: 327–42.

11 Jefferis T (2007) Selection for specialist training: what can we learn from other countries? *British Medical Journal*. **334**: 1302–4.

12 Prideaux D, Roberts C, Eva K *et al.* (2011) Assessment for selection for the health care professions and specialty training: consensus statement and recommendations from the Ottawa 2010 Conference. *Medical Teacher*. **33**(3): 215–23.

13 Eva KW and Reiter HI (2005) Reflecting the relative values of community, faculty and students in the admissions tools of medical school. *Teaching and Learning in Medicine*. **17**: 4–8.

14 Wiley A and Koenig JA (1996) The validity of the Medical College Admission Test for predicting performance in the first two years of medical school. *Academic Medicine*. **71**: S83–5.

15 Aldous CJ, Leeder SR, Price J, Sefton AE and Teubner JK (1997) A selection test for Australian graduate-entry medical schools. *Medical Journal of Australia*. **166**: 247–50.

16 Tutton P and Price M (2002) Selection of medical students: affirmative action goes beyond the selection process. *British Medical Journal*. **324**: 1170–1.

17 Miller JB, Schaad DC, Crittenden RA, Oriol NE and MacLaren C (2003) Communication between programs and applicants during residency selection: effects of the match on medical students' professional development. *Academic Medicine*. **78**: 403–11.

18 Bell JG, Kanellitsas I and Shaffer L (2001) Selection of obstetrics and gynecology residents on the basis of medical school performance. *American Journal of Obstetrics and Gynaecology*. **186**: 1091–4.

19 Brandenburg S, Kruzick T, Lin CT, Robinson A and Adams LJ (2005) Residency selection criteria: what medical students perceive as important. *Medical Education Online*. **10**: 1–6.

20 Wagoner NE and Gray GT (1979) Report on a survey of program directors regarding selection factors in graduate medical education. *Journal of Medical Education*. **54**: 445–52.

21 Wagoner NE and Suriano JR (1999) Program directors' responses to a survey on variables used to select residents in a time of change. *Academic Medicine*. **74**: 51–8.

22 Adams LJ, Brandenburg S and Blake M (2000) Factors influencing internal medicine program directors decisions about applicants. *Academic Medicine*. **75**: 542–3.

23 Crane JT and Ferraro CM (2000) Selection criteria for emergency medicine residency applicants. *Academic Emergency Medicine*. **7**: 54–60.

24 Travis C, Taylor CA and Mayhew HE (1999) Evaluating residency applicants: stable values in a changing market. *Family Medicine*. **31**: 252–6.

25 Villanueva AM, Kaye D, Abdelhak SS and Morahan PS (1995) Comparing selection criteria of residency directors and physicians' employers. *Academic Medicine*. **70**: 261–71.

26 Grantham JR (1993) Radiology resident selection: results of a survey. *Investigative Radiology*. **28**: 99–101.

27 Wagoner NE and Suriano JR (1992) Recommendations for changing the residency selection process based on a survey of program directors. *Academic Medicine*. **67**: 459–64.

28 Patterson F, Ferguson E, Lane PW, Farrell K, Martlew J and Wells AA (2000) Competency model for general practice: implications for selection, training and development. *British Journal of General Practice*. **50**: 188–93.

29 Patterson F, Ferguson E, Lane P, Farrell K, Martlew J and Wells AA (2000) A competency model for general practice: implications for selection and training. *British Journal of General Practice*. **50**: 188–93.

30 Ferguson E, James D and Madeley L (2002) Factors associated with success in medical school: systematic review of the literature. *British Medical Journal*. **324**: 952–7.

31 Salgado JF, Viswesvaran C and Ones D (2001) Predictors used for personnel selection: an overview of constructs, methods, and techniques. In: Anderson N, Ones DS, Sinangil HK and Viswesvaran C (eds) *Handbook of Industrial, Work and Organizational Psychology*, pp. 165–99. Sage, London.

32 Anastasia A and Urbina S (1997) *Psychological Testing* (7e). Prentice Hall, Upper Saddle River, NJ.

33 Hausknecht JP, Day DV and Thomas SC (2004) Applicant reactions to selection procedures: an updated model and meta-analysis. *Personnel Psychology*. **57**: 639–83.

34 Anderson N, Born M and Cunningham-Snell N (2002) Recruitment and selection: applicant perspectives and outcomes. In: Anderson N, Ones DS, Sinangil HK and Viswesvaran C (eds) *Handbook of Industrial, Work and Organizational Psychology*, pp. 200–18. Sage, London.

35 Campion MA, Palmer DK and Campion JE (1997) A review of structure in the selection interview. *Personnel Psychology.* **50**: 655–702.

36 Lievens F and Thornton IIIGC (2005) Assessment centers: recent developments in practice and research. In: Evers A, Smit-Voskuijl O and Anderson N (eds) *Handbook of Personnel Selection*, pp. 243–64. Blackwell Publishing, Oxford.

37 Salgado JF and Anderson N (2002) Cognitive and GMA testing in the European Community: issues and evidence. *Human Performance.* **15**: 75–96.

38 Campion MA, Pursell ED and Brown BK (1988) Structured interviewing: raising the psychometric properties of the employment interview. *Personnel Psychology.* **41**: 25–42.

39 Goho J and Blackman A (2006) The effectiveness of academic admission interviews: an exploratory meta-analysis. *Medical Teacher.* **28**: 335–40.

40 McDaniel MA, Whetzel DL, Schmidt FL and Maurer S (1994) The validity of employment interviews: a comprehensive review and meta-analysis. *Journal of Applied Psychology.* **79**: 599–615.

41 Wiesner WH and Cronshaw SF (1988) A meta-analytic investigation of the impact of interview format and the degree of structure on the validity of the employment interview. *Journal of Occupational Psychology.* **61**: 275–90.

42 Huffcutt AI and Arthur W Jr (1994) Hunter and Hunter (1984) revisited: interview validity for entry-level jobs. *Journal of Applied Psychology.* **79**: 184–90.

43 Cortina JM, Goldstein NB, Payne SC, Davison HK and Gilliland SW (2000) The incremental validity of interview scores over and above cognitive ability and conscientiousness scores. *Personnel Psychology.* **53**: 325–51.

44 Schmidt FL and Hunter JE (1998) The validity and utility of selection methods in personnel psychology: practical and theoretical implications of 85 years of research findings. *Psychological Bulletin.* **124**: 262–74.

45 Bobko P, Roth PL and Potosky D (1999) Derivation and implications of meta-analytic matrix incorporating cognitive ability, alternative predictors and job performance. *Personnel Psychology.* **52**: 561–89.

46 Huffcutt AI and Roth PL (1998) Racial group differences in employment interview evaluations. *Journal of Applied Psychology.* **83**: 179–89.

47 Posthuma RA, Morgeson FP and Campion MA (2002) Beyond employment interview validity: a comprehensive narrative review of recent research and trends over time. *Personnel Psychology.* **55**: 1–81.

48 Kreiter CD, Yin P, Solow C and Brennan RL (2004) Investigating the reliability of the medical school admissions interview. *Advances in Health Sciences Education: Theory and Practice.* **9**(2): 147–59.

49 Patrick LE, Altmaier EM, Kuperman S and Ugolini K (2001) A structured interview for medical school admission, Phase 1: initial procedures and results. *Academic Medicine.* **76**(1): 66–71.

50 Donnon T, Oddone-Paolucci E and Violato C (2009) A predictive validity study of medical judgment vignettes to assess students' noncognitive attributes: a 3-year prospective longitudinal study. *Medical Teacher.* **31**(4): e148–55.

51 Edwards JC, Johnson EK and Molidor JB (1990) The interview in the admission process. *Academic Medicine.* **65**: 167–77.

52 Weisner WH and Weisner CSF (1998) A meta-analytic investigation of the impact of interview format and degree of structure on the validity of the employment interview. *Journal of Occupational and Organizational Psychology.* **61**: 275–90.

53 Terpstra DE, Mohamed AA and Kethley RB (1999) An analysis of federal court cases involving nine selection devices. *International Journal of Selection and Assessment.* **7**: 26–34.

54 Williamson LG, Campion JE, Malos SB, Roehling MV and Campion MA (1997) Employment interview on trial: linking interview structure with litigation outcomes. *Journal of Applied Psychology.* **82**: 900–12.

55 Quintero AJ, Segal LS, King TS and Black KP (2009) The personal interview: assessing the potential for personality similarity to bias the selection of orthopaedic residents. *Academic Medicine.* **84**(10): 1364–72.

56 Albanese MA, Snow MH, Skochelak SE, Huggett KN and Farrell P (2003) Assessing personal qualities in medical schools admissions. *Academic Medicine.* **78**: 313–21.

57 Cleland J, Dowell J, McLachlan J, Nicholson S and Patterson F (2013) Identifying best practice in the selection of medical students (literature review and interview survey). General Medical Council, London. (http://www.gmc-uk.org/about/research/14400.asp; accessed 22 February 2013).

58 Dowell J, Lynch B, Till H, Kumwenda B and Husbands A (2012) The multiple mini-interview in the U.K. context: 3 years of experience at Dundee. *Medical Teacher.* **34**(4): 297–304.

59 Eva KW, Reiter HI, Rosenfeld J and Norman GR (2004) The ability of the multiple mini-interview to predict preclerkship performance in medical school. *Academic Medicine.* **79**(10): S40–2.

60 Roberts C, Walton M, Rothnie I *et al.* (2008) Factors affecting the utility of the multiple mini-interview in selecting candidates for graduate-entry medical school. *Medical Education.* **42**(4): 396–404.

61 O'Brien A, Harvey J, Shannon M, Lewis K and And Valencia O (2011) A comparison of multiple mini-interviews and structured interviews in a UK setting. *Medical Teacher.* **33**: 397–402.

62 Harris S and Owen C (2007) Discerning quality: using the multiple mini-interview in student selection for the Australian National University Medical School. *Medical Education.* **41**: 234–41.

63 Brownell K, Lockyer J, Collin T and Lemay J-F (2007) Introduction of the multiple mini interview into the admissions process at the University of Calgary: acceptability and feasibility. *Medical Teacher.* **29**(4): 394–6.

64 Hofmeister M, Lockyer J and Crutcher R (2009) The multiple mini-interview for selection of international medical graduates into family medicine residency education. *Medical Education.* **43**(6): 573–9.

65 Gafni N, Moshinsky A, Eisenberg O, Zeigler D and Ziv A (2012) Reliability estimates: behavioural stations and questionnaires in medical school admissions. *Medical Education.* **46**(3): 277–88.

66 Kumar K, Roberts C, Rothnie I, du Fresne C and Walton M (2009) Experiences of the multiple mini-interview: a qualitative analysis. *Medical Education.* **43**: 360–7.

67 Razack S, Faremo S, Drolet F, Snell L, Wiseman J and Pickering J (2009) Multiple mini-interviews versus traditional interviews: stakeholder acceptability comparison. *Medical Education.* **43**(10): 993–1000.

68 Humphrey S, Dowson S, Wall D, Diwakar V and Goodyear HM (2008) Multiple mini-interviews: opinions of candidates and interviewers. *Medical Education.* **42**(2): 207–13.

69 Ann Courneya C, Wright K, Frinton V, Mak E, Schulzer M and Pachev G (2005) Medical student selection: choice of a semi-structured panel interview or an unstructured one-on-one interview. *Medical Teacher.* **27**(6): 499–503.

70 Powis DA and Bristow T (1997) Top school marks don't necessarily make top rated students. *Medical Journal of Australia.* **166**: 613.

71 Parry JM, Mathers JM, Stevens AJ *et al.* (2006) Admissions processes for five year medical courses at English schools: review. *British Medical Journal.* **332**: 1005–9.

72 Reiter HI, Eva KW, Rosenfeld J and Norman GR (2007) Multiple mini-interviews predict clerkship and licensing examination performance. *Medical Education.* **41**(4): 378–84.

73 Eva KW, Reiter HI, Trinh K, Wasi P, Rosenfeld J and Norman GR (2009) Predictive validity of the multiple mini-interview for selecting medical trainees. *Medical Education.* **43**(8): 767–75.

74 Oosterveld P and ten Cate O (2004) Generalizability of a study sample assessment procedure for entrance selection for medical school. *Medical Teacher*. **26**(7): 635–9.

75 Dore KL, Kreuger S, Ladhani M *et al.* (2010) The Reliability and Acceptability of the Multiple Mini-Interview as a Selection Instrument for Postgraduate Admissions. *Academic Medicine*. **85**(10): 60–3.

76 McCarthy JM and Goffin RD (2001) Improving the validity of letters of recommendation: an investigation of three standardized reference forms. *Military Psychology*. **13**: 199–222.

77 Ferguson E, James D, O'Hehir F and Sanders A (2003) A pilot study of the roles of personality, references and personal statements in relation to performance over the 5 years of a medical degree. *British Medical Journal*. **326**: 429–31.

78 Muchinsky PM (1979) The use of reference reports in personnel selection: a review and evaluation. *Journal of Occupational Psychology*. **52**: 287–97.

79 Stedman JM, Hatch JP and Schoenfeld LS (2009) Letters of recommendation for the predoctoral internship in medical schools and other settings: do they enhance decision making in the selection process? *Journal of Clinical Psychology in Medical Settings*. **6**(4): 339–45.

80 IRS Employment Review (2002) Of good character: supplying references and providing access. *IRS Employment Review*. **754**: 34–6.

81 Ryan AM, McFarland L, Baron H and Page R (1999) An international look at selection practices: nation and culture as explanations for variability in practice. *Personnel Psychology*. **52**: 359–93.

82 Bates BP (2002) Selection criteria for applicants in primary care osteopathic graduate medical education. *Medical Education*. **102**(11): 621–6.

83 Peskun C, Detsky A and Shandling M (2007) Effectiveness of medical school admissions criteria in predicting residency ranking four years later. *Medical Education*. **41**(1): 57–64.

84 British Medical Association (BMA) Board of Medical Education (2006) *Selection for Specialty Training*. BMA, London.

85 Benbassat J and Baumal R (2007) Uncertainties in the selection of applicants for medical school. *Advances in Health Sciences Education: Theory and Practice*. **12**(4): 509–21.

86 Ferguson E, Sanders A, O'Hehir F and James D (2000) Predictive validity of personal statements and the role of the five factor model of personality in relation to medical training. *Journal of Occupational and Organizational Psychology*. **73**: 321–44.

87 White JS, Lemay J-F, Brownell K and Lockyer J (2011) "A chance to show yourself" - how do applicants approach medical school admission essays? *Medical Teacher*. **33**(10): e541–8.

88 White J, Brownell K, Lemay J-F and Lockyer JM (2012) "What do they want me to say?" The hidden curriculum at work in the medical school selection process: a qualitative study. *BMC Medical Education*. **12**(1): 17.

89 McManus IC, Powis DA, Wakeford R, Ferguson E, James D and Richards P (2005) Intellectual aptitude tests and A levels for selecting UK school leaver entrants for medical school. *British Medical Journal*. **331**: 555–9.

90 Nicholson S (2005) The benefits of aptitude testing for selecting medical students. *British Medical Journal*. **331**: 559–60.

91 Hayward G, Sturdy S and James S (2005) Estimating the reliability of predicted grades. University and Colleges Admission Service. (http://www.ucasresearch.com/documents/Predicted_Grades_2005.pdf; accessed 22 February 2013).

92 McManus IC and Richards P (1986) Prospective survey of performance of medical students during preclinical years. *British Medical Journal*. **293**: 124–7.

93 Arulampalam W, Naylor RA and Smith JP (2004) A hazard model of the probability of medical school dropout in the United Kingdom. *Journal of the Royal Statistical Society. Series A*. **167**(1): 157–78.

94 McManus IC (1997) From selection to qualification: how and why medical students change. In: Allen I, Brown P and Hughes P (eds) *Choosing Tomorrow's Doctors*, pp. 60–79. Policy Studies Institute, London.

95 McManus IC, Smithers E, Partridge P, Keeling A and Fleming PR (2003) A-levels and intelligence as predictors of medical careers in UK doctors: 20-year prospective study. *British Medical Journal*. **327**: 139–42.

96 Lumb AB and Vail A (2004) Comparison of academic, application form and social factors in predicting early performance on the medical course. *Medical Education*. **38**: 1002–5.

97 Powis DA and Rolfe I (1998) Selection and performance of medical students at Newcastle , New South Wales. *Education for Health*. **11**: 15–23.

98 O'Neill L, Hartvigsen J, Wallstedt B, Korsholm L and Eika B (2011) Medical school dropout-testing at admission versus selection by highest grades as predictors. *Medical Education*. **45**: 1111–20.

99 Bertua C, Anderson N and Salgado JF (2005) The predictive validity of cognitive ability tests: a UK meta-analysis. *Journal of Occupational and Organizational Psychology*. **78**: 387–409.

100 Salgado JF, Anderson N, Moscoso S, Bertua C, de Fruyt F and Rolland JP (2003) A meta-analytic study of general mental ability validity for different occupations in the European community. *Journal of Applied Psychology*. **88**: 1068–81.

101 Murphy KR (2002) Can conflicting perspectives on the role of *g* in personnel selection be resolved? *Human Performance*. **15**: 173–86.

102 Kehoe JF (2002) General mental ability and selection in private sector organizations: a commentary. *Human Performance*. **15**: 97–106.

103 Outtz J (2002) The role of cognitive ability tests in employment selection. *Human Performance*. **15**: 161–71.

104 Cronbach LJ (1984) *Essentials of Psychological Testing* (4e). Harper Row, New York.

105 Ackerman PL and Heggestad ED (1997) Intelligence, personality, and interests: evidence for overlapping traits. *Psychological Bulletin*. **121**: 219–45.

106 Blair C (2006) How similar are fluid cognition and general intelligence? A developmental neuroscience perspective on fluid cognition as an aspect of human cognitive ability. *Behavioral and Brain Sciences*. **29**: 109–60.

107 Wright SR and Bradley PM (2010) Has the UK Clinical Aptitude Test improved medical student selection? *Medical Education*. **44**: 1069–76.

108 Julian ER (2005) Validity of the Medical College Admission test for predicting medical school performance. *Medical Education*. **80**(10): 910–7.

109 Donnon T, Paolucci EO and Violato C (2007) The predictive validity of the MCAT for medical school performance and medical board licensing examinations: a meta-analysis of the published research. *Academic Medicine*. **82**(1): 100–6.

110 Callahan CA, Mohammadreza H, Veloski J, Erdmann JB and Gonnella JS (2010) The predictive validity of three versions of the MCAT in relation to performance in medical school, residency, and licensing examinations: a longitudinal study of 36 classes of Jefferson Medical College. *Academic Medicine*. **85**(6): 980–7.

111 Emery JL, Bell JF and Vidal Rodeiro CL (2011) The BioMedical Admissions Test for medical student selection: issues of fairness and bias. *Medical Teacher*. **33**(1): 62–71.

112 McManus IC, Ferguson E, Wakeford R, Powis D and James D (2011) Predictive validity of the Biomedical Admissions Test: an evaluation and case study. *Medical Teacher*. **33**: 53–7.

113 Barrick MR, Mount MK and Judge TA (2001) Personality and performance at the beginning of the new millennium: what do we know and where do we go next? *International Journal of Selection and Assessment*. **9**: 9–30.

114 Knights JA and Kennedy BJ (2006) Medical school selection: screening for dysfunctional tendencies. *Medical Education.* **40**(11): 1058–64.

115 Knights JA and Kennedy BJ (2007) Medical school selection: impact of dysfunctional tendencies on academic performance. *Medical Education.* **41**(4): 3.

116 Lumsden MA, Bore M, Millar K, Jack R and Powis D (2005) Assessment of personal qualities in relation to admission to medical school. *Medical Education.* **39**(3): 258–65.

117 Haight SJ, Chibnall JT, Schindler DL and Slavin SJ (2012) Associations of medical student personality and health/wellness characteristics with their medical school performance across the curriculum. *Academic Medicine.* **87**(4): 476–85.

118 Lievens F, Coetsier P, De Fruyt F and De Maeseneer J (2002) Medical students' personality characteristics and academic performance: a five-factor model perspective. *Medical Education.* **36**: 1050–6.

119 Sefcik DJ, Prerost FJ and Arbet SE (2009) Personality types and performance on aptitude and achievement tests: implications for osteopathic medical education. *Journal of the American Osteopathic Association.* **109**(6): 296–301.

120 Dowell J, Lumsden MA, Powis D *et al.* (2011) Predictive validity of the personal qualities assessment for selection of medical students in Scotland. *Medical Teacher.* **33**(9): e485–8.

121 Lievens F, Ones DS and Dilchert S (2009) Personality scale validities increase throughout medical school. *Journal of Applied Psychology.* **94**(6): 1514–35.

122 Tett RP, Jackson DN, Rothstein M and Reddon JR (1999) Meta-analysis of bi-directional relations in personality-job performance research. *Human Performance.* **12**: 1–29.

123 Murphy KR and Dzieweczynski JL (2005) Why don't measures of broad dimensions of personality perform better as predictors of job performance? *Human Performance.* **18**: 343–57.

124 Birkeland SA, Manson TM, Kisamore JL, Brannick MT and Smith MA (2006) A meta-analytic investigation of job applicant faking on personality measures. *International Journal of Selection and Assessment.* **14**: 317–35.

125 Rosse JG, Stecher MD, Miller JL and Levin RA (1998) The impact of response distortion on pre-employment personality testing and hiring decisions. *Journal of Applied Psychology.* **83**: 634–44.

126 Scarpello VG, Ledvinka J and Bergmann TJ (1995) *Human Resource Management, Environments and Functions* (2e). South-Western College Publishing, Cincinnati, OH.

127 Hough LM, Eaton NK, Dunnette MD, Kamp JD and McCoy RA (1990) Criterion related validities of personality constructs and effect of response distortion on those validities. *Journal of Applied Psychology.* **75**: 581–95.

128 Li A and Bagger J (2006) Using the BIDR to distinguish the effects of impression management and self-deception on the criterion validity of personality measures: a meta-analysis. *International Journal of Selection and Assessment.* **14**: 131–41.

129 Chartered Institute of Personnel and Development (2004) *Recruitment, Retention and Turnover, a Survey of the UK and Ireland.* CIPD, London.

130 IRS Employment Review (2005) Graduate Recruitment 2004/05: upturn and optimism. *IRS Employment Review.* **811**: 40–8.

131 Patterson F, Ferguson E, Lane P and Norfolk T (2001) A new competency based selection system for general practitioners. Paper presented at The 10th International Conference of the International Society for the Study of Individual Differences. Edinburgh, July.

132 Patterson F, Ferguson E, Norfolk T and Lane P (2005) A new selection system to recruit general practice registrars: preliminary findings from a validation study. *British Medical Journal.* **330**: 711–4.

133 Randall R, Davies H, Patterson F and Farrell K (2006) Selecting doctors for postgraduate training in paediatrics using a competency based assessment centre. *Archives of Disease in Childhood.* **91**: 444–8.

134 Randall R, Stewart P, Farrell K and Patterson F (2006) Using an assessment centre to select doctors for postgraduate training in obstetrics and gynaecology. *Obstetrician and Gynaecologist.* **8**: 257–62.

135 Gale TCE, Roberts MJ, Side PJ *et al.* (2010) Predictive validity of a selection centre testing non-technical skills for recruitment to training in anaesthesia. *British Journal of Anaesthesia.* **105**(5): 603–9.

136 Kidd J, Fuller J, Patterson F and Carter Y (2006). Selection Centres: initial description of a collaborative pilot project. *Proceedings for the Association of Medical Education in Europe (AMEE) Conference, Genoa, Italy.*

137 Ziv A, Rubin O, Moshinsky A *et al.* (2008) MOR: a simulation-based assessment centre for evaluating the personal and interpersonal qualities of medical school candidates. *Medical Education.* **42**(10): 991–8.

138 ten Cate O and Smal K (2002) Educational assessment center techniques for entrance selection in medical school. *Academic Medicine.* **77**(7): 737.

139 Damitz M, Manzey D, Kleinmann M and Severin K (2003) Assessment center for pilot selection: construct and criterion validity and the impact of assessor type. *Applied Psychology: An International Review.* **52**: 193–212.

140 Lievens F, Van Keer E and De Witte M (2005) Assessment centers in Belgium: the results of a study on their validity and fairness [French]. *Psychologie du Travail et des Organisations.* **11**: 25–33.

141 Schmitt N, Gooding RZ, Noe RA and Kirsch M (1984) Meta-analyses of validity studies published between 1964 and 1982 and the investigation of study characteristics. *Personnel Psychology.* **37**: 407–22.

142 Dayan K, Kasten R and Fox S (2002) Entry-level police candidate assessment center: an efficient tool or a hammer to kill a fly? *Personnel Psychology.* **55**: 827–49.

143 Krause DE, Kersting M, Heggestad E and Thornton GC (2006) Incremental validity of assessment center ratings over cognitive ability tests: a study at the executive management level. *International Journal of Selection and Assessment.* **14**: 360–71.

144 Lievens F, Harris MM, Van Keer E and Bisqueret C (2003) Predicting cross-cultural training performance: the validity of personality, cognitive ability, and dimensions measured by an assessment center and a behavior description interview. *Journal of Applied Psychology.* **88**: 476–89.

145 Macan TH, Avedon MJ, Paese M and Smith DE (1994) The effects of applicants' reactions to cognitive ability tests and an assessment center. *Personnel Psychology.* **47**: 715–38.

146 Rynes SL and Connerley ML (1993) Applicant reactions to alternative selection procedures. *Journal of Business and Psychology.* **7**: 261–77.

147 Woodruffe C (2000) *Development and Assessment Centres: Identifying and Developing Competence.* Institute of Personnel and Development, London.

148 Patterson F, Ashworth V, Zibarras L, Coan P, Kerrin M and O'Neill P (2012) Evaluations of situational judgement tests to assess non-academic attributes in selection. *Medical Education.* **46**: 850–68.

149 Lievens F, Peeters H and Schollaert E (2008) Situational judgment tests: a review of recent research. *Personnel Review.* **37**(4): 426–41.

150 Christian MS, Edwards BD and Bradley JC (2010) Situational judgement tests: constructs assessed and meta-analysis of criterion-related validities. *Personnel Psychology.* **63**: 83–117.

151 McDaniel MA and Nguyen NT (2001) Situational judgment tests: a review of practice and constructs assessed. *International Journal of Selection and Assessment.* **9**: 103–13.

152 McDaniel MA, Morgeson FP, Finnegan EB, Campion MA and Braverman EP (2001) Use of Situational Judgment Tests to predict

job performance: a clarification of the literature. *Journal of Applied Psychology.* **86**(4): 730–40.

153 Ployhart RE and Ehrhart MG (2003) Be careful what you ask for: effects of response instructions on the construct validity and reliability of situational judgment tests. *International Journal of Selection and Assessment.* **11**(1): 1–16.

154 McDaniel MA, Hartman NS, Whetzel DL and Grub W (2007) Situational judgement tests, response instructions, and validity: a meta-analysis. *Personnel Psychology.* **60**: 63–91.

155 Patterson F, Ashworth V, Kerrin M and O'Neill P (2013) Situational judgement tests represent a measurement method and can be designed to minimise coaching effects. *Medical Education.* **47**: 219–21.

156 Ahmed H, Rhydderch M and Matthews P (2012) Can knowledge tests and situational judgement tests predict selection centre performance? *Medical Education.* **46**(8): 777–84.

157 Connell MSO, Hartman NS, Mcdaniel MA, Lee W, Iii G and Lawrence A (2007) Incremental validity of situational judgment tests for task and contextual job performance. *International Journal of Selection and Assessment.* **15**(1): 19–29.

158 Clevenger J, Pereira GM, Weichmann D, Schmitt N and Schmidt Harvey V (2001) Incremental validity of Situational Judgment Tests. *Journal of Applied Psychology.* **86**(3): 410–7.

159 Koczwara A, Patterson F, Zibarras L, Kerrin M, Irish B and Wilkinson M (2012) Evaluating cognitive ability, knowledge tests and situational judgement tests for postgraduate selection. *Medical Education.* **46**(4): 399–408.

160 Chan D and Schmitt N (1997) Video-based versus paper-and-pencil method of assessment in situational judgment tests: subgroup differences in test performance and face validity perceptions. *Journal of Applied Psychology.* **82**(1): 143–59.

161 Plint S and Patterson F (2010) Identifying critical success factors for designing selection processes into postgraduate specialty training: the case of UK general practice. *Postgraduate Medical Journal.* **86**: 323–7.

162 Patterson F, Tavabie A, Denney M *et al.* (2013) A new competency model for general practice: implications for selection, training and careers. *British Journal of General Practice.* **63**: 331–8 .

163 Skarlicki PD and Folger R (1997) Retaliation in the workplace: the roles of distributive, procedural and interactional justice. *Journal of Applied Psychology.* **82**: 434–43.

164 Ackerman PL (1996) A theory of adult intellectual development: process, personality, interests and knowledge. *Intelligence.* **22**: 227–57.

29 Career progression and support

Caroline Elton[1] and Nicole J Borges[2]
[1] Health Education North West London and Health Education South London, UK
[2] Wright State University Boonshoft School of Medicine, USA

KEY MESSAGES

- The effectiveness of careers support is enhanced if both the provider and recipient work from a shared framework.

- A four-stage model of self-assessment, career exploration, decision-making and implementation planning provides an effective framework for the provision of careers support.

- Contemporary practice highlights the potential limitations of offering directive careers advice. Instead, a more facilitative stance is favoured.

- The literature on personality and medical specialty choice suggests that there is more variation in personality within than between different specialties

- Any psychometric measurement should be complemented by qualitative self-assessment activities.

- Career planning skills are not only useful to guide specialty choice, but are essential throughout a medical career, up to and including retirement.

Introduction

Drawing on medicine-specific and more general careers research, this chapter provides an evidence-based approach to the provision of careers support to medical students and junior doctors. Some of the different career decisions that one might encounter over the length of a medical career are described and a practical model for the provision of careers support is outlined. The literature on the role of psychometric testing is examined in detail in order to make recommendations on how best to incorporate psychometric test results into a career discussion. Some of the potential limitations of adopting an overly directive approach to the provision of careers support are described. The chapter works from the premise that for the majority of students and trainees, the provider of careers support will be a senior clinician, but situations in which a referral to a specialist careers service is indicated are also discussed. Throughout the chapter, the argument is made that medical careers research and practice needs to draw more heavily on contemporary developments in vocational psychology.

Need for support in medical careers

Until the introduction of a raft of major reforms in postgraduate medical education in 2005, designated careers support services for junior doctors in the UK were not widely available. Since the introduction of *Modernising Medical Careers* (MMC), junior doctors have had to make significant career decisions about specialty choice less than 18 months into their postgraduate training.(1) Yet it is known that prior to MMC, many junior doctors had not yet

chosen their final specialty so soon after leaving medical school,(2–4) with women being less likely to be confident about early specialty choices than men.(5) In response to this new, condensed career trajectory, the need for appropriate careers support services was recognised, and subsequently embedded into the reforms. Today, all regions in the UK have established careers support services for junior doctors, and all of the UK medical schools now have a named careers adviser, often linked to a university careers service.(6)

In the USA where the majority of medical schools have postgraduate entry, medical students choose their specialty on exit from medical school. Since 1999 the Association of American Medical Colleges (AAMC) Careers in Medicine web-based resource offers online help for students in career planning, as well as for training faculty in how best to use the resource with their students.(7) However, earlier studies suggested minimal careers advice provision in American medical schools.(8)

In part, the reason for the earlier lack of careers support offered during medical training may be an unstated assumption that a medical degree is a vocational training so career choices have already been made, rendering further careers support superfluous. Yet in all medical training systems it is clear that this assumption is unjustified as career-related decisions are made from the point of application to medical school. For example, medical schools in the UK differ in the ways in which they integrate the clinical and non-clinical training, in the extent of exposure to primary care, in opportunities for studying for an intercalated degree and in the range of student-selected components. Studies have indicated that factors such as opting for an intercalated degree,(9,10) participating in research(11) or studying medicine as a postgraduate(12) can have an impact on final career decisions. In the USA, medical students choose their specialty during the final year prior to graduating. As a result, the final year is largely comprised of electives and is regarded as an important part of testing one's suitability for an intended specialty and also as a way of improving one's chance of a given residency application being successful. So, it is clear that medical students are making career-related decisions during medical school.

Whether decisions about specialty choice are made during medical school (as in the USA and Canada) or after completing a generic junior doctor programme (as in the UK and Australia), there are a large number of different specialties from which to choose. For example, in the UK, on completion of the foundation programme, trainees have a choice of 20 different training programmes, as well as deciding if they want to apply for an academic training pathway which would allow them to combine clinical training with opportunities to complete a research degree. In subsequent years further specialty options branch out from these 20 different post-foundation options and in total in 2013 there are 65 specialties from which to choose (with opportunities for further sub-specialisation in 35 sub-specialties).(13) In Australia there are 80 specialties but no sub-specialties,(13) reflecting differences between medical training systems in whether a given training pathway is considered a specialty in its own right or a sub-specialty.

It is also apparent that career decision-making does not end once the specialty/sub-specialty choice phase has been successfully navigated. For example, decisions have to be made about continuing with research, or fellowship training, about whether to take a leading role in clinical management or clinical education or whether to switch to part-time work. Seen in this way, medical career decision-making is a process that begins before entry to medical school and continues up to the point of retirement.

Provision of effective careers support

Concerns about the quality of careers support that doctors receive are not new.(14–17) More recently, but prior to the implementation of the UK MMC reforms, a national survey on the availability and quality of careers support within medical training recommended that there was a need for high-quality careers information, for the development of self-assessment and career planning tools, for trained advisers who could provide expert careers advice and for national coordination of the careers support available across the UK.(18) Six years later a further survey reported that at least in terms of medical school provision, there was little evidence that these recommendations had been implemented.(6)

MMC recognised that the previous inattention given to the provision of careers support for doctors needed to be remedied, and for the first time in the UK a comprehensive careers support strategy for medical students and junior doctors was produced.(19) This report also recognised that certain groups of doctors, such as those with childcare responsibilities, international medical graduates and doctors with significant health issues, may need specialist careers support.

However, it could also be argued that this initiative was something of a missed opportunity. Given the absence in the policy of any linkage to an underlying theoretical framework of career support, there was no understanding embedded in the recommendations that it can be helpful if both the providers and recipients of careers support share a common framework for the overall career planning process. Yet a large-scale study has clearly demonstrated that sharing an underlying framework enhances the effectiveness of career discussions.(20) This lack of an underpinning theoretical framework also meant that insufficient attention was given to the fact that when providing support for career planning, some tasks come before others and it is important to map these different tasks across the length of the medical training continuum. In effect MMC was perhaps characteristic of the tendency highlighted by Petrides and McManus for developments in medical careers support to become divorced from broader developments in occupational psychology.(21)

Who should provide careers support?

In the UK, national guidance for postgraduate training recommends that the responsibility for the provision of careers support should fall within the remit of the educational supervisor.(22) It is also recognised that some students/junior doctors with more complex career needs (e.g. those with significant health concerns) may need specialist input from trained careers advisers or occupational psychologists.

This notion that, in the main, careers support will be provided by senior clinicians tallies with the trainees' own expectations. For example, in a survey of specialty trainees, Lloyd and Becker reported that study participants looked for careers advice and support from their educational supervisors, rather than from careers professionals.(23)

Improving the quality of careers support

In the non-medical context, an extensive survey of the components of effective career discussions in the workplace identified the importance of both parties having a simple shared framework to structure the discussion.(20) This finding has been incorporated into the approach to careers support described below and the specific framework is the four-stage model of careers guidance that is used throughout the higher education sector, namely:

1. Self-assessment
2. Career exploration
3. Decision-making
4. Plan implementation.

Evidence for this approach comes from an international review of best practice in career development.(24) The Careers in Medicine programme devised by the Association of American Medical Colleges, and used throughout medical schools in the USA, uses the four-stage approach. In turn, the NHS-funded medical careers web resource, which was based on Careers in Medicine, is also structured around the four stages.

BOX 29.1 The parallel between clinical decision-making and career decision-making

Clinical decision-making		Career decision-making
Taking a history	>	Self-assessment
Examining the patient/ investigations	>	Career exploration
Formulating a diagnosis	>	Decision-making
Implementing the treatment plan	>	Implementing the career plan

When using this approach in the medical education context, it is also possible to draw a parallel between career decision-making and clinical decision-making (*see* Box 29.1).

A number of important points can be drawn from this parallel. First, it would make no clinical sense to start with the treatment plan, then formulate a diagnosis and continue working backwards to the history; it is just so with career decision-making where it is not helpful to concentrate on the details of implementing one's career plan if one has not done adequate preparatory work in terms of self-assessment or exploring different options. There is of course one exception and that is in the context of a clinical emergency where one may have to implement a treatment plan before formulating the diagnosis, carrying out investigations or taking a history. But here too there is a career correlate in that sometimes the overriding need is to get any job as a holding position, before working out one's career in the longer term, which requires self-assessment, career exploration, etc.

A further point highlighted by the parallel is that in both clinical and career decision-making, the first two stages are linked. The particular details of the patient history will inform the examination/investigation stage. Similarly, the results of the self-assessment stage inform not only the specific career options that are explored in greater depth, but also the specific questions that should be researched. Furthermore, with both career decision-making and clinical decision-making there may be to-ing and fro-ing between the first two stages: clinically something found on examination may necessitate asking a more detailed history on certain points, and in career decision-making, something that the person discovers when they are exploring a particular option might lead them to go back and rethink the self-assessment stage.

However, whilst the parallel is useful in highlighting a systematic approach to career planning, it also has limitations. In clinical decision-making the aim (although it is not always achieved) is to make a definitive diagnosis. In career decision-making, the notion of a definitive diagnosis can be unhelpful if it is taken to suggest that each doctor could be happy in only one specialty. Instead, the literature suggests that each doctor is likely to be suited to more than one particular specialty.(25)

Two further limitations also need to be discussed. The parallel with clinical decision-making should not be taken to imply that it is pathological to grapple with a career decision. The suggested framework is one that anybody can use in any career situation and it is an approach that applies equally to somebody who is having difficulty deciding what to do next as to somebody who has firmly decided, but wants to maximise their chances of success.

Perhaps the final limitation of the parallel is the most important, and that is the key difference in the locus of decision-making. In clinical decision-making it is for the clinician to make the diagnosis (although in the move to patient-centred care, the ensuing treatment plan will be derived through discussion with the patient). In career decision-making it is for the recipient of careers support to make the decision, although the provider of careers support has a role in helping the recipient structure their passage through the four stages, and challenging them where necessary (see below).

Specialty choice

A vast literature spanning decades of research exists on factors influencing medical specialty choice. Hutt identified six areas on which the literature on career choice in medicine has focused, including background, personality and attitude, educational system, career, working conditions and intrinsic differences within specialties.(26) Other factors associated with specialty choice cited in the literature range from internal, personal or individual characteristics, including personality, values and interests,(27,28) to external factors related to lifestyle,(29,30) such as work hours and income, clinical experiences during medical school(31,32) and exposure to positive and negative role models.(33,34)

The concept of a 'controllable lifestyle' has been referenced for several decades but can be traced back to the work of Schwartz *et al.* in 1989.(30) Recent trends in this literature(35) illuminate lifestyle factors as major influences in the current generation's choice of medical specialty. In the USA, controllable lifestyle specialties, such as anaesthesiology, dermatology, emergency medicine, pathology, psychiatry and radiology, are on the rise as popular medical specialties and as a result it is increasingly competitive for students to gain residency in these specialities. Specialties referred to as 'uncontrollable' in lifestyle include surgery as well as primary care specialties of family medicine, internal medicine and paediatrics. Currently these specialties may be less competitive and all residency match slots may not fill.

A recent study carried out by the Royal College of Physicians(36) concluded that women were drawn to choosing specialties that offered a more controllable lifestyle. These authors also point out that given that the number of female medical students exceeds that of male students, the issue of shying away from specialties that have considerable out-of-hours commitments is likely to have a significant impact on future medical workforce planning.

In considering this area, two further points must be made. First, due to the ways in which a given specialty is practised in different health-care systems, a career choice such as family medicine may be perceived as offering poor control of lifestyle in the USA, but good control in the UK. Second, research has emphasised that the issue of controllable lifestyle is not only of importance to female doctors.(37,38)

More recently researchers in the USA have investigated the relation between medical school debt to choice of specialty, yielding mixed results. Phillips *et al.* found no overall relationship between anticipated debt upon graduating from medical school, but did find that medical students from middle-income households who anticipated more debt were less likely to consider a career in a primary care specialty.(39) Rosenblatt and Andrilla found demographic factors mediated their finding that medical students with more debt were less likely to enter primary care specialties.(40) In their longitudinal study (data from 1997–2006), medical students with higher debt were less likely to choose internal medicine and paediatrics.(41) The issue of the impact of student debt on specialty choice may become increasingly important in the UK context given the rise in university fees that took place in 2011.

Much of the literature on specialty choice has focused on students choosing primary care versus non-primary care careers, and researchers such as Fincher *et al.*,(42) Bland *et al.*(43) and Senf *et al.*,(44) have made important contributions to help medical educators understand the factors related to primary care specialty choice. In particular, the theoretical model developed by Bland *et al.*, although over 15 years old, contains many of the factors related to specialty choice that researchers continue to investigate today.(43) Caution is needed however when applying research findings from the USA to the UK context because specialties such as paediatrics and internal medicine are regarded as primary care specialties in the USA, but secondary care ones in the UK.

Although much of the literature focuses on factors related to specialty choice and how to predict medical specialty choice, a more novel approach comes from the work of Reed *et al.* who posit using decision theory to understand medical specialty choice and focus on the *process* of medical specialty choice decision-making rather than the actual content of the decision.(45) While theoretical, these models have applicability for careers professionals as they help highlight the complexity of medical specialty decision-making and may thereby normalise the experience of a student/trainee who is experiencing difficulty with making a decision. In addition, these models highlight the fact that career decision-making is a developmental task that unfolds over time, and there is therefore a need to prepare students and junior doctors over a period of time, rather than just before the point that they have to make a specialty choice decision.

One might predict that after decades and decades of research the factors associated with choosing a specialty would be well articulated and no longer require further investigative inquiry. To borrow the words of Barzanky, 'What much research has revealed, however, is that the simplicity of the question is deceptive.'(46, p.197) Researchers would agree that understanding medical specialty choice is a complex process affected by a host of factors, and that the factors vary from individual to individual. This contributes to the difficulty in synthesising and summarising the literature.

Psychometric testing

In the USA where specialty choices have to be made by the end of the fourth year of medical school, a number of medical schools offer psychometric testing to assist medical students with their specialty choice decisions. A review of the relevant literature carried out by Borges and Savickas(25) suggested that the Myers–Briggs Type Indicator(47) was the most frequently used psychometric instrument in helping medical students/junior doctors choose their specialty. However, other researchers have constructed medicine-specific indicators, such as the Medical Specialty Preference Inventory(48,49) developed in the USA and Sci45/59,(50) which is a specialty choice inventory developed in the UK.

The Myers–Briggs Type Indicator

The Myers–Briggs Type Indicator (*see* Box 29.2) is a self-report measure of normal personality that assesses differences in how people perceive information, and differences in how they use that information.(47) The inventory assesses the individual's preferences on four dichotomous scales, Extraversion/Intraversion (E/I); Sensing/Intuition (S/N); Thinking/Feeling (T/F) and Judging/Perceiving (J/P). In this way each individual's personality can be categorised into one of 16 different four-letter 'types' (e.g. ESTJ; ISTJ, etc.).

Since the 1950s, Myers and others have researched whether there are consistent relationships between MBTI personality type and the choice of particular medical specialties.(51–54) Based on these studies, some American career resources, such as *The Ultimate Guide to Choosing a Specialty*(55) and the Careers in Medicine website,(7) give information about MBTI codes that are frequently associated with particular specialties. So, for example, Freeman(55) using data from McCaulley(51) lists specialties frequently associated with 'ESTJ' as obstetrics/gynaecology, general practice, general surgery, orthopaedic surgery and paediatrics.

An initial problem associated with the use of personality type to choose a medical specialty thus immediately becomes apparent: this list of specialties commonly associated with this one particular MBTI type covers a broad range of different specialties, spanning both primary and secondary care and surgical/non-surgical specialties. Borges and Savickas,(25) in a comprehensive review of the relevant literature, highlight two further points. First, links between personality and specialty type do not necessarily remain constant over time. For example, there are some American data to suggest that different personality types were attracted to family medicine in the 1970s compared to those in the 1980s. This finding strongly suggests that one needs to be cautious about over-reliance on suggested links between MBTI preferences and specific specialties based on data that may have initially been collected over 30 years ago.

BOX 29.2 FOCUS ON: The Myers–Briggs Type Indicator(47)

Extraversion/Intraversion (E/I)

People who prefer *Extraversion* tend to focus on the outer world of people and external events.

People who prefer *Introversion* tend to focus on their own inner world of ideas and experiences.

Sensing/Intuition (S/N)

People who prefer *Sensing* like to take in information through their senses to find out what is actually happening in the present.

People who prefer *Intuition* like to take in information by seeing the big picture and grasping patterns.

Thinking/Feeling (T/F)

People who prefer to make judgements using *Thinking* tend to look at the logical consequences of a choice.

People who prefer to make judgements using *Feeling* tend to consider what is important to them and other people.

Judging/Perceiving (J/P)

People who prefer to orientate themselves to the outer world using *Judging* live in a planned orderly way.

People who prefer to orientate themselves to the outer world using *Perceiving* live in a flexible, spontaneous way.

The second point to emerge from the Borges and Savickas review is that there is actually more variation in personality type (using both the MBTI and other personality measures) *within* each specialty than *between* specialties.(25) They therefore conclude that all personality types appear in all specialties (although some types are more common than others) and that more than one particular specialty will fit the personality of any particular medical student or doctor.

However, on the basis of their review, Borges and Savickas do not conclude that personality assessment has no role in supporting trainees through the process of specialty choice. Instead, they argue that personality assessment should be viewed as one of a number of different factors that trainees should consider when choosing a specialty. Furthermore, they recommend that if a personality test such as MBTI is carried out, it should be used to increase self-knowledge (*see* Box 29.2) rather than used as a simple diagnostic process that makes a link between a particular personality type and a particular specialty.

Medical Specialty Preference Inventory

The original version of the Medical Specialty Preference Inventory (MSPI)(48) was a 199-item questionnaire that assessed medical students' interest in 40 areas of medical practice and preferences for six specialties: family practice, internal medicine, obstetrics and gynaecology, paediatrics, psychiatry and surgery. Whilst Zimny(49) described predictive validity of the instrument to be in the region of 50%, Savickas *et al.*,(56) found predictive validity indices in the

range of 59% and Glavin *et al.* found that the MSPI predicts medical specialty choice 58% of the time.(57) In a more recent study, however, Borges *et al.* reported that the questionnaire correctly predicted the preferred specialty in only 33% of their sample.(58) In addition, these latter authors also reported that nearly half of their sample (47%) chose specialties not listed in the six specialty fields included in the MSPI. So, clearly both the accuracy of prediction and the breadth of specialties included in the inventory are problematic.

The MSPI has undergone revisions since it original version. In 2009 Sodano and Richard reduced the MSPI down from 38 to 18 factors.(59) Additional research in 2010 supported an expanded number of specialty scales.(60) The Revised MSPI(61) consists of a 150-item scale predicting specialty choice in 16 specialties, and reports two additional studies in which predictive validity was 52% and 46%. The 18 Medical Interest Scales relate interest in different activities to medicine. However, caution is needed when using the instrument with students/trainees outside of the USA because aspects of a particular specialty (e.g. typical patterns of working hours or financial rewards) may differ significantly in different countries.

Sci59 Specialty Choice Inventory

The Sci59 Specialty Choice Inventory is a 130-item questionnaire designed in the UK to help medical students and junior doctors with the task of choosing an appropriate specialty. The first version of the questionnaire included 45 specialties,(50) but the current version now contains additional options, hence the change of name from Sci45 to Sci59. Having completed the questionnaire, respondents are provided with a computer-generated print-out that lists the 10 specialties to which there is greatest fit and the 10 to which there is the least fit. In addition, the print-out also contains a graph showing how the respondent has scored on 12 different underlying subscales, such as 'action orientation', 'coping with uncertainty', 'need for assertiveness', etc.

Sci59 is currently widely available and, in addition to access through the British Medical Association (BMA) website for BMA members, a number of medical schools also offer the instrument. It is therefore of more than academic interest to provide a critical appraisal of the use of Sci59 for helping medical students or junior doctors with the task of identifying an appropriate specialty.

In terms of the instrument design, although the original list of items considered for inclusion in the questionnaire was drawn from interviews with consultants and principals in general practice (GP), in drawing up the final list of items, the questionnaire was actually calibrated using responses from junior doctors who had not yet embarked on higher specialty training. The authors point out that the validity of the scale therefore rests on the assumption that the junior doctors 'had insight into the properties of work in their specialty and of consultant or principal posts and into the skills needed to occupy them'.(50) Yet these authors provide no evidence of the validity of this fundamental assumption (i.e. that a junior's understanding of the nature of work as a consultant or GP principal accords closely with that of the consultant or GP principal who actually occupies these posts).

Another concern is that of the predictive validity of the questionnaire. The original paper in which the design of the questionnaire is described(50) does not include data on predictive validity, and there is only one report in a peer-reviewed journal that examines this question.(62) This was a study of Foundation Year 2 (F2) doctors who filled out the Sci45 questionnaire within the first 2 months of their F2 year, and then again in the last 2 months of the programme, and it reported that 30% of the doctors were successfully appointed to a specialty predicted by their initial Sci45 scores. However, given the design of the study, it is impossible to tease out the different possible explanations for this low predictive validity, such as the questionnaire failing to identify the specialties that most interested the trainee; the interests of the trainee changing over the F2 year; and the trainees applying for, but not being accepted into, the specialties predicted by the Sci45 questionnaire.

Using psychometric test results to help with specialty choice

Given the complexity of factors that may impact on specialty choice, it is not surprising that studies using instruments such as Sci59 or the Revised MSPI often report relatively low predictive validity. In turn, given this low predictive validity, it is clear that caution is needed when using test results to help a medical student or junior doctor choose his or her future career. In other words, the fact that a particular career is listed as appropriate does not 'prove' that the respondent is well suited to that particular specialty. The appropriate use of any set of test results is to view it as a stimulus for further discussion. Examples of the types of issues that a supervisor could discuss with a medical student or trainee are given in Box 29.3. Used in this way, psychometric testing undoubtedly has a role to play in helping the trainee consider possible implications of aspects of their personality, offering reassurance that they might be suited to an emerging area of interest or broadening the range of specialties that they might research further.

 BOX 29.3 HOW TO: Ask questions that explore the implications of psychometric test results

Examples:

What have you learnt about yourself from completing the particular questionnaire?

To what extend do the results accord with the results of assessments that you have carried out during your training, or feedback you have received from your supervisors?

Are there any surprises: How do you account for these?

Which specialities might you be interested in researching further on the basis of the questionnaire results?

Deciding on a career in academic medicine

Another major area of concern in the medical careers literature is the question of what factors predict whether individuals will choose an academic career pathway. In the USA, typically individuals first decide on the vocation of medicine, then render a specialty choice, followed by deciding on whether they wish to pursue an academic pathway. In the UK, it is possible to pursue the academic route alongside medical training (in the small number of MBBS/PhD programmes), as part of foundation training, during the early years of post-foundation training or at some later point.

In the USA, Strauss *et al.* sought to understand factors impacting academic medicine as a career choice.(63) Their systematic review revealed the following as influential in pursuing a career in academic medicine: (i) completion of a graduate degree or fellowship in addition to obtaining a MD degree; (ii) being involved in research and publishing while a student or resident; and (iii) an interest in teaching and/or the intellectual stimulation that the academic career path provides. An academic role model or mentor was also found to have a significant influence on decision-making. Additional factors cited in the literature include perceived status of career in academic medicine,(64) work–life balance(65) and autonomy.(66)

Satisfaction with academic medicine is a growing area of concern in the literature. In their study of medical school faculty, Lowenstein *et al.*(67) found that 42% were considering leaving academic medicine. More recently, another study suggested that about one-quarter of current faculty from 26 US medical schools have considered leaving their careers in academic medicine.(68) They identify factors associated with dissatisfaction (i.e. incongruence in values, lack of institutional support), as well as factors that were unrelated (i.e. gender, faculty rank and lack of mentoring). In the UK, lack of mentoring has been identified as one of a number of factors that contribute to the under-representation of women in senior academic positions alongside difficulty pursuing an academic career when working part-time or flexibly.(69)

The literature on careers in academic medicine tends to be mostly focused in specialty areas rather than a collective assessment of this pathway in general. Two recent articles, however, sought to summarise the literature and address the question of choice of academic medicine as a career pathway.(70,71) Findings by Borges *et al.*(71) suggest that, at least for women, a career in academic medicine tended to happen serendipitously and, as medical students, women knew little if anything about this career path. The authors suggest that medical schools and residency programmes provide specific programming and opportunities to expose their trainees at various stages of their education to academic medicine as a career path.

Contemporary developments in vocational psychology

The vast literature on specialty choice demonstrates the breadth of factors that influence medical specialty decisions. The conceptual models currently available in the medical education literature are primarily focused on factors influencing specialty choice and largely were developed by medical educators. While they serve an important purpose, they may be limited in scope and fail to address the complexity of medical specialty decision-making. Future work in the field may benefit from incorporating developments in vocational psychology, in order to guide both research and careers interventions. For example, from the vocational psychology literature, Rogers *et al.*(72) have applied Social Cognitive Career Theory (SCCT) to the development of a measure of specialty choice. The SCCT model of career decision-making(73) proposes that personal, contextual and experiential factors are responsible for shaping experiences that lead to self-efficacy beliefs, outcome expectations and career goals. In turn, these beliefs and expectations underpin career interests and choices. Even though SCCT is not specifically focused on medical career and specialty choice, the complexity of the theory offers multiple pathways to explore significant factors in career planning with medical students.

Currently in the wider world of vocational psychology there is also considerable interest in bringing together qualitative and quantitative forms of career assessment. So, for example, in a key article in a leading vocational psychology journal, Walsh advocated expanding career assessment beyond traditional psychometric methods 'to consider idiographic, qualitative, and other creative approaches to assessing multiple aspects of both people and contexts'.(74) In the American context researchers are already exploring the possible relevance of qualitative assessment methods in assisting medical students with career choice, to sit alongside more traditional quantitative psychometric methods.(75)

Some UK medical schools have developed excellent career handbooks that encourage students to reflect on their potential suitability for particular specialties as they complete their undergraduate 'firms' in that speciality. Other methods of qualitative assessment in medical school include a compulsory reflective exercise on career planning linked to the undergraduate elective.(76) Undoubtedly these and other comparable initiatives are crucially important, and they are congruent with the recommendation for a greater emphasis on career planning in the undergraduate years.(77)

At the postgraduate level in the UK, some foundation schools use resources such as 'Windmills'(78) or 'ROADS to Success',(79) whilst in the USA, the Careers in Medicine resource incorporates both objective psychometric testing and more subjective qualitative assessments.(7) Navarro, Taylor and Pokorny have also described three innovative ways of incorporating Careers in Medicine resources into the undergraduate curriculum.(80)

One further trend in vocational psychology that could usefully be incorporated into medical careers support is the switch from methods that concentrate on helping individuals make a one-off career decision, to an approach that emphasises the inevitability of change.(81,82) Seen in this way, the task of careers support is to equip individuals with career planning skills so they can become more adept at navigating their way through the decisions that they will face throughout their career.

Helping those whose career plans appear unrealistic

This aspect of the supervisor's role could be paraphrased as 'how to help the student/trainee make best use of the feedback that they have received in order to develop realistic career plans'. In effect the supervisor's role in this situation is to facilitate the trainee's reflection on the *implications* of the feedback for their career plans. So, for example, if an individual wants to pursue a surgical career yet feedback from relevant work-based assessments does not indicate particular surgical aptitude, what careers advice should the trainee be given?

Whilst there is a paucity of literature on this question in the medical education field, it is an issue that is described at length in the generic careers counselling literature.(83,84) This broader literature would suggest that the supporting clinician should focus on posing the sorts of questions outlined in Box 29.4 and avoid directive advice. We caution against giving such advice for a number of reasons. First, telling somebody what career to follow removes responsibility for the decision from the person. This is contradictory to the educational ethos of most medical training curricula which emphasise the importance of developing the trainee's responsibility for their own learning and professional development. Second, directive advice – 'If I were you, I would ditch surgery' – is not the most effective way of getting somebody to take on board the key points. There

BOX 29.4 HOW TO: Ask questions of those whose career plans may be unrealistic

1. Based on the feedback you have received in this post (and previously), what do you see as your key strengths?

2. Based on the feedback you have received in this post (and previously), what do you see as the areas that you find more difficult?

3. What are the key competences that will be assessed for recruitment into your specialty of interest?

4. Who have you talked to/what have you read in order to assess the competitiveness of the particular specialty you are interested in?

5. If the specialty is highly competitive and you have been getting average or below average assessments in relevant areas of your work, what gives you confidence that your career plans are realistic?

6. Going back to review the areas of performance that you seem to perform better in, are there other specialties that might make a better match? Have you also looked at the specialties that in previous years seemed to be shortage specialties? Might any of these specialties suit your particular strengths?

are parallels here with the health behaviour literature, which consistently reports a high degree of non-compliance with directive advice. Third, in giving directive advice it is very easy for personal preferences to seep in inadvertently. For example, it is easy to omit options in which one is not particularly interested, or of which one has little knowledge. Finally, the person giving the directive advice may be in error. For example, the trainee may know that something in their private life is having a seriously detrimental effect on the quality of their work, but they do not want to discuss this with their supervisor. The trainee however knows that previously they have received excellent feedback on areas of their work that are currently causing concern.

It is for these sorts of reasons that professional training courses in careers support suggest that careers practitioners should be wary of giving directive advice about which career paths somebody should follow. A wariness about advice is also congruent with the conclusion reached by Woolf and McManus advocating that the senior clinician should concentrate on 'listening to the needs of students and trainees, understanding their points of view, and encouraging them to make their own decisions'.(85)

Other sources of careers support

A senior clinician who is trying to provide careers support to a student or doctor in postgraduate training whose career plans they believe to be unrealistic might feel that the suggestions made above are insufficient. Where clear constructive feedback has been given but the trainee insists on sticking to their plans, the educational supervisor can suggest that the trainee discuss their career plans with a more senior member of the educational faculty who has overall responsibility for the training programme. In this situation, the educational supervisor can write a brief summary outlining their concerns about the robustness of the trainee's proposed plans and give a copy to the trainee and to the person providing the additional careers support.

The suggestion can also be made that the trainee could consult with somebody from the local medical careers advisory service. In the UK people occupying these roles are qualified careers professionals, and therefore have had relevant training in how to approach delicate careers discussions. In addition, some trainees may find it easier to be more open with careers advisers (as opposed to the clinicians who supervise them) about their career concerns as careers advisers are not involved in carrying out assessments or writing references, or sitting on future interview panels. But here too, the trainee may persist in holding on to their intended plan, which might in the long run turn out well – or it might not. Just as all patients cannot always be helped from making poor health decisions (continuing to smoke, drink too much, etc.), providers of careers support need to be aware that it is not always possible to stop someone from making poor career decisions.(86)

Leaving medicine

Senior clinicians may also be uncertain how to respond when a student or trainee for whom they are responsible tells them that they are considering leaving the profession. Concern about doctors leaving the profession is not new; in 1997 an editorial in the *Journal of the Royal Society of Medicine* was entitled 'Why do young doctors leave the profession?'.(87) However, what is striking is the fact that despite reports of disillusionment amongst junior doctors, the actual proportion of doctors leaving the profession is remarkably low. This was a conclusion reached in the 1997 editorial mentioned above and a review of more recent studies would concur with this position. For example, studies undertaken by the UK Medical Careers Research Group in Oxford suggest that, although quite high levels of dissatisfaction can be expressed, the actual numbers of UK medical graduates intending to leave the profession are low; less than 3% in one study(88) and less than 1% in another.(3)

One possible explanation for the anxiety about loss to the medical workforce despite the figures suggesting that actual rates of leaving the profession are remarkably low could be the difference between expressed rates of dissatisfaction and actual rates of leaving medicine. Rittenhouse *et al.* reported that although physician dissatisfaction had a strong association with expressed intention to leave clinical practice, it was not associated with actual departure from practice.(89) These authors therefore concluded that self-reported intention to leave practice may be more of a proxy for dissatisfaction than a reliable predictor of actual behaviour.

In terms of underlying reasons for leaving the profession a qualitative follow-up study by the BMA of 14 doctors who had left the profession reported that the main reasons were that they felt that they were not valued or supported and that medicine involved an unacceptable work–life balance.(90) It would seem that there is a need for further studies to explore these issues in more depth, but these preliminary findings suggest that these three issues could usefully be explored when faced with a trainee who reports that they are considering switching career. This BMA study also reported high levels of distress amongst the sample together with regrets that they had been unable to access adequate careers support. This might suggest that students or doctors who are considering leaving the profession should be made aware of professional careers support services that could assist them with the major life decision to leave the profession, or to remain working as a doctor.

Conclusions

Students and trainees tend to look to the senior clinicians who supervise them for careers support. The approach outlined in this chapter suggests that caution is needed when giving directive careers advice. Instead, the recommended model is based on a structured approach to careers support that emphasises the importance of thorough self-assessment (using both quantitative and qualitative methods) and careful exploration of options. Furthermore, career decision-making is not over when a specialty/sub-specialty choice has been made, but instead will re-occur up to the point of retirement and the careers support model can be used at any point in one's working life. Some students or trainees whose career decisions are complicated by health or performance issues, or who are considering leaving medicine entirely, may benefit from a referral to a specialist careers support service. Historically, research and interventions in the medical careers field have tended to be divorced from wider developments in vocational psychology and closer collaboration between the two disciplines is recommended.

References

1 Department of Health (2004) *Modernising Medical Careers: The Next Steps*. Department of Health, London.

2 Edwards C, Lambert TW, Goldacre MJ *et al.* (1997) Early medical career choices and eventual careers. *Medical Education*. 31: 237–42.

3 Lambert TW, Goldacre MJ and Turner G (2006) Career choices of the United Kingdom medical graduates of 2002: questionnaire survey. *Medical Education*. 40: 514–21.

4 Goldacre MJ, Laxton L and Lambert TW (2010) Medical graduates' early career choices of specialty and their eventual specialty destinations: UK prospective cohort studies. *British Medical Journal*. 341: c3199.

5 McManus IC and Goldacre MJ (2008) Predicting career destinations. In: Carter Y and Jackson N (eds) *Education and Training: From Theory to Delivery*, pp. 59–78. Oxford University Press, Oxford.

6 Tapper-Jones L, Prout H, Grant A *et al.* (2009) An evaluation of the sources and availability of careers advice in UK medical schools. *British Journal of Hospital Medicine*. 70: 588–91.

7 Association of American Medical Colleges. (2013) Careers in medicine. (http://www.aamc.org/students/cim; accessed 3 February 2013).

8 Zimny GH and Senturia AG (1973) Medical specialty counseling: a survey. *Journal of Medical Education*. 48: 336–42.

9 Nguyen-Van-Tam JS, Logan RFA, Logan SAE *et al.* (2001) What happens to medical students who complete an honours year in public health and epidemiology? *Medical Education*. 35: 134–6.

10 McManus IC, Richards P and Winder BC (1999) Intercalated degrees, learning styles and career preferences: prospective longitudinal study of UK medical students. *British Medical Journal*. 319: 542–6.

11 Lloyd T, Phillips B and Aber RC (2004) Factors that influence doctors' participation in clinical research. *Medical Education*. 38: 848–51.

12 Goldacre MJ, Davidson JW and Lambert TW (2007) Career preferences of graduate and non-graduate entrants to medical schools in the United Kingdom. *Medical Education*. 41: 349–61.

13 General Medical Council (2013) Approved curricula and assessment systems. (http://www.gmc-uk.org/education/A-Z_by_specialty.asp; accessed 3 February 2013).

14 Allen I (1988) *Doctors and Their Careers*. Policy Studies Institute, London.

15 Dillner L (1993) Senior House Officers: the lost tribes. *British Medical Journal*. 307: 1549–51.

16 Lambert TW, Goldacre MJ and Evans J (2000) Views of junior doctors about their work: survey of qualifiers of 1993 and 1996 from United Kingdom medical schools. *Medical Education*. 34: 348–54.

17 Lambert TW and Goldacre MJ (2007) Views of doctors in training on the importance and availability of career advice in UK medicine. *Medical Education*. 41: 460–6.

18 Jackson C, Ball J, Hirsh W *et al.* (2003) *Informing Choices: The need for Career Advice in Medical Training*. National Institute for Careers Education and Counselling, Cambridge, UK.

19 Department of Health (2005) *Career Management: An Approach for Medical Schools, Deaneries, Royal Colleges and Trusts*. MMC Working Group for Career Management, London.

20 Hirsh W, Jackson C and Kidd J (2001) *Straight Talking: Effective Career Discussions at Work*. National Institute for Careers Education and Counselling, Cambridge.

21 Petrides KV and McManus IC (2004) Mapping medical careers: questionnaire assessment of career preferences in medical school applicants and final year students. *BMC Medical Education*. 4: 18.

22 Department of Health (2010) A reference guide to postgraduate specialty training in the UK. (http://www.mmc.nhs.uk/pdf/Gold%20Guide%202010%20Fourth%20Edition%20v08.pdf; accessed 3 February 2013).

23 Lloyd BW and Becker D (2009) Paediatric specialist registrars' views of educational supervision and how it can be improved: a questionnaire study. *Journal of the Royal Society of Medicine*. 100: 375–8.

24 Richard GV (2005) International best practices in career development: review of the literature. *International Journal for Educational and Vocational Guidance*. 5: 189–201.

25 Borges NJ and Savickas ML (2002) Personality and medical specialty choice: a literature review and integration. *Journal of Career Assessment*. 3: 362–80.

26 Hutt R (1976) Doctors' career choice: previous research and its relevance for policy making. *Medical Education*. 10: 463–73.

27 Smith AW, Glenn RC, Williams V *et al.* (2007) What do future (female) paediatricians value. *Journal of Pediatrics*. 151: 443–4.

28 Taber BJ, Hartung PJ and Borges NJ (2011) Personality and values as predictors of medical specialty choice. *Journal of Vocational Behavior*. 78: 202–9.

29 Newton DA, Grayson MS and Thompson LF (2005) The variable influence of lifestyle and income on medical students' career specialty choices: data from two U.S. medical schools, 1998–2004. *Academic Medicine*. 80: 809–14.

30 Schwartz RW, Jarecky RK, Strodel WE *et al.* (1989) Controllable lifestyle: a new factor in carer choice by medical students. *Academic Medicine*. 64: 606–9.

31 Ellsbury KE, Carline JK, Irby DM *et al.* (1998) Influence of third-year clerkships on medical student specialty preferences. *Advances in Health Sciences Education: Theory and Practice*. 3: 177–86.

32 Paiva RE, Vu NV and Verhulst SJ (1982) The effect of clinical experiences in medical school on specialty choice decisions. *Journal of Medical Education*. 57: 666–74.

33 Campus-Outcalt D, Senf J, Watkins AJ *et al.* (1995) The effects of medical schools curricula, faculty role models and biomedical research support on choice of generalist physician careers: a review and quality assessment of the literature. *Academic Medicine*. 70: 611–9.

34 Chang JC, Odrobina MR and McIntyre-Seltman K (2010) Residents as role models: the effect of the obstetrics and gynecology clerkship on medical students' career interest. *Journal of Graduate Medical Education*. 2(3): 341–5.

35 Dorsey ER, Jarjoura D and Rutecki GW (2003) Influence of controllable lifestyle on recent trends in specialty choice by US medical students. *Journal of the American Medical Association*. 290: 1173–8.

36 Royal College of Physicians (2009) *Women and Medicine: The Future*. Royal College of Physicians, London.

37 Gray SF (2004) Women in medicine: doctors of both sexes are seeking balance between life and work. *British Medical Journal*. 329: 742–3.

38 Lambert EM and Holmboe ES (2005) The relationship between specialty choice and gender of U.S. medical students, 1990–2003. *Academic Medicine*. 80: 797–802.

39 Phillips JP, Weismantel DP, Gold KJ *et al.* (2010) Medical student debt and primary care specialty intentions. *Family Medicine*. 42: 616–22.

40 Rosenblatt RA and Andrilla CH (2005) The impact of US medical students' debt on their choice of primary care careers: an analysis of data from the 2002 medical school graduation questionnaire. *Academic Medicine.* **80**: 815–9.

41 Jeffe DB, Whelan AJ and Andriole DA (2010) Primary care specialty choices of United States medical graduates 1997–2006. *Academic Medicine.* **85**(6): 947–58.

42 Fincher RM, Lewis LA and Rogers LQ (1992) Classification model that predicts medical students choices of primary care or non-primary care specialties. *Academic Medicine.* **67**: 324–7.

43 Bland CJ, Meurer LN and Maldonado G (1995) Determinants of primary care specialty choice: a non-statistical meta-analysis of the literature. *Academic Medicine.* **70**: 620–41.

44 Senf JH, Campos-Outcalt D, Watkins AJ *et al.* (1997) A systematic analysis of how medical school characteristics relate to graduates' choices of primary care specialties. *Academic Medicine.* **72**: 524–33.

45 Reed VA, Jernstedt GC and Reber ES (2001) Understanding and improving medical student specialty choice: a synthesis of the literature using decision theory as a referent. *Teaching and Learning in Medicine.* **13**: 117–29.

46 Barzansky B (2000) Commentray: research on specialty choice: a challenge is in the details. *Education for Health.* **13**: 197–2000.

47 Myers IB, McCaulley MH, Quenk NL *et al.* (1998) *MBTI Manual: A Guide to the Development and Use of the Myers-Briggs Type Indicator* (3e). Consulting Psychologists Press, Palo Alto, CA.

48 Zimny GH (1977) *Manual for the Medical Specialty Preference Inventory.* St Louis University School of Medicine, St Louis, MO.

49 Zimny GH (1980) Predictive validity of the Medical Specialty Preference Inventory. *Medical Education.* **14**: 414–8.

50 Gale R and Grant J (2002) Sci45: the development of a specialty choice inventory. *Medical Education.* **36**: 659–66.

51 McCaulley MH (1977) *The Myers Longitudinal Medical Study (Monograph II).* Center for Applications of Psychological Type, Gainesville, GA.

52 Taylor AD, Clark C and Sinclair AE (1990) Personality types of family practice residents in the 1980s. *Academic Medicine.* **65**: 216–8.

53 Wallick M, Cambre K and Randall H (1999) Personality type and medical specialty choice. *Journal of the Louisiana State Medical Society.* **151**: 463–9.

54 Stilwell NA, Wallick MM, Thal SE *et al.* (2000) Myers-Briggs type and medical specialty choice: a new look at an old question. *Teaching and Learning in Medicine.* **12**: 14–20.

55 Freeman B (2004) *The Ultimate Guide to Choosing a Medical Specialty.* Lange Medical Books/McGraw Hill, New York.

56 Savickas ML, Brizzi JS, Brisbi LA *et al.* (1988) Predictive validity of two medical specialty preference inventories. *Measurement and Evaluation in Counseling and Development.* **21**: 106–12.

57 Glavin KW, Richard GV and Porfeli EJ (2009) Predictive validity of the Medical Specialty Choice Inventory. *Journal of Vocational Behavior.* **74**: 128–33.

58 Borges MJ, Gibson DD and Karnani RM (2005) Job satisfaction of physicians with congruent versus incongruent specialty choice. *Evaluation and the Health Professions.* **28**: 400–13.

59 Sodano SM and Richard GV (2009) Construct validity of the Medical Specialty Preference Inventory: a critical analysis. *Journal of Vocational Behavior.* **74**: 30–7.

60 Porfeli EJ, Richard GV and Savickas ML (2010) Development of specialization scales for the MSPI: a comparison of empirical and inductive strategies. *Journal of Vocational Behavior.* **77**: 227–37.

61 Richard GV (2011) *Medical Specialty Preference Inventory, Revised Edition (MSPI-R), Technical Manual.* Association of American Medical Colleges, Washington, DC.

62 O'Donnell ME, Noad R, Boohan M *et al.* (2010) The effect of Modernising Medical Careers on foundation doctor career orientation in the Northern Ireland Foundation School. *Ulster Medical Journal.* **79**: 62–9.

63 Straus SE, Straus C, Tzanetos K; International Campaign to Revitalise Academic Medicine. (2006) Career choice in academic medicine: systematic review. *Journal of General Internal Medicine.* **21**: 1222–9.

64 Kelly WN and Stross JK (1992) Faculty tracks and academic success. *Annals of Internal Medicine.* **116**: 654–9.

65 Sanders AB, Fulginiti JV, Witzke DB *et al.* (1994) Characteristics influencing career decisions of academic and non-academic emergency physicians. *Annals of Emergency Medicine.* **23**: 81–7.

66 Bilbey JH, Fache JS and Burhenne HJ (1992) Are there predictors for future academic radiologists: a Canadian survey. *Canadian Association of Radiologists Journal.* **43**: 369–73.

67 Lowenstein SR, Fernandez G and Crane LA (2007) Medical school faculty discontent: prevalence and predictors of intent to leave academic careers. *BMC Medical Education.* **7**: 37.

68 Pololi LH, Krupat E, Civian JT *et al.* (2012) Why are a quarter of faculty considering leaving academic medicine? A study of their perceptions of institutional culture and intentions to leave at 26 representative U.S. medical schools. *Academic Medicine.* **87**: 1–11.

69 Women in Academic Medicine (2007) *Developing equality in governance and management for career progression.* Women in Academic Medicine Project, London.

70 Borges NJ, Narvarro AM, Grover A *et al.* (2010) Academic medicine careers: a literature review. *Academic Medicine.* **85**: 680–6.

71 Borges NJ, Navarro AM and Grover A (2012) Women physicians: choosing a career in academic medicine. *Academic Medicine.* **87**: 105–14.

72 Rogers ME, Creed PA and Searle J (2009) The development and initial validation of social cognitive career theory instruments to measure choice of medical specialty and practice location. *Journal of Career Assessment.* **17**: 324–37.

73 Lent RW, Brown SD and Hackett G (1994) Toward a unifying social cognitive theory of career and academic interest, choice and performance. *Journal of Vocational Behavior.* **45**: 79–122.

74 Walsh WB (2001) The changing nature of the science of vocational psychology. *Journal of Vocational Behavior.* **59**: 262–74.

75 Hartung PJ and Borges NJ (2005) Toward integrated career assessment: using story to appraise carer dispositions and adaptability. *Journal of Career Assessment.* **13**: 439–51.

76 Elton C and Newport M (2008) The reflective elective: using the elective to develop medical students' skills in career planning. *British Journal of Hospital Medicine.* **69**: 409–11.

77 Tooke J (2008) *Aspiring to excellence: final report of the independent inquiry into Modernising Medical Careers.* MMC Inquiry, London.

78 Hawkins P (2005) *The Art of Building Windmills.* GIEU, The University of Liverpool, Liverpool.

79 Elton C and Reid J (2010) *The ROADS to Success: A Practical Approach for Career Planning for Medical Students, Foundation Trainees and Their Supervisors* (3e). Kent, Surrey and Sussex Deanery, London.

80 Navarro AM, Taylor AD and Pokorny AP (2011) Three innovative curricula for addressing medical students' career development. *Academic Medicine.* **86**: 1–5.

81 Mitchell KE, Levin AS and Krumboltz JD (1999) Planed happenstance: constructing unexpected career opportunities. *Journal of Counseling and Development.* **77**: 115–25.

82 Bright JEH and Pryor RGL (2008) Shiftwork: a chaos theory of careers agenda of careers agenda for change in career counselling. *Australian Journal of Career Development.* **17**: 63–72.

83 Nathan R and Hill L (2006) *Career Counselling* (2e). Sage, London.

84 Ali L and Graham B (1996) *The Counselling Approach to Career Guidance.* Routledge, London.

85 Woolf K and McManus IC (2010) Predicting and guiding career success in medicine. In: Dornan T, Mann K, Scherpbier A and Spencer J (eds) *Learning Medicine: A Text Linking Theory and Practice for Graduate Students and Educators Wanting to Beyond the Basics.* Elsevier, London.

86 Kidd JM (2006) *Understanding Career Counselling: Theory Research and Practice*. Sage, London.

87 Paice E (1997) Why do young doctors leave the profession? *Journal of the Royal Society of Medicine*. **90**: 417–8.

88 Moss PJ, Lambert TW, Goldacre MJ *et al.* (2004) Reasons for considering leaving UK medicine: questionnaire study of junior doctors' comments. *British Medical Journal*. **329**: 1263.

89 Rittenhouse DR, Mertz E, Keane D *et al.* (2004) No exit: an evaluation of physician attrition. *Health Services Research*. **39**: 1571–88.

90 British Medical Journal (2004) *Why do Doctors Leave the Profession?* British Medical Association, Health Policy and Economic Research Unit, London.

Further reading

Cochran L (1997) *Career Counseling: A Narrative Approach*. Sage, London.

Hirsch G (1999) *Strategic Career Management for the 21st Century Physician*. American Medical Association, Chicago, IL.

Nathan R and Hall L (2006) *Career Counselling* (2e). Sage, London.

30 Managing remediation

Deborah Cohen, Melody Rhydderch and Ian Cooper
School of Medicine, Cardiff University, UK

> **KEY MESSAGES**
>
> - Performance is a function of ability, motivation, personality and organisational issues.
> - Performance must be considered in the context of the individual's health, well-being and the educational system they function within.
> - Moving into 'action' – providing solutions and fixing problems – too early may lead to disengagement, a loss of
>
> ownership and reduced chance of successfully achieving change.
> - High-quality records should be kept throughout the remediation process.

Approaches to identifying and assessing performance issues in doctors and medical students are well documented. However, less certain is how best to approach remediation for this group.

In this chapter we explore how best to approach remediation and do so having made two key assumptions. Firstly, that performance is a function of not only ability but also of motivation, personality and organisational issues. Secondly, that performance is also a function of health, well-being and the educational system. We argue for a holistic approach that takes account of all relevant biopsychosocial factors and suggest that educational supervisors have a crucial role to play in helping the remediation process run smoothly. We note that moving into 'action' – providing solutions and fixing problems – too early may lead to disengagement, a loss of ownership and reduced chance of successfully achieving change. Throughout we highlight some key principles, including the following:
- getting the right system in place
- personalised remediation
- engagement and motivation
- taking account of organisational culture
- clarity of roles and boundaries.

We have tried to guide educational supervisors through the process of dialogue with the struggling doctor, exploring the problems, note-keeping and some ideas for how to explore health and other issues in a sensitive way. A case study is used to explore possible pathways for remediation and towards the end of the chapter, we signal some common pitfalls.

Introduction

The management of performance issues in doctors continues to pose considerable challenges to employing organisations, educational and regulatory bodies. The problem is complex and goes beyond a simple question of *ability*, since personality, motivation and organisational factors all impact on individual performance.[1] Models of performance assessment are now well researched and have evolved with a consistent approach worldwide. Models of remediation, however, do not yet have a consistency of approach. Some examples of good practice do exist,[2–8] but evidence of long-term outcomes is harder to establish.[9]

Early literature and methods of remediation often considered performance separately from an individual's health and well-being. More recently, a more broad and holistic approach has been recognised as most effective, where health and the quality of the learning or organisational environment are considered alongside specific performance indicators.

Alongside this it is now recognised that a more proactive approach to remediation is important. Medical students and doctors should be encouraged to seek help early before health, well-being or educational issues impact on performance. Literature has also been published on *why* doctors find it so difficult to seek help. This has led to an improved understanding of the obstacles doctors and medical students face, such as poor provision of support, lack of accessibility and uncertainty about confidentiality.[10] This chapter seeks to reflect evolving thinking and put this work

Understanding Medical Education: Evidence, Theory and Practice, Second Edition. Edited by Tim Swanwick.
© 2014 The Association for the Study of Medical Education. Published 2014 by John Wiley & Sons, Ltd.

in context of revalidation for doctors and associated legislative responsibilities in the UK.(11) However, we are aware that for many readers simply having ideas about how to approach conversations with those who appear to be struggling is still of value, and so the focus of this chapter remains the educational supervisor and the notion that performance is more than simply a function of ability.

The aim is to provide a practical guide for educational supervisors and others faced with the challenge of providing support when confronting a performance issue. We aim to offer advice on how to navigate and manage the process of remediating performance issues and outline principles that underpin good practice. Whilst much of what has been written below has been drafted with an educational supervisor and trainee doctor in mind, the principles and approaches suggested will also be of value to those working with medical students, general practitioners (family physicians), consultant specialists and other non-training grade doctors. For ease of writing, we will refer to the individual providing support as an *educational supervisor* throughout the chapter.

From assessment to remediation

Assessment activity is the mechanism against which individual performance is judged.(12) Historically, the focus of standardised assessment has been targeted at the small minority of doctors whose performance gives substantial rise for concern. In the UK, such doctors were typically referred to the General Medical Council (GMC) and, since 2001, the National Clinical Assessment Service (NCAS). However, with the arrival of *Modernising Medical Careers*(13) and *Good Doctors, Safer Patients*,(14) routine performance assessments have increased, paralleled by a decreased tolerance for poor performance. This situation created a pressing need for educational supervisors to develop their remediation skills in order to respond effectively to the needs of doctors (and indeed students) for whom they are responsible.

Remediation is an intervention, or suite of interventions, required in response to assessment against threshold standards of performance. To deliver effective remediation, educational supervisors must be sensitive to the assessment process and provide a flexible response. They must be able to offer personalised support and direction to the individual, whilst being sensitive and responsive to the organisation(s) in which they work. The problem may often lie in the organisational structure and culture, rather than solely with the individual referred.(15,16) The educational supervisor must consider health and well-being, alongside personality, motivation to change, and organisational and social issues.(1,17,18) Rising to these challenges is no easy task. Identifying that a doctor may be struggling with their performance is complex. Some early workplace signs are contained in Box 30.1.

Perhaps the first and maybe most important task for supervisors is to consider the principles and beliefs that shape the approach of their employing organisations

BOX 30.1 FOCUS ON: Identifying the doctor in difficulty

The doctor who is struggling has many different faces. Paice(19) describes certain 'early warning signs' of the trainee in difficulty. Some of the attributes she describes include the following:

- the doctor who is often difficult to find (*The disappearing act*)
- the doctor who is always at work but achieves less than their colleagues (*Low work rate*)
- the doctor who is quick to lose their temper (*Ward rage*)
- the doctor who is inflexible and has difficulty prioritising (*Rigidity*).

Other doctors she describes as displaying problems with their career choice or having difficulty obtaining their required exams (*Career problems*), while others lack insight and reject constructive criticism (*Insight failure*). Finally, there are those who find ways of sidelining the difficult doctor (*Bypass syndrome*).

or educational institutions, when working with those doctors who require remediation. What follows are some principles that we believe to be fundamental to successful remediation.

Principles to guide remediation

Getting the right system in place

This is perhaps the biggest challenge. Many performance concerns are a function of social, financial and health issues,(17) as well as educational issues, and these must all be addressed if remediation is to be successful and sustainable. The provision of proactive systems that offer help and support is powerful and encourages early help-seeking. The key features of good systems include the following:

- well-defined pathways and systems – for seeking help
- guidance for educational supervisors – as to what to do if they suspect a performance issue
- thoughtful separation of roles – between those who identify there may be a problem or provide an assessment role to those who can provide more in depth remedial input
- transparency – particularly around information sharing as perceptions of what happens to personal information influences whether someone will seek help
- a proactive system – encouraging early help-seeking and prevention through well-being education.

One challenge that remains, notably for doctors undertaking speciality training, is a lack of clarity around the interface between workplace procedures for support and those provided by their educational institution. This can leave both the educational supervisor and the doctor confused as to the process.

Personalised remediation

The purpose of personalised remediation is to match provision closely to individual need and to take health, personality and motivation to change into account. It is not about a standard prescription. Personalised remediation can and should be tailored to different learning styles. Thus educational supervisors need to be aware of the ways in which other disciplines such as occupational health, occupational psychology and language experts can contribute to remediation. A key skill for educational supervisors is knowing when and how to involve and seek advice from others. A challenge for educational supervisors is the availability of these resources either within their workplace or via the educational institution. General practitioners (GPs) in particular have historically not had access to occupational health provision. Revalidation and appraisal processes are prompting a need for a more cohesive approach to identifying expertise to support those with performance issues.

Engagement and motivation

Goulet *et al.*'s(3) work on personalised remediation within the Canadian health system suggested that a doctor's motivation may initially be low, but that the involvement of a licensing authority had a positive effect on their motivation and co-operation. However, whilst the high stakes may motivate a person to agree to attend for remediation, it is not always enough to stimulate genuine engagement. Using techniques and a process to engage doctors and motivate them towards change requires careful planning. Our own preferred evidence-based method for behaviour change is based on 'motivational interviewing'.(18,20) The key message for educational supervisors is to highlight that it is important to access evidence-based methods for engaging and stimulating behaviour change, when supporting doctors whose performance gives rise for concern.

Organisational issues

Organisational factors may both trigger and perpetuate individual poor performance. Unsupportive work environments in the form of high work demands, role ambiguity, poor team working and punitive cultures can all serve to undermine a doctor striving to maintain newly acquired behaviours. In our experience, there is also a pattern of behaviour among a subset of doctors who demonstrate a tendency to 'rage against the machine'. This group continues to fight and blame the whole system, rather than considering the relevant importance of each battle and indeed which battles are worth fighting. Organisational issues and the ways in which they enhance and inhibit individual performance present one of the greatest challenges for educational supervisors.

Clarity of roles and boundaries

Finucane *et al.*(12) have previously argued that performance assessment impacts upon three distinct groups: patients, doctors and employers. These authors also argued that whilst these groups may have conflicting beliefs and expectations of assessment, the process must be acceptable for all. Transparency of the process – being clear 'whose side you are you on' – is key to the doctor engaging and

trusting the system. Educational supervisors cannot consider themselves to be entirely independent in their role. They are in effect an instrument of their educational or employing institution. Thus for educational supervisors being explicit about which hat they are wearing and being clear with the doctor about the boundaries that they work within are imperative to help build engagement and trust.

Getting started

Providing support to a doctor who might be underperforming requires careful consideration. The doctor's career might be at risk, and they may often be resentful of the predicament they find themselves in. They may lack insight into the issues raised or have underlying health, personality or social issues that may have precipitated performance issues. The aim for the educational supervisor is to help guide the individual through what can often be a painful and stressful process. Having considered some general principles, let's now turn to some ideas for managing interactions and conversations with the doctor concerned.

What type of conversation?

Several factors will impact upon the kind of conversation that an educational supervisor may have with a doctor. These include the following:

* the relationship between the supervisor and doctor
* the process in place that determines when an issue should be managed locally or elsewhere
* the extent to which the conversation is considered to be formal or informal
* the nature of the performance issue itself.

Educational supervisors often complain that they are not informed about a doctor's previous performance issues. However, doctors who have experienced performance issues argue that they should be allowed to start afresh and that unnecessarily sharing information about themselves with new colleagues can cause bias or mistrust. Those in educational institutions with responsibility for overseeing management of placements need to be clear with workplaces, supervisors and doctors about the extent of information exchange and sharing. As far as formality of conversations about performance goes, keeping written records of any dialogue, however informal, is important. Clarifying the recording of information and where information is stored helps with transparency and therefore engagement. The formal processes around the interviews and information-recording, although at times difficult, are important to an overall robust and fair process for both the individual doctor and their educational supervisor.

Planning the first discussion

Regardless of the type of conversation, careful planning is required to ensure that all the information is at hand to manage the meeting with confidence. Basic information required includes a summary of the exact nature of the concern and evidence of significant events or complaints. General concerns about performance without details are unhelpful. If acting as the educational supervisor, you will need to be clear about your role, ensure you have all the necessary documentation to hand, structure the meeting and set your objectives before starting. Setting the agenda at the beginning of the meeting and agreeing this with the doctor will reduce misunderstandings. The discussion should aim to cover the presenting problem, factors leading up to the problem, a review of any significant event(s) and relevant past workplace experience. If the doctor does not agree with the planned process for the discussion, the educational supervisor should explore this and negotiate the best way forward.

Exploring the problem

It is important that a doctor under review is given time to discuss their views on any problems that have been raised and their understanding of how such problems might have arisen. Giving the doctor time to speak openly and without prejudice is an important part of the engagement process. Discussion about the details of critical incidents and the doctor's views on events starts to allow ownership of a process which the doctor often feels at odds with. It will need time and a slow pace. In our experience it can take two hours or more, and doctors sometimes take a while to begin to relax and talk freely.

Allowing the doctor to tell their story is often the best starting point for any conversation about performance. The doctor will often describe strong feelings of injustice and misunderstandings, and have their own answers as to what has happened and why. Active listening (*see* Box 30.2) will allow you to guide them through this process.[20] Careful listening and reflection leads to engagement. Engagement is the first step towards a joint understanding of the problem and a move towards behaviour change.[19]

Knowing when to respect a doctor's privacy is as equally important as encouraging them to talk. There may come a point in the conversation where the educational supervisor suspects that there may be a personal or health issue compounding or contributing to the performance issue. Rather than encouraging the doctor to discuss this in detail, it is important for the educational supervisor to signpost to other resources such as occupational health. One point of concern often voiced by supervisors is that although they suggest that a referral to occupational health may be helpful, sometimes a doctor decides not to pursue this. 'We can't *make* them go' is the cry. The same issue often arises with suggestions about seeing their general practitioner (GP), family physician or specialist. It is true, you can't make people seek help, but raising the issue in an environment of support and concern for an individual's well-being can provide an opportunity for the doctor to reflect and consider their next steps. It can take time for a doctor to act on a suggestion – seeking help does not come easily. However, at least the supervisor should document that the suggestion was made and perhaps revisit this at a later stage.

We talked about the importance of having an evidence base to guide conversations. We use behaviour change counselling. This approach evolved from the work of Carl Rogers[21] and was defined first by Miller and Rollnick.[18,20] Behaviour change counselling is a client-centred

---

> ### BOX 30.2 FOCUS ON: Active listening
>
> Active listening is a client-centred technique expounded and developed by Carl Rogers,[21] ensuring that cues are recognised and explored. Rollnick, Butler and McCambridge[20] describe 'three styles' of communication that can enhance this process.
>
> *Instruct:* Give information or advice. Other activities associated with this style include directing, informing, leading, educating, telling and using one's expertise. It is used when there is information one wants to provide that hopefully the person wants to receive.
>
> *Guide:* Encourage the person to set his or her own goals and find ways of achieving them. Other activities associated with this style include coaching, negotiating, encouraging, mobilising and motivating. It is used when the person is facing change, having to make decisions and to act upon them.
>
> *Follow:* Understand the person's experience. Other activities used include gathering information, following, eliciting, attending and empathising. It is used when one wishes to understand how the person feels or what has happened to him or her.

approach to discussing lifestyle changes. Rollnick describes it as: 'Ways of structuring a conversation to maximise the individual's freedom to talk and think about change in an atmosphere free of coercion and the provision of premature solutions'.[18, p. 203] By working carefully through a detailed history of events, a picture of behavioural patterns often starts to emerge. By allowing the doctor ownership of the story, it is our experience that they will often be quite open in providing you with information about difficulties and problems they have encountered in the past. The first discussion can provide great insights into how and why the doctor might be struggling.

Obtaining background information

The nature of the conversation will dictate the information required prior to the meeting. The supervisor will need clear and complete documentation of concerns that have been raised, by whom and an idea of the timescale of events, if they are to be able to conduct the meeting with confidence. Sources of information commonly used to provide such information about workplace behaviour include significant event reviews, records from the appraisal process and annual reviews.

To gain the doctor's confidence in the process they must be clear as to:

- what information has already been collected
- what will happen to previous and new information collected
- how it might be used
- where it will be stored
- who might have access to it, now or in the future.

Significant events should be recorded in detail, continually checking your understanding of the doctor's perspective. Move away from confrontation. An educational supervisor may have some details of events, but challenging the doctor with the content of these at this stage can lead to resistance and difficulty with engagement. Try to get them to recount any other past significant events. This should extend to previous employment and time as a student. Do not focus just on the present situation. This often will help elicit an emerging pattern of behaviour. Useful questions to guide the review include the following.

- What led up to the event?
- What actually happened?
- Was the way you managed the interaction effective or ineffective and why?
- On reflection, how else could it have been handled?

Other sources of information include 360-degree (multi-source) feedback, information available through e-portfolios and information from previous employment or training placements. Whilst educational supervisors can pick up the phone to access details about performance issues from those who have previously worked with the doctor, it is advisable to seek advice about how best to proceed. Seeking off the record uncorroborated information can alienate the doctor and expose the supervisor and those providing information to the risk of having their own integrity questioned.

Where next?

The first discussion is likely to provide a wealth of information about the events leading up to performance issues. If conducted effectively, from a neutral position and with a commitment to explore the doctor's own perspectives without judgement, then the groundwork has been laid towards effective engagement. At this stage, as the educational supervisor, you might suspect that you need more detailed information about one or more of the following:

- past medical history
- personal issues
- personality
- language skills
- cultural issues.

Some of this information is sensitive to access. There is a strong argument that the educational supervisor might not be the right person to seek or discuss all the above factors with the individual doctor, unless the doctor volunteers it freely. This may be a challenge for the educational supervisor whose everyday work as a clinician is to ask patients questions and for intimate details about their personal history. However, a key message at this point is to understand that there are experts whose legitimate professional role is to assess the potential relationship between each of the above factors and work performance. The 'Chinese wall' created by referring an individual doctor to other professionals to discuss issues associated with health, personality, language and culture, which may or may not be related to performance, ensures that irrelevant but potentially deeply personal information can remain private to the individual doctor. The tension for the educational supervisor is maintaining the right balance and knowing when to refer on.

From the above discussion it can be seen that performance problems are often multi-factorial in nature – biological, psychological and social. This first discussion allows the educational supervisor to start to understand how each of these elements might impact on the doctor's performance. Therefore dialogue between the educational supervisor and doctor should tentatively explore whether the individual's health and social background merits review by an occupational health physician or their GP. The presentation as a doctor in difficulty can also often mask underlying mental health problems. Doctors are known to have significantly higher rates of common mental health disorders than the general population. What at face value might present as aggressive or bullying behaviour might on careful evaluation suggest underlying depression, anxiety or more serious conditions such as bipolar disorder or cognitive impairment. Physical ill health may also be an issue. Finally, developing a clear understanding of the individual's social environment and placing this in the context of the problems that they are now facing is important in perhaps understanding *why* the doctor has started to develop difficulties at this point. Box 30.3 provides a framework for understanding how these potential factors may lead up to and perpetuate a doctor's underperformance.

To conclude, the challenge for the educational supervisor is to determine the nature of the problem and the possible causes. In addition, the educational supervisor at this stage will need to decide whether more information is required from other sources, such as occupational health, occupational psychology, psychiatry or communication and language skills assessment. What follows is a description of the kinds of information that supervisors might expect other professionals to be able to provide.

Digging deeper

Occupational health assessments

The impact that physical and mental ill health can have on a doctor's performance is well recognised.(23) The (English) Chief Medical Officer's report on medical regulation, *Good Doctors, Safer Patients*, recognised deficiencies in the provision of care to doctors impaired by mental health and addiction problems, and recommended that services be created to offer appropriate support.(14) *Invisible Patients*(10) adds to our knowledge and understanding of doctors' health behaviours and possible support structures for the future. What is also accepted in both reports is that doctors do present a special case in relation to the need for workplace support.

Employers and educational institutions should look towards close collaboration with occupational health providers for advice and support in the assessment and possible management of doctors who are seen to be underperforming.

An occupational health physician would perform a detailed medical history and look at that history in the

BOX 30.3 Biopsychosocial factors and stages in a doctor's underperformance (adapted from Sharpe and Wilks(22))

Factors	Biological	Psychosocial	Social
Predisposing	Underlying mental or physical disease	Personality Family	Cultural Family
Precipitating	Acute ill health events	Interactions at work	Economic factors Social isolation The culture of the organisation
Perpetuating	Chronic disease	Lack of insight by organisation or individual	Economic Cultural Organisational

context of the workplace and workplace issues that have been raised. For instance, a doctor who presented with poor team management and prioritisation might on detailed questioning admit to a previous head injury or cerebrovascular accident that could indicate a neuropsychological impairment. A doctor presenting with aggressive or inappropriate behaviour might display features suggestive of underlying mental health issues such as depression, addiction or personality disorder. Once a problem has been identified, onward referral for specialist opinion can be made, where appropriate.

Management of health issues in the workplace requires specialist advice and support. So when constructing a programme of support for a doctor with health issues, advice from an occupational health physician should be sought. Some doctors may have a disability that has impacted on their performance and relevant legislation must be considered in supporting them back into the workplace.(24) Once again, an occupational health physician can support any remediation programme in terms of providing advice on 'reasonable adjustments' to the workplace.

Advising the doctor to seek (or providing access to) appropriate occupational health support should always be considered. This will allow liaison with the family doctor or a general practitioner (with the client's consent) and can hasten recovery or, in some instances, provide secondary opinions and advice. The educational supervisor working closely with the occupational health and other specialist can help co-ordinate, rather than *deliver* timely and appropriate support and interventions.

Behavioural assessments

Understanding individual behavioural habits can help to establish effective individualised remediation. Behaviour is a function of personality, learnt behaviour and situational drivers in the organisation. The purpose of this section is to indicate to the educational supervisor the kind of information an occupational psychologist could bring to understanding the relationship between personality and performance. It also distils some key messages about the impact of personality on remediation.

BOX 30.4 WHERE'S THE EVIDENCE: Personality and performance

Since the early 1990s many different personality tests and performance in many different jobs have been investigated. Overall, it has been concluded that personality can be reliably measured using appropriate tests, and for most jobs, certain personality traits can predict job performance.(25) Research has shown that in a large number of occupations job performance, and indeed success at medical school, can be predicted by the big five personality factors;(26,27):

- extraversion
- agreeableness
- emotional stability
- openness
- conscientiousness.

Barrick *et al.*(28) suggest that although not all of the big five personality factors predict generalisable job performance, they do predict success in specific occupations.

The link between personality and performance has been studied for many years, and research has mostly been conducted in an attempt to help the selection procedures. Research up to the late 1980s suggested that there was little, if any, association between personality and performance. However, this theory was dismissed with the emergence of the five-factor model of personality (*see* Box 30.4).(25–28)

Competency and curricula frameworks worldwide stress a number of different aspects that are required of a doctor, including the importance of good communication skills, being able to work well with colleagues and patients, technical competence and general skills.(29–31) General skills include managing one's time, prioritising, being self-critical, problem solving and analysing numerical data The strategies individuals adopt to manage these skills are personality-dependent.

One popular personality indicator that is widely used in health care organisations for personal development and growth is the Myers-Briggs Type Indicator (MBTI).(32) If used correctly – and one reason for the MBTI's popularity is that anyone with an interest in coaching, whatever their background, can be trained to use it – MBTI has the ability to help individuals understand why they behave the way they do, and why they find certain situations difficult. Most importantly, it helps them explore a range of behavioural choices for different situations. Another useful psychometric tool is the Hogan Development Survey, which identifies personality-based performance risks and 'derailers' of interpersonal behaviour(33) and can be extremely useful in highlighting to individuals how they will tend to respond to pressure and stress.

In our experience, it is important to work with the 'grain' of an individual's personality; using behavioural assessments helps remind the doctor and us that 'one size does not fit all'. Any suggested strategies for change are best sustained if they are close to the way an individual tends to normally do things. We believe in the power of a small but sustainable shift in behaviour.

Communication and language assessments

Whilst occupational health services and behavioural assessments are widely available on a national basis, the same cannot be said of communication and language assessments. Yet this type of information can provide an invaluable baseline for working with individual doctors. What follows is a description of these types of assessments. We would suggest that it is invaluable and possible for local trainers and educational supervisors to undertake this activity in some shape or form whether performance problems seem related to patient communications or not. Simply observing a doctor consult can provide many insights for those who are trying to support remediation.

Clinical communication

Poor communication with patients is frequently cited as a core indicator of performance problems. Using observed simulated patient consultations offers the opportunity for the doctor to evaluate their own consulting style and behaviour alongside models of good practice in a non-judgemental manner, allowing the doctor to develop some insight into their own practice.(34) It can provide a good baseline indicator of their active listening and shared decision-making skills, as well as being an indicator of their likely approach to communicating with colleagues.

It is important to note that the object of the exercise is to continue to engage the doctor while making an assessment of their 'needs'. This exercise is not meant to serve as a challenge to the doctor, so it should not include challenging scenarios of, for instance, breaking bad news or dealing with someone who is angry. It is intended to provide a baseline only. In other words, the activity here is to understand which skills the doctor relies on in everyday situations.

Self-evaluation is intended to be descriptive and diagnostic, rather than summative, and providing the doctor with some sort of structure for this is useful. This could, for instance, be a rating scale adapted from standardised forms used in an Objective Structure Clinical Examinations. Using something standardised also provides the opportunity to reflect on progress at a later stage by repeating the exercise.

Language

The assessment of a doctor's language skills is not a novel undertaking. In many countries it has been a requirement for international medical graduates for some years. However, understanding how an individual's language skills impact on a doctor's performance is a relatively new area.

For the doctor, assessing language may present certain problems with regard to engagement. They may have lived and practised in the country for some time. In the UK, they may have already jumped through the requisite hoops such as the International English Language Testing System (IELTS), and Professional and Linguistic Assessment Board (PLAB) to demonstrate competence in communicating in English. In the case of doctors recruited from the European Economic Area, they will not have been required to submit to a language competence test.

For some doctors, particularly those who qualified overseas, one of the factors linked to performance problems may be their use of language. Use should be understood differently from usage. The latter relates more to 'correctness': accuracy of grammar, spelling and pronunciation. 'Use' relates more to the ability to communicate clearly, coherently and appropriately with another person with the range of language knowledge and skill at one's disposal. Of course, there may be some overlap between use and usage, for instance, in the selection of vocabulary.

It is important to look at language use in context: in the workplace, socially and in comparison to country of origin. To this end, the assessment needs to be open-ended, qualitative and exploratory. As with other areas of the assessment the objective is to agree with the doctor possible areas for remediation, and the assessor's role is to provide expertise in helping them to identify and address those areas.

In our experience, assessing language is a highly specialised field but adds significant value to the assessment and the remedial plan. If looking to develop assessment in language, we would suggest that this comprise of two broad parts: a semi-structured interview and a task. The focus of the interview is the doctor's experience of language learning and language use. Here, it is important to explore the doctor's own perception of their language skills and language use, comparing what they learnt with experience 'on the ground' in this country. The tasks could involve the doctor performing some form of extended speaking, for example, explaining something or giving a presentation. On occasions, the issues may be to do with written language. In this case, the doctor should bring samples of reports or correspondence.

During the assessment, the assessor observes the doctor's language use. The aim is to highlight evidence of fluency and 'disfluency', to explore the range and appropriateness of lexis used by the doctor. This assessment is also interested in phonological features (pronunciation, stress, rhythm and intonation, discourse management, grammatical range and accuracy). In particular, the purpose of the tasks is to enable an exploration of the doctor's ability to convey meaning clearly, to present complex information with suitable guidance following rules of coherence and cohesion, to guide the listener and to use appropriate rhetorical devices.

Delivering remediation

However assessment of underlying issues is carried out, by this point a picture of the doctor should have emerged. The process should have provided an understanding of the doctor's health issues, if any, personality and the way they communicate, thus paving the way for the development of a tailored programme of support.

A key challenge for the educational supervisor will be to consider their role in the remedial process. Depending on the services available, supervisors may have to occupy a combination of roles. During the assessment phase you might be acting as the case manager, have an initial dialogue with the doctor and then maybe referring on to some of the specialist services, as described above. However, as time goes on, the educational supervisor may also have to take on the role of the remediator. This might also include acting as an assessor at the end of the process. We have written what follows with the idea in mind that you are likely to take all three roles in some form or other during the remediation process.

Case review

The remedial plan will be dependent on the complexity of the situation. A complex case may require bringing together the individuals who have supported the educational supervisor in undertaking assessment activity, often through the performance support unit from the local deanery or medical school. These professionals will not only provide varying perspectives on the problems raised, but also bring robustness to the review. A multidisciplinary approach will enhance the rigour of the process. This is important if decisions are challenged at a later stage. It may be, for instance, that an opinion from a specialist, such as a psychiatrist, is requested by occupational health. This will add to the robust process of assessment and remediation planning and delivery. Recording of all documentation should be rigorous. Once all the documentation is collated, the next stage is to discuss the evidence with the team and decide what the remedial plan should look like. We call this activity 'case review'. The exact form that this activity takes will be depending on local processes and infrastructures. In essence, the questions should be: what interventions are required? In what order they should be delivered? Who should deliver them? What is the desired outcome? Finally, what are the most appropriate time lines for review? Below we describe such a process with reference to the case of Dr J (*see* Box 30.5).

The remedial plan

The case review should give the educational supervisor an overall picture of the major issues that need to be addressed.

> ### BOX 30.5 Case study
>
> Dr J is in his fourth year of specialist training in obstetrics and gynaecology and has been referred following his annual assessment. He was noted to have somewhat erratic and unpredictable behaviour. His referral described someone who shouted at the nurses and the junior staff when under stress and who most recently had thrown equipment around the operating theatre. On a day-to-day basis he was known for being a social and friendly character, although in his 360-degree appraisal he has been criticised for being overly jocular with staff.
>
> An initial assessment was conducted. This reveals that Dr J is married with one child, a boy aged 5, who suffers with autism. Dr J moved schools five times as a child. He participated in team sports at medical school and was a high achiever. His father died when he was 16. When asked about his strategy for getting things done, his belief is that it is 'OK to tell it as it is'. His consultation video revealed a tendency not to listen to patients, and there was also a lack of clarity in the way he gave and explained information. During his videoed doctor–doctor consultation, where he was asked to provide feedback to a more junior trainee who had persistent performance problems, he became quite agitated when the junior doctor questioned his judgement.
>
> He gave an indication during all three assessments that he was angry to have been referred, as he felt strongly that he was a good doctor, cared about his patients and had no problems with his clinical skills. He had to contend with a very difficult work environment that was riddled with poor practice.

In relation to Dr J the team came to the conclusion that he was quite extrovert in nature, so 'spoke before he thought'. He had strongly held beliefs about what was right and wrong in terms of the quality of medical practice and felt he was justified in airing his views. However, he seemed to lack insight into organisational issues around his team and the hospital in which he worked. Finally, underlying this there were issues around lack of self-confidence in both the workplace and being able to support his wife with their son's disability.

Therefore for Dr J, the issues that required support were around learning to reflect on his practice, developing his negotiating skills and work on organisational issues. These three threads would aim to develop more insight into his behaviour and provide him with some skills and strategies to manage more challenging situations. Thus the interventions used are likely to require a blend of behavioural and cognitive approaches. This in turn might help him develop more confidence in thinking about how he might manage his personal situation.

Mustering resources

A key decision at this point is to consider who will be involved in the remediation process and how that will be resourced. Those institutions responsible for medical education vary with regard to the specific arrangements that exist to undertake remedial work. Thus what follows is a general description of remediation activity, some of which may be undertaken by an educational supervisor and some of which may be undertaken by others. However, the educational supervisor is likely to play a role in ensuring that continuity exists between remediation activities. In each of the activities described below, we use the term 'remediator' to cover the individual who is working with the doctor at that moment, acknowledging that a combination of different remediators may be used.

Structuring the interventions

Once the remedial plan has been outlined, the educational supervisor will need to decide which interventions to use and how to link them. Ordering the interventions requires careful consideration. The correct order will allow the doctor to move forward in a manner that provides a sense of autonomy over the process. By allowing the doctor a sense of control and the ability to work initially in their comfort zone the process starts to move the doctor from engagement into action.

Starting out

Understanding the individual's personality and what is of 'high importance' suggests pathways for initiating the process. So for Dr J, starting with a session that explores real events in a way that might use role-play and video feedback would probably feel acceptable given his preference for practical, action-based learning. Using actors who are trained in giving feedback is especially helpful in this role. Thus, setting up the actor as someone with a similar personality to Dr J would be a useful starting point. Dr J would probably not find this too stressful as like personalities often respond well to each other. The remediator can then coach Dr J around 'what he did', 'how it felt' and what he 'might want to do better'. The remediator might anticipate that reflection is less comfortable for Dr J. This would be predicted by personality questionnaire feedback and reinforced by work on learning styles. The actor can respond in role about how they felt, what worked and what did not work. This is often the first step for the doctor in gaining insight into their normal behavioural pattern. It starts the reflection into daily practice that might not come easily to someone like Dr J.

Coaching could follow on from such an activity. This session could focus on some of the activities and responses discussed in the first role-play session. Starting with such a session for Dr J may have led to resistance, as this is not a natural path for him. Finally, further interactive role-play with a more difficult case, and sessions building on organisational issues is a pathway we have found to lead to increasing self-confidence and change. Had Dr J been a more introvert individual, starting with reflection and critical incident analysis with a coach might have been a more natural pathway.

Coaching

Coaching in this context describes an activity whereby remediation is based on a method or methods for stimulating change. It is important that the methods and approaches chosen have an evidence base. It is also important that the acquisition of practical behavioural skills takes place within a wider framework whereby the individual is encouraged to think about their beliefs and strategies. It is our view that remediation has behavioural and cognitive components. The purpose of coaching is to create a context whereby the individual can acquire new behavioural skills and cognitive strategies side by side. At this stage, active listening skills help guide the individual to discover insights into the conditions under which they might be prepared to change, and thus its emphasis is on the cognitive. Rooting the development of new skills in a context whereby the individual is discovering a new way of interpreting what is going on around them prepares the individual for getting ready to acquire new skills.

Role-playing newly learned skills

A typical tipping point comes with the realisation by the doctor that their current approach is not working or does not always work, or simply that they could become more effective. The question asked by the doctor then centres around how they can become more effective. If shouting at the nurses does not result in the correct equipment being given to Dr J when he needs it, what else can he do? One common pathway is that a doctor such as Dr J, who is usually extroverted and expressive, becomes uncharacteristically quiet and unsure about how best to assert himself. Equally, he finds this strategy frustrating because it is not his preferred way of behaving. He feels it also achieves nothing, but at least he perceives that it keeps him out of trouble or beyond criticism.

Role-play creates a situation whereby the new skills can be practised and improved. Using constructive feedback from the remediator and actor, combined with video review and self-assessment, can be powerful and effective in engaging the doctor. Some doctors question the extent to which role-play in this context can really simulate the organisational context. Central to our approach is the use of events from the doctor's own experiences, particularly those significant events that contributed to the referral. The doctor is asked to retell the story of the event or events. The actor will often be present to allow a clear picture to be constructed. This type of intervention is used to explore memories of interpersonal interactions. It provides a structure to examine not just actual communication and language skills, but also beliefs about influencing, negotiation and leadership.

Setting goals and time lines

Remediation should be set apart from counselling or other forms of therapy that the individual may require and seen as a clearly defined set of interventions that have a manageable time line. Counselling or therapy might sit alongside the remedial process, but they are not one and the same thing. Setting time lines should be seen as part of the agenda-setting process.

Consideration of how many sessions should be provided and when progress should be reviewed adds structure and helps guide the remediator(s) and the doctor. Review dates should be considered at the outset. There are also external constraints to consider when setting time lines, such as in-training assessments, hospital reviews or professional regulatory hearings. Sharing an understanding with the doctor that the remedial process sits alongside these time lines helps engagement and reduces anxiety. Understanding the doctor's work and social environment is also important. For instance, if Dr J was a trainee working in a nearby hospital with a review of their progress in four months, then the majority of the work should be completed in single sessions lasting two–t- three hours over a period of three months. If, however, Dr J was a trainee who has a long distance to travel, it might be more applicable to run a two-day intensive workshop for him with a review one month later, whilst keeping a reflective diary that he would email to his supervisor every week and offering him the opportunity to use Skype™ or other social media methods to keep in contact. Setting clear objectives at this stage helps set out the plans and reviews that will guide the process at a later stage.

Reviewing progress

The amount of time taken to see progress appears to vary as a function of individual differences. The proxy measures for progress in this context are as follows:

- engagement with remediation, that is, turning up for appointments
- willingness and ability to engage in reflective conversation
- insight into the nature of the problem(s) and their causes
- ability to work with the remediator to generate alternative strategies and skills
- active participation in practising new skills
- ability to discuss the use of acquired skills and strategies and how these have been applied in the workplace.

With regard to the process of review, it is difficult to be prescriptive in setting review points for each doctor when the programme is individualised. However, the educational supervisor in the role of case manager should bring the remediation team together to routinely review progress and will need to be sensitive to particular tipping points, such as reaching a judgement about:

- when a doctor has made enough progress such that remediation can stop
- whether a doctor has reached a plateau in their progress such that further remediation is unlikely to achieve additional improvement
- whether the doctor is likely to benefit from individualised support at all.

Knowing when to stop trying in the face of no improvement is probably the most difficult decision of all, and one of the most frequently asked questions by educational supervisors with regard to this topic. There is no one definitive right answer, but having a defined approach to assessment, a clear pathway for remediation and the involvement of different individuals such as performance support units, training programme directors and experienced remediators, means that the decision about when to stop is much more robust.

Measuring success

Success is hard to measure, and at present there are few validated tools that help provide hard evidence. Success might be seen as improved feedback from colleagues and the remediator(s). It may be passing exams that have been repeatedly failed. It might be achieving success at interview where the individual had failed for many months previously. It might also be an end to the patient complaints. Success might also be the doctor recognising their own limitations, whether due to behaviour or underlying health issues, and leaving their chosen career path. However, developing insight and changing behaviour takes time. The remedial process should give the individual space to move from a position of resistance to a place where they are ready to change. It should guide the doctor to develop an understanding of how his or her behaviour has impacted on their performance and offer solutions in the form of strategies and skills.

The role of insight

In our experience, underperformance is complex, such that it is not possible to conclude that any one personality profile is more at risk than any other. However, we have seen common patterns of behaviour that appear to trigger and perpetuate episodes of underperformance. More importantly perhaps with regard to remediation, some patterns of behaviour stand out as indicating the stage of development that a doctor may be at.

We have recognised the following specific patterns.

- The doctor recognises the problem behaviour as an area for development, but does not know how to develop an alternative set of skills.
- The doctor recognises the problem, but focuses on justifying why that behaviour pattern is important.
- The doctor does not recognise that a particular behaviour pattern is negative.

Kruger and Dunning[35] described how poor performers have less insight into their inadequacies than high performers. The more competent they become, the lower they self-rate their own performance. Kruger and Dunning conclude that perhaps insight in some doctors can be achieved with training.

Evaluation

As in other educational settings, such as assessment and development centres, evaluation is concerned to a large extent with the utility of the process. The reason evaluation in this context remains a challenge is that whilst multiple sources of evidence and/or methods are often used, they are typically fragmented and not always conducted in a pre-planned way in the workplace. Even where they are pre-planned, such as in the case in the UK of National Clinical Assessment Service (NCAS) assessments, it can be difficult to bring together evidence conducted by different professionals, often over many months. Thus evaluation of remediation services is in its infancy and needs to be further developed. However, educational supervisors should strive to develop some system of evaluating the individual doctors they work with that fits within their organisational structure.

Pitfalls and problems

The process of remediation is high stake. Ensuring clarity at all stages is important.

Legal and ethical issues

The nature of the remediation service provided must be carefully considered prior to entering into any agreement with an individual or organisation. The ethical and legal implications of a training-led service providing support for a trainee will be different from a hospital offering independent services to an employed consultant. Understanding where the responsibilities to the individual doctor and the referring organisation may lie and the nature of the information that can be imparted to third parties should be carefully considered before entering into any process. Areas to review when setting up a service should include the following.

- *Written reports*: confirming whether these fall within the Access to Medical Reports Act (1988).
- *Patient safety*: if there is evidence of risk to patient safety, then there must be a pathway in which serious concerns can be raised with the referring organisation.
- *Consent*: the individual doctor should be aware of the contract they are entering into when they attend for remediation.
- *Case notes*: ownership of the notes and how they are stored and held, along with access to the case files.

Blurring of boundaries

Good communication between stakeholders at the outset is key to delivering a successful service. Managing the expectations of both the educational institution and the individual doctor reduces the risk of misunderstanding later on. Such communication might include:

- outlining the roles of the remediation process with the doctor at the outset
- specifying what the remediation can offer and its limitations
- clarity of what the content of any progress report might look like
- patient safety and duty of care of the educational supervisor to the referring doctor and the organisation.

Record-keeping

It is advisable to keep records to the same standard as any clinical records. A good maxim is that 'if it isn't written down, it hasn't happened'.

Inappropriate referrals

The package of remediation offered should centre on the areas of expertise that are available locally or knowing where and how to refer on for further support. Setting referral criteria for onward referral is crucial to reducing the risk of inappropriate referrals (*see* Box 30.6).

Conclusion

To conclude, the primary purpose of this work is to return a doctor to effective practice where possible, by taking a

---

> ### BOX 30.6 FOCUS ON: When to refer on (UK)
>
> The General Medical Council's (GMC) key concern is whether a doctor is fit to practise. It is not involved with general complaints of a minor nature, nor of performance problems that are capable of being resolved locally. It can take action when:
>
> - a doctor has been convicted of a criminal offence
> - there is an allegation of serious professional misconduct
> - a doctor's professional performance may be seriously deficient
> - a doctor with health problems continues to practise whilst unfit and patient safety is compromised.
>
> If there is evidence that patients may be at risk, the GMC can suspend or restrict a doctor's registration as an interim measure. *See* the 'Concerns about doctors' section of the GMC's website (http://www.gmc-uk.org/concerns/index.asp).
>
> A National Clinical Assessment Service (NCAS) assessment is likely to be appropriate where:
>
> - concern(s) are substantiated: from the evidence available there is confidence that expressed concerns are accurate statements
> - concern(s) are significant: the actions about which concerns are expressed fall well short of what would be expected from another doctor in similar circumstances
> - concern(s) are repetitious: ongoing problems and/or problems on at least two separate occasions are identified
> - concern(s) do not appear to be sufficiently serious to warrant an immediate referral to the GMC
> - local procedures have failed to resolve the problem or are not appropriate
> - a NCAS performance assessment appears to offer a likely way forward in enabling the case to move towards a resolution.

---

holistic approach to understanding the nature of the performance issue, its triggers and impacts. At the heart of this chapter is the argument that it is important for those involved to take a holistic approach, one that takes account of health, personal and social factors and that places the doctor's well-being at the centre of remediation. We have argued that the educational supervisor has a crucial role to play in helping to support doctors who run into difficulty, but highlighted that they cannot do so effectively without knowing what is expected of them, understanding what resources to call upon and being clear about when to ask for help. Seeing a doctor return to performing well, contributing to their team and enjoying work is a rewarding experience and well-designed evidence-based remediation can make a difference to supervisor confidence, doctor performance and well-being, and ultimately patient care.

References

1 Cohen D and Rhydderch M (2006) Measuring a doctor's performance: personality, health and well-being. *Occupational Medicine.* **56**: 38–40.

2 Cohen D, Rollnick S, Smail S *et al.* (2005) Communication, stress and distress: evolution of an individual support programme for medical students. *Medical Education.* **39**(5): 76–81.

3 Goulet F, Jacques A and Gagnon R (2003) An innovative approach to remedial continuing medical education, 1992–2002. *Academic Medicine.* **80**: 553–40.

4 Joesbury H, Mathers N and Lane P (2001) Supporting GPs whose performance gives cause for concern: the North Trent experience. *Family Practice.* **18**(2): 123–30.

5 Bahrami J (1997) Remediation. *British Medical Journal.* **315**: 2.

6 Burrows P, Khan A, Bowden R *et al.* (2004) The fresh start simulated surgery. *Education for Primary Care.* **15**: 328–35.

7 Firth-Cozens J and King J (2006) The role of education and training. In: Cox J, King J, Hutchinson A *et al.* (eds) *Understanding Doctors' Performance*, pp. 61–77. Radcliffe Publishing in association with National Clinical Assessment Service of the National Patient Safety Agency, Oxford.

8 Paice E (2006) The role of education and training. In: Cox J, King J, Hutchinson A *et al.* (eds) *Understanding Doctors' Performance*, pp. 78–90. Radcliffe Publishing in association with National Clinical Assessment Service of the National Patient Safety Agency, Oxford.

9 Hauer KE, Ciccone A, Henzel TR *et al.* (2009) Remediation of the deficiencies of physicians across the continuum from medical school to practice: a thematic review of the literature. *Academic Medicine.* **84**(12): 1822–32.

10 Department of Health (2010) Invisible Patients, Report of the Working Group on the Health of Health Professionals. Department of Health, London.

11 Swanwick T and Whiteman J (2013) Remediation: where does the responsibility lie? *Postgraduate Medical Journal.* **89**: 1–3.

12 Finucane PM, Barron SR, Davies HA *et al.* (2002) Towards an acceptance of performance appraisal. *Medical Education.* **36**: 959–64.

13 Department of Health (2003) *Modernising Medical Careers.* Department of Health, London.

14 Department of Health (2006) *Good Doctors, Safer Patients: Proposals to Strengthen the System to Assure and Improve the Performance of Doctors and to Protect the Safety of Patients.* Department of Health, London.

15 Murphy KR and Cleveland JN (1995) *Understanding Performance Appraisal: Social, Organisational and Goal-Based Perspectives.* Sage Publications, Thousand Oaks, CA.

16 Leape L and Fromson JA (2006) Problem doctors: is there a system level solution. *Annals of Internal Medicine.* **144**: 107–15.

17 Harrison J (2006) Illness in doctors and dentists and their fitness for work – are the cobblers children getting their shoes at last? *Occupational Medicine.* **56**: 75–6.

18 Miller W and Rollnick S (2002) *Motivational Interviewing: Preparing People to Change* (2e). Guilford Press, New York.

19 Paice E and Orton V (2004) Early signs of the trainee in difficulty. *Hospital Medicine.* **65**: 238–40.

20 Rollnick S, Butler CC, McCambridge J *et al.* (2005) Consultations about changing behaviour. *British Medical Journal.* **331**: 961–3.

21 Rogers CR (1951) *Client Centered Therapy.* Houghton-Mifflin, Boston.

22 Sharpe M and Wilks D (2002) ABC of psychological medicine: fatigue. *British Medical Journal.* **325**: 480–3.

23 Firth-Cozens J (2006) A perspective on stress and depression. In: Cox J, King J, Hutchinson A and McAvoy P (eds) *Understanding Doctors' Performance*, pp. 22–37. Radcliffe Publishing in association with National Clinical Assessment Service of the National Patient Safety Agency, Oxford.

24 UK Government (2010) Equality Act 2010 c.15. (http://www.legislation.gov.uk/ukpga/2010/15/contents; accessed 22 December 2012).

25 Kierstead J (1998) Personality and job performance: a research overview. (http://www.psagency-agencefp.gc.ca/research/personnel/personality_e.asp; accessed 22 December 2012).

26 Dudley N, Orvis KA, Lebiecki JE *et al.* (2006) A meta-analytic investigation of conscientiousness in the prediction of job performance. *Journal of Applied Psychology.* **91**: 40–57.

27 Ferguson E, James D and Madeley L (2002) Learning in practice: factors associated with success in medical school. *British Medical Journal.* **324**: 952–7.

28 Barrick MR, Mount M and Judge T (2001) Personality and performance at the beginning of the new millennium. *International Journal of Selection and Assessment.* **9**: 9–30.

29 General Medical Council (2009) *Tomorrow's Doctors.* GMC, London. 9.

30 Frank JR (ed.) (2005) *The CanMEDS 2005 Physician Competency Framework. Better Standards. Better Physicians. Better Care.* The Royal College of Physicians and Surgeons of Canada, Ottawa, ON.

31 Association of American Medical Colleges Liaison Committee on Medical Education (2012) Functions and structure of a medical school: standards for accreditation of medical education programs leading to the M.D. degree. (http://www.lcme.org/functions.pdf; accessed 22 December 2012).

32 Myers IB, McCaulley MH, Quenk NL *et al.* (1998) *MBTI Manual. A Guide to the Development and Use of the Myers Briggs Type Indicator* (3e). Consulting Psychologists Press, Menlo Park, CA.

33 Hogan Assessment Systems (2012) Hogan Development Survey. (http://www.hoganassessments.com/sites/default/files/assessments/pdf/HDS_Brochure.pdf; accessed 23 December 2012).

34 Lane C and Rollnick S (2007) The use of simulated patients and role-play in communication skills training: a review of the literature to August 2005. *Patient Education and Counselling.* **67**: 13–20.

35 Kruger J and Dunning D (1999) Unskilled and unaware of it: how difficulties in recognising one's own incompetence lead to inflated self-assessments. *Journal of Personality and Social Psychology.* **77**: 1121–34.

Further reading

Cox J, King J, Hutchinson A *et al.* (eds) (2006) *Understanding Doctors' Performance.* Radcliffe Publishing, Oxford.

Firth-Cozens J (2006) A perspective on stress and depression. In: Cox J, King J, Hutchinson A and McAvoy P (eds) *Understanding Doctors' Performance*, pp. 22–37. Radcliffe Publishing in association with National Clinical Assessment Service of the National Patient Safety Agency, Oxford.

Jackson N, Jamieson A and Khan A (eds) (2007) *Assessment in Medical Education and Training: A Practical Guide.* Radcliffe Publishing, Oxford.

The National Clinical Assessment Service (http://www.ncas.npsa.nhs.uk) provides advice to trusts and training organisations. The website is packed with comprehensive and informative resources, including toolkits, publications and practical advice.

31 Dealing with diversity

Antony Americano[1] and Dinesh Bhugra[2]
[1]University of London, UK
[2]Institute of Psychiatry, King's College London, UK; Maudsley Hospital, UK

 KEY MESSAGES

- Competence in diversity requires an awareness of differing styles, values, beliefs and practices.
- Diversity includes areas covered by legislation, other stratifications in society and the differences that make us all unique.
- Social inclusion is a key political priority.
- Understanding disability and different approaches to it is very important for clinicians.

- Barriers in diversity are linked to language, stereotypes and cultural bias.
- Lack of awareness of diversity affects all levels of training.
- Societies of origin influence personality traits and expectations.
- Training in diversity can be integrated with teaching and supervision.

Introduction

Theory and a growing body of evidence suggest that competence in diversity is central to a successful relationship between clinician and patient. This interaction is based on a power differential that is reliant on education, social status and other factors, which will vary according to culture, gender, disability, location of the interaction (e.g. home visit or outpatient clinic) and geography (e.g. rural or urban). Similarly, belief systems, religious factors and cultural expectations play a role in acceptance of, and adherence to, treatment, in which again the clinician–patient encounter becomes central. Paralleling this interaction in health care education is the relationship between clinician-teacher and learner. An understanding of diversity is therefore essential in the teaching and practice of medicine, as well as for personal and professional growth. However, diversity is not a straightforward concept, and confusion surrounds its meaning and aims. Diversity is complex, multifactorial and its value contested. The aim of this chapter is to help the reader understand this complexity, specifically as it relates to clinical education. As the authors are UK-based, specific legislative examples are necessarily domestic in nature. The majority of the key messages are, however, internationally generalisable.

Defining diversity

The terms *diversity* and *equalities* (sometimes *equality* or *equal opportunities*) often appear together and may be used interchangeably. But whilst similar, the foci for these terms

are different. The *diversity* approach is concerned with valuing the contributions of everyone in society, embracing individual differences and encompassing the full range of social groupings. It has a broad scope and covers issues such as personality traits and type, learning style, accent, class and professional background, as well as a number of societal subgroups recognised in law. Whilst diversity recognises *group* issues, the emphasis is on the *individual*.

Equalities on the other hand – although concerned with the same general principle of inclusion – has a greater focus on legislation or groups experiencing officially recognised social exclusion or injustice. Because there is legislative force behind much of equalities, it has a greater emphasis on policies, monitoring and targets than diversity. The emphasis is on the level of the group.

The concepts of diversity and equalities are not fixed and immutable; they vary across geography: Northern Ireland, for socio-political reasons, addressed discrimination on the grounds of religion years before the rest of the UK, and across time, sex and race discrimination legislation have been on the statute in the UK for over 30 years, while age was not added until 2006. Similarly, the way diversity is medicalised (or pathologised) changes over time. For example, until the 1970s homosexuality was a mental illness to be found in the *Diagnostic and Statistical Manual (DSM II) of Psychiatric Disorders*. Once it was removed, homosexuality was no longer an illness, and gay men and lesbian women are now afforded legal protection from discrimination.

These examples demonstrate that the concepts of diversity and equalities are socially constructed and reflect the concerns of particular groups of people at particular points

Understanding Medical Education: Evidence, Theory and Practice, Second Edition. Edited by Tim Swanwick.
© 2014 The Association for the Study of Medical Education. Published 2014 by John Wiley & Sons, Ltd.

or periods in time.(1,2) As society is heterogeneous, there will always be dissent about what, or who, is to be included or excluded. At this point, it is helpful to consider a taxonomy of diversity developed by Jehn *et al.*(3)

Social category diversity

Social category diversity is concerned with demographic differences like gender and ethnicity, core equalities concerns in medical education. Jehn *et al.* theorised that difficulties in this factor would impact on group communication and cohesion, which of course are essential to effective clinical practice.

Informational diversity

Also known as 'organisational diversity', this refers to background diversity such as knowledge, education, experience, tenure and functional background. Medicine is recognised as a distinct 'tribe' among other health care 'tribes' such as those in nursing, pharmacy and physiotherapy. A similar situation is replicated within medicine itself, where there are many distinct subgroups. These types of difference were theorised by Jehn *et al.* to affect group communication and cohesion as well as generate higher task-related conflict.

Value diversity

This refers to differences in personality and attitudes and in some ways is the richest source of difference with the potential to impact on individual, team and organisational life. This factor raises issues of 'team fit' and personality clashes, as well as fundamentally different belief systems. If this difference cannot be managed, it can lead to conflict within teams, across professional groups and with patients and carers.

Jehn's taxonomy helps us to understand the complexity of diversity, because no single element will define an individual's unique contribution as they will differ within and across the three domains.

Fairness

The complexity of different belief systems is then at the very heart of diversity. But why is it necessary to take such an approach? Why, specifically, is the commonsensical notion of *fairness* not acceptable to all? We can see why not by looking at three different approaches to fairness: equity, equality and need. To illustrate these approaches we use the example of selection, which could be into training, or higher education.

Equity

An applicant considers his or her own merits and selection outcome compared with a referent other's input-to-output ratio. If the referent other is deemed to be getting more for the same input or the same for less input, then unfairness will be perceived. This is in line with the principle of meritocracy and is individualistic in nature. Fairness is therefore judged by whether the person who has done most (studied, gained prizes, etc.) gets the job.(4)

Equality

Here, an applicant will take a more social view looking for equal chance and representation for groups within society. In particular, this has been relevant when considering the employment position of minority ethnic groups, women and disabled people, and more recently in relation to age, sexual orientation and religion. Fairness in selection is judged by the presence or absence of discriminated-against groups in the workforce, for example, at the consultant level or within training programmes.

Need

This approach goes further in applying the principle of social justice allocating employment on the basis of need, for example, economic in respect of the unemployed or social with regard to the child-rearing responsibilities of single parents. Fairness is judged by meeting the needs of those who have nothing or not enough, for example, refugee doctors needing support to restart their career.

These three different approaches help to explain why any move to make a given process fairer is likely to be met with approval from some and disapproval from others, depending on the values they bring(5) and their own conceptualisation of fairness. This analysis is applicable to any situation where access to limited resources or to desired goals are in play. At the same time, it should be recognised that human motivation can be more complex than this simple model proposes and that people can be more selfless and selfish than assumed.

Diversity in organisations

Impact

How does diversity impact, positively or negatively, on group performance and behaviour? It has been theorised that effective management of diversity is good for group and organisational performance, and conversely that poor management of diversity is damaging.(6)

An evidence base for this assertion exists but is generally inconclusive. Different studies show a complex range of results that are hard to generalise, in part due to the limitations of the studies themselves and the difficulty in controlling for variables. Additionally, it is theorised that the value of diversity to group performance may depend on the type of task. The value may be particularly high when understanding of a particular social category is a benefit, but less, or negatively so, when tasks do not require such input.(3) One study proposing a positive benefit looked at 486 British companies and found that promoting diversity reduced recruitment costs, increased employee motivation and staff retention, and improved employer image.(7)

Whatever the questions about the evidence base, there is a socio-legal reality to be faced. A well-established body of legislation and new legal responsibilities for promoting race, gender and disability equality in the public sector make some aspects of diversity a must-do (*see* 'The Sociopolitical Context').

Furthermore, bad publicity on diversity can be damaging to an organisation and may alienate sections of the com-

BOX 31.1 FOCUS ON: The evolution of terminology

You can be forgiven for being confused about some of the terminology used when discussing diversity. The language used differs from place to place and has changed over time. For example, *Asian* in the UK refers to Indian, Bangladeshi, Pakistani and other similarly located peoples. In the USA, this refers mainly to people of Chinese and Far Eastern origin.

Whilst it is important to try to use acceptable terminology, particularly if the group concerned has requested this, using the correct terms does not, by itself, achieve equality, and using the wrong term unknowingly is not a cardinal sin. Otherwise fear of offending takes over from having an open dialogue on the issues. The dialogue is what matters. The following explains some terms and how they have evolved over time.

Black

A common term 20 years ago, 'black' was used as a generic, political term to describe all non-white minority ethnic groups. The aim was to emphasise solidarity among those who shared a common experience of discrimination because of skin colour. Currently, it is not common to describe skin colour in this broad way. Mainly this is because many people did not feel that this term adequately considered the diversity of culture and experience present. The term 'black and minority ethnic groups' (BME) has come into common use recently.

Ethnic minorities

This term refers to groups that are not the major ethnic group in a country or particular geography. There is a growing preference for using the term '*minority ethnic* group' as opposed to 'ethnic minority group'. The reason for this is that the former emphasises the minority aspect rather than the ethnicity. It reminds us that everyone has an ethnicity and therefore ethnicity should not be demonised or made to be exotic. Additionally, minority ethnic groups can be predominantly white, for example, Irish.

Disability

There are a number of conflicting models of disability (*see* Box 31.3). Disability is often used to refer to an individual's impairment – the medical model. However, many disabled people see their disability as being caused by the attitude of society and the organisational arrangements (services, etc.) made by society – the social model. Thus *disabled person*, rather than 'person with a disability', is preferred.

Equalities

Equalities are often misinterpreted as being concerned with treating everyone the same. In reality the equality, or equal opportunities, is concerned with 'opportunity' rather than treatment. Outcomes are the important measures of *equal opportunities*. We do not start on a level playing field and social exclusion is inevitable if differences are not recognised.

Institutional racism

New words and phrases emerge all the time from the general socio-political milieu, sometimes from a single event. One example is the term *institutional racism*, which was coined following an enquiry into the handling of the investigation (by the Metropolitan Police) of the killing of black teenager Stephen Lawrence. The Macpherson report defined institutional racism as: 'The collective failure of an organisation to provide an appropriate and professional service to people because of their colour, culture or ethnic origin which can be seen or detected in processes; attitudes and behaviour which amount to discrimination through unwitting prejudice, ignorance, thoughtlessness and racist stereotyping which disadvantages minority ethnic people'. (8, para. 6.34)

---

munity it serves. The findings of institutional racism (*see* Box 31.1 for definition) against the Metropolitan Police as a result of the Stephen Lawrence Inquiry(8) are a good example of the damaging impact of failing to manage diversity adequately.

Competence

There are five essential elements that contribute to a system's ability to become more diversity competent and compliant. These principles are based on those for organisational cultural competency. The system should:

- value diversity
- have the capacity for diversity self-assessment
- be conscious of the dynamics inherent when cultures and diversities interact
- institutionalise diversity knowledge about its client group
- develop adaptations to delivering what is required and expected by reflecting an understanding of diversity.

These five elements must be manifested in every level of the organisation through policy, structures and services.

As cultural competence is a developmental process,(9) so diversity competence can be conceived along a continuum. These developmental stages of an organisation's competence in diversity are depicted in Figure 31.1. It is essential that organisations assess where they are on the continuum because it will allow them to put ameliorative measures, such as appropriate staff training, in place.

Clinical teachers may also need to determine where they are along the continuum of diversity competency so they can choose what steps are required to further develop their needs (*see* Box 31.2). Clinical teachers should check their own responses to other cultures, strategies for coping with these and their ability to understand and help students

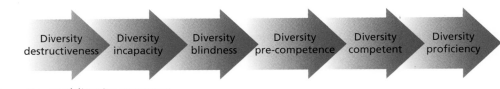

Figure 31.1 The continuum of diversity competence.
Source: Cross *et al.*(9)

BOX 31.2 Diversity competence: A framework

Knowledge
- Understanding of culture, conflict and potential problems
- Knowledge of history, language, religion, customs, values
- Knowledge of medical models predominant
- Understanding of social, political, economic, institutional factors
- Knowledge of support and services
- Knowledge of local diversity and differences

Professional skills
- Techniques for learning and teaching about diversity
- Ability to communicate clearly and accurately
- Ability to openly discuss diversity issues
- Ability to recognise issues to do with conflict
- Ability to recognise and combat racism
- Ability to plan culturally appropriate teaching
- Ability to evaluate skills

Personal attributes
- Empathy and flexibility in attitudes
- Acceptance of differences due to diversity
- Willingness to work with diverse clients
- Openness to new experiences and people
- Awareness of differences and similarities across diverse groups

---

from diverse backgrounds. The consequences of a lack of awareness of broad diversity-related issues are many, and may mean that trainers are unable to train trainees appropriately, who in turn may then ignore these issues in their patients and carers.

The socio-political context

Everyone in society will come into contact with the health care system, whether directly or via family and friends. The effectiveness of that contact can make a difference in the quality and duration of a person's life. Health care is therefore rightly a political issue and at times, more problematically, an ideological battlefield. Medical education cannot shield itself from this reality and the current political priori-

ties of ending social exclusion. This includes fair selection and promotion in the medical profession for people from all backgrounds, as well as fair access to health care and equality of outcomes. To this end, organisations such as the Higher Education Funding Council for England have set clear targets to promote access to higher education. In some areas, such as gender, the student profile has changed dramatically, with many more women getting into medical school. In other areas, such as disability participation and social class, much work remains to be done.

As key political issues, diversity and social inclusion have seen themselves incorporated into plans to modernise the UK's National Health Service (NHS) over the last ten years. The Department of Health's Corporate Plan 2012-13 commits to:

> Better health: strengthening our public health system, protecting people's health and wellbeing to improve health outcomes and tackle health inequalities across all ages.(10)

Disparity between different groups (for example, gender, ethnic and social class) can be found in health, income, education, employment, housing and community safety, and in many aspects of day-to-day life. Health professionals should have an interest in all aspects of social inequality as they all have an impact on health.

Despite significant advances in medicine and higher spending on health, profound social inequalities persist across the world, even within the most developed nations. In the UK, for example, there are marked differences between the health outcomes of people from different socio-economic groups and ethnic backgrounds on key health outcomes such as infant mortality and life expectancy.(11) In London alone, there is a difference of seven years in life expectancy to be found by simply travelling eight stops on a local rail link.(12) Such differences in health outcomes are very real and demand attention.

Governments use the law as a key method of tackling these concerns. Accordingly, we have seen 40 years of developing law and case law concerning equality, inclusion and inalienable human rights. First tackling gender and race issues, legislation and case law has grown to include human rights, disability, age, religion, gender reassignment and sexual orientation. These have not only had a fundamental influence on organisational policy but also on clinical practice.

The influence on policy and behaviour in the public sector has recently been increased with the introduction of equalities duties, first covering race, closely followed by disability and gender. The UK Equality Act 2010 consolidated existing legislation and introduced the Public Sector Equality Duty, extending coverage to age, religion or belief, gender reassignment and sexual orientation. The aim of the duty is to make equalities part of the day-to-day business of public bodies.(13) Such legislative requirements apply across the board and in medical education will impact on the postgraduate as well as undergraduate arena. Both will need to show their ability to comply with this duty through strong leadership, clear policies and clear evidence of compliance. Education and training are central to managing this process successfully. This is particularly challenging for postgraduate medical education where trainees learn on the job and as employees. All organisations involved in postgraduate medical education must show leadership, if the aims of diversity are to be achieved.

Regulatory frameworks tend to mirror these broader concerns. The UK General Medical Council's (GMC) guidance document *Good Medical Practice*(14) lays out the professional standards expected of all doctors. This includes a diversity statement in that doctors must not discriminate against colleagues because of their views on culture, beliefs, race or colour. To address this standard and ensure legal compliance, the teaching of cultural competence has become increasingly common in undergraduate medicine. Less is understood about cultural competence training in postgraduate education, where it competes with organisational and service priorities and training in clinical competencies.

More generally, concerns about *adverse impact* in medical education have been raised for over 25 years now. Adverse impact is where a particular group performs or succeeds noticeably below the norm. There have been concerns about the success rate of minority ethnic candidates gaining entry into UK medical schools(15–17) and in relation to age and socio-economic background.(18) The concern about adverse impact extends to the career progression of women and minority ethnic groups through the junior doctor grades.(19,20) Black minority ethnic groups are most likely to end up working in unpopular specialties or in career-grade posts.(21) Further concerns encompass leadership and academic roles, with women and minority ethnic groups found to be under-represented in these areas too.(22,23) A similar situation can be found in the US. Although minority groups comprise 30 per cent of the US population, only 13 per cent of medical students, 6 per cent of practising physicians, and 3 per cent of faculty are members of an under-represented minority group.(24) Similar international concerns regarding the representation of women are documented with horizontal segregation (women concentrated in certain areas) and vertical segregation (women under-represented in higher levels of the profession) common.(25)

Adverse impact does not equate to unlawful discrimination. It does, however, challenge us to look at the reasons for the differences and consider the consequences for social equity that this disparity causes.

Disability

Among diversity themes, disability merits specific mention as it is frequently misunderstood.(26) Inevitably, the following section can only function as an overview of a complex area, and again, the UK legislative framework is taken as the example. The Medical Act 1983 has long allowed the GMC to tailor training to enable disabled students to become qualified. More recent moves to competency-based assessment will also help with this approach. The focus of training can change from an individual being required to carry out particular tasks/procedures in order to progress. Instead, the underlying competencies can be identified and demonstrated in alternative ways, where it is safe to do so.

Developing legislative coverage introduced the Special Education Needs and Disability Act 2001 (SENDA) to protect students, including higher education students, from disability discrimination. Its scope includes examinations and assessments, short courses, arrangements for work placements, and libraries and learning resources. SENDA amended the Disability Discrimination Act 1995 (DDA), which had a broader view of disability discrimination. Under the terms of the DDA (which have now been incorporated into the Equality Act 2010) it is illegal to treat people less favourably in the provision of goods, facilities and services; in offering and during employment; and in education. All three areas are key, as postgraduate medical education occurs within an employment framework and whilst providing essential services to patients. To ignore these aspects is therefore to miss the reality of what the student is being trained to do.

In October 2004, the DDA was further extended to cover organisations that confer, renew or extend a professional or trade qualification – for example, GMC and General Dental Council. Therefore a qualifications body cannot unlawfully discriminate against a disabled person when it is awarding, renewing, extending or withdrawing a professional or trade qualification. Again, these provisions have been incorporated into the Equality Act 2010.

Despite such legislation, disabled people are under-represented among medical graduates, when compared with other disciplines. The number of disabled applicants accepted into UK degree courses rose from just under 5 per cent to 5.5 per cent between 2001 and 2006. The figure for medicine and dentistry stands at 2 per cent.(27) There remains a significant stigma around disability in medical careers, with a study suggesting that medical students associated disability with predominantly depersonalised or negative words.(28) These associations improved with training. A medicalised model of disability is often prevalent in discussions around the education of health care professionals, whereas a social model is preferred by disabled people (*see* Box 31.3).

Cultural diversity

The concept of *culture* cuts across all three categories of Jehn's typology,(3) referring to the 'inherited ideas, beliefs, values and knowledge which constitute the shared bases of social action'.(30) Often, we have inherited multiple cultures within us – for example, the culture of a particular university or organisation; and values related to religion,

---

BOX 31.3 Models of disability. *Source*: Americano(29)

	Medical model	Charitable model	Social model
The individual	Individual is a patient/dependent	Individual is a charity case/hero (dependent or exceptional)	Individual is a distinct member of society with rights/independent
Source of problem	Medical condition	Impairment	Attitudes in and organisation of society
Solution/approach	Medical intervention/conditions to be treated/controlled	Provide help. Cases to be pitied/made heroic	Change society, ensure individuals' rights
Locus of power	Responsibility held by clinical staff	Responsibility held by 'charitable' staff/volunteers	Responsibility held by disabled people

---

gender or sexual orientation often compete within an individual and influence his or her interactions with others. As a result, cultural identity is evolutionary, and changes with time and place. Diversity can be as great within a culture as it is across cultures, since not all beliefs, values, attitudes or behaviours will be shared, even within the same cultural group. Culture, again, needs to be distinguished from *race*, which is defined as a group of people with common ancestry with identifiable inherited physical attributes, and from *ethnicity*, which is usually a self-ascription reliant on common ancestral characteristics and cultural traditions, including religion and language.

Cultural competence

Cultural competence relies on a sophisticated awareness of these cultural beliefs, values and practices, yet it is somehow expected to emerge if the racial and ethnic mix of the workforce is representative of the local population. In reality this is not the case, and as the working practices of health professionals are theoretically the same, because of a common education or job description, understanding of differences in how those practices are acted out, through training in cultural competence,(31) becomes essential.

Training in cultural competence then bridges a number of social, cultural and economic factors. Undergraduate curricula often incorporate lectures and course work on cultural competency in health care provision. In a review, Bhui *et al.*(31) noted that the importance ascribed to training and education in cultural competence was high, but limited information was available on the contents or learning methods. Furthermore, there was no information on whether groups of health professionals required similar or different approaches. The authors also argued that cultural competence, including attention to organisational values, training and communication must be embedded in the organisational infrastructure and ethos.

Cultural competence has been defined as the ability of individuals to:
- look beyond their own cultural interpretations
- to maintain objectivity when dealing with individuals from other cultures

- demonstrate an ability to understand behaviours without passing judgement.

The acceptance of, and respect for, difference, coupled with self-assessment and an attention to the dynamics of difference and resources available, form part of the cultural competence. Culturally competent individuals incorporate skills, knowledge, attitudes and competencies to address the needs of service users, whose cultural values and expectations are different.

As doctors or other health care professionals, one of the main vehicles for the expression of cultural competence is how we communicate with others. And it is to issues of cross-cultural communication that we turn next.

Cross-cultural communication

Cultural communication refers to the process of exchanging ideas using culturally appropriate idioms that can be understood in the context of culture, gender, previous experience and education. Barriers to cross-cultural communication are linked to language, non-verbal communication, stereotypes of other cultures and the tendency to evaluate behaviour from the other culture as good or bad based on one's own cultural bias. Stress related to cross-cultural encounters and filters may prevent one from accurately understanding what others are trying to communicate and may lead to culture clash.(32) The key components of all interpersonal communication are verbal and non-verbal, the two working in synergy to convey a message. Where an interpreter is present, additional complexities are created as verbal and non-verbal messaging is routed, fully, or partially, through a third party.

Verbal communication

Both verbal and non-verbal types of communication are influenced by cultural norms and values. Culture has language as a key component and using verbal skills to communicate with those from different cultural and linguistic backgrounds may need adequate adjustment. Individuals who speak two or more languages may often have a primary language, which is the language they think in. They may hide communication problems in the guise of reverting to primary language or they may revert to it when feeling anxious or distressed. This may be particularly important at the time of examinations and assessments. It is worth bearing in mind that some words are particularly specific to some cultures, for example, *schadenfreude* (broadly interpreted as pleasure derived from the misfortunes of others), and cannot easily be translated. Thus concepts that are meaningful in one language may not exist in another. Poor skills in English language are sometimes mistaken for low intelligence quotient or slowness. Furthermore, an understanding of English language in social settings may not translate into understanding medical terminology or vice versa.

Non-verbal communication

It has been argued that over two-thirds of communication is non-verbal. Non-verbal communication includes gestures, eye contact, touching, facial expressions, body language, proximity, style of speaking and emotional tone. Non-verbal communication refers to the way we look, move, feel, sound or smell.

Gesturing can vary across cultural settings and extra gestures should not be misinterpreted as agitation unless there are clear reasons for this assessment and other signs support this view. Similarly, in some cultures close proximity to the teacher may be sought, whereas in others it may be frowned upon, and therefore being close and making eye contact may be seen as hostile. In some cultures avoiding direct eye-to-eye contact and looking at the floor may be a sign of deference and respect, rather than an insult or ignoring the individual. The physical distance between two people is also a result of cultural norms and values. Close proximity and touching may be a sign of warmth in some cultures, whereas in others it may be seen as a representation of sexual interest. Lack of close contact or touching may be seen as cold and hostile in some cultures. Similarly, speaking at a louder level is acceptable in some cultures, but seen as aggressive in others. Furthermore, cutting across conversations is common in some cultures but not others, and thus may be interpreted as rude and intrusive. Silence, in some cultures, may be seen as approval and agreement, whereas in others it may be hostile. In summary, non-verbal communication:

- conveys personal attitudes – respect, being interested, liking the speaker or person being spoken to, etc.
- expresses emotional states – cultures determine when and how disappointment, anger, etc. are shown
- manages conversation – by encouraging or discouraging, exchanging rituals and regulating self-presentation.

Non-verbal communication can be improved by increased sensitivity to the student's body language, demeanour, eye contact, gestures, emotional tone, physical distance and an awareness of what may be normal in the culture.

Working with interpreters

Interpreters are generally professional individuals (but not always) who are proficient in at least two languages and therefore can act as a bridge and a communicator between two individuals. Their task is to facilitate the exchange of information in a non-biased manner. Bearing in mind both

BOX 31.4 FOCUS ON: Cultural distance

Hofstede *et al.*(33) point out that although cultures differ, they all meet the same five basic problems of social life. However, each culture develops its own solutions. These basic problems include issues of identity, hierarchy and power distance, gender, truth and virtue. An awareness of these will empower and enable the teacher in managing education across cultures.

Different cultures adopt different positions on a spectrum of social participation between *individualism* and *communitarianism*. According to Hampden-Turner and Trompenaars,(34) individualism is characterised by competition, self-reliance, self-interest, and personal growth and fulfilment, whereas communitarianism (equated with sociocentrism or collectivism) relies on social concern, altruism, co-operation, and public service and societal legacy. Extremes at both ends of the scale can be destructive in organisations. In teaching, consideration needs to be given to how these cultural differences affect whether some issues are better addressed in groups or with individuals.

verbal and non-verbal communication, a good interpreter should be able to interpret both without taking sides. Frequent errors in interpretation include distortion, deletion, omission, blocking of messages that may be seen as against the culture, incorrect translation, inadequate interpretation and difficulty in finding equivalent words for concepts that cannot be translated. Translation can be literal or conceptual. There is an equal danger in underestimating someone's language skills as in overestimating them. The gender and age of the interpreter may be important, as is preparation before any interpreted session, especially in relation to difficult words. During the session, it is important to ensure that the role of the interpreter is clearly defined, and after the session, a period of debriefing is usually very helpful to explore technical problems, cultural nuances (*see* Box 31.4) and share information in preparation for future contacts.

Diversity in medical education

Students and trainees in the health care professions come from a variety of cultural backgrounds and bring their own set of experiences, prejudices and expectations with them. In teaching and training, these can be worked with to develop diversity awareness and overcome prejudice. This is (literally) vital as patients' exposure to actual and 'perceived' beliefs about prejudice and related acts influences their own and their carers' expectations of health care professionals and the health service. A patient's readiness to seek help from any particular health care professionals will depend on their overt or tacit appraisal of the professional's competence and knowledge,(35) and that will include their assessment of the individual's cultural competence. On the other side of the desk, insensitivity to diversity in the process of diagnosis and management has been often blamed for over-diagnosis of certain conditions(36,37) and pathways to care experienced by ethnic minority patients.(38)

The training of students can take place in different settings using different models. Training in diversity can be delivered by students themselves, the voluntary sector, academics and professional experts from different backgrounds, using experiential, cognitive or knowledge-based models in small groups, lectures, large groups or through policy changes.

Training and education in diversity can also be provided in the postgraduate sector through in-service training. This will include knowledge-based learning – keeping up to date with changes in local laws pertaining to equalities; however, to develop and improve the co-ordination of agencies and professions, a team-based learning approach is required, allowing team members to learn from each other and hone their own skills. Core skills may be shared across disciplines within the team; the training is therefore both multi- and interdisciplinary.

Similarly, although clinical teachers in medical schools may be aware of cultural and diversity issues, social services and the voluntary sector appear to be much better at training their staff for cross-cultural (and diversity) encounters and in the implementation of equal opportunities practice.(39) Theoretical models used for training can be reflexive, experiential, motivational change, cognitive or based on belief systems. Role-play, small groups, observations, knowledge and attitudes can be used to explore learning.

The exact formats for teaching diversity can be multilevel and multifaceted. These can be developed according to the interest and resources available. Courses may be day release or weekend, organised in teams or groups, and at the local, regional or national level. Further top-up sessions can be provided by e-learning or distance-learning packages. Each student can thus work at both an individual and a group level.

It will be apparent from the above that diversity is a subject that is best dealt with in groups. This may take different forms, and in the section that follows we describe some possible models.

Teaching and training

The basic principle for diversity training is to have a structured framework. The components of the framework will be dictated by the resources available, curricula requirements, time allocated and the specific needs of students. Any approach that deals with diversity has to place diversity at the source and centre of the expected behaviours and past expectations. Group exercises will allow students to explore their own attitudes to diversity without feeling overawed. Throughout the process, skilled feedback is extremely important and the facilitators must be keenly aware of their own world view.

Learning about diversity can take place in a number of sessions, with identification of barriers in communication, building on existing knowledge, awareness of different types of messages and legal issues. Diversity profiles of the national and local populations can provide a useful introduction and information on setting up the right targets in teaching. Using role play and real scenarios can open up the possibility of exploring personal experiences. The trainees can identify changes in attitudes, behaviour and knowledge, built on discussions with additional written information. Web-based learning can contribute to the consolidation of attitudinal changes. A follow-up session a few months later can help in identifying changes in clinical practice, attitudes, skills and knowledge, and perceptions of the learning.

A number of models for the delivery of diversity training are suggested here, modified from Bhui and Bhugra.(35)

Developing specialists in the team

Training is team-based, and each member of the group takes on the responsibility of liaising with one cultural or diverse group and becomes the educator for the team. The role of educators will depend on their skills and interests, and the focus for teaching may be, for example, policy, legal status or the development of services. As a result of this exercise, the individual becomes a cultural 'specialist' and his or her skills and knowledge can then be communicated to other team members. The major advantage in this approach is the ownership of change within the team, and the liaising person becomes the repository of information. A major disadvantage is that the individual may feel isolated and burdened if the rest of the team choose not to acquire necessary knowledge and skills.

Liaison with voluntary and independent providers

Here, voluntary and independent service providers act as liaison resources and brokers to provide delivery of training and supervision. The advantage of such a joint approach is mutual learning, support and respect. The service providers will also be seen as acceptable by users and carers. A key disadvantage is that the voluntary or independent sector may feel overwhelmed and compromised. Working with independent providers may be seen as unacceptable and unorthodox. These organisations may also appear to be less aware of evidence-based practice in relation to diversity. It may also be difficult in practice to match up the two sets of values.

Using cultural brokers

A cultural broker is an individual from a specific culture who can provide a link between the services and the community. Such an individual educates both sides – one side on cultural norms and mores, and the other side about the availability of services. Thus training and supervision can be two-way. The key advantage of such an approach is that the links with community are strengthened and learning is at the place of work. Its disadvantages include perceived situations where such an individual is seen as taking sides and may be wrongly aligned in the community's mind with the services.

Consulting expert panels

The use of expert advisory panels is another model(40) that has been successfully adopted in the assessment of health needs with North American Indian communities. This approach allows participation in identifying health needs by various diverse groups, who can sanction appropriate treatments and provide directive guidance on taboos. This model can provide ongoing education for both qualified professionals and their trainees, and has the advantage of having committee liaison rather than a single individual being responsible. However, competing interests may create a multitude of problems and be cumbersome.

Supervision and diversity

Cassimir and Morrison(41) suggest that the therapist must try to assume the internal frame of reference of the client and perceive the world as the client sees it, as well as seeing the client as they see themselves. Trainees and students can be viewed in the same light and trained in turn to see their patients in the same way. Even with adequate training and knowledge, the health professional's skills and competencies need to be updated regularly with ongoing service-based training that reflects the demographic shifts. Initial training is therefore usefully supplemented by high-quality supervision for which various models have been described.(35) For students and trainees, such supervision may need to be based in their clinical settings, when they are established as part of the team providing services.

In some situations supervision itself can raise complex diversity issues. For example, a student with a physical impairment may feel that his or her non-disabled supervisor is unable to understand issues to do with the barriers he or she faces. Similarly, if further aspects of identity are taken into account, there may be additional problems. For example, a visually impaired, female, Asian student may feel she is not being dealt with appropriately by a non-disabled, male, white supervisor.

In supervision settings the power relationship between teacher/trainer and student is unequal, and this may become further exaggerated by diversity matters. These unequal variables will include disability, ethnicity, gender and sexual orientation, as well as experiences and status differences. The supervisor/trainer should be able to set clear boundaries on the duration, type of supervision and the physical location of such an interaction. Supervision sessions will, and indeed must, involve discussion of feelings related to transference and counter-transference, which will include factors related to age, gender, ethnicity, sexual orientation and disability. Even though these are not specifically therapeutic sessions, sharing of experiences, some exploration of the feelings on both sides and discussions about future plans may all contribute to feelings of anger, frustration or contentment on either side. Students or trainees may hesitate in rebelling or transmitting their feelings in such a session. These interactions are rarely straightforward and can sometimes lead to sabotaging the session, miscommunication or subversion of the supervisor's task.

Conclusions

Although dealing with diversity may be daunting, the use of existing knowledge, classification of attributes and building on skills, can enable and empower teachers in dealing with students from diverse backgrounds with diverse needs. Identifying personal world views and using training methods at the individual and group levels will yield positive results. Students and trainees will have varying needs. Taking steps to understand and address those needs will help maximise learning outcomes and thus be positive for patient care. How organisational diversity impacts performance in the workplace and thus the quality of health care is not yet fully understood. It will also be subject to multiple stakeholder viewpoints, many of which will conflict. What is clear is that in an increasingly multicultural society with its expectations of social equality, a failure to engage with the broad range of issues that diversity raises is damaging to the credibility of both the organisation and the individual professional. Dealing with diversity is difficult, but diversity must be dealt with.

References

1 Brockner J, Chen Y-R, Mannix EA, Leung K and Skarlicki DP (2000) Culture and procedural fairness: when the effect of what you do depends on how you do it. *Administrative Science Quarterly.* **45**: 138–59.

2 Steiner DD and Gilliland SW (1996) Fairness reactions to personnel selection techniques in France and the United States. *Journal of Applied Psychology.* **81**: 134–41.

3 Jehn KA, Northcraft GB and Neale MA (1999) Why differences make a difference: a field study of diversity, conflict and performance in work groups. *Administrative Science Quarterly.* **44**: 741–63.

4 Adams JS (1963) Toward an understanding of inequity. *Journal of Abnormal and Social Psychology.* **67**: 422–36.

5 Arvey RD and Sackett PR (1993) Fairness in selection: current developments and perspectives. In: Schmitt N and Borman WC (eds) *Personnel Selection in Organizations.* Jossey-Bass, San Francisco, CA.

6 Bagshaw M (2004) Is diversity divisive? A positive training approach. *Industrial and Commercial Training.* **36**: 153–7.

7 Rajan A and Harris S (2003) The business impact of diversity. *Personnel Today.* 9(February): 18.

8 MacPherson W (1999) The Stephen Lawrence Enquiry. Report of an inquiry by Sir William MacPherson of Cluny. The Stationery Office, London. (http://www.archive.official-documents.co.uk/document/cm42/4262/sli-00.htm; accessed 9 June 2013).

9 Cross TL, Barzon BJ, Dennis KW and Isaacs MR (1989) *Towards a Culturally Competent System of Care: A Monograph on Effective Services for Minority Children Who are Severely Emotionally Disturbed.* CASSP Technical Assistance Center, Georgetown University Child Development Center, Washington, DC.

10 Department of Health (2012). Corporate Plan 2012–13, pp. 6–8. Department of Health 290090. (https://www.gov.uk/government/publications/department-of-health-corporate-plan-2012-to-2013; accessed 8 June 2013).

11 Marmott M (2010) *Fair Society, Healthy Lives: Strategic Review of Health Inequalities in England.* UCL Institute of Health Equity, London.

12 Darzi A (2007) Healthcare for London: a framework for action. NHS, London.(http://www.londonhp.nhs.uk/publications/a-framework-for-action/; accessed 9 June 2013).

13 Equality and Human Rights Commission (2012). The Essential Guide to the Public Sector Equality Duty. EHRC Third edition, January 2012. (http://www.equalityhumanrights.com/uploaded_files/EqualityAct/PSED/essential_guide_update.pdf;; accessed 9 June 2013).

14 General Medical Council (2006, Updated March 2009) *Good Medical Practice*. GMC, London. ISBN: 978-0-901458-24-7.

15 McKenzie KJ (1995) Racial discrimination in medicine (Editorial). *British Medical Journal*. **310**: 478–9.

16 Collier J and Broke A (1986) Racial and sexual discrimination in the selection of students for London medical schools. *Medical Education*. **20**: 86–90.

17 McManus IC, Richards P and Maitlis SL (1989) Prospective study of the disadvantage of people from ethnic minority groups applying to medical schools in the United Kingdom. *British Medical Journal*. **298**: 723–6.

18 McManus IC (1998) Factors affecting likelihood of applicants being offered a place in medical schools in the United Kingdom in 1996 and 1997: retrospective study. *British Medical Journal*. **317**: 1111–7.

19 McKeigue PM, Richards JDM and Richards P (1990) Effects of discrimination by sex and race on early careers of British medical graduates during 1981–7. *British Medical Journal*. **301**: 961–4.

20 Commission for Racial Equality (1996) *Appointing NHS Consultants and Senior Registrars: Report of a Formal Investigation*. CRE, London.

21 Coker N (2001) *Racism in Medicine: An Agenda for Change*. King's Fund, London.

22 Royal College of Physicians (2001) Career Choices and Opportunities. A report of a working party of the Federation of Royal Colleges of Physicians. RCP, London..

23 Price EG, Gozu A, Kern DE *et al.* (2005) The role of cultural diversity climate in recruitment, promotion and retention of faculty in academic medicine. *Journal of General Internal Medicine*. **20**: 565–71.

24 Kripalani S, Bussey-Jones J, Katz MG *et al.* (2006) A prescription for cultural competence in medical education. *Journal of General Internal Medicine*. **21**: 1116–20.

25 Kilminster S, Downes J, Gough B *et al.* (2007) Women in medicine – is there a problem? A literature review of the changing gender composition, structures and occupational cultures in medicine. *Medical Education*. **41**: 39–49.

26 Melville C (2005) Discrimination and health inequalities experienced by disabled people. *Medical Education*. **39**: 122–6.

27 University Colleges and Admissions Services (2013) Statistical Services. (http://www.ucas.ac.uk/about_us/stat_services/stats_online/; accessed 9 June 2013).

28 Byron M, Cockshott Z, Brownett H *et al.* (2005) What does disability mean for medical students? An exploration of the words medical students associate with the term 'disability. *Medical Education*. **39**: 176–83.

29 Americano A (2006) Illness and disability. In: Hastie A (ed.) *Flexible Working and Training for Doctors and Dentists*, pp. 173–89. Radcliffe Publishing, Oxford.

30 *Collins English Dictionary* (2007) HarperCollins, London.

31 Bhui K, Warfa N, Edonya P, McKenzie K and Bhugra D (2007) Cultural competence in mental health care: a review of model evaluations. *BMC Health Services Research*. **7**: 15.

32 Barma L (1982) Stumbling blocks in intercultural communication: exercises, stories and syntheticultures. In: Samovar L and Porter R (eds) *Intercultural Communication: A Reader*, pp. 330–8. Wadsworth, Belmont, CA.

33 Hofstede GJ, Pedersen PB and Hofstede G (2002) *Exploring Culture: Exercises, Stories and Syntheticultures*. Intercultural Press, Yarmouth, ME.

34 Hampden-Turner C and Trompenaars F (2000) *Building Cross-cultural Competence*. Yale University Press, New Haven, CT.

35 Bhui K and Bhugra D (1998) Training and supervision in effective cross-cultural mental health services. *Hospital Medicine*. **59**: 861–5.

36 Bhugra D, Leff J, Mallet R *et al.* (1997) Incidence and outcome of schizophrenia in whites, African-Caribbeans and Asians in London. *Psychological Medicine*. **27**: 791–8.

37 Bhui K (1997) London's ethnic minorities and the provision of mental health services. In: Johnson S, Ramsay R, Thornicroft G and Brooks L (eds) *London's Mental Health Services*, pp. 143–66. King's Fund Institute, London.

38 Bhugra D, Harding C and Lippett R (2004) Pathways into care and satisfaction for black patients in south London. *Journal of Mental Health*. **13**: 171–83.

39 Gray P (1998) Voluntary organisations. In: Bhugra D and Bahl V (eds) *Ethnicity: An Agenda for Mental Health*, pp. 202–10. Gaskell, London.

40 Timpson J (1984) Indian mental health: changes in the delivery of care in North Western Ontario. *Canadian Journal of Psychiatry*. **29**: 234–41.

41 Cassimir G and Morrison BJ (1993) Re-thinking work with multicultural population. *Community Mental Health Journal*. **29**: 547–9.

Further reading

Americano A (2005) Educating doctors for diversity. In: Hastie A, Hastie I, Jackson N *et al.* (eds) *Postgraduate Medical Education and Training: A Guide for Primary and Secondary Care*, pp. 97–109. Radcliffe Publishing, Oxford.

Americano A (2006) Illness and disability. In: Hastie A (ed.) *Flexible Working and Training for Doctors and Dentists*, pp. 173–89. Radcliffe Publishing, Oxford.

Bhugra D and Bhui K (2007) *Textbook of Cultural Psychiatry*. Cambridge University Press, London.

Kandola R and Fullerton J (1998) *Diversity in Action: Managing the Mosaic*. CIPD, London.

Tseng W-S and Streltzer D (eds) (2004) *Cultural Competence in Clinical Psychiatry*. American Psychiatric Publishing, Washington DC and London.

Web-based resources

Advisory Conciliation and Arbitration Service (ACAS), http://www.acas.org.uk. Helpline: +44 (0)845 747 4747

Chartered Institute of Personnel & Development, http://www.cipd.co.uk

Commission for Equality and Human Rights, http://www.equalityhumanrights.com

Department of Health (type in 'diversity' or 'inequalities' in the search engine), http://www.dh.gov.uk

Equality and Diversity Forum, http://www.edf.org.uk

GLADD – site for lesbian, gay, bisexual and transgender doctors and dentists, http://www.gladd.co.uk/index.htm

32 Developing medical educators: A journey, not a destination

Yvonne Steinert
Faculty of Medicine, McGill University, Canada

 KEY MESSAGES

- The term 'medical educator' describes a number of roles, including that of teacher, curriculum planner and evaluator, educational leader and administrator, researcher and scholar.
- There are many ways in which to develop as a medical educator. 'Formal' staff development activities are only one way to achieve this goal. Other approaches include 'learning on the job', belonging to a community of educators, mentorship and role-modelling, and organisational support and development.
- The content of staff development activities should move beyond the enhancement of teaching effectiveness and target

leadership abilities, the promotion of scholarship, and organisational change and development.
- Staff development activities should be guided by knowledge of core competencies for medical educators.
- Students and residents should be introduced to staff development activities early in their careers.
- Medical education is a social endeavour and the idea of community – and communities of practice – is fundamental to the development of medical educators.

Introduction

The Latin origin of the word 'doctor' (*doceo*) translates as 'I teach', but the majority of doctors, although expert in *what* they teach, have had little or no training in *how* to teach.(1) Doctors are also minimally prepared for the many and various roles that are subsumed under the term 'medical educator'. As Jason and Westberg state, 'The one task that is distinctively related to being a faculty member is teaching; all the other tasks can be pursued in other settings. Paradoxically, the central responsibility of faculty members is typically the one for which they are least prepared'.(2)

In the past, it was assumed that intelligent people who have been students for many years have learnt – or can automatically learn – to be successful faculty members, and little or no support for staff development was provided.(3) This is no longer true. Increasing attention has been placed on the design and development of staff development programmes, in diverse contexts and settings.(4–7) Moreover, in recent years, a number of regulatory and international bodies have started to pay attention to the accreditation of teachers and teaching,(8–10) and they have highlighted the importance of staff development in the certification of educators.(11) In the UK, for example, the role of teacher is increasingly recognised as a core professional activity for all doctors, and one that cannot be left to chance, aptitude or inclination.(12)

The goal of this chapter is to focus on the development of medical educators. To achieve this objective, we will try to define what is meant by a *medical educator*, describe the required core competencies and examine different ways of developing medical educators. Moreover, as staff development is one of the most common ways to achieve this objective, much of this chapter will examine what is known about formal staff development programmes. However, we will also address the role and importance of work-based learning, communities of practice, mentorship and role-modelling, and organisational support and development.

What is a medical educator?

The medical education literature tends to use the terms 'teacher' and 'medical educator' interchangeably, with no clear definitions. To inform this paper, we conducted a series of semi-structured interviews with 12 medical educators at McGill to ascertain their definitions and conceptions of being a medical educator.(13) Definitions included a broad range of conceptualisations, some of which are highlighted below:

> The medical educator is someone who critically reflects on the quality of the educational experience and tries to innovate and improve on what they have done.

Medical educators have a passion, not just an interest, but a passion for bringing out the best, or finding ways to bring out the best, in students and learners that they work with to help develop the best physicians that we can . . .

A medical educator is someone who uses theories and principles of education in their activities. This includes teaching, scholarship, curricular design and evaluation, and research across the educational continuum . . .

What is striking in these definitions is the emphasis on reflection, passion, innovation and informed practice across a continuum of tasks and activities.

In this chapter, the term 'medical educator' will encompass a broad spectrum of roles that include teaching, curriculum design and evaluation, educational leadership and innovation, and research and scholarship. Moreover, medical educators, whether in the clinical or classroom setting, will refer to individuals who actively *reflect* on what they do, using experience and available evidence to *inform* their educational practice and to *enhance* the teaching and learning of future health care professionals: [We] continually ask ourselves how we can do this better: 'How can we get [our students] to be the best that they can be' . . . 'If my program is working, can I still make it better? If it is not working, why not and how can I improve it?'(13) 'Either explicitly, or implicitly, we use what we have learnt about education over the years to inform our teaching . . .'.(13)

What is faculty development?

Staff development, or faculty development, as it is often called, has become an increasingly important component of medical education. Faculty development activities have been designed to improve teacher effectiveness at all levels of the educational continuum (e.g. undergraduate, postgraduate and continuing medical education), and diverse programmes have been offered to health care professionals in many settings.(14) In this chapter, staff development will refer to that broad range of activities that institutions use to *renew* or *assist* faculty in their multiple roles.(15) That is, staff development is a planned programme designed to prepare institutions and faculty members for their various roles(16) and to improve an individual's knowledge and skills in the areas of teaching, research and administration.(17) The term 'staff' or 'faculty' connotes no particular employment relationship but applies to all those involved in the processes of medical education on behalf of an educational institution. The goal of staff development is to teach faculty members the skills relevant to their institutional and faculty role and to sustain their vitality, both now and in the future.

Faculty development can provide medical educators with knowledge and skills about teaching and learning, curriculum design and delivery, student assessment and programme evaluation, and leadership and administration, as well as research and scholarship. It can also reinforce or alter attitudes or beliefs about education and scholarly activity, provide a conceptual framework for what is often performed on an intuitive basis, and introduce clinicians and basic scientists to a community of medical educators interested in medical education and the enhancement of teaching and learning for students, patients and peers.

In addition, staff development can serve as a useful instrument in the promotion of organisational change.(5,18) That is, staff development can help build consensus, generate support and enthusiasm, and implement a change initiative; it can also help change the culture within the institution by altering the formal, informal and hidden curriculum(19,20) and by enhancing organisational capacities.(21) As Swanwick(22) states, staff development should be: 'An institution-wide pursuit with the intent of professionalizing the educational activities of teachers, enhancing educational infrastructure, and building educational capacity for the future . . .'.(22)

In many ways, staff development can play an important role at both the *individual* and the *organisational* level.(23) Moreover, although staff development activities predominantly focus on teaching and instructional effectiveness, there is a critical need for these activities to also address the other roles of medical educators, including that of curriculum designer, educational leader and administrator, and scholar.

A curriculum for staff development?

Attributes and behaviours of effective clinical teachers have been identified in the literature. For example, Irby(24) reports that students value the following characteristics in their teachers:
- enthusiasm
- a positive attitude towards teaching
- rapport with students and patients
- availability and accessibility
- clinical competence
- subject matter expertise.

A number of core teaching skills have also been identified. These include the following:
- the establishment of a positive learning environment
- the setting of clear objectives and expectations
- the provision of timely and relevant information
- the effective use of questioning and other instructional methods
- appropriate role-modelling
- the provision of constructive feedback and objective-based evaluations.(25)

It is interesting to note, however, that many staff development programmes have been developed independently of a curriculum for teachers and educators. As Purcell and Lloyd-Jones state, 'Faculties have developed a plethora of teacher training programmes for medical teachers. But what is good medical teaching? Unless we know what it is, how can we develop it?'(12)

The literature provides us with some examples of developing core competencies for teachers. For example, Bland *et al.*(16) define an extensive set of essential skills, goals and objectives for successful medical faculty in five domains, as follows:
- education
- administration

- research
- written communication
- professional academic skills.

More recently, the UK-based Academy of Medical Educators[26] has developed *Professional Standards* for medical educators that are divided into core values of medical educators and five domains, outlining 'detailed outcomes in terms of understanding, skills and behaviour required of medical educators'. The suggested core values include the following:

- professional integrity
- educational scholarship
- equality of opportunity and diversity
- respect for the public
- respect for patients
- respect for learners
- respect for colleagues.

Importantly, these core values are seen to underpin the professional practice and development of medical educators and serve as the foundation for the following five domains of educational practice:

- the design and planning of learning activities
- teaching and supporting learners
- assessment and feedback to learners
- educational research and evidence-based practice
- educational management and leadership.

Each of these domains further describes a set of standards that are expected of medical educators and can serve as a useful tool for self-assessment as well as programme development.

Other researchers have compared student and faculty perceptions of effective clinical teaching. For example, Buchel and Edwards[27] asked residents and faculty members to rate the attributes of effective teachers. Both residents and faculty agreed that clinical competence is one of the most important attributes of an effective clinical teacher. They also agreed that better educators were those who demonstrated enthusiasm for their educational responsibilities. At the same time, residents commented that it was important for a quality educator to respect their autonomy and independence as clinicians, whereas faculty members reported that this was one of the least important traits of an effective teacher. In addition, faculty felt that serving as a role-model worth emulating was essential, a factor stressed by previous authors.[28] Residents, however, did not believe that this was an important attribute and ranked it at the bottom of their list. Clearly, the perceptions of residents and faculty members are not always congruent, although an 'evidence-based' set of attitudes and behaviours should guide the development of staff development programmes.

It should also be noted that much less has been written about the roles of educational *leader* and *scholar*, roles that are often subsumed under the term 'medical educator'. In an interesting study, Bordage *et al*.[29] surveyed deans and associate deans to identify the educational and leadership skills required of 'programme directors with major educational and leadership responsibilities'. Their results indicate the importance of nine key skill areas, as follows:

- oral communication
- interpersonal abilities

- clinical competence
- educational goal definition
- educational design
- problem-solving and decision-making
- team-building
- written communication
- budgeting and financial management.

Spencer and Jordan[30] also highlight the fact that educational change requires leadership and that we need to equip our colleagues to implement change. Clearly, the development of medical educators should address leadership competencies, as well as those that promote scholarship in its broadest sense.

Boyer[31] identifies the following four categories of scholarship:

- discovery
- integration
- application
- teaching.

Roughly considered, scholarship in education can involve the discovery of new knowledge (i.e. research), the integration or application of existing knowledge to new areas, and teaching.[32] Scholarship also provides a common ground for assessing the diverse roles and contributions of faculty members to the mission of the medical school and can take on many forms. For example, peer-reviewed publications and grants are products of the *scholarship of discovery*, which has been synonymous with research in the traditional sense. The *scholarship of integration* has been defined as making connections across the disciplines, illuminating data in a revealing way, whereas the *scholarship of application* has been likened to 'service' in one's own field of knowledge, to the application of theory into practice.

In medical education, fellowship programme development and web-based instructional materials are examples of the *scholarship of integration* and *application*. The *scholarship of teaching* involves the capacity to effectively communicate one's own knowledge, skills and beliefs. Moreover, teaching becomes scholarship when it is made public, is available for peer review and critique and can be reproduced and built on by other scholars.[33] The promotion of scholarship, and helping educators foster scholarly activities among their colleagues, are important factors in the development of medical educators, and yet ones that are often neglected.

As this discussion suggests, the development of a curriculum for medical educators merits attention. At the same time, it would also be worth focusing on a better understanding of the teacher's experience. In an interesting study, Higgs and McAllister[34] studied the 'experience of being a clinical educator' and discovered that this experience consisted of six interactive and dynamic dimensions, as follows:

- a sense of self (or self-identity)
- a sense of relationship with others
- a sense of being a clinical educator
- a sense of agency, or purposeful action
- seeking dynamic self-congruence
- the experience of growth and change.

Based on this research, and our experience at McGill, it would be worthwhile to take a more careful look at the 'lived experience' of being an educator and to use this experience as a framework for training: 'My pride as a medical educator comes from watching the light go on in my students' eyes and knowing why the light goes off . . .'(13) 'When I see junior colleagues work and demonstrate excellence in patient care, going the extra mile . . . I know that I have had an impact'.(13)

In summary, medical teachers and educators need to be prepared for complex(35) and demanding roles that include teaching, leadership and administration, and scholarship in its broadest meaning.

How can we develop medical educators?

'Formal' approaches to developing medical educators

The most common staff development formats have included workshops and seminars, short courses, sabbaticals and fellowships.(36) Other methods include degree programmes, peer coaching, augmented feedback and online learning. A brief description of some of these formats follows.

Workshop, seminars and short courses

Workshops are popular because of their inherent flexibility and promotion of active learning. In particular, teachers value a variety of teaching methods within this format, including interactive lectures, small-group discussions and exercises, role-plays and simulations, and experiential learning.(36) Workshops are commonly used to promote skill acquisition (e.g. lecturing or small-group teaching skills),(37,38) prepare for new curricula (e.g. problem-based learning)(39,40) or help faculty adapt to new teaching environments (e.g. teaching in the ambulatory setting).(41,42) Workshops on leadership styles and skills(43) and/or curriculum design and innovation(44) can also help prepare educators for their leadership roles, whereas short courses on research methods(45) and writing for publication(46) can help prepare clinicians and basic scientists for their scholarly work.

To date, the majority of staff development programmes have focused on teaching improvement. That is, they aim to improve teachers' skills in clinical teaching, small-group facilitation, feedback and evaluation.(36) A number of programmes also target specific core competencies (e.g. the teaching and evaluation of communication skills; professionalism) and the use of technology in teaching and learning. Less attention has been paid to the personal development of health care professionals, educational leadership and scholarship, and organisational development and change. Although instructional effectiveness at the individual level is critically important, a more comprehensive approach is needed.(14) We clearly need to develop individuals who will be able to provide leadership to educational programmes, act as educational mentors, and design and deliver innovative educational programmes. As Cusimano and David(47) state, there is an enormous need

for more health care professionals trained in methods of educating others so that medical education will continue to be responsive to driving forces of change. As previously stated, staff development also has an important role to play in promoting teaching as a scholarly activity and in creating an educational climate that encourages and rewards educational leadership, innovation and excellence.

Fellowships and other longitudinal programmes

Fellowships of varying length, format and emphasis have been utilised in many disciplines.(48–50) More recently, integrated, longitudinal programmes have been developed as an alternative to fellowship programmes or sabbaticals. These programmes, in which faculty commit 10–20 per cent of their time over one-to-two years, allow health care professionals to maintain most of their clinical, research and administrative responsibilities, whilst furthering their own professional development. Programme components typically consist of a variety of methods, including university courses, monthly seminars, independent research projects and participation in staff development activities. Integrated longitudinal programmes, such as a *Teaching Scholars Program*,(51–54) have particular appeal because teachers can continue to practise and teach while improving their educational knowledge and skills. Also, these programmes allow for the development of educational leadership and scholarly activity in medical education.(55)

In summary, although fellowship and other longitudinal programmes vary in structure, duration and content, they all enable the acquisition of expertise and excellence in teaching, curricular design and evaluation, and educational leadership. Many of them also provide assistance in academic and career development(56,57) and help create a community of teachers and educators. In addition, they encourage the dissemination of new knowledge and understanding to further the field of medical education.

Degree programmes

Certificate or degree programmes are becoming increasingly popular in many settings. In part, this is due to what some authors have termed the 'professionalisation' of medical education.(11,12) Several authors and organisations have argued for the need to certify medical educators and thereby ensure global standards; others do not agree and worry about disenfranchising keen and committed educators (*see* Box 32.1).

Cohen *et al.*(60) provided an update on Master's degrees in medical education and reported on 21 different programmes in Holland,(1) Canada,(3) Australia,(3) the USA(6) and the UK.(8) As these authors suggest, an advanced degree in medical education offers essential grounding in educational theory and practice and can provide the foundation for educational research and scholarship. Another review of Master's degrees in medical education was conducted by Tekian and Harris,(61) who highlighted an increased proliferation of Master's level programmes for health professions education. These authors described the commonalities (e.g. focus, content, educational requirements) and differences (e.g. structure, organisation) of 71 programmes and argued for the need to establish accredita-

BOX 32.1 FOCUS ON: The professionalisation of medical educators

One of the Dutch terms for staff development is *Docentprofessionalisering*, which loosely translates as the 'professionalisation' of teaching. This is of particular interest as we witness the professionalisation of medical education in a number of venues. For example, in the UK, the Dearing Report makes a number of recommendations about faculty in higher education, including the following which is pertinent in this context:

We recommend that institutions of higher education begin immediately to develop or seek access to programmes for teacher training of their staff, if they do not have them, and that all institutions seek national accreditation of such programmes from the Institute for Learning and Teaching in Higher Education.(58)

The UK General Medical Council's *Good Medical Practice* states that:

Teaching, training, appraising and assessing doctors and students are important for the care of patients now and in the future. You should be willing to contribute to these activities . . . If you are involved in teaching you must develop the skills, attitudes and practices of a competent teacher.(8)

As noted earlier, the Academy of Medical Educators in the UK(26) has developed a series of standards for medical educators, organised into five domains. The Academy has also contributed to the development of a framework for the approval of trainers, which has been adopted by the General Medical Council as national policy. In addition, the World Federation of Medical Educators has articulated a *Staff Activity and Development Policy* which states the following:

The medical school **must** formulate and implement a staff activity and development policy which: allows a balance of capacity between teaching, research and service functions; ensures recognition of meritorious academic activities, with appropriate emphasis on teaching, research and service qualifications; ensures that clinical service functions and research are used in teaching and learning; ensures sufficient knowledge by individual staff members of the total curriculum; and includes teacher training, development, support and appraisal.(10)

In a similar vein, the International Association of Medical Colleges has stated that 'opportunities for professional development must be provided to enhance faculty members' skills and leadership abilities in education and research'.(9) More specifically, their basic standard states that 'the medical school must have a staff policy which addresses a balance of capacity for teaching, research and service functions, and ensures recognition of meritorious academic activities, with appropriate emphasis on both research attainment and teaching qualifications'.

Although the emphasis on accreditation for teaching and standards for teaching has not received the same attention in Canada or the USA, there is clearly a movement towards increased accountability and accreditation of teaching, one of the roles of the medical educator.(59) Moreover, as Eitel *et al.*(11) suggest, staff development is one of the prerequisites for certification leading to the professionalisation of medical educators.

tion processes, based on common criteria and methods for evaluating these programmes. In addition, they suggested that there is a need to address the geographic maldistribution of advanced degree programmes. Pugsley *et al.*(62) also commented on the variability in content and quality among Master's programmes in medical education and argued for increased standards and quality assurance. Nonetheless, despite these concerns, most universities in the UK now require staff to undertake a university certificate in teaching and learning, and many medical schools, in partnership with National Health Service (NHS) trusts, are providing opportunities for advanced educational training.(63) Degree programmes can be particularly helpful to individuals interested in educational leadership, administration or research.

Peer coaching

Peer coaching as a method of staff development has been described extensively in the education literature. Key elements of peer coaching include the identification of individual learning goals (e.g. improving specific teaching skills), focused observation of teaching by colleagues, and the provision of feedback, analysis and support.(64) This under-utilised approach, sometimes called *co-teaching* or *peer observation*, has particular appeal because it occurs in the teacher's own practice setting, enables individualised learning and fosters collaboration.(65) It also allows health care professionals to learn about each other, as they teach together and, in this way, can nurture the development of medical educators.

'Informal' approaches to developing medical educators

Although staff development programmes are a popular way of developing medical educators, a number of alternative approaches should also be considered. Box 32.2 describes how medical educators at McGill University started the 'journey' of becoming a medical educator. For many, it started with their 'job responsibilities' and slowly evolved into a career path. The following section describes four of these important pathways.

Work-based learning

Work-based learning, often defined as learning *for* work, learning *at* work and learning *from* work,(22) is fundamental to the development of medical educators, for whom 'learning on the job' is often the first entry into teaching and education. In fact, it is in the everyday workplace – where educators conduct their clinical, research and teaching activities, and interact with faculty, colleagues and students – that learning most often takes place. It would therefore be extremely worthwhile to help medical educators see their everyday experiences as 'learning experiences' and encourage them to reflect with colleagues and students on learning that has occurred in the clinical or classroom setting. It would also help bring staff development to the workplace.

It is interesting that staff development activities have traditionally been conducted away from the educator's workplace, requiring participants to take their 'lessons

BOX 32.2 Ways of becoming a medical educator

Colleagues at the Centre for Medical Education at McGill University identified the following ways of 'becoming a medical educator'.(13)

- **By the nature of my responsibilities** – *One of the nice things about medical education is that you can often have an administrative position that allows you to have a lab. I was undergraduate program director for quite a while . . . by doing that it's given me a lab to try various innovations and evaluate them.*

- **By participating in staff development and other training opportunities** – *Participating in faculty development workshops introduced me to a community of educators and got me 'hooked' . . . I haven't stopped learning since.*

- **By pursuing an advanced degree** – *My advanced degree allowed me to look at things with education glasses on. It also gave me the opportunity to immerse myself in a group with similar interests and needs.*

- **By wanting to** – *I had the interest and the desire. I have always wanted to be a teacher and I was good at teaching . . . I followed my passion.*

- **By belonging to a community (of experts)** – *For me the most valuable part has been meeting regularly with a group of like-minded individuals committed to excellence and scholarship in medical education . . . I have become immersed in the culture.*

- **By being mentored and through role-modelling** – *I could not have done this alone. . . .*

- **By** *doing* **medical education** – *I have learned by doing – and using, either explicitly, or implicitly, what I have learned over the years to inform my teaching.*

learnt' back to their own contexts. Perhaps it is time to reverse this trend and think about how we can enhance the learning that takes place in the work environment.(66) By working together and participating in a larger community, clinicians and basic scientists can build new knowledge and understanding and develop approaches to problems faced in teaching and learning.(67)

Communities of practice

Closely related to 'learning at work' is the concept of situated learning and communities of practice. In my own setting, medical educators have commented on the role and value of a community of medical educators, brought together by a common interest in the enhancement of teaching and learning for students across the educational continuum and involvement in scholarly work in medical education, as a critical factor in their own development: 'For me it has been beneficial to be immersed in a group which is actually physically removed from where I do my clinical work . . . where I come to regularly and am forced to engage in the discussions and try out new ideas'.(13)

Barab *et al.*(68) define a community of practice as a 'persistent, sustaining, social network of individuals who share

and develop an overlapping knowledge base, set of beliefs, values, history and experiences focused on a common practice and/or mutual enterprise'. Clearly, formal staff development programmes can play a pivotal role in developing communities of practice. At the same time, belonging to such a community can play a critical role in the development of medical educators.

Lave and Wenger(67) suggest that the success of a community of practice depends on the following five factors:
- the existence and sharing by the community of a common goal
- the existence and use of knowledge to achieve that goal
- the nature and importance of relationships formed among community members
- the relationships between the community and those outside it
- the relationship between the work of the community and the value of the activity.

In his later work, Wenger(69) also adds the notion that achieving the shared goals of the community requires a shared repertoire of common resources, including language, stories and practices (*see* Box 32.3).

In many ways, centres and/or departments of medical education, as well as the newer forms of academies,(71–73) can offer a setting for 'communities of practice' to develop. They can also help nurture and support both new and experienced teachers and educators. These centres and academies, which have been described in the literature and are increasing in number, can also help develop and sustain medical education as an academic discipline.(59) Critical to their success is a common purpose, open communication and opportunities for dialogue, guidance and institutional support.

Mentorship and role-modelling

Mentoring is a common strategy to promote the development, socialisation and maturation of academic medical faculty.(16,74) However, although several formal mentorship programmes have been described,(75,76) this is an under-utilised approach for staff development, especially with regard to academic and career development. Daloz(77) describes a mentorship model that balances three key elements: support, challenge and a vision of the individual's future career. This model can also serve as a helpful framework in staff development. Given the importance of mentoring for socialisation into the profession, the development of meaningful academic activities, career satisfaction and the development of close collaborative relationships,(76) we must work to promote and recognise mentorship as a way of developing medical educators.

Role-modelling, on the other hand, is instrumental in the development of all medical educators' roles, although it is not usually recognised as such. In our setting, educators have commented on the value of mentors and the importance of role-modelling in their formation: 'Medical education involves risks. Without the support of my mentors and role-models, I would not have had the courage to accomplish what I did'.(13)

Learning from role-models occurs through observation and reflection and is a complex mix of conscious and

BOX 32.3 FOCUS ON: Cultivating communities of practice

Wenger *et al.*(70) describe seven principles for cultivating communities of practice that have direct relevance for the development of medical educators. They include the following:

- *Design for evolution* – Communities should build on pre-existing personal networks and allow for natural growth and development. Design elements should be catalysts for the community's natural evolution.(70)

- *Open a dialogue between insider and outsider perspectives* – Good community design requires an insider's perspective to lead the discovery of what the community is about; however, an outside perspective is often needed to help members' see untapped possibilities.

- *Invite different levels of participation* – People participate in communities for different reasons (e.g. because the community provides value; for personal connections; to enhance skill development). Different levels of engagement (e.g. core, active, peripheral) are to be expected and encouraged. Successful communities often 'build benches' for those on the side lines.(70)

- *Develop both public and private community spaces* – Most communities have public events where members gather to exchange ideas, solve problems or explore new concepts. However, communities are more than their 'calendar of events'.(70) The heart of the community is the one-on-one networking that occurs informally. All communities require both public and private interactions.

- *Focus on value* – Communities thrive because they deliver value to the organisation, to the teams on which community members serve and to the community members themselves. Articulation of its value helps a community to develop and grow.

- *Combine familiarity and excitement* – Successful communities offer the 'familiar comforts of a hometown' but also provide enough interest and variety to keep new ideas and new people cycling into the community.(70)

- *Create a rhythm for the community* – There are many rhythms in a community (e.g. the syncopation of familiar and exciting events, the frequency of private interactions, the ebb and flow of people from the side lines into active participation and the pace of the community's overall evolution). The rhythm of a community is the strongest indicator of its being alive.

unconscious activities.(78) Whilst we are all aware of the conscious observation of observed behaviours, understanding the power of the unconscious component is essential to effective role-modelling. We should also remember that role-models differ from mentors.(79) Role-models inspire and teach by example – often whilst they are doing other things; mentors have an explicit relationship with a colleague over time.(80)

Organisational support and development

A recent survey of faculty members' needs for faculty development(81) highlights the necessity to look at staff development as 'development, orientation *and/or* support'. Interestingly, most programmes focus on the 'development' part. Much less has been written about faculty orientation and/or support.

Support for medical educators can take different forms, including managerial and organisational support, provision of information, recognition of teaching excellence and consideration of educational scholarship in promotion and tenure. As an example, support systems and materials are available in various areas of medical education(82) and range from textbooks tailored to the needs of those responsible for training doctors(83) to flexible and open learning materials and resources. Organisational support also includes the following:

- the development of institutional policies that support and reward excellence in teaching(11)
- a re-examination of the criteria for academic promotion and increased credit for educational initiatives(84)
- an increase in training and mentoring programmes
- enhanced resources for training teachers and junior faculty members.

In my own setting, the need for an orientation programme for 'new' faculty members has been expressed as follows: 'You have to know how to navigate the system and there are certain expectations and if somebody doesn't make that explicit to you, it's very hard to figure out . . .'(85)

As staff developers and medical educators, we often tend to focus on the individual teacher and overlook the importance of organisational support and development.(18)

How can we start early?

Although the primary focus of this chapter addresses the development of faculty members as medical educators, many authors have expressed the view that staff development should start at entry to medical school.(86) As frequently observed, medical students teach in a variety of settings and participate regularly in peer-assisted learning.(87) Residents also play a critical role in the teaching of other residents and students,(88) and in fact, it has been estimated that residents spend as much as 25 per cent of their time in teaching activities, including the supervision, instruction, and evaluation of medical students and more junior residents.(89) At the same time, residents have identified teaching as an important part of their responsibilities(90) and value learning about their educational roles.(91)

In examining the role of undergraduate medical students, Dandavino *et al.*(86) outline a number of reasons why medical students should learn about teaching. On the one hand, medical students will become future residents and faculty members, and many of them will take on significant teaching roles. In addition, teaching is an essential component of the doctor-patient relationship and it is hypothesised that medical students will become more efficient communicators as a result of teacher training. It is also hoped that medical students will become better learners as a result of increased knowledge about teaching and learning. Studies have indicated that students are enthusiastic about their role in education,(92) interested in learning about teaching,(93) and often rated as effective teachers.(94) Similar observations have been made about residents. For example, studies have shown that residents contribute significantly to the education of medical students,(88,95) and that medical students perceive them as playing a critical role in their training,(96,97) especially as residents are closer to the students' experiences and able to draw upon their own teaching and learning practices. Some have also wondered whether improved teaching can increase residents' clinical competence,(98,99) but this question merits further investigation.

Within the context of promoting students and residents as teachers, a number of programmes have been described. (100–104) Some of these programmes include short workshops and seminars for students. For example, Bardach *et al.*(105) described four one-hour 'How to Teach' sessions for final-year students, whereas Nestel and Kidd(106) reported on the evaluation of a workshop designed to prepare students for their role as peer tutors. In both examples, students believed that formal instruction in teaching should become a required part of their experience; they also felt that they could use what they had learnt in their educational contexts. A number of schools also offer student-as-teacher programmes,(101) whereas others have described elective activities in medical education, usually with a small number of students.(107) Elective experiences range in duration from one to four weeks and most students reported that the elective had imparted valuable knowledge and skills. Interestingly, however, very few medical schools seem to incorporate teaching skills into their undergraduate curricula in a systematic (or routine) fashion.(92) At the same time, many institutions offer opportunities for students and residents to serve as teachers through peer and near-peer teaching. For example, students can assume the role of tutors in student-led programmes(108,109) or teaching assistants in specific courses.(110) As Peluso and Hafler(92) have said, peer and near-peer teaching opportunities are valuable in allowing students to develop educational sessions, organise tutoring programmes or provide discrete teaching opportunities to more junior colleagues. However, they are limited by 'the confines of a pre-existing curriculum and minimal control over the timing, content and format of the teaching activities'.(92)

A variety of resident-as-teacher programmes have also been described. The format of these activities mirror many of those designed for students and faculty members, and include workshops, seminars and teaching retreats.(88) The value of integrated curricula to improve teaching skills,(111) and the role of chief resident as preparation for becoming a medical educator,(112) has also been noted. The majority of available programmes are rated positively by residents, with noted changes in knowledge and attitudes towards teaching.(88) In addition, residents value the experiential nature of activities, the role of feedback and support for their roles as teachers, and the learning that occurs 'on the job'.

Looking forward, staff development programmes for students and residents should be considered an essential component of core curricula and include content about adult learning principles, as well as the broad array of teaching techniques that can be used during case presentations, formal lectures and informal team discussions.(86) They should also be evaluated in a rigorous and systematic fashion. In addition, we should remember that medical students and residents can gain valuable experience as future educators from their lived experiences, including participation in peer-teaching, course design, relevant committees, and ongoing educational research activities.(92) Early and intentional exposure can help students and residents better appreciate the role of physicians as teachers and perhaps even encourage a career as a medical educator.

Although most of the relevant literature focuses on students and residents as teachers, the need to prepare learners for leadership and management roles has been highlighted by some authors.(113,114) As Ackerly *et al.* have stated, 'The active cultivation of future leaders is [urgently] required'.(115) Although the specific focus of described programmes does not specifically address leadership for medical educators, the learning formats resemble those of faculty members with an emphasis on the value of experiential learning, the role of mentorship and the benefit of longitudinal projects.(115) In addition, special pathways(116,117) and joint MD-MBA programmes(118,119) have been created to promote leadership development at an early stage, and irrespective of the programme, a skill-based approach that exposes learners to different career paths of physician leaders is encouraged.(116) It should also be noted that leadership (or management) is included as a core competency in different educational frameworks,(120,121) and as a result, training in this area aligns well with both curricular expectations and health care needs. The same can be said of learners' roles as researchers and scholars. The importance of developing students and residents as researchers has also been highlighted in the literature, although integrating research skills into the role of becoming a future medical educator is more limited. Nonetheless, some valuable examples can be identified, including a research rotation for internal medicine residents,(122) the completion of a scholarly project during residency,(123) participation in research ethics boards for undergraduate students(124) and student electives in medical education.(125) As is the case with faculty members, faculty development in this area must address the multiple roles that a medical educator can play.

What is known about effectiveness?

Research on the impact of staff development activities has shown that overall satisfaction with programmes is high, and that participants recommend these activities to their colleagues. Teachers also report a positive change in attitudes towards teaching, as well as self-reported changes in knowledge about educational principles and specific teaching behaviours.(36) Other benefits include increased personal interest and enthusiasm, improved self-confidence, a greater sense of belonging to a community, and educational leadership and innovation. In our setting, participants in staff development activities have commented on the value of meeting like-minded colleagues and feeling a renewed sense of commitment and enthusiasm about teaching. As one participant reflected: 'I leave rejuvenated and ready to go out and teach a thousand students again!'(51)

Others have identified the value of conceptual frameworks for what they do intuitively, as illustrated in the following quote: 'I was given new tools to teach. Not only were they described to me in words, but they were also used in front of me and I was part and parcel of the demonstration'.(51)

In 2006, as part of the Best Evidence in Medical Education (BEME) collaboration, an international group of medical educators systematically reviewed the faculty development literature to ascertain the impact of faculty development initiatives on teaching effectiveness in medical education.(36) The results of this review indicate that the majority of the interventions targeted practising clinicians and included workshops, seminar series, short courses, longitudinal programmes and 'other' interventions, such as peer coaching, augmented feedback and site visits. The 53 reviewed articles included six randomised controlled trials and 47 quasi-experimental studies, of which 31 used a pre-test/post-test design. Box 32.4 summarises the findings of this review.

Despite numerous descriptions of staff development programmes, there has been a paucity of research demonstrating the effectiveness of most faculty development activities.(5,36) Few programmes have conducted comprehensive evaluations to ascertain what effect the programme is having on faculty, and data to support the efficacy of these initiatives have been lacking. Of the studies that have been conducted in this area, most have relied on the assessment of participant satisfaction; some have assessed the impact on cognitive learning or performance and several others have examined the long-term impact of these interventions. In addition, most of the research has relied on self-report, rather than objective outcome measures or observations of change. More specifically, methods to evaluate staff development programmes have included the following:

- end-of-session evaluations
- follow-up survey questionnaires
- pre- and post-assessments of cognitive or attitudinal change
- direct observations of teaching behaviour
- student evaluations
- faculty self-ratings of post-training performance.
Common problems have included the following:
- lack of control or comparison groups
- heavy reliance on self-report measures of change
- small sample sizes.

There is clearly a need for more rigorous research designs and a greater use of qualitative and mixed methods to capture the complexity of faculty development interventions. The use of newer methods of performance-based assessment, incorporating diverse data sources, is also indi-

---

BOX 32.4 WHERE'S THE EVIDENCE: Results of a systematic review

The Best Evidence in Medical Education (BEME) review of faculty development initiatives designed to improve teaching effectiveness in medical education(36) reported the following outcomes.

- *High satisfaction with staff development programmes* – Participants' overall satisfaction with staff development programmes was high. Moreover, they consistently found programmes to be acceptable, useful and relevant to their objectives. They also valued the methods used, especially those with a practical and skills-based focus.

- *Changes in attitudes towards teaching and staff development* – Participants reported positive changes in attitudes towards staff development and teaching as a result of their involvement in these activities. They cited a greater awareness of personal strengths and limitations, increased motivation and enthusiasm for teaching and learning, and a notable appreciation of the benefits of professional development.

- *Gains in knowledge and skills* – Participants reported increased knowledge of educational principles and strategies as well as gains in teaching skills. Where formal tests of knowledge were used, significant gains were shown.

- *Changes in teaching behaviour* – Self-perceived changes in teaching behaviours were consistently reported. While student evaluations did not always reflect participants' perceptions, observed changes in teaching performance were also detected.

- *Changes in organisational practice and student learning* – Although changes in organisational practice and student learning were not frequently investigated, changes did include greater educational involvement and establishment of collegial networks.

---

cated, as is the value of process-oriented studies comparing different faculty development strategies and the maintenance of change over time.

What theoretical frameworks can guide the development of medical educators?

MacDougall and Drummond(125) point out that there is no clear theoretical framework to describe how medical teachers and educators develop. In fact, despite an emphasis on educational 'know how' and practice, theory is noticeably absent from the staff development literature. In common with medical education itself, it would seem that a number of educational theories can be applied to faculty development and the development of medical educators. Many of these theoretical perspectives are covered in detail elsewhere in this book, notably in Chapter 2; however, three theoretical frameworks are particularly relevant: situated learning,(126) Knowles' principles of adult learning(127,128) and Kolb and Fry's experiential learning cycle.(129)

Situated learning

Situated learning is based on the notion that knowledge is *contextually situated* and fundamentally influenced by the *activity*, *context* and *culture* in which it is used.(126) This view of knowledge as *situated* in *authentic contexts* has important implications for our understanding of staff development and the design and delivery of instructional activities for faculty members. Situated learning theory brings together the cognitive base and experiential learning that is needed to facilitate the acquisition of new behaviours. That is, it bridges the gap between the 'know what' and the 'know how' of teaching and learning by embedding learning in authentic activities. It also helps transform knowledge from the abstract and theoretical to the useable and useful.(130) The proponents of situated learning suggest that there should be a balance between the explicit teaching of a subject and the activities in which the knowledge learnt is used in an authentic context – both essential principles in staff development.

Some of the key components of situated learning include 'cognitive apprenticeship', collaborative learning, reflection, deliberate practice and articulation of learning skills.(131)

Cognitive apprenticeship, a fundamental element of situated learning, has particular relevance to staff development. Apprenticeship is a familiar and pervasive method of learning in medicine.(132) Cognitive apprenticeship differs from a more traditional approach in that the process of carrying out the task that is to be learnt is not always observable; learning is not always situated in the workplace; and transfer of skills to new situations is required. Thus, to translate the model of traditional apprenticeship to cognitive apprenticeship, teachers need to:

- identify the processes of the task and make them visible, or explicit, to the student
- situate abstract tasks in authentic contexts, so that students understand the relevance of the work
- vary the diversity of learning situations
- articulate common aspects so that students can transfer their new knowledge and learning to new situations.(132)

Collaborative learning is another important feature of situated learning and cognitive apprenticeship. Brown *et al.*(126) identify the following strategies to promote collaborative learning:

- collective problem-solving
- displaying and identifying multiple roles
- confronting ineffective strategies and misconceptions
- developing collaborative work skills.

Small-group work, peer teaching and group projects can also facilitate the acquisition of collaborative skills. As teamwork is a fundamental component of health care delivery, collaborative learning is essential in staff development.

Reflection, an essential ingredient of situated learning, has received increasing attention in the medical literature. In practice, there are three kinds of reflective activity. Schön(133) describes a spontaneous reaction (i.e. 'thinking on your feet') as 'reflection *in* action'. This type of reflection, which is frequently described as a subliminal process of which the participant is only partially aware, most likely involves pattern recognition; as well, it is usually triggered by recognition that 'something doesn't seem right'.(133,134) Thinking of a situation after it has happened and initiating the ability to re-evaluate the situation is referred to as 'reflection *on* action'. This type of reflection, in which the participant is fully aware of what has occurred, allows the participant to mentally reconstruct the experience, paying particular attention to context. Reflection on action also forms a bridge between the re-lived situation and knowledge retrieved from internal memory or other external sources.(134)

Whilst the development of the capacity to reflect 'in' and 'on' action has become an important feature of medical practice, 'reflection *for* action'(135) forms an additional avenue for professional training and improvement of practice, as it involves planning for the next step. As Lachman and Pawlina have observed, 'The benefits of reflective practice, whilst meeting the objectives of new and revised curricula, extend beyond the construct of a medical curriculum. The process of reflection and its basis of critical thinking allows for the integration of theoretical concepts into practice, increased learning through experience, enhanced critical thinking and judgment in complex situations and the encouragement of student-centred learning'.(135) Clearly, all of these benefits are of vital importance in the development of medical educators.

Practice is another central component of situated learning. Repeated practice serves to test, refine and extend skills into a web of increasing expertise in a social context of collaboration and reflection.(131) It also enables skills to become deeply rooted and 'automatically' mobilised as needed. The notion of experiential learning is closely tied to the concept of practice.

Articulation includes two aspects.(131) First, it refers to the concept of articulating or separating out different component skills in order to learn them more effectively. An example of this is effective communication with peers. Second, articulation refers to the goal of getting individuals to articulate their knowledge, reasoning or problem-solving processes in a specific domain. By articulating problem-solving processes, learners come to better understand their thinking processes, and they are better able to explain things to themselves and to others. Articulation also helps to make learning – and reflection – visible.

Closely tied to the notion of situated learning is the concept of 'legitimate peripheral participation'.(67) This social practice, which combines 'learning by doing' (also known as 'experiential learning') and apprenticeship into a single theoretical perspective, is the process by which a novice becomes an expert. That is, from a situated learning perspective, learners build new knowledge and understanding through gradual participation in the community of which they are becoming a part. As learners, they begin at the edge – or periphery – of the community, where because of their status as learners, they have what is called 'legitimate peripheral participation'.(136)

In many ways, teachers go through a similar process. A key element of participation in the community is the opportunity to see and participate in the framing of problems and understand how knowledge is structured. According to Wenger,(69) social participation within the community is the key to informal learning. It is also embedded in the practices and relationships of the workplace and helps create identity and meaning. In addition, it complements, and can substitute for, formal learning mechanisms. Informal learning is often not acknowledged as learning within organisations; rather, it is typically regarded as being 'part of the job'. However, learning at work is a key component of the development of medical educators, and there is value in rendering this learning as visible as possible so that it can be valued as an important component of staff development.

Principles of adult learning

Although some have argued that adult learning is not a theory(137) but merely a description of the adult learner, others believe that Knowle's principles of adult learning, also referred to as andragogy,(127,128) form an important theoretical construct.(138) In either case, andragogy captures essential characteristics of adult learners and offers important guidelines for planning staff development programmes. Key principles include the following.

- Adults are independent.
- Adults come to learning situations with a variety of motivations and expectations about particular learning goals and teaching methods.
- Adults demonstrate different learning styles.
- Much of adult learning is 'relearning' rather than new learning.
- Adult learning often involves changes in attitudes as well as skills.
- Most adults prefer to learn through experience.
- Incentives for adult learning usually come from within the individual.
- Feedback is usually more important than tests and evaluations.

Clearly, the incorporation of these principles into the design of any educational programme will enhance receptivity, relevance and engagement. An understanding of these principles can also influence pacing, meaning and motivation.

Experiential learning

Kolb and Fry(129) provide a description of the learning cycle that highlights the role of experience in the learning process. More specifically, they describe how experience is translated into concepts, which in turn guide the choice of new experiences.(139) In this model, which should be considered in the design of all instructional events, learning is viewed as a four-stage cycle (*see* Figure 2.2). Immediate, concrete experience is the basis for observation and reflection; observations are then assimilated into a personal theory, from which new implications for action can be deduced, and all of these steps eventually lead to new experiences. According to Kolb and Fry,(129) learners need opportunities to experience each step of the learning cycle. That is, they need the ability to:

- experience diverse situations (in both the classroom and the clinical setting)

- observe and reflect on what they have learnt (often in a large group session)
- develop their own theory and understanding of the world
- experiment new ways of being in order for learning to occur.

Attention to the experiential learning cycle will facilitate teaching *and* learning and ensure that different learning styles are respected and nurtured in any staff development programme.

How should we set about designing a staff development programme?

As formal staff development programmes are one of the most common ways of developing medical educators, this section will highlight some general guidelines that have been previously described and can be of use to staff developers.(14)

Understand the organisational culture

Staff development programmes take place within the context of a specific institution or organisation. It is imperative to understand the culture of that institution and to be responsive to its needs. Staff development programmes should also capitalise on the organisation's strengths and work with the leadership to ensure success. In many ways, the cultural context can be used to promote or enhance staff development efforts. For example, as some authors have suggested, 'staff development during times of educational or curricular reform can take on added importance'.(140) It is also important to assess institutional support for staff development activities, ascertain available resources and lobby effectively. Clearly, staff development cannot occur in a vacuum.(14)

Determine appropriate goals and priorities

As with the design of any programme, it is imperative to define goals and priorities carefully. What are we trying to achieve – and why is it important to do so? It is equally important to determine programme objectives as they will influence our target audience, choice of programme, overall content and methodology. Determining priorities is not always easy, and it often involves consultations with key stakeholders. However, it is always essential to balance individual *and* organisational needs.

Conduct needs assessments to ensure relevant programming

As stated earlier, staff development programmes should base themselves on the needs of the individual as well as the institution. Student needs, patient needs and societal needs may also help direct relevant activities.(14) Assessing needs is necessary to refine goals, determine content, identify preferred learning formats and assure relevance. It is also a way of promoting early 'buy-in'. Common methods include:

- written questionnaires or surveys
- interviews or focus groups with key informants (e.g. participants, students, educational leaders)

- observations of teachers 'in action'
- literature reviews
- environmental scans of available programmes and resources.(141,142)

Whenever possible, we should try to gain information from multiple sources and distinguish between 'needs' and 'wants'. Clearly, an individual teacher's perceived needs may differ from those expressed by their students or peers. Needs assessments can also help further translate goals into objectives, which will serve as the basis for programme planning and evaluation of outcome.

Develop different programmes to accommodate diverse needs

Different staff development formats have been described in an earlier section. Clearly, we must design programmes that accommodate diverse goals and objectives, content areas, and the needs of the individual and the organisation. For example, if our goal is to improve our colleagues' lecturing skills, a half-day workshop on interactive lecturing might be the programme of choice. On the other hand, if we wish to promote educational leadership and scholarly activity among our peers, a teaching scholars programme or educational fellowship might be the preferred method.(14) In this context, it is also helpful to remember that staff *development* can include development, orientation, recognition and support, and different programmes are required to accommodate diverse objectives.

Incorporate principles of adult learning and instructional design

As previously mentioned, adults come to learning situations with a variety of motivations and expectations about teaching methods and goals. Incorporation of these principles into the design of a staff development programme is clearly needed, as physicians demonstrate a high degree of self-direction and possess numerous experiences that should serve as the basis for learning.(14)

Principles of instructional design should also be followed. For example, it is important to develop clear learning goals and objectives, identify key content areas, design appropriate teaching and learning strategies, and create appropriate methods of evaluation of both the students and the curriculum. It is equally important to integrate theory with practice(143) and to ensure that the learning is perceived as relevant to the work setting and to the profession. Learning should be interactive, participatory and experientially based, using the participants' previous learning and experience as a starting point. Detailed planning and organisation involving all stakeholders is critical, as is the creation of a positive learning environment. However, although theory should inform practice, staff development initiatives must remain relevant and practical (*see* Box 32.5).

Offer a range of diverse educational methods

In line with principles of adult learning, staff development programmes should try to offer a variety of educational methods that promote experiential learning, reflection, feedback and immediacy of application. Common learning

BOX 32.5 WHERE'S THE EVIDENCE: Key features of staff development

The BEME review of faculty development initiatives designed to improve teaching effectiveness in medical education(36) found that the following 'key features' contribute to the effectiveness of staff development activities.

- *Experiential learning* – This includes the importance of applying what had been learned, practising skills and receiving feedback on these skills.
- *Provision of feedback* – The role of feedback in promoting change is important, as is the use of feedback as a specific intervention strategy.
- *Effective peer and colleague relationships* – This includes the value of peers as role-models, the mutual exchange of information and ideas and the importance of collegial support to promote and retain change.
- *Well-designed interventions following principles of teaching and learning* – Adherence to principles of instructional design and principles of adult learning promote effective learning and skill acquisition.
- *Use of multiple instructional methods to achieve intended objectives* – This includes a diversity of educational methods within single interventions to accommodate learning styles and preferences.

methods include interactive lectures, case presentations, small-group discussions and individual exercises, role-plays and simulations, videotape reviews and live demonstrations. Practice with feedback is also key, as is the opportunity to reflect on personal values and attitudes. Computer-aided instruction, debates and reaction panels, journal clubs and self-directed readings are additional methods to consider. In line with our previous example, a workshop on interactive lecturing might include interactive plenary presentations, small group discussions and exercises, and opportunities for practice and feedback. A fellowship programme might include group seminars, independent projects and structured readings. Whatever the method, the needs and learning preferences of the participants should be respected, and the method should match the objective. Health care professionals learn best 'by doing', and experiential learning should be promoted whenever possible.(14)

Promote buy-in and market effectively

The decision to participate in a staff development programme or activity is not as simple as it might at first appear. It involves the individual's reaction to a particular offering, motivation to develop or enhance a specific skill, being available at the time of the session and overcoming the psychological barrier of admitting need.(140) As faculty developers, it is our challenge to overcome reluctance and to market our 'product' in such a way that resistance becomes a resource to learning. In our context, we have seen the value of targeted mailings, professionally designed brochures and 'branding' of our product to promote interest. Continuing education credits, as well as free and flexible programming, can also help facilitate motivation and attendance. Buy-in involves agreement on importance, widespread support and dedication of time and resources at both the individual and the system level and must be considered in all programming initiatives.(144)

Work to overcome commonly encountered challenges

Common challenges faced by faculty developers include the following:

- lack of institutional support and resources for programme planning
- defining goals and priorities
- assessing needs and balancing individual and organisational needs
- motivating faculty to participate
- obtaining faculty buy-in
- promoting a 'culture change' that reflects renewed interest in teaching and learning.

Staff developers must inevitably work to overcome these problems through a variety of means that can include creative programming, skilled marketing and the delivery of high-quality activities. Flexible scheduling and collaborative programming, which address clearly identified needs, can also help ensure success at the system level.

Prepare staff developers

The recruitment and preparation of staff developers is rarely reported. However, it is important to recruit carefully, train effectively, partner creatively and build on previous experiences.(144) Medical educators can be involved in a number of ways: as co-facilitators, as programme planners or as consultants. In our own setting, we try to involve new faculty members in each staff development activity and conduct a preparatory meeting (or 'dry run') to review content and process, solicit feedback and promote 'ownership'. We also conclude each activity with a 'debriefing' session to discuss lessons learnt and plan for the future. Whenever possible, staff developers should be individuals who are well respected by their peers and have some educational expertise and experience in facilitating groups. It has been said that 'to teach is to learn twice'; this principle is clearly one of the main motivating factors for staff developers.

Evaluate – and demonstrate – effectiveness

The need to evaluate staff development programmes and activities is clear. In fact, we must remember that the evaluation of staff development is more than an academic exercise, and our findings must be used in the design, delivery and marketing of our programmes. It has also been stated earlier that staff development must strive to promote education as a scholarly activity; we must role-model this approach in all that we do.(5)

In preparing to evaluate a staff development programme or activity, we should consider the goal of the evaluation (e.g. programme planning versus decision-making, policy formation versus academic inquiry), available data sources (e.g. participants, peers, students or residents), common methods of evaluation (e.g. questionnaires, focus groups, objective tests, observations), resources to support assessment (e.g. institutional support, research grants) and models of programme evaluation (e.g. goal attainment, decision facilitation). Kirkpatrick's levels of evaluation(145) are also helpful in conceptualising and framing the assessment of outcome. They include the following:

- *reaction* – participants' views on the learning experience
- *learning* – change in participants' attitudes, knowledge or skills
- *behaviour* – change in participants' behaviour
- *results* – changes in the organisational system, the patient or the learner.

At a minimum, a practical and feasible evaluation should include an assessment of utility and relevance, content, teaching and learning methods, and intent to change. Moreover, as evaluation is an integral part of programme planning, it should be conceptualised at the beginning of any programme. It should also include qualitative and quantitative assessments of learning and behaviour change using a variety of methods and data sources. For more on evaluation methods *see* Chapter 27.

Conclusion

As the demands for accountability in higher education gain momentum, pressures to change professional conduct in medical education will continue to grow.(11) Moreover, as the emphasis on global standards in medical education increases,(10,146) so will the need for the professional development of medical educators. As Glicken and Merenstein(20) aptly state, faculty members often come to medical teaching with the 'wisdom and experience that dictates what their students need to know', although they have not been trained for the job at hand. Clearly, it is our responsibility to enable this training, either through formal or informal approaches.

We also need to remember that medical education is a social endeavour. Faculty members at McGill University have identified core attributes (including reflection, passion, enthusiasm and pride) and skills (such as the ability to maintain multiple perspectives, situate learning, work with others and see the 'big picture') needed to become a medical educator.(13) They have also highlighted the benefit of a community of scholars in the formation of medical educators (as outlined in Box 32.2). In many ways, these suggestions can serve as a road map for developing medical educators, as each of us finds joy and satisfaction in this journey of discovery: 'To me a medical educator is someone who devotes part of their career and time and interests towards medical teaching and education. It is not the title that counts. It is more the effort and the amount of time and the process and the products that get produced that defines the level of medical educator we become'.(13) 'You become a medical educator once you add the intangible – the passion and the commitment, the dedication and the creativity . . .'(13)

Acknowledgements

I would like to thank Dr Peter McLeod, Dr Linda Snell and Dr Peter Cantillon for their helpful comments on an earlier version of this chapter. I would also like to gratefully acknowledge my colleagues at the Centre for Medical Education and the Faculty of Medicine at McGill University for their continued participation, insights and feedback on our faculty development programmes and activities. My own understanding of this complex process would not have been possible without this 'community of practice'. Some of the material used in this chapter has been published previously in a contribution by the author to *A Practical Guide for Medical Teachers*(14) and to *Teaching Medical Professionalism*(147) and is reproduced here with permission.

References

1 Miller G (1980) *Educating Medical Teachers*. Harvard University Press, Cambridge, MA.

2 Jason H and Westberg J (1982) *Teachers and Teaching in US Medical Schools*. Appleton-Century-Crofts, New York.

3 Harris D, Krause K, Parish D and Smith M (2007) Academic competencies for medical faculty. *Family Medicine*. **39**: 343–50.

4 Skeff KM, Stratos GA, Bergen MR *et al.* (1999) Regional teaching improvement programs for community-based teachers. *American Journal of Medicine*. **106**: 76–80.

5 Steinert Y (2000) Faculty development in the new millennium: key challenges and future directions. *Medical Teacher*. **22**: 44–50.

6 Clark JM, Houston TK, Kolodner K *et al.* (2004) Teaching the teachers: national survey of faculty development in departments of medicine of US teaching hospitals. *Journal of General Internal Medicine*. **19**: 205–14.

7 McLean M, Cilliers F and Van Wyk JM (2008) Faculty development: yesterday, today and tomorrow. *Medical Teacher*. **30**: 555–84.

8 General Medical Council (2006) Good medical practice. (http://www.gmc-uk.org; accessed 10 December 2012).

9 International Association of Medical Educators (2012) Composite standards. (http://www.iaomc.org/cs.htm; accessed 10 December 2012).

10 World Federation for Medical Education (2007) Global standards programme. (http://www.wfme.org; accessed 10 December 2012).

11 Eitel F, Kanz KG and Tesche A (2000) Training and certification of teachers and trainers: the professionalization of medical education. *Medical Teacher*. **22**: 517–26.

12 Purcell N and Lloyd-Jones G (2003) Standards for medical educators. *Medical Education*. **37**: 149–54.

13 Steinert Y (2008) From teacher to medical educator: the spectrum of medical education. Unpublished report, Centre for Medical Education, Montreal.

14 Steinert Y (2005) Staff development. In: Dent J and Harden R (eds) *A Practical Guide for Medical Teachers*, pp. 390–9. Elsevier Churchill Livingstone, Edinburgh.

15 Centra JA (1978) Types of faculty development programs. *Journal of Higher Education*. **49**: 151–62.

16 Bland C, Schmitz C, Stritter F, Henry R and Aluise J (1990) *Successful Faculty in Academic Medicine: Essential Skills and How to Acquire Them*. Springer Publishing Company, New York.

17 Sheets KJ and Schwenk TL (1990) Faculty development for family medicine educators: an agenda for future activities. *Teaching and Learning in Medicine*. **2**: 141–8.

18 Steinert Y, Cruess RL, Cruess SR *et al.* (2007) Faculty development as an instrument of change: a case study on teaching professionalism. *Academic Medicine*. **82**: 1057–64.

19 Hafferty FW (1998) Beyond curriculum reform: confronting medicine's hidden curriculum. *Academic Medicine*. **73**: 403–7.

20 Glicken AD and Merenstein GB (2007) Addressing the hidden curriculum: understanding educator professionalism. *Medical Teacher*. **29**: 54–7.

21 Bligh J (2005) Faculty development. *Medical Education*. **39**: 120–1.

22 Swanwick T (2008) See one, do one, then what? Faculty development in postgraduate medical education. *Postgraduate Medical Journal*. **84**: 339–43.

23 Wilkerson L and Irby DM (1998) Strategies for improving teaching practices: a comprehensive approach to faculty development. *Academic Medicine*. **73**: 387–96.

24 Irby DM (1994) What clinical teachers in medicine need to know. *Academic Medicine*. **69**: 333–42.

25 Copeland HL and Hewson MG (2000) Developing and testing an instrument to measure the effectiveness of clinical teaching in an academic medical center. *Academic Medicine*. **75**: 161–6.

26 Academy of Medical Educators (2012) Professional standards. (http://www.wfme.org, accessed 10 December 2012).

27 Buchel TL and Edwards FD (2005) Characteristics of effective clinical teachers. *Family Medicine*. **37**: 30–5.

28 Wright SM and Carrese JA (2002) Excellence in role modeling: insight and perspectives from the pros. *Canadian Medical Association Journal*. **167**: 638–43.

29 Bordage G, Foley R and Goldyn S (2000) Skills and attributes of directors of educational programmes. *Medical Education*. **34**: 206–10.

30 Spencer J and Jordan R (2001) Educational outcome and leadership to meet the needs of modern health care. *Quality in Health Care*. **10**: ii38–45.

31 Boyer E (1990) *Scholarship Reconsidered: Priorities of the Professoriate*. Princeton University Press, Princeton, NJ.

32 Simpson D and Fincher R (1999) Making a case for the teaching scholar. *Academic Medicine*. **74**: 1296–9.

33 Glassick CE (2000) Boyer's expanded definitions of scholarship, the standards for assessing scholarship and the elusiveness of the scholarship of teaching. *Academic Medicine*. **75**: 877–80.

34 Higgs J and McAllister L (2007) Educating clinical educators: using a model of the experience of being a clinical educator. *Medical Teacher*. **29**: e51–7.

35 Fraser SW and Greenhalgh T (2001) Coping with complexity: educating for capability. *British Medical Journal*. **323**: 799–803.

36 Steinert Y, Mann K, Centeno A *et al.* (2006) A systematic review of faculty development initiatives designed to improve teaching effectiveness in medical education: BEME guide No. 8. *Medical Teacher*. **28**: 497–526.

37 Nasmith L and Steinert Y (2001) The evaluation of a workshop to promote interactive lecturing. *Teaching and Learning in Medicine*. **13**: 43–8.

38 Nasmith L, Steinert Y, Saroyan A *et al.* (1997) Assessing the impact of a faculty development workshop: a methodological study. *Teaching and Learning in Medicine*. **9**: 209–14.

39 Nayer M (1995) Faculty development for problem-based learning programs. *Teaching and Learning in Medicine*. **7**: 138–48.

40 Olmesdahl PJ and Manning DM (1999) Impact of training on PBL facilitators. *Medical Education*. **33**: 753–5.

41 Quirk ME, DeWitt T, Lasser D *et al.* (1998) Evaluation of primary care futures: a faculty development program for community health center preceptors. *Academic Medicine*. **73**: 705–7.

42 Wilkerson L and Sarkin RT (1998) Arrows in the quiver: evaluation of a workshop on ambulatory teaching. *Academic Medicine.* **73**: s67–9.

43 Steinert Y, Nasmith L and Daigle N (2003) Executive skills for medical faculty: a workshop description and evaluation. *Medical Teacher.* **25**: 666–8.

44 Steinert Y, Cruess S, Cruess R and Snell L (2005) Faculty development for teaching and evaluating professionalism: from programme design to curriculum change. *Medical Education.* **39**: 127–36.

45 Baldwin CD, Goldblum RM, Rassin DK and Levine HG (1994) Facilitating faculty development and research through critical review of grant proposals and articles. *Academic Medicine.* **69**: 62–4.

46 Steinert Y, McLeod PJ, Liben S and Snell L (2008) Writing for publication in medical education: the benefits of a faculty development workshop and peer writing group. *Medical Teacher.* **30**: e280–5.

47 Cusimano MD and David MA (1998) A compendium of higher education opportunities in health professions education. *Academic Medicine.* **73**: 1255–9.

48 Hitchcock MA, Lamkin BD, Mygdal WK et al. (1986) Affective changes in faculty development fellows in family medicine. *Journal of Medical Education.* **61**: 394–403.

49 Searle NS, Hatem CJ, Perkowski L and Wilkerson L (2006) Why invest in an educational fellowship program? *Academic Medicine.* **81**: 936–40.

50 Gruppen LD, Simpson D, Searle NS et al. (2006) Educational fellowship programs: common themes and overarching issues. *Academic Medicine.* **81**: 990–4.

51 Steinert Y, Nasmith L, McLeod PJ and Conochie L (2003) A teaching scholars program to develop leaders in medical education. *Academic Medicine.* **78**: 142–9.

52 Steinert Y and McLeod PJ (2006) From novice to informed educator: the teaching scholars program for educators in the health sciences. *Academic Medicine.* **81**: 969–74.

53 Rosenbaum ME, Lenoch S and Ferguson KJ (2005) Outcomes of a teaching scholars program to promote leadership in faculty development. *Teaching and Learning in Medicine.* **17**: 247–52.

54 Muller JH and Irby DM (2006) Developing educational leaders: the teaching scholars program at the University of California, San Francisco, School of Medicine. *Academic Medicine.* **81**: 959–64.

55 Steinert Y, Naismith L and Mann K (2012) Faculty development initiatives designed to promote leadership in medical education. A BEME systematic review: BEME guide No. 19. *Medical Teacher.* **34**: 483–503.

56 Wilkerson L, Uijtdehaage S and Relan A (2006) Increasing the pool of educational leaders for UCLA. *Academic Medicine.* **81**: 954–8.

57 Hatem CJ, Lown BA and Newman LR (2006) The academic health centre coming of age: helping faculty become better teachers and agents of educational change. *Academic Medicine.* **81**: 941–4.

58 Dearing R (1997) *Higher Education in the Learning Society: report of the National Committee of Inquiry into Higher Education.* HMSO, London.

59 Walsh K (2007) Professionalism in medical education: could an academy play a role? *Medical Teacher.* **29**: 425–6.

60 Cohen R, Murnaghan L, Collins J and Pratt D (2005) An update on master's degrees in medical education. *Medical Teacher.* **27**: 686–92.

61 Tekian A and Harris I (2012) Preparing health professions education leaders worldwide: a description of masters-level programs. *Medical Teacher.* **34**: 52–8.

62 Pugsley L, Brigley S, Allery L and Macdonald J (2008) Counting quality because quality counts: differing standards in master's in medical education programmes. *Medical Teacher.* **30**: 80–5.

63 Hesketh EA, Bagnall G, Buckley EG et al. (2001) A framework for developing excellence as a clinical educator. *Medical Education.* **35**: 555–64.

64 Flynn SP, Bedinghaus J, Snyder C and Hekelman F (1994) Peer coaching in clinical teaching: a case report. *Family Medicine.* **26**: 569–70.

65 Orlander JD, Gupta M, Fincke BG et al. (2000) Co-teaching: a faculty development strategy. *Medical Education.* **34**: 257–65.

66 Boud D and Middleton H (2003) Learning from others at work: communities of practice and informal learning. *Journal of Workplace Learning.* **15**: 194–202.

67 Lave J and Wenger E (1991) *Situated Learning: Legitimate Peripheral Participation.* Cambridge University Press, New York.

68 Barab SA, Barnett M and Squire K (2002) Developing an empirical account of a community of practice: characterizing the essential tensions. *The Journal of the Learning Sciences.* **11**: 489–542.

69 Wenger E (1998) *Communities of Practice: Learning, Meaning and Identity.* Cambridge University Press, New York.

70 Wenger E, McDermott R and Snyder W (2002) *Cultivating Communities of Practice.* Harvard Business School Press, Boston.

71 Bligh J and Brice J (2007) The Academy of Medical Educators: a professional home for medical educators in the UK. *Medical Education.* **41**: 625–7.

72 Cooke M, Irby DM and Debas HT (2003) The UCSF academy of medical educators. *Academic Medicine.* **78**: 666–72.

73 Irby DM, Cooke M, Lowenstein D and Richards B (2004) The academy movement: a structural approach to reinvigorating the educational mission. *Academic Medicine.* **79**: 729–36.

74 Bligh J (1999) Mentoring: an invisible support network. *Medical Education.* **33**: 2–3.

75 Morzinski J, Diehr S, Bower DJ and Simpson DE (1996) A descriptive, cross-sectional study of formal mentoring for faculty. *Family Medicine.* **28**: 434–8.

76 Pololi LH, Knight SM, Dennis K and Frankel RM (2002) Helping medical school faculty realize their dreams: an innovative, collaborative mentoring program. *Academic Medicine.* **77**: 377–84.

77 Daloz L (1986) *Effective Teaching and Mentoring.* Jossey-Bass, San Francisco.

78 Epstein RM, Cole DR, Gawinski BA et al. (1998) How students learn from community-based preceptors. *Archives of Family Medicine.* **7**: 149–54.

79 Ricer RE (1998) Defining preceptor, mentor, and role model. *Family Medicine.* **30**: 328.

80 Paice E, Heard S and Moss F (2002) How important are role models in making good doctors? *British Medical Journal.* **325**: 707–10.

81 Steinert Y and Walsh A (2006) *A Faculty Development Program for Teachers of International Medical Graduates.* Association of Faculties of Medicine of Canada, Ottawa.

82 Grant J (1998) Offering training and support to trainers. In: Paice E (ed.) *Delivering the New Doctor.* Association for the Study of Medical Education, Edinburgh.

83 Jolly B and Grant J (1997) *The Good Assessment Guide: A Practical Guide to Assessment and Appraisal for Higher Specialist Training.* Joint Centre for Education in Medicine, London.

84 Azer SA (2005) The qualities of a good teacher: how can they be acquired and sustained? *Journal of the Royal Society of Medicine.* **98**: 67–9.

85 Steinert Y, McLeod P, Boillat M et al. (2008) Faculty development: a Field of Dreams? *Medical Education.* **43**: 42–9.

86 Dandavino M, Snell L and Wiseman J (2007) Why medical students should learn how to teach. *Medical Teacher.* **29**: 558–65.

87 Topping KJ (1996) The effectiveness of peer tutoring in further and higher education: a typology and review of the literature. *Higher Education.* **32**: 321–45.

88 Hill AG, Yu TC, Barrow M and Hattie J (2009) A systematic review of resident-as-teacher programmes. *Medical Education.* **43**: 1129–40.

89 Seely AJE (1999) The teaching contributions of residents. *Canadian Medical Association Journal.* **161**: 1239–41.

90 Busari JO, Prince KJ, Scherpbier AJ, Van Der Vleuten CP and Essed GG (2002) How residents perceive their teaching role in the clinical setting: a qualitative study. *Medical Teacher.* **24**: 57–61.

91 Thomas PS, Harris P, Rendina N and Keogh G (2002) Residents as teachers: outcomes of a brief training programme. *Education for Health.* **15**: 71–8.

92 Peluso MJ and Hafler JP (2011) Medical students as medical educators: opportunities for skill development in the absence of formal training programs. *The Yale Journal of Biology and Medicine.* **84**: 203–9.

93 Bing-You RG and Sproul MS (1992) Medical students' perceptions of themselves and residents as teachers. *Medical Teacher.* **14**: 133–8.

94 Haist SA, Wilson JF, Brigham NL, Fosson SE and Blue AV (1998) Comparing fourth-year medical students with faculty in the teaching of physical examination skills to first-year students. *Academic Medicine.* **73**: 198–200.

95 Edwards JC, Friedland JA and Bing-You R (2002) *Residents' Teaching Skills.* Springer, New York.

96 Sternszus R, Cruess SR, Cruess RL *et al.* (2012) Residents as role models: impact on undergraduate trainees. *Academic Medicine.* **87**: 1282–7.

97 Walton JM and Patel H (2008) Residents as teachers in Canadian paediatric training programs: a survey of program director and resident perspectives. *Paediatrics and Child Health.* **13**: 675–9.

98 Busari JO and Scherpbier AJ (2004) Why residents should teach: a literature review. *Journal of Postgraduate Medicine.* **50**: 205–10.

99 Seely AJ, Pelletier MP, Snell LS and Trudel JL (1999) Do surgical residents rated as better teachers perform better on in-training examinations? *American Journal of Surgery.* **177**: 33–7.

100 Busari JO, Scherpbier AJ, van der Vleuten CP and Essed GG (2006) A two-day teacher-training programme for medical residents: investigating the impact on teaching ability. *Advances in Health Sciences Education: Theory and Practice.* **11**: 133–44.

101 Pasquinelli LM and Greenberg LW (2008) A review of medical school programs that train medical students as teachers (MEDSATS). *Teaching and Learning in Medicine.* **20**: 73–81.

102 Pasquale SJ and Pugnaire MP (2002) Preparing medical students to teach. *Academic Medicine.* **77**: 1175–6.

103 Soriano RP, Blatt B, Coplit L *et al.* (2010) Teaching medical students how to teach: a national survey of students-as-teachers programs in U.S. medical schools. *Academic Medicine.* **85**: 1725–31.

104 Wamsley MA, Julian KA and Wipf JE (2004) A literature review of 'Resident-as-Teacher' curricula. Do teaching courses make a difference? *Journal of General Internal Medicine.* **19**: 574–81.

105 Bardach NS, Vedanthan R and Haber RJ (2003) 'Teaching to teach': enhancing fourth year medical students' teaching skills. *Medical Education.* **37**: 1031–2.

106 Nestel D and Kidd J (2002) Evaluating a teaching skills workshop for medical students. *Medical Education.* **36**: 1094–5.

107 Craig JL and Page G (1987) Teaching in medicine: an elective course for third-year students. *Medical Education.* **21**: 386–90.

108 Schaffer JL, Wile MZ and Griggs RC (1990) Students teaching students: a medical school peer tutorial programme. *Medical Education.* **24**: 336–43.

109 Walker-Bartnick LA, Berger JH and Kappelman MM (1984) A model for peer tutoring in the medical school setting. *Journal of Medical Education.* **59**: 309–15.

110 Evans DJ and Cuffe T (2009) Near-peer teaching in anatomy: an approach for deeper learning. *Anatomical Sciences Education.* **2**: 227–33.

111 Morrison EH, Rucker L, Boker JR *et al.* (2004) The effect of a 13-hour curriculum to improve residents' teaching skills: a randomized trial. *Annals of Internal Medicine.* **141**: 257–63.

112 Moser EM, Kothari N and Stagnaro-Green A (2008) Chief residents as educators: an effective method of resident development. *Teaching and Learning in Medicine.* **20**: 323–8.

113 Berkenbosch L, Bax M, Scherpbier A, Heyligers I, Muijtjens AM and Busari JO (2013) How Dutch medical specialists perceive the competencies and training needs of medical residents in healthcare management. *Medical Teacher.* **35**: e1090–102.

114 Blumenthal DM, Bernard K, Bohnen J and Bohmer R (2012) Addressing the leadership gap in medicine: residents' need for systematic leadership development training. *Academic Medicine.* **87**: 513–22.

115 Ackerly DC, Sangvai DG, Udayakumar K *et al.* (2011) Training the next generation of physician-executives: an innovative residency pathway in management and leadership. *Academic Medicine.* **86**: 575–9.

116 Kuo AK, Thyne SM, Chen HC *et al.* (2010) An innovative residency program designed to develop leaders to improve the health of children. *Academic Medicine.* **85**: 1603–8.

117 Paller MS, Becker T, Cantor B and Freeman SL (2000) Introducing residents to a career in management: the Physician Management Pathway. *Academic Medicine.* **75**: 761–4.

118 Larson DB, Chandler M and Forman HP (2003) MD/MBA programs in the United States: evidence of a change in health care leadership. *Academic Medicine.* **78**: 335–41.

119 Sherrill WW (2000) Dual-degree MD-MBA students: a look at the future of medical leadership. *Academic Medicine.* **75**: S37–9.

120 Accreditation Council for Graduate Medical Education (2012) Competency evaluation system. (http://www.acgme.org/acgmeweb/; accessed 10 December 2012).

121 Frank J (2005) The CanMEDS 2005 physician competency framework. (http://www.royalcollege.ca/portal/page/portal/rc/common/documents/canmeds/resources/publications/framework_full_e.pdf; accessed 10 December 2012).

122 Kanna B, Deng C, Erickson SN *et al.* (2006) The research rotation: competency-based structured and novel approach to research training of internal medicine residents. *BMC Medical Education.* **6**: 52.

123 Rivera JA, Levine RB and Wright SM (2005) Completing a scholarly project during residency training: perspectives of residents who have been successful. *Journal of General Internal Medicine.* **20**: 366–9.

124 Walton NA, Karabanow AG and Saleh J (2008) Students as members of university-based Academic Research Ethics Boards: a natural evolution. *Journal of Academic Ethics.* **6**: 117–27.

125 MacDougall J and Drummond M (2005) The development of medical teachers: an enquiry into the learning histories of 10 experienced medical teachers. *Medical Education.* **39**: 1213–20.

126 Brown JS, Collins A and Duguid P (1989) Situated cognition and the culture of learning. *Educational Researcher.* **18**: 32–42.

127 Knowles M (1984) *Andragogy in Action.* Jossey-Bass, San Francisco.

128 Knowles M (1980) *The Modern Practice of Adult Education: From Pedagogy to Androgogy.* Cambridge Books, New York.

129 Kolb D and Fry R (1975) Towards an applied theory of experiential learning. In: Cooper C (ed.) *Theories of Group Processes.* John Wiley, London.

130 Cruess RL and Cruess SR (2006) Teaching professionalism: general principles. *Medical Teacher.* **28**: 205–8.

131 McLellan H (1996) *Situated Learning Perspectives.* Educational Technology Publications, Englewood Cliffs, NJ.

132 Mann K (2006) Learning and teaching in professional character development. In: Kenney N (ed.) *Lost Virtue: Professional Character Development in Medical Education.* Elsevier, New York.

133 Schön D (1983) *The Reflective Practitioner: How Professionals Think in Action.* Basic Books, New York.

134 Hewson MG (1991) Reflection in clinical teaching: an analysis of reflection-on-action and its implications for staffing residents. *Medical Teacher.* **13**: 227–31.

135 Lachman N and Pawlina W (2006) Integrating professionalism in early medical education: the theory and application of reflec-

tive practice in the anatomy curriculum. *Clinical Anatomy.* **19**: 456–60.

136 Robertson K (2005) Reflection in professional practice and education. *Australian Family Physician.* **34**: 781–3.

137 Norman GR (1999) The adult learner: a mythical species. *Academic Medicine.* **74**: 886–9.

138 Merriam SB (1996) Updating our knowledge of adult learning. *Journal of Continuing Education in the Health Professions.* **16**: 136–43.

139 Boud D, Keogh R and Walker D (1985) *Reflection: Turning Experience into Learning.* Kogan Page, London.

140 Rubeck RF and Witzke DB (1998) Faculty development: a field of dreams. *Academic Medicine.* **73**: S32–7.

141 Grant J (2002) Learning needs assessment: assessing the need. *British Medical Journal.* **324**: 156–9.

142 Lockyer J (1998) Needs assessment: lessons learned. *Journal of Continuing Education in the Health Professions.* **18**: 190–2.

143 Kaufman D, Mann K and Jennett P (2000) *Teaching and Learning in Medical Education: How Theory can Inform Practice.* Association for the Study of Medical Education, Edinburgh.

144 Steinert Y (2005) Staff development for clinical teachers. *The Clinical Teacher.* **2**: 104–10.

145 Kirkpatrick D (1994) *Evaluating Training Programs: The Four Levels.* Berrett-Koehler Publishers, San Francisco.

146 Karle H (2007) European specifications for global standards in medical education. *Medical Education.* **41**: 924–5.

147 Steinert Y (2009) Educational theory and strategies for teaching and learning professionalism. In: Cruess R, Cruess S and Steinert Y (eds) *Teaching Medical Professionalism*, pp. 31–52. Cambridge University Press, New York.

33 Educational leadership

Judy McKimm[1] and Tim Swanwick[2]
[1]College of Medicine, Swansea University, UK
[2]Health Education North Central and East London, UK

 KEY MESSAGES

- Leadership is a social construct that reflects the preoccupations of the time.
- Leadership and strategic management are inextricably intertwined.
- Leadership is, first and foremost, about change.
- The most effective leaders have well-developed self-insight coupled with knowledge and awareness of the strengths and abilities of their 'followers'.

- Effective health care education leaders have to work across multiple boundaries; organisational, cultural and professional.
- Educational leadership in health care occurs within complex environments.
- Effective leadership requires deep contextual awareness and the ability to scan the horizon
- Leadership is about being and doing; leaders need to 'walk the walk'.

Introduction

Education leaders in medical and other health professions carry a 'double burden'. They have to manage and lead universities and other educational institutions in a rapidly changing global environment while working in close collaboration with a range of health care delivery partners with their own financial and service-driven agendas. The complexity and pace of change in health care means that the need for effective leaders and leadership development has never been so important; however, in a sector that is continually focused on the achievement of targets and balancing budgets, training and development are not always given the highest priority.

Nationally, health care education is driven by key governmental health and educational policy initiatives that set the context for educational leaders. These include aspirational policies, such as 'widening access' and expanding higher education, as well as an inexorable drive towards greater public accountability – a problematic area for leaders who work in universities traditionally run on collegial models of participative but autonomous decision-making and consensus.

Bush[1] notes that it is vital for education leaders to maintain 'education' as their central concern. This is difficult to achieve in the health care sector, where there are inherent tensions between the purposes of *education*, the demands of *vocational training*, which has as its goal the production of a competent, safe future workforce and the demands of delivering a high quality service to patients and communities. Funding for the different stages and parts of medical education is often misaligned and, depending on the health

and education structure in different countries, derived from different places: the public sector (e.g. government departments), private and voluntary sectors, charities, endowments and non-governmental organisations.

In many countries, leadership development in the health services has been intrinsically linked to service redesign, improvements and delivery. For example, in the UK, the NHS Institute for Innovation and Improvement, has been responsible for developing the *NHS Leadership Qualities Framework*,[2] a series of *Improvement Leaders' Guides* and more recently, a *Medical Leadership Competency Framework*.[3] Leadership in the NHS is firmly sited in service improvement, and the newly formed NHS Leadership Academy (http://www.leadershipacademy.nhs.uk/) lays out an underpinning philosophy about leadership development – one that assumes that leadership skills can be learned, aligns leadership qualities with management capabilities, locates leadership and leadership development at all levels within the organisation and aims to create an empowerment culture based on supporting people, the transformation of followers into leaders and the development and creation of a shared vision.[4] (*See* Figure 33.1.)

In higher (or tertiary) education, which educates and trains the medical and health care workforce of the future at pre-registration level, public sector service improvement does not have the same priority, and policy agendas differ. Most higher education strategies focus on delivering a high quality student experience, ensuring equity of access and outcome, enhancing research outputs and ensuring graduates are fit for employment or further study. Performance indicators use various metrics to identify and reward universities and colleges for achieving these aims. There are

Understanding Medical Education: Evidence, Theory and Practice, Second Edition. Edited by Tim Swanwick.
© 2014 The Association for the Study of Medical Education. Published 2014 by John Wiley & Sons, Ltd.

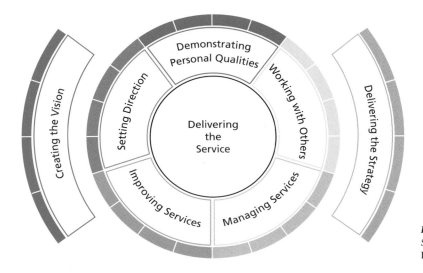

Figure 33.1 Leadership Framework.
Source: The Leadership Framework is ©NHS
Leadership Academy, 2011.(4) All rights reserved.

some inherent tensions and contradictions in leading change in today's public sector organisations. For health care education, this is exacerbated by differences between health service and education policies, values, systems and practices.

Another unique feature that faces health care educators is the challenge of leading education across professional boundaries. Leaders in health care education have to be aware of the needs and demands of multiple stakeholders in the current drive to produce competent health care practitioners, open to working in a flexible way. Working with academics, clinicians, health care managers and professionals with differing values and education systems means that leaders need to quickly establish credibility with different stakeholders, use and develop sound interpersonal skills and demonstrate effective management capabilities.

Leadership training and development is often patchy and not easy to access for more junior staff. Higher education has traditionally been focused on developing the management skills of heads of departments and more senior management rather than forming part of succession planning and developing leadership capacity at all levels. Changes in skills mix and professional roles, changes in funding and commissioning arrangements and emerging organisational changes such as mergers, collaborations and partnerships will mean that tomorrow's health care education leaders will require higher-level leadership and management skills than ever before.

Leadership and management

There are many definitions of leadership. Leadership theory looks not only at individuals but also at the relationship between leaders and followers and the context or situation in which they operate. In recent years, many theorists have found it useful to distinguish between *management* and *leadership*, and although there is considerable overlap and interdependency, differentiating between the two concepts will help us begin to explore what leadership is and

some of the assumptions made about, and expectations of, people working in educational settings.

For Bennis and Nanus, 'managers are people who do things right and leaders are people who do the right thing'.(5) Managers are often described as performing *functions* in organisations, usually holding a particular formal title or fulfilling a particular role. Management is concerned with planning, organising, coordinating, commanding or controlling the activities of staff.(6) Leaders, by contrast, aim to influence and guide others into pursuing particular objectives or visions of the future and to motivate them into wanting to follow. Yukl suggests that 'leadership is the process of influencing others to understand and agree about what needs to be done and how it can be done effectively and the process of facilitating individual and collective efforts to accomplish the shared objectives'.(7)

Kotter(8) contrasts leadership and management and suggests that whereas leadership sets a direction and develops a vision for the future, that is, producing change and movement, management is more concerned with planning and with providing order and consistency in organisations rather than the process of producing change. Covey *et al.* put a slightly different slant on this, suggesting that managers work within an existing 'paradigm', solve problems and manage people, whereas leaders create new paradigms, challenge systems, seek new opportunities and lead people.(9)

The differences between leadership and management identified by many authors over the years are succinctly summarised by Northouse(10) (*see* Box 33.1). However, contemporary leadership theory, for example, Blagg and Young,(11) Yukl(7) and Storey,(12) suggests that in practice it is often the same person who operates in both capacities and that the most effective people in organisations are both managers and leaders.

Furthermore, in universities, administrators are often distinguished from academics, reflecting the way in which university systems have developed. The terms 'leaders' and 'managers' are not so widely used, although individuals clearly fulfil management and leadership functions. In

BOX 33.1 Management versus leadership
(adapted from Northouse(10))

Management	Leadership
Produces order and consistency through:	*Produces change and movement through:*
• Planning and budgeting	• Setting direction
• Problem-solving	• Problem defining
• Organising and staffing	• Building commitment
• Controlling and monitoring	• Motivating and sustaining

practice, the barriers and constructs that often worked to place academics and administrators seemingly in opposition to one another are breaking down, as educational organisations are becoming more aware of the need to operate efficiently and effectively in an increasingly competitive global market. Educational leaders can no longer rely wholly on formal positional authority but must seek to develop and display appropriate leadership characteristics and qualities, and it is increasingly recognised that people at all levels in an organisation have the potential to perform and display leadership.

A brief history of leadership

The next two sections consider leadership models and theories, charting their development and unpicking the contribution that they make in enhancing our understanding of what leaders do and what leadership is. It is important to remember that leadership is a social construct; theories and models of leadership tend therefore, to be of their time and reflect the prevailing public 'mood' and the preoccupations of (largely North American) enterprise. Leadership theories and models can be broadly divided into three overlapping categories, as follows:
- those which focus on the personal qualities or personality of the leader as an individual
- those which relate to the interaction of the leader with other people
- those which seek to explain leadership behaviours in relation to the environment or system.(13)

In the first half of the 20th century, leadership theory revolved around personal qualities, an approach based on the assumption that leaders are born rather than made. This gave rise to the pervasive idea of the 'great man' or 'heroic' leader who will be a leader under any circumstances. The 'great man' theories emphasised characteristics such as intelligence, energy and dominance, but several major reviews of the literature failed to consistently identify personality traits that differentiated leaders from non-leaders. Interestingly, trait theory has made a comeback in recent years with the emotional intelligence theories of Goleman,(14) and research on the influence of personality traits on leadership behaviours.(15) From the 1950s onwards, attention shifted from personal characteristics of

leaders to their behaviours, in particular, how their *style* and behaviours impacted on groups. Blake and Mouton,(16) for instance, consider the differences between 'task-focused' and 'people-focused' leaders and argue that high levels of concern for both is what is required, while authors such as Tannenbaum and Schmidt(17) argued for a range of leadership styles involving varying degrees of delegated autonomy, from the 'autocratic' to the 'abdicatory'.

While these models introduce the idea of leadership as a group of behaviours, they give little indication as to what sort of behaviours worked best in what circumstances. This was addressed through the work of, among others Fiedler(18) and Hersey and Blanchard.(19) who describe a range of 'contingency theories'. The latter achieved widespread popularity through the *One Minute Manager* series with their explication of *situational* leadership. Hersey and Blanchard's argument is that leaders need to adapt their style to variations in the competence and commitment of followers. The four styles identified are: directing, coaching, supporting and delegating. A situational approach to leadership is also adopted by Adair in his 'three circles' model.(20) Adair recommends that, depending on the circumstances, the focus of a leader's attention should be distributed flexibly between the *task*, the *individual* and the *team*.

It became apparent in the 1980s that none of the existing leadership theories offered advice on how to cope in environments of continuous change. Various authors highlighted that the models described so far were effectively managerial or transactional which helped people plan, order and organise at times of stability but were inadequate at describing how people or organisations might be led through periods of significant change. A new paradigm emerged – that of *transformational* leadership:(21) leadership through the transformation of the willingness of others to work towards the goal of some future desired state.

A fusion of the transformational notion of social influence and leadership trait theory led, in the 1980s and 1990s, to the emergence of *charismatic* leadership as a solution to organisational problems. Effective leaders were viewed as dominant personalities brimming with self-confidence and offering a clearly articulated ideology. They offered a strong role model and had high expectations of followers. However, it quickly became apparent that this culture of organisational 'heroes' was both unhealthy and unsustainable, and more recently there has been a shift towards thinking that emphasises the thoughtful, value-led leader, highlighting the notion of followership and relational leadership;(22,23) bringing to the fore ideas of *distributed*,(24) *engaging*(25) and *collaborative*(26) leadership. More recent considerations of leadership emphasise that leaders need to be aware of and responsive to the complexity of the systems and organisations in which they work.(27,28) From these perspectives, models such as adaptive or eco-leadership have emerged.(29)

However, as many authors, including Bryman(30) and Storey,(12) have noted, these stages signal a change in emphasis – not a shift away – from previous models. Like the abominable snowman, a definitive model of leadership remains an elusive thing to track down.

Educational management and leadership

Writers and researchers who have focused on educational leadership and management, as opposed to general theories of leadership, tend to locate phenomena associated with educational leadership within various paradigms,(31) perspectives,(32) models(1) or metaphors.(33) All these terms tend to be applied in similar ways rather than reflect significant differences in meaning, and we will use them interchangeably here.

National education policies emphasise the centrality of educational leadership and management. There is no shortage of leadership advice from government, consultants, academics and education authorities to leaders in schools, colleges and universities, but as Bush notes, 'many of these prescriptions are atheoretical in the sense that they are not underpinned by explicit values or concepts'.(34) Although leadership and management are practical activities, theories can help inform and influence practice by suggesting new ways and frameworks in which events, interrelationships and situations can be seen. Pragmatic decisions might appear to be common sense, but 'common sense' is grounded in assumptions, limitations, a view about an organisation and a particular frame of reference. 'Theory-for-practice'(35) encourages us to look at organisations and relationships in a different light, helping us interpret and make sense of complexity and ambiguity and make relevant and informed management and leadership decisions.

Most of the theory and research on educational management and leadership relates to the context of schools and colleges with very little in the context of the education of health professionals. However, the broader research is useful in helping us look at the organisations and relationships involved in delivering medical education.

Bush and Glover(36) describe a typology of management models, building on previous work by Leithwood *et al.*(37) This framework, with its parallel grouping of leadership theories, is shown in Box 33.2. As discussed above, we believe that effective leadership is inextricably intertwined with strategic management, and for the remainder of this section shall consider general leadership theories alongside their analogous management paradigms. On the way, we will also consider the applicability of each model to the leadership and management of health professions' education.

Formal management: managerial leadership

Formal management models view educational organisations as hierarchical, bounded bureaucratic systems with an official structure – often represented by an organisational chart – and relationships characterised by virtue of the legitimate authority vested in them. Managerial decisions are seen as objective, rational and goal oriented. Leaders have positional power over those beneath them but are accountable to internal and external bodies or committees, such as the senate, councils or boards.

Theories drawn from structural or system sociology underpin these managerial models, most notably the concept of *bureaucracy*. Weber(38) describes a bureaucratic

---

BOX 33.2 Typology of management and leadership models (adapted from Bush and Glover(36))

Management model	Leadership model
Formal	Managerial
Collegial	Participative
	Transformational
	Interpersonal
	Distributed
	Collaborative
Political	Transactional
Subjective	Post-modern
Ambiguity	Contingent
Cultural	Value-driven

---

organisation as existing to achieve established purposes, with work best achieved through specialisation, division of labour, coordination and control, a description that sits well with contemporary education organisations.

In *managerial leadership*, leaders are responsible for:

- setting goals and ensuring the organisation reaches the goals
- maintaining the integrity of the educational structure and working within it using power and authority to the organisation's advantage
- 'bounding' the system in alignment with how the organisation sees the relationship with the external environment.

In these models, leaders are often seen, and revered, as holding much of the organisation's power and are expected to make decisions based on their own knowledge and expertise. In practice, most organisations invest power and authority across a senior management team rather than in a single leader, thus ensuring that the hierarchy stays in place and that the formal systems, structures and procedures are maintained. These 'Apollonian'(39) structures can provide a platform for the 'hero' leader; indeed, in education, such a figure may actively be sought out. Universities, for instance, often invest a huge amount of time, energy and resources in seeking out the best new vice-chancellor. Storey notes that in a managerial organisation, 'The need for leadership is often addressed in terms of the "reputational capital" that a celebrated leader can bring . . . this is very interesting and revealing because it highlights the importance of stakeholder perception'.(12)

In reality, modern educational organisations are complex and 'messy'; professional staff expect to be consulted and involved in decision making; goals are difficult to state and measure, as many of them are long term; and individuals do not necessarily behave in a prescribed way. In medical and health care education, additional areas of conflict arise because many individuals have authority and power in one arena – for instance, in their role as a consultant clinician – but may have little organisational power or authority in an academic setting. This, coupled with traditional power discrepancies between the professions in terms of authority, accountability, status and reward, means that there are additional tensions in health care education organisations that do not exist in schools, colleges or other university departments.

So, while it is recognised that bureaucracy may be an appropriate organisational model for educational management,(40) inherent weaknesses exist – predominantly a tendency for the organisation to become preoccupied with the maintenance of its own structure and processes (rules, regulations and procedures), thus forgetting its original educational purposes or relegating them to a position of subordinance.(41) Another general criticism is that bureaucracies are deprofessionalising, stripping away the autonomy of practitioners,(42) an issue explored in more detail by Mintzberg.(43) If the leader focuses too much on the system, and forgets to balance this with paying attention to the teams and individuals that work in the organisation, then there is risk of over-management and lack of creativity and responsiveness to change.

Minztberg dissects organisations into five generic components and in doing so identifies a simple organisational taxonomy, namely, organisations as:

- a machine bureaucracy
- a professional organisation
- an entrepreneurial start-up
- an adhocracy.

A *machine bureaucracy* can be conceptualised a factory or production line, pumping out a standardised product under instructions from management. In the *entrepreneurial start-up*, the owner-manager takes the strategic decisions while remaining hands-on in the day-to-day business of the organisation. The *adhocracy* is an ambiguous and organic form in which structural elements combine, disassociate and recombine to address complex problems. Health care education tends to be structured in *professional bureaucracies*, and this has profound implications for management and leadership.

In a professional organisation, Mintzberg(43) suggests that a small *strategic apex*, assisted by a supportive *technostructure* and *staff*, manages through a small *middle line* a large *operating core* of professionals. For the coordination of its work, a professional bureaucracy relies on the standardisation of skills through training and indoctrination, and although the operating professionals have considerable control, the standards to which they perform are set outside the structure of the organisation, usually by a self-governing association of fellow professional organisations. The professional tends to resist rationalisation of their skills as this drives the structure towards that of a machine bureaucracy, thus destroying professional autonomy. Organisational strategy in the professional organisation is represented by the cumulative effect over time of multiple projects or initiatives undertaken by its members. As a consequence of these characteristics, the professional organisation tends to be rather inflexible, good at producing a standard unchanging product but ill suited to adaptation. Response to change is slow – evolution as opposed to revolution – and 'top-down' calls for reform are usually resisted.

In a professional organisation operating in a *collegial* management model, leaders and managers are seen to sit 'alongside' colleagues rather than manage from 'above'.(44) even though the organisational charts may portray otherwise. Collegiality assumes a common set of values, an authority of expertise and decisions reached through a process of discussion leading to consensus. Collegiality has been shown in mainstream education to improve the quality of decision making, to bring about more effective implementation and, perhaps most importantly, to be the type of management teachers want.(45)

Unfortunately, as will be apparent, collegial management in the public sector is in conflict with the prevailing bureaucratic culture, a conflict heightened by governmental pressures for increased output and greater public accountability.

Collegial management: transformational, interpersonal and distributed leadership

The collegial management model is normative; it is believed that members of the organisation share beliefs, values and norms and that decision making is made democratically. However, this belief is often illusory rather than grounded in reality, and leaders need to spend time ensuring that consultation and participation in decision making is real. They need to seek out and clearly define the beliefs and values that individuals and groups from different professional backgrounds share. Collegial decisions are founded on expert authority.

The collegial model is highly appropriate for small professional organisations. Larger units, such as universities, also retain many elements of collegiality in that they have extensive committee structures to facilitate representation and participation, and academic autonomy and freedom are valued at the 'bottom-up' approach. However, there has always been a separation between academic and non-academic staff and the right to participation in decision making that these roles enjoy. More recently, universities have been described as moving towards a more 'top-down', managerial model, partly in response to increased competition in a global marketplace. This shift also enables clear organisational goals that 'fit' all disciplines and professional groups within the educational organisation to be agreed. It has also led Hargreaves to describe the emergence of a phenomenon widespread in the public sector, that of 'contrived collegiality'(45) consultation without the possibility of control.

The management model of collegiality sits with participative, transformational, relational and distributed/shared leadership models, all of which rest on the notion of the leader as 'first among equals',(46) utilising the skills of influencing, negotiation, listening, facilitation and consensus building rather than acting in the role of a commanding and controlling hero leader. Such leaders are aware of the complexity and interactivity of decision-making processes and are able to recognise and harness the expertise of the professionals whom they lead, as well as demonstrate sensitivity towards the 'informal codes of professional practice which govern expectations' between the leader and his or her staff.(47)

A number of what have come to be known as 'new paradigm' models of leadership(30) emerged in the 1980s. Transformational, charismatic and visionary leaders define organisational reality through the articulation of a clear vision and its supporting values. Thus new paradigm models depict leaders as managers of meaning rather than in terms of the way they influence processes. In the public sector, and notably in the NHS, transformational leadership has been seen as the key to addressing some of the limitations of a transactional approach, and the NHS leadership frameworks for example contain an interesting amalgam of the two paradigms where 'empowering others' can be found nestling alongside 'holding to account'.

Leadership has experienced a major re-interpretation from representing an authority relationship (now referred to as management or transactional leadership which may or may not involve some form of pushing or coercion) to a process of influencing followers or staff for whom one is responsible, by inspiring them, or pulling them to a vision of some future state . . . this new form of leadership is called transformational leadership because such individuals transform followers.(48)

Transformational leadership is characterised by the '4 Is' of Bass and Avolio:(21)
- idealised influence
- inspirational motivation
- individualised consideration
- intellectual stimulation.

Transformational leadership and its near relatives, *interpersonal* and *relational leadership*,(1) are rooted in the philosophical belief that meaning is socially constructed. Grint describes the 'constitutive approach' as one in which leaders not only mould followers' interpretation of the environment but also present it as being the correct interpretation.(49) Here lies one of the critiques of transformational leadership, in that leaders may be tempted to manipulate meaning to suit their own ends. Writers such as Maccoby(50) highlight that there is a dark side to such charismatic leadership, that of the narcissistic leader, who can challenge change and disrupt the status quo but also can be arrogant and grandiose, thriving on risk and seeking power, glory and admiration. A wave of corporate scandals over the last twenty years has served to highlight the dangers of a narcissistic leader. Further on in this chapter, we shall see how the concepts of 'value-led' or 'servant' leadership help to compensate for some of the possibly negative aspects of the transformational approach.

Another post-charismatic model of leadership is described by Fullan,(51) a model based around embedded learning, devolved leadership in teams, and learning as a product of confrontation, mistakes and experimentation. Practice is made public in a collaborative culture. *Distributed leadership* or 'leadership at all levels' is currently receiving considerable attention in education and the health care sector(52) though not without critical challenge.(53,54)

The case for distributed leadership is made on the basis of the following:
- a belief in leadership teams: a team being a more effective unit than an individual

- the fact that as organisations become more complex places to manage and lead, there is a need for leadership at all levels, with 'coherence making'(28) as everyone's responsibility
- the development of pools of talent, from which tomorrow's leaders may be drawn.

A related model is that of *collaborative leadership*, focussing on a commitment to partnership working for the good of service users, draws on many of the approaches outlined above. However, it also demands a specific set of qualities and behaviours. Collaborative leadership too, shares the burden but also the power and resources. This requires that 'collaborative leaders are personally mature. They have a solid enough sense of self that they do not fear loss of control'.(55) Above all, collaborative leaders must listen, and be seen to do so. As van Zwanenberg notes: 'The person in a position of leadership who is not open to actively listening, questioning and reflecting in a very conscious way will be judged as a hypocrite if they continue to talk the language of partnership . . .'(56).

All of the above models value human capital and the development of sustainable organisations, and for leaders and managers this has a clear message. An effective organisation will align the motivational goals of the individual employee with its own needs, not only to motivate employees but to avoid risk. A strong organisation is resilient and (through the people involved in its activities) can respond appropriately to internal and external change. The consequences of poor role/person fit are profound, and Argyris(57) found that over time, frustration intensified, leading to absenteeism, psychological withdrawal, restriction of output, feather bedding, sabotage and formation of power groups to redress the balance. The alternative strategy was to climb the hierarchy to, what was perceived to be a better job and perpetuate the whole process.

To summarise a wealth of literature on the human side of organisations, successfully led organisations *empower* employees and *invest* in people (*see* Box 33.3).

Political management: transactional leadership

Power flows in educational organisations through three main conduits, as follows:
- bureaucratic processes (boards, committees, management hierarchies)
- collegiality (consensual decision making informed by expert knowledge)
- micro-politics(58) (negotiation, bargaining, conflict, subterfuge).

The potential sources of power in organisations have been analysed by a number of theorists.(59,60) Hoyle,(35) for instance, has distinguished four main types, as follows:
- *structural* – power as the property of office
- *personality* – charisma and 'the aura of authority'
- *expertise* – which includes access to information as well as specialised knowledge
- *opportunity* – power through the occupancy of key administrative roles.

BOX 33.3 Leading through people

Empower employees	Invest in people
• Redesign work	• Hire the right people
• Provide autonomy	• Reward them well
• Encourage participation	• Promote from within
• Focus on job enrichment	• Train and educate
• Emphasise teamwork	• Share the wealth
• Ensure upward influence	

Politics then is ultimately about the deployment of such resources through the wielding and yielding of power, and the day-to-day interactions of people and their ideologies. Sometimes, considerable power resides in the lowliest of roles, such as the hospital laundry worker or switchboard operator. Authority(61) is a related concept, differentiated from power in Box 33.4. Baldridge's work on universities in the USA(46) highlights the role that interest and pressure groups have on influencing decision making and forcing change. His model of how policies emerge is iterative and dynamic: competition for scarce resources leading to formal and informal grouping jostling and positioning themselves for control, with power accruing to dominant coalitions. Personal and professional interests feed into the melee, the former in relation to status, working conditions and reward, and the latter to gain commitment to particular ways of working, curricular models, teaching and learning methods or student groupings.(36)

Hoyle describes how educational leaders can adopt political strategies to achieve their aims.(36) These include *dividing and ruling, co-optation, displacement, controlling information,* and *controlling meetings,* the last of these strategies achieved through the dubious strategies of rigging agendas, losing recommendations, lobbying members of the group, invoking outside bodies or massaging minutes.

The exercise of power is also a major preoccupation of *transactional leadership,* a leadership model based on the following four assumptions:

- people are motivated by reward and punishment
- social systems work best with a clear chain of command
- authority resides within line management
- subordinates are there to do what their manager tells them.

Leadership of the transactional variety starts then to look very much like management, a similarity emphasised by Kotter,(62) who asserts that transformational leadership is about strategy and people, whereas transactional leadership revolves around systems and resources. Kotter though, is also clear that both leadership paradigms are needed in an effective organisation.

> Leadership is different from management, but not for the reason people think. Leadership isn't mystical and mysterious. It has nothing to do with having charisma or other exotic personality traits. It's not the province of the chosen few. Nor is leadership necessarily better than management or a replace-

BOX 33.4 FOCUS ON: Power and authority

The relationship between power and authority is not straightforward. It is perfectly possible to have one without the other. Power, as has been described, is about the control and manipulation of scarce resources – whether they be physical, economic, knowledge-based or to do with personal qualities.(5) Authority relates to the right, or perceived right, to exercise power.

According to the economist and sociologist Max Weber,(61) all leaders are surrounded in a myth of superiority that derives from three forms of legitimate authority: charismatic, traditional and rational–legal domination.

Charismatic domination derives from the personal qualities of the leader. Many religious leaders, and some political ones, derive their authority from this form of domination.

Traditional domination relates to positions that preserve long-established values and social relationships. In the UK, the Royal Family carry authority, not because of charisma but because an otherwise meritocratic society allows them to continue to adopt that social position derived purely from inheritance.

Rational or legal domination is the most advanced, and relates to authority as a function of delegated power within a bureaucraticy. Those in authority give orders (and expect to be obeyed) because their office gives them the right to give orders. However, there is a context-specific element to this, and orders are only to be obeyed if they are relevant to the situation in which they are given. The head of your department or school has rational–legal authority, and who knows, may also have charisma . . .

Power in educational institutions may go hand in hand with authority, such as those budgetary decisions made by the dean, head, principal or executive board. However, power in organisations is often wielded without authority through a process of 'influence' and micro-politics.

ment for it: rather leadership and management are two distinctive and complementary activities. Both are necessary for success in an increasingly complex and volatile business environment.(8, p. 103)

Subjective management: post-modern leadership

Bush(1) describes subjective management models as those which 'assume that organisations are the creations of people within them'. Participants are thought to interpret situations in different ways, and these individuals' perceptions are derived from their background and values. In this socially constructed view, organisations' structures, people and activities have different meanings for each of their members and exist only in the experience of those members. Different writers vary in the emphasis they put

---

BOX 33.5 Leadership that gets results:(14) The leadership styles

	Coercive	Authoritative	Affiliatative	Democratic	Pace-setting	Coaching
What the leader does	Demands immediate compliance	Mobilises people towards a vision	Creates harmony and builds bonds	Forges consensus through participation	Sets high standards for performance	Develops people for the future
When it works best	In a crisis	When a clear direction is needed	To heal rifts and motivate people in stressful circumstances	To get buy-in from valuable employees	To obtain quick results from a well-motivated team	To help an employee improve their performance
Overall effect on climate	–	++	+	+	–	+

---

on individuals rather than the organisation; some see the tension between the individual perspective and organisational collective as a 'chasm', whereas others see it more like a dialectic, with interdependence between constantly changing individual and collective meanings.

Post-modern leadership is a relatively undefined concept; it has similarities to the subjective model in that different actors are seen as bringing multiple meanings and realities to any organisation or situation. 'Situations must be understood at local level with particular attention to diversity';(63) this emphasises the fluid and 'chaotic' nature of contemporary society in which power is *enacted* (ibid) through all members, thus leading to empowerment. Leaders need to rely on their skills as interpreters of meaning articulated in different ways by multiple stakeholders. The hero visionary does not fit in the post-modern world; leaders need to listen to, and focus on, people as individuals with their own world views.

Ambiguity management: contingent leadership

Ambiguity models emphasise organisational change, uncertainty and unpredictability. Organisational goals, systems and processes are seen as unclear and not well understood, and participation in decision making is fluid as individuals opt in and out. Organisations are characterised by fragmentation and 'loose coupling',(64) particularly educational organisations in which members have a high degree of autonomy and discretion. The most famous of the models is the 'garbage can' model described by Cohen and March(65) in their research into colleges and universities, identifying that decisions are the result of fluid processes in which problems, solutions, participants and choice opportunities all interact to generate outcomes or decisions.

Gilbert(66) defines *situational* or *contingent leadership* as 'an approach based on the commonsensical idea that there will be interactions in most situations between the leader's attitude and attitudes, the tasks to be undertaken, the strengths and weaknesses of the team and the environment in which the leader and team have to operate'. Contingency leadership models see leaders as having to adapt their

stance and style to the particular situation rather than seeing one leadership approach as being the 'right' one. Peck *et al.*(67) note, for example, that 'transformational characteristics may be more appropriate in the earlier stages of a transition process, with the transactional characteristics required to stabilise transformational change'. It is not that one is superior or inferior to the other but rather that effective leaders appear to be able to utilise many styles and select those appropriate to the specific situation.

What are those styles? A Hay-McBer study identified six drivers of organisational climate or working atmosphere(14) (*see* Box 33.5). Effective leaders used all styles flexibly dependent on the situation, with the *authoritative* leadership style found to have the most positive effect on business performance of the six.

In the complex world of medical and health care education, effective leaders will be those who can respond to different situations in a measured way, selecting the appropriate leadership style to suit the situation. This point is particularly relevant for those who are coming from one leadership role (e.g. in clinical practice) into another (e.g. academia), as Gilbert(66) highlights: 'Success in one environment does not necessarily translate to another'. However, being able to adopt different styles of leadership is not the same as changing one's personality. Followers value authenticity and consistency in leaders very highly, these behaviours generate trust which is a key element of high-performing teams.

Cultural management: value-led leadership

Cultural models of management are very influential in mainstream education, and they emphasise the importance of informal modes of influence and of the centrality of values, beliefs and ideologies. Individuals are seen as actors who bring their ideas and values to their relationships with others. In turn, this influences the way in which an organisation develops norms and traditions – 'the way we do things around here'(68) – which are reinforced by symbols, ceremonies and rituals. Symbols are central to the construction of meaning, and in medical and health care education these abound as part of the undergraduate (pre-registration) socialisation process and continue throughout professional life. The importance of understanding the meaning ascribed to linguistic, behavioural and visual or physical symbols cannot be underestimated by leaders, particularly those who want to work inter-professionally or across organisations.

A strong organisational culture enables people to identify themselves and their aspirations with the purpose of the organisation and can heighten faith and confidence in an organisation in the midst of environmental turbulence and adversity. Organisational culture can be influenced in a variety of ways. The academic trappings (gowns, maces, medals, crests, etc.) adopted by many professional organisations in medicine are good examples of how cultural expression serves to define, or brand, an organisation. Small changes in culture make big differences, and it is the leader's responsibility to pay attention to the detail as well as the big picture. Quite often, the solution to an underperforming organisation is not to undertake a massive restructuring exercise but to change the organisational culture which again requires leadership at all levels.

Leaders also need to be aware of how changing demographics and widening participation impact on organisational and professional cultures; issues concerning gender, race, ethnicity and class can lead to a need to reframe cultural norms and values. Leaders may well have to deal with uncomfortable moments as once-dominant ideologies and positions are challenged and come under scrutiny.

Leaders with a strong ethical and value-led approach, which acknowledges cultural shifts and responds appropriately, will be more effective than those who operate merely on exchange transactions. Such values-driven or moral leaders need to ensure that their central values accord with those in the educational organisation, or there will be dissonance and discomfort for all those involved. In times of financial hardship and competing agendas, maintaining integrity and an ethical stance can sometimes be very difficult, particularly so if we do not fully know ourselves. Such self-knowledge features large in the writings of Daniel Goleman on emotional intelligence. Goleman[69] argues that in order to be successful in dealing with others, it is important to have effective awareness, control and management of your own emotions and a deep understanding of your own goals, responses and behaviour patterns.

Personal values and concern for others are also at the heart of Greenleaf's[70] *servant leadership*, where, as Collins puts it, 'professional will is seen alongside personal self-effacement'.[71] The difference between the servant leader and other forms of leadership is that the servant leader 'is servant first . . . It begins with the natural feeling that one wants to serve, to serve first. Then conscious choice brings one to aspire to lead'.[69] The primacy of serving a higher purpose has made Greenleaf's approach popular in the church and not-for-profit sectors and the central concept of 'stewardship' sits easily alongside the drive to develop sustainable organisations and embed succession planning through the diffusion of leadership throughout the organisation.

One particular value-led approach that is particularly relevant to medical education is that of *instructional leader-ship* which Bush describes as 'focussing on the direction rather than the process of leadership . . . with a firm emphasis on the purpose of education and the need to focus on teaching and learning as the prime purpose of educational institutions'.[1] Although this model emerged out of school leadership, in professional education increasingly there is a renewed focus on teaching and learning and in supporting teachers' professional development. Examples of instructional leadership can be seen in the establishment of bodies such as the Academy of Medical Educators[72] in the UK, and in the appointment of senior managers in health care organisations and in universities with named responsibilities for 'teaching and learning' or education.

Leading teams

Recent thinking then has shifted the leadership focus back from whole organisations to distributed leadership involving small groups and teams.[52,73] *Team building* has long been a part of organisational and professional development activities. Manz and Sims suggest that a new management style will be needed for team-based organisations – *superleadership* – with the locus of control shifting from the leader to the team.[74]

Teachers use team-leading and team-building concepts all the time when they are managing groups of students and trainees, and the majority of teacher training programmes include small-group teaching, looking at the role of the teacher as facilitator in helping a group achieve its outcomes in terms of both task and process. In educational leadership, aspiring or existing leaders can draw on their educational expertise and use their skills in a transferable way with the teams they are leading.

Recent research by the UK Government's Performance and Innovation Unit[75] suggests that the climate within a given team can account for up to 30 per cent of its performance and that the leader of the team has a primary role in creating the appropriate climate. The climate of a team is difficult to break down into its component parts but includes elements such as levels of personal autonomy, adequate reward and recognition, and clarity of roles and boundaries. An effective leader then will need an understanding of the nature of teams and the necessary conditions for them to function well. Adair[20] proposes that a team leader should strive to maintain a balance between three key areas of need in order to achieve team and organisational objectives in a sustainable way. It would be difficult to imagine any situation where a perfect balance between the three needs is always achieved, but the task of the leader is to attempt to maintain balance and also to manage the situation when one of the three (usually task) takes precedence over the others.

Team leaders need to have certain behaviours that facilitate teamworking. Kozlowski *et al.*[76] identify the following helpful behaviours:
- developing shared knowledge among team members
- acting as a mentor
- instructing others
- facilitating group processes

- providing information
- monitoring performance
- promoting open communication
- providing goals
- allocating resources efficiently.

Other skills include the ability to lead participative meetings, listening skills, the ability to handle conflict, group-centred decision-making skills, team-building skills, and coaching and developing skills.

Teams are dynamic units that are constantly evolving, and this evolution involves a number of identifiable stages famously identified by Tuckman.(77) The stage at which a team finds itself – forming, storming, norming or performing – is directly related to the quality and quantity of its output. A team leader needs to know which stage his or her team is at and support the team through its various transitions.

For a team to achieve its potential, it is also essential that the operational roles of its members are matched as closely as possible to their individual working and social style. People function within teams in different ways, but these can be identified and roles can be allocated accordingly to ensure that the team reaches its full potential. Belbin(78) famously classifies individual behaviours in teams into nine distinct 'roles' – observable tendencies of individuals to relate with their colleagues and contribute to the team (*see* Box 33.6).

A number of tools are available to help analyse the membership of the team. However, the ability of the leader to identify preferred roles using a degree of intuition should not be underestimated. It must also be borne in mind that team roles are tendencies, not fixed patterns, and most team members will have at least one secondary tendency. Not every team will have all roles at its disposal, but Belbin's research found that teams that did, tended to perform more effectively. If there are elements missing, it falls on the leader to find ways to address the shortfall.

Perhaps the most important caveats that should accompany such an approach, particularly in the context of higher education, are that no single team role is more important than another and that the potential weaknesses of each role should be seen as allowable. Successful teams thrive on their diversity and allow members to play on their strengths. Attempting to change behaviours may be counterproductive and stifle individuality. The task of the leader is to exploit the strengths, allow for the weaknesses and exploit the natural motivation that an understanding of the needs and capacities of everyone in the team engenders.

Leading change

Like leadership, change is an elusive concept, and literature on change and change management is vast.(79–81) As a working definition, change can be considered as the transformation of an individual or a system from one state to another, a process that may be initiated by internal factors or external forces or both. An understanding of the nature of change and change management is essential for any educational leader, none more so than those who work in

> **BOX 33.6 Belbin team roles**(78)
>
> **Plant:** an 'ideas person'. Thoughtful, creative, brilliant, radical. Better at thinking than communicating. Not interested in details.
>
> **Co-ordinator:** the 'chairperson'. A good team captain. Involves all team members and plays a mediator role in discussions. Co-ordinates work rather than doing it.
>
> **Monitor evaluator:** the 'critic'. Evaluates everything carefully, seeing both sides of every argument. Cold and objective. Can be perceived as negative and/or unenthusiastic.
>
> **Implementer:** a 'doer'. A reliable worker who puts ideas into action and gets on with it. May not be very imaginative or flexible.
>
> **Completer finisher:** the conscientious details person. Pays attention to detail and completes the job. Can be a worrier.
>
> **Resource investigator:** the 'networker'. The group's ambassador and detective, making friends and tracking down information and resources. Initial enthusiasm can fade before the project is completed.
>
> **Shaper:** the 'driver'. Pushes through ideas and keeps projects moving, enjoying the cut and thrust of the action. Can upset others as they do this.
>
> **Teamworker:** the 'peacemaker'. Lubricates the team with diplomacy and helps keep the team working effectively. Everybody's friend. Can be indecisive.
>
> **Specialist:** the 'expert'. Provides technical or other specialist knowledge to the team. Input is usually restricted to their own specialism.

the health sector. Behind every effort to lead change is a set of assumptions or theories, whether implicit or explicit, about how to bring that change about. In considering recent developments in health care education, we wish to emphasise a shift in the conceptualisation of change and change management that has occurred in recent years.

Mintzberg(82) summarises this shift in thinking in arguing that change can be thought of as either a pre-planned and predictable event or alternatively as an open-ended, ongoing and unpredictable process aimed at aligning and realigning in response to a changing environment. Early attempts at delineating change, such as that of Lewin,(83) focused on defining phases or stages of the process that might be managed before moving on to the next. Lewin's model describes unfreezing the present situation, moving to a new situation and refreezing. Bullock and Batten(84) similarly define a four-stage model of exploration–planning–action–integration. Implicit in both, and indeed in many other models, is the constancy of both the existing and the new state and the assumption that, given the appropriate skills and resources, the movement to the new state can be brought about in a controlled manner. Yet more models of change emphasise the problem-solving approach of problem identification, solution generation, choice of solution, implementation and evaluation,(85,86) again stressing a rational, linear progression through the change process.

More recently, there has been twofold acceptance that a rational approach to change will only get you so far and that it is change, not stability, that is the steady state.

House(32) notably outlines a trilogy of perspectives on educational change: *technological, cultural* and *political*. Not only does this provide a useful model for the analysis of change events but it acknowledges the importance of issues other than the innovation itself, particularly how innovations are interpreted and integrated into their destination social fabric (the cultural perspective) and how power, authority and competing interests are played against each other (the political perspective). That is not to say that a techno-rational approach to change is wrong, but as we have discussed, having multiple perspectives or frames through which to examine problems enables a richer repertoire of management strategies to be deployed.

The second emerging theme is the acceptance that change is here to stay. Furthermore, as Fullan points out, 'it is a mug's game to hope for the speed of change to slow down'.(87) Change and reform in education, and indeed the health service, have become a way of life. In recent years, seemingly disconnected and often conflicting policies have rained down on health and education professionals with increasing rapidity as politicians attempt to make their mark in a rapidly revolving political cycle. However, this is not a new phenomenon, and Baker has concluded after a lifetime of study of educational reform that: 'Planned change for (educators) is not the cumulative development of a comprehensive strategy. Rather, it is "one dammed thing after another"'.(88)

Leading complex systems

Multiple perspectives on change and the 'acceleration of just about everything'(89) are then acknowledged features of our social era, a period that has been labelled variously as postmodernity,(90) late capitalism,(91) and the informational society.(92) These key features have led naturally to an interest in complex systems by social scientists. Indeed, Hargreaves *et al.*(93) adds a fourth 'post-modern' perspective to House's original typology acknowledging *complexity* – alongside two other characteristic elements of late capitalism, consumerism and diversity – as a key feature of 21st-century educational change. New paradigms of change management are developing, borne out of the language of chaos and complexity theory, a relatively new area of scientific enquiry, a little more than 15 years old, which offers insights into the behaviour of large-scale physical, biological and social systems. Complexity theory arises from the observation that order will often spontaneously emerge out of what appears to be chaos. Complexity deals with the nature of emergence, innovation, learning and adaptation.(94)

Human systems have a tendency to avoid the onset of chaos if at all possible. Sometimes, this occurs to such a great extent in organisations that stability and equilibrium set in, leading to stereotypical patterns of behaviour and poor change responsiveness. However, the environment is sufficiently chaotic and elements within in it sufficiently inter-related not to allow the state to persist for long, and an oscillation sets in between the twin pulls of the urge to maintain integrity (autopoeisis) and the impulse to explore and adapt to the changing environment.

In social systems, stasis occurs where there is a high level of agreement and an equally high level of certainty. Chaos ensues when there is neither agreement nor certainty. Between these two extremes lies an area of variable agreement and variable certainty, and this is the zone of complexity where anything is possible, the 'swampy lowlands'(95) wherein lie the really important problems worth grappling with.

Businesses,(96) schools(45) and health care organisations(97,98) have all been viewed as 'complex adaptive systems' where 'order is not totally predetermined and fixed, but the universe (however defined) is creative, emergent (through iteration, learning and recursion), evolutionary and changing, transformative and turbulent'.(79) Despite this constant disequilibrium, the complex adaptive system strives to create order out of chaos, constantly reorganising in response to the changing environment. Complex adaptive systems display 'perpetual novelty'(99) and a propensity for problem solving. So what does complexity mean for educational leadership?

Broadly, the literature identifies a spectrum of possible ways that leaders might interact with a complex system ranging from the descriptive to the manipulative.(98) (*See* Figure 33.2.) At the interactionist end of this spectrum are the systems thinkers of the 1980s who position themselves outside the system, recommending influencing it through judicious and thought-through interventions.(100) More nihilistic are academics such as Stacey(101) who see the leader's role as one of articulating emerging themes and making tentative suggestions about what might be going on. Axelrod and Cohen(102) occupy some of the middle ground in their advice for those that seek to influence, to pay attention to internal processes, particularly those that foster variation, encourage interaction of system agents and promote selection pressures. Alongside them, Johnson and Scholes(103) are two of a number of authors who advocate concentration on developing a culture in which more-or-less the right thing is then likely to happen, more of the time.

Across the spectrum, the message is the same, essentially a non-directive approach to change management, as Mintzberg and colleagues advise: 'The best way to manage change is to allow for it to happen, to be pulled by the concerns out there rather than being pushed by the concepts in here'.(103)

Pascale *et al.*(104) similarly advocate perturbing the system and standing back to observe the results. Fullan(28) too countenances, 'never a check list – always complexity' but does set out a series of observations on complex change (*see* Box 33.7), which provide useful guidance for the instigators of educational reform. Importantly though, in addition to recognising the self-determination of complex systems, Fullan also emphasises the importance of leadership to the change process.

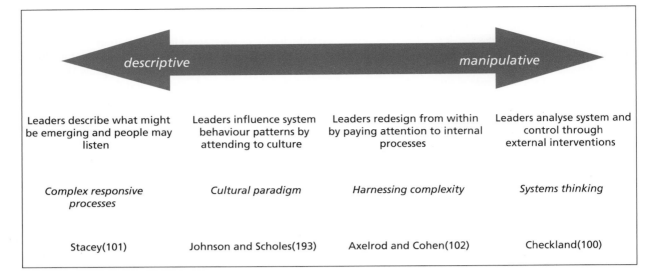

Leaders describe what might be emerging and people may listen	Leaders influence system behaviour patterns by attending to culture	Leaders redesign from within by paying attention to internal processes	Leaders analyse system and control through external interventions
Complex responsive processes	*Cultural paradigm*	*Harnessing complexity*	*Systems thinking*
Stacey(101)	Johnson and Scholes(193)	Axelrod and Cohen(102)	Checkland(100)

Figure 33.2 Leading in complex systems.

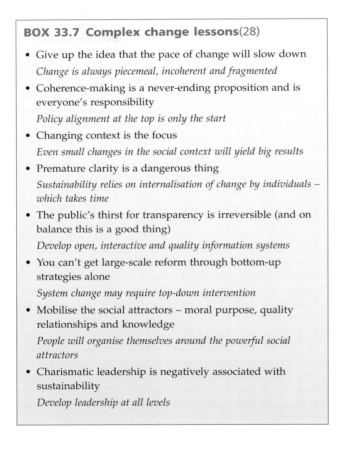

BOX 33.7 Complex change lessons(28)

- Give up the idea that the pace of change will slow down
  Change is always piecemeal, incoherent and fragmented
- Coherence-making is a never-ending proposition and is everyone's responsibility
  Policy alignment at the top is only the start
- Changing context is the focus
  Even small changes in the social context will yield big results
- Premature clarity is a dangerous thing
  Sustainability relies on internalisation of change by individuals – which takes time
- The public's thirst for transparency is irreversible (and on balance this is a good thing)
  Develop open, interactive and quality information systems
- You can't get large-scale reform through bottom-up strategies alone
  System change may require top-down intervention
- Mobilise the social attractors – moral purpose, quality relationships and knowledge
  People will organise themselves around the powerful social attractors
- Charismatic leadership is negatively associated with sustainability
  Develop leadership at all levels

Fraser and Greenhalgh(105) summarise a number of complexity concepts applicable to education and training, a follows.

- Neither the system nor its external environment is, or ever will be, constant.
- Individuals within a system are independent and creative decision makers.
- Uncertainty and paradox are inherent within the system.
- Problems that cannot be solved can nevertheless be 'moved forward'.
- Effective solutions can emerge from minimum specification.
- Small changes can have big effects.
- Behaviour exhibits patterns (that can be termed 'attractors').
- Change is more easily adopted when it taps into attractor patterns.

Both Fraser and Greenhalgh and Fullan acknowledge the complex nature of educational change and that self-organisation of an educational system can occur given minimal direction. Both also acknowledge the importance of *attractors* or traits within systems that set the direction for this self-organisation. Values, principles, goals, theories and leadership can all act as attractors, pulling together ideas, information, people and energy in generating new and emergent patterns.

Setting direction

As we identified earlier, one of the key features of leadership, as opposed to management, is the setting of direction through the articulation of a vision and the development of a strategy.

Strategy, though, is a word that has multiple meanings concisely summarised by Mintzberg *et al.*,(106) namely:

- *a plan* – a guide to take one along a path from a current state to some future state
- *a pattern* – a consistent pattern of behaviour
- *a position* – the location of a particular product in a market
- *a perspective* – a way of interacting
- *a ploy* – a tactic designed to outwit a competitor.

Also, one, some or all of these constructions may be employed in the process of strategic planning.

Strategic planning has a number of functions. It sets direction, focuses effort, defines the organisation and provides a consistency of approach and behaviour. However, there are downsides, as a strategic plan, beautifully written and long in gestation, may encourage 'groupthink', blinding the leadership of an organisation to new opportunities. Consistency, too, is not always desirable, as it may serve to overlook the rich diversity within any organisation. A strategic plan needs therefore to be flexible enough to take into account changes in the environment or new ideas and ways of doing things that emerge during the plan's lifetime.

The classic model of strategic planning traces a journey from a vision (often expressed as 'purpose' or a 'mission'), through aims, objectives and action plans, to monitoring arrangements (*see* Figure 33.3). It is a pathway underpinned by the expressed and (one hopes) lived values of the organisation.

To be successful, strategic planning needs to take account of the views of all stakeholders. For a medical school department, these might include the university, students, teachers and tutors, the hospital, the local postgraduate organisation, other medical schools, patient groups, professional bodies and regulators. Taking people with you is key, and to settle on a strategic direction too early in the process is fraught with danger. In Claxton's words, 'slow knowing' is the key: 'One needs to be able to soak up experience of complex domains – such as human relationships – through one's pores, and to extract subtle, contingent patterns that are latent within it. And to do that one needs to be able to attend to a whole range of situations patiently without comprehension; to resist the temptation to foreclose on what that experience may have to teach'.(107, p. 192)

Strategic planning should therefore have at its heart a reiterative process of evaluative analysis, a gauging and regauging of the operating environment of the organisation, canvassing the views of stakeholders, understanding trends and developing an awareness of the shaping forces at work. Through this process, leaders may also act to 'seize the future'(2) as they work outside their own organisation to shape the key uncertainties that lie ahead. A number of approaches may be used to gather information to inform a strategic plan, and some of these are illustrated in Box 33.8.

Having articulated a vision and, through an iterative process, agreed on a number of strategic aims or broad statements of intent, organisational objectives can be defined. To be effective, objectives should be SMART: specific, measurable, achievable, realistic, time bounded. Tactics and action plans can then be developed to meet the stated objectives and plans put in place for monitoring and evaluation. This is now the arena of project management about which, much has been written.(108) but we will not dwell on here. Throughout this iterative process, the leader needs to ensure that at all levels, the strategic plan is concordant with the organisation's agreed values. Without a strong backbone of values, a strategic plan becomes meaningless, and commitment will be lacking. In order to keep organisational values fresh and meaningful, they themselves should be reviewed and rearticulated on a regular basis.

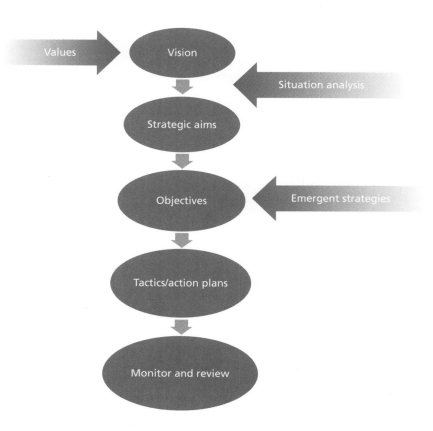

Figure 33.3 Strategic planning.

BOX 33.8 HOW TO: Develop a strategic plan

A number of tools may assist the process of strategic planning.

SWOT analysis

SWOT enables the organisation to identify its specific competencies, and alongside consideration of its values ensures that there is good alignment between the external environment and internal situation. The mnemonic stands for: the organisation's internal Strengths; the organisation's Weaknesses; the Opportunities presented by the external environment; and Threats in the external environment.

Gap analysis

Gap analysis is done to map the gap that exists between implied and specified future requirements and the existing situation. Gap analysis highlights services and/or functions that have been accidentally left out, deliberately eliminated or are yet to be developed or procured. The underlying method is simple and revolves around two simple questions: Where are we now, i.e. where will we be if we don't change anything? Where do we want to be, i.e. what does the environment demand of us?

PEST analysis

PEST provides a means of identifying possible futures facing an organisation and is useful for broadening perspectives on future strategy. The four PEST headings are: Political, Economic, Social and Technological.

Porter's 'Five Forces'

Another model developed by Michael Porter of the Harvard Business School(109) is designed to aid an analysis of the organisation's environment and the attractiveness of the industry. The five forces are the:

- risk of new competitors
- threat of substitute products
- bargaining power of buyers
- bargaining power of providers
- degree of competitive rivalry between existing institutions.

Through choosing an appropriate strategy, the organisation can alter the impact of these forces to its advantage, e.g. by collaborating, rather than competing with rivals.

Stakeholder analysis

Stakeholder analysis provides a tool to explore how the views of others might affect the implementation of your strategy. All individuals or groups that might have an interest in your plan are listed and defined as 'opposed', 'neutral' or 'supportive'. How far would you have to move an individual or group for the plan to succeed? It may be enough just to shift some stakeholders to neutral, but essential to obtain the active support of others. How might the plan be presented differently to meet the needs of each group (think politically here) and/or what changes might you have to make in order to make it acceptable or desirable?

Scenario-planning

Traditional forecasting methods often fail to predict significant changes, particularly when the environment is turbulent and unpredictable. Scenario-planning enables us not to predict the future, but to devise a number of possible futures for the organisation concerned. A strategy can then be developed that would best equip the organisation to survive in those possible worlds. Scenario-planning is best carried out by a group that includes representation from all walks of the organisation, as the idea is to devise scenarios that take into account as many different perspectives as possible.

Leading for improvement

Donald Berwick, one of the great contemporary thinkers on health care improvement, defined what he called the 'central law of improvement',(110) namely, that *every system is perfectly designed to achieve the results it achieves*. From this, he developed the idea that real improvement can only occur from changing systems, not changing within systems. Effective leaders of improvement then, rather than exhorting or cajoling people to work harder within a system, challenge the very system itself and provide a vision of a superior alternative.

A simple model for achieving change that results in improvement – and change and improvement are not necessarily the same thing – asks three basic questions:(111)
- What are we trying to achieve?
- How will we know if a change leads to an improvement?

- What changes could we make that we think will result in improvement?

There are several leadership elements to these questions. Clarity about what is to be achieved is an absolute obligation on the leader, to set the aims and mission of the organisation and to communicate these clearly. The more clearly aims are articulated, the greater the chance of them being realised.

The second of the questions relates to the measurement of outcomes, not as a way of instituting punishment or reward (e.g. star ratings and league tables) but as a means to learn. If we introduce this new assessment system, how will we know that it makes a difference? How will we know whether a problem-based learning curriculum will lead to better doctors?

Also, in an educational field full of self-determining professionals, a third key leadership task is to provide an environment that encourages innovation and experimentation. Constant small improvements that involve everyone in the organisation expand the available 'gene pool' of ideas and potential solutions. The 'never-ending proposition' of 'coherence making'(87) then becomes everyone's responsibility.

Change-adept organisations empower their members and build capacity through personal professional development. In a change-responsive organisation, blame is eliminated, innovation is encouraged, and there is an open environment of continuous improvement. In schools, promoting the professional development of colleagues has been found to be central in helping teachers cope with and instigate change.(112) In addition, Lomax(113) suggests that a research perspective is needed, encouraging all staff to think critically about their work. In this way, a professional learning community can be developed.

In developing a climate of continuous learning and improvement, we are in effect building a *learning organisation*. Learning organisations concern themselves with learning at all levels and place a high value on both individual and organisational development. As such, they are said to be quicker to adapt to change.(114)

Improvement as described becomes predominantly a developmental issue and one of getting the organisational culture right. What if things go wrong? As discussed in the section on human resources above, rewarding people well, both materially and through positive feedback, is important in terms of motivation. However, there is a flip side to this. The leader who does not intervene when performance is slipping or praises contributions that are substandard, as well as those that are excellent, cheapens their positive regard and will lose the respect of their followers. Without clear and consistent standards to which followers are held accountable, praise and reward will have no value.

Challenges for health care education leaders

Leading in medical and education, especially at senior level, can lead to particular issues and challenges not encountered by those working in other educational disciplines or contexts. One of the main reasons is that medical education is developed and delivered across professional, subject discipline and organisational boundaries. The organisations involved are bound by their own structures, systems, funding mechanisms, cultures, norms and values, and it is often difficult to straddle the clinical–academic 'divide'.

McKimm(115) carried out interviews with a small number of established leaders in medical and health care education in the UK and identified a set of issues and challenges consistently noted by the interviewees. Similar issues were also noted by Lieff and Albert(116) in their research on Canadian medical education leaders.

Personal issues
- Maintaining an appropriate work–life balance is difficult, especially for those with domestic commitments.

- The culture of senior management practice in both clinical and academic life has impact on career progression for those with domestic responsibilities.
- Some women noted the existence of the 'glass ceiling' and impact of taking career breaks.
- Leaders who had trained as clinicians had to make decisions on how to manage both clinical and academic careers and when/if to leave clinical practice.
- Leaving clinical practice is tied in with maintaining leadership credibility.
- Aspiring leaders with non-traditional career backgrounds feel that they will be overlooked in consideration for senior management positions, especially at medical schools.

Organisational and cultural issues
- Many organisational barriers to leadership exist; leaders need to understand the culture and anthropology of their own organisation to succeed.
- Some leaders felt that their profession, discipline or clinical specialty is perceived in a stereotyped or 'less serious' way by others, and this has impeded career development.
- Clinicians from some specialties may be better able to cope with the dual demands of clinical and academic life than those from others.

Balancing competing agendas
- An overwhelming issue identified is working within a rapidly changing and complex health care system.
- Dual demands of working in higher education (which is highly accountable) and the NHS (which is subject to rapid change) put a strain on health care education leaders not found in other sectors of higher education.
- Tensions between management styles, cultures, values and demands of higher education and the NHS – a 'crowded stage' with multiple task masters.

The wider agenda
- Health care education leaders need to be aware of their influential role in changing and improving health care systems.
- Senior medical education leaders need an accessible forum for discussion of high level educational change.
- Leaders need to be aware of the wider educational and health care agendas and help drive issues such as interprofessional learning and collaboration, promoting diversity and innovation in educational management and leadership.

The issues and challenges raised by the leaders in the study highlight that most leaders in medical and health care education will at some point have to make decisions about their leadership direction and whether that lies predominantly in higher education, a clinical setting, undergraduate or postgraduate education. Many opportunities exist for leading at various levels and in different contexts in medical education. Becoming aware of the opportunities available and matching this to experience and capabilities are a part of the leadership journey, often revisited many times during a career.

Leadership development

As Storey points out: 'the public sector has ... addressed the leadership development agenda in a particularly high profile and emphatic way'.(12) In parallel with the shifting perspectives on leadership itself from trait and style, through task versus people and transformational and other 'new paradigm' approaches, to the current position that explores what McDermott(117) calls 'leadership from within' (emphasising reflection, emotions, values and openness to experience), traditional approaches to learning leadership from 'experts' have given way to experiential and learner-centred approaches. Learning capability is now seen as a key strategic resource, and leadership is seen as central to the development of 'learning organisations'.(118,119)

In addition to the management and leadership programmes offered by universities and the health care sector, different professional groups have taken different approaches to leadership development, and there is a range of leadership development programmes on offer to health care educators. Some of these emphasise the value of leadership development in an inter-professional context (learning from and with other professionals), but most are focused either on clinical leadership or strategic management and leadership development in higher education. There are very few programmes that are discipline based or that specifically aim to cross the health care and higher education divide.

Aspiring or current educational leaders can access a range of programmes to support their ongoing professional development. The most effective of these provide a mixture of strategic management, organisational and leadership theory coupled with practical exercises geared to the context in which the leader is or will be working. Many programmes use tools and exercises designed to deepen self-awareness and reflection and encourage support for individuals in the form of action learning sets, coaching or mentoring. However, effective programmes need also to be longitudinal and oriented around individuals and the organisations in which they work.(13) For this to happen, management and leadership development must be embedded in the culture of every educational organisation.

Summary

Leadership is one of those concepts that seems very easy to define, until you try to do so. This chapter offers an overview of the way in which leadership theory has developed over the past 50 or so years, illuminating some of the most influential concepts and indicating how these might apply to the health care education leaders of today and tomorrow. We have not had room to do justice to all the ideas surrounding leadership nor have we explored some of the pressing issues facing leaders of diverse organisations, such as those concerned with gender or race. In some sections, we have focused on developments in the UK and the close relationship between higher education and the NHS, but the theoretical concepts are applicable to a wider international audience.

We hope that this brief guide to leadership highlights what health care education might require of its leaders of the future: what kind of leader and what attributes, skills and qualities those leaders might need to demonstrate. If we are to develop a health care workforce capable of delivering high-quality services, then we will need to develop excellence in health care education, and this in turn will require educational leaders at all levels who can manage as well as lead, and who can work effectively and collaboratively across boundaries.

References

1 Bush T (2003) *Theories of Educational Management and Leadership.* Sage, London.

2 NHS Leadership Centre (2003) *NHS Leadership Qualities Framework.* NHS Leadership Centre, London.

3 Academy of Medical Royal Colleges and NHS Institute for Innovation and Improvement (2008) *Medical Leadership Competency Framework.* Academy of Medical Royal Colleges, London.

4 NHS Leadership Academy (2012) Leadership framework. (http://www.leadershipacademy.nhs.uk/; accessed 2 January 2013).

5 Bennis W and Nanus N (1985) *Leaders: The Strategies for Taking Charge.* Harper & Row, New York.

6 Fayol H (1949) *General and Industrial Management.* Pitman Publishing, London.

7 Yukl G (2002) *Leadership in Organisations* (5e). Prentice Hall, Upper Saddle River, NJ.

8 Kotter JP (1990) What leaders really do. *Harvard Business Review.* **May/Jun**: 103–11.

9 Covey S, Merrill AR and Merrill RR (1994) *First Things First.* Simon & Schuster, New York.

10 Northouse P (2004) *Leadership: Theory and Practice* (3e). Sage, London.

11 Blagg D and Young S (2001) What makes a good leader? *Harvard Business School Bulletin.* (http://www.alumni.hbs.edu/bulletin/2001/february/leader.html; accessed 9 June 2013).

12 Storey J (ed.) (2004) *Leadership in Organisations: Current Issues and Key Trends.* Routledge, London.

13 Swanwick T and McKimm J (2013) Faculty development for leadership and management. In: Steinert Y (ed.) *Faculty Development in the Health Professions.* Springer Publications, New York.

14 Goleman D (2000) Leadership that gets results. *Harvard Business Review.* **Mar/Apr**: 78–90.

15 Judge TA, Bono JE, Ilies R and Gerhardt MW (2002) Personality and leadership: a qualitative and quantitative review. *Journal of Applied Psychology.* **87**(4): 765–80.

16 Blake R and Mouton J (1964) *The Managerial Grid.* Gulf, Houston, TX.

17 Tannenbaum R and Schmidt W (1958) How to choose a leadership pattern: should a leader be democratic or autocratic or something in between? *Harvard Business Review.* **36**: 95–101.

18 Fiedler F (1964) A contingency model of leadership effectiveness. In: Berkowitz L (ed.) *Advances in Experimental Social Psychology,* pp. 149–90. Academic Press, New York.

19 Hersey P and Blanchard K (1988) *Management of Organizational Behaviour.* Prentice Hall, Englewood Cliffs, NJ.

20 Adair J (1973) *Action-Centred Leadership.* McGraw-Hill, New York.

21 Bass B and Avolio B (1994) *Improving Organizational Effectiveness through Transformational Leadership.* Sage, Thousand Oaks, CA.

22 Kellerman B (2007) What every leader needs to know about followers. *Harvard Business Review.* **85**(12): 84–91.

23 Vanderslice V (1988) Separating leadership from leaders: an assessment of the effect of leader and follower roles. *Human Relations.* **41**: 677–96.

24 Bolden R (2010) Leadership, management and organisational development. In: Thorpe R, Gold J and Mumford A (eds) *Gower Handbook of Leadership and Management Development* (5e), pp. 117–32. Gower, Farnham.

25 Alimo-Metcalfe B and Alban-Metcalfe J (2006) More (good) leaders for the public sector. *International Journal of Public Sector Management.* **19**(4): 73–95.

26 McKimm J (2011) Collaborative leadership. In: Swanwick T and McKimm J (eds) *ABC of Clinical Leadership.* Wiley-Blackwell, Oxford.

27 Mennin S (2010) Self-organisation, integration and curriculum in the complex world of medical education. *Medical Education.* **44**: 20–30.

28 Fullan M (2001) *Leading in a Culture of Change.* Jossey-Bass, San Francisco, CA.

29 Western S (2011) An overview of leadership discourses. In: Preedy M, Bennett N and Wise C (eds) *Educational Leadership: Context, Strategy and Collaboration.* The Open University, Milton Keynes.

30 Bryman A (1996) Leadership in organisations. In: Clegg SR, Harvey C and Nord WR (eds) *Handbook of Organisational Studies*, pp. 276–92. Sage, London.

31 Boyd W (1992) The power of paradigms: reconceptualising educational policy and management. *Educational Administration Quarterly.* **28**(4): 504–28.

32 House E (1981) Three perspectives on innovation: technological, political and cultural. In: Lehming R and Kane M (eds) *Improving Schools: Using What We Know*, pp. 42–114. Sage, Beverley Hills, CA.

33 Morgan G (1998) *Images of Organization: The Executive Edition.* Berrett-Kochler Publications, San Francisco, CA and Sage, Thousand Oaks, CA.

34 Bush T (1999) Crisis or crossroads? The discipline of educational management in the late 1990s. *Educational Management and Administration.* **27**(3): 239–52.

35 Hoyle E (1986) *The Politics of School Management.* Hodder & Stoughton, London.

36 Bush T and Glover D (2002) *School Leadership: concepts and evidence.* National College for School Leadership, Nottingham.

37 Leithwood K, Jantzi D and Steinbach R (1999) *Changing Leadership for Changing Times.* Open University Press, Buckingham.

38 Weber M (1947) *The Theory of Social and Economic Organization.* Free Press, New York.

39 Handy C (1995) *Gods of Management: The Changing Work of Organizations.* Doubleday, New York.

40 Lungu G (1985) In defense of bureaucratic organization in education. *Educational Management and Administration.* **13**: 172–8.

41 Osborne A (1990) The nature of educational management. In: West-Burnham J (ed.) *Education Management for the 1990s*, pp. 9–10. Longman, Harlow.

42 Bush T (1995) *Theories of Educational Management* (2e). Paul Chapman, London.

43 Mintzberg H (1992) *Structure in Fives: Designing Effective Organisations.* Prentice Hall, Harlow.

44 Bush T (2002) Educational management: theory and practice. In: Bush T and Bell L (eds) *The Principles and Practice of Education Management*, pp. 15–31. Paul Chapman, London.

45 Hargreaves A (1994) *Changing Teachers, Changing Times: Teachers' Work and Culture in a Postmodern Age.* Cassell, London.

46 Baldridge JV, Curtis DV, Ecker G and Riley GL (1978) *Policy Making and Effective Leadership.* Jossey-Bass, San Francisco, CA.

47 Coulson A (1986) *The Managerial Work of Headteachers.* Sheffield City Polytechnic, Sheffeld.

48 Alimo-Metcalfe B (1998) *Effective Leadership.* Local Government Management Board, London.

49 Grint K (1995) *Management: A Sociological Introduction.* Polity Press, Oxford.

50 Maccoby M (2000) Narcissistic leaders: the incredible pros, the inevitable cons. *Harvard Business Review.* **Jan/Feb**: 69–77.

51 Fullan M (2001) *The New Meaning of Educational Change* (3e). Routledge Falmer, London.

52 Bennett N, Wise C, Woods PA and Harvey JA (2003) Distributed leadership: a review of literature. National College for School Leadership. (http://oro.open.ac.uk/8534/1/bennett-distributed-leadership-full.pdf, accessed 2 January 2013).

53 Gronn P (2008) The future of distributed leadership. *Journal of Educational Administration.* **46**(2): 141–58.

54 Bolden R, Petrov G and Gosling J (2009) Distributed leadership in higher education: rhetoric and reality. *Educational Management Administration and Leadership.* **37**: 2.

55 Turning Point Leadership Development National Excellence Collaborative (2002) Academics and practitioners on collaborative leadership. (http://www.turningpointprogram.org/Pages/pdfs/lead_dev/LDC_panels_lowres.pdf;; accessed 9 June 2013).

56 Van Zwanenberg Z (2003) *Modern Leadership for Modern Services.* Scottish Leadership Foundation, Alloa.

57 Argyris C (1964) *Integrating the Individual and the Organization.* Wiley, New York.

58 Ball S (1987) *The Micropolitics of the School: Towards a Theory of School Organisation.* Methuen, London.

59 Hales C (1997) Power, authority and influence. In: Harris A, Preedy M and Bennett N (eds) *Organizational Effectiveness and Improvement in Education*, pp. 22–30. Open University Press, Buckingham.

60 Handy C (1993) *Understanding Organisations* (4e). Penguin Books, London.

61 Weber M (1998) The types of legitimate domination. In: Roth G and Wittich C (eds) *Economy and Society*, pp. 215–54. University of California Press, Berkeley, CA.

62 Kotter J (1996) *Leading Change.* Harvard Business School Press, Boston.

63 Keough T and Tobin B (2001) Postmodern leadership and the policy lexicon: from theory, proxy to practice. Paper presented at the Pan-Canadian Education Research Agenda Symposium, Quebec.

64 Weick K (1976) Educational organizations as loosely coupled systems. *Administrative Science Quarterly.* **21**(1): 1–19.

65 Cohen MD and March JG (1976) *Leadership and Ambiguity: The American College President.* Harvard Business School Press, Boston.

66 Gilbert P (2005) *Leadership: Being Effective and Remaining Human.* Russell House Publishing, Lyme Regis.

67 Peck E, Dickinson H and Smith J (2006) Transforming or transacting? The role of leaders in organisational transition. *British Journal of Leadership in Public Services.* **2**(3): 4–14.

68 Deal TE (1985) The symbolism of effective schools. *Elementary School Journal.* **85**(5): 601–20.

69 Goleman D (1996) *Emotional Intelligence.* Bloomsbury, London.

70 Greenleaf RK (1977) *Servant Leadership: A Journey into the Nature of Legitimate Power and Greatness.* Paulist Press, Mahwah, NJ.

71 Collins J (2001) *Good to Great.* Random House, London.

72 Bligh J and Brice J (2007) The Academy of Medical Educators: a professional home for medical educators in the UK. *Medical Education.* **41**(7): 625.

73 Alimo-Metcalfe B and Alban-Metcalfe J (2004) Leadership in public sector organisations. In: Storey J (ed.) *Leadership in Organisations: Current Issues and Key Trends*, pp. 173–202. Routledge, London.

74 Manz CC and Sims HP (1991) Super-leadership: beyond the myth of heroic leadership. *Organisational Dynamics.* **19**: 18–35.

75 Performance and Innovation Unit (2000) Strengthening leadership in the public sector. (http://www.cabinet-office.gov.uk/innovation; accessed 11 September 2006).

76 Kozlowski SWJ, Gully SM, Salas E and Cannon-Bowers JA (1995) Team leadership and development: theory, principles, and guidelines for training leaders and teams. Third Symposium on Work Teams, University of North Texas, Dallas, TX.

77 Tuckman B (1965) Developmental sequence in small groups. *Psychological Bulletin.* **63**: 384–9.

78 Belbin RM (1991) *Management Teams: Why They Succeed or Fail.* Heinemann, London.

79 Morrison K (1998) *Management Theories for Educational Change.* Paul Chapman, London.

80 Handy C (1989) *The Age of Unreason.* Business Books, London.

81 Iles V and Sutherland K (2001) *Organisational Change: a review for healthcare managers, researchers and professionals.* National Coordinating Centre for NHS Service Delivery and Organisation, London.

82 Mintzberg H (1987) Crafting strategy. *Harvard Business Review.* **Mar/Apr**(2): 66–75.

83 Lewin K (1958) Group decisions and social change. In: Swanson G, Newcomb T and Hartley L (eds) *Readings in Social Psychology,* pp. 459–73. Rinehart & Winston, New York.

84 Bullock R and Batten D (1985) It's just a phase we're going through: a review and synthesis of OD phase analysis. *Group & Organization Studies.* **10**: 383–412.

85 Buchanan D and Boddy D (1992) *The Expertise of the Change Agent.* Prentice Hall, Harlow.

86 Bank J (1992) *The Essence of Total Quality Management.* Prentice Hall, Harlow.

87 Fullan M (2003) *Change Forces with a Vengeance.* Routledge Falmer, London.

88 Baker P, Curtis D and Beneson W (1991) Structures and processes of planned change. *The School Community Journal.* **Fall/Winter**(1): 11–9.

89 Gleick J (1999) *Faster: The Acceleration of just about Everything.* Pantheon, New York.

90 Harvey D (1989) *The Condition of Postmodernity.* Polity Press, Cambridge, MA.

91 Jameson F (1991) *Postmodernism, or, the Cultural Logic of Late Capitalism.* Verso, London.

92 Castells M (1996) *The Rise of the Network Society.* Blackwell, Oxford.

93 Hargreaves A, Earl L and Schmidt M (2002) Perspectives on alternative assessment reform. *American Educational Research Journal.* **39**(1): 69–95.

94 Battram A (1998) *Navigating Complexity.* The Industrial Society, London.

95 Schön D (1983) *The Reflective Practitioner: How Professionals Think in Action.* Basic Books, New York.

96 Lewin R and Regine B (2000) *The Soul at Work.* Simon & Schuster, New York.

97 Plesk P and Greenhalgh T (2001) The challenge of complexity in health care. *British Medical Journal.* **323**: 625–8.

98 Kernick D (2002) Complexity and healthcare organisation. In: Sweeney K and Griffiths F (eds) *Complexity and Healthcare: An Introduction,* pp. 93–121. Radcliffe, Oxford.

99 Waldrop M (1992) *Complexity: The Emerging Science at the Edge of Order and Chaos.* Penguin, Harmondsworth.

100 Checkland P (1981) *Systems Thinking, Systems Practice.* Wiley, Oxford.

101 Stacey R (2001) *Complex Responsive Processes in Organisations.* Routledge, London.

102 Axelrod R and Cohen MD (2000) *Harnessing Complexity.* Basic Books, New York.

103 Johnson G and Scholes K (1997) *Exploring Corporate Strategy.* Prentice-Hall, Harlow.

104 Pascale R, Milleman M and Gioja L (2000) *Surfing the Edge of Chaos.* Crown Business Publishing, New York.

105 Fraser S and Greenhalgh T (2001) Coping with complexity: educating for capability. *British Medical Journal.* **323**: 799–803.

106 Mintzberg H, Ahlstrand B and Lampel J (1998) *Strategy Safari: A Guided Tour through the Wilds of Strategic Management.* Free Press, New York.

107 Claxton G (1997) *Hare Brained and Tortoise Mind.* Fourth Estate, London.

108 Nokes S, Greenwood A and Goodman M (2003) *The Definitive Guide to Project Management: The Fast Track to Getting the Job Done on Time and on Budget* (Financial Times series). Pearson Education, Edinburgh.

109 Porter ME (1980) *Competitive Strategy: Techniques for Analyzing Industries and Competitors.* 1 Edition. The Free Press, New York.

110 Berwick D (1996) A primer on the improvement of systems. *British Medical Journal.* **312**: 619–22.

111 Langley GJ, Nolan KM and Nolan TW (1992) *The Foundation of Improvement.* API Publishing, Silver Spring, MD.

112 Moyles J, Suchuitsky W and Chapman L (1998) *Teaching Fledglings to Fly: Report on Mentoring in Primary Schools.* Association of Teachers and Lecturers, London.

113 Lomax P (1990) *Managing Staff Development in Schools: An Action Research Approach,* BERA Dialogues 3. Multilingual Matters, Clevedon.

114 Senge P (1990) *The Fifth Discipline: The Art and Practice of the Learning Organization.* Doubleday, New York.

115 McKimm J (2004) *Case Studies in Leadership in Medical and Health Care Education: special report 5.* Higher Education Academy Subject Centre for Medicine, Dentistry and Veterinary Medicine, Newcastle-upon-Tyne.

116 Lieff S and Albert M (2010) The mindsets of medical education leaders; how do they conceive of their work? *Academic Medicine.* **85**(1): 57–62.

117 McDermott GR (1994) Partnering with God: ignatian spirituality and leadership in groups. In: Conger JA (ed.) *Spirituality at Work: Discovering the Spirituality in Leadership,* pp. 132–61. Jossey-Bass, San Francisco, CA.

118 Shewhart WA (1931) *Economic Control of Manufacturing Product.* Van Nostrand, New York.

119 Drath WH and Palus CJ (1994) *Making Common Sense: Leadership as Meaning Making in a Community of Practice.* Center for Creative Leadership, Greensboro, NC.

Further reading

Adair J (2002) *Effective Strategic Leadership.* Macmillan, London.

Belbin R (1999) *Management Teams: Why They Succeed or Fail.* Butterworth Heinneman, Oxford.

Bolden R (2004) What is leadership? University of Exeter Leadership South West Research Report. (http://www.leadershipsouthwest.com; accessed 20 April 2006).

Bush T and Bell L (eds) (2002) *The Principles and Practice of Education Management.* Paul Chapman, London.

Fullan M (2005) *Leadership and Sustainability: Systems Thinkers in Action.* Corwin Press (Sage), Thousand Oaks, CA.

Hoyle E and Wallace M (2005) *Educational Leadership: Ambiguity, Professionals and Managerialism.* Sage, London.

Iles V and Sutherland K (1997) Organisational Change A review for healthcare managers, professionals and researchers. National Co-ordinating Centre for NHS Service Delivery and Organisation, London. (http://www.netscc.ac.uk/hsdr/files/project/SDO_FR_08-1001-001_V01.pdf; accessed 8 January 2013).

Kotter J (1990) *A Force for Change: How Leadership Differs from Management.* Free Press, New York.

Kydd L, Anderson A and Newton W (eds) (2003) *Leading People and Teams in Education*. Sage, London.

Lewin R (1993) *Complexity: Life on the Edge of Chaos*. Phoenix, London.

Mullins LJ (1999) *Management and Organisational Behaviour* (5e). Financial Times Pitman Publishing, London.

Open University (2005) *Systems Thinking and Practice – a primer*. Open University, Milton Keynes.

Rost JC (1991) *Leadership for the 21st Century*. Praeger, New York.

Swanwick T and McKimm J (2010) *The ABC of Clinical Leadership*. Wiley-Blackwell, Oxford.

Sweeney K and Griffiths F (eds) (2002) *Complexity and Healthcare: An Introduction*. Radcliffe Publishing, Oxford.

Index

Understanding Medical Education: Evidence, Theory and Practice, Second Edition. Edited by Tim Swanwick.
© 2014 The Association for the Study of Medical Education. Published 2014 by John Wiley & Sons, Ltd.